A Textbook of

Neurology

A Textbook of
Neurology

SIXTH EDITION

H. HOUSTON MERRITT, M.D.

Henry L. and Lucy Moses
Professor of Neurology, Emeritus
Columbia University;

Consultant in Neurology,
Presbyterian Hospital in the City of New York;

Vice President, Emeritus, in Charge of Medical Affairs and
Dean Emeritus of the Faculty of Medicine,
Columbia University

Lea & Febiger • 1979 • Philadelphia

First Edition, 1955
Reprinted, 1955, 1957

Second Edition, 1959
Reprinted, 1959, 1961

Third Edition, 1963
Reprinted, 1964, 1966

Fourth Edition, 1967
Reprinted, 1968, 1969, 1970

Fifth Edition, 1973
Reprinted, 1974, 1975, 1977

Sixth Edition, 1979

Library of Congress Cataloging in Publication Data

Merritt, Hiram Houston, 1902–
  A textbook of neurology.

  Includes bibliographies and index.
  1. Nervous system—Diseases.   2. Neurology.
I. Title.   [DNLM: 1. Nervous system diseases. WL100.3 M572t]
RC346.M4   1979   616.8   78-24403
ISBN 0-8121-0629-6

Published in Great Britain by Henry Kimpton Publishers, London

PRINTED IN THE UNITED STATES OF AMERICA

Print Number: 4   3   2   1

To

M. C. M.

Preface

The first edition of this text on neurology, or, more properly, diseases of the nervous system, was published in 1955.

Its general acceptance is attested to by the fact that over 30,000 copies of the fifth edition were published, as well as editions in Spanish, Portuguese and Japanese, and English editions were published in India and China.

The volume is intended for medical students, residents and interns in internal medicine, neurology, neurosurgery, orthopedics and other surgical specialties related to neurology.

The diseases are considered according to etiology. An attempt was made to make the discussion complete but concise, covering incidence, pathology and symptomatology, diagnosis and therapy.

The first editions of the text were written almost entirely by the original author. It soon became obvious that the subject matter became too complex an assignment for a single author.

Again, I am indebted to many of my friends who have provided illustrations for the new edition. I am also greatly indebted to the authors who contributed new material to the text.

H. Houston Merritt

Contributors

Dr. Joao Lobo Antunes
Department of Neurosurgery
Neurological Institute
New York, New York

Dr. Arnold Friedman
Tucson, Arizona 85712

Dr. Gilbert Glaser,
Chairman
Department of Neurology
Yale University School of
    Medicine
New Haven, Connecticut

Dr. Donald H. Harter
Chairman
Department of Neurology
The Medical School
Northwestern University
Chicago, Illinois

Dr. Robert Katzman
Chairman
Department of Neurology
Albert Einstein School of
    Medicine
Bronx, New York

Dr. Charles Poser
Chairman
Department of Neurology
University of Vermont
College of Medicine
Burlington, Vermont

Dr. Roger N. Rosenberg
Professor and Chairman
Department of Neurology
The University of Texas
Health Science Center
Southwestern Medical School
Dallas, Texas

Dr. Lewis P. Rowland
Chairman
Department of Neurology
Neurological Institute
New York, New York

Dr. James F. Toole
Chairman
Department of Neurology
The Bowman Gray School of
    Medicine
Winston-Salem, North Carolina

Dr. Harry H. White
Menninger Foundation
Topeka, Kansas

Dr. Melvin D. Yahr
Chairman
Department of Neurology
Mt. Sinai School of Medicine
New York, New York

Contents

CHAPTER 7 • METABOLIC DISEASES 643
Harry H. White

CHAPTER 8 • DISEASES OF THE MYELIN SHEATH 767
Charles M. Poser

CHAPTER 9 • PAROXYSMAL DISORDERS 825
Arnold P. Friedman

Chapter 1

Infections

DONALD H. HARTER, and H. HOUSTON MERRITT

The parenchyma, the coverings and the blood vessels of the nervous system may be invaded by practically all of the pathogenic microorganisms. It is customary, for convenience of description, to divide the syndromes produced according to the chief site of the involvement. This division is an arbitrary one because the inflammatory process not infrequently involves more than one of these structures.

INFECTIONS OF THE MENINGES

Involvement of the meninges by pathogenic microorganisms is known as leptomeningitis. These cases are subdivided into two groups, acute and subacute meningitis according to the severity of the inflammatory reactions, which in part is related to the nature of the infecting organism.

Acute Purulent Meningitis

Microorganisms may gain access to the ventriculo-subarachnoid space by way of the blood stream in the course of a septicemia or as a metastasis from infection of the heart, lung and other viscera. The meninges may be invaded by direct extension from a septic focus in the skull, spine or parenchyma of the nervous system. Organisms may gain entrance to the subarachnoid space through compound fractures of the skull and fractures through the nasal sinuses or mastoid. They may be introduced by lumbar puncture performed for the removal of fluid or the injection of sera, air, contrast media, anesthetics and the like. Neonatal meningitis is frequently due to genitourinary infections in the mother. The pathology, symptomatology and clinical course of patients with acute purulent meningitis are similar regardless of the causative organisms. The diagnosis and program of therapy depend on the isolation and identification of the organism and the determination of the source of the infection.

Table 1. Frequency of the Various Forms of
Acute Purulent Meningitis
(Data Collected from Literature)

Causative Organism	No. of Cases	%
Meningococcus	2039	30
No organism isolated	1719	26
Hemophilus influenzae	1209	18
Pneumococcus	1076	16
Miscellaneous	501	7
Streptococcus	206	3
Total	6750	100

Table 2. The Incidence and The Mortality Rate of Various Forms of
Acute Purulent Meningitis at the Columbia-Presbyterian Medical
Center in the Pre- and Post-antibiotic Eras

1930–1939

Etiology	No. of Cases	% of Total	No. Died	% Died
Pneumococcus	79	28	78	99
Meningococcus	62	22	30	48
Streptococcus	48	17	46	96
H. influenzae	42	15	36	86
Unknown	21	8	11	52
Staphylococcus	14	5	14	100
Gram-negative bacilli	12	4	9	75
Others	2	1	2	100
Total	280	100	226	81

1953–1962

Etiology	No. of Cases	% of Total	No. Died	% Died*
H. influenzae	80	28	8	10
Unknown	65	22	13	20
Pneumococcus	51	18	16	31
Gram-negative bacilli	40	14	23	58
Meningococcus	22	8	1	5
Staphylococcus	21	7	10	48
Streptococcus	7	2	4	57
Others	3	1	1	33
Total	289	100	76	26

*These figures have been further reduced in the past two decades by the use of more effective antimicrobial agents.

Pathogenesis. Acute purulent meningitis may be the result of infection with almost any of the pathogenic bacteria. Isolated examples of infection by the uncommon forms are recorded in the literature, but most frequently the meningococcus, pneumococcus, streptococcus and the influenza bacillus are the causative organisms. The frequency of the occurrence of the common forms of acute purulent meningitis is shown in Table 1. In recent years there has been an increase in the incidence of infection with the influenza bacillus, pneumococcus, staphylococcus, and coliform gram-negative bacteria. There has also been an increase in the incidence of cases in which no organism can be isolated. This is probably due to the administration of therapy prior to admission to the hospital and the performance of lumbar puncture. In infants and young children Hemophilus influenzae is the cause of purulent meningitis in approximately one third of the patients. In the neonatal period E. coli, Group B streptococci, Staphylococcus aureus and Listeria monocytogenes are the most common causative agents.

The beneficial effect of antibiotic treatment is shown by the fact that the mortality rate of all forms of bacterial meningitis at the Columbia-Presbyterian Medical Center was 81% in the decade 1930–39, as compared to 26% in 1953–62 (Table 2). There have been further reductions in the mortality rate in the past two decades as the result of the introduction of more effective antimicrobial agents.

For convenience sake, special features of the common forms of acute purulent meningitis are described separately.

Meningococcal Meningitis

Meningococcal meningitis or acute cerebrospinal fever was described by Vieusseux in 1805 and the causative organism was identified by Weichselbaum in 1887. It occurs almost constantly in sporadic form and at irregular intervals in epidemic form. Epidemics are especially apt to occur when there are large shifts in population as in time of war.

Pathogenesis. The meningococci (Neisseria meningitidis) may gain access to the meninges directly from the nasopharynx through the cribriform plate or by way of the blood stream. The fact that organisms can be cultured from the blood or from cutaneous lesions before the appearance of meningitis is strong evidence that the infection takes place through the blood stream by way of the choroid plexus in many, if not all, cases. In addition, it has been shown that the ventricular fluid may be teeming with organisms before infection of the meninges is evident.

Pathology. In acute fulminating cases death may occur before there are any significant pathological changes in the nervous system. In the usual case where death does not occur for several days after the onset of the disease, there is an intense inflammatory reaction in the meninges. The inflammatory reaction is especially severe in the subarachnoid spaces over the convexity of the brain and around the cisterns at the base of the brain and it may extend a short distance along the perivascular spaces into the substance of the brain and spinal cord. Rarely the inflammatory reaction breaks into the parenchyma. Meningococci, both intra- and extracellularly, are found in the meninges and the fluid from the ventricles and subarachnoid space. With progress of the infection the pia-arachnoid becomes thickened and adhesions may form. Adhesions at the base may interfere with the flow of cerebrospinal fluid from the fourth ventricle and produce hydrocephalus. Inflammatory reaction and fibrosis of the meninges along the roots of the cranial nerves are thought to be the cause of the cranial nerve palsies which occasionally develop. This is not the only mechanism for such paralyses, however. Damage to the auditory nerve often occurs suddenly, and the auditory defect is usually permanent. This may be explained as the result of extension of the infection to the inner ear or to thrombosis of the nutrient artery. In addition, facial paralysis not infrequently occurs after the meningeal reaction has subsided and is best explained on another, perhaps allergic, basis. Signs and symptoms of parenchymatous damage, hemiplegia, aphasia, or cerebellar signs are infrequent and are probably due to the formation of infarcts as the result of thrombosis of inflamed arteries or veins. Damage to the spinal cord, myelitis, is explained on a similar basis. Myelitis or damage to the roots of the cauda equina is rare in the absence of intrathecal treatment with serum or chemicals and it is probable that the latter substances play an important role in the production of these complications.

With efficient treatment, and in some cases without treatment, the inflammatory reaction in the meninges subsides and no evidence of the infection may be found at autopsy in patients who die some months or years later.

Incidence. The meningococcus is the causative organism in approximately one fourth of all cases of purulent meningitis. While both the sporadic and epidemic forms of the disease may attack individuals of all ages, children are predominantly affected. In many large epidemics over 75% of the cases were under ten years of age. Males appear to be slightly more susceptible than females. The normal habitat of the meningococcus is the nasopharynx and the disease is spread by carriers or by individuals with the disease. An effective polysaccharide vaccine for Groups A and C meningococci is available. Its use has reduced the incidence of meningococcal infection among military recruits.

Symptomatology. The onset of meningococcal meningitis, similar to that of other forms of meningitis, is accompanied by chills and fever, headache, nausea and vomiting, pain in the back, stiffness of the neck, and prostration. The occurrence of herpes simplex, conjunctivitis and a petechial or hemorrhagic skin rash is common with meningococcal infections. At the onset, the patient is irritable and in children there is frequently a characteristic sharp shrill cry (meningeal cry). With progress of the disease, the sensorium becomes clouded and stupor or coma may develop. Occasionally the onset may be accompanied by deep coma. Convulsive seizures are not infrequently an early symptom, but focal neurological signs are uncommon. Acute fulminating cases with severe circulatory collapse are relatively rare.

Signs. The patient appears acutely ill, and may be confused, stuporous or semi-comatose. The temperature is elevated to 101° or 103° F, but occasionally it may be normal at the onset. The pulse is usually rapid and the respiratory rate is increased. Blood pressure is normal except in acute fulminating cases when there may be a severe degree of hypotension. There is rigidity of the neck with positive Kernig and Brudzinski signs. The reflexes are often decreased but occasionally they may be increased. Cranial nerve palsies and focal neurological signs are uncommon. These complications usually do not develop until several days after the onset of the infection. The optic discs are normal, but choking may develop if the meningitis persists for more than a week.

Laboratory Data. The white blood cells in the peripheral blood are increased with counts usually in the range of 10,000 to 30,000 per cu mm, but they occasionally may be within normal limits or higher than 40,000 per cu mm. The urine may contain albumin, casts and red blood cells. Meningococci can be cultured from the nasopharynx in practically all cases, from the blood in over one half of the cases in the early stages, and from the skin lesions when these are present.

The cerebrospinal fluid is under increased pressure, usually between 200 and 500 mm of water. The fluid is cloudy or purulent and contains a large number of cells, predominantly polymorphonuclear leukocytes. The cell count in the fluid is usually between 2,000 and 10,000 per cu mm. Occasionally it may be less than 100 and infrequently more than 20,000 per cu mm. The protein content is increased. The sugar content is decreased, usually to levels below 20 mg per 100 ml. Organisms can be seen intra-and extracellularly in stained smears of the fluid and they can be cultured on the appropriate media in over 90% of untreated cases. Counter-current immunoelectrophoresis may demonstrate meningococcal antigen in spinal fluid.

Complications and Sequelae. The complications and sequelae include those commonly associated with an inflammatory process in the meninges and its blood vessels (convulsions, cranial nerve palsies, focal cerebral lesions, damage to the spinal cord or nerve roots, hydrocephalus), and those which are due to involvement of other portions of the body by meningococci such as panophthalmitis and other types of ocular infection, arthritis, purpura, pericarditis, endocarditis, myocarditis, pleurisy, orchitis, epididymitis, albuminuria or hematuria, and adrenal hemorrhage. Disseminated intravascular coagulation may complicate the meningitis. In addition there may be complications arising as the result of intercurrent infection of the upper respiratory tract, middle ear and lungs. Any of the above complications may leave a permanent residual but the most common sequelae are due to injury of the nervous system. These include deafness, ocular palsies, blindness, changes in mentality, convulsions and hydrocephalus.

With the methods of treatment available at the present time, complications and sequelae of the meningeal infection are rare and the complications due to the involvement of other parts of the body by the meningococci or other intercurrent infections are more readily controlled. In 300 sulfonamide-treated cases, reported by Farmer in 1945, neurological complications occurred in less than 9% and a permanent residual in less than 2%. Sixth nerve palsy developed early in the course of the disease in 3% and completely disappeared within a few weeks. Seventh nerve palsy occurred as a late complication in 3% of the cases. It usually developed between the fifth and fourteenth day, at a time when the cerebrospinal fluid was relatively cell-free. Recovery from the facial paralysis, either unilateral or bilateral, was usually complete within a few months. Eighth nerve palsy, usually bilateral, was present in 2% and was followed by permanent deafness. Focal neurological signs—convulsions, hemiplegia and aphasia—were present in only 1%, and in all of these the signs and symptoms were transient. Similar findings were reported by Dodge and Swartz in 1965, but the frequency has greatly decreased in recent years.

Diagnosis. The diagnosis of meningococcal meningitis can be made with certainty only by the isolation of the organism from the cerebrospinal fluid. However, the diagnosis can be made with relative certainty before the organisms are isolated in a patient with headache, vomiting, chills and fever, stiffness of the neck, and a petechial cutaneous rash, especially if there is an epidemic of meningococcal meningitis or if there has been exposure to a known case of meningococcal meningitis.

In establishing the diagnosis of meningococcal meningitis, cultures should be made of the skin lesions, nasopharyngeal secretions, blood and cerebrospinal fluid. Since meningococci are particularly sensitive to chilling and freezing it is important that inoculation of the appropriate media be made promptly, preferably directly from the lumbar puncture needle. In addition, a tube containing 5 to 10 ml of fluid can be incubated for subculture after a few hours. The diagnosis can be established in the majority of cases by examination of smears of the sediment of the cerebrospinal fluid, which have been stained by the Gram stain.

Prognosis. The mortality rate of untreated meningococcal meningitis varied widely in different epidemics, but was usually between 50 and 90%. There is little evidence to indicate that the older forms of therapy, particularly that in which immune serum was injected intravenously and intrathecally, had any appreciable effect on the course of the disease. With present-day therapy, however, the mortality rate is less than 5% and the incidence of complications and sequelae is low.

Features of the disease which influence the mortality rate are the age of the patient, the presence of bacteremia, type of meningococcus, day of treatment, complications, and general condition of the patient. The lowest fatality rates are seen in patient between the ages of five and ten years, and in patients without bacteremia who are treated early in the course of the disease. The highest mortality rates occur in infants, in elderly, debilitated individuals, in those who are treated late in the course of the disease and in those with extensive hemorrhages into the adrenal gland.

Treatment. Aqueous penicillin G or ampicillin administered intravenously is the treatment of choice. If the patient is allergic to penicillin, chloramphenicol is the preferred alternative drug. The duration of treatment should be seven to ten days. The cerebrospinal fluid should be examined twenty-four hours after the initiation of treatment in order to assess the effectiveness of the treatment and reexamined after the full course has been given.

The state of the fluid balance and hydration should be carefully monitored by the measurement of central venous pressure. Dehydration is common and fluids should be replaced by intravenous administration. Hyponatremia, which is not uncommon, may be due to excessive fluid intake or the inappropriate secretion of antidiuretic hormone. It can be relieved by the restriction of water intake.

Increased intracranial pressure can usually be controlled by removal of cerebrospinal fluid. The development of cerebral edema may require the use of osmotic diuretics such as intravenous mannitol solution or the administration of dexamethasone.

Diphenylhydantoin, diazepam, or phenobarbital can be used to control recurrent convulsive seizures.

If hypovolemic shock occurs, volume expansion with isotonic electrolyte solution is indicated. Isoproterenol or dopamine may be required. Heparinization should be considered if there is evidence of intravascular clotting.

Persons who have had intimate contact with meningococcal meningitis patients may be given rifampin or minocycline for three to four days as a prophylactic measure.

Pneumococcal Meningitis

The pneumococcus (Streptococcus pneumoniae) is next in frequency to the meningococcus and influenza bacillus as a cause of meningitis. Meningeal infection is usually a complication of otitis media, mastoiditis, sinusitis, fractures of the skull, upper respiratory infections and infections of the lung (Table 3). Alcoholism, asplenism, sickle cell disease and multiple myeloma predispose patients to developing pneumococcal meningitis. The infection may occur at any age, but over 50% of the cases are less than one or over fifty years of age. The two sexes are about equally involved.

The clinical symptoms, physical signs and laboratory findings in pneumococcal meningitis are the same as those of other forms of acute purulent meningitis. The diagnosis is usually made without difficulty because the cerebrospinal fluid contains large numbers of the organisms. When gram-positive diplococci are seen in smears of the fluid or its sediment, a positive Neufeld reaction will serve to identify both the pneumococcus and its type. Counter-current immunoelectrophoresis of spinal fluid and serum may be helpful in demonstrating pneumococcal antigen. When the meningitis is secondary to mastoid or nasal sinus infection, the type III pneumococcus is most common; in postpneumonic infections pneumococci of types I and II are most common; in meningitis following fracture of the skull the organisms are usually of higher types and correspond to strains of lesser virulence which are normally present in the nose and throat. Prior to the introduction of sulfonamides the mortality rate in pneumococcal meningitis was almost 100% and at the present time it is still in the neighborhood of 30%. The prognosis for recovery is best in cases which follow fractures of the skull and those with no known source of infection. The mortality rate is especially high when the meningitis

Table 3. Primary Focus of Infection in 275 Cases of Pneumococcal Meningitis

(Modified from Appelbaum and Abler, New York State J. Med. 1958.)

Type of Focus	No. of Cases	%
None known	66	24
Upper respiratory infection	40	15
Otitis media with or without mastoiditis	92	33
Pneumonia	52	19
Sinusitis	8	3
Head injury	14	5
Cellulitis	3	1
Total	275	100

follows pneumonia, empyema, lung abscess, or when there is a persisting bacteremia indicating the presence of an endocarditis.

Aqueous benzyl penicillin or ampicillin given intravenously is the drug of choice in the treatment of pneumococcal meningitis. The treatment should be continued for twelve to fifteen days. The primary focus of infection should be eradicated by surgery if necessary. Persistent cerebrospinal fluid fistulas following fractures of the skull must be closed by craniotomy and suturing of the dura. Otherwise the meningitis will almost certainly recur.

Staphylococcal Meningitis

The staphylococcus is a relatively infrequent cause of meningitis. Meningitis may develop as a result of spread from furuncles on the face or from staphylococcal infections elsewhere in the body. It is not infrequently a complication of cavernous sinus thrombosis, epidural or subdural abscess and neurosurgical procedures involving shunting to relieve hydrocephalus. Intravenous methicillin or nafcillin is the preferred treatment. Therapy must be continued for two to four weeks. Complications such as ventriculitis, arachnoiditis and hydrocephalus may occur. The original focus of infection should be eradicated. Laminectomy should be performed immediately when a spinal epidural abscess is present and cranial subdural abscess should be drained through craniotomy openings.

Streptococcal Meningitis

Infection with the streptococcus accounts for approximately 6% of all cases of meningitis. Streptococcal meningitis is usually caused by group A organisms. The symptoms are not distinguished from other forms of meningitis. Occasionally, members of other groups may be isolated from spinal fluid. It is always secondary to some septic focus, most commonly in the mastoid or nasal sinuses. Treatment is the same as outlined for the treatment of pneumococcal meningitis together with surgical eradication of the primary focus.

Influenzal Meningitis

Infections of the meninges by Hemophilus influenzae were reported as early as 1899. At the present time it is the third most common type of acute purulent meningitis (Table 1) and accounts for 18% of all cases of meningitis. In infants and children influenzal meningitis is usually primary. In adults it is more commonly secondary to acute sinusitis, otitis media, fracture of the skull, and associated with spinal fluid rhinorrhea, agammaglobulinemia, diabetes mellitus or alcoholism. It is predominantly a disease of infancy and early childhood, over 50% of the cases occurring within the first two years of life and 90% before the age of five. The disease affects the two sexes equally and is more prevalent in the winter months.

The pathology of influenzal meningitis does not differ from that of other forms of acute purulent meningitis, except in cases with a protracted course where localized pockets of infection in the meninges or cortex, internal hydrocephalus, degeneration of cranial nerves and focal loss of cerebral substance secondary to thrombosis of vessels may be found.

The symptoms and physical signs of influenzal meningitis are similar to those of other forms of acute bacterial meningitis. The disease usually lasts ten to twenty days. Occasionally it may be fulminating, and not infrequently it is protracted and extends over a period of several weeks or months.

The cerebrospinal fluid changes are similar to those described for the other acute meningitides. The organisms can be cultured from the cerebrospinal fluid. Blood cultures are positive in a high percentage of cases in the early stage of the disease.

Complications and sequelae are common in untreated cases due to the protracted course of the disease. These include: Paralysis of extraocular muscles, deafness, blindness, hemiplegia, recurrent convulsions and mental deficiency.

The mortality rate in untreated cases in influenzal meningitis in infants is over 90%. The prognosis is not so grave in adults in whom spontaneous recovery is more frequent. Adequate treatment has reduced the mortality rate to less than 5%, but sequelae are not uncommon.

The diagnosis of influenzal meningitis is based on the isolation of the organisms from the cerebrospinal fluid and blood on Fildes' or Leventhal's medium. The type of organism can be determined by means of capsular swelling with specific rabbit antiserum. Hemophilus influenzae antigen may be demonstrated in spinal fluid by counter-immunoelectrophoresis. Although there are six known types, the vast majority of the infections in infants are due to type G. The emergence of ampicillin resistant Hemophilus influenzae strains has made it necessary to begin treatment with both ampicillin and chloramphenicol given intravenously by separate injections. As soon as the antibiotic sensitivity of the recovered bacterium is known, one of the two antibiotics should be stopped and the other continued for ten to fourteen days until the patient is well, the spinal fluid cell count less than 50 per cu mm and the spinal fluid glucose normal.

Subdural effusion, which may occur in infants with any form of meningitis, is most commonly seen in connection with influenzal meningitis. Persistent vomiting, bulging fontanelles, convulsion, focal neurological signs and persistent fever should lead to consideration of this complication. Prompt relief of the symptoms usually follows evacuation of the effusion by tapping the subdural space through the fontanelles. Persistent or secondary fever without worsening of meningeal signs may be due to an extracranial focus of infection, such as a contaminated urinary or venous catheter, or to drug administration.

Meningitis Due to Other Bacteria

Meningitis in the newborn infant is most often caused by coliform gram-negative bacilli, especially E. coli, group B hemolytic streptococci, Staphylococcus aureus and Listeria monocytogenes. It often accompanies septicemia and may show none of the typical signs of meningitis in children and adults. Instead, the infant shows irritability, lethargy, anorexia and bulging fontanelles. Meningitis due to gram-negative enteric bacteria also occurs frequently in immunosuppressed or chronically ill, hospitalized patients or persons with penetrating head injuries, congenital defects or diabetes mellitus.

Gentamicin is the drug of choice in meningitis due to enterobacteria. Intrathecal, as well as intramuscular or intravenous therapy may be necessary, while spinal fluid cultures remain positive because of the drug's poor penetration into the spinal fluid.

Meningitis due to Listeria monocytogenes may occur in immunosuppressed adults as well as in infants. A laboratory report of "diphtheroids" seen on Gram stain or isolated in culture should suggest the possible presence of Listeria monocytogenes. The treatment of choice for Listeria monocytogenes meningitis is ampicillin or benzyl penicillin.

Gonococcal meningitis usually presents in patients with other accompanying signs and symptoms of gonorrhea. It most often occurs in pregnancy or during menses.

Acute Purulent Meningitis of Unknown Etiology

Occasionally a patient may present clinical symptoms indicative of an acute purulent meningitis but with atypical cerebrospinal fluid findings. These patients have usually manifested nonspecific symptoms and have been treated for several days with some form of antimicrobial therapy in dosages sufficient to modify the cerebrospinal abnormalities, but not sufficient to eradicate the infection. In these cases the pleocytosis in the cerebrospinal fluid is usually only of a moderate degree (500 to 1,000 cells per cu mm with predominance of polymorphonuclear leukocytes) and the sugar content is normal or only slightly decreased. Organisms are not seen on stained smears and are cultured with difficulty. Repeated lumbar puncture may be helpful in arriving at the correct diagnosis. Antibiotics should be selected on the basis of epidemiologic or clinical factors. The age of the patient and the setting in which the infection occurred are the primary considerations. Therapy should be modified if an organism different from that originally suspected is isolated or the clinical response is less than optimal.

REFERENCES

Balagtas, R. D., et al.: Secondary and Prolonged Fevers in Bacterial Meningitis, J. Pediatr., 77, 957, 1970.
Benson, P., Nyhan, W. L., and Shimizu, H.: The Prognosis of Subdural Effusions Complicating Pyogenic Meningitis, J. Pediatr., 57, 670, 1960.
Carpenter, R. R. and Petersdorf, R. G.: The Clinical Spectrum of Meningitis, Am. J. Med., 33, 262, 1962.
Converse, G. M., et al.: Alteration of Cerebrospinal Fluid Findings by Partial Treatment of Bacterial Meningitis, J. Pediatr., 83, 220, 1973.
Dodge, P. R., and Swartz, M. N.: Bacterial Meningitis—A Review of Selected Aspects, N. Engl. J. Med., 272, 725, 779, 842, 898, 954, and 1003, 1965.
Edwards, E. A., Muehl, P. M., and Peckinpaugh, R. O.: Diagnosis of Bacterial Meningitis by Counter-immunoelectrophoresis, J. Lab. Clin. Med., 80, 449, 1972.
Farmer, T. W.: Neurologic Complications during Meningococcic Meningitis Treated With Sulfonamide Drugs, Arch. Intern. Med., 76, 201, 1945.
Feigin, R. D. and Shackelford, P. G.: Value of Repeat Lumbar Puncture in the Differential Diagnosis of Meningitis, N. Engl. J. Med., 289, 571, 1973.
Feigin, R. D., et al.: Prospective Evaluation of Treatment of Hemophilus Influenzae Meningitis, J. Pediatr., 88, 542, 1976.
Feigin, R. D., and Dodge, P. R.: Bacterial Meningitis: Newer Concepts of Pathophysiology and Neurologic Sequelae, Pediatr. Clin. North Am., 23, 541, 1976.
Harter, D. H., and Petersdorf, R. G.: A Consideration of the Pathogenesis of Bacterial Meningitis: Review of Experimental and Clinical Studies, Yale J. Biol. Med., 32, 280, 1960.
Hodges, G. R., and Perkins, R. L.: Acute Bacterial Meningitis: An Analysis of Factors Influencing Prognosis, Am. J. Med. Sci., 270, 427, 1975.
Lavetter, A., et al.: Meningitis Due to Listeria Monocytogenes, N. Engl. J. Med., 285, 598, 1971.
Overall, J. C., Jr.: Neonatal Bacterial Meningitis, J. Pediatr., 76, 499, 1970.
Qadri, S. M. H., Berotte, J. M., and Wende, R. D.: Incidence and Etiology of Septic Meningitis in a Metropolitan County Hospital, Am. J. Clin. Pathol., 4, 550, 1976.
Richter, R. W., and Brust, J. C. M.: Pneumococcal Meningitis at Harlem Hospital, N.Y. State J. Med., 71, 2747, 1971.
Sell, S. H. W., et al.: Long Term Sequelae of Hemophilus Influenzae Meningitis, Pediatrics, 49, 206, 1972.
Tramont, E. C.: Management of Bacterial Meningitis, Milit. Med., 141, 589, 1976.
Weiss, W., et al.: Prognostic Factors in Pneumococcal Meningitis, Arch. Intern. Med., 120, 517, 1967.

Subacute Meningitis

Subacute meningitis is usually due to infection with tubercle bacilli or mycotic organisms. The clinical syndrome differs from that of acute purulent meningitis in that the onset of symptoms is usually less acute, the degree of inflammatory reaction less severe, the course more prolonged, and relapses are apt to occur, especially with mycotic infection.

Tuberculous Meningitis

Tuberculous meningitis differs from that caused by most of the other common bacteria in that the course is more prolonged, the mortality rate is higher, the changes in the cerebrospinal fluid are less severe, and the treatment is less effective.

Pathogenesis. Tuberculous meningitis is always secondary to tuberculosis elsewhere in the body. The primary focus of infection is most commonly in the lungs, but it may be in the lymph glands, bones, nasal sinuses, gastrointestinal tract or any other organ in the body. The onset of meningeal symptoms may coincide with signs of acute miliary dissemination or there may be clinical evidence of activity in the primary focus, but not infrequently the meningitis is the only manifestation of activity of the disease.

It has been claimed that the meningitis is practically always secondary to rupture of a cerebral tubercle into the ventriculo-subarachnoid spaces. Tubercles in the nervous system of any appreciable size are a rarity in the United States. This fact does not prove, however, that the meningitis may not result from dissemination of the bacteria from minute or microscopic tubercles near the meningeal surfaces. In a number of cases the meningitis may be a manifestation of an acute miliary dissemination of the disease from other viscera, suggesting that the meningitis is due to lodgment of bacteria directly in the meninges or choroid plexus.

Pathology. The older literature contains many reports of diffuse or circumscribed granulomatous involvement of the meninges by tuberculosis. This form of the infection is distinctly rare and the appearance of the brains of patients who have died in the acute stages of tuberculous meningitis is not very different from that seen in other forms of meningitis. The meninges on the surface of the brain and the spinal cord are cloudy and thickened but the process is often most intense at the base of the brain. In fatal cases which are kept alive for some weeks by inadequate therapy, this process may be so intense that it forms a thick collar of fibrosis around the optic nerves, cerebral peduncles and basilar surface of the pons and midbrain. The ventricles are moderately dilated and the ependymal lining is covered with exudate or appears roughened (granular ependymitis). Minute tubercles may be visible in the meninges, choroid plexus or cerebral substances. On microscopic examination the exudate in the thickened meninges is composed chiefly of mononuclear cells, lymphocytes, plasma cells, macrophages and fibroblasts with an occasional giant cell. The inflammatory process may extend for a short distance into the cerebral substance where minute granulomas may also be found. Proliferative changes are frequently seen in the inflamed vessels of the meninges producing a panarteritis similar to the Heubner type seen in chronic syphilitic meningitis. These arteritic changes may lead to thrombosis of the vessel and formation of infarcts in the cerebral substance.

Incidence. Tuberculous meningitis was formerly the most common form of meningitis except for that due to meningococcus. With the advent of effective methods of therapy for tuberculosis, the incidence of meningitis due to this organism has decreased, but meningitis still remains the most serious complication and the most common cause of death in tuberculous children. Although tuberculous meningitis may occur at any age, it is most common in childhood and early adult life. Approximately one third of the cases develop before the age of ten and over 85% occur before the age of forty (Table 4). It is rare below the age of six months. The incidence in the two sexes is approximately equal.

Symptoms. The onset is usually subacute, with headache, vomiting, fever, apathy and irritability as the most prominent symptoms. Stiffness of the neck and vomiting become evident within a few days. Convulsive seizures are not uncommon in children during the first days of the disease. The headache becomes progressively more severe and in infants there is bulging of the fontanelles. The pain often results in a peculiarly shrill cry (meningeal cry). With progress of the disease patients become stuporous or comatose. Blindness and signs of damage to other cranial nerves may appear or there may be convulsive seizures or focal neurological signs.

Physical Findings. The physical findings in the early stages are those associated with meningeal infection, *i.e.,* fever, irritability, stiffness of the neck and Kernig's sign. The deep reflexes may be exaggerated or depressed. Signs of increased intracranial pressure and focal damage to the nervous system are rarely present at the onset. The initial irritability is gradually replaced by apathy and stupor. Choking of the discs,

Table 4.   The Age Incidence of 84 Cases of Tuberculous Meningitis

Age in Years	No. of Cases	%
½ to 9	26	31
10 to 19	11	13
20 to 29	24	29
30 to 39	12	14
Over 40	11	13
Total	84	100

cranial nerve palsies and focal neurologic signs are common in the latter stages of the disease. Clinical evidence of tuberculosis elsewhere in the body may or may not be present.

The temperature, which is only moderately elevated (100° to 102° F) in the early stages, rises to high levels before death. The respiratory and pulse rates are increased. In the terminal stages respirations become irregular and of the Cheyne-Stokes type.

Diagnosis. The diagnosis of tuberculous meningitis can be established only by culturing the organisms from the cerebrospinal fluid or by results of inoculation of guinea pigs. The cerebrospinal fluid findings are, however, quite characteristic and a presumptive diagnosis can be made when the typical abnormalities are present. These include: An increased pressure; a slightly cloudy or ground-glass appearance to the fluid with formation of a clot on standing; a moderate pleocytosis varying from 25 to 500 cells per cu mm, with lymphocytes as the predominating cell type; increased protein content; decreased sugar content with values in the range of 20 to 40 mg per 100 ml; a negative serological test for syphilis; and absence of growth when the fluid is inoculated on routine culture media. While no one of the above abnormalities is diagnostic, their occurrence in combination is almost pathognomonic, and is sufficient evidence to warrant intensive therapy until the diagnosis can be confirmed by stained smears of the sediment or pellicle, by culture of the fluid or by guinea pig inoculation. Other diagnostic aids include a thorough search for a primary focus including roentgenograms of the chest and tuberculin skin tests. The latter is of value chiefly in infants or young children.

Differential Diagnosis. Tuberculous meningitis must be differentiated from other forms of acute and subacute meningitis, viral infections, and meningeal reactions to septic foci in the skull or spine.

Acute purulent meningitis is characterized by a high cell count and the presence of the causative organisms in the cerebrospinal fluid. Preliminary antibiotic therapy of purulent meningitis may cause the spinal fluid findings to mimic those of tuberculous meningitis.

The cerebrospinal fluid in syphilitic meningitis may show changes quite similar to those of tuberculous meningitis. The normal or relatively normal sugar content and the positive serological reactions make the diagnosis of syphilitic meningitis relatively easy.

The clinical picture and cerebrospinal fluid findings in cryptococcus meningitis may be identical with those of tuberculous meningitis. The differential can be made by finding the budding yeast organisms in the counting chamber, in stained smears, or by culture on Sabouraud's medium.

Meningeal involvement in the course of viral infections such as mumps, lymphocytic choriomeningitis and the various forms of viral encephalitis may give a clinical picture similar to that of tuberculous meningitis. In these cases the cerebrospinal fluid sugar content is almost always normal.

Diffuse involvement of the meninges by metastatic tumors (carcinoma or sarcoma) or by gliogenous tumors may produce mental confusion and meningeal signs. The cerebrospinal fluid may contain a number of lymphocytes and polymorphonuclear leukocytes and a reduced sugar content. The protracted course or the finding of neoplastic cells in the cerebrospinal fluid exclude the diagnosis of tuberculous meningitis.

Prognosis and Course. Tuberculous meningitis is a highly fatal disease. Prior to the advent of streptomycin and isoniazid there was no effective therapy. A few cases were reported in the literature in which there was apparently a spontaneous cure. The diagnosis in most of such cases is open to doubt. For all practical purposes the disease can be considered as 100% fatal and death usually occurs within three to four weeks of the onset. There was a considerable reduction in the mortality rate when streptomycin was first used, and now with the administration of isoniazid, alone or in combination with other drugs, the mortality rate is less than 20%. Falk reported a mortality rate of 73% in 171 adults treated with streptomycin alone. This rate was reduced to 20% in the 129 patients treated with streptomycin, isoniazid and para-aminosalicylic acid. The prognosis is influenced considerably by the age of the patients. Weiss and his associates obtained a cure in 81% of 16 children under the age of eleven years, 53% of 32 patients aged eleven to forty-one years, and in only 14% of 22 patients over forty-one years of age. The presence of active tuberculosis in other organs or of miliary tuberculosis does not significantly affect the prognosis if isoniazid is given. Relapses occasionally occur after a period of months or even years in apparently cured cases.

Sequelae. Minor or major sequelae occur in approximately one fourth of the patients who recover. These vary from minimal degree of facial weakness to severe intellectual and physical disorganization. In the 100 children reported by Lorber, physical sequelae were found in 23, and an intelligence quotient of less than 80 in 21. Physical defects included deafness (6 cases), convulsive seizures (8 cases), blindness (3 cases), hemiplegia (7 cases), paraplegia (3 cases) and quadriplegia (1 case). Intracranial calcifications were found in the roentgenograms of 45 of the patients. These calcifications usually appeared between two and three years after the onset of the disease, and were commonly seen in the meninges at the base of the skull and rarely in the substance of the brain. Falk reported neurological residuals in 54 of 235 adults (23%) who were living one year or more after the start of therapy.

Treatment. Treatment should be started immediately in a patient with the characteristic clinical symptoms and cerebrospinal findings without waiting for bacteriological confirmation of the diagnosis. It is generally agreed that the prognosis for recovery and freedom from sequelae is directly related to the promptness of the initiation of therapy. As initial form of therapy, isoniazid supplemented with rifampin and ethambutol is used and continued for eighteen to twenty-four months. Intramuscular injections of streptomycin may be used. Corticosteroids may prove beneficial in the early phases of the disease when there is evidence of impending subarachnoid block or cerebral edema. Peripheral neuropathy secondary to isoniazid treatment can be prevented by giving pyridoxine. Intrathecal therapy is not indicated.

REFERENCES

Bobrowitz, I. D.: Ethambutal in Tuberculous Meningitis, Chest, 61, 629, 1972.
Falk, A.: U. S. Veterans Administration—Armed Forces Cooperative Study on the Chemotherapy of Tuberculosis, XIII. Tuberculous Meningitis in Adults with Special Reference to Survival, Neurological Residuals and Work Status, Am. Rev. Respir. Dis., 91, 823, 1965.
Kocen, R. S., and Parsons, M.: Neurological Complications of Tuberculosis: Some Unusual Manifestations, Q. J. Med., 39, 17, 1970.
Lincoln, E. M., Sordillo, V. R., and Davies, P. A.: Tuberculous Meningitis in Children, J. Pediatr., 57, 807, 1960.
Lorber, J.: Long-Term Follow-up of 100 Children Who Recovered from Tuberculous Meningitis, Pediatrics, 28, 778, 1961.
McKendrick, G. D. W., and Grose, R. J.: Tuberculous Meningitis, J. Neurol., Neurosurg. Psychiatry, 20, 198, 1957.
Merritt, H. H., and Fremont-Smith, F.: The Cerebrospinal Fluid in Tuberculous Meningitis, Arch. Neurol. Psychiatry, 33, 516, 1935.
Osuntokun, B. O., Adeuja, A. O. G. and Familusi, J. B.: Tuberculous Meningitis in Nigerians. A study of 194 Patients, Trop. Geogr. Med., 23, 225, 1971.
Steiner, P., and Portugaleza, C.: Tuberculous Meningitis in Children. A Review of 24 Cases Observed Between the Years 1965 to 1970 at the Kings County Medical Center of Brooklyn with Special Reference to the Problem of Infection with Primary Drug-resistant Strains of M. Tuberculosis, Am. Rev. Respir. Dis., 107, 22, 1973.
Sumaya, C. V., et al.: Tuberculous Meningitis in Children During the Isoniazid Era, J. Pediatr., 87, 43, 1975.
Udani, P. M., Parekh, U. C., and Dastur, D. K.: Neurological and Related Syndromes in CNS Tuberculosis, J. Neurol. Sci., 14, 341, 1971.
Weiss, W., and Flippin, H. F.: The Prognosis of Tuberculous Meningitis in the Isoniazid Era, Am. J. Med. Sci., 242, 423, 1961.

Brucellosis

Brucellosis (undulant fever) is a disease with protean manifestation due to infection with short, slender, rod-shaped gram-negative micro-organisms. The infection is transmitted to man from animals, usually cattle or swine. An acute febrile illness is characteristic of the early stages of the disease. This is followed by the subacute and chronic stages in about 15 to 20% of the cases with localized infection of the bones, joints, lungs, kidney, liver, lymph nodes and other organs.

Involvement of the nervous system is rare. A few cases have been reported with symptoms and signs of a meningoencephalitis, meningomyelitis, or neuritis.

The cerebrospinal fluid in the reported cases was under increased pressure, with a pleocytosis varying from a few to several hundred cells. The protein content was moderately to greatly increased and the sugar content decreased.

In a few cases with central nervous system involvement that have come to autopsy, there was a subacute meningitis with perivascular infiltration and thickening of the vessels in the brain and spinal cord, degenerative changes in the white and gray matter. Organisms have been cultured from the spinal fluid of a few cases.

The diagnosis is made from a history of previous symptoms of the disease, culture of the organism from the blood or cerebrospinal fluid, and agglutination tests.

Treatment is with tetracycline and streptomycin. Ampicillin may also be effective.

REFERENCES

Busch, L. A., and Parker, R. L.: Brucellosis in the United States, J. Infect. Dis., 125, 289, 1972.
Fincham, R. W., Sahs, A. L., and Joynt, R. J.: Protean Manifestations of Nervous System Brucellosis, J.A.M.A., 784, 269, 1963.
Mushinski, J. F., Taniguchi, R. M., and Stiefel, J. W.: Guillain-Barre Syndrome Associated with Ulceroglandular Tularemia, Neurology, 14, 877, 1964.
Williams, E.: Brucellosis, Br. Med. J., 1, 791, 1973.

Fungal Meningitis

The meninges and the central nervous system are occasionally invaded in the course of infection by any of the pathogenic fungi. In recent years there has been an increase in the incidence and severity of this type of infection. This has been attributed to two factors; new antimicrobial agents have destroyed the normal nonpathogenic bacterial flora which are presumably of importance in preventing the growth of fungi; and the widespread use of corticosteroids. It has become apparent that the use of these steroids has increased the incidence of infections with fungi of low pathogenicity to man and greatly increased the severity of infections with the more pathogenic organisms, particularly in patients with Hodgkin's disease, leukemia or in other diseases which interfere with the immune reactions. The administration of immunosuppressive agents to patients with kidney or other organ transplants or as a method of treatment for presumably autoimmune diseases may be followed by systemic infection with fungi.

The lungs, skin, hair and other organs are usually the primary site of involvement by the pathogenic fungi but involvement of the nervous system has been reported in most of them. This involvement usually takes the form of a meningitis, but there may also be granuloma or abscess formation in the meninges or in the parenchyma of the nervous system. Involvement of the nervous system is relatively uncommon in infections with actinomycosis, aspergillus, blastomycosis of the North American type, candida, coccidioidomycosis, histoplasmosis, maduromycosis and nocardiosis. It is quite common in cryptococcosis, where primary involvement of the nervous system sometimes occurs. In mucormycosis extension of the infection from the nasal sinuses and eye to the brain is a common event.

Diagnosis of fungal infections is often difficult and depends on the alertness of the physician to the possibility of this type of disease. The characteristic findings in the roentgenograms of the lungs and other organs, skin tests, serological tests and isolation of the organisms from the lesions are important aids in establishing the diagnosis.

Treatment of fungal infections in man is at best unsatisfactory. The administration of penicillin and the other commonly used antimicrobial agents is usually not only useless but may also lead to the spread of the infection, with the exception of infection by actinomycosis and nocardiosis. The former is curable by either the tetracycline antibiotics or penicillin and the latter by the sulfonamides. Hydroxystilbamidine is effective in the treatment of blastomycosis. Some success has been obtained in the treatment of other fungal infections by antifungal agents, particularly amphotericin B and 5-fluorocytosine.

REFERENCES

General

Bennett, J. E.: Chemotherapy of Systemic Mycoses, N. Engl. J. Med., 290, 30, 1974.
Codish, S. D., and Tobias, J. S.: Managing Systemic Mycoses in the Compromised Host, J.A.M.A., 235, 2132, 1976.
Furcolow, M. L.: The Use of Amphotericin B. in Blastomycosis, Cryptococcosis and Histoplasmosis, Med. Clin. North Am., 47, 1119, 1963.
Louria, D. B.: Deep-seated Mycotic Infections, Allergy to Fungi and Mycotoxins, N. Engl. J. Med., 227, 1065, 1126, 1967.
Rifkind, D., et al.: Systemic Fungal Infections Complicating Renal Transplantation and Immunosuppressive Therapy, Am. J. Med., 43, 28, 1967.
Vandevelde, A. G., et al.: 5-Fluorocytosine in the Treatment of Mycotic Infections, Ann. Intern. Med., 77, 43, 1972.
Rowsell, H. C.: Mycotic Infections of Animals Transmissible to Man, Am. J. Med. Sci., 245, 333, 1963.
Vorreith, M.: Mycotic Encephalitis, Acta Neuropathol., 11, 55, 1968.

Actinomycosis

Bolton, C. F., and Ashenhurst, E. M.: Actinomycosis of the Brain, Case Report and Review of the Literature, Can. Med. Assoc. J., 90, 922, 1964.
Brown, J. R.: Human Actinomycosis, A Study of 181 Subjects, Hum. Pathol., 4, 319, 1973.

Aspergillosis

Gowing, N. F., and Hamlin, I. M.: Tissue Reactions to Aspergillus in Cases of Hodgkin's Disease and Leukemia, J. Clin. Pathol., 13, 396, 1960.

Groevic, N., and Matthews, W. F.: Pathologic Changes in Acute Disseminated Aspergillosis, Particularly Involvement of the Central Nervous System, Am. J. Clin. Pathol., 32, 536, 1959.

Hedges, T. R., and Leung, L. S. E.: Parasellar and Orbital Apex Syndrome Caused by Aspergillosis, Neurology, 26, 117, 1976.

Kaufman, D. M., Thal, L. J., and Farmer, P. M.: Central Nervous System Aspergillosis in 2 Young Adults, Neurology, 26, 484, 1976.

Young, R. C., et al.: Aspergillosis: The Spectrum of Disease in 98 Patients, Medicine, 49, 147, 1970.

Blastomycosis

Curtis, A. C., and Bocobo, F. C.: North American Blastomycosis, J. Chronic Dis., 5, 404, 1957.

Loudon, R. G., and Lawson, R. A., Jr.: Systemic Blastomycosis, Recurrent Neurological Relapse in a Case Treated with Amphotericin B, Ann. Intern. Med., 55, 141, 1961.

Rainey, R. L., and Harris, J. R.: Disseminated Blastomycosis with Meningeal Involvement, Arch. Intern. Med., 117, 745, 1966.

Candida (Moniliasis)

Black, J. T.: Cerebral Candidiosis: Case Report and Review of Literature, J. Neurol. Neurosurg. Psychiatry, 33, 864, 1970.

Louria, D. B., Stiff, D. P., and Bennett, B.: Disseminated Moniliasis in the Adult, Medicine, 41, 307, 1962.

Roessmann, U., and Friede, R. L.: Candida Infection of the Brain, Arch. Pathol., 84, 495, 1967.

Coccidioidomycosis

Abud-Ortega, A. F., Harris, L., and Rozdilsky, B.: Chronic Coccidioidal Meningitis, Can. Med. Assoc. J., 105, 613, 1971.

Caudill, R. G., Smith, C. E., and Reinarz, J. A.: Coccidioidal Meningitis, Am. J. Med., 49, 360, 1970.

Perry, D. M. and Kirby, W. M. M.: Acute Disseminated Coccidioidomycosis. Two Cases Treated with Amphotericin B, Arch. Intern. Med., 105, 929, 1966.

Winn, W. A.: Coccidioidomycosis and Amphotericin B., Med. Clin. North Am., 47, 1131, 1963.

Histoplasmosis

Sprofkin, B. E., Shapiro, J. L., and Lux, J. L.: Histoplasmosis of the Central Nervous System, J. Neuropathol. Exp. Neurol., 14, 288, 1955.

Vanek, J., and Schwartz, J.: The Gamut of Histoplasmosis, Am. J. Med., 50, 89, 1971.

White, H. H., and Fritzlen, T. J.: Cerebral Granuloma Caused by Histoplasma Capsulatum, J. Neurosurg., 19, 260, 1962.

Maduromycosis

Aronson, S. M., Benham, R., and Wolf, A.: Maduromycosis of the Central Nervous System, J. Neuropathol. Exp. Neurol., 12, 158, 1953.

Nocardiosis

Carlile, W. K., Holley, K. E., and Logan, G. B.: Fatal Acute Disseminated Nocardiosis in a Child, J.A.M.A., 184, 477, 1963.

Larsen, M. C., Diamond, H. D., and Collins, H. S.: Nocardia Asteroides Infection, Arch. Intern. Med., 103, 712, 1959.

Murray, J. F., et al.: The Changing Spectrum of Nocardiosis, Am. Rev. Respir. Dis., *83,* 315, 1961.
Turner, E. and Whitby, J. L.: Nocardial Brain Abscess: Successfully Treated with Aspiration and Sulfonamides, J. Neurosurg., *31,* 227, 1969.
Welsh, J. D., Rhoades, E. R., and Jaques, W.: Disseminated Nocardiosis Involving Spinal Cord, Arch. Intern. Med., *108,* 73, 1961.

Cryptococcosis

Cryptococcosis is the most common form of fungal infection of the nervous system. The disease may simulate tuberculous meningitis, tumor of the brain, encephalitis, and various psychoses.

Pathogenesis. The infecting organism is Cryptococcus neoformans. Infections with this organism have been previously described in the literature under various terms such as torulosis, yeast meningitis, and European blastomycosis. The respiratory tract is considered to be the usual portal of entry of the organism. Less common sites of inoculation in man are the skin and mucous membranes. Pathogenic strains of C. neoformans are contained in the droppings from pigeons and other birds and it is presumed that they are inhaled by man.

The incidence of infection is higher in patients with malignant diseases of the reticuloendothelial system such as Hodgkin's disease, lymphosarcoma and leukemia. Subjective and objective evidence of involvement of other organs of the body may or may not be present in the patients with central nervous system infection.

Pathology. The changes in the nervous system include infiltration of the meninges with mononuclear cells and the microorganisms. The organisms may be scattered diffusely through the parenchyma of the nervous system with little or no inflammatory reaction in the tissues. Rarely there is an abscess in the brain or large granulomas may be formed in the meninges of the brain or spinal cord.

Symptoms and Signs. The onset of symptoms of involvement of the nervous system is subacute. Meningeal symptoms usually predominate but occasionally focal neurologic signs or mental symptoms are in the foreground. The clinical picture in the usual case is that of a subacute meningitis or encephalitis. The diagnosis of tuberculous meningitis is usually entertained until attention is directed to the correct diagnosis by the peculiar appearance of some of the "cells" in the cerebrospinal fluid. The diagnosis of yeast meningitis is then established by culture of the organisms on Sabouraud's medium.

The syndrome in the cases with a large granuloma in the cerebrum, cerebellum or brain stem is the same as that of other expanding lesions in these sites. The diagnosis of a granuloma has rarely been made in such cases before operation. It can be made only when meningeal involvement is also present and the organisms are recovered from the cerebrospinal fluid.

Laboratory Data. The cerebrospinal fluid findings in infections with cryptococci (Table 5) are similar to those of tuberculous meningitis. The fluid is usually under an increased pressure. There is a slight or moderate pleocytosis varying between 10 and 500 cells per cu mm. The protein content is increased. The sugar content is decreased, with values commonly between 15 and 35 mg. The diagnosis is made by the

Table 5.   The Cerebrospinal Fluid from Two Patients with Cryptococcal Meningitis (Necropsy Proven)

Case	Date	Pressure	Cells	Protein	Sugar
1	8–30–28	210	20	228	36
	10–13–28	500	96	190	39
2	7– 5–30	170	140	133	19
	12–29–31	320	204	228	46
	6–20–32	120	420	231	32
	8– 8–33	...	30	618	13

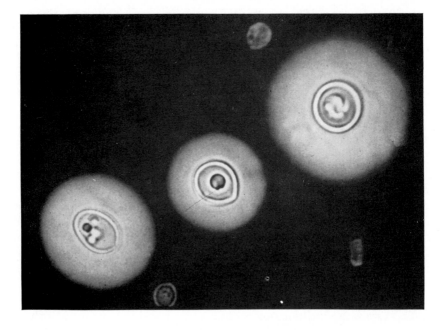

Figure 1.   Cryptococcus neoformans meningitis. Fresh preparation of sediment from spinal fluid stained with India ink. The capsule is three times the diameter of the cell. (Courtesy Dr. Margarita Silva.)

findings of the organisms in the counting chamber or centrifuged sediment of the fluid (Fig. 1), by growth on Sabouraud's medium or by the results of animal inoculations. The organisms may also be cultured from the urine, blood, stool, sputum and bone marrow. Rarely the organism cannot be seen on smear or grown in cultures. The diagnosis can be established by the immunological detection of cryptococcal antigen in serum and cerebrospinal fluid.

Course. The disease in untreated cases is usually fatal within a few months but occasionally the course may extend over several years (Fig. 2) with recurring periods of remissions and exacerbations. We have seen several cases with yeast organisms in the cerebrospinal fluid for three or more years (see Case 2, Table 5). Spontaneous cure has been reported in a few cases. Treatment with amphotericin B has a definite beneficial effect. Butler and his associates reported improvement in 31 of 36 treated cases. Seventeen of the 31 patients who showed improvement remained well, 3 died of unrelated causes and 11 had one or more relapses of meningitis.

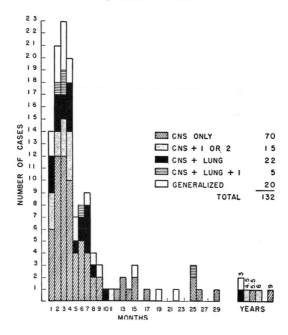

DURATION IN MONTHS FROM ONSET
OF SYMPTOMS TO DEATH

Figure 2.   Duration of life in 132 cases of cryptococcal meningitis. The stippled area referred to as 1 and 2 in the figure indicates cases in which skin or bones were also involved. (Courtesy Dr. Charles Carton.)

Treatment. The commonly used antimicrobial agents have no appreciable effect on the course of the infection. Some successes have been reported with the administration of amphotericin B and 5-fluorocytosine. Combined treatment must be used to prevent failure due to emergence of fluorocytosine resistance. Amphotericin B administration by cisternal injection or into the cerebral ventricles by an Ommaya reservoir has been used. Sterility of the spinal fluid is probably the best end point of successful treatment. The course of treatment should be repeated if there is a relapse.

Side effects of the administration of amphotericin B include thrombophlebitis, nausea and vomiting, fever, anemia, hypokalemia and elevation of the blood urea level. Aspirin, antihistamines, blood transfusions and temporary reduction in the dosage of the drug are of value in the control of these side effects.

REFERENCES

Butler, W. T., et al.: Diagnostic and Prognostic Value of Clinical and Laboratory Findings in Cryptococcal Meningitis. A Follow-up of Forty Patients, N. Engl. J. Med., *270*, 59, 1964.
Diamond R. D., and Bennett, J. E.: Prognostic Factors in Cryptococcal Meningitis, Ann. Intern. Med., *80*, 176, 1974.
Edwards, V. E., Sutherland, J. M., and Tyrer, J. H.: Cryptococcosis of the Central Nervous System, J. Neurol. Neurosurg. Psychiatry, *33*, 415, 1970.
Lewis, J. L. and Rabinovitch, S.: The Wide Spectrum of Cryptococcal Infections, Am. J. Med., *53*, 315, 1972.
Littman, M. L. and Zimmerman, L. E.: *Cryptococcosis*, New York, Grune & Stratton, 1956, 205 pp.
Littman, M. L., and Walter, J. E.: Cryptococcosis: Current Status, Am. J. Med., *45*, 922, 1968.
McDonald, R., Greenberg, E. N., and Kramer, R.: Cryptococcal Meningitis, Arch. Dis. Child., *45*, 417, 1970.
Snow, R. M. and Dismukes, W. E.: Cryptococcal Meningitis: Diagnostic Value of Cryptococcal Antigen in Cerebrospinal Fluid, Arch. Intern. Med., *135*, 1155, 1975.
Swanson, H. S. and Smith, W. A.: Torula Granuloma Simulating Cerebral Tumors, Arch. Neurol. Psychiatry, *51*, 426, 1944.

Mucormycosis

Mucormycosis is a disease caused by certain fungi, especially Rhizopus, that are common contaminants of laboratory cultures and not ordinarily pathogenic. Cases have been reported in all parts of the United States, Canada and England and the disease is probably world-wide. It usually occurs as a complication of diabetes mellitus and blood dyscrasias, particularly the leukemias. The use of antibiotics and corticosteroids may also be predisposing factors. The fungi enter the nose and in susceptible persons they produce sinusitis and orbital cellulitis, penetrate arteries to produce thrombosis of the ophthalmic and internal carotid arteries, and later invade veins and lymphatics.

There are ocular, cerebral, pulmonary, intestinal and disseminated forms of the disease.

Proptosis, ocular palsies, and hemiplegia are the common neurological signs associated with involvement of the orbit and the internal carotid artery. The organisms may invade the meninges and produce a meningitis or they may extend into the brain and produce a mycotic encephalitis.

The diagnosis is made by examination of the sputum, spinal fluid or exudate from the nasal sinuses. Culture of Rhizopus is corroborative, but not diagnostic because it is a common contaminant.

The disease is highly fatal and death is almost inevitable when the nervous system is invaded. Death usually occurs within one day to several weeks after the onset of infection. Clinical recovery has been reported when only the sinus or orbit is involved.

Treatment consists of the administration of amphotericin B and control of the diabetes. The use of corticosteroids and bacterial antibiotics should be discontinued.

REFERENCES

Goss, J. S.: Acute Orbital Mucormycosis, Arch, Ophthalmol., 65, 214, 1961.

Hoagland, R. J., et al.: Mucormycosis, Am. J. Med. Sci., 242, 415, 1961.

Landau, J. W. and Newcomer, V. D.: Acute Cerebral Phycomycosis (Mucormycosis), J. Pediatr., 61, 363, 1962.

McBride, R. A., Corson, J. M., and Dammin, G. J.: Mucormycosis, Am. J. Med., 28, 832, 1960.

Sandler, R., et al.: Successfully Treated Rhinocerebral Phycomycosis in Well-Controlled Diabetes, N. Engl. J. Med., 285, 1180, 1971.

Smith, H. W., and Kirchner, J. A.: Cerebral Mucormycosis, Arch. Ophthalmol., 68, 715, 1958.

Sarcoidosis

Sarcoidosis (Besnier-Boeck-Schaumann disease) is a generalized disease of unknown etiology which is characterized by the development of small nodules (follicles or tubercles). Numerous clinical syndromes result depending upon the organ involved. The lungs, skin, lymph nodes, bones, eye and parotid glands are most commonly the site of the lesions. The nervous system is only occasionally invaded. The peripheral or cranial nerves, the meninges or any portion of the brain or spinal cord may be involved. The seventh cranial nerve is frequently affected in conjunction with uveitis and parotitis (uveoparotid fever). Involvement of the muscles has been reported in a few cases.

Etiology and Pathology. The etiology of sarcoidosis is as yet unknown. Many observers are of the opinion that it is an atypical form of

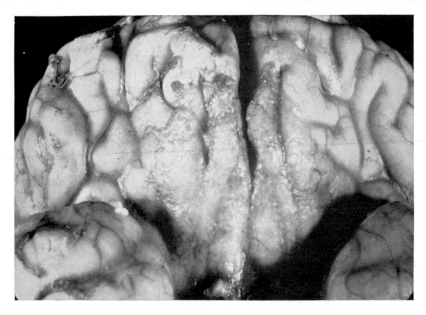

Figure 3.   Sarcoidosis. Lesions in the meninges at the base of the
frontal lobe. (Courtesy Dr. Abner Wolf.)

infection with the tubercle bacillus. The characteristic lesions (Fig. 3)
are small nodules composed of lymphocytes, endothelial and giant
cells. Tubercle bacilli are not found in the lesions except when active
tuberculosis develops in patients with sarcoidosis. In these cases,
tubercle bacilli may be found in the pre-existing sarcoid lesion.

Incidence. Sarcoidosis may occur at any period of life but it is most
common between the ages of fifteen and forty. All races are affected but
in the United States there is an apparent predilection for the Negro. The
sexes are equally affected. The exact incidence of involvement of the
nervous system is not known. Mayock and his associates found
evidence of involvement of the peripheral or central nervous system in
23 of 145 patients (16%), but in their review of the literature they found
that the nervous system was reported to be affected in only 32 of 625
cases (5.1%).

Symptoms and Signs—Cranial Nerves. The cranial nerves are the
most common site of involvement of the nervous system in sarcoidosis.
Facial paralysis, either unilateral or bilateral, occurred in over 50% of
the reported cases. This was usually in association with uveitis and
parotitis. The facial paralysis is not necessarily related to swelling of
the parotid gland, because it may precede the development of the
parotitis or occur independently of any swelling of the gland. In

addition, the taste fibers are involved in a number of cases. The facial paralysis usually clears entirely but occasionally there may be contractures or facial spasm.

Optic neuritis, optic atrophy or swelling of the optic discs, recorded in approximately 25% of the cases with involvement of the nervous system, may occur as the result of direct involvement of the nerve or from pressure on the nerve by lesions in the infundibular region. Visual field defects and diabetes insipidus have also been reported. Other ocular lesions in addition to the uveitis include chorioretinitis, perivasculitis and choroidal atrophy.

Involvement of one or more of all the remaining cranial nerves has been reported.

Peripheral Nerves. Any of the peripheral nerves may be affected alone or in combination with other peripheral or cranial nerves, with resulting weakness and atrophy of the muscles and cutaneous sensory loss in the distribution of the affected nerve.

Meningitis. Signs of meningitis or meningoencephalitis are accompanied by cerebrospinal fluid abnormalities of the type commonly seen in a subacute meningitis. In these cases the pressure is increased, there is a mild pleocytosis (10 to 200 cells, mainly lymphocytes), an increased protein content and changes in the colloidal gold reaction in the first or mid zone. The sugar content of the fluid may be decreased (15 to 40 mg per 100 ml) but no organisms are recovered. A slight pleocytosis and increased protein content in the cerebrospinal fluid may be found in the absence of any symptoms of meningeal involvement. The gamma globulin content of the spinal fluid may be increased.

Chronic adhesive arachnoiditis or nodule formation may develop in the dura or arachnoid, especially in the posterior fossa.

Brain and Spinal Cord. In addition to the occurrence of parenchymal lesions secondary to involvement of the meninges, single or multiple lesions may develop in the cerebral hemisphere, basal ganglia, brain stem, cerebellum or spinal cord. The appropriate focal neurological symptoms and signs are present in these cases and, in addition, convulsive seizures and choked discs may develop when there are large lesions in the cerebellum or cerebral hemispheres.

Muscles. Involvement of the muscles may be found on biopsy without any clinical symptoms. Occasionally, however, this may be manifested by a moderate or severe degree of weakness and muscular atrophy. The tendon reflexes may be reduced or absent in the involved muscles.

Laboratory Data. Fever of a moderate degree is an inconstant feature. A mild leukocytosis with eosinophilia is present in approximately one third of the cases. Anemia may occur and an elevation of the serum globulin is found in about one half of the cases. The serum calcium content is moderately or greatly increased in about 15% of the cases. The tuberculin reaction in the skin is negative. The cerebrospinal fluid findings have been discussed previously under meningeal involvement.

Diagnosis. The diagnosis of sarcoidosis as the cause of neurological signs and symptoms is usually made without difficulty when the latter occur in association with cutaneous or glandular manifestations of the disease, and the diagnosis can be confirmed by biopsy of the nodules. Granulomas may also be found in tissue obtained by muscle or liver biopsy. In addition, the ocular manifestations and the roentgenographic appearance of the lesions in the lungs and bones are sufficiently characteristic to be of value in the differential diagnosis. In the absence of active manifestations of the process in other organs of the body, the diagnosis cannot be definitely established. Usually, however, there will be a history of the previous occurrence of uveitis or some of the other manifestations of the disease. The Kveim test is of value in establishing the diagnosis in doubtful cases.

According to Israel and Goldstein the Kveim-antigen test is associated with lymphadenopathy. It is most likely to be positive in sarcoidosis when the lymph nodes are involved, but it is also occasionally positive in patients with lymphadenopathy from other causes.

The differential diagnosis includes epidemic parotitis, Hodgkin's disease, leprosy, syphilis, cryptococcosis, and tuberculosis. These conditions can usually be excluded by the clinical picture, biopsy of the nodules, the x-ray findings and other laboratory tests.

Facial palsy is extremely rare in epidemic parotitis and uveitis is not a part of the clinical picture of the disease. In the cases with meningeal involvement, cryptococcosis is excluded by the failure to recover the organisms from the cerebrospinal fluid and tuberculous meningitis by the chronic course as well as by the absence of tubercle bacilli.

Course and Prognosis. Sarcoidosis is in general a benign disease, tending to involve one or more systems of the body in the course of several or many years, and then to subside spontaneously. As a rule, there is a slow recovery of function of the palsies which result from lesions in the peripheral or cranial nerves. There may also be a remission of the signs of meningeal or parenchymatous involvement. Death may result from increased intracranial pressure. Active tuberculosis may develop at any time in patients with sarcoidosis and prove fatal.

Treatment. No specific therapy is known. There is no evidence to indicate that the antibiotics have any effect on the disease. ACTH and the adrenal steroids have a beneficial effect on the lesions in the central nervous system as well as in other organs.

REFERENCES

Cares, R. M., Gordon, B. S., and Kreuger, E.: Boeck's Sarcoid in Chronic Meningo-Encephalitis. Organic Psychosis with Massive Softening due to Boeck's Disease, J. Neuropathol. Exp. Neurol., *16*, 544, 1957.

Colover, J.: Sarcoidosis with Involvement of the Nervous System, Brain, *71*, 451, 1948.

Cromptom, M. R., and MacDermot, V.: Sarcoidosis Associated with Progressive Muscular Wasting and Weakness, Brain, *84*, 62, 1961.

Day, A. L., and Sypert, G. W.: Spinal Cord Sarcoidosis, Ann. Neurol., *1*, 79, 1977.

Douglas, A. C., and Maloney, A. F. J.: Sarcoidosis of the Central Nervous System, J. Neurol. Neurosurg. Psychiatry, *36*, 1024, 1973.

Gaines, J. D., Eckman, P. B., and Remington, J. S.: Low CSF Glucose in Sarcoidosis Involving the Central Nervous System, Arch. Intern. Med., *125*, 333, 1970.

Herring, A. B., and Urich, H.: Sarcoidosis of Central Nervous System, J. Neurol. Sci., *9*, 405, 1969.

Hinterbuchner, C. N., and Hinterbuchner, L. P.: Myopathic Syndrome in Muscular Sarcoidosis, Brain, *87*, 355, 1964.

Matthews, W. B.: Sarcoidosis of the Nervous System, J. Neurol. Neurosurg. Psychiatry, *28*, 23, 1965.

Mayock, R. L., et al.: Manifestations of Sarcoidosis, Am. J. Med., *35*, 67, 1963.

Mitchell, D. N., and Scadding, J. G.: Sarcoidosis, Am. Rev. Respir. Dis., *110*, 774, 1974.

Pennell, W. H.: Boeck's Sarcoid with Involvement of the Central Nervous System, Arch. Neurol. Psychiatry, *66*, 728, 1951.

Siltzbach, L. E., et al.: Course and Prognosis of Sarcoidosis Around the World, Am. J. Med., *57*, 847, 1974.

Teirstein, A. S., Wolf, B. S., and Siltzbach, L. E.: Sarcoidosis of the Skull, N. Engl. J. Med., *265*, 65, 1961.

Wiederholt, W. C., and Siekert, R. G.: Neurological Manifestations of Sarcoidosis, Neurology, *15*, 1147, 1965.

Behcet's Syndrome

A syndrome of unknown etiology, characterized by the occurrence of relapsing uveitis, recurrent genital and oral ulcers, was described by Behcet in 1937. Since that time more than one thousand cases have been reported in the literature. It is now known that the disease may involve the nervous system, skin, joints, peripheral blood vessels and other organs. Evidence of central nervous system involvement is present in approximately 25%. Pathological confirmation of cerebral involvement has been obtained in a few cases. The disease appears to have a predilection for young adult males.

Etiology and Pathology. The etiology of the disease is unknown. Sezer isolated a virus from the eye of one patient. Evans, Pallis and Spillane recovered a virus from the brain and cerebrospinal fluid of one patient and showed that neutralizing antibodies were present in 11 clinical cases of Behcet's syndrome. However, the absence of inclusion bodies and the negative results of animal inoculations cast doubt on the virus etiology of this disease.

In cases that have been studied at necropsy, there was a mild inflammatory reaction in the meninges and in the perivascular spaces of the cerebrum, basal ganglia, brain stem and cerebellum and degenerative changes in the ganglion cells. Inflammatory changes were also found in the iris, choroid, retina and optic nerve.

Incidence. As noted above the number of reported cases is fairly large. The disease has been reported from Europe, particularly in the countries bordering on the Mediterranean Sea, America and Japan. The age of onset is in the third to sixth decade of life and men are more frequently affected than women. The exact incidence of neurological symptoms is not known, but it is probably less than 10% of the affected individuals.

Symptoms and Signs. The ocular signs include keratoconjunctivitis, iritis, hypopyon, uveitis and hemorrhage into the vitreous. These may progress to total blindness in one or both eyes. The cutaneous lesions are in the nature of painful recurrent and indolent ulcers, which are most commonly found on the genitalia or the buccal mucosa. Joint effusions, furunculosis, erythema nodosum, thrombophlebitis, and nonspecific skin sensitivity are also common. The liver may be enlarged.

Any portion of the nervous system may be affected. Cranial nerve palsies are common. Other symptoms and signs include papilledema, convulsions, mental confusion, coma, aphasia, hemiparesis, quadriparesis, pseudobulbar palsy, and evidence of involvement of the basal ganglia, cerebellum or spinal cord.

Laboratory Data. A low-grade fever is common during the acute exacerbations of the disease. This may be accompanied by an elevation of the sedimentation rate, anemia and a slight leukocytosis in the blood. A polyclonal increase of serum gamma globulin may be present with elevated levels of IgA and IgM. Coagulation profile may disclose elevated levels of clotting factors.

The cerebrospinal fluid pressure may be slightly increased. There is a pleocytosis in the fluid of a mild or moderate degree, and a moderate increase in the protein content. Spinal fluid sugars, when reported, have been normal. The serological tests for syphilis are negative in the blood and cerebrospinal fluid. Spinal fluid cultures have been negative. Mild diffuse abnormalities may be found on the electroencephalogram.

Diagnosis and Differential Diagnosis. The diagnosis is based on the occurrence of signs of a meningoencephalitis in combination with the characteristic cutaneous and ocular lesions. Syphilis is excluded by the negative serological tests and sarcoidosis by the absence of other signs of this disease and a negative Kveim test.

Course. The course of the disease is characterized by a series of remissions and exacerbations extending over a number of years. During the period of remission there may be great improvement in all of the symptoms. Unilateral amblyopia or complete blindness may result from the ocular lesions and residuals of the neurological lesions are not uncommon.

Knowledge of the disease is too recent to state the ultimate fate of the affected individuals. Death has occurred from the disease chiefly when the central nervous system became involved. Permanent remission of symptoms has not been reported.

Treatment. Various antibiotics, chemotherapy, and corticosteroids have been used in the treatment but there is no evidence that any of these forms of therapy have any effect on the course of the disease.

REFERENCES

Alema, G., and Bignami, A.: Involvement of the Nervous System in Behcet's Disease. Pages 52 to 66 in *International Symposium on Behcet's Disease.* Basel and New York, S. Karger, 1966.
Chajek, T., and Fainaru, M.: Behcet's Disease. A Report of 41 Cases and a Review of the Literature, Medicine, *54*, 179, 1975.
Evans, A. D., Pallis, C. A., and Spillane, J. D.: Involvement of the Nervous System in Behcet's Syndrome. Report of Three Cases and Isolation of Virus, Lancet, *2*, 349, 1957.
Kalbian, V. V., and Challis, M. T.: Behcet's Disease. Report of Twelve Cases with Three Manifesting as Papilledema, Am. J. Med., *49*, 823, 1970.
Kawakita, H., et al.: Neurological Aspects of Behcet's Disease, J. Neurol. Sci., 5, 417, 1967.
McMenemey, W. H., and Lawrence, B. J.: Encephalomyelopathy in Behcet's Disease: Report of Necropsy Findings in Two Cases, Lancet, *2*, 353, 1957.
Norman, R. M., and Campbell, A. M. G.: The Neuropathology of Behcet's Disease. Pages 67–78 in *International Symposium on Behcet's Disease.* Basel and New York, S. Karger, 1966.
O'Duffy, J. D., and Goldstein, N. P.: Neurologic Involvement in Seven Patients with Behcet's Disease, Am. J. Med., *61*, 170, 1976.
Rubinstein, L. J., and Urich, H.: Meningoencephalitis of Behcet's Disease: Case Report with Pathological Findings, Brain, *86*, 151, 1963.
Wolf, S. M., Schotland, D. L., and Phillips, L. L.: Involvement of Nervous System in Behcet's Syndrome, Arch. Neurol., *12*, 315, 1965.

Uveomeningoencephalitic Syndrome

A relatively rare disease characterized by uveitis, retinal hemorrhages and detachment, depigmentation of the skin and hair, and signs of involvement of the nervous system has been reported by Vogt, Harada and Koyanagi. The clinical course is divided into three phases: meningeal, ophthalmic and convalescent.

Involvement of the nervous system is present in practically all of the cases. The neurological symptoms are due to an inflammatory adhesive arachnoiditis. Deafness, delirium, diabetes insipidus, hemiplegia, ocular palsies and psychotic manifestations may occur. The cerebrospinal fluid is under increased pressure. There is a moderate degree of lymphocytic pleocytosis and increased protein content in the fluid.

The period of activity of the process lasts for six to twelve months and is followed by a recrudescence of the ophthalmic and neurological signs.

The cause of the disease is unknown. It has been suggested that it is due to a viral infection, but proof for this is lacking. The eye lesions are similar to those of sympathetic ophthalmia.

There is no specific therapy, but there are reports in the literature which suggest that the administration of corticosteroids may be of value.

REFERENCES

Harada, E.: Clinical Study of Nonsuppurative Choroiditis, Acta Soc. Ophth. Japan., *30*, 356, 1926.
Koyanagi, Y.: Dysacousia, Alopecia, and Poliosis with Severe Uveitis of Non-traumatic Origin, Klin. Monatsbl. f. Augenh., *82*, 194, 1929.
Pattison, E. M.: Uveomeningoencephalitic Syndrome (Vogt-Koyanagi-Harada), Arch. Neurol., *12*, 197, 1965.
Reed, H.: Uveo-Encephalitis, World Neurol., *1*, 173, 1960.
Riehl, J-L., and Andrews, J. M.: Uveomeningoencephalitic Syndrome, Neurology, *16*, 603, 1966.

ASEPTIC MENINGEAL REACTION

Aseptic meningeal reaction (sympathetic meningitis) is a term used to describe those cases with evidence of a meningeal reaction in the cerebrospinal fluid in the absence of any infecting organism. There are two general classes of cases which fall into this category: (1) Those in which the meningeal reaction is due to a septic or necrotic focus within the skull or spinal canal; and (2) those in which the meningeal reaction is due to the introduction of foreign substances into the subarachnoid space (air, dyes, drugs, sera, blood and the like).

The symptoms which are present in the patients in the first group are those associated with the infection or morbid process in the skull or spinal cavity, and only occasionally are there any symptoms and signs of meningeal irritation.

In the second group of patients, where the meningeal reaction is due to the introduction of foreign substances into the subarachnoid space, there may be fever, headache and stiffness of the neck. The appearance of these symptoms leads to the suspicion that an actual infection of the meninges has been produced by the inadvertent introduction of pathogenic organisms. The normal sugar content of the fluid and the absence of organisms on culture establish the nature of the meningeal reaction.

The findings in the cerebrospinal fluid characteristic of an aseptic meningeal reaction are an increase in pressure (200 to 600 mm of water), a varying degree of pleocytosis (10 to 4,000 cells per cu mm), a slight or moderate increase in the protein content, a normal sugar content and the absence of organisms on culture. With a severe degree of meningeal reaction, the fluid may be purulent in appearance and contain several thousand cells per cu mm with a predominance of polymorphonuclear leukocytes. With a lesser degree of meningeal reaction, the fluid may be normal in appearance or only slightly cloudy and contain a moderate number of cells (10 to several hundred per cu mm), with lymphocytes the predominating cell type in the fluids with less than 100 cells per cu mm. The pathogenesis of the changes in the cerebrospinal fluid is not clearly understood. The septic foci in the head which are more commonly associated with an aseptic meningeal reaction are septic thrombosis of the intracranial venous sinuses, osteomyelitis of the spine or skull, extradural, subdural or intracerebral abscesses, or septic cerebral emboli. Nonseptic foci of necrosis are only rarely accompanied by an aseptic meningeal reaction. Occasionally patients with an intracerebral tumor or cerebral hemorrhage which is near to the ventricular walls may show the typical changes in the cerebrospinal fluid.

The diagnosis of an aseptic meningeal reaction in patients with a septic or necrotic focus in the skull or spinal cord is important in that it directs attention to the presence of this focus and the necessity for appropriate surgical and medical therapy before the meninges are actually invaded by the infectious process or other cerebral or spinal complications develop.

REFERENCE

Merritt, H. H., and Fremont-Smith, F.: The Cerebrospinal Fluid, Philadelphia, W. B. Saunders Co., 1938. 333 pp.

MENINGISM

Coincidental with the onset of any of the acute infectious diseases in childhood or young adult life, there may be headache, stiffness of the neck, Kernig's sign and, rarely, delirium, convulsions or coma. The appearance of these symptoms may lead to the tentative diagnosis of an acute meningitis or preparalytic poliomyelitis.

The occurrence of meningeal signs in the absence of meningitis, which has been variously described as serous meningitis or meningism, is due to a disturbance in the osmotic relationship between the blood and the cerebrospinal fluid. At the onset of acute infectious diseases (pneumonia, typhoid fever, the acute exanthemata and so forth), there is a retention of fluid in the body and dilution of the blood. This dilution of the blood makes it hypotonic to the cerebrospinal fluid. In an attempt to re-establish an equilibrium, water is transferred to the

cerebrospinal fluid through the choroid plexus. This results in a more
rapid formation of fluid than can be normally absorbed. The intracranial pressure rises and the cerebrospinal fluid is diluted. This dilution
explains the reduction in the protein and chloride content of the fluid.
The characteristic findings on lumbar puncture are a slight or moderate
increase in pressure, a clear, colorless fluid which contains no cells,
and a moderate reduction in the protein and chloride content of the
fluid.

This state of abnormal relationship between the osmotic pressure of
the blood and the cerebrospinal fluid is a transient one and clears up
with diuresis or when sufficient time has elapsed for an equilibrium
between the rate of formation and absorption of the cerebrospinal fluid
to be established. When this occurs, the symptoms disappear. Spinal
puncture, which is usually performed as a diagnostic measure in these
cases, is the only therapy necessary for the relief of the symptoms. The
reduction of pressure by the removal of fluid results in the disappearance of symptoms. Only rarely is more than one puncture necessary.

REFERENCES

Fremont-Smith, F., Dailey, M. E., and Thomas, G. W.: Dilution of Blood and Cerebrospi-
    nal Fluid in Fever, J. Clin. Invest., 6, 9, 1928–29.
Quincke, H.: Ueber Meningitis serosa, Sammlung, klin. Vortr. v.Volkmann, 1893, 67.

SUBDURAL AND EPIDURAL INFECTIONS
Cerebral Subdural Empyema

A collection of pus between the dura and the arachnoid of the brain is
known as subdural abscess or empyema.

Etiology. Subdural empyema may result from the direct extension of
infection from the middle ear, the nasal sinuses or meninges. It may
develop as a complication of compound fractures of the skull, or in the
course of septicemia. The infection is most commonly due to streptococci but may be caused by any of the pyogenic bacteria. The
mechanism of the formation of an abscess in the subdural space
following compound fractures of the skull is easily understood, but the
factors which lead to subdural infection rather than leptomeningitis or
cerebral abscess in patients with infections of the nasal sinuses or
mastoids are less clear. Chronic infection of the mastoid or paranasal
sinuses with thrombophlebitis of the venous sinuses or osteomyelitis
and necrosis of the cranial vault commonly precedes the development
of the subdural infection. Subdural effusions with or without bacteria
are a common complication of influenzal and other meningitides in
infancy.

Pathology. The findings depend upon the mode of entry of the infection into the subdural space. In traumatic cases there may be osteomyelitis of the overlying skull, with or without accompanying foreign bodies. When the abscess is secondary to infection of the nasal sinuses or middle ear, thrombophlebitis of the venous sinuses or osteomyelitis of the frontal or temporal bone is a common finding. Free pus or granulations may be present on the outer surface of the dura. The exudate lies free in the subdural space and covers the major portion of the hemisphere. In older cases there may be beginning organization of the exudate in a thin layer on the inner surface of the dura, but the infection is never encapsulated. The brain beneath the pus is molded in a manner similar to that seen in cases of subdural hematoma. Thrombosis or thrombophlebitis of the superficial cortical veins, especially in the frontal region, is common and produces a hemorrhagic softening of the gray and white matter drained by the thrombosed vessels. The subarachnoid spaces beneath the subdural empyema are filled with a purulent exudate but there is no generalized leptomeningitis in the initial stage.

Incidence. Subdural empyema is a relatively rare form of intracranial infection, occurring less than half as frequently as brain abscess. In 10,000 autopsies Courville and Nielsen found intracranial extension of otitis or sinusitis in 903 cases, divided as follows: Leptomeningitis 817 cases, brain abscess 54 cases, and subdural empyema 32 cases. Kubik and Adams reported intracranial suppurative complications of ear or nasal sinus disease in 79 of 1,600 autopsies. There were 11 cases of subdural empyema, 10 complicating sinusitis and 1 of otitic origin, 27 brain abscesses and 41 cases of leptomeningitis.

Subdural empyema may develop at any age but is most common in children or young adults. Males are much more frequently affected than females.

Symptoms and Signs. The symptomatology includes those associated with the focus of origin of the infection and those due to the intracranial extension. Local pain is present in the region of the infected nasal sinus or ear and there is tenderness on pressure over these regions. Orbital swelling is usually present when the infection is secondary to frontal sinus disease. Chills, fever, and severe headache are common initial symptoms of the intracranial involvement. Stiffness of neck and Kernig's sign are present. With progress of the infection the patient lapses into a confused, somnolent or comatose state. Thrombophlebitis of the cortical veins is signalized by jacksonian or generalized convulsions and by the appearance of focal neurological signs, such as hemiplegia, aphasia, paralysis of conjugate deviation of the eyes or cortical sensory loss. In the late stages the intracranial pressure is increased and the optic discs may be choked.

Laboratory Data. The white blood count is increased to 20,000 to 40,000. Roentgenograms of the skull may show evidence of infection of the mastoid or nasal sinuses or of osteomyelitis of the skull. The cerebrospinal fluid is under increased pressure. It is usually clear and colorless and there is a moderate pleocytosis, varying from 25 and 500 cells per cu mm with 10 to 80% polymorphonuclear leukocytes. The protein content is increased, with values commonly in the range of 75 to 150 mg per 100 ml. The sugar content is normal and the fluids are sterile unless the subdural infection is secondary to a purulent lep-tomeningitis.

Diagnosis. The diagnosis of subdural empyema should be considered whenever meningeal symptoms or focal neurological signs develop in patients presenting evidence of a suppurative process in nasal sinuses, mastoid or other cranial structures. Computed tomography (CT) scan and angiography are of aid in establishing the diagnosis.

Differential Diagnosis. Subdural empyema must be differentiated from other intracranial complications of infections in the ear or nasal sinus. These include extradural abscess, sinus thrombosis and brain abscess. The presence of focal neurological signs and stiffness of the neck are against the diagnosis of extradural abscess. In addition, patients are not as acutely ill with an infection limited to the extradural space.

The differential diagnosis between subdural abscess and septic thrombosis of the superior longitudinal sinus is difficult because focal neurological signs and convulsive seizures are common to both conditions. In fact, thrombosis of sinus or its tributaries is a frequent complication of subdural abscess. Factors in favor of the diagnosis of sinus thrombosis are a septic temperature and the absence of signs of meningeal irritation. Subdural empyema can also be confused with viral encephalitis or various types of meningitis. The diagnosis may be obscured by early antibiotic therapy.

Brain abscess can be distinguished by the relatively insidious onset and the protracted course.

Clinical Course. The mortality rate is high because of failure to make the diagnosis. If untreated, death commonly follows the onset of focal neurological signs within three to six days. With prompt evacuation of the pus and chemotherapy recovery is possible, even after focal neurological signs have appeared. Gradual improvement of the focal neurological signs is to be expected after recovery from the infection.

Treatment. The treatment of subdural abscess is surgical evacuation of the pus through trephine operation, carefully avoiding passage through the infected nasal sinuses. Penicillin and other antibiotics should be given before and after the operation. Irrigation of the subdural space with bacitracin has also been recommended.

REFERENCES

Bhandari, Y. S., and Sarkari, N. B. S.: Subdural Empyema. A Review of 37 Cases, J. Neurosurg., *32*, 35, 1970.
Coonrod, J. D., and Dans, P. E.: Subdural Empyema, Am. J. Med., *53*, 85, 1972.
Courville, C. B., and Nielsen, J. M.: Fatal Complications of Otitis Media with Particular Reference to Intracranial Lesions in a Series of 10,000 Autopsies, Arch. Otolaryngol., *19*, 451, 1934.
Hitchcock, E., and Andreadis, A.: Subdural Empyema: A Review of 29 Cases, J. Neurol. Neurosurg. Psychiatry, *27*, 422, 1964.
Kubik, C. S., and Adams, R. D.: Subdural Empyema, Brain, *66*, 18, 1943.

Spinal Epidural Abscess

Infections of the spinal epidural space are accompanied by fever, headache, pain in the back, weakness of the lower extremities and finally a complete paraplegia.

Etiology. Infections may reach the fatty tissue in the spinal epidural space by one of three routes: (1) Direct extension from inflammatory processes in adjacent tissues, such as decubitus ulcers, carbuncles or perinephric abscesses; (2) perforating wounds or lumbar puncture; and (3) metastasis through the blood stream from infections elsewhere in the body. The latter method of infection accounts for the vast majority of cases. The primary site of infection is often a furuncle on the skin but septic foci in the tonsils, uterus or elsewhere in the body may metastasize to the epidural fat. It is thought by some that vertebral osteomyelitis always precedes infection of the epidural space.

The organism is practically always the Staphylococcus aureus, but cases have been reported which were due to pneumococcus, streptococcus, typhoid bacillus or Gram-negative enteric bacteria.

Pathology. No region of the spine is immune to infection, but the mid-dorsal vertebrae are most frequently affected. The character of the osteomyelitis in the vertebra is similar to that encountered in other bones of the body. The laminae are most commonly involved but any part of the vertebra, including the body, may be the seat of the infection. The infection in the epidural space may be acute or chronic. In acute cases, which are by far the most common, there is a purulent necrosis of the epidural fat extending over several segments or the entire length of the cord. The pus is almost always posterior to the spinal cord, but it may be on the anterior surface. When the infecting organism is of low virulence, the infection may become localized and assume a granulomatous nature.

The lesions in the spinal cord depend on the extent to which the infection has progressed before treatment is instituted. Necrosis in the periphery of the cord may result from pressure of the abscess or myelomalacia of one or several segments may occur when the veins or arteries are thrombosed. There is ascending degeneration above and descending degeneration below the level of the necrotic lesion. Rarely, the substance of the spinal cord may be infected by extension through the meninges, with the formation of a spinal cord abscess.

Incidence. Spinal epidural abscess is rare. Two hundred and ten cases were recorded in the literature before 1937 (Browder and Myers) and 69 cases were collected by Grant between 1937 and 1945. The total of 279 cases were divided as follows: Acute, 200; subacute, 8; and chronic, 71. The infection may occur at any age.

Symptoms and Signs. The symptoms of acute spinal epidural abscess develop suddenly, several days or weeks following an infection of the skin or other parts of the body. Occasionally the preceding infection may be so slight that it is overlooked. Severe pain in the back or in the legs is usually the presenting symptom. This is followed within a few days by stiffness of the neck, headache, malaise and fever. If untreated, paralysis of the lower extremities may develop suddenly.

In chronic cases where the infection is localized and there is granuloma formation, the signs are those of cord compression which differ in no way from those of other extradural tumors.

In acute cases the patient is lethargic or irritable, the temperature varies from 101° to 104° F and is of the septic type. The pulse rate is increased. There is stiffness of the neck and a Kernig sign. The deep reflexes may be increased or decreased and the plantar responses may be extensor in type. With thrombosis of the spinal vessels there is a flaccid paraplegia with complete loss of sensation below the level of the lesion and paralysis of the bladder or rectum. Immediately following the onset of the paraplegia, the deep and superficial reflexes are absent in the paralyzed extremities.

In chronic cases the neurological signs are similar to those which are seen with other types of extradural tumors.

Laboratory Data. In acute cases there is a leukocytosis in the blood and the cerebrospinal fluid findings are constant and characteristic. Lumbar puncture should be performed with caution in any case where the diagnosis of acute spinal epidural abscess is considered. The needle should be introduced slowly and suction applied with a syringe as the epidural space is approached. If the infection has extended to the level of the puncture, pus may be withdrawn from the epidural space. If this occurs, the needle should be withdrawn without entering and possibly infecting the subarachnoid space. The pressure is normal or increased and there is complete or almost complete subarachnoid block. The fluid is xanthochromic or cloudy in appearance. There is usually a slight or moderate pleocytosis in the fluid, varying from a few to several hundred cells per cu mm. The protein content is increased with values commonly between 100 and 1500 mg per 100 ml. The sugar content of the fluid is normal and cultures of the fluid are sterile unless meningitis has developed.

In chronic cases there is complete or almost complete spinal block. The protein content of the fluid is increased and there is an inconstant pleocytosis.

Myelography is almost invariably abnormal, most often demonstrating complete block suggestive of extradural compression.

Diagnosis. The diagnosis of acute spinal epidural abscess is established with certainty only by the withdrawal of pus from the epidural space. A presumptive diagnosis can be made when subarachnoid block is found in a patient with pains in back and lower extremities of acute onset together with signs of meningeal irritation. This is especially true when there is a history of recent pyogenic infection. The diagnosis should be made before signs of a complete or incomplete transection of the cord develop.

The diagnosis of chronic granulomatous infection is rarely made before operation. The signs are those of cord compression. Operation is indicated by the presence of these signs and evidence of spinal subarachnoid block.

Differential Diagnosis. Acute spinal epidural abscess must be differentiated from acute or subacute meningitis, acute anterior poliomyelitis and acute multiple sclerosis. The findings at spinal puncture are sufficient to differentiate between these conditions.

Chronic epidural abscess can be differentiated from epidural tumors only by operation.

Course and Prognosis. If treatment is delayed in acute spinal epidural abscess, complete or incomplete transverse myelitis almost invariably develops. Flaccid paraplegia, sphincter paralysis and sensory loss below the level of the lesion persist throughout the life of the individual. With the passage of time, deep reflexes return in the paralyzed extremities and withdrawal or defense reflexes may appear.

Death may occur in the acute case as a direct result of the infection or secondary to complications. The mortality rate in the 72 acute cases tabulated by Browder and Myers in 1937 was 61%. In contrast, the mortality rate in the 15 chronic granulomatous cases was only 20%. A reduction in the mortality rate to 31% in the acute cases and 10% in the chronic cases has resulted from familiarity with the clinical syndrome which leads to early diagnosis and treatment.

Treatment. The treatment of spinal epidural abscess is prompt surgical drainage by laminectomy. Antibiotics should be administered before and after the operation. Delay in draining the abscess will result in permanent paralysis. Little improvement can be expected in acute cases with signs of transverse myelitis if the operation is performed after they occur because these signs are due to softening of the spinal cord secondary to thrombosis of the spinal vessels. In chronic cases where compression of the cord is playing a role in the production of the signs, considerable improvement in the neurological symptoms and signs may be expected after the operation.

REFERENCES

Altrocchi, P. H.: Acute Spinal Epidural Abscess vs. Acute Transverse Myelopathy, Arch. Neurol., 9, 17, 1963.
Arzt, P. K.: Abscess within the Spinal Cord, Arch. Neurol. Psychiatry, 51, 533, 1944.
Baker, A. S., et al.: Spinal Epidural Abscess, N. Engl. J. Med., 293, 463, 1975.
Browder, J., and Myers, R.: Infections of the Spinal Epidural Space, Am. J. Surg., 37, 4, 1937.
Enberg, R. N., and Kaplan, J. R.: Spinal Epidural Abscess in Children, Clin. Pediatr., 13, 247, 1974.
Grant, F. C.: Epidural Spinal Abscess, J.A.M.A., 128, 509, 1945.
Schiller, F., and Shadle, O. W.: Extrathecal and Intrathecal Suppuration, Arch. Neurol., 7, 33, 1962.

CEREBRAL VEINS AND SINUSES

Lesions of the small cerebral veins are uncommon. They may be affected by extension of an infectious or thrombotic process in the large dural sinuses and, rarely, they are the site of a primary phlebitis. Occlusion of the cortical and subcortical veins may cause focal neurological symptoms and signs.

The large dural sinuses may become thrombosed when they are infected or when there is infection in the epidural or subdural spaces. Thrombosis of the dural sinuses may also occur in infants when there is severe dehydration or marasmus. In adults they may be occluded by trauma, tumor masses or by the formation of clots in polycythemia and other conditions. The dural sinuses which are most frequently thrombosed are the lateral, cavernous and superior sagittal. Less frequently affected are the straight sinus and the vein of Galen.

Lateral Sinus

Thrombosis of the lateral sinus is usually secondary to otitis media and mastoiditis. Lateral sinus thrombosis is now a clinical rarity. Infants and children are most commonly affected. The thrombosis may occur coincidental with the acute attack of otitis and mastoiditis or it may be delayed to the chronic stage of the infection.

Symptoms and Signs. Involvement of the sinus is usually heralded by the advent of a septic fever and chills, but occasionally the thrombosis is not accompanied by a febrile reaction. Septicemia, most commonly with hemolytic streptococcus, is present in about half the cases. Petechiae in the skin and mucous membranes, septic embolism of the lungs, joints and muscles are infrequent complications of the septicemia.

The classical symptoms of lateral sinus thrombosis are fever, headache, nausea and vomiting. The latter signs are due to an increase in the intracranial pressure and are most apt to occur when the right sinus is occluded. This is due to the fact that the anatomical configuration of the sinuses in most individuals is such that the right sinus drains the greater portion of blood from the brain. Local signs of thrombosis of the sinus are usually absent but occasionally there is swelling over the mastoid region, distention of the superficial veins in this region and tenderness over the course of the jugular vein in the neck.

Papilledema develops in approximately half of the cases as the result of increased intracranial pressure. This is usually bilateral, but occasionally it may be on only one side, possibly as result of extension of the process to the cavernous sinuses. The increased intracranial pressure may cause separation of the sutures or bulging of the fontanelles in infants.

Drowsiness and coma are not uncommon symptoms. Convulsive seizures may also occur but focal neurological symptoms are rare. A few cases have been reported with jacksonian convulsive seizures followed by a hemiplegia, possibly due to extension of infection into the veins draining the lateral surface of the hemisphere. These signs, however, usually indicate the presence of an abscess in the cerebral hemisphere. Diplopia may result from injury to the sixth cranial nerve by increased intracranial pressure or from involvement of the nerve by extension of the infection in the petrous bone. The latter may be accompanied by pain in the face as the result of damage to the fifth nerve (Gradenigo's syndrome). Rarely there may be signs of damage to the ninth, tenth and eleventh nerves. These are presumed to be due to pressure on these nerves as they pass through the jugular foramen by the distended jugular vein. It is more probable, however, that they are the result of extension of the infection into the bone (osteomyelitis) surrounding these structures.

Laboratory Data. There is a leukocytosis in the blood and, as previously noted, the organism may be recovered from the blood in 50% of the cases. The cerebrospinal fluid shows the changes characteristic of an aseptic meningeal reaction (p. 32). The pressure is increased. The fluid is usually slightly turbid or cloudy and contains several to many hundred leukocytes. The sugar content of the fluid is normal and cultures are sterile unless an actual bacterial meningitis has developed.

Diagnosis. The diagnosis of lateral sinus thrombosis is made on the basis of signs of increased intracranial pressure in a patient with an acute or chronic otitis and mastoiditis. The only other diagnosis which may cause difficulty is abscess of the temporal lobe or other parts of the cerebral hemisphere. The development of a hemiplegia, aphasia or hemianopia is in favor of the latter diagnosis and the possibility of an intracerebral abscess should be excluded by CT brain scan or angiography, if necessary, in all cases with these focal signs.

Course and Prognosis. The mortality rate is high in untreated cases of lateral sinus thrombosis. Occasionally the infected thrombus may heal by complete organization, but more commonly death will result from septicemia, meningitis, extension of the infection to the cavernous or longitudinal sinus, or abscess of the brain.

In the treated cases which recover, intracranial pressure may continue to be elevated for some months, especially if the jugular vein on the right side is ligated.

Treatment. The occurrence of a thrombosis of the lateral sinus should be prevented by the prompt treatment of infections of the middle ear. The treatment of the thrombosis, when it does occur, is by antibiotics and surgical drainage. Infected bone should be removed, the sinus exposed and drained, and the jugular vein ligated if deemed necessary.

Cavernous Sinus

Cavernous sinus thrombosis is usually secondary to suppurative processes in the orbit, nasal sinuses or upper half of the face. The infective process, which commonly involves only one sinus at the onset, rapidly spreads via the circular sinus to the opposite side. One or both may be secondarily involved by extension of infection from one of the other dural sinuses. Nonseptic thrombosis of the cavernous sinus is extremely rare. The sinus may be partially or totally occluded by tumor masses, trauma or arteriovenous aneurysms.

Symptoms and Signs. The onset of symptoms of a septic thrombosis is usually sudden and dramatic. The patient appears acutely ill and there is a septic type of febrile reaction. There is pain in the eye and the orbits are painful to pressure. The bulbs are proptosed and there is edema and chemosis of the conjunctivae and eyelids. Diplopia ensues as the result of unequal protrusion of the two eyes or involvement of the oculomotor nerves. Ptosis may be present and obscured by the exophthalmos. The optic discs are swollen and there are numerous small or large hemorrhages around the disc when the orbital veins are occluded. The corneae are cloudy and ulcers may develop. The pupils may be dilated or small. The pupillary reactions are preserved in some cases and in others they are lost. Visual acuity may be normal or moderately impaired.

The above train of signs is present when the infection spreads to the sinus from the face or nasal sinuses. It is subject to some modification when the infection originates in the throat, sphenoids or the ear. In these cases the evolution of symptoms is subacute and there is a lesser degree of engorgement of the orbit.

Laboratory Data. The laboratory findings in patients with cavernous sinus thrombosis are similar to those in patients with lateral sinus thrombosis.

Diagnosis. Cavernous sinus thrombosis must be distinguished from other conditions which produce exophthalmos and congestion in the orbit. These include orbital tumors, meningiomas and other tumors in the region of the sphenoid, malignant exophthalmos and arteriovenous aneurysms. The differential diagnosis should not be diffcult because the evolution of symptoms is slow in all of the latter conditions except arteriovenous aneurysms. Arteriovenous aneurysm can be differentiated by the pulsating exophthalmos, the presence of a bruit, and recession of the exophthalmos when the carotid artery is occluded by digital pressure.

Treatment. Septic thrombosis of the cavernous sinus was until recent years almost invariably fatal because of the development of an acute meningitis. Cures have been effected with the use of antibiotics with or without anticoagulants.

Superior Sagittal Sinus

The superior sagittal sinus is less commonly the site of an infective thrombosis than either the lateral or cavernous sinus. Infections may reach the superior sagittal sinus from the nasal cavities or as secondary extensions from the lateral or cavernous sinuses. The superior sagittal sinus may also be occluded by the extension of infection from osteomyelitis or from epidural or subdural infection.

The superior sagittal sinus is the most common site of nonseptic sinus thrombosis associated with dehydration and marasmus in infancy. It may also be occluded by trauma or by tumors (meningiomas). Sagittal sinus thrombosis has also been associated with the use of oral contraceptives, pregnancy, hemolytic anemia, sickle cell trait, thrombocytopenia, ulcerative colitis, diabetes and a variety of other diseases. Occasionally nonseptic thrombosis of the sinus may occur in adults without any obvious cause.

Symptoms and Signs. The general signs are prostration, fever, headache and choked discs. Local signs include edema of the forehead and anterior part of the scalp and engorgement of the veins in the neighborhood of the anterior or posterior fontanelles, with the formation of a caput medusae.

Focal neurological signs and symptoms may be entirely absent in the nonseptic type of thrombosis with increased intracranial pressure as the only presenting sign. Extension of the clot into the larger cerebral veins is, however, almost always accompanied by the onset of dramatic signs as a result of hemorrhage into the cortical white and gray matter. Extension into these veins is common in the septic type of thrombosis and it also occurs in a high percentage of the nonseptic type. Convulsive seizures, often unilateral, hemiplegia, aphasia or hemianopia may occur.

Laboratory Data. The laboratory findings in patients with septic thrombosis of the superior sagittal sinus are similar to those in patients with lateral sinus thrombosis. In the nonseptic type, the cerebrospinal fluid is under increased pressure but there is no evidence of an aseptic meningeal reaction in the fluid in the nature of a pleocytosis. Occasionally the cerebrospinal fluid is bloody or xanthochromic as the result of cortical and meningeal hemorrhage.

Diagnosis. The diagnosis of superior longitudinal sinus thrombosis should be considered in all patients with a septic focus in the head when there are jacksonian convulsive seizures and focal neurological signs. The diagnosis of nonseptic thrombosis should be considered in all infants who develop signs of increased intracranial pressure and cerebral symptoms during the course of severe anemias, nutritional disturbances and cachexia. The diagnosis can be established by angiography. The dye can be introduced into the sinus through the fontanelles in infants or after trephination in adults.

Prognosis. The prognosis for life is poor in patients with a septic thrombosis. Death usually results from meningitis or hemorrhagic lesions in the brain. Occasionally, cases in which the diagnosis seemed fairly well established have survived, some with residuals in the form of hemiplegia, mental deficiency, and recurrent convulsive seizures.

The prognosis is less grave in patients with a nonseptic thrombosis. Symptoms may recede after a period of months, possibly as the result of recanalization of the sinus or the development of collateral circulation.

Treatment. Antibiotics should be administered to the patients with septic thrombosis. Craniotomy with evacuation of subdural or epidural abscess should be performed when these are present. There is no satisfactory treatment of the nonseptic type. Ray reported improvement after incision of the sinus and removal of the clot from an adult in whom the diagnosis had been made by the introduction of radiopaque dye directly into the sinus.

Other Dural Sinuses

Thrombosis of the inferior longitudinal sinus, the straight sinus, the petrosals or the great vein of Galen rarely occurs alone. They are usually involved by secondary extension of a septic or nonseptic thrombosis of the lateral, superior sagittal or cavernous sinuses. Any signs or symptoms which may be produced by thrombosis of the inferior longitudinal, straight or petrosal sinuses are usually masked by those resulting from involvement of the more important sinuses. Thrombosis of the great vein of Galen may cause hemorrhages in the central white matter of the hemispheres or in the basal ganglia and lateral ventricles.

REFERENCES

Bailey, O. T., and Haas, G. M.: Dural Sinus Thrombosis in Early Life. I. Clinical Manifestations and Extent of Brain Injury in Acute Sinus Thrombosis, J. Pediatr., 77, 755, 1937.
————: Dural Sinus Thrombosis in Early Life: Recovery from Acute Thrombosis of Superior Longitudinal Sinus and Its Relation to Certain Acquired Cerebral Lesions in Childhood, Brain, 60, 293, 1937.
Bailey, O. T.: Results of Long Survival after Thrombosis of the Superior Sagittal Sinus, Neurology, 9, 741. 1959.
Brown, P.: Septic Cavernous Sinus Thrombosis, Bull. Johns Hopkins Hosp., 109, 68, 1961.
Gettelfinger, D. M., and Kokmen, E.: Superior Sagittal Sinus Thrombosis, Arch. Neurol., 34, 2, 1977.
Greer, M.: Benign Intracranial Hypertension. I. Mastoiditis and Lateral Sinus Obstruction, Neurology, 12, 472, 1962.
Holmes, G., and Sargent, P.: Injuries of the Superior Longitudinal Sinus, Br. Med. J., 2, 493, 1915.
Hubert, L.: Thrombosis of the Lateral Sinus, J.A.M.A., 117, 1409, 1941.
Kalbag, R. M., and Woolf, A. L.: Cerebral Venous Thrombosis, London, Oxford University Press, 1967.
Kinal, M. E., and Jaeger, R. M.: Thrombophlebitis of Dural Venous Sinuses Following Otitis Media, J. Neurosurg., 17, 81, 1960.
Krayenbühl, H. A.: Cerebral Venous and Sinus Thrombosis, Clin. Neurosurg., 14, 1, 1966.
Ray, B. S., and Dunbar, H. S.: Thrombosis of the Superior Sagittal Sinus as a Cause of Pseudotumor Cerebri: Methods of Diagnosis and Treatment, Tr. Am. Neurol. A., 75, 12,1950.

Malignant External Otitis

Involvement of the bones at the base of the skull by infectious processes may be accompanied by osteomyelitis with or without abscess formation. Infections of the mastoid or temporal bone may cause cranial nerve palsies, particularly of the facial and acoustic nerve. Paralysis of the lower cranial nerves develops when the occipital bone is affected.

In recent years a number of cases have been reported with infection of external auditory canal by Pseudomonas aeruginosa with spread to the local subcutaneous tissues, the parotid gland, the temporomandibular joint, the masseter muscle and the temporal bone. A necrotizing osteitis of the temporal bone develops. The high mortality rate (40%) has led to the use of the term "malignant" for this form of osteitis.

The symptoms and signs include pain in the ear, with or without a purulent discharge, swelling of the parotid gland, trismus and paralysis of the sixth, seventh, eighth, tenth and eleventh nerves. Fatality is usually related to the development of meningitis.

Debridement of the infected bone and the administration of gentamicin or carbamicillin have resulted in arrest or cure of the disease in a number of cases.

REFERENCE

Schwarz, G. A.: Neurologic Complications of Malignant External Otitis, Neurology, 21, 1077, 1971.

BRAIN ABSCESS

Encapsulated or free pus in a substance of the brain tissue following an acute purulent infection is known as brain abscess. Abscesses may vary in size from a microscopic collection of inflammatory cells to an area of purulent necrosis involving the major part of one hemisphere. Abscess of the brain has been known for over two hundred years but the surgical treatment started with Macewen in 1880.

Etiology. Brain abscesses arise either as direct extension from infections within the cranial cavity (mastoid, nasal sinuses, osteomyelitis of the skull), from infections secondary to fracture of the skull, or as metastases from infection elsewhere in the body. Infections in the middle ear or mastoid may spread to the cerebellum or temporal lobe through involvement of the bone and meninges or by way of the blood vessels or nerves, with or without extradural or subdural infection or thrombosis of the lateral sinus. Rarely infection from the mastoid may metastasize through the blood stream to other portions of the brain, thus explaining the occurrence of an abscess in one hemisphere secondary to disease in the contralateral mastoid. Infection in the frontal, ethmoid or, rarely, the maxillary sinuses spreads to the frontal lobes through erosion of the skull. Subdural or extradural infection or thrombosis of the venous sinuses may or may not be present in addition.

Metastatic abscesses of the brain are commonly secondary to suppurative processes in the lungs (bronchiectasis or lung abscess). Less frequently they may follow bacterial endocarditis. Other sources of infection include the tonsils and upper respiratory tract, in which cases the infection may reach the brain along the carotid sheath. Infections elsewhere than in the heart or lungs occasionally metastasize to the brain. The route of infection in such cases is not clear. Brain abscess occurs in about 2% of patients with congenital heart disease. It is generally believed that metastatic brain abscesses are usually multiple, but Eagleton states that in approximately 45% of the cases only one abscess is present.

Abscesses of the brain secondary to cranial trauma are due to the introduction of infected missiles or tissues into the brain substance through compound fractures of the skull. These are far less common than in former years.

The infecting organism may be any of the common pyogenic bacteria, but Staphylococcus aureus, Streptococcus viridans, hemolytic streptococcus, Enterobacteriaceae and anaerobes such as Bacteroides are most commonly found. Pneumococci, meningococci and Hemophilus influenzae are rarely recovered from brain abscesses. Not infrequently the abscess will be sterile by the time operation is performed. Brain abscess is an infrequent complication of infection with the Entamoeba histolytica.

Pathology. The pathological changes in brain abscess (Fig. 4) are similar regardless of whether the infection extends to the brain directly

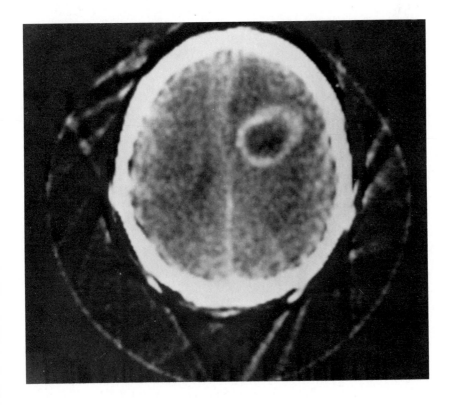

Figure 4. Brain abscess, from A.F.I.P. Collection.
(Courtesy Dr. Jan Leestma.)

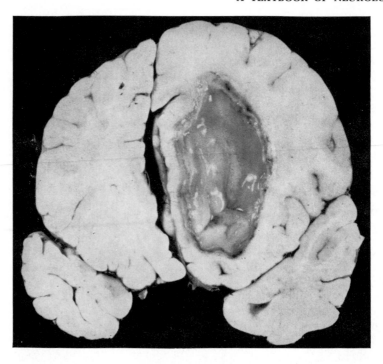

Figure 5.   Brain abscess. Fresh abscess in frontal lobe secondary to pulmonary infection.
(Courtesy Dr. Abner Wolf.)

from an epidural or subdural infection, by a retrograde thrombosis of
veins or by metastasis through the arterial system. In the first stage
there is a suppurative necrosis of brain tissue (purulent encephalitis).
When immunological forces control the spread of the infection the
macroglia and fibroblasts proliferate in an attempt to surround the
infected and necrotic tissue. The success of the body in limiting the
spread of infection and the density of the capsule are the main factors
in the final outcome. Edema of the adjacent portion of the cerebrum or
of the entire hemisphere is a common finding (Fig. 5).

   Incidence. Brain abscesses were quite common in the early decades
of this century, but the introduction of effective therapy for purulent
infection of mastoid and nasal sinuses has greatly reduced the incidence of all intracranial complications of these infections including
brain abscess. Brain abscesses are relatively rare and constitute less
than 2% of the patients who are referred to a neurosurgeon for
intracranial surgery. Brain abscess may occur at any age but it is more
common in the first to third decades of life, due to the high incidence of
mastoid and nasal sinus disease at this period. The figures for 658 cases

collected by Atkinson were: First decade, 11%; second decade, 38%; third decade, 30%; and all later decades together, only 21%. Males are slightly more frequently affected than are females.

Symptoms. The symptoms of brain abscess are essentially the same as those of any expanding lesion in the brain. Symptoms of infection are lacking unless the focus which gave rise to the abscess is still active. Chills and fever at the onset of the invasion of the nervous system are said to be present in some cases but are distinctly rare except in cases where there is an embolic lesion in the brain secondary to acute endocarditis.

Since edema of neighboring brain tissue is common, increased intracranial pressure develops rapidly. Thus headache, nausea and vomiting are early symptoms. Convulsions, focal or generalized, are common.

Signs. The body temperature is normal or subnormal except when it is elevated as the result of other complications or activity of the septic focus which was the source of the abscess. The pulse and respiratory rates are normal unless the intracranial pressure is greatly increased. The optic discs are choked in over 50% of the cases, depending to some extent upon the site of the abscess. Inequality in the degree of the choking in the two eyes has no lateralizing value. Signs of injury to the third or sixth cranial nerve as a result of increased intracranial pressure are occasionally seen. Focal signs include: Hemiparesis or hemiplegia when the abscess is in the cerebral hemispheres; torpidity and mental confusion are especially prominent with abscesses in the frontal lobe; hemianopia and aphasic disturbances, particularly anomia, when the temporal or parieto-occipital lobes are involved; ataxia, intention tremor, nystagmus and other symptoms of cerebellar and vestibular dysfunction when the abscess is in the cerebellum. Not infrequently, however, the signs of an abscess in the cerebrum or cerebellum are limited to those resulting from increased intracranial pressure.

Abscesses in the brain stem are distinctly rare, and the diagnosis is usually established at necropsy. Fever, headache, cranial nerve palsies, hemiparesis, dysphagia and vomiting were the common symptoms in the 38 patients collected from the literature by Weickhardt.

Laboratory Data. Examination of the blood and urine is normal unless there is activity in the septic focus or unless complications are present.

The changes in the cerebrospinal fluid are related to the size, location and stage of development of the abscess and to the presence or absence of acute meningitis. When the latter is present, the cerebrospinal fluid findings are those commonly seen in acute purulent meningitis. The discussion here will be confined to those cases in which bacterial infection of the meninges is absent. They are essentially those of an expanding intracranial lesion (increased pressure) plus those which accompany an aseptic meningeal reaction. The pressure is elevated in almost all cases. In our series it was over 200 mm in 70% and greater than 300 mm in 60%. The fluids are usually clear and colorless but they may be cloudy or turbid in the early stages and a fine clot may form in fluids with a high cell count. The cell count is directly related to the stage of encapsulation of the abscess and its nearness to the meningeal or ventricular surfaces. The cell count varies from normal to a thousand or more cells per cu mm. In early unencapsulated abscesses near the ventriculo-subarachnoid space the cell count is great, with a high percentage of polymorphonuclear leukocytes. The cell count is normal or only slightly increased when the abscess is firmly encapsulated. The cell count in 34 cases examined at various stages of the disease varied between 4 and 800 cells with an average of 135 cells per cu mm. Extension of the abscess to the meninges or ventricles is accompanied by an increase in the cell count and other findings of acute meningitis. Rupture of an abscess into the ventricles is signalized by a sudden rise of pressure and the presence of free pus in the cerebrospinal fluid with a cell count of 20,000 to 50,000 per cu mm. The protein content is moderately increased (between 45 and 200 mg) in about 75% of the cases. The sugar content of the fluid is normal. A decrease in sugar content below 40 mg indicates that the meninges have been invaded by bacteria.

The electroencephalographic changes are similar to those which are found in cases with other space-occupying lesions. Radionuclide scan is usually positive, but false negative results have been reported.

Roentgenograms of the skull may show separation of sutures in infants or children and an increase in the convolution markings. Widening of the sella turcica, thinning of the clinoid processes and displacement of the pineal gland may occur in adults. Computerized tomography (CT) scan with contrast enhancement permits accurate determination of capsule formation and precise localization of the abscess (Fig. 4).

Diagnosis. The diagnosis of a brain abscess can be made without difficulty when convulsions, focal neurological signs or increased intracranial pressure develop in a patient with an acute or chronic infection in the middle ear, mastoid, nasal sinuses, heart or lungs or with congenital heart disease. In the absence of any obvious focus of infection, the diagnosis may be very difficult and may require computerized tomography or cerebral angiography.

Differential Diagnosis. The common differential diagnoses which must be considered are brain tumor, extradural or subdural abscess, sinus thrombosis, encephalitis and meningitis. Most of these conditions can usually be differentiated by the history of the development of symptoms and the results of roentgenography of the skull, electroen-cephalogram and CT brain scan.

The diagnosis of meningitis is readily established by examination of the cerebrospinal fluid. The differential between brain tumor and abscess cannot be made before operation in many instances. The presence of an active focus of infection in the mastoid or nasal sinuses and a pleocytosis in the cerebrospinal fluid are strong evidence for the diagnosis of an abscess. Subdural, or rarely, epidural infections in the frontal regions may give signs and symptoms exactly the same as those of an abscess in the frontal lobe and in many the differential diagnosis cannot be made. Exploratory operation is indicated in both conditions.

Thrombosis of the lateral sinus often follows middle ear or mastoid infection and may be accompanied by convulsions and signs of increased intracranial pressure, making the differentiation between this condition and abscess of the temporal lobe or cerebellum difficult. The presence of focal neurological signs, hemiplegia, hemianopia or aphasia, are in favor of the diagnosis of an abscess. Similarly, chronic increased intracranial pressure may follow thrombosis or ligation of the lateral sinus. This condition is often described under the terms otitic hydrocephalus or hypertensive meningeal hydrops. The increased intracranial pressure with choked discs which occurs in these cases is due to interference with the drainage of blood from the brain.

Prognosis. The outcome of untreated brain abscess is, with rare exceptions, fatal. The mortality in surgically treated cases varies depending upon various factors: Location and degree and encapsula-tion of the abscess, site of the original infection, presence of complica-tions and whether there are single or multiple abscesses. The mortality rate in the 99 cases reported by Loeser and Scheinberg, and in the 100 cases reported by Northcroft and Wyke was approximately 45%. Mortality in more recently reported series varies from 35 to 55%. The highest mortality rate was in the cases where the primary infection was in the lungs.

Treatment. The treatment of brain abscess is surgical evacuation of the pus. The operation is usually delayed until the abscess is firmly encapsulated. Computerized tomography now makes it possible to determine when this stage has been reached.

The surgical treatment of brain abscess varies from complete extirpa-tion to repeated drainage through a trephine opening. Other methods include marsupialization of the cavity, packing the cavity, and various forms of incision and drainage. The ideal treatment is complete removal of the abscess within its capsule. Any method of surgical treatment should be combined with the administration of antibiotics in full therapeutic doses both pre- and postoperatively.

The sequelae of brain abscess include recurrence of the abscess, the development of new abscess if the primary focus still exists, residual focal neurological defects, and the development or continuation of recurrent convulsive seizures. Prophylactic treatment with phenobarbital or diphenylhydantoin should be given for at least a year to all patients who have been treated for an abscess in the cerebral hemisphere.

REFERENCES

Atkinson, E. M.: *Abscess of the Brain; Its Pathology, Diagnosis and Treatment*, London, Medical Publications, Ltd., 1934, 289 pp.

Brewer, N. S., MacCarty, C. S., and Wellman, W. E.: Brain Abscess. A Review of Recent Experiences, Ann. Intern. Med., *82*, 571, 1975.

Bellar, A. J., Sahar, A., and Praiss, I.: Brain Abscess. Review of 89 Cases Over a Period of 30 years, J. Neurol. Neurosurg. Psychiatry, *36*, 757, 1973.

Carey, M. E., Chou, S. N., and French, L. A.: Experience with Brain Abscesses, J. Neurosurg., *36*, 1, 1972.

Courville, C. B., and Nielsen, J. M.: Fatal Complications of Otitis Media, with Particular Reference to Intracranial Lesions in a Series of 10,000 Autopsies, Arch. Otolaryngol., *19*, 451, 1934.

Eagleton, W. P.: *Brain Abscess*, New York, Macmillan, 1922, 297 pp.

Loeser, E., Jr., and Scheinberg, L.: Brain Abscesses. A Review of Ninety-Nine Cases, Neurology, *7*, 601, 1957.

Macewen, W.: *Pyogenic Infective Diseases of the Brain and Spinal Cord, Meningitis, Abscess of Brain, Infective Sinus Thrombosis*, Glasgow, James Maclehose & Sons, 1893, 354 pp.

Matson, D. D., and Salam, M.: Brain Abscess in Congenital Heart Disease, Pediatrics, *27*, 772, 1961.

Morgan, H., Wood, M. W., and Murphey, F.: Experience with 88 Consecutive Cases of Brain Abscess, J. Neurosurg., *38*, 698, 1973.

New, P. F. J., Davis, K. R., and Ballantine, H. T., Jr.: Computed Tomography in Cerebral Abscess, Radiology, *121*, 641, 1976.

Northcroft, G. B., and Wyke, B. D.: Seizures Following Surgical Treatment of Intracranial Abscesses. A Clinical and Electroencephalographic Study, J. Neurosurg., *14*, 249, 1957.

Shaw, M. D. M., and Russell, J. A.: Value of Computed Tomography in the Diagnosis of Intracranial Abscess, J. Neurol. Neurosurg. Psychiatry, *40*, 214, 1977.

Turner, A. L., and Reynolds, F. E.: *Intracranial Pyogenic Disease. A Pathological and Clinical Study of the Pathways of Infection from the Face, Nasal and Paranasal Air-cavities*, London, Oliver, 1931, 271 pp.

Weickhardt, G. D., and Davis, R. L.: Solitary Abscess of the Brainstem, Neurology, *14*, 918, 1964.

Wright, R. L., and Ballantine, T. J.: Management of Brain Abscesses in Children and Adolescents, Am. J. Dis. Child., *114*, 113, 1967.

VIRAL INFECTIONS

Although rabies has been known since ancient times and acute anterior poliomyelitis was recognized as a clinical entity in 1840, our knowledge of the role of viruses in the production of neurological disease is of recent origin. In 1804, Zinke showed that rabies could be produced in a normal dog by inoculation of saliva from a rabid animal, and in 1909, Landsteiner and Popper produced a flaccid paralysis in monkeys by the injection of an emulsion of spinal cord from a fatal case of poliomyelitis. In 1930 a filtrable virus was recovered and definitely proven to be the causal agent of encephalitis in man. With the use of electron microscopic, tissue culture and immunological techniques over the past years, many additional viruses which infect the nervous system have been recovered and characterized.

Although the list of viruses which may affect man in epidemic or sporadic forms is extensive, viral infections are not a common cause of disease of the nervous system in man. Many of the diseases which will be considered have occurred in the form of local epidemics or as the result of laboratory infection. Caution should be exercised in considering a wide variety of neurological diseases to be caused by viruses without definitive proof.

Classification. Viruses are classified according to their nucleic acid content, size, sensitivity to lipid solvents, morphology and mode of development in cells. The principal division is made as to whether the virus contains RNA or DNA. Members of almost every major animal virus groups have been implicated in the production of neurological

Table 6. Viral Infections of the Nervous System

RNA-Containing Viruses:	Representative Viruses Responsible for Neurological Disease
Picornavirus (enterovirus)	Poliovirus Coxsackie virus ECHO virus
Togavirus (arbovirus)	Equine Encephalomyelitis (Eastern, Western, Venezuela) St. Louis Encephalitis Japanese Encephalitis Tick-borne Encephalitis Rubella
Bunyavirus	California
Orthomyxovirus	Influenza
Paramyxovirus	Measles (subacute sclerosing panencephalitis) Mumps
Arenavirus	Lymphocytic choriomeningitis
Rhabdovirus	Rabies
DNA-Containing Viruses:	
Herpesviruses	Herpes simplex Varicella-zoster Cytomegalovirus
Papovavirus	Progressive multifocal leukoencephalopathy
Poxvirus	Vaccinia

illness in animals or man (Table 6). The nature of the lesions produced varies with the virus and the experimental conditions. They may include neoplastic transformation, system degeneration or congenital defects, such as cerebellar agenesis and aqueductal stenosis, as well as the inflammatory and destructive changes often considered typical of viral infection. In addition, the concept of viral infection producing only an acute illness following within days after introduction of the agent has been challenged by demonstration that in "slow" viral infections illness may not appear until many years after exposure to the responsible virus. The development of subacute sclerosing panencephalitis many years after original exposure to measles virus is an example of this.

The distinction between neurotropic and non-neurotropic viruses according to whether or not the nervous system is the primary or secondary site of the disease's attack may be largely artificial. Most viruses which affect the nervous system as a target organ do so after they have multiplied in other organs. Dissemination to the nervous system occurs by the hematogenous route or by spread along nerve fibers.

Common biologic properties of members of a specific virus group may well dictate how they attack the central nervous system and the type of disease they produce. For example, individual picornaviruses, such as poliovirus and the ECHO virus, cause somewhat similar clinical syndromes. Members of specific virus groups also show different predilections for cell types or regions of the nervous system. Thus, members of the myxovirus group attack ependymal cells and herpes simplex virus shows preference for frontal and temporal lobes.

The tendency for a disease to appear in an epidemic or sporadic form may also be related to the virus' biological properties. Most epidemic forms of encephalititis or myelitis are due to infection with picornaviruses or togaviruses. Many togaviruses require a multiplication phase in mosquitoes or ticks before they can infect man; human epidemics occur when climatic and other conditions favor a large population of infected insect vectors. Neurological diseases due to members of other virus groups usually occur sporadically or as isolated instances complicating viral infections of other organs or systems.

Diagnosis. Acute viral infection of the nervous system can manifest itself clinically in two forms—viral ("aseptic") meningitis or encephalitis (Table 7). Viral meningitis is usually a self-limited illness characterized by signs of meningeal irritation such as headache, photophobia and neck stiffness. Encephalitis entails involvement of parenchymal brain tissue as indicated by convulsive seizures, alterations in the state of consciousness and focal neurological abnormalities. When both meningeal and cortical findings are present, the

Table 7. Specific Etiology of CNS Syndromes of Viral Etiology
(Walter Reed Army Institute of Research 1958–1963)*

	Aseptic Meningitis	Encephalitis	Paralytic Disease	Total
Mumps	28	11	1	40
LCM†	7	0	0	7
H. simplex	2	7	0	9
Poliovirus	18	5	66	89
Coxsackie A	18	1	0	19
Coxsackie B	71	4	0	75
ECHO	55	3	1	59
Arbovirus	3	5	0	8

*After Buescher, et al., Res. Publ. Assn. Nerv. Ment. Dis. 44, 147, 1968.
†Lymphocytic choriomeningitis.

term "meningoencephalitis" may be used. The cerebrospinal fluid findings in viral meningitis and viral encephalitis may be similar, consisting of an increase in pressure, pleocytosis of varying degree, a moderate protein elevation and a normal sugar content.

Knowledge of whether the illness is occurring in an epidemic setting and of the seasonal occurrence of the various forms of acute viral infections may indicate the methods to be used in detecting the infective agent. Infection with the picornaviruses or arboviruses tends to occur in the summer and early fall months while other viruses, such as mumps, occur in the late winter or spring.

The diagnosis in non-fatal cases can be made by a combination of serological tests and by the inoculation of blood, nasopharyngeal washings, feces, or cerebrospinal fluid into susceptible animals and tissue culture systems. Since infectious virus particles in human fluids and tissues are usually few in number and since many viruses are easily disrupted and inactivated even at room temperature, tissues and fluids to be used for virus isolation studies should be frozen as soon as they are obtained and transported to the laboratory in the frozen state.

The ability to recover virus from the cerebrospinal fluid varies according to the nature of the agent. Certain viruses, such as mumps virus, frequently can be isolated from the spinal fluid while other viruses, such as poliovirus, are rarely recovered. Recovery of virus from tissues or fluids in which it may be normally found is inconclusive. In this case, demonstration of development of antibodies by the patient is essential to establishing an etiologic diagnosis.

Serological tests are applicable to all known acute viral diseases of the nervous system. The most commonly used method is the complement fixation test, but hemagglutination-inhibition, immunofluorescence or neutralization reactions may be used. In the performance of the tests it is necessary that the blood be collected under aseptic precautions. Serum should be removed from the clot as soon as possible, frozen and kept at a low temperature until the tests are made. The diagnosis of a viral infection and the establishment of the type of virus rest upon the development of antibodies to the infection. It is therefore necessary to show that antibodies are not present or are present only in low titer in the early stage of the illness and that they are present in a high titer at a proper interval following the onset of symptoms. Since several to many days are usually required for the development of antibodies, serum removed in the first few days of the illness can serve as the control and serum withdrawn in the convalescent stage, three to six weeks after the onset of the illness, may be used to determine whether antibodies have developed. If the antibodies are present in equal titer in both specimens, it can be stated that the acute illness was not due to the virus which is being tested. The positive tests merely indicate that the individual has had at some time in the past an infection with this type of virus.

If brain tissue from the patient is available either in fatal cases or by brain biopsy, further studies to define the responsible virus can be done. Brain sections can be stained by the fluorescence antibody method to determine if specific viral antigen can be detected. Electron microscopic studies may indicate the presence of virus particles or components of specific morphology. Suspensions of brain and spinal cord can be injected into susceptible animals and tissue culture cell lines. In special instances, tissue cultures can be initiated from brain tissue itself. Such brain cell cultures can then be examined for the presence of viral antigens or infective virus. If an agent is recovered, final identification can be made by neutralization with known specific antiserum.

Treatment. There is as yet no fully adequate therapy for the majority of viral infections of the nervous system. The single exception may be the use of the DNA inhibitors in the treatment of herpesvirus and papovavirus infections.

Immunization procedures with either live attenuated vaccines or inactivated virus are available for rabies, poliomyelitis, mumps, rubella and measles. Immunization against the arboviruses has not been given adequate trial in man and has been used mainly to protect laboratory workers.

Although one can anticipate that effective antiviral chemotherapeutic agents will become available in the future, vector control and mass immunization appear to be the most practical means for effective control at the present time.

REFERENCES

Andrews, C., and Pereira, H. G.: *Viruses of Vertebrates*, 3rd Ed., Baltimore, Williams & Wilkins, 1972, 451 pp.

Fenner, F., et al.: *The Biology of Animal Viruses*, 2nd Ed., New York, Academic Press, 1974, 834 pp.
Fenner, F., and White, D. O.: *Medical Virology*, 2nd Ed., New York, Academic Press, 1976, 487 pp.
Fields, W. S., and Blattner, R. L.: *Viral Encephalitis*, Springfield, Charles C Thomas, 1958, 225 pp.
Fucillo, D. A., et al.: Slow Virus Diseases, Ann. Rev. Microbiol., *28*, 231 1974.
Gajdusek, D. C.: Slow-Virus Infections of the Nervous System, N. Engl. J. Med., *276*, 392–400, 1967.
Gajdusek, D. C., Gibbs, C. J. Jr., and Alpers, M.: *Slow, Latent and Temperate Virus Infections*, Washington , D.C., Government Printing Office, 1965, NINDB Monograph No. 2, PHS Pub. No. 1378.
Illis, L. S. (Ed.): *Viral Diseases of the Central Nervous System*, Baltimore, Williams & Wilkins, 1975, 226 pp.
Johnson, R. T., and Mims, C. A.: Pathogenesis of Virus Infections of the Nervous System, N. Engl. J. Med., *278*, 23, 84, 1968.
Landsteiner, K., and Popper, E.: Uebertragung der Poliomyelitis acuta auf Affen, Zischr. f. Immunitätsforsch, u. exper. Therap., *2*, 377, 1909.
Meulen, V. ter, and Katz, M. (Eds): *Central Slow Virus Infections of the Central Nervous System*, New York, Springer Verlag, 258 pp.
Lennette, E. H., Magoffin, R. L., and Knouf, E. G.: Viral Central Nervous System Disease. An etiologic study conducted at the Los Angeles County General Hospital, J.A.M.A., *179*, 687–695, 1962.
Lennette, E. H., and Schmidt, N. J., eds.: *Diagnostic Procedures for Viral and Rickettsial Disease*, 4th ed., New York, Amer. Public Health Assoc. Inc., 1969.
Lepow, M. L., et al.: A Clinical Epidemiologic and Laboratory Investigation of Aseptic Meningitis During the Four-year Period, 1955–1958. I. Observations Concerning Etiology and Epidemiology, N. Engl. J. Med., *266*, 1181, 1962.
Lepow, M. L., et al.: A Clinical Epidemiologic and Laboratory Investigation of Aseptic Meningitis during the Four-year Period, 1955–1958. II. The Clinical Disease and its Sequelae, N. Engl. J. Med., *266*, 1188, 1962.
Meyer, H. M., Jr., et al.: Central Nervous System Syndromes of "Viral" Etiology. A Study of 713 Cases, Am. J. Med., *29*, 334, 1960.
Rhodes, A. J., and van Rooyen, C. E.: *Textbook of Virology*, 5th Ed., Baltimore, Williams & Wilkins, 1969, 966 pp.
Zimmerman, H. M., ed.: *Infections of the Nervous System*. Volume 44, Publ. Assoc. Res. Nerv. & Ment. Dis., Baltimore, Williams & Wilkins, 1968.

Picornavirus Infections

Picornaviruses are small, non-enveloped RNA viruses which multiply in the cytoplasm of cells. They are the smallest RNA viruses, therefore the name "pico (small) RNA virus." The group can be divided into two subgroups: the enteroviruses which are found primarily in the gastrointestinal tract and the rhinoviruses which are found in the nasopharynx. The enteroviruses are made up of in turn the polioviruses, Coxsackie viruses and ECHO viruses, all of which are capable of producing inflammation in the central nervous system.

The picornaviruses are usually stable to inactivation by most agents. The enteroviruses are resistant to the acid and bile of intestinal contents and may survive for long periods in sewage or water. Picornaviruses grow only in primate cells and are highly cytocidal. Virus particles may form crystalline arrays in the cytoplasm of cells which are recognized as acidophilic inclusions in histological preparations.

Poliomyelitis

Acute anterior poliomyelitis (infantile paralysis, Heine-Medin disease) is an acute generalized disease caused by poliovirus infection characterized by destruction of the motor cells in the spinal cord and brain stem, and the appearance of a flaccid paralysis of the muscles innervated by the affected neurons.

Although the disease has probably occurred for many centuries, the first clear description was given by Jacob Heine in 1840 and the foundation of our knowledge of the epidemiology of the disease was laid by Medin in 1890. The studies of Landsteiner, Popper, Flexner, Lewis and others in the first decade of this century proved that the disease was caused by a virus.

Invasion of the nervous system occurs as a relatively late manifestation of the disease. Orally ingested virus appears to multiply initially in the pharynx and ileum, probably in lymphoid tissue of the tonsils and Peyer's patches. The virus then spreads to cervical and mesenteric lymph nodes and can be detected in the blood shortly thereafter. Viremia is accompanied by no symptoms or a brief minor illness. There is still dispute as to how the virus gains access to the nervous system in paralytic cases. The possibilities include direct spread from the blood stream or by way of peripheral sympathetic or sensory ganglia at the sites of multiplication in the gastrointestinal tract or other extraneural tissues.

The virus has a predilection for the large motor cells, causing chromatolysis with acidophilic inclusions and necrosis of the cells. The necrotic cells are phagocytized by leukocytes. Degeneration of the neurons is accompanied by an inflammatory reaction in the adjacent meninges and in the perivascular spaces and by secondary proliferation of the microglia. Recovery may occur in partially damaged cells, but the severely damaged cells are phagocytized and removed. The degenerative changes are most intense in the ventral horn cells, and the motor cells in the medulla, but the neurons in the posterior horn, the posterior root ganglion and elsewhere in the central nervous system are involved to a lesser degree. The inflammatory reaction is also present in the white matter (Fig. 6). Although the pathological changes are most intense in the spinal cord and medulla, any portion of the nervous system may be affected, including the midbrain, cerebellum, basal ganglia and cerebral cortex. The selective affinity of the virus for the large motor cells is again manifest by the predominance of the involvement of the motor area of the cerebral cortex. Degeneration of the peripheral nerves follows destruction of the motor cells. With subsidence of the destructive process the inflammatory reaction disappears. The macroglia proliferate in an attempt to fill the defect caused

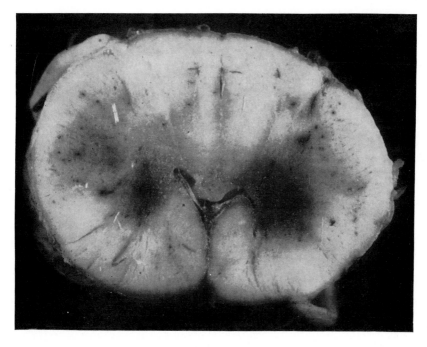

Figure 6. Acute anterior poliomyelitis. Congestion and inflammation in gray and white matter of cervical cord. (Courtesy Dr. Abner Wolf.)

by the loss of nerve cells. This is often incomplete and there may be shrinkage of the spinal cord or cyst formation in the ventral horns.

Epidemiology. Acute anterior poliomyelitis is worldwide in distribution but is more prevalent in temperate climates. It may occur in sporadic, endemic or epidemic form at any time of the year but it is most common in the fall months.

Acute anterior poliomyelitis was formerly the most common form of viral infection of the nervous system. Prior to 1956 there were approximately 25,000 to 50,000 cases annually in the United States.

Since the advent of an effective vaccine, the incidence of the disease has dramatically decreased in the United States as well as in other countries. In fact paralytic poliomyelitis is becoming a clinical rarity except for isolated cases and small epidemics in areas where the population has not been vaccinated. Figure 7 taken from the United States Public Health Service poliomyelitis surveillance reports shows the magnitude of the decrease of incidence of reported cases of poliomyelitis in the United States in the years between 1935 and 1964 which has persisted up to date. A similar decrease has been reported in

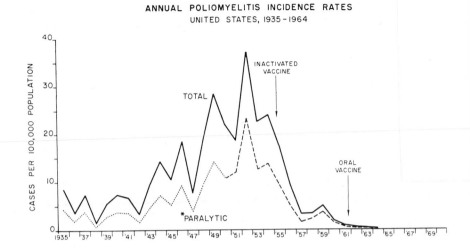

ANNUAL POLIOMYELITIS INCIDENCE RATES
UNITED STATES, 1935 – 1964

Figure 7.

*Paralytic cases prior to 1951 assumed to be 50% of total. Since 1951, cases reported as unspecified were prorated among paralytic and nonparalytic cases. SOURCE: National Morbidity Reports

other countries in which vaccination has been practiced on a large scale.

In 1975, 8 cases of paralytic poliomyelitis were reported in the United States; none of the patients had received an adequate course of poliovirus vaccination.

Three antigenically distinct types of poliovirus have been defined. All three types can cause paralytic poliomyelitis or viral meningitis, but type I appears to be most often associated with paralytic disease.

The disease may occur at any age, but the majority of cases are in infants and children under the age of ten. It is rare before the age of six months. There is some variation in the age incidence in different epidemics, but approximately 10% occur before the age of one, 80 to 90% before the age of ten and 5% after the age of twenty. In recent years there has been an increase in the incidence of the disease in young adults. Males are slightly more frequently affected than females.

The virus is present in the oropharynx during the first week of the disease. It can be demonstrated in the feces for a longer period and has been isolated from them as long as nineteen days before the onset of paralytic symptoms, as well as in healthy contacts during an epidemic. In fatal human cases, the virus has been recovered regularly from the brain and spinal cord. It can be detected in the pharyngeal wall, but much more readily in the intestinal wall and its contents.

Prophylaxis. Oral vaccination with live attenuated virus (Sabin) is remarkably effective in the prevention of paralytic infections. Antibody response is dependent on multiplication of attenuated virus in the gastrointestinal tract. Significant antibody levels develop more rapidly and persist longer than those which follow immunization with formalized polioviruses (Salk). Live attenuated vaccine is also capable of spreading and thus immunizing contacts of vaccinated individuals. It is recommended that three immunizing doses of trivalent oral vaccine be given within the first year of life beginning at six to twelve weeks of age. A fourth dose may be given before entering school. Immunization with live vaccine is best carried out in the winter months.

Symptoms. The symptoms at the onset of poliomyelitis are similar to those of any acute infection. In about a fourth of the cases these initial symptoms subside in thirty-six to forty-eight hours and the patient is apparently well for two to three days until there is a secondary rise in temperature (dromedary type) accompanied by symptoms of meningeal irritation. In the majority of cases, this second phase of the illness follows directly upon the first without any intervening period of freedom from symptoms. The headache increases in severity and muscle soreness appears in various parts of the body, most commonly in the neck and back. Drowsiness or stupor occasionally develops, but when the patients are aroused they are irritable and apprehensive. Convulsions are occasionally seen at this stage in infants.

Paralysis, when it occurs, usually develops between the second and fifth day after the onset of signs of involvement of the nervous system but it may appear as the initial symptom of the disease or in rare instances may be delayed for as long as two or three weeks. After the onset of paralysis, there may be extension of the motor loss for three to five days. Further progress of signs and symptoms rarely occurs after this time. The fever lasts for four to seven days and subsides by lysis. The temperature may return to normal before the development of paralysis or while the paralysis is advancing.

Acute cerebellar ataxia has also been observed in poliovirus-infected children.

The muscles of the extremities are usually involved but in severe cases respiratory and cardiac muscles may be affected.

Laboratory Data. There is a leukocytosis in the blood. The cerebrospinal fluid pressure may be increased and there is a pleocytosis in the fluid which develops in the period before the onset of the paralysis and persists for a varying length afterwards. The protein content is slightly elevated except in the cases with a severe degree of paralysis where it may be elevated to 100 to 300 mg and persist for several weeks.

Diagnosis. The diagnosis of acute anterior poliomyelitis can be made without difficulty in the majority of cases by the acute development of an asymmetrical flaccid paralysis accompanied by the characteristic changes in the cerebrospinal fluid. A presumptive diagnosis can be made in the preparalytic stage and in nonparalytic cases during an epidemic. The diagnosis can be suspected in patients who have not been vaccinated or have defects in their immune response. The diagnosis of poliovirus infection can be established with certainty by recovery of the virus from stool, throat washings, cerebrospinal fluid or blood. Recovery of virus from feces requires the additional demonstration of a four-fold rise in the patient's antibody level in complement fixation or neutralization tests before a specific viral diagnosis can be made.

Prognosis. Death in the majority of cases is due to respiratory failure or pulmonary complications. The mortality rate is highest in the bulbar form of the disease where it is often greater than 50%. The prognosis is poor when the paralysis is extensive or when there is a slow progress of paralysis with exacerbations and involvement of new muscles over a period of days.

The prognosis with regard to return of function in paralyzed or weak muscles depends on whether the ventral horn cells have been destroyed or only partially damaged.

Treatment. The treatment in the preparalytic stage is essentially supportive in nature. Paralysis of muscles which results in stretching or malposition may require the application of removable splints. Fluid, vitamin and electrolyte intake should be maintained by intravenous injection if indicated. When the muscle tenderness has subsided, gentle massage, together with active and passive movements, is given for the purpose of relaxing muscles and preventing contractures. These procedures should not be carried to the point where they produce pain or fatigue the patient. Attention should be given to the bladder and bowel. Catheterization may be necessary for a few days and enemas are advisable if the abdominal muscles are weakened.

Treatment of patients with paralysis of respiratory muscles or bulbar involvement requires great care. The patient should be watched carefully for signs of respiratory embarrassment and as soon as these become apparent, mechanical respiratory assistance should be given immediately. The development of anxiety in a patient who has previously been calm is a serious warning of cerebral anoxia and may precede labored breathing or cyanosis. When patients are reassured and given artificial respiratory assistance, the chances of recovery are greatly increased. The use of the respirator should be continued in bulbar cases until the respiratory centers have recovered. If the respiratory difficulty is due to paralysis of intercostal muscles and the diaphragm, the patient may need the aid of a respirator for varying periods daily for many months.

Treatment of the patient in the convalescent stage and thereafter consists of physiotherapy, muscle re-education, application of appropriate corrective appliances and orthopedic surgery. Rehabilitation of the severely paralyzed patient requires facilities available only in special institutes for rehabilitation, the ingenuity of the physician and great courage and persistence on the part of the patient.

REFERENCES

Horstmann, D. M.: Epidemiology of Poliomyelitis and Allied Diseases, Yale J. Biol. Med., 36, 5, 1963.
Horstmann, D. M., et al.: Immunization of Preschool Children with Oral Poliovirus Vaccine (Sabin), J.A.M.A., 178, 693, 1961.
Horstmann, D. M., McCallum, R. V., and Maseola, A. D.: Viremia in Human Poliomyelitis, J. Exp. Med., 99, 355, 1954.
Koprowski, H.: Live Poliomyelitis Virus Vaccines, J.A.M.A., 178, 1151, 1961.
Mendez-Cashion, D., Sanchez-Longo, L. P., Valcarcel, M., and Rosen, L.: Acute Cerebellar Ataxia in Children Associated with Infection by Poliovirus 1, Pediatrics, 29, 808, 1962.
Paul, J. R.: History of Poliomyelitis, New Haven, Yale Univ. Press. 1971. (Yale Studies in the History of Science and Medicine.)
———: Status of Vaccination against Poliomyelitis with Particular Reference to Oral Vaccination, N. Engl. J. Med., 264, 651, 1961.
Sabin, A. B.: Pathogenesis of Poliomyelitis. Reappraisal in the Light of New Data, Science, 123, 1151, 1956.
———: Eradication of Poliomyelitis, Ann. Intern. Med., 55, 353, 1961.
Salk, J. E.: Persistence of Immunity after Administration of Formalin-treated Poliovirus Vaccine, Lancet, 2, 715, 1960.

Coxsackie Viruses

In 1948 Dalldorf and Sickles inoculated specimens obtained from patients with suspected poliomyelitis into the brains of newborn mice and discovered the Coxsackie viruses. Coxsackie viruses have the structural and biological features of the picornavirus group. Two subgroups, A and B, can be distinguished by their effects on suckling mice. In mice, group A viruses cause myositis leading to flaccid paralysis and death. Group B viruses cause encephalitis, myocarditis, pancreatitis and necrosis of brown fat; animals develop tremors, spasms and paralysis before death. Twenty-four group A and six group B serotypes are currently recognized.

When they involve the human nervous system, both group A and group B Coxsackie viruses most frequently cause so-called aseptic meningitis. Occasionally, Coxsackie infection results in paralytic illness or encephalitis. Coxsackie viruses are also known to produce herpangina, pericarditis and myocarditis and epidemic myalgia (Bornholm disease). Coxsackie A4 virus has been recovered from the brains of infants with the syndrome of "sudden unexpected death."

The symptoms and signs of meningeal involvement are similar to those which follow infection with any of the other known viruses. The onset may be acute or subacute with fever, headache, malaise, nausea and abdominal pain. Stiffness of the neck and vomiting usually have their onset twenty-four to forty-eight hours after the initial symptoms. There is a mild or moderate elevation of the body temperature. Muscular paralysis, sensory disturbances or reflex changes are rare. Muscular paralyses, when present, are mild and transient. Occasionally meningeal symptoms occur in combination with myalgia, pleurodynia or herpangina.

The cerebrospinal fluid pressure is normal or slightly increased. There is a mild or moderate pleocytosis in the fluid, ranging from 25 to 250 per cu mm with 10 to 50% polymorphonuclear cells. The protein content is normal or slightly increased and the sugar content is normal.

Diagnosis of infection with Coxsackie virus can be established only by recovery of the virus from the feces, throat washings or cerebrospinal fluid and by demonstrating an increase in viral antibodies in the serum. Meningitis due to one of the Coxsackie viruses cannot be distinguished from the other viral agents which cause the so-called aseptic meningitis except by laboratory studies. It is differentiated from meningitis due to pyogenic bacteria and yeast by the relatively low cell count and the normal sugar content in the cerebrospinal fluid.

REFERENCES

Curnen, E. C.: The Coxsackie Viruses, Pediatr. Clin. North Am., 7, 903, 1960.
Dalldorf, G., and Sickles, G. M.: An Unidentified Filterable Agent Isolated From the Feces of Children with Paralysis, Science, 108, 61, 1948.
Feldman, W., and Larke, R. P. B.: Acute Cerebellar Ataxia Associated with Isolation of Coxsackievirus Type A9, Can. Med. Assn. J., 106, 1104, 1972.
Gordon, R. B., Lennette, E. H., and Sandrock, R. S.: The Varied Clinical Manifestations of Coxsackie Virus Infections, Arch. Intern. Med., 103, 63, 1959.
Heathfield, K. W. G., et al.: Coxsackie B5 Infections in Essex, 1965, with Particular Reference to the Nervous System, Q. J. Med., 36, 579, 1967.
Horstmann, D. M. and Yamada, N.: Enterovirus Infections of the Central Nervous System, Res. Publ. Ass. Nerv. & Ment. Dis., 44, 236, 1968.
Kibrick, S.: Current Status of Coxsackie and ECHO Viruses in Human Disease, Progr. Med. Virol., 6, 27, 1964.
McLean, D. M., et al.: Coxsackie B5 Virus as a Cause of Neonatal Encephalitis and Myocarditis, Can. Med. Ass. J., 85, 1046, 1961.
McLeod, D. G., et al.: Clinical Features of Aseptic Meningitis Caused by Coxsackie B Virus, Lancet, 2, 701, 1956.
Syverton, J. T., et al.: Outbreak of Aseptic Meningitis Caused by Coxsackie B5 Virus, Laboratory, Clinical and Epidemiologic Study, J.A.M.A., 164, 2015, 1957.

ECHO Viruses

This group of picornaviruses were originally isolated in cell culture from the feces of apparently normal persons. They were considered "orphans" because they lacked a parent disease. The designation

ECHO was derived from the first letters of the term Enteric Cytopathogenic Human Orphans. Thirty-three serotypes are now recognized. Many strains cause hemagglutination of human type O erythrocytes.

The ECHO viruses have now been shown to produce gastroenteritis, macular exanthema and upper respiratory infections. When the nervous system is infected, the syndrome of aseptic meningitis results. Types 4, 6 and 9 are particularly common causes of viral meningitis.

The clinical picture of infection with the ECHO viruses is similar to that of nonparalytic poliomyelitis. Children are more frequently affected than adults. The main features of the disease are fever, coryza, sore throat, vomiting and diarrhea. A rubelliform rash is present in a number of the cases. Headache, stiffness of the neck, lethargy, irritability and slight muscular weakness are the symptoms which indicate involvement of the nervous system and suggest the possibility of acute anterior poliomyelitis. The disease usually runs a benign course with subsidence of the symptoms in one or two weeks.

Cerebellar ataxia has been reported in children as the result of ECHO virus infection. The onset of ataxia is acute; the course is benign with remission of the symptoms within a few weeks. Oculomotor nerve paralysis with pupillomotor fiber sparing has been observed in conjunction with ECHO virus infection.

The spinal fluid pleocytosis may vary from several hundred to a thousand or more cells per cu mm, but is usually less than 500 per cu mm. Early in the infection there may be as many as 90% polymorphonuclear leukocytes; within forty-eight hours, however, the response becomes completely mononuclear. The protein content of the fluid is normal or slightly elevated. The sugar content remains normal.

The ECHO viruses are commonly recovered from feces, throat swabs or cerebrospinal fluid. Human or simian monkey kidney cells are used in virus isolation. Virus typing is carried out by neutralization or hemagglutination-inhibition tests. Neutralizing antibodies are present in the serum one week after the onset of illness and persist for several months.

REFERENCES

Boissard, G. P. B., et al.: Isolation of Viruses Related to ECHO Virus Type 9 from Outbreaks of Aseptic Meningitis, Lancet, 1, 500, 1957.

Hayes, R. E., Cramblett, H. G., and Kronfol, H. J.: ECHO Virus and Meningoencephalitis in Infants and Children, J.A.M.A., 208, 1657, 1969.

Hertenstein, J. R., et al.: Acute Unilateral Oculomotor Paralysis Associated with ECHO 9 Viral Infections, J. Pediatr., 89, 79, 1976.

Karzon, D. T., et al.: Aseptic Meningitis Epidemic due to ECHO 4 Virus. Am. J. Dis. Child., 101, 610, 1961.

———: An Epidemic of Aseptic Meningitis Syndrome due to ECHO Virus Type 6. II. A Clinical Study of ECHO 6 Infection, Pediatrics, 29, 418, 1962.

McAllister, R. M., Hummeler, K., and Coriell, L. L.: Acute Cerebellar Ataxia. Report of a
Case with Isolation of Type 9 ECHO Virus from the Cerebrospinal Fluid, N. Engl. J.
Med., *261*, 1159, 1959.
Sanford, J. P., and Sulkin, S. E.: The Clinical Spectrum of the ECHO-Virus Infection, N.
Engl. J. Med., *261*, 1113, 1959.
Wenner, H. A.: The ECHO Viruses, Ann. N.Y. Acad. Sci., *101*, 398, 1962.

Togaviruses

The togaviruses or arboviruses (*arthropod-borne*) are small, spherical, ether-sensitive viruses which contain RNA. Over 200 serologically distinct arboviruses are currently recognized. These viruses develop within the cytoplasm of infected cells often within vacuoles. The virus particle contains an electron-dense core surrounded by a lipoprotein envelope which has projections. Many togaviruses agglutinate erythrocytes of newborn chicks or adult geese within restricted pH ranges. Togaviruses can be divided into groups on the basis of their cross-reactivity in hemagglutination-inhibition or complement-fixation tests.

Most togaviruses are capable of multiplication in a blood-sucking arthropod vector. In their natural environment these viruses alternate between an invertebrate vector and a vertebrate mammal. Mosquitoes and ticks are the most common vectors. Birds appear to be the principal natural hosts, but wild snakes and some rodents are probably a secondary reservoir. Man and horse are incidental hosts and infection of man or horse appears to terminate the chain of infection.

Approximately 80 arboviruses are known to cause human disease. The spectrum of disease produced is broad, ranging from hemorrhagic fevers (yellow fever), arthralgias with or without rash (dengue) and encephalitis.

Arboviruses are difficult to isolate in the laboratory. Virus may be recovered from blood during the early phases (two to four days) of the illness. In non-fatal cases, the diagnosis usually depends on the demonstration of a four-fold rise in antibodies during the course of the illness. The virus may be isolated from the tissues of fatal cases by the intracerebral inoculation of infant mice and susceptible tissue culture cells.

Arbovirus infection of the nervous system may result in viral meningitis or in an encephalitis of moderate or severe nature. Diseases due to arboviruses typically occur in late summer and early fall months.

Equine Encephalomyelitis

Etiology. Three distinct types of equine encephalomyelitis are now recognized to occur in the United States. They are due to three serologically distinct Group A arboviruses: Eastern equine encephalitis (EEE), Western equine encephalitis (WEE) and Venezuelan equine encephalitis (VEE). Infection with these viruses was considered to be exclusively limited to horses until 1932 when Meyer reported an unusual type of encephalitis in three men who were working in close contact with affected animals. The first cases in which EEE virus was recovered from human brain tissue were reported from Massachusetts in 1938 by Fothergill and his co-workers. Many arboviruses take their name from the location in which they were first isolated. They are not confined, however, by specific geographic boundaries. WEE virus infection is now known to occur in virtually all parts of the United States, and cases of EEE have been reported in regions west of the Mississippi River, as well as in eastern South America and the Philippines.

Pathology. In EEE the brain appears congested and there are widespread degenerative changes in the nerve cells. The meninges and perivascular spaces of the brain are intensely infiltrated with polymorphonuclear leukocytes and round cells. In places the accumulation of these cells is so great that they give the appearance of small abscesses. Destruction of myelin is not prominent except in the neighborhood of the necrotic foci. The lesions are found in both the white and gray matter and are most intensive in the cerebrum and brain stem, but they may also be present in the cerebellum and spinal cord.

In contrast to EEE, the pathology of WEE is characterized by a less severe degree of inflammatory reaction, a paucity of changes in the nerve cells, more extensive areas of demyelinization and greater frequency of petechial hemorrhage.

Incidence. Equine encephalomyelitis is a rare infection in man, tending to occur as isolated cases or in small epidemics. Epizootics in horses may precede the occurrence of human cases by several weeks. Equine encephalomyelitis affects mainly infants, children and adults over fifty years of age. There is no sex preponderance. Inapparent infection is common in all age groups.

Symptomatology. Infection with the EEE virus is characterized by the sudden onset of drowsiness, stupor or coma with convulsive seizures, headache, vomiting, stiffness of the neck and high fever. Cranial nerve palsies, hemiplegia and other focal neurologic signs are common.

The symptoms of infection with WEE and VEE are less severe. The onset is acute, with general malaise and headache followed occasionally by convulsions and nausea and vomiting. The temperature is moderately elevated. The headaches increase in severity and drowsiness or lethargy appears. There is stiffness of the neck, generalized motor weakness and depression of the reflexes, but cranial nerve palsies and focal neurologic signs are uncommon.

Laboratory Data. There is a leukocytosis in the blood, especially in infections with EEE where counts as high as 35,000 have been reported.

The cerebrospinal fluid changes are greatest in EEE where the pressure is always moderately or greatly increased. The fluids are cloudy or purulent, containing 500 to 3,000 cells per cu mm with a predominance of polymorphonuclear leukocytes. The protein content is increased but the sugar content is normal. With subsidence of the acute stage the cell count drops, lymphocytes become the predominating cell type and there is a greater increase in the protein content.

The changes in the cerebrospinal fluid in WEE and VEE are less severe. The pressure is usually normal and the cellular increase is moderate, with counts varying from normal to 200 cells, and mononuclears the predominating cell type.

Diagnosis. Isolation of equine encephalomyelitis viruses from blood and spinal fluid of patients during life has been accomplished infrequently in the early phases of the disease. It cannot be considered a practical diagnostic method. The hemagglutination-inhibition, complement-fixation or neutralization tests are the serologic methods of choice in cases that recover. In fatal cases, the diagnosis can be established by isolation of the virus from brain. Togavirus particles have been recognized in brain specimens examined by electron microscopy.

Differential Diagnosis. Equine encephalomyelitis must be differentiated from the other acute infectious diseases of the nervous system including acute and subacute meningitides, encephalomyelitis following the acute exanthemata, aseptic meningeal reaction associated with infections in the skull, brain abscess and other virus infections of the nervous system.

The acute and subacute meningitides are excluded by the normal sugar content and the absence of bacteria in the cerebrospinal fluid. Encephalomyelitis following acute exanthemata, aseptic meningeal reaction accompanying infections in the skull, and brain abscess are excluded by the absence of the usual associated findings in these conditions. Differentiation from other virus encephalomyelitides can only be made by isolation of the virus or by serological tests.

Course and Prognosis. The mortality rate in EEE is over 50%. The duration of the disease varies from less than one day in fulminating cases to over four weeks in less severe cases. In patients who recover sequelae such as mental deficiency, cranial nerve palsies, hemiplegia, aphasia and convulsions are common. Children under ten years of age have greater likeliness to survive the acute infection, but also have the greatest chance of being left with severe neurological disability.

The fatality rate in WEE is less than 5%. Sequelae among young infants are frequent and severe, but are uncommon in adults who recover from the illness. The mortality rate in VEE is less than 0.5%; nearly all deaths have occurred in young children.

Treatment. Treatment in the acute stage of the disease is entirely supportive. Vaccines against the equine encephalomyelitis viruses have been produced; their use should be confined to laboratory workers and others whose occupations occasion unusual exposure to the virus. Vaccination on a large-scale community program is not indicated because of the low incidence of the disease.

REFERENCES

Aguilar, M. J., Calanchini, P. R., and Finley, K. H.: Perinatal Arbovirus Encephalitis and Its Sequelae, Res. Publ. Ass. Nerv. Ment. Dis., 44, 216, 1968.

Altman, R. M., Goldfield, M., and Sussman, O.: The Impact of Vector-borne Viral Diseases in the Middle Atlantic States, Med. Clin. North Am., 51, 661, 1967.

Ayres, J. C., and Feemster, R. F.: The Sequelae of Eastern Equine Encephalomyelitis, N. Engl. J. Med., 240, 960, 1949.

Baker, A. B., and Noran, H. H.: Western Variety of Equine Encephalitis in Man, Arch. Neurol. & Psychiat., 47, 565, 1942.

Bastian, F. O., et al.: Eastern Equine Encephalomyelitis: Histopathologic and Ultrastructural Changes with Isolation of the Virus in a Human Case, Am. J. Clin. Pathol., 64, 10, 1975.

Chamberlain, R. W.: Arboviruses, the Arthropod-borne Animal Viruses, Current Topics Microbiol. Immunol., 42, 38, 1968.

Ehrenkranz, N. J., Sinclair, M. C., Buff, E., and Lyman, D. O.: The Natural Occurrence of Venezuelan Equine Encephalitis in the United States, N. Engl. J. Med., 282, 298, 1970.

Farber, S., Hill, A., Connerly, M. L., and Dingle, J. H.: Encephalitis in Infants and Children Caused by the Virus of the Eastern Variety of Equine Encephalitis, J.A.M.A., 114, 1725, 1940.

Finley, K. H., et al.: Western Encephalitis and Cerebral Ontogenesis, Arch. Neurol., 16, 140, 1967.

Fothergill, L. D., Dingle, J. H., Farber, S., and Connerly, M. L.: Human Encephalitis Caused by Virus of Eastern Variety of Equine Encephalomyelitis, N. Engl. J. Med., 219, 411, 1938.

Meyer, K. F.: Equine Encephalomyelitis, Ann. Intern. Med., 6, 645, 1932.

Noran H. H., and Baker, A. B.: Sequels of Equine Encephalomyelitis, Arch, Neurol. & Psychiat., 49, 398, 1943.

————: Western Equine Encephalitis; Pathogenesis of the Pathological Lesions, J. Neuropathol. Exp. Neurol., 4, 269, 1945.

Rozdilsky, B., Robertson, H. E., and Charney, J.: Western Encephalitis: Report of Eight Fatal Cases. Saskatchewan Epidemic, 1965, Can. Med. Assoc. J., 98, 79, 1968.

Sellers, R. T., Bergold, G. H., Suárez, O. M., and Morales, A.: Investigations During Venezuelan Equine Encephalitis Outbreaks in Venezuela—1962–1964, Am. J. Trop. Med., 14, 460, 1965.

St. Louis Encephalitis

The first outbreak of acute encephalitis in which a virus was definitely established as the etiologic agent was the epidemic which occurred in St. Louis in 1933. This type of encephalitis had probably existed in this area prior to 1933 since sporadic cases of encephalitis had occurred in St. Louis in July and August during the previous fourteen years, and a small epidemic (38 cases) of encephalitis occurred in Paris, Illinois, in 1932. Neutralization tests on the serum of recovered cases of this epidemic proved it to be due to a virus identical with that of the St. Louis epidemic of 1933. Since 1933 repeated outbreaks have occurred in the United States with increasing frequency and widening geographic distribution. St. Louis encephalitis is the most common form of arbovirus encephalitis in the United States.

The virus responsible for St. Louis encephalitis is a mosquito-transmitted Group B arbovirus (flavivirus). Epidemics follow two epidemiological patterns. In the west, mixed outbreaks of St. Louis and Western equine encephalitis have occurred in rural areas. The second pattern of infection has appeared in recent epidemics in the Midwest, New Jersey, Florida and Texas. In this form, the disease occurs in cities and has a tendency to affect older persons. As with other arboviruses, disease in man usually appears in the midsummer to early fall. There is no sex predominance.

Pathology. Grossly there is a mild degree of vascular congestion and there are occasional petechial hemorrhages. The characteristic microscopic changes are a slight infiltration of the meninges and blood vessels of the brain and spinal cord with mononuclear cells, focal accumulation of inflammatory and glial cells in the substance of the brain, and degenerative changes in the neurons. Both gray and white matter are involved, but the nuclear masses of the thalamus and midbrain are more affected than the cortex.

Symptoms and Signs. Infection with St. Louis encephalitis virus most frequently results in inapparent infection. Symptoms in these abortive cases are so mild that they are diagnosed only by the development of viral antibodies.

Approximately three fourths of patients with clinical manifestations have encephalitis; the remaining have aseptic meningitis or nonspecific illness. Almost all patients over forty years of age develop encephalitic signs.

The onset of neurological symptoms may be abrupt or may be preceded by a prodromal illness of three or four days' duration, characterized by headache, myalgia, fever, sore throat or gastrointestinal symptoms. The headache increases in severity, and stiffness of the neck develops. Other common signs include increase or diminution of the deep tendon reflexes, moderately coarse intention tremor of the fingers, lips and tongue, reduction in the size of the pupils, and absence of abdominal skin reflexes. In the more severe cases there may be delirium, coma or stupor, disturbance of vesical and rectal sphincters, focal neurologic signs and, rarely, cranial nerve palsies.

The temperature is elevated (100° to 104° F) from the onset and falls by lysis or crisis in ten days to two weeks. The pulse is increased in proportion to the fever. Rarely there is a bradycardia.

Laboratory Data. There is a mild to moderate leukocytosis in the blood. The cerebrospinal fluid is usually abnormal. The fluid is clear and colorless. There is a mild pleocytosis in the majority of cases, averaging approximately 100 cells per cu mm. Cell counts as high as 500 or more have been reported. Lymphocytes are the predominating cell type, although a few polymorphonuclear cells may be found early in the disease. The sugar content of the fluid is normal.

Diagnosis and Differential Diagnosis. The diagnosis of encephalitis due to infection with the St. Louis virus can be made only by isolation of the virus from blood, spinal fluid or brain tissue or by the development of antibodies. It must be differentiated from the subacute meningitides and other forms of viral encephalitis. The differential from tuberculous and other meningitides can be made from the examination of the cerebrospinal fluid. Differentiation from other forms of viral encephalitis depends upon the results of serological tests.

Course and Prognosis. The disease runs an acute course in the majority of cases and results in death or recovery within two to three weeks. Occasionally the symptoms may be of longer duration. The mortality rate in the 1933 epidemic in St. Louis was 20%. The mortality varied from 2 to 12% in subsequent epidemics. Cranial nerve palsies, hemiplegia and other local neurologic signs are more common in the cases with prolonged coma or confusion.

Sequelae. Minor nonspecific complaints such as headaches, insomnia, easy fatigability and nervousness occurring three to five months after the illness appear to be the most common aftereffects. Residuals of cranial nerve palsies, hemiplegia and aphasia are found in a small percentage of cases. Epileptiform attacks or behavior changes in children are rare.

Treatment. There is no specific treatment of the encephalitis due to the St. Louis virus.

REFERENCES

Barrett, F. F., Yow, M. D. and Phillips, C. A.: St. Louis Encephalitis in Children During the 1964 Epidemic, J.A.M.A., *193*, 381, 1965.
Beckmann, J. W.: Neurologic Aspects of the Epidemic of Encephalitis in St. Louis, Arch. Neurol. & Psychiat., *33*, 732, 1935.
Brody, J. A., Burns, K. F., Browning, G., and Schattner, J. D.: Apparent and Inapparent Attack Rates for St. Louis Encephalitis in a Selected Population, N. Engl. J. Med., *261*, 644, 1959.
Hempelmann, T. C.: The Symptoms and Diagnosis of Encephalitis; 1933 St. Louis Epidemic, J.A.M.A., *103*, 733, 1934.
Luby, J. P., Sulkin, S. E. and Sanford, J. P.: The Epidemiology of St. Louis Encephalitis (SLE): a Review, Ann. Rev. Med., *20*, 329, 1969.
McCordock, H. A., Collier, W., and Gray, S. H.: The Pathologic Changes of St. Louis Type of Acute Encephalitis, J.A.M.A., *103*, 822, 1934.
Powell, K. E., and Blakey, D. L.: St. Louis Encephalitis: The 1975 Epidemic in Mississippi, J.A.M.A., *237*, 2294, 1977.
Riggs, S., Smith, D. L. and Phillips, C. A.: St. Louis Encephalitis in Adults During the 1964 Houston Epidemic, J.A.M.A., *193*, 284, 1965.

Southern, P. M. Jr., Smith, J. W., Luby, J. P. et al.: Clinical and Laboratory Features of Epidemic St. Louis Encephalitis, Ann. Intern. Med., 71, 681, 1969.
Weil, A.: Histopathology of the Central Nervous System in Epidemic Encephalitis (St. Louis Epidemic), Arch. Neurol. & Psychiat., 31, 1139, 1934.

Japanese Encephalitis

Japanese encephalitis was first identified as a distinct disease after a large epidemic in 1924, although a form of encephalitis had appeared in Japan almost every summer and had been recognized as a clinical entity as early as 1871. The etiologic agent is a mosquito-transmitted Group B arbovirus. The disease has a characteristic seasonal occurrence, with the worst outbreaks in hot, dry weather. It is most common in Japan but is also found in neighboring regions. The changes in the nervous system include degeneration of the ganglion cells in the cerebellum, cerebral cortex, basal ganglia and substantia nigra and to a lesser extent the medulla and spinal cord. The leptomeninges are infiltrated with lymphocytes and the vessels in the substance of the nervous system are surrounded by monocytes and macrophages. Focal necrosis and glial nodules are not uncommon.

The clinical picture and laboratory findings are similar to those of equine encephalomyelitis. The disease is most common in children and the mortality rate in some epidemics has been as high as 60%. This figure is undoubtedly high because the majority of the mild cases are not admitted to a hospital.

Severe neurological residuals and mental defects may be present in the recovered cases but the typical sequelae of encephalitis lethargica do not develop. The diagnosis may be established by isolation of the virus from the blood, cerebrospinal fluid or cerebral tissue and by appropriate serologic tests. There is no specific treatment. Formalized vaccines for protection of humans have been widely used but are of questionable value.

REFERENCES

Dickerson, R. B., Newton, J. R., and Hansen, J. E.: Diagnosis and Immediate Prognosis of Japanese B Encephalitis, Am. J. Med., 12, 277, 1952.
Haymaker, W., and Sabin, A. B.: Topographic Distribution of Lesions in Central Nervous System in Japanese B Encephalitis, Arch. Neurol. & Psychiat., 57, 673, 1947.
Ketel, N. B., and Ognibene, A. J.: Japanese B Encephalitis in Vietnam, Am. J. Med. Sci., 261, 271, 1971.
Lewis, L., et al.: Japanese B Encephalitis, Arch. Neurol. & Psychiat., 57, 430, 1947.
Pieper, S. J., Jr., and Kurland, L. T.: Sequelae of Japanese B and Mumps Encephalitis. Recent Follow-up of Patients Affected in 1947–1948 Epidemic on Guam, Am. J. Trop. M. Hyg., 7, 481, 1958.
Richter, R. W., and Shimojyo, S.: Neurologic Sequelae of Japanese B Encephalitis, Neurology, 11, 553, 1961.
Zimmerman, H. M.: Pathology of Japanese B Encephalitis, Am. J. Pathol., 22, 965, 1946.

California Virus Encephalitis

Human neurological disease associated with California encephalitis virus was first recognized in the early 1960s. Infection has subsequently been shown to occur in Midwestern states and along the Eastern Seaboard and is now known to be an important cause of encephalitis in the United States. California virus is now classified among the bunyaviruses, a group of enveloped viruses with segmented, circular ribonucleoproteins.

The virus is transmitted by the mosquito. The disease occurs in the late summer and early fall and nearly all cases have occurred in children. Infants under one year of age and adults are rarely affected. Headache, nausea and vomiting, changes in sensorium, meningeal irritation and upper motor neuron signs have been commonly reported. The peripheral blood count is usually elevated. The cerebrospinal fluid contains an increased number of lymphocytes and shows the other findings typical of viral meningitis or encephalitis.

The case fatality is low. Recovery usually occurs within seven to ten days. Emotional lability, learning difficulties and recurrent seizures have been reported as sequelae.

The diagnosis can be established by serological studies. Neutralizing and hemagglutination-inhibition antibodies appear shortly after the onset of the disease; complement-fixing antibodies can be detected ten to twelve days after initial symptoms.

REFERENCES

Balfour, H. H., Jr., et al.: California Arbovirus (La Crosse) Infections, Pediatrics, 52, 680, 1973.
Chun, R. W. M., Thompson, W. H., Grabow, J. D. and Mathews, C. G.: California Arbovirus Encephalitis in Children, Neurology, 18, 369, 1968.
Cramblett, H. G., Stegmiller, H. and Spencer, C.: California Encephalitis Virus Infections in Children: Clinical and Laboratory Studies, J.A.M.A., 198, 108, 1966.
Hilty, M. D., et al.: California Encephalitis in Children, Am. J. Dis. Childh., 124, 530, 1972.
Thompson, W. H. and Evans, A. S.: California Encephalitis Virus Studies in Wisconsin, Amer. J. Epidem., 81, 230, 1965.
Young, D. J.: California Encephalitis Virus: a Report of Three Cases and a Review of the Literature, Ann. Intern. Med., 65, 419, 1966.

Mumps Meningitis and Encephalomyelitis

Etiology. Mumps is a disease due to a paramyxovirus which has predilection for the salivary glands, mature gonads, pancreas, breast and the nervous system. The virus causes hemagglutination of erythrocytes of fowls, man and other species, produces hemolysis and contains complement-fixing components. There is only one serotype. Like other paramyxoviruses, mumps virus develops from the cell surface by a budding process.

Clinical evidence of involvement of the nervous system occurs in the form of a mild meningitis or encephalitis in a small percentage of the cases. Other neurological complications of mumps include an encephalomyelitis with cranial and peripheral nerve palsies, myelitis and peripheral neuritis. It is not clear whether these neurological complications of mumps are due to direct action of the virus or whether they are due to allergic or other factors as is thought to be the case with similar complications following vaccination and various infectious diseases (postinfectious encephalomyelitis).

Pathology. The pathology of mumps meningitis and encephalitis has not been clearly elucidated because of the low mortality rate. The pathologic changes are limited to an infiltration of the meninges and cerebral blood vessels with lymphocytes and mononuclear cells. The morbid changes in cases of encephalomyelitis following mumps are exactly the same as those which are found following other infectious diseases, namely, a perivenous demyelinization with infiltration of the vessels of the brain and spinal cord by lymphocytes and phagocytic microglia.

Incidence. The incidence of neurological complications of mumps varies greatly in different epidemics. The statistics cited by Wesselhoeft show an incidence varying between a low of less than 1% in several large epidemics of over 2,500 cases each and a high of 9% in the 1,705 cases of Dopter, 10% in the 210 cases of Steinberg and 11% in the 100 cases reported by Heeren. A slight pleocytosis may be found in the cerebrospinal fluid with little or no clinical evidence of meningitis, and a few cases have been reported in which meningeal symptoms were the only indication of infection (mumps sine parotide). Holden and his associates performed a lumbar puncture on the fourth day in 100 consecutive cases of mumps. The diagnosis of mumps meningitis was made in 33 of the 100 cases on the basis of the presence of headache, drowsiness and stiffness of the neck. A pleocytosis greater than 10 cells per cu mm was present in all but 5 of their 33 cases. In 4 additional cases there was a pleocytosis in the cerebrospinal fluid without any neurological symptoms.

Although the two sexes are equally susceptible to mumps, neurological complications are much more frequent in the male. Children are commonly affected but epidemics may occur in young adults living under community conditions best exemplified by Army camps. The majority of cases of mumps encephalitis is the United States appear to occur in the late spring and early summer months.

Symptoms. In the vast majority of cases the symptoms of involvement of the nervous system are those of a mild meningitis, i.e., headache, drowsiness and stiffness of the neck. These symptoms commonly appear two to ten days after the onset of the parotitis. Rarely, they may precede the onset of the swelling of the salivary glands. These symptoms are benign and disappear within a few days.

Complications. Deafness is the most common sequel of mumps. The loss of hearing, which is unilateral in over two thirds of the cases, may develop gradually or it may have an abrupt onset accompanied by vertigo and tinnitus. The cause of the deafness which follows mumps is not known. It is usually presumed to be due to damage to the labyrinth.

Myelitis, polyneuritis, encephalitis, optic neuritis and other cranial nerve palsies may develop seven to fifteen days after the onset of the parotitis. These complications are similar to those which develop after other infectious diseases and are considered to be an example of so-called post-infectious encephalomyelitis.

Laboratory Data. In mumps meningitis the blood usually shows a relative lymphocytosis and a slight leukopenia. The cerebrospinal fluid is under a slightly increased pressure. The fluid is clear and colorless except in the fluid with a high cell count when it may be slightly opalescent. The cell count is increased (Table 8), usually in the range of 25 to 500 cells but occasionally the counts may be as high as 3,000 cells per cu mm. Lymphocytes usually constitute 90 to 96% of the total, even in fluids with a high cell count, but rarely polymorphonuclear leukocytes may predominate in the early stages. The degree of pleocytosis is not related to the severity of symptoms and it may persist for thirty to sixty days. Inclusions of viral nucleocapsid-like material have been recognized by electron microscopic observation of spinal fluid cells from patients with mumps meningitis. The protein content is normal or moderately increased. The sugar content is normal. In a few rare instances, the spinal fluid of patients with mumps meningitis may show a moderate reduction in the sugar content. Mumps virus can be recovered from the spinal fluid in a significant number of cases.

Diagnosis. The diagnosis of mumps meningitis is made on the basis of meningeal symptoms and a pleocytosis in the cerebrospinal fluid in a

Table 8. The Cerebrospinal Fluid Findings in Four Cases of Mumps Meningitis

Case	Pressure	Cells Number	% Lympho-cytes	Protein mg./100 ml	Sugar mg./100 ml	Colloidal Gold
1	. . .	500	98	44	48	1112321100
2	260	27	100	20	83	0110000000
3	190	120	90	. .	60	0122100000
4	80	310	100	17	48	0000000000

patient with mumps. The diagnosis in patients who develop neurologi-cal symptoms during an epidemic of mumps without evidence of involvement of the salivary glands cannot be made with certainty unless the virus can be recovered from the cerebrospinal fluid or there is a significant increase in the complement fixation antibodies in the serum.

Differential Diagnosis. Mumps meningitis must be differentiated from other forms of meningitis, especially tuberculous. The normal sugar content and the absence of organisms in the cerebrospinal fluid are important in excluding acute purulent or tuberculous meningitis.

REFERENCES

Azimi, P. H., Cramblett, H. G. and Haynes, R. E.: Mumps Meningoencephalitis in Children, J.A.M.A., 207, 509, 1969.

Herndon, R. M.: Ependymitis in Mumps Virus Meningitis: Electronmicroscopic Studies of Cerebrospinal Fluids, Arch. Neurol., 30, 475, 1974.

Holden, E. M., Eagles, A. Y., and Stevens, J. E., Jr.: Mumps Involvement of the Central Nervous System, J.A.M.A., 131, 382, 1946.

Johnstone, J. A., et al.: Meningitis and Encephalitis Associated with Mumps Infection: A 10 Year Study, Arch. Dis. Childh., 47, 647, 1972.

Levitt, L. P., et al.: Central Nervous System Mumps: A Review of 64 Cases, Neurology, 20, 829, 1970.

McLean, D. M., et al.: Mumps Meningoencephalitis. Toronto, 1963, Can. Med. Assoc. J., 90, 458, 1964.

Riffenburgh, R. S.: Ocular Manifestations of Mumps, Arch. Ophth., 66, 739, 1961.

Schwarz, G. A., Yang, D. C., and Noone, E. L.: Meningoencephalo-myelitis with Epidemic Parotitis, Arch. Neurol., 11, 453, 1964.

Taylor, F. B., Jr., and Torenson, W. E.: Primary Mumps Meningo-encephalitis, Arch. Intern. Med., 112, 216, 1963.

Wilfert, C. M.: Mumps Meningoencephalitis with Low Cerebrospinal-fluid Glucose, Prolonged Pleocytosis and Elevation of Protein, N. Engl. J. Med., 280, 855, 1969.

Subacute Sclerosing Panencephalitis

Subacute sclerosing panencephalitis (inclusion body encephalitis, subacute progressive encephalitis in children and adolescents) is a disease associated with infection by measles virus or a measles-like virus characterized by progressive dementia, incoordination, ataxia, myoclonic jerks and other focal neurological signs. The disease was first described by Dawson in 1934 and felt to be of viral origin because of the presence of intranuclear inclusions of Type A which are morphologically indistinguishable from those seen in herpes simplex encephalitis. Numerous cases have been reported since that date, but recovery of a viral agent was not possible until the advent of specialized techniques of viral isolation. Most authors are of the opinion that the cases reported by Van Bogaert in 1945 under the title of subacute sclerosing leukoencephaltitis belong to the entity, although intranuclear inclusions were not a prominent feature of his cases.

In the severe, long-standing cases the brain may feel unduly hard. There is a perivascular infiltration in the cortex and white matter with plasma and other mononuclear cells. There are patchy areas of demyelinization and gliosis in the white matter and deeper layers of the cortex. The neurons of the cortex, basal ganglia, pons and inferior olives show degenerative changes. Intranuclear and intracytoplasmic inclusion bodies are found in neurons and glial cells. When examined with the electron microscope, these inclusions have been found to be composed of hollow filaments such as those seen in tissue culture cells infected with paramyxoviruses (Fig. 8). When stained by the fluorescence antibody method, positive staining reaction for measles virus is obtained.

Children under the age of twelve are predominantly affected, although a few cases in adults have been reported. Males are more often affected than females, and some epidemiological reports have indicated that cases occur more often in rural than in urban settings. The

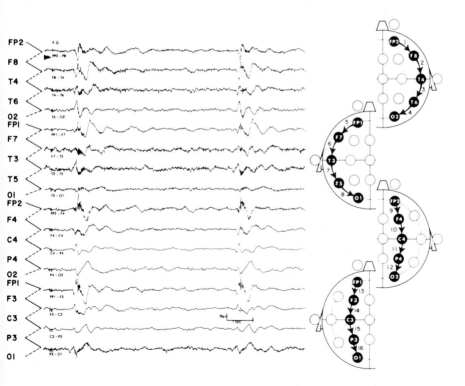

Figure 8. Subacute sclerosing panencephalitis. Multiphasic long duration sharp wave discharges repeat every 7 seconds in a 14 year old boy. In this condition, periodic discharges recur regularly at 4 to 8 second intervals.

disease has a gradual onset without fever. Forgetfulness, inability to keep up with school work and restlessness are common early symptoms. These are followed in the course of weeks or months by incoordination, ataxia, myoclonic jerks of the muscles of the trunk and extremities, apraxia and loss of speech. Vision and hearing are preserved until the terminal stage, in which there is a rigid quadriplegia simulating complete decortication. Cranial nerve palsies may appear and patches of chorioretinitis have been reported in occasional cases. Cases of coincidental infectious mononucleosis and subacute sclerosing panencephalitis have been reported.

Elevated levels of measles antibody can be found in serum and cerebrospinal fluid. The spinal fluid is under normal pressure and the cell count is normal or only slightly increased. The protein content is normal, but a striking increase in the cerebrospinal immunoglobulin content is found even in an otherwise normal fluid. Homogeneous IgG bands representing measles virus-specific antibodies can be demonstrated by agarose electrophoresis of spinal fluid. The electroencephalogram usually shows a widespread abnormality of the cortical activity with bursts of wave and spike complexes occurring at a rate of 2 to 4 per second synchronous with or independent of the myoclonic jerks (Fig. 8).

Virus isolation was accomplished by establishing tissue culture cell lines from brain biopsies obtained from patients with the disorder. These cultures contained measles virus antigen as demonstrated by fluorescence antibody staining and could be made to shed an infectious virus serologically indistinguishable from measles virus by co-cultivation with other established tissue culture cell lines. Although measles virus or a closely related viral agent appears clearly involved in the etiology of the disease, its pathogenesis is still uncertain. Well-documented cases of the disease apparently following immunization with live attenuated measles vaccine strains have been reported. There is suggestive evidence that patients who develop this disorder have had clinical measles earlier in life than normal populations.

The course of the disease is prolonged, usually lasting a number of months in younger children and many months to several years in the adolescent group.

There is as yet no proven effective therapy.

REFERENCES

Agnarsdóttir, G.: Subacute Sclerosing Panencephalitis, Recent Advances in Clinical Virology, Number One. A. P. Waterson, Ed., Churchill Livingston, Edinburgh, 1977, pp. 21–49.
Brain, W. R., Greenfield, J. G., and Russell, D. S.: Subacute Inclusion Encephalitis (Dawson Type), Brain, 71, 365, 1948.

Cape, C. A., et al.: Adult Onset of Subacute Sclerosing Panencephalitis, Arch. Neurol., 28, 124, 1973.

Clark, N. S., and Best, P. V.: Subacute Sclerosing (Inclusion Body) Encephalitis, Arch. Dis. Child., 39, 356, 1964.

Connolly, J. H., Allen, I. V., Hurwitz, L. J., and Millar, J. H. O.: Measles-virus Antibody and Antigen in Subacute Sclerosing Panencephalitis, Lancet, 1, 542, 1967.

Dawson, J. R.: Cellular Inclusions in Cerebral Lesions of Epidemic Encephalitis, Arch. Neurol. & Psychiat., 31, 685, 1934.

Feorino, P. M., et al.: Mononucleosis Associated with Subacute Sclerosing Panencephalitis, Lancet, 3, 530, 1975.

Font, R. L., Jenis, E. H., and Tuck, K. D.: Measles Maculopathy Associated with Subacute Sclerosing Panencephalitis, Arch, Pathol., 96, 168, 1973.

Freeman, J. M.: The Clinical Spectrum and Early Diagnosis of Dawson's Encephalitis, Pediatrics, 75, 590, 1969.

Horta-Barbara, L., Fuccillo, D. A., Sever, J. L. and Zeman, W.: Subacute Sclerosing Panencephalitis: Isolation of Measles Virus from a Brain Biopsy, Nature (London), 221, 974, 1969.

Jabbour, J. T., et al.: Epidemiology of Subacute Panencephalitis (SSPE). A Report of the SSPE Registry, J.A.M.A., 220, 959, 1972.

Meulen, V. ter, et al.: Subacute Sclerosing Panencephalitis: A review, Curr. Top. Microbiol., Immunol., 57, 1, 1972.

Morgan, B., et al.: Ocular Manifestations of Subacute Sclerosing Panencephalitis, Am. J. Dis. Child., 130, 1019, 1976.

Payne, F. E., Baublis, J. V., and Itabashi, H. H.: Isolation of Measles Virus from Cell Cultures of Brain from a Patient with Subacute Sclerosing Panencephalitis. N. Engl. J. Med., 281, 585, 1969.

Sever, J. L., and Zeman, W., eds.: Measles Virus and Subacute Sclerosing Panencephalitis, Neurology, 18, No. 1, Part 2, 1968.

Tellez-Nagel, J., and Harter, D. H.: Subacute Sclerosing Leukoencephalitis: Ultrastructure of Intranuclear and Intracytoplasmic Inclusions, Science, 154, 899, 1966.

Van Bogaert, L.: Une Leuco-encéphalite sclerosante subaigue, J. Neurol. Neurosurg. Psychiat., 8, 101, 1945.

Vandirk, B., and Norrby, E.: Oligoclonal IgG Antibody Response in the Central Nervous System to Different Measles Antigens in Subacute Sclerosing Panencephalitis, Proc. Nat. Acad., 70, 1060, 1973.

Rabies

Rabies (hydrophobia, lyssa, rage) is an acute viral disease of the central nervous system which is transmitted to man by the bite of a rabid animal. It is characterized by a variable incubation period, restlessness, hyperesthesia, convulsive phenomena, laryngeal spasms, widespread paralysis and almost invariably death.

Etiology. Rabies virus is an enveloped bullet-shaped virus which contains single-stranded RNA. Because of its characteristic morphology, rabies is classed among the rhabdo (rod-shaped) viruses. Hemagglutination with goose erythrocytes occurs under special conditions. The virus appears capable of infecting every warm-blooded animal. Rodents are used for laboratory investigations, and the virus has been shown to replicate in a number of tissue culture cell lines. The virus can be recovered from brain by intracerebral inoculation into suckling mice. The virus of rabies is present in the saliva of infected animals and is transmitted to man through bites or abrasions of the skin. After inoculation, the virus travels to the central nervous system by way of the nerves. The disease is usually caused by the bite of a rabid dog, but it may be transmitted by cats, wolves, foxes, jackals, skunks, and other domestic or wild animals. Cases have been reported in which the infection was transmitted by the vampire bat.

The incubation period usually varies between one to three months with extremes of twelve days to more than a year. In general, the incubation period is directly related to the severity of the bite or bites and their location. The period is shortest when the wound is on the face and longest when the leg is bitten.

Pathology. The pathology of rabies is that of a generalized encephalitis and myelitis. There is a diffuse perivascular infiltration of the entire central nervous system with lymphocytes and to a less extent with polymorphonuclear leukocytes and plasma cells. There are diffuse degenerative changes in the neurons. Characteristic, but not pathognomonic, of the disease is the presence of acidophilic inclusion bodies in the neurons (Fig. 9). These are most commonly found in the ganglion cells of the Ammon's horn, but they may be seen in neurons of the cortex, cerebellum and other portions of the central nervous system, as well as in the spinal ganglia. These inclusions contain rabies virus antigen as demonstrated by immunofluorescence. Virus particles simi-

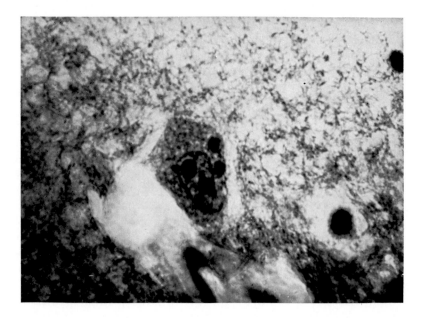

Figure 9.   Rabies: Inclusion bodies in cytoplasm of ganglion cell of cerebral cortex.

lar to those of rabies virions have been found in electron microscopic studies of the inclusion bodies. Occasionally these inclusion bodies are absent. There are proliferative changes in the microglia with the formation of rod cells which may be collected into small nodules (Babes tubercles). The degenerative changes in the neurons may be quite severe with little or no inflammatory reaction. This is especially apt to occur in cases with a long incubation period.

Incidence. The incidence of rabies is directly proportional to the diligence of public health authorities in the control of rabid animals. The disease is almost nonexistent in Great Britain where strict regulations are enforced. It is becoming a clinical rarity in the United States and most of the countries of Central Europe, but it is quite prevalent in Southeastern Europe and Asia.

The incidence of the disease in individuals who have been bitten by rabid dogs is low (5 to 10%) but it is high (40%) when the bite is inflicted by a rabid wolf. The incidence is highest when the wounds are severe and near the head. It is low when the bite is inflicted through clothing, which cleans some or most of the infecting saliva from the teeth.

Symptomatology. The onset of the disease is usually signalized by pain or numbness in the region of the bite, soon followed by apathy, drowsiness, headache and anorexia. This period of lethargy passes rapidly into a state of excitability in which all external stimuli are apt to produce localized twitchings or generalized convulsions. There may be delirium with hallucinations. There is a profuse flow of saliva and spasmodic contractions of the pharynx and larynx occur. The latter are precipitated by any attempt to take liquid or solid food. As a result the patient violently refuses to accept any liquids, hence the name hydrophobia. The body temperature is usually elevated and may reach 105° to 107° F in the terminal stages. The stage of hyperirritability gradually passes over into a state of generalized paralysis and coma. Death results from paralysis of respiration.

Occasionally the disease may have its onset with paralysis (paralytic form), without convulsive phenomena or laryngeal spasm. The paralysis is a flaccid type and may start in one extremity and spread rapidly to involve the others. Rarely, the symptoms and signs of a transverse myelitis may develop.

Complications. Encephalomyelitis and polyneuritis can be complications of antirabic therapy.

Laboratory Data. There is a leukocytosis in the blood and albumin may be present in the urine. The cerebrospinal fluid is under normal pressure and there is an inconstant lymphocytic pleocytosis, varying from 5 to several hundred per cu mm. The protein content may be increased.

Diagnosis. The diagnosis of rabies is made from the appearance of the characteristic symptoms after the bite of a rabid animal.

Course and Prognosis. The disease is almost always fatal and usually runs its course in two to five days. Death within twenty-four hours of the onset of symptoms has been reported. A few cases with recovery have been reported.

Treatment. There is no specific anti-viral therapy. Treatment is therefore entirely prophylactic, and includes both passive antibody and vaccine. Passive immunization is by use of human immune rabies globulin. Immune globulin is infiltrated into the wound and given intramuscularly. If human gamma globulin is not available, equine rabies antiserum can be used after appropriate tests for horse serum sensitivity. If the animal is rabid, the administration of globulin or serum should be followed by a full course of active immunization with duck embryo vaccine.

Serum sickness is common after the injection of the horse serum and should be treated with antihistamines. Neurological complications are rare with the duck-embryo vaccine.

REFERENCES

Babes, V.: *Traite de la Rage*, Paris, J. B. Bailliere, 1912.
Bhatt, D. R. et al.: Human Rabies, Am. J. Dis. Child., 129, 862, 1974.
Corey, L. and Hattwick, M. A. W.: Treatment of Persons Exposed to Rabies, J.A.M.A., 232, 272, 1975.
Dupont, J. R., and Earle, K. M.: Human Rabies Encephalitis, a Study of Forty-nine Fatal Cases with a Review of the Literature, Neurology, 15, 1023, 1965.
Hurst, E. W., and Pawan, J. L.: An Outbreak of Rabies in Trinidad, Without History of Bites, and with Symptoms of an Acute Ascending Myelitis, Lancet, 2, 622, 1931.
Kaplan, M. M.: Epidemiology of Rabies, Nature, 221, 421, 1969.
Koprowski, H.: Rabies, Pediatr. Clin. North Am., 2, 55, 1955.
Kent, J. R. and Finegold, M.: Human Rabies Transmitted By the Bite of a Bat, N. Engl. J. Med., 263, 1058, 1960.
Lowenberg, K.: Rabies in Man, Arch. Neurol. & Psychiat., 19, 638, 1928.
Miller, A. and Nathanson, N.: Rabies: Recent Advances in Pathogenesis and Control, Ann. Neurol., 2, 511, 1977.
Porras, C., et al.: Recovery from Rabies in Man, Ann. Intern. Med., 85, 44, 1976.
Sung, J. H., et al.: A Case of Human Rabies and Ultrastructure of the Negri Body, J. Neuropathol. Exp. Neurol., 35, 541, 1976.
Warrell, D. A., et al.: Pathophysiology Studies in Human Rabies, Am. J. Med., 60, 180, 1976.
Webster, L. T.: *Rabies*, New York, The Macmillan Co., 1942. 168 pp.

Lymphocytic Choriomeningitis

Lymphocytic choriomeningitis (benign lymphocytic meningitis) is a relatively benign viral infection of the meninges and central nervous system. The clinical features of the disease were described by Wallgren in 1925 (under the term aseptic meningitis). The disease is of historical importance because it was the first in which a virus was proven to be the cause of a benign meningitis with a predominance of lymphocytes in the cerebrospinal fluid.

Etiology and Incidence. Armstrong and Lillie in 1934 recovered a hitherto undescribed virus from the brain of a patient who had died of encephalitis during the St. Louis epidemic in 1933. This virus produced an infiltration of round cells in the meninges and choroid plexus of experimental animals and was designated by them as the virus of experimental lymphocytic choriomeningitis. In 1935, Traub found that this same virus was carried by apparently healthy mice. The role of the virus in human disease was established by Rivers and Scott in 1935 when they isolated it from the cerebrospinal fluid of 2 patients with the clinical syndrome described by Wallgren. Recent electron microscopic studies have demonstrated that the lymphocytic choriomeningitis virus particle has surface projections and contains 1 to 10 electron-dense granules. On the basis of this distinctive morphology, the virus is now classified among the RNA-containing arena ("sandy") viruses. It is now clear that lymphocytic choriomeningitis virus is the cause of only a small percentage of the cases which have been described by the terms benign lymphocytic or acute aseptic meningitis. The vast majority of such cases are due to infection of the meninges by picornaviruses, mumps or other viruses.

The portal of entry is probably through the respiratory tract. Virus multiplication first occurs in the respiratory epithelium. Some patients develop symptoms of an upper respiratory illness or an influenza-like illness. Mice are the major reservoir of the virus and are implicated as the intermediate host. Hamsters may be a source of infection. The illness has occurred in laboratory workers having contact with hamsters and individuals who keep pet hamsters.

Although the virus of lymphocytic choriomeningitis is a rare cause of meningitis, immunological studies suggest that infection without symptomatic involvement of the meninges is common since 11 per cent of 2,000 sera tested by Armstrong and Lillie contained neutralizing antibodies against the virus.

The virus attacks all races and individuals of all ages but is most common between the ages of fifteen and forty. The two sexes are equally affected. The disease is most common in the spring and fall months.

Pathology. The pathology of the disease has not been adequately studied because of the low mortality rate. In addition, the majority of the reports in the literature lack confirmatory viral studies. Changes found in fatal cases include infiltration of the meninges and choroid plexus with lymphocytes, perivascular infiltration in the brain substance and degenerative changes in the ganglion cells. Proliferation of the arachnoid with the formation of an adhesive arachnoiditis (Barker and Ford) and focal lesions in the brain and spinal cord (Howard) have been reported.

Symptoms and Signs. Invasion of the blood stream by the virus of lymphocytic choriomeningitis may produce symptoms of a systemic infection with or without evidence of involvement of the central nervous system. Onset of the infection is characterized by headache, malaise, generalized pains, fever and symptoms of upper respiratory infection or pneumonia. The meningeal symptoms commonly develop within one week after the onset. Occasionally there is a remission in the prodromal symptoms and the patient is apparently in good health when meningeal symptoms develop.

Severe headache, nausea and vomiting mark the beginning of the meningeal phase. Drowsiness or stupor develops within twenty-four to forty-eight hours. The temperature is moderately elevated (99° to 104° F). The usual signs of meningitis, stiff neck, Kernig's sign, and depressed or hyperactive reflexes, are present. In rare cases the parenchyma of the nervous system may be involved (encephalitic forms). Choked discs, oculomotor and facial palsies and signs of focal lesions in the brain or a transverse lesion of the spinal cord have been reported. In the encephalitic form convalescence is prolonged, but there is considerable restoration of function in the damaged tissue.

Laboratory Data. The peripheral leukocyte count is often normal, but may be elevated with a predominance of polymorphonuclear leukocytes. The cerebrospinal fluid is under increased pressure. It is clear and colorless but a fine fibrin clot may form. The fluids contain an excess of cells, varying from less than a hundred to several thousand per cu mm. Lymphocytes constitute almost 100% of the cells. The protein content is increased. The sugar content is normal.

Diagnosis. A presumptive diagnosis of lymphocytic choriomeningitis can be made on the basis of the characteristic history (prodromal symptoms followed by meningitis) and the cerebrospinal fluid findings. A definitive viral diagnosis may be made by recovery of the virus from blood or spinal fluid. In most cases the diagnosis is made by seroconversion. Complement-fixing antibodies are usually detectable one to two weeks after the onset of disease; neutralizing antibodies appear after six to eight weeks.

Differential Diagnosis. Lymphocytic choriomeningitis must be differentiated from other diseases which are associated with a lymphocytic pleocytosis in the cerebrospinal fluid, including tuberculous meningitis, syphilitic meningitis, meningitis caused by enteroviruses, mumps meningitis, herpes zoster, infectious mononucleosis, and meningeal reactions to septic foci in the skull. The differential diagnosis can be made without difficulty in the majority of these conditions by the presence of the characteristic clinical and cerebrospinal findings and by the results of serological tests.

Course and Prognosis. The duration of the meningeal symptoms varies from one to four weeks with an average of three weeks. The mortality rate is low and complete recovery is the rule except in the rare cases with encephalitis where residuals of focal lesions in the brain or spinal cord may be present.

Treatment. There is no specific treatment.

REFERENCES

Armstrong, C., and Lille, R. D.: Experimental Lymphocytic Choriomeningitis of Monkeys and Mice Produced by a Virus Encountered in Studies of the 1933 St. Louis Encephalitis Epidemic, Pub. Health Rep., *49*, 1019, 1934.
Barker, L. F., and Ford, F. R.: Chronic Arachnoiditis Obliterating Spinal Subarachnoid Space, J.A.M.A., *109*, 785, 1937.
Colmore, J. P.: Severe Infections with the Virus of Lymphocytic Choriomeningitis, J.A.M.A., *148*, 1199, 1952.
Farmer, T. W., and Janeway, C. A.: Infections with Virus of Lymphocytic Choriomeningitis, Medicine, *21*, 1, 1942.
Howard, M. E.: Infection with the Virus of Choriomeningitis in Man, Yale J. Biol. & Med., *13*, 161, 1940.
Rivers, T. M., and Scott, T. F. M.: Meningitis in Man Caused by a Filtrable Virus, Science, *81*, 439, 1935.
Vanzee, B. E., et al.: Lymphocytic Meningitis in University Hospital Personnel: Clinical Features, Am. J. Med., *58*, 803, 1975.
Warkel, R. L., et al.: Fatal Acute Meningoencephalitis, Due to Lymphocytic Choriomeningitis Virus, Neurology, *23*, 198, 1973.

Rubella

Rubella (German measles) is the cause of an exanthematous disease which can produce marked neurological damage in the unborn child of a mother infected during pregnancy. Gregg, an Australian ophthalmologist, was the first to correlate the occurrence of congenital cataracts among newborn babies with maternal rubells infection during the first trimester of pregnancy. Congenital rubella is now known to produce a variety of defects including deafness, mental retardation and cardiac abnormalities. The frequency of congenital defects is highest in the first trimester of pregnancy and falls as gestation advances.

Rubella virus was originally isolated by demonstrating that monkey-kidney cells infected with the virus became resistant to superinfection with picornaviruses. Subsequently the virus was shown to grow and produce cytopathogenic changes in a number of continuous cell lines, making it possible to characterize the virus' properties and develop a vaccine. The virus has many of the properties associated with the togaviruses. It is an enveloped virus which contains RNA and agglutinates erythrocytes from pigeons, geese and one-day-old chicks.

Rubella virus induces a chronic persistent infection in the fetus. Infants may shed virus for long periods of time after birth from the nasopharynx, eye or spinal fluid. Virus production continues despite the development of neutralizing and hemagglutinating antibodies by the infected child.

The lesions in the nervous system are those of a chronic leptomeningitis with infiltration of mononuclear cells, lymphocytes and plasma cells. Small areas of necrosis and glial cell proliferation are seen in the basal ganglia, midbrain, pons and spinal cord. Microscopic vasculitis and perivascular calcification can also occur.

The infant with rubella encephalitis is usually lethargic, hypotonic, or inactive at birth or within the first few days or weeks after birth. Within the next several months, the child may develop restlessness, head retraction, opisthotonic posturing and rigidity. Seizures and a meningitis-like illness may occur. The anterior fontanelle is usually large and microcephaly is common. The child may have other associated defects such as deafness, cardiac anomalies and congestive heart failure, cataracts, thrombocytopenia and areas of hyperpigmentation about the navel, forehead and cheeks. Improvement of varying degrees may be noted after the first six to twelve months of life.

The cerebrospinal fluid contains an increased number of cells as well as a moderately increased protein content. Rubella virus can be recovered from the spinal fluid of approximately one fourth of the cases and may persist in the spinal fluid for as long as eighteen months after birth.

Specific diagnosis can be made by recovery of the virus from throat swab, urine, spinal fluid, leukocytes, bone marrow and lens. Evidence of past infection can be made by serologic tests.

The primary method of treatment is prevention of fetal infection. Live rubella vaccine should be given to all children between one year and puberty. Adolescent girls and non-pregnant women should be given vaccine if shown susceptible to rubella by serological testing.

A chronic progressive encephalitis developing in the second decade of life occurs in patients with congenital rubella. Deterioration of motor and mental functions begins after a stable period of ten or more years. The cerebrospinal fluid has an increased cell count, protein content and IgG level. High titers of antibody to rubella virus are present in both serum and spinal fluid. Rubella virus can be recovered from brain by cell co-cultivation methods. Patients with this condition develop dementia, myoclonic seizures, abnormal involuntary movements and spasticity. The course of the disease is one of progressive deterioration.

REFERENCES

Desmond, M. M., et al.: Congenital Rubella Encephalitis, J. Pediatr., 71, 311, 1967.
Gregg, N. M.: Congenital Cataract Following German Measles in the Mother, J. Ophth. Soc. Australia, 3, 35, 1941.

Naeye, R. L., and Blanc, W.: Pathogenesis of Congenital Rubella. J.A.M.A., *194*, 109, 1965.
Rorke, L. B. and Spiro, A. J.: Cerebral Lesions in Congenital Rubella Syndrome, J. Pediatr., *70*, 243, 1967.
Townsend, J. J., et al.: Progressive Rubella Panencephalitis: Late Onset after Congenital Rubella., N. Engl. J. Med., *292*, 990, 1975.
————: The Neuropathology of Progressive Rubella Panencephalitis of Late Onset, Brain, *99*, 81, 1976.
Weil, M. L., et al.: Chronic Progressive Panencephalitis Due to Rubella. Virus Simulating Subacute Sclerosing Panencephalitis, N. Engl. J. Med., *292*, 994, 1975.

Herpesvirus

The herpesvirus group is composed of DNA-containing viruses which contain a lipid envelope and multiply in the nucleus of the cell. Members of this group share the common feature of establishing latent infections. Herpesviruses may remain quiescent for long periods of time being demonstrable only sporadically or not at all until a stimulus triggers reactivated infection. Within cells, accumulations of virus particles can often be recognized in the nucleus in the form of acidophilic inclusion bodies. Members of the herpesvirus group which are associated with neurological disease include herpes simplex, varicella-zoster, cytomegalovirus and the Epstein-Barr (EB) virus.

Herpes Simplex Encephalitis

Although encephalitis due to herpes simplex virus was once considered to be a relatively infrequent occurrence, improvements in virus isolation techniques have led to recognition of the virus' role in encephalitis and it is now felt to be the single most important cause of fatal sporadic encephalitis in the United States.

Two antigenic types of herpes simplex virus (herpesvirus hominis) are distinguished by serological testing. The type 1 strains are responsible for almost all cases of herpes simplex encephalitis and meningitis in adults. Type 2 strains appear to effect the genitalia. In the neonatal period, herpetic meningitis or encephalitis is related to type 2 infection probably by spread of the virus during delivery.

Approximately 20% of patients with herpes simplex infection of the nervous system show signs of an aseptic meningitis which is indistinguishable from that syndrome which is caused by other viruses. Herpes simplex infection constitutes approximately 1 to 2% of patients with the syndrome of viral meningitis. In most instances, herpes simplex causes encephalitis. All age groups are affected, and there is no seasonal incidence.

Type 2 herpes simplex virus, the cause of genital herpes, is associated with a generalized herpetic infection in infants and occasional cases of viral meningitis in adults.

In fatal cases there is an intense meningitis and widespread destructive changes in the parenchyma of the brain and spinal cord. Necrotic, inflammatory or hemorrhagic lesions may be found. There is often an unusual degree of cerebral edema accompanying the necrotic lesions and a predilection for involvement of the frontal and temporal lobes. These inclusions containing viral antigen and herpes virus particles have been recognized in diseased brain on electron microscopic examination.

The disease may occur at any age, but more than one half of the cases occur in patients over twenty years of age. Herpes simplex encephalitis has been reported in patients with Hodgkin's disease, probably on the basis of an impaired host immune response. The most common early signs in herpes simplex encephalitis are fever and headache. The onset of the disease is most often abrupt and is ushered in by a major motor seizure. In a significant number of patients, however, the encephalitis may evolve more slowly with expressive aphasia, paresthesias or mental changes preceding more severe neurological signs. Most patients have a temperature in the range of 101° to 104° F at the time of admission; pyrexia tends to prove refractory to antipyretic treatment. Nuchal rigidity or other signs of meningeal irritation are often found. Localized neurological signs in the form of focal paralysis or hemiplegia are often present. Herpetic skin lesions are seen in only a few of the reported cases.

There is a moderate leukocytosis in the blood. The cerebrospinal fluid pressure may be moderately or greatly increased. The pleocytosis in the fluid varies from less than 10 to 700 cells per cu mm; lymphocytes or polymorphonuclear leukocytes may predominate. Red blood cells may be found in a few cases. The spinal fluid sugar content may be low in some cases. The electroencephalogram is usually abnormal with focal or generalized changes; periodic complexes against a slow-wave background may be seen.

The diagnosis can be established only by recovery of or demonstration of viral antigen in brain. Since patients may show a rise in antibody titer with recurrent herpes simplex cutaneous lesions or with inapparent infection, a four-fold rise in the antibody titer to herpesvirus may occur in patients with encephalitis from other causes. Fluctuations in antibody level may also occur with reactivated infection, and there may be uncertainty about the significance of a positive serologic response. The diagnosis can be made, in a fair proportion of patients, by examining tissue obtained by brain biopsy. The presence of characteristic intranuclear inclusions, a positive staining reaction of brain cells by fluorescence antibody staining or the finding of typical herpes virions on electron microscopic examination may indicate herpesvirus infection. More recently, a solid phase radioimmune assay has been developed for the demonstration of herpesvirus antigen in brain. Inoculation of brain biopsy suspensions into susceptible rodents and tissue cultures may result in recovery of the virus. Since herpes simplex encephalitis carries a high mortality and since therapy with the DNA inhibitors has been used with some success, diagnostic measures leading to the demonstration of the virus should be initiated as soon as possible when the disease is suspected.

The disease appears fatal in approximately 70% of the cases. Recovery may be complete in mild cases, but patients who survive the acute disease are usually left with severe neurological residuals. Measures to decrease intracranial pressure, including the administration of adrenal corticosteroids, may be indicated. In 1966, Breeden, Hall and Tyler first used systemic treatment with the DNA inhibitor, iododeoxyuridine. The efficacy of this drug in the treatment of herpes simplex encephalitis has not been established. Contolled studies of the drug had to be terminated because of its marked toxicity. Therapeutic benefit from the use of adenine arabinoside (Vidarabine), a DNA inhibitor less toxic than iododeoxyuridine, has been described.

REFERENCES

Breeden, C. J., Hall, T. C., and Tyler, H. R.: Herpes Simplex Encephalitis Treated with Systemic 5-iodo-2'deoxyuridine, Ann. Intern. Med., 65, 1050, 1966.
Johnson, K. P., Rosenthal, M. S., and Lerner, P. I.: Herpes Simplex Encephalitis, The Course in Five Virologically Proven Cases, Arch. Neurol., 27, 103, 1972.
Johnson, R. T., Olson, L. C., and Buescher, E. L.: Herpes Simplex Virus Infections of the Central Nervous System: Problems in Laboratory Diagnosis, Arch. Neurol., 18, 260, 1968.
Longson, M., and Bailey, A. S.: Herpes Encephalitis. Recent Advances in Clinical Virology, Number One, A. P. Waterson, Ed., Edinburgh, Churchill Livingston, 1977, pp. 1–19.
Longson, M.: Acute Necrotizing Encephalitis and Other Herpes Simplex Virus Infections, Postgrad. Med. J., 49, 371, 1973.
Miller, J. K., Hesser, F., and Tompkins, V. N.: Herpes Simplex Encephalitis. Report of 20 Cases, Ann. Intern. Med., 64, 92, 1966.
Olson, L. C., et al.: Herpesvirus Infections of the Human Central Nervous System, New Engl. J. Med., 277, 1271, 1967.
Price, R., et al.: Herpes Simplex Encephalitis in an Anergic Patient, Am. J. Med., 54, 222, 1973.
Rexman, J. H. W.: The Angiographic and Brain Scan Features of Acute Herpes Simplex Encephalitis, Br. J. Radiol., 47, 179, 1974.
Sarubbi, F. A., Jr., et al.: Herpesvirus Hominis Encephalitis Virus Isolation from Brain Biopsy in Seven Patients and Results of Therapy, Arch. Neurol., 29, 268, 1973.
Swanson, J. L., Craighead, J. E., and Reynolds, E. P.: Electron Microscopic Observations on Herpesvirus Hominis (Herpes Simplex Virus) Encephalitis in Man, Lab. Invest., 15, 1966, 1966.
Whitley, R. J., et al.: Adenine Arabinoside Therapy of Biopsy-Proven Herpes Simplex Encephalitis. National Institute of Allergy and Infectious Diseases Collaborative Antiviral Study, N. Engl. J. Med., 297, 289, 1977.

Herpes Zoster

Herpes zoster (shingles) is a viral disease which produces inflammatory lesions in the posterior root ganglia and is characterized clinically by the appearance of pain and a skin eruption in the

distribution of the affected ganglia. Signs and symptoms of involvement of the motor roots or the central nervous system are also present
in a small percentage of the cases.

Etiology. The virus of herpes zoster is identical to varicella virus
which is the causative agent of chickenpox. The varicella-zoster virus
is a large enveloped DNA-containing virus which has the same structure as other herpesviruses. The agent can be cultured in human tissue
culture cells where it tends to remain bound to cells. Varicella virus
recovered from chickenpox patients is identical to herpes zoster virus
recovered from patients with shingles by all serological tests. Children
can catch chickenpox from exposure to adults with shingles, but adults
are subject to zoster only if they have had chickenpox earlier in life.
Such epidemiologic considerations led Hope-Simpson to speculate
that zoster infection represents re-activation of latent varicella-zoster
virus originally acquired during a childhood attack of chickenpox.
Although varicella-zoster virus is able to remain latent within tissues in
the same manner as herpes simplex virus, there is no antigenic
similarity between the two viruses.

Herpes zoster frequently occurs in connection with systemic infections, immunosuppressive therapy, and localized lesions of the spine
or nerve roots (acute meningitides, tuberculosis, Hodgkin's disease,
metastatic carcinoma and trauma to the spine). In some cases the
cutaneous eruption is at the same segment as the localized lesion of the
spine, but in others it is at an entirely different level. It is most probable
that systemic disease or local lesions of the spine or nerve roots merely
serve to activate the infection.

Pathology. Although the symptoms are commonly confined to the
distribution of one or two sensory roots, the pathological changes are
usually more widespread. The affected ganglia of the spinal or cranial
nerve roots are swollen and inflamed. The inflammatory reaction is
chiefly of a lymphocytic nature but a few polymorphonuclear leukocytes or plasma cells may also be present. Some of the cells of the
ganglion are swollen and others are degenerated. The inflammatory
process commonly extends to the meninges and into the root entry
zone (posterior poliomyelitis). Not infrequently there is some inflammatory reaction in the ventral horn and in the perivascular space of the
white matter of the spinal cord. The pathological changes in the
ganglia of the cranial nerves and in the brain stem are similar to those
in the spinal root and spinal cord.

Incidence. Herpes zoster is a relatively common disease but
symptoms of involvement of the nervous system, with the exception of
pain, are rare. The disease is more common in the female than in the
male and may occur at any time of life. It is most common in middle or
later life. There is a tendency for the disease to be more prevalent in the
spring and fall.

Symptoms and Signs. The disease may have its onset with headache and fever but more commonly the initial symptom is a neuralgic pain in the distribution of the affected roots. The pain is followed in the course of three to four days by reddening of the skin and appearance of clusters of vesicles in part of the area supplied by the affected roots. These vesicles, which contain clear fluid, may be discrete or they may coalesce. Within ten days to two weeks the vesicles are covered with a scab, which after desquamation leaves a pigmented scar. These scars are usually replaced by normally colored skin in the ensuing months. Permanent scarring may occur if there is ulceration or infection of the vesicles. Coincidentally with the eruption there is swelling of the lymph nodes which drain the affected area. This adenopathy is usually painless and subsides with the skin rash.

Herpes zoster is primarily an infection of the spinal ganglion but the cranial ganglia are affected in about 20% of the cases. The thoracic, lumbar, cervical and sacral segments are involved in descending order of frequency. The involvement is almost always unilateral but both sides may be involved in one or more segments.

Among the less common symptoms are impairment of cutaneous sensation and muscular weakness in the distribution of the affected root, headache, stiffness of the neck, or confusion. The latter symptoms are an indication of involvement of the meninges. Motor weakness in the intercostal muscles may be present and not be noted. Involvement of the cervical or lumbar segments may be accompanied by weakness and subsequent atrophy of isolated muscle groups in the upper or lower extremity. Paralysis of the facial muscles with involvement of the otic ganglion and oculomotor palsies with involvement of the ophthalmic ganglion may also occur.

Ophthalmic Zoster. Involvement of the gasserian ganglion occurs in approximately 20% of the cases. Any division of the ganglion may be involved but the first division is most commonly affected. The seriousness of the involvement of this ganglion is due to the changes which develop in the eyes secondary to panophthalmitis or scarring of the cornea. There may be a temporary or permanent paresis of the muscles supplied by the oculomotor nerves.

Geniculate Herpes. Involvement of the otic and geniculate ganglia (Ramsay Hunt syndrome) although rare, assumes prominence because of the appearance of paralysis of the facial muscles. The cutaneous rash is usually confined to the tympanic membrane and the external auditory canal. At times it may spread to involve the outer surface of the lobe of the ear and when combined with cervical involvement, vesicles are found on portions of the neck. The facial paralysis is exactly similar to that of so-called Bell's palsy. Partial or complete recovery is the rule. Involvement of the ganglia of Corti and Scarpa is accompanied by tinnitus, vertigo, nausea and loss of hearing.

Other Symptoms. Although there is a lymphocytic pleocytosis in the cerebrospinal fluid, meningeal symptoms are uncommon. Signs of involvement of the tracts of the spinal cord in the form of a Brown-Séquard syndrome or an incomplete transverse lesion of the spinal cord have been reported. Mental confusion, ataxia and focal cerebral symptoms have been attributed to involvement of the brain by the varicella-zoster virus (herpes zoster encephalitis). Polyneuritis of the so-called infectious or Guillain-Barré type has been reported as a sequel of herpes zoster.

Complications. The complications of herpes zoster include injury to the eyes, scarring of the skin, facial or other palsies and post-herpetic neuralgia. The latter is most common in elderly debilitated patients and affects chiefly the ophthalmic or intercostal nerves. The pains are persistent and are sharp and shooting in nature. The skin is sensitive to touch. These pains may persist for months or years and are often refractory to all forms of treatment.

Laboratory Data. The abnormalities in the laboratory findings are confined to the cerebrospinal fluid. There is an inconstant lymphocytic pleocytosis, which may be found before the onset of the cutaneous rash. The fluid is normal in many of the cases with symptoms of involvement of only one thoracic segment but it is practically always abnormal when there is involvement of cranial ganglia or when paralysis or other neurological signs are present. The cell count in the fluid varies from 10 to several hundred per cu mm with lymphocytes as the predominating cell type. The protein content is normal or moderately increased. The sugar content of the fluid is normal.

Diagnosis. The diagnosis of herpes zoster is made without difficulty when the characteristic rash is present. In the pre-eruptive stage the pain may lead to the erroneous diagnosis of disease of the abdominal or thoracic viscera. The possibility of herpes zoster should be considered in all patients with root pains of sudden onset which have existed for less than four days. Difficulties in diagnosis may also be encountered when the vesicles are very widespread or when they are scant or entirely absent (zoster sine herpete). It is possible that herpes zoster, for example, may cause intercostal neuralgia or facial palsy without any cutaneous eruption, but a careful search will usually reveal a few vesicles.

If necessary, varicella-zoster virus may be isolated from vesicle fluid by inoculation into susceptible human or monkey cells and identified by serological means. Antibody determinations on paired sera may also be of help in establishing the diagnosis.

Treatment. There is still no effective specific antiviral treatment. In the immunosuppressed host with herpes zoster, adenine arabinoside has shown some promise of effectiveness. Zoster immune globulin is useful in prophylaxis, but is not helpful in clinical therapy. A variety of medications can be used locally for the skin eruption. Although antibiotics have no effect on the virus, they may be indicated to control secondary infection particularly in ophthalmic zoster or myelitis with secondary infection.

Postherpetic neuralgia is difficult to treat. Section of the affected posterior roots has not always been successful in bringing about relief of pain. X-ray irradiation of the affected segments may be effective in some cases.

REFERENCES

Aleksic, S. N., Budzilovich, G. N., and Lieberman, A. N.: Herpes Zoster Oticus and Facial Palsy (Ramsay Hunt Syndrome): Clinico-pathologic Study and Review of Literature, J. Neurol. Sci., 20, 149, 1973.

Anastasopoulos, G., Routsonis, K., and Ierodiakonou, C. S.: Ophthalmic Herpes Zoster with Contralateral Hemiplegia, J. Neurol. Neurosurg., & Psychiat., 21, 210, 1958.

Applebaum, E., Kreps, S. I., and Sunshine, A.: Herpes Zoster Encephalitis, Am. J. Med., 32 25, 1962.

Gold, E.: Serologic and Virus-isolation Studies of Patients with Varicella or Herpes Zoster Infection, N. Engl. J. Med., 274, 181, 1966.

Grant, B. D., and Rowe, C. R.: Motor Paralysis of the Extremities in Herpes Zoster, J. Bone & Joint Surg., 43–A, 885, 1961.

Hogan, E. L, and Krigman, M. R.: Herpes Zoster Myelitis: Evidence for Viral Invasion of Spinal Cord, Arch. Neurol., 29, 309, 1973.

Hunt, J. R.: The Sensory Field of the Facial Nerve: a Further Contribution to the Symptomatology of the Geniculate Ganglion, Brain, 38, 418, 1915.

Knox, J. D. E., Levy, R., and Simpson, J. A.: Herpes Zoster and the Landry-Guillain-Barré Syndrome, J. Neurol., Neurosurg. & Psychiat., 24, 167, 1961.

McAlpine, D., et al.: Acute Demyelinating Disease Complicating Herpes Zoster, J. Neurol., Neurosurg. & Psychiat., 22, 120, 1959.

McCormick, W. F., et al.: Varicella-zoster Encephalomyelitis: a Morphologic and Virologic Study. A.M.A. Arch. Neurol., 21, 559, 1969.

Norris, F. H., Jr., et al.: Herpes-zoster Meningoencephalitis, J. Infect. Dis., 122, 335, 1970.

Schimpff, S., et al.: Varicella Zoster Infection in Patients with Cancer, Ann. Intern. Med., 76, 241, 1972.

White, H. H.: Varicella Myelopathy, N. Engl. J. Med., 266, 772, 1962.

Whitley, R. J.: Adenine Arabinoside Therapy of Herpes Zoster in the Immunosuppressed, NIAID Collaborative Antiviral Study, N. Engl. J. Med., 294, 1193, 1976.

Cytomegalic Inclusion Body Disease

Cytomegalic inclusion body disease is an infection which occurs in utero by transplacental transmission. The responsible agent is cytomegalovirus, a member of the herpesvirus group which is among the common parasites of man. The virus can only be grown in cultured human cells. Multiplication is slow and much of the newly formed virus remains cell-associated. Cytomegalovirus infection results in the appearance of large, swollen cells often containing large acidophilic intranuclear and cytoplasmic inclusions.

Intrauterine infection of the nervous system may result in stillbirth or prematurity. The cerebrum is affected by a granulomatous encephalitis with extensive subependymal calcification. Hydrocephalus, hydranencephaly, microcephaly, cerebellar hypoplasia, or other types of developmental defects of the brain may be found. Convulsive seizures, focal neurological signs and mental retardation are common in infants that survive. Jaundice with hepatosplenomegaly, purpuric lesions and hemolytic anemia may be present. Periventricular calcification is often seen in roentgenograms of the skull. Affected infants often succumb in the neonatal period but prolonged periods of survival are possible.

The disease may also occur in adults producing a mononucleosis-like syndrome, but involvement of the nervous system is uncommon in the adult form of the disease. Infection with cytomegalovirus in 12 of 34 patients who died following renal transplantation and immunosuppression was reported by Schneck. Fatal cytomegalovirus encephalitis has been noted in immunosuppressed patients. Cytomegalovirus infection has been implicated as a cause of infectious polyneuritis.

Cytomegalovirus can be recovered from urine, saliva or liver biopsy specimens. Complement-fixation and neutralization tests are available. A presumptive diagnosis can be made by looking for typical cytomegalic cells in stained preparations of urinary sediment or saliva. There is no known effective therapy for the infection.

REFERENCES

Courville, C. B.: Cerebral Lesions in Cytomegalic Inclusion Disease, Bull. Los Angeles Neurol. Soc., 26, 9, 1961.
Crome, L.: Cytomegalic Inclusion-body Disease, World Neurology, 2, 447, 1961.
Dorfman, L. J.: Cytomegalovirus Encephalitis in Adults, Neurology, 23, 136, 1973.
Schneck, S. A.: Neuropathological Features of Human Organ Transplantation. Probable Cytomegalovirus Infection, J. Neuropathol. Exp. Neurol., 24, 415, 1965.
Schnitz, H., and Enders, G.: Cytomegalovirus as a Frequent Cause of Guillain-Barré Syndrome, J. Med. Virol., 1, 21, 1977.
Weller, T. H.: The Cytomegaloviruses: Ubiquitous Agents with Protean Clinical Manifestations, N. Engl. J. Med., 285, 203, 267, 1971.

Infectious Mononucleosis

Infectious mononucleosis (glandular fever) is a systemic disease that is of viral origin with involvement of the lymph nodes, spleen, liver, skin and occasionally the central nervous system. It occurs sporadically and in small epidemics. It is most common in children and young adults. The usual symptoms and signs are headaches, malaise, sore throat, fever, enlargement of the lymph nodes in the cervical region, occasionally enlargement of the spleen and changes in the blood. Unusual manifestations include a cutaneous rash, jaundice and symptoms of involvement of the nervous system.

Henle and his co-workers demonstrated that patients with heterophil-positive infectious mononucleosis develop antibodies to the Epstein-Barr (EB) virus during the course of their illness. EB virus is a herpesvirus originally isolated from African children with Burkitt's lymphoma. These findings suggest that the EB virus is the etiologic cause of infectious mononucleosis.

Although neurological complications rank second as a cause of death after splenic rupture, autopsy studies of the brain in fatal cases of infectious mononucleosis have been few in number. Acute cortical inflammation similar to that seen in other viral infections has been observed. Atypical cells, probably lymphocytes, have been found in the inflammatory exudate. The pathological changes in cases which died following the onset of a severe polyneuritis are similar to those of so-called infectious polyneuritis.

The exact incidence of involvement of the nervous system is unknown but it is probably less than 1%. A lymphocytic pleocytosis in the cerebrospinal fluid may be found in the absence of any neurological symptoms or signs. Severe headache and stiffness of the neck are the initial symptoms of cerebral involvement. Delirium, convulsions, coma and focal neurological signs are rare manifestions. Optic neuritis, paralysis of the facial or oculomotor nerves, acute autonomic neuropathy and a generalized polyneuritis have been reported in a few cases. The latter is indistinguishable from the syndrome of infectious polyneuritis. Cerebellar involvement has also been associated with infectious mononucleosis.

The central nervous system manifestations may appear early in the course of the disease in the absence of any other findings or their onset may be delayed to the convalescent stage. The prognosis is excellent with complete remission of symptoms in all cases except those with respiratory paralysis in severe polyneuritis.

In the laboratory examination the important findings are a leukocytosis in the blood with an increase in the lymphocytes and the appearance of abnormal mononuclear cells. With involvement of the meninges there is a lymphocytic pleocytosis in the cerebrospinal fluid (10 to 600 cell per cu mm) with or without a slight increase in protein content. The sugar content of the fluid is normal and the serologic tests for syphilis are negative in the cerebrospinal fluid. False positive tests for syphilis are occasionally obtained on the serum.

The diagnosis is established by the appearance of neurological symptoms in patients with other manifestations of the disease. The differential diagnosis includes mumps and other virus diseases which cause a lymphocytic meningeal reaction. The differential can be made by a study of the blood, the heterophil antibody reaction and measurement of the antibody response to EB virus antigens. Oropharyngeal excretion of EB virus can also be determined. These tests should be performed on all cases of lymphocytic meningitis in which the diagnosis is obscure.

There is no specific therapy. Treatment with steroids may be indicated in certain patients with severe pharyngotonsillitis or other complications.

REFERENCES

Bonynge, T. W., and Von Hagen, K. O.: Severe Optic Neuritis in Infectious Mononucleosis, J.A.M.A., 148, 933, 1952.
Davie, J. C., Ceballos, R., and Little, S. C.: Infectious Mononucleosis with Fatal Neuronitis, Arch. Neurol., 9, 265, 1963.
Gautier-Smith, P. C.: Neurological Complications of Glandular Fever (Infectious Mononucleosis), Brain, 88, 323, 1965.
Grose, C., et al.: Primary Epstein-Barr Virus Infections in Acute Neurologic Disease, N. Engl. J. Med., 292, 392, 1975.
Henle, G., Henle, W., and Diehl, V.: Relation of Burkitt's Tumor-Associated Herpes-type Virus to Infectious Mononucleosis, Proc. Nat. Acad. Sci. U.S.A., 59, 94, 1968.
Lange, B. J., et al.: Encephalitis in Infectious Mononucleosis: Diagnostic Considerations, Pediatrics, 58, 877, 1976.
Ricker, W., Blumberg, A., Peters, C. H., and Widerman, A.: The Association of the Guillain-Barré Syndrome with Infectious Mononucleosis, Blood, 2, 217, 1947.
Schnell, R. G., et al.: Infectious Mononucleosis: Neurologic and EEG Findings, Medicine, 45, 51, 1966.
Silverstein, A., Steinberg, G., and Nathanson, M.: Nervous System Involvement in Infectious Mononucleosis. The Heralding and/or Major Manifestations, Arch. Neurol., 26, 353, 1972.
Sworn, M. J., and Urich, H.: Acute Encephalitis in Infectious Mononucleosis, J. Path., 100, 210, 1970.

Progressive Multifocal Leukoencephalopathy

In the past decade attention has been called to the occurrence of areas of demyelination in the cerebrum, brain stem and spinal cord of patients suffering with malignant neoplasms. Cases have been reported in association with carcinoma of the lungs, breast and other organs and in patients with chronic lymphatic or myelogenous leukemia, Hodgkin's disease, lymphosarcoma and other tumors of the reticuloendothelial system. The disease has also been reported in association with granulomatous inflammation and transplantation and treatment with immunosuppressive agents. A few cases occurring in the apparent absence of a primary disease have been described.

The pathologic condition is characterized by the presence of multiple, in part confluent, areas of demyelination in various parts of the nervous system, accompanied by mild or moderate degree of perivascular infiltration. Hyperplasia of astrocytes into bizarre giant forms which may resemble neoplastic cells is found. Eosinophilic intranuclear inclusions are seen in oligodendroglial cells. Electron microscopic studies have shown that these inclusions are composed of virus-like particles which are structurally similar to the polyoma, SV40, and K virus subgroup of the papovaviruses (Fig. 10). It is postulated that the demyelination is due to destruction of oligodendroglia by the virus. A new and serologically distinct papovavirus, called JC virus, has been recovered from human fetal glial cells inoculated with brain extracts. JC virus has been repeatedly isolated from progressive multifocal leukoencephalopathic brains. Its presence in brain can also be demonstrated by immune electron microscopy.

The clinical manifestations of the disease are quite diverse and are related to the location and number of the lesions. Hemiplegia, other focal signs and mental symptoms are common in the patients with lesions in the cerebral hemispheres; cranial nerve palsies and other brain stem symptoms in patients with lesions in that area; and incomplete or complete transverse myelitis when the spinal cord is involved. The symptoms and signs are progressive and death ensues in a few months.

There have been reports of treatment with DNA inhibitors, such as cytosine arabinoside and adenine arabinoside, but the results remain inconclusive.

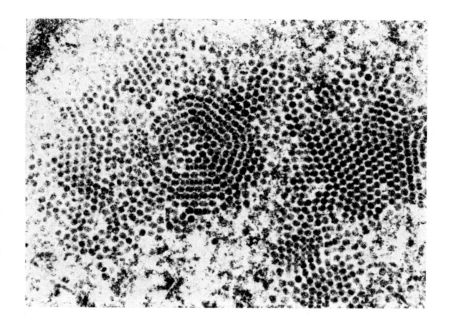

Figure 10.   Papovavirus-like particles present in glial nucleus in progressive multifocal leukoencephalopathic brain. (×65,000) (Courtesy of Dr. G. M. Zu Rhein.)

REFERENCES

Astrom, K. E., Mancall, E. L., and Richardson, E. P., Jr., Progressive Multifocal Leukoencephalopathy; a Hitherto Unrecognized Complication of Chronic Lymphatic Leukemia and Hodgkin's Disease, Brain, 81, 93, 1958.
Gardner, S. D.: The New Papovaviruses: Their Nature and Significance. Recent Advances in Clinical Virology, Number One, A. P. Waterson, Ed., Edinburgh, Churchill Livingston, 1977, pp. 93–115.
Howatson, A. F., Nagai, M., and Zu Rhein, G. M.: Polyoma-like Virions in Human Demyelinating Brain Disease, Can. Med. Assoc. J., 93, 379, 1965.
Manz, H. J., Dinsdale, H. B., and Morrin, P. A. T.: Progressive Multifocal Leukoencephalopathy After Renal Transplantation, Ann. Intern. Med., 75, 77, 1971.
Padgett, B. L.,et al.: Cultivation of Papova-like Virus from Human Brain with Progressive Multifocal Leucoencephalopathy, Lancet, 1, 1257, 1971.
Richardson, E. P., Jr.: Progressive Multifocal Leucoencephalopathy, N. Engl. J. Med., 265, 815, 1961.
Silverman, L., and Rubinstein, L. J.: Progressive Multifocal Leucoencephalopathy, J. Ultrastruct. Res., 13, 567, 1965.
Weiner, L. P., et al.: Isolation of Virus Related to SV40 from Patients with Progressive Multifocal Leukoencephalopathy, N. Engl. J. Med., 286, 385, 1972.
Zu Rhein, G. M., and Chou, S.: Particles Resembling Papova Viruses in Human Cerebral Demyelinating Disease, Science, 148, 1477, 1965.

Transmissible Spongiform Encephalopathies

There is a group of diseases of man and animals which shows common neuropathological findings and appears to be due to transmissible infectious agents with unique properties. The animal diseases are scrapie of sheep and mink encephalopathy. The agent responsible for scrapie has been most extensively studied. Although it is difficult to separate or purify the scrapie agent from diseased tissue, the agent appears so unusually resistant to x-irradiation, ultraviolet exposure or chemical treatment that several workers have felt that the agent does not contain nucleic acid and is not truly a virus. Another peculiarity of these agents is that they do not provoke antibodies in the host after either natural or laboratory infection. The two neurological diseases of man which may be caused by similar agents are kuru and Creutzfeldt-Jakob disease.

Kuru. This progressive and fatal neurologic disorder occurs exclusively among natives of the New Guinea Highlands. It is manifested by incoordination of gait, cerebellar dysfunction, abnormal involuntary movements resembling myoclonus, athetosis or chorea, convergent strabismus and dementia. The illness terminates fatally in four to twenty-four months. Eighty per cent of adults afflicted are women. Cannibalism has been considered as a possible mode of transmission. Neuropathological changes include widespread neuronal loss and intense astrocytic and microglial proliferation. Perivascular inflammatory changes are rarely observed. The similarity between the neuropathological changes of kuru with those seen in scrapie-afflicted sheep led Gadjusek and Gibbs to attempt to infect higher primates with kuru brain suspensions. Inoculation of chimpanzees was followed by the appearance of a kuru-like disease eighteen to twenty-one months later and subpassage to other chimpanzees produced a similar neurological disease.

Creutzfeldt-Jakob disease (spastic pseudosclerosis, cortico-striato-spinal degeneration). Creutzfeldt and Jakob described in 1920 and 1921 a progressive disease of the cortex, basal ganglia and spinal cord which developed in middle-aged or elderly adults. The disease is relatively rare. The report of Siedler and Malamud would indicate that its frequency is one half of that of Pick's disease, and one fifth that of Alzheimer's disease. These authors were able to find 57 well-documented cases in the literature in addition to the 15 studied by them.

The pathologic condition is essentially degenerative in nature with loss of the nerve cells in the cortex, basal ganglia and spinal cord (Table 9). The clinical features include familial and sporadic incidence, onset in middle or late life, but occasionally in early adult life, gradual development of pyramidal signs (weakness and stiffness of the ex-

Table 9. Frequency of Involvement of Various Portions of the Nervous System in 72 Cases of Creutzfeldt-Jakob's Disease
(After Siedler and Malamud, J. Neuropathol. Exp. Neurol., 1963)

Location	No. of Cases	%
Cortex	72	100
Basal ganglia	65	90
Corticospinal tracts	24	33
Motor neurons	27	38
Thalamus	48	67
Cerebellum	38	53

Table 10. Frequency of Symptoms and Signs in 72 Cases of Creutzfeldt-Jakob's Disease
(After Siedler and Malamud, J. Neuropathol. Exp. Neurol., 1963)

Signs and Symptoms	No. of Cases	%
Dementia	72	100
Basal ganglia	52	72
Upper motor neuron	50	69
Lower motor neuron	20	28
Aphasia	20	28
Myoclonus	33	46
Other seizures	15	21
Visual loss	16	22

tremities with accompanying reflex changes) and the superimposition
of extra-pyramidal signs (tremors, rigidity, dysarthria and slowness of
movements). Mental deterioration and psychotic manifestations are
common. Muscular atrophy is present when the motor cells of the
medulla and spinal cord are affected. Myoclonus and convulsive
seizures occur in a large percentage of the cases. In some cases signs
and symptoms of cerebellar dysfunction may predominate (Table 10).
Paroxysmal burst of spike or slow wave activity intervals of 0.6 to 1.8
seconds is characteristic of the electroencephalogram in the late stages
of the disease (Fig. 11). The disease runs a rapid course with death
occurring within a few months or years in the majority of the cases.
There is no specific treatment.

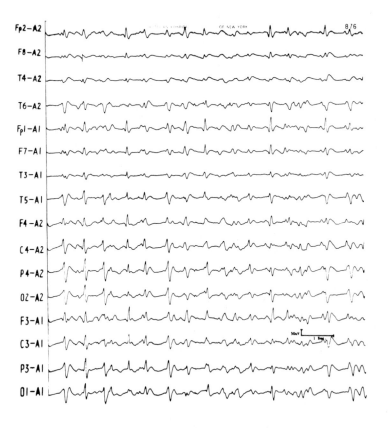

Figure 11. Creutzfeldt-Jakob Disease. Record of a 65 year old man shows spikes or
sharp waves at intervals of 0.7 of a second throughout the recording. Such periodicity
with .6 to 1.8 second intervals occur late and may be absent in the early stages of the
disease.

It has been possible to produce a neurological illness in chimpanzees by the inoculation of brain suspensions prepared from the brains of Creutzfeldt-Jakob patients. The neuropathological changes found in these chimpanzees resemble those observed in patients with Creutzfeldt-Jakob disease. It is also possible to transmit the illness experimentally to a variety of simian species as well as cats, hamsters and guinea pigs.

Inadvertent man-to-man transmission has also been reported following corneal transplantation and the use of inadequately sterilized stereotactic brain electrodes. Caution must be exercised in operating or pathology suites when handling a tissue from suspected Creutzfeldt-Jakob patient.

REFERENCES

Bernouilli, C., et al.: Danger of Accidental Person-to-Person Transmission of Creutzfeldt-Jakob Disease by Surgery, Lancet, 1, 478, 1977.

Brownell, B., and Oppenheimer, D. R.: An Ataxic Form of Subacute Presenile Polioencephalopathy (Creutzfeldt-Jakob Disease), J. Neurol., Neurosurg., & Psychiat., 28, 350, 1965.

Burger, L. J., Rowan, A. J., and Goldensohn, E. S.: Creutzfeldt-Jakob Disease. An Electroencephalographic Study, Arch. Neurol., 26, 428, 1972.

Duffy, P. et al.: Possible Person-to-Person Transmission of Creutzfeldt-Jakob Disease, N. Engl., J. Med., 290 692, 1974.

Gajdusek, D. C.: Unconventional Viruses and the Origin and Disappearance of Kuru, Science, 197, 943, 1977.

Gajdusek, D. C. et al.: Precautions in Medical Care of, and in Handling Materials from, Patients with Transmissible Virus Dementia (Creutzfeldt-Jakob Disease), N. Engl. J. Med., 297, 1253, 1977.

Gajdusek, D. C., and Zigas, V.: Kuru. Clinical, Pathological and Epidemiological Study of an Acute Progressive Degenerative Disease of the Central Nervous System among Natives of the Eastern Highlands of New Guinea, Am. J. Med., 26, 442, 1959.

Gibbs, C. J., Jr., et al.: Creutzfeldt-Jakob Disease (Spongiform Encephalopathy) Transmission to the Chimpanzee, Science, 161, 388, 1968.

Gibbs, C. J., Jr., and Gajdusek, D. C.: Experimental Subacute Spongiform Virus Encephalopathies in Primates and Other Laboratory Animals, Science, 182, 67, 1973.

Kirschbaum, W. R.: Creutzfeldt-Jakob Disease, New York, American Elsevier, 1968, pp. 251.

Matthews, W. B.: Creutzfeldt Disease as a Transmissable Encephalopathy. Recent Advances in Clinical Virology: Number One, A. P. Waterson, Ed., Edinburgh, Churchill Livingston, 1977, pp. 51–60.

Roos, R., Gajdusek, D. C., and Gibbs, C. J., Jr.: The Clinical Characteristics of Transmissable Creutzfeldt-Jakob Disease, Brain, 96, 1, 1973.

Siedler, H., and Malamud, N.: Creutzfeldt-Jakob's Disease. Clinicopathologic Report of 15 Cases and Review of the Literature, J. Neuropath. & Exper. Neurol., 22, 381, 1963.

Postvaccinal and Postinfectious Encephalomyelitis

An acute encephalomyelitis may occur in the course of various infections, particularly the acute exanthematous disease of childhood, and following vaccination against smallpox and rabies. The clinical symptoms and the pathological changes are similar in all of these cases, regardless of the nature of the acute infection, and they are therefore all considered together.

The list of diseases which may be accompanied or followed by signs and symptoms of an encephalomyelitis is probably not complete as yet, but at present it includes: typhoid, measles; rubella, varicella-zoster; smallpox; mumps, influenza, infectious mononucleosis or other obscure febrile disease; and vaccination against smallpox or rabies. Reactions in the nervous system may also follow inoculations with typhoid vaccine and with sera—particularly that against tetanus. In these latter conditions, the clinical picture is apt to be that of a mononeuritis or generalized polyneuritis.

Etiology. The etiology of postvaccinal and postinfectious encephalomyelitis is not known. Since the condition occurs in the course of diseases which are known to be of viral origin or follows vaccination against viral diseases, it was natural to assume that the changes in the nervous system were due to direct involvement by either the virus of the disease itself or by some other virus activated by the infection. Against this theory, however, is the fact that virus has been isolated from only a few of the cases. The virus of vaccinia, measles, varicella-zoster and mumps have been isolated from the brain or cerebrospinal fluid, and cytoplasmic or nuclear inclusion bodies have been found in the neurons in fatal cases associated with measles and varicella-zoster.

Other theories include damage by a toxin elaborated by the virus or an allergic reaction. There is no definite proof for either of these theories but the temporal coincidence of the onset of neurological symptoms and the appearance of antibodies in the blood against the infection is advanced by some authors as evidence in favor of an allergic factor.

Pathology. There is little or no change in the external appearance of the brain or spinal cord. On sectioning there are many small yellowish-red lesions in the white matter of the cerebrum, cerebellum, brain stem and spinal cord. The characteristic feature of these lesions is a loss of myelin, with relative sparing of the axis cylinders. The lesions in the brain are oval or round and usually surround a distended vein. In cross sections of the spinal cord, they tend to extend in a radial manner from the gray matter to the periphery of the cord (Fig. 12). The lesions are usually found in large numbers in almost all parts of the central nervous system, but in some cases they may be concentrated in the white matter of the cortex and in others the cerebellum, brain stem or spinal cord may be most severely affected. On microscopic examination of appropriately stained specimens there is complete or incomplete destruction of myelin sheaths within the lesions, with a fairly sharp margin between the affected and normal areas. Axis cylinders are

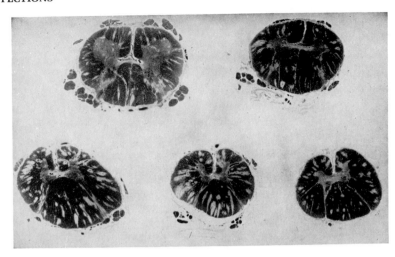

Figure 12. Acute postinfectious encephalomyelitis. Radial streaks of demyelination in spinal cord. (Myelin sheath stain.)

affected to much less extent than the myelin sheaths. Within the lesion and in the perivascular space of adjacent vessels there is an accumulation of phagocytic microglial cells. A few lymphocytes are found in the perivascular spaces and in the meninges. Although the lesions are concentrated in the white matter, a few patches may be found in the gray matter. Nerve cells in these areas may be destroyed or show various degenerative changes.

Incidence. The frequency of encephalomyelitis following vaccination against smallpox has not been accurately established. The statistics given by Gorter for over a half million vaccinations in various countries of the world give figures which vary from 0.2 to 4.5 per 10,000 vaccinations. Greenberg reported that 45 cases of encephalitis with 4 deaths followed the vaccination of 5,000,000 people in New York City in one month in 1947. According to these figures the incidence would be less than 1 in 100,000. Reactions are more frequent following primary than secondary vaccination. No age group is exempt, but neurological complications are extremely rare in infants and are uncommon after the age of thirty years. The two sexes are equally affected. The time of onset of neurological symptoms is remarkably constant. In the vast majority of cases the onset occurs ten to twelve days after vaccination. Extremes vary from four to thirty days.

The incidence of encephalomyelitis following vaccination against rabies is estimated as 1 in 600. The figure, together with the mortality rate (11%), is sufficiently high to contraindicate indiscriminate use of this vaccine. The incidence has been greatly reduced since the introduction of the use of vaccine prepared from duck embryo.

Damage to the nervous system with the acute exanthemata occurs most commonly following measles, where the incidence in different epidemics varied from 1 per 400 to 1 per 1,000 cases. It is much less frequent following varicella-zoster, rubella, mumps and smallpox.

Symptoms and Signs. The symptoms and signs of encephalomyelitis following vaccination or the acute exanthemata are related to the portion of the nervous system which is most severely damaged and are not dependent on the type of vaccination or the nature of the exanthematous disease.

Since any portion of the nervous system may be affected, it is not surprising that variable clinical syndromes may occur. In some cases there are signs and symptoms of generalized involvement of the nervous system, but more commonly one or more portions of the neuraxis suffers the brunt of the damage resulting in various fairly clear-cut clinical syndromes: Meningeal; encephalitic; brain stem; spinal cord; and neuritic.

Symptoms of involvement of the meninges—headaches, stiffness of the neck and drowsiness—are common early in the course of all types. In a number of cases there are no further symptoms. In others these initial signs and symptoms may be followed by evidence of damage to the cerebrum. In the encephalitic form there may be convulsions; stupor, coma, hemiplegia, aphasia or other signs of focal cerebral involvement. Cranial nerve palsies or signs and symptoms of cerebellar dysfunction predominate in a few cases. More common than brain stem or cerebellar involvement, however, are signs and symptoms of injury to the spinal cord. This may take the form of an acute transverse myelitis, a Brown-Séquard lesion, or focal damage to gray and white matter at some level of the cord.

Peripheral nerve involvement is rare in the encephalomyelitides following smallpox vaccination or the acute exanthemata. It is more frequent, however, following antirabic vaccine, where an acute ascending paralysis of the Landry type is not uncommon.

Paralyses of the muscles innervated by axillary and long thoracic nerves are the usual neurological complications of antitetanus vaccine, but any of the nerves of the brachial plexus may be affected. Rarely there may be a generalized polyneuritis but isolated involvement of the lumbosacral or cranial nerves is exceedingly rare.

Laboratory Data. The only significant laboratory findings are in the cerebrospinal fluid and the electroencephalogram. The cerebrospinal fluid pressure is usually normal but it may be slightly elevated. There is a mild or moderate increase in the white cells, 15 to 250 cells per cu mm with lymphocytes as the predominating cell type. The protein content is normal or slightly elevated (35 to 150 mg per 100 ml). Sugar and chloride content are within normal limits. The electroencephalogram is abnormal in practically all cases. There is an increase in the number of slow frequencies, and often 4- to 6-per-second waves become prominent. The abnormalities are usually generalized and symmetrical on the two sides of the head, but focal or unilateral changes may be found. The abnormalities persist for several weeks after apparent clinical recovery. Persisting abnormalities correlate well with permanent neurologic damage or convulsive disorders.

Diagnosis and Differential Diagnosis. Since there is no specific diagnostic test, the diagnosis of postinfectious or postvaccinal encephalomyelitis should be considered when neurological signs develop four to eighteen days following vaccination or the onset of one of the acute exanthemata. The differential diagnosis includes practically all of the acute diseases of the nervous system, particularly the acute or subacute meningitides.

Prognosis and Course. The mortality rate is high (10 to 30%) in the cases with severe involvement of the nervous system in measles or after rabies vaccination. It is low in the cases with involvement only of the peripheral nerves. Death may occur as a result of cerebral damage in the acute stage or following intercurrent infections, bedsores or urinary sepsis in late stages. In patients who survive, there is usually a surprising degree of improvement of the neurological signs. There may be residual palsies, but complete recovery is not uncommon. Postencephalitic sequelae, such as parkinsonism, do not occur and as a rule there are no new symptoms after recovery from an acute attack. Behavior disorders, mental deterioration or convulsive seizures may occur as sequelae in children. A few cases have been reported in which the clinical syndrome of multiple sclerosis, with remissions and exacerbation of symptoms, has followed postinfectious or postvaccinal encephalomyelitis but this is an extreme rarity.

Treatment. There are a number of reports which suggest that the administration of corticosteroids reduces the severity of the neurological defects.

REFERENCES

Ambler, M., et al.: Focal Encephalomyelitis in Infectious Mononucleosis: A Report with Pathological Description, Ann. Intern. Med., 75, 579, 1971.

Angulo, J. J., Pimenta-de-Campos, E., and De Salles-Gomes, L. F.: Post-vaccinal Meningo-Encephalitis. Isolation of the Virus from the Brain, J.A.M.A., 187, 151, 1964.

Appelbaum, E., Greenberg, M., and Nelson, J.: Neurological Complications Following Antirabies Vaccination, J.A.M.A., 151, 188, 1953.

Ferraro, A., and Roizin, L.: Hyperergic Encephalomyelitis Following Exanthematic Diseases, Infectious Diseases and Vaccination, J. Neuropath. & Exper. Neurol., 16, 423, 1957.

Gorter, E.: Postvaccinal Encephalitis, J.A.M.A., *101*, 1871, 1933.

Greenberg, M.: Complications of Vaccination Against Smallpox, Am. J. Dis. Child., *76*, 492, 1948.

Harter, D. H. and Choppin, P. W.: Possible Mechanisms in the Pathogenesis of "Post-infectious" Encephalomyelitis, Res. Publ. Ass. Nerv. Ment. Dis., *49*, 342, 1971.

Hoyne, A. L, and Slotkowski, E. L.: Frequency of Encephalitis as Complications of Measles, Am. J. Dis. Child., *73*, 554, 1947.

La Boccetta, A. C., and Tornay, A. S.: Measles Encephalitis, Am. J. Dis. Child., *107*, 247, 1964.

Levy, L. L., and Roseman, E.: Electroencephalographic Studies of the Encephalopathies. III Serial Studies in Measles Encephalitis, Am. J. Dis. Child., *88*, 5, 1954.

Meulen, V. ter, et al.: Isolation of Infectious Measles Virus in Measles Encephalitis, Lancet, *2*, 1172, 1972.

Miller, H. G., Stanton, J. B., and Gibbons, J. L.: Para-infectious Encephalomyelitis and Related Syndromes, Quart. J. Med., *25*, 427, 1956.

Prussin, G., and Katabi, G.: Dorsolumbar Myelitis Following Antirabies Vaccination with Duck Embryo Vaccine, Ann. Intern. Med., *60*, 114, 1964.

Ramachandran, S., et al.: Acute Disseminated Encephalomyelitis in Typhoid Fever, Br. Med. J., *1*, 494, 1975.

Sherman, F. E., Michaels, R. H., and Kenny, F. M.: Acute Encephalopathy (Encephalitis) Complicating Rubella, J.A.M.A., *192*, 675, 1965.

Spillane, J. D., and Wells, C. E. C.: The Neurology of Jennerian Vaccination. A Clinical Account of the Neurological Complications which Occurred During the Smallpox Epidemic in South Wales in 1962, Brain, *87*, 1, 1964.

Williams, H. W., and Chafee, F. H.: Demyelinating Encephalomyelitis in a Case of Tetanus Treated with Antitoxin, N. Engl. J. Med., *264*, 489, 1961.

Encephalitis Lethargica

Encephalitis lethargica (sleeping sickness, von Economo's disease) is a disease of unknown etiology, which occurred in epidemic form in the years 1916 and 1926. Clinically, the disease was characterized by signs and symptoms of diffuse involvement of the brain and by the development of various sequelae in a large percentage of the recovered cases. Although the disease spread rapidly over the entire world, it is practically extinct at the present time. The disease is of importance since patients who are suffering from its sequelae are still living and, in addition, there is always the possibility that it may occur in epidemic form again.

Epidemiology, The first cases of encephalitis lethargica appeared in Vienna in the winter of 1916 and 1917. It was recognized in England in 1918 and in the United States in 1919. The exact number involved is unknown. The Matheson survey collected 42,998 cases from 1919 to 1927, but this figure represents only a small percentage of the total.

The disease was fairly evenly distributed through all the decades of life and affected the two sexes evenly. All races and occupations were affected. Familial incidence was uncommon and it was not possible to trace the spread of the disease by contact with an affected individual.

Etiology. The etiology of encephalitis lethargica is unknown. Some workers claimed that they were able to transmit the disease to animals and that they had isolated a virus from brain tissue of fatal cases. It is now agreed that the disease was due to a virus but proof is lacking.

Pathology. In the acute stages there was a diffuse inflammatory reaction in the meninges and around the blood vessels of the brain and spinal cord, and acute degenerative changes in the neurons. The inflammatory changes were greatest in the brain stem, basal ganglia and cerebellum, but the cortex and subcortical white matter are involved, as are also both the gray and white matter of the spinal cord.

Symptoms and Signs. The symptoms were usually of acute or subacute onset. Fever was usually present at the onset but it sometimes did not develop until later. It was commonly of mild degree and lasted only a few days. In fatal cases there was often a rise to 107° F or greater in the terminal stages.

Headache was present in a large percentage of cases reported. Lethargy was one of the most common of the early symptoms. It lasted only a few days in some cases, but in others persisted for weeks or months. Occasionally the lethargy alternated with insomnia and delirium, or there was a reversal in the sleep rhythm.

Disorders of eye movements, the most frequent sign of localized damage to the nervous system, were present in approximately 75% of the cases. They varied from a transient diplopia to a complete paralysis of one or more ocular muscles.

Although hemiplegia or monoplegia was occasionally seen, the most frequent motor symptoms were those associated with disease of the basal ganglia. Choreiform, athetoid, dystonic, myoclonic and tic-like movements were present in the acute stages in a number of cases. Rigidity and alternating tremors, sometimes present at this stage, were more commonly a sequel of the disease. Intention tremor and other cerebellar symptoms were present in a few cases.

Delirium, depression, euphoria, manic excitement, and psychic disturbances characteristic of an acute organic psychosis were not uncommon symptoms in the acute state. Convulsions were distinctly rare. Other cortical signs including aphasia, apraxia, and agnosia were present in a few patients. Evidences of autonomic dysfunction were occasionally present.

Laboratory Data. There was an inconstant leukocytosis in the blood during the first few weeks of the disease. The laboratory data were otherwise normal except for changes in the cerebrospinal fluid. A lymphocytic pleocytosis was generally present during the first few weeks, but it usually disappeared within two months of the onset. The protein content was normal in approximately half the cases. Values greater than 100 mg per 100 ml were rare.

Diagnosis. The diagnosis of encephalitis lethargica is, for all practical purposes, never justified at the present time. In the light of present knowledge, all that can be said is that the diagnosis may be justified in any case with signs and symptoms of a generalized disturbance of the nervous system with the special features of disturbed sleep rhythm and diplopia during the acute stage and the development of signs of injury to the basal ganglia at that time or in subsequent years.

Course and Prognosis. In the average case the duration of the acute stage was about four weeks. Not infrequently the acute stage was much longer and merged gradually into the so-called postencephalitic phase of the disease. The mortality rate varied in different countries and from year to year in any one country. In most of the large series the mortality rate was approximately 25% and was highest in infants and in the elderly. The frequency of residuals or sequelae is unknown because long-term follow-up of any large series of cases is lacking.

Aftereffects or Sequelae. There has been a great deal of discussion as to the pathogenesis of the symptoms which develop in patients who recover from an acute attack of encephalitis lethargica. In some instances these symptoms were merely a continuation of those which were present in the acute state. In others, the symptoms developed after an interval of several months or even many years during which the patient was apparently well.

The parkinsonian syndrome which develops after encephalitis lethargica is similar to that of the idiopathic type (paralysis agitans) and in many cases a differential diagnosis is not possible. There are, however, a number of features which, if present, point to postencephalitic origin. These include the development of parkinsonism in childhood or early adult life and the presence of symptoms which are uncommon in other forms of parkinsonism, such as grimaces, torticollis, torsion spasms, myoclonus, oculogyric crises, facial and respiratory tics, and bizarre postures and gaits.

Behavior disorders and emotional instability without evidence of intellectual impairment were common sequelae in children. They occurred in approximately one third of the cases, the majority of whom had no evidence of parkinsonism, and tended to remit with the passage of years.

REFERENCES

Association for Research in Nervous and Mental Disease. *Acute Epidemic Encephalitis (Lethargic Encephalitis),* New York, Paul B. Hoeber, Inc., 1921, 258 pp.
Hall, A. J.: *Epidemic Encephalitis (Encephalitis Lethargica),* New York, William Wood & Co., 1924, 229 pp.
Neal, J. B., et al.: *Encephalitis,* New York, Grune & Stratton, 1942, 563 pp.
Riley, H. A.: Epidemic Encephalitis, Arch. Neurol. & Psychiat., 24, 574, 1930.
von Economo, C.: Encephalitis Lethargica, Wien. klin. Wcshr., 30, 581, 1917.

RICKETTSIAL INFECTIONS

Microorganisms known as rickettsiae, which are intermediate in character between bacteria and viruses, are capable of producing disease in man. These organisms are readily visible in microscopic preparations as pleomorphic coccobacillary forms. They multiply only within certain cells of susceptible species and are found in various arthropods in nature. Diseases due to rickettsiae are divided into five groups on the basis of clinical features, epidemiologic aspects, and serologic and immunologic characteristics as follows: (1) Typhus group: (a) louse-borne, (b) flea-borne, (c) Brill's disease; (2) spotted fever group (tick-borne); (3) scrub typhus (mite-borne); (4) Q fever; (5) trench fever. The last two groups (Q fever and trench fever) differ from the other three in that the organisms pass through the Berkefeld filter and the Weil-Felix reaction is negative. Invasion of the nervous system is common only in infections with organisms of the first three groups.

Typhus Fever

Three types of infection in man with rickettsiae of the typhus group are recognized: (1) The classical epidemic or European type which is transmitted to man by the bite of the body louse; (2) murine type which is endemic throughout the world and is transmitted to man by the bite of fleas from rats; (3) Brill's disease, the name given to cases that occurred sporadically in immigrants to the United States from South-western Europe, and not associated with body lice. It was thought to be an infection with the murine type but according to Zinsser it represents a recurrence of typhus in individuals who had been infected previously in Europe.

Pathology. The pathological changes are most severe in the skin, but the heart, lungs and central nervous system are also involved. The brain is edematous and minute petechial hemorrhages are present. The characteristic microscopic lesions are small, round nodules composed of elongated microglia, lymphocytes and endothelial cells. These are scattered diffusely throughout the nervous system in close relation to the smaller vessels. Vessels in the center of the lesions show severe degenerative changes. The endothelial cells are swollen and the lumen may be occluded. In addition to the microglia nodules, there is a mild degree of perivascular infiltration in the meninges and parenchyma.

Incidence. Since its recognition as a disease entity in the sixteenth century, typhus has been known as one of the great epidemic diseases of the world. It is especially prevalent in war times or whenever there is a massing of people in camps, prisons and ships.

The louse-borne type (R. prowazeki) is endemic to Central Europe, Russia, Ireland, Spain, Turkey, North Africa, Japan, Northern China, Mexico and South America. In the epidemic form all age groups are affected. In some epidemics both sexes are equally affected, in others it is more common in the male.

Murine typhus (R. mooseri) is world-wide in distribution. It is apparently on the increase in the United States, where 332 cases were reported in 1931 and 5,193 in 1945. The disease is most prevalent in Southern and Southwestern states and among individuals whose occupations bring them into rat-infested premises. The disease is most common in the late summer and fall months. The freedom of the population from lice explains the absence of epidemics in the United States.

Symptoms and Signs. The incubation period lasts from ten to fourteen days. The onset of symptoms is abrupt, with fever, prostration and muscular aches and pains. The skin eruption appears on the third to seventh day as pink, erythematous macules, profusely scattered over the trunk and extremities. Symptoms of involvement of the nervous system are present in practically all cases. Headache, stiffness of the neck and delirium are early manifestations. Later there may be various degrees of coma, convulsive seizures and signs of focal damage to the cerebrum, spinal cord or cranial and peripheral nerves.

Laboratory Data. The white cell count in the blood is usually normal. The serum proteins are lowered. The urine is concentrated and contains albumin. Oliguria, as the result of dehydration, is common and the blood urea may be greatly elevated. The Weil-Felix reaction is positive in the serum after the fifth day. The cerebrospinal fluid pressure is usually normal but it may be slightly increased. The fluid is clear but contains a small or moderate number of white cells (25 to 200 per cu mm), usually lymphocytes. The protein is slightly increased, but the sugar is normal.

Diagnosis. A presumptive diagnosis of typhus fever can be made on the basis of the characteristic skin rash and signs of involvement of the nervous system. The diagnosis is established by the Weil-Felix reaction which becomes positive in the fifth to eighth day of the disease. The titer rises in the first few weeks of the convalescence and then falls. The organism can be recovered by inoculation of blood or ground clot into guinea pigs, other rodents or into fertile hens' eggs. Meningococcus meningitis with septicemia is excluded by the sterile blood culture and the findings in the cerebrospinal fluid. The differential between louse-borne and murine types is made by means of the complement fixation test. The differential diagnosis between typhus and spotted fever can be made by complement fixation and virus neutralization tests.

Course and Prognosis. The course of typhus fever usually extends over a period of two to three weeks. In patients who recover there is improvement in general condition after about ten to twelve days. The fever becomes remittent and subsides in a few days. Complications include bronchitis and bronchopneumonia, myocardial degeneration, gangrene of the skin or extremities and thrombosis of large abdominal, pulmonary or cerebral vessels.

The mortality rate in epidemics of louse-borne typhus has varied greatly, from over 50% to less than 5. In childhood the disease is mild and the mortality rate below the age of twenty years is low. After this age there is a steady increase in mortality with each decade. Death is usually due to the development of pneumonia. The mortality rate in murine typhus in the United States is low, under 5%. There are no neurological residuals in patients who recover.

Treatment. Chloramphenicol and tetracycline antibiotics are effective agents in the treatment of all of the rickettsial infections. Seriously ill patients will require intravenous administration of antibiotics.

General nursing care is of great importance in the management of patients with epidemic typhus. Codeine may be needed to combat headache. Cold packs should be administered when the temperature rises above 104° F. The vector must be removed from patients by appropriate measures.

Spotted Fever

Rocky Mountain spotted fever is an acute endemic febrile disease produced by infection with the Rickettsia rickettsii. It is transmitted to man through the medium of various ticks, the most common of which are the Dermacentor andersoni in the Rocky Mountain and Pacific Coast states and Dermacentor variabilis (dog tick) in the East and South. Rabbits, squirrels and other small rodents serve as hosts for the ticks and are responsible for maintaining the infection in nature. Diseases of the Rocky Mountain fever group are present throughout the world and include boutonneuse fever of the Mediterranean area, Brazilian spotted fever, Tobia fever of Colombia, Choix or penta fever of Mexico, Kenya fever, South African tick-bite fever, rickettsial pox and some of the rickettsioses of India, Russia and Australia.

Pathology. The lesions of spotted fever are similar to those of typhus. In addition to the glial nodules and perivascular infiltration, minute areas of focal necrosis in the nervous system are common as the result of thrombosis of small arterioles.

Incidence. Until 1930, it was thought that Rocky Mountain spotted fever was confined to the mountainous regions of the Northwest portion of the United States. In recent years the disease has been reported from Canada, South America and every state in the United

States except Maine, Vermont, Rhode Island and Connecticut. Approximately 500 cases are reported annually in the United States mostly from rural areas. The seasonal prevalence of the disease corresponds to the tick seasons of the locality concerned, that is the spring and summer months in the United States. Adult males are most frequently infected in the West. In the East a high percentage of infections is in children and women due in part to the fact that the vector in the East infests the dog, a household pet.

Symptoms and Signs. The clinical picture is similar to that of typhus, the chief differential points being the duration of fever and the time of appearance and location of the rash. The rash which appears on the third or fourth day resembles the slight mottling of measles. This fades and is followed by rose-red, maculopapular lesions on the ankles and wrists. The rash rapidly spreads to the legs, arms and chest. Neurological symptoms occur early and are frequently a prominent feature. Delirium or coma alternating with restlessness is present during the height of the fever. Tremors, convulsions, opisthotonos and muscular rigidity may occur. Retinal venous engorgement, retinal edema, papilledema, retinal exudates and choroiditis may occur. Deafness, visual disturbances, slurred speech and mental confusion may be present and persist for a few weeks following recovery.

Laboratory Data. The laboratory findings are similar to those of typhus fever, except that leukocytosis in the blood is more common. Proteinuria and hematuria are commonly found. The Weil-Felix reaction is positive. The cerebrospinal fluid is usually normal. A few patients have a mild to moderate spinal fluid pleocytosis.

Diagnosis. The diagnosis is made on the basis of the development of the characteristic rash and other symptoms of the disease four to six days following exposure to ticks. Clinical distinction from typhus fever may be impossible. The onset of the rash in distal parts of the extremities is in favor of spotted fever. In rare instances, however, neurological signs may present before the rash appears. Final diagnosis depends on the results of neutralization and complement fixation tests.

Course and Prognosis. In cases that recover the fever falls by lysis at about the end of the third week, although mild cases may become afebrile before the end of the second week. Convalescence may be slow and residuals of damage to the nervous system may persist for several months.

The virulence of the infection varies with the locality. It is highest in the Bitter Root Valley of Montana where the death rate for non-vaccinated adults averages about 80% and for children about 37%. The over-all mortality rate in the South and East (20%) is approximately the same as that for other sections of the Northwest.

Treatment. Control measures include personal care and vaccination.

Tick infested areas should be avoided. If exposure is necessary, the wearing of high boots, leggings or socks outside the trouser legs is indicated. Body and clothing should be inspected after exposure and attached ticks should be removed with tweezers or with a piece of paper held between the fingers. The hands should be carefully washed after handling the ticks. Workers whose occupations require constant exposure to tick-infested regions should be vaccinated yearly just before the advent of the tick season.

The treatment of Rocky Mountain spotted fever is with the tetracyclines or chloramphenicol.

Scrub Typhus (Tsutsugamushi Disease)

Scrub typhus is an infectious disease caused by Rickettsia tsutsugamushi which is transmitted to man by the bite of a mite. It resembles the other rickettsial diseases and is characterized by sudden onset of fever, cutaneous eruption and the presence of an ulcerative lesion (eschar) at the site of attachment of the chigger.

Epidemiology. The disease was originally described from the Northwestern part of Honshu Island. At the beginning of World War II, scrub typhus was known to occur in India, Indochina, New Guinea, Australia, the Malay States and Dutch East Indies. The causative organism, R. tsutsugamushi, is transmitted to man by the bite of the larval form of the mite, popularly known as "harvest mite," "red bug," or "chigger." Although many types of vertebrates serve as hosts for the mites, only rodents have been demonstrated to harbor the R. tsutsugamushi in nature.

Pathology. The histopathology of scrub typhus is basically disseminated focal vasculitis and perivasculitis with conspicuous involvement of the vessels in the skin, lungs, heart and brain. There may be an associated parenchymal involvement of these organs.

In the brain there is a vasculitis and perivasculitis similar to those found in other organs. In addition, there is lymphocytic infiltration of the meninges, perivascular cuffing in the parenchyma and the formation of glial nodules similar to those of epidemic or murine typhus.

Incidence. The disease has a scattered or focal distribution in those areas in which it is endemic. Infection is related to exposure to the type of terrain suitable for both rodent population and the specific mite vector. In Japan the disease tends to have a seasonal incidence, but it is prevalent throughout the year in the tropics.

Symptoms and Signs. The disease begins abruptly, following an incubation period of ten to eighteen days, with fever and headache. The headache increases in intensity and may become quite severe. Conjunctival congestion, lymphadenitis, deafness, apathy and anorexia are

common symptoms. Delirium, coma, restlessness and muscular twitchings are present in severe cases. A primary lesion, the eschar, is seen in
nearly all cases and represents the former site of attachment of the
infected mite. Multiple eschars may be present. The cutaneous rash
appears between the fifth and eighth day of the disease. The eruption is
macular or maculopapular and non-hemorrhagic. The trunk is involved
first with later extension to the extremities.

Laboratory Data. The white blood count may be normal or low in the
early stages, but a slight leukocytosis is not uncommon in the second
week. Plasma proteins may be lowered and there is a reduction in the
serum chloride content. There is a moderate pleocytosis and an
increase in protein content of the cerebrospinal fluid.

Diagnosis. The diagnosis is made on the basis of the development of
typical symptoms, the presence of the characteristic eschar and the
positive Weil-Felix reaction in the serum. The agglutinins reach a
maximum titer by the end of the third week and decline rapidly, often
disappearing by the fifth or sixth week. The diagnosis can be confirmed
by recovering the causal rickettsia from white mice which have been
injected with blood removed from a patient during the febrile period.

Course and Prognosis. The mortality rate varies greatly with local
epidemics, the rate ranging from 40 to 60% in Japan and from 5 to 20%
in Burma and Malaya. During World War II approximately 6,685 cases
of scrub typhus were reported among United States personnel, with
284 deaths (mortality rate 4%). In fatal cases, death usually occurs in
the second or third week as a result of pneumonia, cardiac failure or
cerebral involvement.

In cases that recover, the temperature begins to fall at the end of the
second or third week. Permanent residuals are not common but the
period of convalescence may extend over several months.

Treatment. The treatment of scrub typhus is the same as that
described for typhus fever.

REFERENCES

Ahlm, C. E., and Lipshutz, J.: Tsutsugamushi Fever in the Southwest Pacific Theater,
    J.A.M.A., *124*, 1095, 1944.
Aikawa, J. K.: *Rocky Mountain Spotted Fever.* Springfield, Charles C Thomas, 1966.
Bell, W. E., and Lascari, A. D.: Rocky Mountain Spotted Fever. Neurological Symptoms in
    the Acute Phase, Neurology, *20*, 841, 1970.
Harrell, G. T.: Rickettsial Involvement of the Nervous System, Med. Clin. North Am., *37*,
    395, 1953.
Herman, E.: Neurological Syndromes in Typhus Fever, J. Nerv. Ment. Dis., *109*, 25, 1949.
Holmgren, B., et al.: Tick-borne Meningoencephalomyelitis in Sweden, Acta Med.
    Scand., *164*, 507, 1959.
McReynolds, E. W., and Roy, S., III,: An Epidemic of Tick-borne Typhus in Children, Am.
    J. Dis. Child., *126*, 779, 1973.
Miller, E. S., and Beeson, P. B.: Murine Typhus Fever, Medicine, *25*, 1, 1946.

Miller, J. Q., and Price, T. R.: The Nervous System in Rocky Mountain Spotted Fever, Neurology, *22*, 561, 1972.
Murray, E. S., et al.: Brill's Disease. I. Clinical and Laboratory Diagnosis, J.A.M.A., *142*, 1059, 1950.
Peters, A. H.: Tick Borne Typhus (Rocky Mountain Spotted Fever) Epidemiologic Trends, J.A.M.A., *216*, 1003, 1971.
Ripley, H. S.: Neuropsychiatric Observations on Tsutsugamushi Fever (Scrub Typhus), Arch. Neurol. Psychiat., *56*, 42, 1946.
Wolbach, S. B., Todd, J. L., and Palfrey, F. W.: *The Etiology and Pathology of Typhus, Being the Main Report of the Typhus Research Commission of the League of Red Cross Societies to Poland,* Cambridge, Harvard University Press, 1922. 222 pp.
Woodward, T. E.: Rickettsial Diseases in the United States, Med. Clin. North Am., *43*, 1507, 1959.

OTHER MICROORGANISMS

Cerebral Malaria

Involvement of the nervous system occurs in less than 2% of patients with malaria and is most common in infections with the malignant tertian form (Plasmodium falciparum, estivo-autumnal).

Pathology and Pathogenesis. The neurological symptoms are due to occlusion of capillaries with pigment-laden cells and parasites (Fig. 13), and the presence of multiple petechial hemorrhages. Areas of

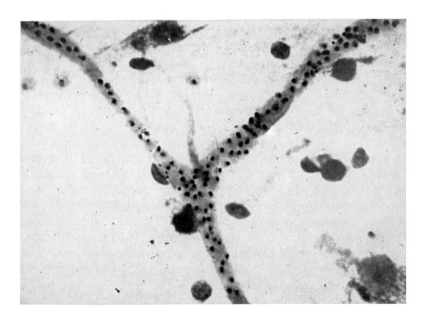

Figure 13.   Cerebral malaria. Cortical vessels congested with plasmodia.
(Courtesy Dr. Abner Wolf.)

softening as a result of thrombotic occlusion of vessels are rare and it is probable that the pathological changes in the nervous system are reversible.

Symptoms and Signs. The neurological symptoms usually appear in the second or third week of the illness but they may be the initial manifestation. The onset of cerebral symptoms has no relationship to the height of the fever. Headache, photophobia, vertigo, convulsions, delirium and coma are the most common symptoms. There may be stiffness of the neck, transient paralyses, aphasia, hemianopia or cerebellar ataxia. Myoclonus, chorea and intention tremors have been observed. Cranial nerve palsies and choked disc rarely occur. Psychic manifestations, delirium, disorientation, amnesia, negativeness or combativeness are present in a large percentage of the cases.

Laboratory Data. The laboratory findings include anemia and the presence in the red blood cells of great numbers of parasites, usually of the malignant tertian type. The cerebrospinal fluid may be under increased pressure. The fluid may be slightly xanthochromic and contain a small or moderate number of lymphocytes. The protein content may be moderately increased. The sugar content is normal. The serological tests for syphilis may be positive in the blood but are negative in the cerebrospinal fluid.

Diagnosis. The diagnosis of cerebral malaria is made from the appearance of cerebral symptoms and the findings of the organisms of P. falciparum in the blood. Delirium, convulsions or coma may occur as symptoms of general infection in patients with Plasmodium vivax in the absence of cerebral involvement. The symptoms in these cases are transient and respond readily to antimalarial therapy.

Prognosis. The mortality rate is approximately 30 to 40% in all cases of cerebral malaria. It is highest (80%) when there is a combination of coma and convulsions. There are few or no residuals in the patients who recover.

Treatment. Cerebral malaria is a true medical emergency. In critically ill patients, treatment includes chloraquine phosphate by intramuscular injection, pyrimethamine and sulfadiazine by nasogastric tube, and quinine sulfate intravenously. Diphenylhydantoin should be given to control seizures. Transfusions of whole blood or plasma may be required. Dexamethasone has been recommended to reduce cerebral edema. Sedation with paraldehyde may be necessary in excited or delirious patients. Daily lumbar punctures may be done to relieve increased intracranial pressure.

REFERENCES

Arieti, S.: Histopathologic Changes in Cerebral Malaria and Their Relation to Psychotic Sequels, Arch. Neurol. & Psychiat., 56, 79, 1946.

Boshes, B.: Neuropsychiatric Manifestions during the Course of Malaria; Experiences in the Mediterranean Theater in World War II, Arch. Neurol. & Psychiat., *58*, 14, 1947.
Daroff, R. B., et al.: Cerebral Malaria, J.A.M.A., *202*, 679, 1967.
Hill, G. J., II, Knight, V., Coatney, G. R., and Lawless, D. K.: Vivax Malaria Complicated by Aphasia and Hemiparesis, Arch. Intern. Med., *112*, 863, 1963.
Rigdon, R. H., and Fletcher, D. E.: Lesions in Brain Associated with Malaria; Pathologic Study on Man and on Experimental Animals, Arch. Neurol. & Psychiat., *53*, 191, 1945.
Simpson, W. M., and Sagebiel, J. L.: Symposium on First Year of Activities at U.S. Naval Base Hospital; Cerebral Malaria, U.S. Naval Med. Bull., *41*, 1596, 1943.

Trichinosis

Involvement of the central nervous system in patients with trichinosis, estimated to occur in 10 to 17% of the cases, may be manifested by confusion, delirium and focal neurological signs.

Pathology. The pathological changes in the nervous system include the presence of filiform larvae in the cerebral capillaries and in the parenchyma, perivascular inflammation, petechial hemorrhages and granulomatous nodules.

Symptoms and Signs. Neurological symptoms may develop any time within the first few weeks of the infection. There may be a severe encephalitis with confusion, coma, and evidence of focal damage to the cerebrum or cerebellum, with monoplegia, hemiplegia, quadriplegia, cerebellar ataxia or bulbar palsy. Edema of the optic nerve and meningeal signs may also occur. Loss of the reflexes, which may occur in the absence of other neurological symptoms, is probably due to the muscular involvement.

The most significant laboratory finding is a leukocytosis and eosinophilia in the blood. The cerebrospinal fluid may be normal or there may be a slight lymphocytic pleocytosis but occasionally a few eosinophils may be present. The parasites have been found in the cerebrospinal fluid of a few cases.

Diagnosis. The diagnosis is usually not difficult when neurologic symptoms appear in one or more of a group of individuals who have eaten infected pork and show the other manifestations of the disease (gastrointestinal symptoms, tenderness of the muscles and edema of the eyelids). Difficulty is encountered in the isolated cases where the infection results from the ingestion of meat preparations which supposedly contain no pork, or where the other manifestations of the infection are lacking. Trichinosis should be considered as an etiological factor in all patients with an encephalitis of obscure nature. Repeated examination of the blood for eosinophilia, biopsy of the muscles and the specific skin test and precipitin test for infection with trichina should establish the diagnosis.

Prognosis. Recovery within a few days or weeks is the rule except when there is profound coma or evidence of severe damage to the cerebrum. The disease has been reported to have a 10% mortality. Recovery is usually accompanied by complete or almost complete remission of the neurologic signs. Recurrent convulsive seizures have been reported as a late sequel of the cerebral infection.

Treatment. The treatment is symptomatic. The administration of corticosteroids and thiabendazole have been recommended.

REFERENCES

Barr, R.: Human Trichinosis. Report of Four Cases with Emphasis on Central Nervous System Involvement, Can. Med. J., 95, 912, 1966.
Dalessio, D., and Wolff, H. G.: Trichinella Spiralis Infection of the Central Nervous System, Arch. Neurol., 4, 407, 1961.
Gould, S. E.: *Trichinosis*, Springfield, Ill., Charles C Thomas, 1945, 356 pp.
Kramer, M. D., and Aita, J. F.: Trichinosis with CNS Involvement, Neurology, 22, 485, 1972.
Leitner, M. J., and Grynkewich, S. E.: Encephalopathy Associated with Trichinosis. Treatment with ACTH and Cortisone, Am. J. Med. Sci., 236, 546, 1958.
Merritt, H. H., and Rosenbaum, M.: Involvement of the Nervous System in Trichiniasis, J.A.M.A., 106, 1646, 1936.
Most, H., and Abeles, M. M.: Trichiniasis Involving the Nervous System; Clinical and Neuropathologic Review, Arch. Neurol. Psychiatry, 37, 589, 1937.

Schistosomiasis

Involvement of the nervous system by the ova of trematodes is rare. In the majority of the reported cases the lesions were associated with infection with S. japonicum, but isolated cases of S. haematobium and S. mansoni have also been recorded. The mechanism by which the ova are deposited in the nervous system is not understood. S. japonicum has a predilection for the cerebral hemispheres, while S. haematobium and S. mansoni more frequently affect the spinal cord.

Pathology. The presence of the ova in the nervous system causes an inflammatory exudate containing eosinophils and giant cells, necrosis of the parenchyma and deposition of calcium. The juxtaposition of numerous small lesions may result in formation of a large granulomatous tumor.

Incidence. Schistosomiasis is a disease occurring mainly in the Orient and in the tropics. World War II gave occasion to observe it in United States troops. The onset of symptoms may occur within a few months of exposure or it may be delayed for one to two years. Relapses may occur several or many years after the original infection. The central nervous system is involved in approximately 3 to 5% of the cases.

Symptomatology. Headaches, jacksonian or generalized convulsive seizures, hemiplegia and other focal neurological signs are common when the cerebrum is involved. Large lesions may cause an increase in the intracranial pressure with papilledema. The clinical picture in the cerebral cases may simulate meningitis, encephalitis or a tumor. Granulomatous masses in the spinal cord may produce signs and symptoms of an incomplete transverse lesion, with or without spinal subarachnoid block depending on the size of the lesion.

Laboratory Data. There is a leukocytosis with an increase in the eosinophils in the blood. The cerebrospinal fluid pressure may be increased with large intracerebral lesions, and partial or incomplete subarachnoid block may occur with spinal lesions. There may be a slight or moderate pleocytosis in the fluid (sometimes with eosinophils) and an increased protein content. Spinal cord lesions are demonstrated by myelography.

Diagnosis. The diagnosis is established from the history of gastrointestinal upset, eosinophilia in the blood and the presence of ova in the stools. Skin tests, complement fixation tests and biopsy of the rectal mucosa are also of value in the establishment of the diagnosis.

Treatment. Niridazole and antimony preparations are used as specific therapy. Oral steroids may also be of benefit. Anticonvulsive drugs should be given to control the seizures. Surgical excision of the large granulomatous lesions may be required.

REFERENCES

Bird, A. V.: Acute Spinal Schistosomiasis, Neurology, 14, 647, 1964.
Blankfein, R. J., and Chirico, A. M.: Cerebral Schistosomiasis, Neurology, 15, 957, 1965.
Budzilovich, G. N., Most, H., and Feigin, I.: Pathogenesis and Latency of Spinal Cord Schistosomiasis, Arch. Pathol., 77, 383, 1964.
Hammarsten, J. F.: Diagnosis of Cerebral Schistosomiasis, Arch. Neurol. Psychiat., 79, 132, 1958.
Kane, C. A., and Most, H.: Schistosomiasis of Central Nervous System: Experiences in World War II, Arch. Neurol. Psychiat., 59, 141, 1948.
Lechtenberg, R., and Vaida, G. A.: Schistosomiasis of the Spinal Cord, Neurology, 27, 55, 1977.
Marcial-Rojas, R. A., and Fiol, R. E.: Neurologic Complications of Schistosomiasis, Ann. Intern. Med., 59, 215, 1963.
Tillman, A. J. B.: Schistosomiasis Japonica with Cerebral Manifestations, Arch. Intern. Med., 79, 36, 1947.
Watson, C. W., Murphey, F., and Little, S. C.: Schistosomiasis of the Brain Due to Schistosoma Japonicum, Arch. Neurol. Psychiat., 57, 199, 1947.

Echinococcus (Hydatid Cysts)

Echinococcus granulosus is a helminth parasite of the dog family. There is an intermediate phase of development with hydatid cyst formation in other mammals. Sheep and cattle are usually the intermediate hosts, but man may be affected. The disease is most common in sheep-raising countries and is quite rare in the United States.

The cysts are most commonly found in the liver and the lungs. If the embryos pass the pulmonary barrier, cyst formation may occur in any organ. The brain is involved in about 2% of the cases and neurological symptoms may develop in patients with cysts in the skull or spine.

Cerebral cysts are usually single. They are most common in the cerebral hemispheres but may develop in the ventricles or cerebellum. The infestation may occur at any age but is most common in children from rural areas.

The signs and symptoms which develop with cysts in the brain are similar to those of tumor in the affected region. The diagnosis of hydatid cyst as the cause of cerebral symptoms is rarely made before operation. Computerized tomography scanning and angiography rather than ventriculography should be used in localizing the lesions, because of the danger of puncturing the cyst.

Treatment is surgical removal *in toto* without puncturing the cyst.

REFERENCES

Anderson, M., Bickerstaff, E. R., and Hamilton, J. C.: Cerebral Hydatid Cysts in Britain, J. Neurol. Neurosurg. Psychiatry, *38*, 1104, 1975.
Araná-Iniguez, R., and San Julián, J.: Hydatid Cysts of the Brain, J. Neurosurg., *12*, 323, 1955.
Ayres, C. M., Davey, L. M., and German, W. J.: Cerebral Hydatidosis, J. Neurosurg., *20*, 371, 1963.
Malloch, J. D.: Hydatid Disease of the Spine, Br. Med. J., *1*, 633, 1965.

Cysticercosis

Cysticercosis is the result of encystment of the larvae of Taenia solium or Taenia saginata in the tissues. In the human, Taenia solium is by far the most common.

In the 450 cases followed by Dixon and Lipscomb, clinical evidence of involvement of the nervous system was found in more than 70% of the cases. In the 47 cases which came to autopsy, cysticerci were found in the nervous system as follow: cerebrum 44, cerebellum 8, spinal cord 2, and meninges 22. The cysts in the nervous system are usually multiple and of small size.

Cysticercus of the brain is extremely rare in the United States. None was encountered in Cushing's series of over 2000 intracranial tumors. They are common in the Middle East, India and South America. Arana and Asenjo found 25 cases of brain cysticercosis in 202 intracranial tumors at the Central Neurological Institute in Santiago in a period of three and one half years. Cysticerci in the meninges or cerebrum usually become encapsulated but those in the ventricular cavity do not.

Symptoms usually develop within four years of the infestation, with ranges varying from a few months to many years. Convulsive seizures occur in over 90% of the cases. Symptoms of increased intracranial pressure, mental disturbances and focal neurological signs are present in a small percentage of the cases.

The diagnosis should be suspected whenever convulsive seizures or other signs of intracranial lesions develop in an individual who has resided in a region where the disease is endemic. Eosinophilia may or may not be present in the blood. A pleocytosis varying from a few cells to a thousand or more develops in the cerebrospinal fluid when the meninges are involved. Eosinophils have been found in the fluids of some of the cases.

Calcified nodules are seen in the roentgenograms of the muscles in a high percentage of the cases and to a lesser extent in the intracranial cavity. The diagnosis can be established by biopsy of subcuticular nodules, which can be found by careful examination in most of the cases. Immunological tests have been developed but their reliability is questionable. The prognosis is less serious than is commonly considered. Death occurs in about 10% of the cases as result of status epilepticus, increased intracranial pressure or meningitis. In the cases that survive disability is mainly related to the severity of the convulsive disorder.

Niclosamide, paromycin, dichlorophen, or quinacrine can be used to clear the intestinal tract of the parasites, but will probably have no effect on the encysted larvae. Anticonvulsive drugs should be given to control the seizures. When the cysts are multiple or when they occur in the meninges or as a grape-like cluster in the fourth ventricle, surgical removal is not possible. Single cysts in the cerebral hemispheres have been removed with complete relief of symptoms.

REFERENCES

Arseni, C., and Cristescu, A.: Epilepsy Due to Cerebral Cysticercosis, Epilepsia, 13, 253, 1972.
Bickerstaff, E. R., et al.: The Racemose Form of Cerebral Cysticercosis, Brain, 75, 1, 1952.
Dixon, H. B. F., and Lipscomb, F. M.: Cysticercosis: An Analysis and Follow-up of 450 Cases, Medical Research Council Special Report Series No. 299, London, Her Majesty's Stationery Office, 1961.
Hesketh, K. T.: Cysticercosis of the Dorsal Cord, J. Neurol. Neurosurg. Psychiatry, 38, 445, 1965.
Nieto, D.: Cysticercosis of the Nervous System. Diagnosis by Means of the Spinal Fluid Complement Fixation Test, Neurology, 6, 725, 1956.
Obrador, S.: Clinical Aspects of Cerebral Cysticercosis, Arch. Neurol. and Psychiat., 59, 457, 1948.
Stepien, L., and Chórobski, J.: Cysticercosis Cerebri and Its Operative Treatment, Arch. Neurol. and Psychiat., 61, 499, 1949.

Eosinophilic Meningitis

Recent reports in the literature indicate that the nervous system of man may be invaded by the metastrongylid lungworm of rats, Angiostronglyus cantonesis, which uses a molluscan intermediate host and invades the domestic rat and other rodents in the course of its life cycle. Infection in man in usually due to the ingestion of shrimp, crabs and fish which serve as transport hosts. Cases have been reported from Hawaii, Thailand and Southeast Asia.

Involvement of the nervous system in man is characterized by an acute meningeal reaction. In addition to the meningeal reaction there may be an encephalitis or encephalomyelitis. The infection is most common in children. The lesions in the nervous system are due to destruction of tissue by the parasite and to necrosis and aneurysmal dilatation of cerebral vessels resulting in small or large hemorrhages. The disease commonly takes the form of an acute meningitis with a moderate or severe degree of pleocytosis in the cerebrospinal fluid with 10 to 50% eosinophils in the fluid. In the severe cases, death may be the result of small or large hemorrhagic lesions in the brain or spinal cord.

REFERENCES

Char, D. F. B., and Rosen, L.: Eosinophilic Meningitis Among Children in Hawaii, J. Ped., 70, 28, 1967.
Nye, S. W., et al.: Lesions of the Brain in Eosinophilic Meningitis, Arch. Path., 89, 9, 1970.
Panyagupta, S.: Eosinophilic Meningoencephalitis in Thailand, Am. J. Trop. Med., 14, 370, 1965.

Toxoplasmosis

Toxoplasmosis is the term used to describe infection in the human by the protozoan organism, Toxoplasma gondii. The infection, which has a predilection for the central nervous system and the eye, develops most commonly *in utero*, producing encephalitis and chorioretinitis.

Etiology and Pathology. The toxoplasma are minute, about 2 by 3 micra, oval, pyriform, rounded or elongated protoplasmic masses, with a central nucleus. They occur singly or in clusters in the host cells and multiply by binary fission. The organisms invade the walls of blood vessels in the nervous system and produce an inflammatory reaction. Miliary granulomas are formed. They may become calcified or undergo necrosis. The granulomatous lesions are scattered throughout the central nervous system and may be found in the meninges and ependyma. Hydrocephalus may develop from occlusion of the aqueduct of Sylvius by the resulting ependymitis. The microorganisms are present in the epithelioid cells of the granulomas (Fig. 14); they may also be found in the endothelial cells of blood vessels and in the nerve cells. Lesions in the retina are common, and occasionally they are also present in the lungs, kidneys, liver, spleen or skin.

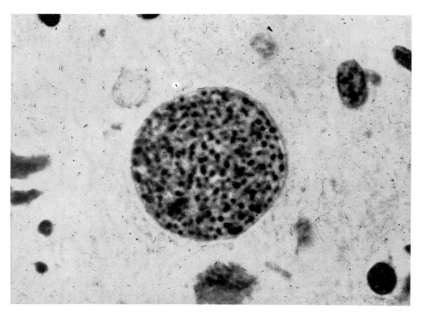

Figure 14.   Toxoplasma parasites within epithelioid cell.
(Courtesy Dr. Abner Wolf.)

Incidence. Toxoplasmosis is a rare disease and did not receive much attention until the studies of Wolf and Cowen and of Sabin. The infection occurs most commonly *in utero* but it may develop in early childhood or adult life.

Symptomatology. In the congenital form the symptoms are evident in the first few days of life. The common manifestations are inanition, convulsions, spasticity of the extremities, opisthotonos, chorioretinitis, microphthalmus or other congenital defects in development of the eye. Optic atrophy is common and there may be an internal hydrocephalus. Symptoms in the infantile form are similar to those of the congenital form but may not make their appearance until the third to fifth years of life. There may be enlargement of the liver and spleen with elevation of the icteric index. The presence of calcified nodules in the nervous system can be demonstrated by roentgenograms of the skull. Cerebral calcifications are not found in postnatally acquired infections.

In the acquired form of the disease, which may occur in children and in adults, the skin, lung and lymph glands are the common sites of involvement, but the eyes and the nervous system may also be involved. Acquired toxoplasmosis generally develops in immunosuppressed patients or patients with severe debilitating diseases. It may resemble infectious mononucleosis or cytomegalovirus disease. Acute meningitis, acute and chronic encephalitis, granuloma formation in the parenchyma of the nervous system, and myositis have been reported as features of the disease in the acquired form.

Laboratory Data. There may be a moderate or severe anemia and a mild leukocytosis or leukopenia. The cerebrospinal fluid may be under increased pressure. The protein content of the fluid is generally increased and there is an inconstant pleocytosis. Cell counts as high as several thousand, mostly lymphocytes, have been recorded.

Diagnosis. The diagnosis is made from the combination of the symptoms of encephalitis, lesions in the eye (chorioretinitis, optic atrophy and microphthalmus), and evidence of calcification in the brain. Toxoplasma can be demonstrated in cerebrospinal fluid sediment with Wright's or Giemsa's stain. The organism can be cultivated from spinal fluid sediment in laboratory mice. Serum antibodies can be demonstrated by dye, immunofluorescence, complement fixation, agglutination and indirect hemagglutination tests. Demonstration of IgM antibodies by immunofluorescence is particularly helpful.

Course and Prognosis. The prognosis is poor in the congenital form, over half of the cases dying a few weeks after birth. Mental and neurological defects are present in the cases that survive. The mortality rate is also high in the infantile form of encephalitis.

Treatment. The sulfonamides (sulfamethazine, sulfapyrazine and sulfadiazine) in combination with daraprim are reported to be effective in the treatment of both the congenital and the acquired forms.

REFERENCES

Beckett, R. S., and Flynn, F. J., Jr.: Toxoplasmosis, N. Engl. J. Med., 249, 345, 1953.
Budzilovich, G. N.: Acquired Toxoplasmosis, Am. J. Clin. Pathol., 35, 66, 1961.
Cowen, D., Wolf, A., and Paige, B. H.: Toxoplasmic Encephalomyelitis, Arch, Neurol. Psychiat., 48, 689, 1942.
Feldman, H. A.: Human Toxoplasmosis, J. Chronic Dis., 10, 488, 1959.
Feldman, H. A.: Toxoplasmosis: An Overview, Bull. N.Y. Acad. Med., 50, 110, 1974.
Ghatak, N. R., Poon, T. P., and Zimmerman, H. M.: Toxoplasmosis of the Central Nervous System in Adults, Arch. Pathol., 89, 337, 1970.
Koch, F. L. P., et al.: Toxoplasmic Encephalomyelitis, Arch. Ophthalmol., 29, 1, 1943.
Remington, J. S., Jacobs, L., and Kaufman, H. E.: Toxoplasmosis in the Adult, N. Engl. J. Med., 262, 180, 1960.
Rowland, L. P., and Greer, M.: Toxoplasmic Polymyositis, Neurology, 11, 367, 1961.
Sabin, A. B.: Toxoplasmic Encephalitis in Children, J.A.M.A., 116, 801, 1941.
Siim, J. G.: Human Toxoplasmosis, Baltimore, Williams & Wilkins, 1960, 211 pp.
Theologides, A., and Kennedy, B. J.: Clinical Manifestations of Toxoplasmosis in the Adult, Arch. Intern. Med., 117, 536, 1966.
Townsend, J. J., et al.: Acquired Toxoplasmosis, Arch, Neurol., 32, 335, 1975.
Wolf, A., Cowen, D., and Paige, B. H.: Toxoplasmic Encephalomyelitis. III. New Case of Granulomatous Encephalomyelitis Due to a Protozoon, Am. J. Pathol., 15, 657, 1939.

Trypanosomiasis (Sleeping Sickness)

Two distinct varieties of infection with trypanosomes are recognized, the African form which is due to infection with T. gambiense or T. rhodesiense and the South American form (Chagas disease) which is endemic in South America and is due to infection by T. cruzi.

Etiology and Pathology. In the African form of the disease the organisms retain their trypanosome form and multiply by longitudinal fission. They are transmitted from man to man by the tsetse fly, occasionally by other flies or insects, and by mechanical contact. The pathological changes in the central nervous system are those of a chronic meningoencephalitis.

The organisms of South American trypanosomiasis (Chagas disease) when found in the blood have an ordinary trypanoform structure. They do not, however, reproduce in the blood but invade tissues and are transformed into typical leishmania parasites. These may later assume the trypanosome form and re-enter the blood stream. The infection is transmitted from an animal host (rodents, cats, opossum, armadillo, etc.) to man by a blood-sucking insect known as Lamus magistus. The pathological lesions in the nervous system consist of miliary granulomata composed of proliferated microglial cells. The organisms are present in glial and nerve cells. The lesions are diffusely scattered throughout the nervous system and are accompanied by a patchy reaction in the meninges and parenchyma.

Symptomatology. The disease in African sleeping sickness passes through two indistinct stages, febrile and lethargic. The incubation period is quite variable. In some cases symptoms may have their onset within two weeks of the infection. In others it may be delayed for months or years. The first stage of the disease is characterized by a remitting fever, chronic adenitis, exanthemata and asthenia. During this period, which may last for several months or years, the organisms are present in the blood. The first stage passes imperceptibly into the second, in which there is an exaggeration of the previous symptoms and evidence of involvement of the nervous system in the form of tremors, incoordination, convulsions, paralyses, mental disturbances, apathy, and somnolence. There are progressive weakness and loss of weight. If untreated, death usually ensues within a year after the appearance of cerebral symptoms.

In South American trypanosomiasis the acute stage generally lasts about one month and is characterized, especially in children, by fever, swelling of the thyroid with myxedema, and enlargement of the lymph nodes, liver and spleen. During this stage trypanosomes are present in the blood and the leishmaniform bodies in the tissue. The secondary stage is characterized by evidence of involvement of the viscera, particularly the thyroid, heart, adrenal and the central nervous system. Various neurological signs have been described, including hemiplegia, diplegia, aphasia and choreo-athetosis. Intelligence is almost always affected, due in part to the cerebral lesion as well as to the thyroid deficiency. Cranial nerve palsies and convulsions may occur. The disease is slowly progressive with occasional acute exacerbations associated with fever. Death usually ensues within a few months or years.

Laboratory Data. Some degree of anemia is common in all forms of trypanosomiasis. There is a lymphocytic pleocytosis in the cerebrospinal fluid, an increased protein content and various changes are seen in the colloidal gold reactions.

Diagnosis. The diagnosis depends upon the development of characteristic symptoms in residents of regions in which various forms of the disease are endemic. The diagnosis is established by the demonstration of the organisms in the blood or cerebrospinal fluid, in material obtained from puncture of an enlarged node, or by the inoculation of these substances into susceptible animals (mice, guinea pigs, rabbits and monkeys). Serologic tests are also available.

Treatment. Melarsoprol, an organic arsenical, is of value in the treatment of central nervous system involvement by T. gambiense and T. rhodesiense infections of the nervous system. No drug treatment is established as safe and effective in chronic Chagas disease. Bayer 2502 (Lampit) is usually effective, however, in the acute stage of infection.

REFERENCES

Hunter, G. W., et al.: *A Manual of Tropical Medicine*, 3rd Ed., Philadelphia, W. B. Saunders Co., 1960, 892 pp.
Lumsden, W. H. R.: Trypanosomiasis, Br. Med. Bull., *28*, 34, 1972.
Manson-Bahr, P. H.: *Manson's Tropical Diseases. A Manual of the Diseases of Warm Climates*, 16th ed., Baltimore, Williams & Wilkins, 1966. 2000 pp.
Mulligan, H. W. (ed.).: *The African Trypanosomiasis*, London: Allen & Irwin, 1970.
Pearce, L.: *The Treatment of Human Trypanosomiasis with Tryparsamide*, New York, The Rockefeller Institute for Medical Research, 1930. 339 pp. (Monographs of the Rockefeller Institute for Medical Research, No. 23.)
Spencer, H. C., Jr., et al.: Imported African Trypanosomiasis in the United States, Ann. Intern. Med., *82*, 633, 1975.

Primary Amebic Meningoencephalitis

It has been known for many years that amoebae may invade the nervous system and produce circumscribed abscess. In recent years, however, there have been numerous reports of the finding of free-living (Naegleria) amoebae in the cerebrospinal fluid in patients with an acute meningitis or meningoencephalitis.

Cases have been reported from the United States, Europe and other parts of the world.

The infection usually occurs in children or young adults who have been swimming in fresh or brackish waters. The onset of symptoms of meningitis or meningoencephalitis is acute. The cerebrospinal fluid is under increased pressure with a moderate or severe degree of pleocytosis in the fluid, an increased protein content, and a decrease in the glucose content. Red blood cells may also be present. Trophozoites may be recognized in a wet preparation of uncentrifuged spinal fluid. No organisms are demonstrated on Gram stain or routine culture. The organism can be cultured on ordinary culture media which has been seeded with coliform bacteria. The disease is rapidly fatal, but recovery has been reported. Amphotericin B has been used as treatment.

REFERENCES

Apley, J., et al.: Primary Amebic Meningoencephalomyelitis in Britain, Br. Med. J., 7, 596, 1970.
Butt, C. C.: Primary Amebic Meningoencephalitis, N. Engl. J. Med., 274, 1473, 1966.
Carter, R. F.: Primary Amoebic Meningoencephalitis: An Appraisal of Present Knowledge, Trans. R. Soc. Trop. Med. Hyg., 66, 193, 1972.
Duma, R. J., et al.: Primary Amebic Meningoencephalitis, N. Engl. J. Med., 281, 1315, 1969.
Neto, J. G. dos Santos: Fatal Primary Amebic Meningoencephalitis, Am. J. Clin. Pathol., 54, 737, 1970.

Leprosy

Leprosy, Hansen's disease, is a chronic disease due to infection by the Mycobacterium leprae which has a predilection for the skin and the peripheral nerves. Two major clinical types are recognized: lepromatous and tuberculoid.

Etiology. Mycobacterium leprae, an acid-fast, rod-shaped organism morphologically similar to the tubercle bacillus, is generally accepted as the direct cause of the disease, although it has not fulfilled Koch's postulates. The organism can be demonstrated in the cutaneous lesion and is sometimes present in the blood stream.

The disease is transmitted by direct contact which must be intimate and prolonged because the contagiousness is low. The portal of entry is probably through abrasions in the skin or mucous membranes. The incubation period is long, averaging three to four years in children and much longer in adults.

Pathology. The affected nerve trunks are diffusely thickened or are studded with nodular swellings. There is an overgrowth of connective tissue with degeneration of the axon and myelin sheath. Bacilli are present in the perineurium and endoneural septa. They have been found in the dorsal root ganglia, the spinal cord and brain but they do not produce any significant lesions within the central nervous system. Degenerative changes in the posterior funiculi of the cord, which are found in some cases, can be attributed to the peripheral neuritis.

Incidence. Leprosy is most common in tropical and subtropical climates, and it is estimated that 10 to 20 million people are infected with the disease. The disease is prevalent in South and Central America, China, India and Africa. It is uncommon in Europe or North America. In the United States the disease is mostly confined to Louisiana, Texas, Florida and Southern California.

Children are especially liable to the disease but it may occur in adults. In childhood, the disease is evenly distributed between the two sexes, but in adult life males are more frequently affected.

Symptoms and Signs. In the majority of cases there is a mixture of cutaneous and nervous lesions. The earliest manifestation of neural leprosy is an erythematous macule, the lepride. This lesion grows by peripheral extension to form an annular macule. The macule has an atrophic, depigmented center which is partially or completely anesthetic. These lesions may attain an enormous size and cover the major portion of one extremity or the torso. Infection of the nerve may result in the formation of nodules or fusiform swelling along its course. Although any of the peripheral nerves may be affected, the disease has a predilection for the ulnar, great auricular, anterior tibial, external popliteal nerves, and the fifth and seventh cranial nerves. Repeated attacks of neuralgic pains often precede the onset of motor weakness or sensory loss.

Cranial Nerves. Involvement of the fifth nerve is manifested by the appearance of patches of anesthesia on the face. Involvement of the entire sensory distribution of the nerve or its motor division is rare. Keratitis and ulceration may ensue as result of injury to the anesthetic cornea. Complete paralysis of the facial nerve is rare but weakness of a portion of one or several muscles is common. The muscles of the upper half of the face are most severely affected. Partial paralysis of the orbicularis and other facial muscles may result in lagophthalmos, ectropion and facial asymmetry. Involvement of the oculomotor or other cranial nerves is rare.

Motor System. Weakness and atrophy develop in the muscles innervated by the affected nerves. In the extremities there is wasting of the small muscles of the hands and feet, with later extension to the forearm and leg, but the proximal muscles are usually spared. Clawing of the hands or feet is common but wrist-drop and foot-drop are late manifestations. Fibrillary twitchings may occur and contractures may develop.

Sensory System. Cutaneous sensation is impaired or lost in the distribution of the affected nerves in a somewhat irregular fashion. Various types of dissociated sensory impairment are seen. The sensory impairment may be of a nerve or root distribution but more commonly it is of a glove-and-stocking type. Deep sensation, pressure pain, the appreciation of vibration and position sense are usually spared or are less severely affected than superficial cutaneous sensation.

Reflexes. Tendon reflexes may be preserved but they are usually reduced or lost with progress of the disease. The abdominal skin reflexes and plantar responses are normal.

Other Signs. Vasomotor and trophic disturbances are almost always present. Anhydrosis and cyanosis of the hands and feet are common. Trophic ulcers develop on the knuckles and on the plantar surface of the feet. There may be various arthropathies as well as resorption of the bones of the fingers, starting in the terminal phalanges and progressing upward. The skin shrinks as digits become shorter and finally the nail may be attached to a small stump.

Laboratory Data. There are no significant changes in the blood or urine, except for the occurence of a positive Wassermann, Kahn or similar tests in the blood in a large percentage of cases. There have been few reports on the examination of the cerebrospinal fluid. The only abnormality reported was a slight increase in the protein content. Hansen's bacillus can be found in the scrapings from the cutaneous lesions and in nerve biopsy specimens.

Diagnosis. The diagnosis of leprosy is made without difficulty from the characteristic skin and neuritic lesions. The clinical picture may occasionally have a superficial similarity to that of syringomyelia, hypertrophic interstitial neuritis or von Recklinghausen's disease. The correct diagnosis is usually not difficult if the possibility of leprosy is kept in mind and scrapings from the lesions are examined for acid-fast bacilli.

Course and Prognosis. The prognosis in the neural form of the disease is less grave than in the cutaneous form, where death within ten to twenty years is the rule. Neural leprosy is not necessarily fatal. The progress of the neuritis is slow and the disease may come to a spontaneous arrest or be controlled by therapy. Incapacitation may result from the paralyses and disfigurements.

Treatment. No specific therapy for leprosy has been discovered. Drugs of the sulfone class such as dapsone (4,4-diamino-di-phenylsulphone) are recommended for their bacteriostatic effect. Patients with sulfone-resistant bacilli are best treated with rifampin, clofazimine or diphenylthiourea.

REFERENCES

Browne, S. A.: Some Less Common Neurological Findings in Leprosy, J. Neurol. Sci., 2, 253, 1965.

Canizares, O.: Diagnosis and Treatment of Leprosy in the United States, Med. Clin. North Am., 49, 801, 1965.

Cochrane, R. G., and Davey, T. F.: Leprosy in Theory and Practice. 2nd Ed. Baltimore, Williams & Wilkins, 1964, 680 pp.
Crawford, C. L.: Neurological Lesions in Leprosy, Leprosy Rev., 39, 9, 1968.
Jamison, D. G.: Modern Trends in Leprosy, Postgrad. Med. J., 45, 408, 1969.
Monrad-Krohn, G. H.: The Neurological Aspect of Leprosy, Chicago, Chicago Medical Book Co., 1923, 79 pp.
Trautman, J. R.: The Management of Leprosy and its Complications, N. Engl. J. Med., 273, 756, 1965.

ACUTE (SYDENHAM'S) CHOREA

Sydenham's chorea (acute chorea, St. Vitus' dance, chorea minor, rheumatic chorea) is a disease of childhood characterized by the occurrence of rapid, irregular, aimless, involuntary movements of the muscles of the extremities, face and trunk. The etiology of the disease is unknown, but it is now generally considered to be a manifestation of rheumatic fever. The course of the disease is self-limited and fatalities are rare except as result of cardiac complications.

Etiology and Pathology. Numerous reports have implicated a streptococcus or diplococcus as the causative organism of acute chorea, but these claims have not received general credence. The close relationship of chorea to rheumatic fever is shown by the fact that approximately three fourths of the cases evidence at some time in their life, either prior to, coincidental with, or following the attack of chorea, other manifestations of the disease in the form of arthritis, myocarditis, endocarditis or pericarditis. Patients with rheumatic chorea have been found to have antibodies which react with subthalamic and caudate nuclei neurons in immunofluorescence assays. Such antibodies also appear to react with antigens shared by Group A streptococcal membranes.

Since uncomplicated acute chorea is rarely fatal, the pathological changes in the nervous system have not been clearly elucidated. Many of the changes which have been reported in fatal cases can be attributed to embolic phenomena and terminal changes. Degenerative changes in the nerve cells of the cortex, basal ganglia and cerebellum, ameboid changes in the glial and proliferative changes in the meningeal and cortical vessels have been reported. A mild degree of inflammatory reaction has been found in a few cases.

Incidence. Acute chorea is almost exclusively a disease of childhood, with over 80% of the cases occurring between the ages of five and fifteen years. Onset before the age of five is rare and the occurrence of the first attack after the age of fifteen is uncommon, except during pregnancy in the late teens and early twenties. All races are affected, although it is said to be uncommon in the Negro. Females are affected over twice as frequently as males. The disease occurs at all times of the year but is less common in summer.

Symptoms and Signs. The characteristic features are involuntary movements, incoordination, muscular weakness and psychic manifestations. The symptoms may be of gradual onset or they may appear suddenly after an emotional upset. The adverse influence of all external stimuli on the symptoms makes it probable that the emotional upset only serves to call attention to preexisting symptoms of a milder degree.

The severity of the symptoms is subject to a great deal of variation. In mild cases, there may be only a general restlessness, facial grimacing and a slight degree of incoordination in the performance of willed movements. In severe cases, the range and extent of the involuntary movements may be so great as to incapacitate the child.

The involuntary movements are quick and are similar to normal willed movements, but they are not performed for any useful purpose. Jerking movements of the upper extremity and flinging movements of the legs may interfere with normal use of the arms and make walking difficult or impossible. Involuntary movements of the facial muscles, tongue and palate produce a dysarthria, which may be so severe that the child ceases to try to talk and is mute. Involuntary movements of the abdominal and trunk muscles may alter the respiratory rate. The involuntary movements are generalized but as a rule they are more severe in the upper extremities than in the lower extremities or the face. In about a third of the cases the movements are greater on one side of the body and, rarely, they may appear to be entirely confined to that side (hemichorea). The severity of the involuntary movements is greatly influenced by emotional factors and external stimuli. The child may lie quietly in bed when undisturbed, but the movements may become quite severe when emotionally excited or subjected to a prolonged examination. The involuntary movements disappear entirely when the patient is asleep and they can be reduced in the waking state by the administration of sedative drugs.

There is weakness of voluntary movements and there is an inability to maintain any sustained effort. The occurrence of involuntary movements in antagonist muscles during the attempt to make voluntary movements produces an incoordination, with the dropping or throwing of objects held in the hand or an awkward stumbling gait. The inability to sustain contractions of the muscles can be demonstrated by a waxing and waning of the force of the pressure when the child grips the hand of the examiner. Rarely the weakness may be so great that one or more limbs appear to be paralyzed (paralytic chorea). There are no muscular atrophies, contractures or fixation in abnormal postures. The appearance of the hands when the arms are held extended in front of the body is, however, quite characteristic. The wrist is sharply flexed and the fingers hyperextended at the proximal and terminal phalanges.

This posture of the hand (Warner's hand) can be imitated only with difficulty by a normal person. Pronation of the forearm when the arms are extended (pronator sign) is also commonly seen. Voluntary movements are often performed rapidly in order to prevent their interruption by involuntary movements. On command, the tongue is protruded quickly and rapidly withdrawn to prevent biting of the tongue by involuntary movements of the jaw muscles.

The cranial nerves are unaffected except for the involuntary movements of the facial, jaw, tongue and palatal muscles. There are no sensory changes. The tendon reflexes may be increased, decreased or temporarily absent. Occasionally, the knee jerks are pendular in character, but more commonly the contraction of the quadriceps muscle on tapping the patellar tendon is maintained for a short interval causing the leg to remain extended ("caught-up" or "hung-up" reflex). The plantar response is usually flexor in type, but occasionally an extensor plantar response is obtained.

Mental changes of a mild or severe degree are frequently present. The child is fretful, irritable or emotionally unstable. Apathy is not uncommon. The involuntary movements may prevent sleep and sleep may be interrupted by nightmares or unpleasant dreams. In severe cases there may be mental confusion, agitation, hallucinations and delusions (chorea insaniens).

Chorea may recur or develop for the first time in young women during pregnancy (chorea gravidarum). The disease is apt to be more severe during pregnancy and mental symptoms are common.

Laboratory Data. The temperature and pulse are normal unless complications develop. The results of the examination of urine and blood including the erythrocyte sedimentation rate and C-reactive protein are often normal. Eosinophilia has been reported and a mild or moderate degree of anemia is not infrequent. The cerebrospinal fluid is usually normal, but a slight pleocytosis has been reported in a few cases. Nonspecific changes may be found in the electroencephalogram. Decrease in the percentage time of the alpha rhythm and the presence of continuous slow wave activity of increased amplitude have been reported.

Complications. Other manifestations of the rheumatic infection may occur during the course of the chorea or may precede or follow it. It is estimated that cardiac complications, usually an endocarditis, occur in approximately 20% of the cases. Myocarditis and pericarditis are less common. Vegetative endocarditis with embolic phenomena may occur, but is quite rare. A previous history of rheumatic polyarthritis is common, but involvement of the joints during the course of the chorea is rare. Other infrequent complications include subcutaneous rheumatic nodules, erythema nodosum and purpura.

Diagnosis. The diagnosis is made without difficulty from the appearance of the characteristic choreiform movements in a child. Tics and habit-spasms may offer some difficulty, but these movements are stereotyped and localized always to the same muscle or groups of muscles.

Some difficulty in diagnosis may be encountered in the case with apparent paralysis of the extremities, but the previous existence or the subsequent development of choreic movements should clarify the diagnosis.

Chorea insaniens may be confused with a manic psychosis, but the character of the involuntary movements should serve to distinguish between these two conditions.

The age of onset, clinical course and the character of the involuntary movements readily differentiate acute chorea from other diseases of the basal ganglia.

Course and Prognosis. Acute chorea is a relatively benign disease with complete recovery as the rule in uncomplicated cases. The mortality rate of approximately 2% is chiefly due to the associated cardiac complications. Death may result from exhaustion from violent movements. The duration of the symptoms is quite variable. In the average case they persist for three to six weeks. Occasionally, the course may be prolonged over several months, and it is not unusual for involuntary movements of a mild degree to persist for many months after recrudescence of the more severe movements. Recurrences after months or several years are reported in approximately one third of the cases.

Treatment. There is no specific treatment for the disease. Symptomatic therapy may be of great value in the control of the movements. In the mild form, bed rest during the period of active movements is sufficient. The room should be quiet and all external stimuli reduced to a minimum. When the severity of the movements interferes with proper rest, sedatives in the form of barbiturates, chloral hydrate or paraldehyde may be needed. Phenothiazines and haloperidol are of value in reducing the severity of the movements. There is no good evidence to show that the termination of pregnancy exerts any influence on the course of chorea of pregnancy.

The prophylactic administration of penicillin is recommended in order to prevent the development of other manifestations of rheumatic fever.

REFERENCES

Aron, A. M., Freeman, J. M., and Carter, S.: The Natural History of Sydenham's Chorea, Am. J. Med., *38*, 83, 1965.
Bird, M. T., Palkes, H., and Prensky, A. L.: A Follow-up Study of Sydenham's Chorea, Neurology, *26*, 601, 1976.

Greenfield, J. G., and Wolfsohn, J. M.: The Pathology of Sydenham's Chorea, Lancet, 2, 603, 1922.
Husby, G., et al.: Antibodies Reacting with Cytoplasm of Subthalamic and Caudate Nuclei Neurons in Chorea and Acute Rheumatic Fever, J. Exp. Med., 144, 1094, 1976.
Jones, T. D., and Bland, E. F.: Clinical Significance of Chorea as Manifestation of Rheumatic Fever, J.A.M.A., 105, 571, 1935.
Willson, P., and Preece, A. A.: Chorea Gravidarum, Arch. Intern. Med., 49, 471, 671, 1932.
Ziegler, L. H.: The Neuropathological Findings in a Case of Acute Sydenham's Chorea, J. Nerv. Men. Dis., 65, 273, 1927.

Syphilis

In view of the rarity of neurosyphilis at the present time and the unlikelihood of its return, the discussion of this entity is curtailed. It is thought wise, however, to review briefly this devastating disease which at one time accounted for 10% of all patients admitted to mental hospitals, with an always fatal disease—dementia paralytica, and was responsible for an even higher percentage of patients admitted to the neurological wards of general hospitals with tabes dorsalis and other crippling forms of neurosyphilis.

Historical Review. The fact that syphilis could affect the nervous system was first recognized in the latter part of the past century. The first description of dementia paralytica was by Bayle in 1882, and tabes dorsalis was described by Erb in 1892. With the discovery of the technique of lumbar puncture by Quincke in 1891, it was possible to demonstrate invasion of the nervous system by the virus of syphilis in the early stages of the disease many years before symptoms became evident but the spirochete was not isolated from the brain by Noguchi and Moore until 1913, and no effective treatment was available until malarial fever was introduced by Wagner von Juaregg in 1918. This treatment was widely used in the fourth and fifth decades of this century. Since then penicillin and other spirocheticidal drugs have been found to be safer and more effective therapy and neurosyphilis has almost entirely been eliminated.

Epidemiology. The development of neurosyphilis in an individual infected with syphilis is related to a number of known factors including race, sex, and the occurrence of acute febrile illness after the primary infection.

Serious (parenchymatous) neurosyphilis is more common in men than in women, and it is much more common in the whites than in the blacks. The lower incidence in the female is related in part to pregnancy, since parenchymatous neurosyphilis is uncommon in women who had a number of pregnancies after being infected.

The fact that a history of the occurrence of an acute febrile illness in the years after contraction of syphilis was rare in patients who developed dementia paralytica led Wagner von Juaregg to the conclusion that febrile illness may play a role in the prevention of dementia paralytica and thus gave him the idea of fever therapy, the first effective treatment for neurosyphilis.

But the most important factor in the prevention of neurosyphilis before the introduction of fever therapy and penicillin was the type of treatment given in the period just after the primary infection. A significant reduction in the incidence of dementia paralytica and tabes dorsalis could be obtained by the long continued administration of the arsphenamines in the primary, secondary and asymptomatic stages of

Table 11.   Classification of Neurosyphilis
(After Merritt, Adams and Solomon, *Neurosyphilis*, Oxford University Press, 1946)

Type	Clinical Symptoms	Pathology
I. Asymptomatic	No symptoms. Cerebrospinal fluid abnormal	Various. Chiefly leptomeningitis; arteritis or encephalitis may also be present
II. Meningeal and vascular A. Cerebral meningeal 1. Diffuse	Increased intracranial pressure and cranial nerve palsies	Leptomeningitis with hydrocephalus. Degeneration of cranial nerves. Arteritis also present.
2. Focal	Increased intracranial pressure and focal cerebral symptoms and signs of slow onset	Granuloma formation (gumma)
B. Cerebral vascular	Focal cerebral symptoms and signs of sudden onset	Endarteritis with encephalomalacia
C. Spinal meningeal and vascular	Paresthesias, weakness, atrophy and sensory loss in extremities and trunk	Admixture of endarteritis and .meningeal infiltration and thickening with degeneration of nerve roots and substance of the cord—myelomalacia
III. Parenchymatous A. Tabetic	Pains, paresthesias, crises, ataxia, impairment of pupillary reflexes, loss of deep tendon reflexes, impairment of proprioceptive sensation, and trophic changes	Leptomeningitis and degenerative changes in posterior roots, dorsal funiculi and in the brain stem
B. Paretic	Personality changes, convulsions and mental deterioration. Physical deterioration in late stages	Meningoencephalitis
C. Optic Atrophy*	Loss of vision, pallor of optic discs	Leptomeningitis and atrophy of optic nerves

*Rarely occurs alone. Usually found in connection with tabetic or paretic neurosyphilis.

the disease. These drugs were of little or no value after the symptoms and signs of neurosyphilis had developed.

Although fever therapy produced by the inoculation of tertian malaria or by fever cabinet was effective in arresting the course of the disease, this type of therapy was accompanied by a significant risk to the patient and it was soon replaced by penicillin.

The widespread use of penicillin in the fifth decade of this century made a drastic change in the incidence of neurosyphilis as well as cardiac syphilis. All forms of neurosyphilis and cardiac syphilis are now clinical rarities. This continues to be true even though there are periodic increases in the incidence of primary syphilis. Penicillin and other antibiotics seem to be capable of eradicating the spirochetes and preventing the development of cardiac or neurosyphilis if they are given for any acute infection. It is now difficult for individuals who are not treated for primary infection with Spirochaeta pallida to escape therapy at some later date with penicillin or one of the antibiotic drugs for gonorrhea or some other acute infection.

The incidence of neurosyphilis in recent years has been almost nil but in the era before the use of penicillin it developed in approximately 30% of the patients affected by primary syphilis.

Pathology. The pathology of neurosyphilis is related to the duration of the infection and the portion of the nervous system affected. In early stages of the disease the meninges are infiltrated with lymphocytes and other mononuclear cells. The inflammatory changes in the meninges affect the cranial nerves resulting in degeneration of the axons. The acute inflammatory process may invade the small vessels in the meninges resulting in proliferation of the endothelial cells and occlusion of small vessels causing areas of softening in the brain and spinal cord. Meningitis and arteritis of spinal vessels may produce demyelination of the white matter in the spinal cord and myelomalacia in the periphery of the cord and occasionally cause an acute transverse myelitis.

The pathological changes in dementia paralytica are of slow evolution. There are inflammatory changes in the meninges. The small cortical vessels are infiltrated with lymphocytes and plasma cells with occasional extension of the inflammation into the substance of the cortex. The inflammation is accompanied by degeneration of cortical neurons and proliferation of the glia cells.

Spirochetes can be found in the cortex of cases of dementia paralytica but only rarely in other forms of neurosyphilis.

In tabes dorsalis the inflammation of the meninges and blood vessels is followed in a number of years by degeneration of the posterior roots and the posterior funiculi of the spinal cord (Fig. 15) and occasionally of the cranial nerves.

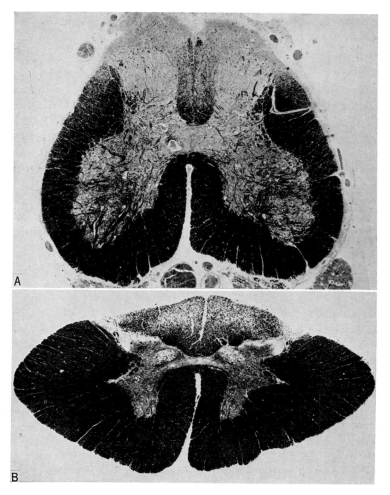

Figure 15. Tabes dorsalis. Degeneration of the posterior column in the sacral and thoracic cord (myelin sheath stain). (Merritt, H. H., Adams, R. D., and Solomon, H. C.: *Neurosyphilis*, Oxford University Press.)

Incidence. There has been a great decrease in the incidence of neurosyphilis in recent years, which is due to the efficacy of the treatment of early syphilis and asymptomatic neurosyphilis by penicillin. All forms of neurosyphilis are clinical rarities on medical and neurological wards and the rate of admission of cases of dementia paralytica to mental hospitals has almost entirely ceased in the past twenty years. For obvious reasons there are no figures for the recent years. As to the incidence of neurosyphilis in the era before the use of penicillin, Turner, on the basis of an analysis of 10,000 cases of syphilis, reported an incidence of neurosyphilis of 39% in the white male, 22% in the white female, 16% in the black male and 7% in the black female. Merritt, Adams and Solomon found syphilis of the nervous system in 29% of 2,263 cases of syphilis, all of whom were examined clinically and serologically (including cerebrospinal fluid) after the secondary stage. The relative incidence of the various forms of neurosyphilis in the prepenicillin era is shown in Table 12. In general, tabetic and asymptomatic neurosyphilis each constituted approximately 30% of all cases of neurosyphilis; paretic neurosyphilis, 12%; and all of the other forms, the remaining 28%.

Asymptomatic Neurosyphilis. The term "asymptomatic neurosyphilis" is used to describe the group of patients who have abnormalities in the cerebrospinal fluid indicating syphilitic infection of the nervous system, but who do not have at that time any clinical symptoms or abnormal signs on neurological examination.

The serious effects of syphilis on the human organism are mainly due to injury to the cardiovascular and central nervous system. There is no satisfactory way of detecting cardiac involvement before the development of clinical signs, but the presence or absence of invasion of the nervous system can be determined early in the course of the disease by examining the cerebrospinal fluid. This makes it imperative that the cerebrospinal fluid be examined in every patient in whom the diagnosis of syphilis is suspected or established. In patients with early syphilis the cerebrospinal fluid should be examined at the end of the course of treatment. If this treatment is given in a short period of time with penicillin, the fluid should be examined again one to two years after the treatment is completed, even if it was negative at the first examination.

The pathology of asymptomatic neurosyphilis is not known. It is presumed that the pathological changes in most cases are confined to the meninges, but in a certain percentage of cases the parenchyma and the vascular system must also be affected. The parenchymatous changes of paretic neurosyphilis, for example, must be present for some months before clinical evidence of this damage is manifest. In such cases, it might be possible that the fortuitous examination of the cerebrospinal fluid in the period immediately preceding the onset of symptoms would lead to the diagnosis of asymptomatic neurosyphilis, although the pathological changes may be characteristic of parenchymatous neurosyphilis.

Incidence of asymptomatic neurosyphilis varies according to the duration of the infection. There is a rapid rise in the incidence in the first two years after infection. After the second year there is a gradual decrease due to the development of symptomatic neurosyphilis or to

Table 12. The Relative Incidence of Various Forms of Neurosyphilis
(After Merritt, Adams and Solomon, *Neurosyphilis*, Oxford University Press, 1946)

Type of Neurosyphilis	No. of Cases	%
Asymptomatic	219	31
Tabetic	203	30
Paretic	78	12
Tabo-paretic	19	3
Vascular	66	10
Meningeal	37	6
Eighth nerve	9	1
Optic neuritis	20	3
Spinal cord	19	3
Miscellaneous	6	1
Total	676	100

spontaneous sterilization of the cerebrospinal fluid. The age incidence follows a curve similar to that of infection by syphilis, with the greatest number of cases in the third to fifth decades.

Cerebral Meningeal Neurosyphilis. Involvement of the cerebral meninges is evidenced by the development of an acute or subacute meningitis, with or without cranial nerve palsies. In a small percentage of the cases focal neurological signs may be added as the result of a concomitant arteritis.

The incubation period between the initial infection and the appearance of the meningeal symptoms varies from a few months to many years. In the vast majority of cases they appear within the first year of the infection and in about 10% they are coincident with the secondary rash.

The symptoms can be divided into three groups: (1) those which are due to increased intracranial pressure resulting from interference with the cerebrospinal fluid circulation (hydrocephalus), (2) those due to damage to the cranial nerves (cranial nerve palsies), and (3) those which are due to thrombosis of small cerebral vessels secondary to inflammation of the meninges.

The disease runs a benign course, but permanent residuals of the cranial nerve palsies may persist. Treatment is important to prevent later development of dementia paralytica or tabes dorsalis.

Cerebral Vascular Syphilis. Involvement of the brain in neurosyphilis usually takes the form of dementia paralytica but occasionally the blood vessels are affected by syphilitic endarteritis producing small cerebral vascular lesions. Cerebral vascular syphilis has been grossly overdiagnosed. It was formerly made in all middle-aged individuals with syphilis who had a cerebral vascular lesion. In the majority of these patients the symptoms were due to cerebral arteriosclerosis.

Meningeal or vascular syphilis (meningomyelitis) of the cord is rare. It occurs in less than 1% of patients with untreated syphilis and is one tenth as frequent as tabes dorsalis. Although the symptoms may appear at any time, they usually have their onset five to thirty years after the initial infection. Most of the cases, therefore, are in young or middle-aged adults. Males are affected four times as frequently as females.

The diagnosis of meningeal or vascular syphilis of the spinal cord is made on basis of symptoms and signs of spinal cord involvement and the characteristic abnormalities in the cerebrospinal fluid. Meningeal and vascular syphilis of the spinal cord must be differentiated from tabes dorsalis and other diseases which affect the spinal cord.

The prognosis in syphilitic meningomyelitis is usually good. With antisyphilitic treatment symptoms improve and there is partial or complete regression of the clinical signs.

The prognosis for life is poor in patients with thrombosis of the spinal arteries. In patients who live, there is usually little improvement in the neurological signs even with intensive antisyphilitic treatment. This is to be expected from the nature of the pathological changes.

Gummas of the spinal cord of hypertrophic pachymeningitis were extremely rare. They did not respond to antisyphilitic treatment and even when a gumma was removed surgically the results were disappointing.

Dementia Paralytica. Dementia paralytica (general paresis of the insane, syphilitic meningoencephalitis, paretic neurosyphilis) is a chronic spirochetal meningoencephalitis which destroys neurons in the cerebral cortex and leads to a general dissolution of mental and physical capacities. The disease is of historical importance because it

Table 13.   Pathology of Dementia Paralytica
(Changes Localized to or Most Severe in the Frontal and Temporal Poles)

Macroscopic
1. Thickening and opacity of the meninges.
2. Widening of cerebral sulci.
3. Dilatation of the cerebral ventricles.
4. Granular ependymitis.

Microscopic
1. Inflammatory reaction—perivascular and meningeal.
2. Degenerative changes in parenchyma.
3. Degenerative and reactive changes (rod cells) in glia.
4. Deposition of iron pigment.
5. Presence of spirochetes.

was one of the first mental disorders for which a definite pathology was established.

Pathology (Table 13). Microscopically the brain is atrophic, particularly in the anterior portion of the frontal and temporal lobes. Over the atrophic area the leptomeninges are opaque, thickened and adherent to the underlying cortex (Fig. 16) and the cerebral sulci are widened and filled with an excess of fluid. On sectioning the brain, the ventricles are studded with fine sand-like granulations (granular ependymitis) (Figs. 17—19).

Symptomatology. The clinical manifestations of dementia paralytica (Table 14) may simulate those of any type of mental disorder of either the functional or organic reaction types and symptom complexes of the minor or major psychoses are encountered.

The course of untreated dementia paralytica usually extends over several years and may be divided into three parts: (1) the incipient

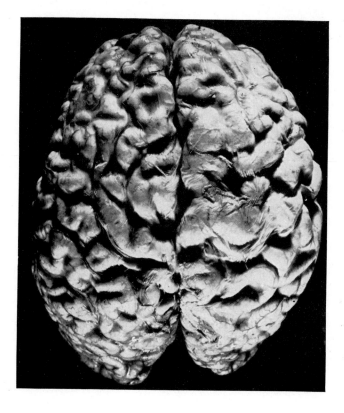

Figure 16.   Dementia paralytica. Thickening of the meninges and atrophy of the cerebral convolutions. (Merritt, H. H., Adams, R. D., and Solomon, H. C.: *Neurosyphilis,* Oxford University Press.)

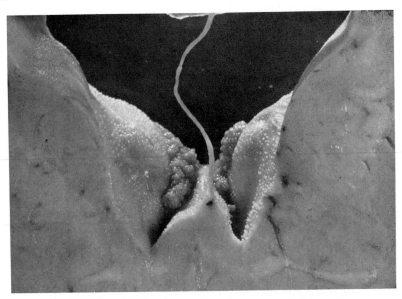

Figure 17.   Dementia paralytica. Granular ependymitis of the floor of lateral ventricles. (Merritt, H. H., Adams, R. D., and Solomon, H. C.: *Neurosyphilis*, Oxford University Press.)

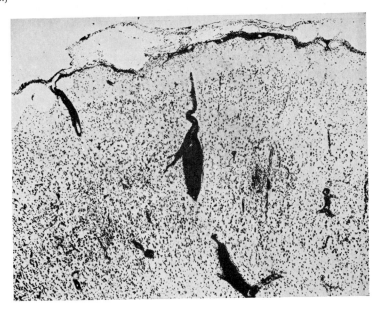

Figure 18.   Dementia paralytica. Inflammatory reaction in the meninges and in the perivascular spaces of the cortical vessels. (Nissl stain) (Merritt, H! H., Adams, R. D., and Solomon, H. C.: *Neurosyphilis*, Oxford University Press.)

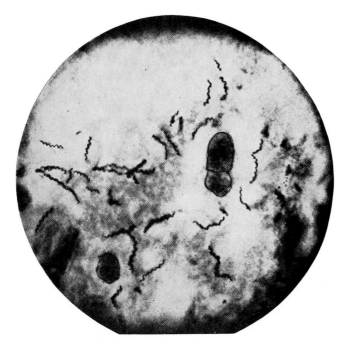

Figure 19. Dementia paralytica. Spirochetes in cortex. (Levaditi stain) (Merritt, H. H., Adams, R. D., and Solomon, H. C.: *Neurosyphilis,* Oxford University Press.)

stage, (2) the period of full development of the psychosis and (3) the period of decline.

The most devastating effect of dementia paralytica is on the mind. Although the psychotic pictures presented by dementia paralytica are multiform and reproduce all known psychoses, there are several fairly characteristic clinical pictures. The most common of these is the simple deteriorated type, characterized by memory defect, impairment of judgment and excessive lability of mood. The gradual dissolution of mental faculties proceeds in all cases to a state comparable to imbecility and idiocy. General motor weakness accompanied by convulsive seizures develops in the terminal stages.

Clinical Course. Untreated the disease is progressive leading to death in three to five years. Penicillin is effective in the treatment of dementia paralytica. The clinical results depend to a great extent upon the nature of the pathology which is present at the time of the start of treatment. If most of the symptoms are due to a disturbance of cerebral function related to the inflammatory reaction, complete cure is to be expected. If, however, there has been a significant degree of degeneration of the

Table 14.   Symptoms of Dementia Paralytica

Early Stage	Late Stage
Irritability	Impaired memory
Fatigability	Defective judgment
Conduct slump	Depression or elation
Personality changes	Lack of insight
Headaches	Confusion and disorientation
Forgetfulness	Poorly systematized delusions
Tremors	Seizures
	Transient paralysis or aphasia

Table 15.   Neurological Signs of Dementia Paralytica

Common

1. Relaxed, expressionless facies
2. Tremors of facial and lingual muscles
3. Dysarthria
4. Impairment of handwriting
5. Hyperactive tendon reflexes

Rare

1. Focal signs—hemiplegia, hemianopia, etc.
2. Optic atrophy
3. Eye muscle palsies
4. Absent reflexes
5. Babinski toe sign

cerebral neurons, the disease process can be arrested but complete cure is not to be expected.

Tabes Dorsalis. Tabes dorsalis or progressive locomotor ataxia is characterized pathologically by degenerative changes in the posterior roots, in the posterior funiculi of the spinal cord and in the brain stem, and clinically by lancinating pains, progressive ataxia, loss of reflexes, varying degrees of loss of proprioceptive sensibility, and functional disorders of bladder, bowels and generative organs.

There is shrinkage of the lumbar and sacral dorsal roots and the dorsal funiculi of the spinal cord. The changes in the posterior funiculi are limited to the column of Goll (Fig. 15) except in rare cases where there is degeneration of the dorsal roots in the cervical region (cervical tabes). The optic or other cranial nerves are shrunken in cases where they are involved. In the early stage of the disease the leptomeninges and the intraspinal portion of the posterior roots are infiltrated with lymphocytes and plasma cells.

Signs. The cardinal signs of tabes dorsalis (Table 16) are loss of tendon reflexes (usually ankle and knee), impairment of vibratory and

Table 16.   Symptoms and Signs in Tabetic Neurosyphilis
Analysis of 150 Cases

Symptoms	%	Signs	%
Lancinating pains	75	Abnormal pupils	94
Ataxia	42	Argyll Robertson	48
Bladder disturbance	33	Other abnormalities	64
Parathesias	24	Reflex abnormalities	
Gastric or visceral crises	18	Absent ankle jerks	94
Visual loss	16	Absent knee jerks	81
Rectal incontinence	14	Absent reflexes	11
Deafness	7	Romberg sign	55
Impotence	4	Impaired sensation	
		Impaired vibratory sense	52
		Impaired vision	43
		Impaired touch and pain	13
		Optic atrophy	20
		Ocular palsy	10
		Charcot joints	7

position sense in the lower extremities and abnormalities in the pupils. To these may be added disorders of cutaneous and deep sensibility, hypotonia, weakness or atrophy of the muscles, disorders of the genital organs, bladder or rectum, optic atrophy, cranial nerve palsies, and so-called trophic disturbances (Charcot joint or mal perforant).

Some degree of pupillary abnormality is the form of inequality or irregularity of the pupils, or impairment of their reaction to light is present in over 90% of the cases. The Argyll-Robertson pupil is found in over 50%.

Tabes dorsalis is, in comparison to dementia paralytica, a relatively benign disease. It is rarely fatal in itself. Death may result from complications of the urinary tract infections due to incontinence or the patient may be incapacitated by blindness or ataxia. As a rule, however, the progress of the disease is halted by treatment or comes to a spontaneous arrest before the patient is incapacitated. Persistence of the ataxia and the lightning pains is not uncommon.

Congenital Neurosyphilis. Although congenital syphilis was recognized in the sixteenth century, congenital dementia paralytica was first described by Clouston in 1877, the congenital tabes dorsalis by Hemak in 1885.

The clinical syndrome and pathological reaction which occur as the result of infection of the fetus by way of the placental circulation are similar to those which develop when the infection is acquired after birth. There are, however, some variations from the adult type of symptoms when the infection is acquired at this early stage of life.

The percentage of children of syphilitic parents who develop syphilis is not known. The incidence of congenital syphilis is related to the duration of infection in the mother. The longer the mother has had syphilis, the less the chance for pregnancy to terminate in the birth of a congenitally syphilitic child. Similarly, adequate treatment of the syphilitic mother during pregnancy greatly decreases the incidence of infection in the child. The frequency of neurosyphilis in children with congenital syphilis is approximately the same as in acquired neurosyphilis. The relative proportion of the various clinical forms of congenital neurosyphilis is similar to that of acquired neurosyphilis except that tabes dorsalis is much less common.

Diagnosis. The fact that the incidence of neurosyphilis is so low and our experience with some of the new tests for syphilis is limited, makes it somewhat difficult to be dogmatic about the diagnosis of neurosyphilis at the present time. It can be said that typical cases of tabes dorsalis are not seen, but there are reports in the literature recording a high incidence of neurosyphilis in some hospitals based on certain serological tests on the blood or spinal fluid or the finding of spirochetes in the aqueous humor. These cases are usually patients with mental symptoms but none of them has been proven by pathological examination to have had dementia paralytica.

No new cases of typical tabes dorsalis have been reported and this form of neurosyphilis was the most common form in the prepenicillin era.

Laboratory Data. The only significant laboratory findings in neurosyphilis are positive tests for syphilis in the blood or cerebrospinal fluid. These are usually positive throughout the course of the disease unless reversed by therapy. In addition, the cerebrospinal fluid had a number of abnormalities, an increase in the number of cells and protein content of the fluid and an increase in the gammaglobulin content with precipitation of colloidal suspensions (colloidal gold curve) particularly in the paretic form of the infection. The changes in the cerebrospinal fluid have resisted therapy with arsenical therapy but are rapidly eliminated by penicillin.

Treatment. Neurosyphilis is readily eliminated by penicillin and the clinical results are dependent on the degree of tissue destruction at the time of the initiation of therapy. The dosage required is small but it is customary to give 10 to 15 million units in divided doses over a period of ten to twenty days.

REFERENCES

Adie, W. J.: Argyll Robertson Pupils, True and False, Brit. Med. J., 2, 136, 1931.
Argyll Robertson, D.: Four Cases of Spinal Miosis with Remarks on the Action of Light on the Pupil, Edinburgh M.J., 15, 487, 1869.

Bayle, A. L. J.: *Recherches sur l'arachnite chronique.* Paris, 1822.

Bruusgaard, E.: Über das Schicksal der nicht spezifische behandelten Leuetiker, Arch. f. Derm. u. Syph., *157*, 309, 1929.

Duchenne, G.: De L'ataxe locomotive progressive, Arch. gën. de Mëd., *12*, 641, 1858–9.

Erb, W. H.: Ueber Syphilitische Spinalparalyse, Neurol. Centralbl., *11*, 161, 1892.

Hahn, R. D., *et al.*: Penicillin Treatment of Asymptomatic Central Nervous System Syphilis. 1. Probability of Progression to Symptomatic Neurosyphilis, Arch. Dermat., *76*, 355, 1956.

Hahn, R. D., *et al.*: Penicillin Treatment of General Paresis (Dementia Paralytica), Arch. Neurol. & Psychiat., *81*, 557, 1959.

Heubner, O.: *Die luetische erkrankung der Hirnarterien,* Leipzig, F. C. W. Vogel, 1874.

Mattauscheck, E., and Pilez, A.: Zweite Mitteilung über 4134 katamnestische verfolgte Fälle von luetische Infektionen, Ztschr. f. d. ges. Neurol. u. Psychiat., *15*, 608, 1913.

Merritt, H. H., Adams, R. D., and Solomon, H. C.: *Neurosyphilis,* New York, Oxford University Press, 1946, 443 pp.

Noguchi, H., and Moore, J. W.: A Demonstration of Treponema Pallidum in the Brain of General Paresis. J. Exper. Med., *17*, 232, 1913.

Sparling, P. F.: Diagnosis and Treatment of Syphilis, New Eng. J. Med., *284*, 642, 1971.

Spielmeyer, W.: Zur Pathogenese der Tabes, Ztschr. f. d. gen. Neurol. u. Psychiat, *84*, 257, 1923; *91*, 67, 1924; *97*, 287, 1925.

Turner, T. B.: The Race and Sex Distribution of the Lesions of Syphilis in 1000 Cases, Bull. Johns Hopkins Hosp., *46*, 159, 1930.

Wagner-Jauregg, J.: Über die Einwirkung der Malaria auf die progressive Paralyse, Psychiat. neur. Wschr., *20*, 132, 1918–19.

Wilner, E., and Brody, J. A.: Prognosis of General Paresis after Treatment, The Lancet, *2*, 1370, 1968.

Chapter 2

Vascular Diseases of Brain and Spinal Cord

JAMES F. TOOLE, M.D.*

INTRODUCTION

The neurons and glia of the brain require for their metabolism an uninterrupted supply of about 150 gm of glucose and 72 liters of oxygen per twenty-four hours. Because it does not store these substances, the brain can function for only a few minutes if they are reduced below critical levels. The arterial blood supplies these and other nutrients; the venous blood removes waste products—principally CO_2, acid metabolites, and heat.

With each contraction the heart thrusts into the ascending aorta about 70 ml of blood, of which about 10 to 15 ml are destined for the brain. The adult brain weighs about 1500 gm and the blood flow allotted to it is in the range of 750 to 1000 ml per minute. Of this total about 350 ml flows through each internal carotid artery and about 100 to 200 ml through the vertebral-basilar system.

Anatomic Considerations

Each cerebral hemisphere is supplied by its own internal carotid artery which rises from the common carotid behind the angle of the jaw and ascends behind the pharynx to enter the cranium through the carotid canal. The two internal carotid arteries travel through the cavernous sinuses beside the sella turcica. Above the sinuses each gives off its ophthalmic anterior choroidal artery and then divides into anterior and middle cerebral arteries. This vascular system supplies the optic nerves and retina, the frontal and parietal lobes, and parts of the temporal lobe.

* I wish to thank Doctors David L. Kelly, J. M. McWhorter, and Jean Angelo for their many helpful suggestions and Dr. Dixon M. Moody for supplying the CT scans and commenting upon the neuroradiologic sections of this chapter.

149

The vertebral and basilar arteries function as a unit. Each vertebral artery arises from a subclavian artery and ascends through a bony canal in the cervical vertebrae to enter the skull through the foramen magnum, where it gives off the posterior inferior cerebellar artery and the anterior median spinal arteries. At the pontomedullary junction, the two vertebral arteries join to form the basilar artery, which has three general groups of branches: paramedian, short circumferential, and long circumferential arteries. The basilar artery ends at the level of the midbrain by dividing into the two posterior cerebral arteries, which in turn supply the medial portions of the temporal lobes and the occipital lobes of the cerebrum. The vertebral-basilar system supplies the upper cervical portion of the spinal cord, the brain stem, cerebellum, thalamus, and the auditory and vestibular apparatuses.

Three varieties of interconnections among the carotid and vertebral-basilar systems help to ensure even distribution of blood to the brain. The first type is entirely extracranial, joining the two external carotid arteries and the external carotid and the vertebral arteries. The second category connects extra- to intracranial vessels, mainly through the orbit. Branches of the external carotid artery, for example, join the ophthalmic artery. The third variety is entirely intracranial and consists mainly of the circle of Willis, which lies at the base of the brain and interconnects the carotid system of one side with that of the other (via the anterior communicating artery) and the vertebral-basilar with the carotid systems (via the posterior communicating arteries). Other anastomoses over the surface of the brain and in the ventricles interconnect the anterior, middle, and posterior cerebral arteries.

As a group, these rich anastomotic networks protect the brain by allowing for alternate routes which can circumvent obstructions in any of the main arteries supplying the brain. For example, an obstruction of the internal carotid artery in the neck may be bypassed by external carotid, ophthalmic, and internal carotid anastomoses. Obstructions of a vertebral artery can be bypassed by interconnections between its external carotid and distal vertebral arteries. As a third example, obstruction to a proximal segment of a middle cerebral artery might be symptomless if there are adequate interconnections between the distal branches of the posterior cerebral and the anterior cerebral arteries (Fig. 20).

The small arteries and arterioles which spring from the surface arteries and penetrate the parenchyma have few interconnections with one another and function as end arteries. When one of these becomes obstructed, the result is tissue ischemia or infarction.

These smaller arteries and arterioles control blood flow within the brain. A well-developed muscular coat gives them the capacity to constrict in response to elevations in blood pressure and to dilate in

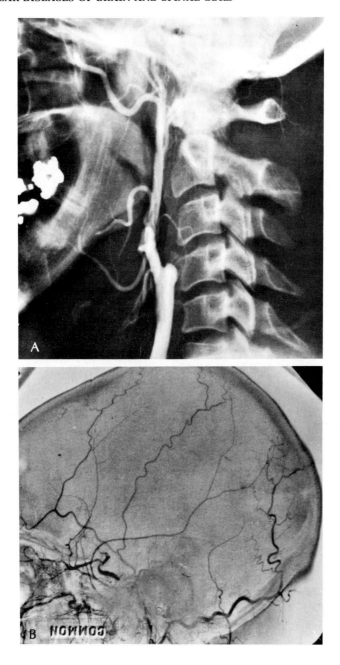

Figure 20.   Occlusion of the proximal internal carotid artery. *A*, Stump of vessel is present posterior to the normally filled external carotid artery. *B*, The ophthalmic artery fills via collaterals from the external carotid and then fills the distal internal carotid artery in a retrograde manner. (Courtesy Dr. Dixon M. Moody.)

response to hypotension. Thus they help to ensure a constant perfusion pressure and blood flow to the capillary networks which they supply.

The capillaries are in close proximity to cell bodies of neurons and are joined to them by protoplasmic astrocytes which are interposed between the two structures, with one extension wrapped around the capillary and another applied to the neuron. Many authorities believe that astrocytes regulate the flow of nutrients and metabolites between the cell body and capillary blood.

Within this system only the arterioles, which are exquisitely sensitive to changes in pCO_2 and pO_2, respond dramatically to pharmacologic agents. When the partial pressure of carbon dioxide in arterial blood is increased, the arterioles dilate and cerebral blood flow increases. When CO_2 is reduced, they constrict and the flow is reduced. Changes in the partial pressure of oxygen have the opposite effect. During cerebral activity increase in metabolism results in concomitant increases in regional flow. In cerebrovascular disease this autoregulation is disturbed generally or focally.

REFERENCES

Fields, W. S., Bruetman, M. E., and Weibel, J.: Collateral Circulation of the Brain, Monographs of the Surgical Sciences, 2, 183, 1965.
Gillilan, L. A.: The Arterial and Venous Blood Supplies to the Forebrain (Including the Internal Capsule) of Primates, Neurology, 18, 653, 1968.
Kaplan, H. A., and Ford, D. H.: The Brain Vascular System, Amsterdam, Elsevier Publishing Company, 1966.
Stephens, R. B., and Stilwell, D. L.: Arteries and Veins of the Human Brain, Springfield, Charles C Thomas, 1969.
Weidner, W., Hanafee, W., and Markham, C. H.: Intracranial Collateral Circulation via Leptomeningeal and Rete Mirabile Anastomoses, Neurology, 15, 39, 1965.

ETIOLOGIC AND PATHOLOGIC CONSIDERATIONS

Cerebrovascular disease is a disorder involving any of the arteries or veins which supply the brain.

The changes which occur in the brain in response to vascular disease can be classified into two general types: ischemic and hemorrhagic.

Ischemia and Infarction

When blood supply is interrupted for thirty seconds ischemia develops and brain metabolism is altered. After a minute neuronal function may cease; after five minutes tissue anoxia initiates an irreversible chain of events leading to cerebral infarction. If the blood supply is restored during the stage of ischemia, no permanent damage results.

Etiology. There are many causes for ischemia, including occlusion of an artery by thrombus or embolus. Ischemia may occur when, despite a patent vascular system, arterial pressure falls below critical levels. It also develops when constituents of the blood are too viscous to be propelled through the system (as in polycythemia dysproteinemia and thrombocytosis) or when the content of glucose or oxygen in the blood is too low to support metabolic activity.

Acute or chronic meningitis, herpetic encephalitis, or arteritis caused by syphilis may cause thrombosis of one or more of the cerebral arteries. Other unusual causes of infarction are thromboangiitis obliterans, polyarteritis nodosa, and occlusion of veins draining the brain. At times neoplasms or edema can compress cerebral vessels and cut off blood supply to brain tissues. Aortocranial arteries may be occluded by dissecting aneurysms, and the vertebral arteries may be compressed by arthritis of the cervical spine. Cerebral arterial spasm is an unusual cause of ischemia, but does occur in migraine syndromes.

Whether occlusive lesions produce symptoms and signs depends upon the collateral circulation with which a person is born or which develops to circumvent gradual occlusion of a primary channel. The adequacy of the collateral circulation depends upon many factors, the principal one being the rate of development of the obstruction.

The most common causes of infarction are atherosclerosis and embolism. Atherothrombosis is presumed to be due to clotting at the site of an ulcerated plaque in the vessel wall (Fig. 21). The clot propagates until it (1) occludes the lumen or (2) sheds microemboli which plug distal arteries. In an autopsy series composed of 142 patients who died soon after cerebral infarction, Moossy found in 78 (55%) an intracranial thrombosis consistent with the clinical picture.

Arteriosclerotic plaques may develop at any point along the carotid and vertebral-basilar system, the most common site being in the carotid sinus at the point where the internal carotid artery arises from the common carotid. Yates and Hutchinson made a careful study of the entire length of the extra- and intracranial arteries in 100 patients whose deaths were attributed to cerebral ischemia or infarction. After excluding the cases in which death resulted from cerebral hemorrhage, tumors, circulatory failure, and the like, they found 35 cases of cerebral infarction. "Significant" stenosis or occlusion of the *intracranial* arteries was found in 19 of these; "significant" stenosis or occlusion of the *extracranial* arteries was present in all but three.

An angiographic evaluation of 221 patients with a cerebral infarction (Table 17) revealed occlusion or stenosis of the internal carotid, the vertebral artery, or one of their major branches in 150 cases. The incidence for the three main cerebral arteries was: anterior cerebral 42, middle cerebral 28, posterior cerebral 1. The proportion of extra- and intracranial vascular pathologic conditions causing stroke varies with racial groups. In Caucasians extracranial lesions are frequent, while in Blacks and Orientals the frequency of intracranial lesions is higher.

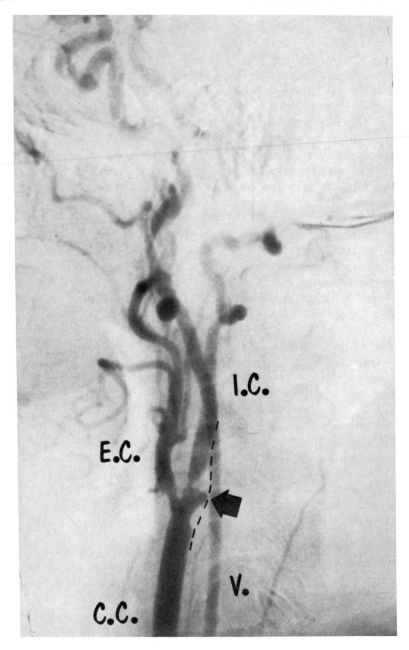

Figure 21. Carotid angiogram (subtraction technique) shows an ulcerated plaque at the origin of the internal carotid artery (arrow). The dotted line shows the position of the vessel wall underlying the plaque. I.C.=internal carotid, E.C.=external carotid, C.C.=common carotid artery, and V.=vertebral artery. (Courtesy Dr. Frank W. Farrell, Jr.)

Table 17. Angiographic Findings in 221 Cases of Infarction

(After Gurdjian, Lindner, Hardy and Thomas, Neurology, *8*, 724, 1961)

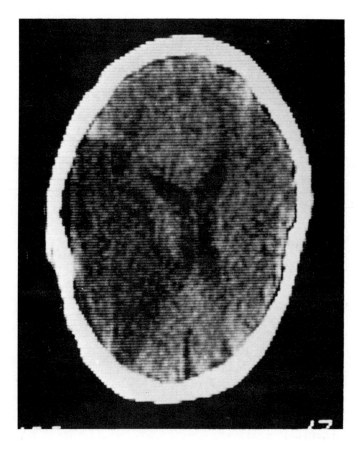

Figure 22. CT brain scan of cerebral infarction five days after occlusion of the middle cerebral artery. Edema in the infarcted area causes radiolucency and swelling with compression of the ipsilateral ventricle. (Courtesy Dr. Dixon M. Moody.)

Pathology. Steps in the evolution of an infarct are: (1) local vasodilatation, (2) stasis of the blood column with segmentation of the red cells, (3) edema (Fig. 22), and (4) necrosis. Although most infarcts are pale, a "red infarct" is occasionally produced by local hemorrhage into the necrotic tissue. There is a propensity for gray matter to have petechial hemorrhages and for white matter to have pale (ischemic) infarction. Such hemorrhage probably occurs when the clot or embolus migrates and flow through the infarcted area is restored. If the interruption is sufficiently prolonged and infarction develops, the tissue first softens, then liquefies, and finally a cavity forms as the debris is removed by the phagocytic microglia. In an attempt to fill the defect, astroglia in the surrounding brain proliferate and invade the softened area, and new capillaries are formed. The glial and vascular scar which eventually results is usually imperfect. If the area is large, the cavity may collapse (Fig. 23) or become the site for the formation of small multilocular cysts filled with clear fluid.

Many patients have multiple infarctions. In a series of 106 autopsied cases of cerebral infarction studied by Aring and Merritt a single lesion was found in 82 cases; two or more softenings of varying age were found in 24 cases.

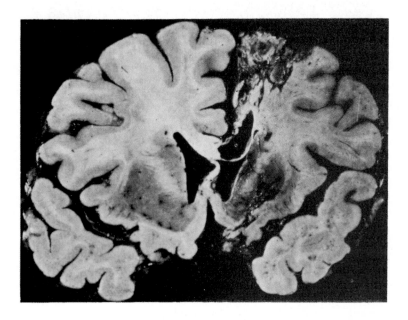

Figure 23.   Infarction in distribution of the anterior cerebral artery with softening of paracentral lobule and cavity formation in corpus callosum. (Merritt, H. H., Adams, R. D., and Solomon, H. C.: *Neurosyphilis,* courtesy Oxford University Press.)

Small cystic infarcts or lacunes are the most common of all forms of infarction. These occur in the basal ganglia, internal capsule, and basis pontis, and less commonly in the centrum semiovale and cerebellum. They result from occlusions of perforating arteries damaged by long-standing hypertension. The lacunar state is discussed on page 195.

Embolism

Cerebral embolism is the term used to describe occlusion of an artery by a fragment of clotted blood, tumor, fat, air, or other foreign substance. The sequence of events is similar to that described for infarction, except that an element of vasospasm may be superimposed. Most emboli are sterile, but those which arise from subacute or acute bacterial endocarditis or septic processes in the lungs may contain bacteria. The result may be arteritis *with* or *without* aneurysm formation (mycotic aneurysm), abscess, localized encephalitis, or meningitis in the area where they lodge.

Etiology. Air embolism may follow injuries or surgical procedures involving the lungs, the dural sinuses or jugular veins or the release of bubbles of nitrogen into the general circulation following a rapid reduction in barometric pressure. Fat embolism is usually associated with bone fracture.

In children, cerebral emboli are commonly associated with valvular heart disease (rheumatic or congenital) with superimposed endocarditis. In adults, embolism is commonly caused by atrial fibrillation or myocardial infarction. Thrombi in the left atrium may dislodge during fibrillation or after cardioversion has restored more forceful and rhythmic contractions. These emboli may be asymptomatic or create the clinical picture of TIA's or of infarction depending upon the rapidity with which blood flow to tissue supplied by the embolized artery is reconstituted. Following myocardial infarction, a portion of the clot which forms on the necrotic endocardium may break off and find its way to a cerebral artery.

Recurrent emboli to the lungs may cause pulmonary hypertension with resultant inversion of the pressure gradient across the foramen ovale. As a consequence, subsequent emboli may traverse the foramen to the left heart and thence to the brain—a paradoxical embolus. Other rare causes of cerebral embolism are atrial myxoma and marantic endocarditis.

The commonest cause of transient ischemic attacks is microembolism from atherosclerotic plaques located in the aortocranial arteries. These plaques form a nidus for clots, which may break off or may ulcerate and discharge their contents of cholesterol and calcium into the blood stream.

Pathology. Tissue supplied by an embolized artery becomes ischemic, and unless the embolus disintegrates or migrates further, infarction which may be hemorrhagic results. Except in cases where the embolus contains bacteria, the pathological changes in the brain tissue are the same as those seen in cerebral infarction due to atherothrombosis. Cerebral emboli are frequently multiple and associated with embolism of the peripheral vessels or with infarcts in the lungs, spleen, kidneys, and other viscera.

Intracerebral Hemorrhage

Hemorrhage may result from rupture of a vessel anywhere within the cranial cavity. Intracranial hemorrhages may be classified according to *location* (extradural, subdural, subarachnoid, parenchymatous, or intraventricular), according to the *nature of the ruptured vessel or vessels* (arterial, capillary, venous), and according to *cause* (traumatic or degenerative). Trauma to the middle meningeal artery or vein produces extradural hematoma, and many subdural hematomas are caused by traumatic rupture of the bridging veins that traverse the subdural space. The vessels most often ruptured in hypertensive patients are intracerebral arterioles. Each of these forms of hemorrhage produces a characteristic clinical and pathological picture. We will consider intracerebral hemorrhage now and the other forms later on in this chapter.

Etiology. The vast majority of parenchymatous hemorrhages result from the rupture of microaneurysms of the arterioles—the end result of chronic arterial hypertension. These microaneurysms are most commonly found in the basal ganglia, particularly the putamen and thalamus.

In other instances, small hamartomas situated in the hemispheres, usually the frontal or temporal lobes, rupture. Other causes are large arteriovenous malformations, blood dyscrasias, various systemic disorders which affect blood coagulation, neoplasms and damage to the cerebral vessels by infections, toxins, and occasionally by administration of therapeutic agents such as anticoagulants. Cerebral hemorrhages may also result from acute leukemia, aplastic anemia, polycythemia, thrombocytopenic purpura, and scurvy. In such cases, the hemorrhages may be multiple and of varied sizes.

Intracerebral bleeding is most commonly attributed to rupture of an artery, but some hemorrhages are venous in origin. The rupture of a vessel may follow softening of surrounding brain tissue; moreover, it is probable that changes in tension in the vessels result from exertion or emotional excitement and changes in the caliber of the vessels (vasodilatation) are factors which contribute to rupture. Hemorrhages deep

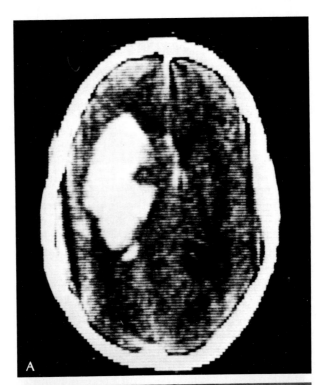

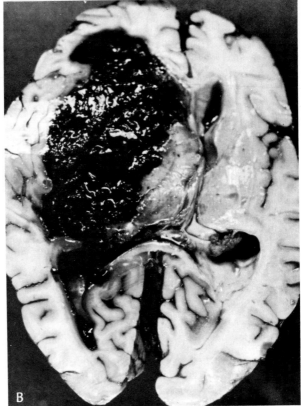

Figure 24. Hypertensive ganglionic hemorrhage. *A,* On CT brain scan the hemorrhage has ruptured into and compresses the ipsilateral ventricle (slit-like white areas medial to hemorrhage). *B,* Cut brain of same patient. (Courtesy Dr. Dixon M. Moody.)

in the substance of the brain, especially in the midbrain or pons, may result from trauma to the head or may occur when pressure above the tentorium cerebelli increases to the point that secondary compression of the uncus and hippocampus occurs at the incisura resulting in venous congestion, edema, and rupture of veins and capillaries.

Pathology. About 80% of hypertensive intracerebral hemorrhages are fatal. At autopsy, it is found that the blood has destroyed and/or displaced a portion of the brain tissue (Fig. 24). If the hemorrhage is a large one, it is often impossible to find the ruptured vessel. By far the most common site for a single hemorrhage is the basal ganglia. Hemorrhages in this location usually originate in the thalamus or the lenticular nucleus and extend to involve the internal capsule; at times the hemorrhage ruptures into the lateral ventricle, then spreads through the ventricular system into the subarachnoid space. Hemorrhages of this magnitude are almost always fatal. Hemorrhage into the lobes of the cerebral hemisphere or into the cerebellum usually remains confined within the brain parenchyma but occasionally ruptures outward into the subarachnoid space and, rarely, into the subdural space as well.

If the patient lives, blood and necrotic brain tissue are removed by phagocytes. The destroyed brain is partially replaced by connective tissue, fibrous tissues, glia and newly-formed blood vessels, leaving a shrunken fluid-filled cavity. Less frequently the blood clot is treated as a foreign body and is surrounded by a thick membrane composed of glial and connective tissue.

Of 113 autopsied cases of hypertensive cerebral hemorrhage Aring and Merritt found only 5 which showed two or more hemorrhages; in the remaining cases, a single hemorrhage was present in the following locations: basal ganglia 70, lobes of the cerebral hemisphere 32, brain stem 4, and cerebellum 2. These figures are similar to those given by other authors, except that cerebellar hemorrhages have been reported to constitute 10% of the cases in some series. In only 7 of all 113 cases was there any evidence of a previous cerebral vascular lesion. In these 7 the appearance of the old lesion was that of softening due to infarction.

The advent of computerized cranial tomography has revolutionized the diagnosis of cerebral hemorrhage. This new technique for imaging the parenchyma of the brain without trauma to the patient is extraordinarily accurate in pinpointing the location and in giving strong clues to the etiology of an acute cerebrovascular episode. It is particularly valuable for the diagnosis of cerebral hemorrhage because of the increased density of blood which shows as a positive image on the CT scan (Fig. 25). Because of this there is developing an increased interest in surgical removal of blood clots during the acute phase of the ictus.

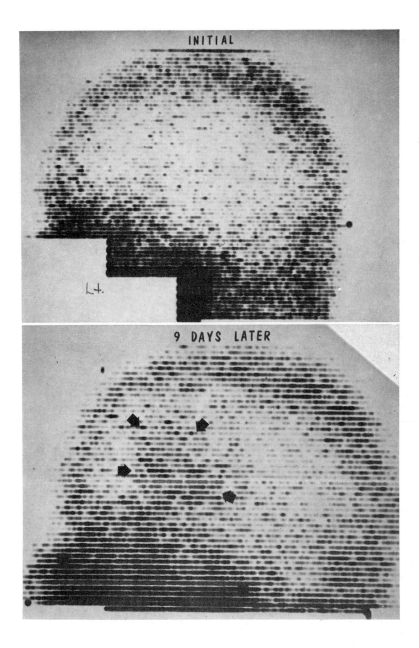

Figure 25. *A*, Acute middle cerebral artery occlusion. ^{99m}Tc isotopic brain scan was normal on day 1 of the ictus. *B*,Repeat scan nine days later shows abnormal uptake in the middle cerebral distribution (arrows). (Courtesy Dr. C. Douglas Maynard.)

Subarachnoid Hemorrhage

Subarachnoid hemorrhage occurs when blood leaks into the sub-arachnoid space either primarily when vessels which traverse the subarachnoid space rupture as in the case of arterial aneurysms of the arterial circle of Willis or secondarily when a hemorrhage into the parenchyma of the brain ruptures through to the subarachnoid space. Subarachnoid hemorrhage is often treated differently from paren-chymatous intracerebral hemorrhage and is due to different etiologies.

REFERENCES

Etiologic and Pathologic Considerations

Adams, G. F. et al.: Cerebral Embolism and Mitral Stenosis: Survival with and without Anticoagulants, J. Neurol., Neurosurg Psych., *37*, 378, 1974.

Aring, C. D., and Merritt, H. H.: Differential Diagnosis Between Cerebral Hemorrhage and Cerebral Thrombosis, Arch. Intern. Med., *56*, 435, 1935.

Baker, A. B., Flora, G. C., Resch, J. A., and Lowenson, R.: The Geographic Pathology of Atherosclerosis; A Review of the Literature with Some Personal Observations on Cerebral Atherosclerosis, J. Chr. Dis., *20*, 685, 1967.

Cole, F. M., and Yates, P. O.: Comparative Incidence of Cerebrovascular Lesions in Normotensive and Hypertensive Patients, Neurology, *18*, 255, 1968.

Fairfax, A. J. et al.: Systemic Embolism in Chronic Sinoatrial Disorder, N. Engl. J. Med., *295*, 190, 1976.

Friedman, G. D., Loveland, D. B., and Ehrlich, S. P.: Relationship of Stroke to Other Cardiovascular Disease, Circulation, *38*, 533, 1968.

Hatano, S., Shigematsu, I., and Strasser, T.: *Stroke Control in the Community*, Proceed-ings of the World Health Organization, Tokyo, WHO, 1976.

Ingvar, D. H., and Lassen, Niels A.: *Brain Work: The Coupling of Function, Metabolism and Blood Flow in the Brain*; Proceedings of the Alfred Benzon Symposium VIII, Copenhagen, Munksgaard, 1975.

Kannel, W. B.: Current Status of the Epidemiology of Brain Infarction Associated with Occlusive Arterial Disease, Stroke, *2*, 295, 1971.

Kannel, W. B., Wold, P. A., Verter, J., and McNamara, P. M.: Epidemiological Assessment of the Role of Blood Pressure in Stroke. The Framingham Study, J.A.M.A., *214*, 301, 1970.

Kurtzke, J. F.: *Epidemiology of Cerebrovascular Disease*, New York, Springer-Verlag, 1969.

Locksley, H. B.: Hemorrhagic Strokes. Principal Causes, Natural History, and Treatment, Med. Clin. N. Am., *52*, 1193, 1968.

Maroon, J. C., and Campbell, R. L.: Atrial Myxoma: A Treatable Cause of Stroke, J. Neurol. Neurosurg. & Psychiat., *32*, 129, 1969.

McCormick, W. F., and Schochet, S. S., Jr.: *Atlas of Cerebrovascular Disease*, Philadel-phia, W. B. Saunders Co., 1976.

Moossy, J.: Cerebral Infarction and Intracranial Arterial Thrombosis, Arch. Neurol., *14*, 119, 1966.

Moossy, J.: Cerebral Atherosclerosis, Intracranial and Extracranial Lesions, in *Pathology of the Nervous System*, v. 2, edited by J. Minkler, New York, McGraw-Hill Book Co., 1971, pp. 1423-1432.

Norris, J. W., et al.: Diagnosis of Cerebral Embolism (letters to Editor), N. Engl. J. Med., *295*, 1017, 1976.

Purves, M. J.: *The Physiology of the Cerebral Circulation*, London, Cambridge University Press, 1972.

Vost, A., Wolochow, D. A., and Howell, D. A.: Incidence of Infarcts of the Brain in Heart Disease, J. Path. Bacteriol., *88*, 463, 1964.

Whisnant, J. P.: Epidemiology of Stroke: Emphasis on Transient Ischemic Attacks and Hypertension, Stroke, *5*,68, 1974.

CLINICAL CONSIDERATIONS

Incidence

Cerebrovascular disease is the most common neurologic disorder in adults, being found in about 25% of all autopsies. Stroke, which occurs in the end stage of cerebrovascular disease, is overwhelmingly the result of atherosclerosis and hypertension. It kills 275,000 and disables 300,000 Americans annually. At any one time 2 million Americans are estimated to be victims and about 30% of these are under sixty-five years of age. Cerebral arteriosclerosis and associated neurologic disability are responsible for about 15% of admissions to institutions for chronic care in the United States.

The frequency of symptomatic cerebrovascular disease depends in part on age, sex, and geographic location, so that it is misleading to be too specific about the incidence of the various forms. In the United States it is generally accepted that in the general population about 70% of strokes are due to atherothrombosis, 20% to hemorrhages of various types, and 10% to embolism. However, embolism is relatively more frequent in younger people and hemorrhage in Negroes. Consequently the incidence of the various forms found in a hospital series depends upon the population served and whether it is a general or a referral hospital.

In Table 18 we have compiled the incidence of strokes due to primary cerebrovascular disorders at the Bowman Gray-Baptist Hospital Medical Center, a 600-bed general hospital.

Although cerebrovascular lesions may occur at any age, in any season, at any time, in either sex, and in all races, each of these factors affects the incidence and prevalence of the various types of cerebrovascular disease. Cerebral hemorrhage and infarction are uncommon before the age of forty. The incidence of cerebral infarction is greatest

Table 18. The Incidence of Various Forms of Cerebral Vascular Lesions*

	Necropsy Diagnosis		Clinical Diagnosis	
	No.	%	No.	%
Cerebral hemorrhage	51	36	157	17
Primary subarachnoid hemorrhage	33	23	177	18
Cerebral atherothrombosis and infarction	58	41	463	49
Cerebral embolus	0	0	149	16
Total	142	100	946	100

* Bowman Gray-North Carolina Baptist Hospital, Winston-Salem, N. C. From July 1966 to June 1971.

Table 19.   The Age Incidence (in Percentages) of Cerebrovascular
Lesions in Autopsy Proven Cases

	Hemorrhage		Infarction	
Age in Years	Intracerebral*	Primary Subarachnoid†	Athero-thrombosis*	Embolism*
Less than 20	1	11	0	9
20 to 29	0	17	0	9
30 to 39	3	19	1	14
40 to 49	21	20	7	14
50 to 59	27	18	24	27
60 to 69	26	10	36	22
70 to 79	20	4	25	0
Over 80	2	1	7	5
Total	100	100	100	100

* After Aring and Merritt.
† After McDonald and Korb.

between sixty and eighty years of age; that of cerebral hemorrhage, between forty and seventy. The incidence of cerebral embolism and primary subarachnoid hemorrhage is more evenly spread, but is highest in the fifth and sixth decades (Table 19). Strokes from all causes are slightly more common in the winter than in summer months.

The Stroke-Prone Profile

Cerebral infarction is not an accidental occurrence, as the commonly used but poorly chosen term *cerebral vascular accident* implies, but is the end result of a chain of events set in motion some decades before the episode occurs. Epidemiologic investigations are now identifying highly susceptible persons and the factors which predispose to stroke, and are providing estimates of the risk associated with each factor, singly and in combination. Known components of the stroke-prone profile are:
1. Transient ischemic attacks; previous cerebral infarction
2. Hypertension
3. Cardiac abnormalities
   a. Electrocardiographic abnormalities indicating left ventricular hypertrophy
   b. Myocardial infarction
   c. Cardiac dysrhythmias—particularly atrial fibrillation
   d. X-ray evidence of cardiac enlargement—particularly if accompanied by EKG evidence of left ventricular hypertrophy
   e. Congestive heart failure
4. Clinical evidence of atherosclerosis
   a. Angina pectoris
   b. Intermittent claudication of legs
   c. Arterial bruits—especially if carotid pulses are absent

5. Diabetes mellitus or any evidence of impaired glucose tolerance
6. Elevated blood lipids
   a. Cholesterol (below age fifty)
   b. Beta lipoprotein and possibly endogenous triglyceride and pre-beta lipoprotein

Other, less well-documented, possible risk factors in thrombotic stroke include:
1. Cigarette smoking
2. Erythrocytosis (high hematocrit)
3. Gout (hyperuricemia)

Premonitory and Initial Symptoms

Although the various types of cerebral vascular disease differ slightly in the mode of onset, symptomatology, and clinical course, it is often difficult on the basis of the clinical data alone to determine the nature of the lesion in any individual case. Therefore, the symptoms of the various types of cerebral vascular lesions will be discussed together.

Patients with cerebral vascular disease are usually asymptomatic until the disorder reaches a late stage. Premonitory symptoms of stroke and cerebral vascular disease are infrequent. When they occur, they may be so nonspecific that they are not recognized as signs of impending stroke. They include headache, dizziness, drowsiness, and mental confusion. One or more of these symptoms is present with many of the cerebral vascular diseases, but it has not yet been determined whether or not they are more common or more severe in the period immediately preceding the stroke.

Focal premonitory symptoms when present usually presage the onset of infarction rather than hemorrhage. In about a third of the cases transient ischemic episodes causing aphasia, paresis, visual field defects, or paresthesias on one side of the body precede the permanent deficit. In most cases these transient attacks are probably due to ischemia associated with microemboli cast off from an atherothrombotic plaque in the carotid or vertebral-basilar arteries. An aneurysm, by compressing one of the cranial nerves, may cause focal signs for several weeks or months before it ruptures.

The following information should be obtained by specific questions in all cases either from the patient or from the family because they may be premonitory events or factors.

1. *Seizures.* If these are present, a detailed history and description of the attacks must be obtained.

2. *Cardiac irregularities.* Does the heart beat irregularly or slowly during attacks (suggesting Stokes-Adams syndrome)?

3. *Headaches.* What are their duration, frequency, type, severity, site, and radiation—and what aggravates or relieves them?

4. *Visual disturbances.* Are they unilateral or bilateral, transient or persistent? Is visual loss partial or total? Does the patient have diplopia, visual hallucinations, or scotomata?

5. *Auditory disturbances.* Does the patient have deafness or tinnitus?

6. *Mental changes.* Have members of the family noted changes in the patient's cerebration, emotional reactions, or memory?

7. *Precipitating factors.* Are any of the symptoms affected by a change in head position or body posture, or by arm exercise? Is there a history of head injury, suggesting the possibility of a subdural hematoma?

8. *Predisposing factors.* Does the patient have hypertension, heart disease, or diabetes? Does he smoke? Is the patient using any medications which could contribute to the problem (e.g., oral contraceptives, hypotensive drugs, anticoagulants, or alcohol)?

9. *Past history.* Has the patient had similar attacks in the past, especially "minor" or transient neurologic disturbances which have cleared spontaneously?

10. *Family history.* Have blood relatives had strokes, seizures, hypertension, or heart attacks?

Onset

In the vast majority of cases the symptoms of a cerebral vascular episode are of sudden onset and reach maximum intensity within minutes or hours. These symptoms may be focal or generalized. Since the *focal* neurologic symptoms (paralysis, sensory loss, speech defects, etc.) are related to the *site* of the hemorrhage or infarct, they are discussed later in connection with the syndromes of the various cerebral arteries. The *generalized* symptoms (which include headache, vomiting, convulsions, and coma) are more common in patients with an intracerebral or subarachnoid hemorrhage. In many cases, confusion, disorientation, and impairment of memory are also present during the period immediately following the ictus. These are in part related to the disturbances of cerebral function associated with the vascular lesion and in part to generalized cerebral vascular disease.

EXAMINATION OF THE PATIENT

General Examination

The patient's head must be examined carefully for evidence of injury. The size and reactions of the pupils should be noted and the optic discs should be examined. The odor of the breath, the character of the respiration and the presence or absence of stiffness of the neck should be noted, and the temperature, pulse rate and blood pressure should be recorded.

If the hemorrhage is small or if a minor vessel is occluded, there may be no change in the *vital signs*. With a large hemorrhage or the occlusion of a major vessel, however, the temperature may be elevated and the heart rate increased. Alterations in the rate and depth of respirations occur in approximately 40% of the cases of cerebral hemorrhage. Abnormalities such as Cheyne-Stokes respirations are present in about 25% of the patients with cerebral embolism and in less than 10% of those with a cerebral infarction. A continued rise in temperature, pulse rate, and respiratory rate indicates that the vaso-motor and thermoregulating centers have ceased to function.

Since arteriosclerosis and hypertension are the most frequent causes of both intracerebral hemorrhage and intracerebral infarction, it is not surprising that cardiac abnormalities, elevation of the blood pressure, and evidence of sclerosis in the peripheral and retinal vessels are common findings in such cases. Whereas the blood pressure is within normal limits in most patients with a cerebral embolism, it is elevated in the vast majority of those with cerebral hemorrhage or infarction, although either of these may occur in the presence of normal blood pressure (Tables 20 and 21). The average systolic and diastolic pressures are slightly higher with hemorrhage. Hypertension and cardiac enlargement are common findings in patients with primary subarachnoid hemorrhage after the age of forty. Atrial fibrillation or clinical signs of cardiac enlargement are present in more than 90% of the patients with a cerebral embolus. Cardiac conduction defects and

Table 20.   The Systolic Blood Pressure* in Autopsy Proven Cases of Cerebral Vascular Lesions (in Percentages)
(After Aring and Merritt)

	Hemorrhage		Infarction	
Blood Pressure (mm Hg)	Intracerebral (107 cases)	Subarachnoid* (30 cases)	Athero-thrombosis (96 cases)	Embolism (19 cases)
80 to 99	1	0	0	16
100 to 139	10	30	11	32
140 to 159	10	13	18	32
160 to 199	39	20	45	15
Over 200	40	37	26	5
Total	100	100	100	100

* Not autopsy controlled.

Table 21.   The Diastolic Blood Pressure* in Autopsy Proven Cases of
Cerebral Vascular Lesions (in Percentages)
(After Aring and Merritt)

	Hemorrhage		Infarction	
Blood Pressure (mm Hg)	Intracerebral (107 cases)	Subarachnoid† (30 cases)	Athero-thrombosis (96 cases)	Embolism (19 cases)
40 to 79	11	17	16	43
80 to 99	23	30	32	31
100 to 139	55	50	43	26
140 to 179	11	3	9	0
Total	100	100	100	100

* Blood pressure taken on admission to hospital.
† Not autopsy controlled.

dysrhythmias as well as acute pulmonary edema occur in some patients
with subarachnoid hemorrhage as a direct result of the trauma to the
cardioregulation centers of the brain.

Neurologic Examination

It is of paramount importance to determine whether hemiplegia is
present. In a comatose patient this can usually be done by careful
observation of the face and examination of the extremities. When one
cheek puffs out with each expiration, that side of the face is paralyzed.
Paralysis of the extremities can be determined by lifting each extremity
and allowing it to fall; the paralyzed limb will fall heavily, while the
unparalyzed limb will gradually sink to the bed. If a patient is in deep
coma, however, all limbs may fall heavily. Vigorous stimulation of the
soles of the feet by a blunt stick or key will cause withdrawal of an
unparalyzed limb, while a paralyzed limb will remain inert unless
there is reflex withdrawal with a Babinski sign.

The type and frequency of pupillary abnormalities in patients with
cerebral vascular lesions vary with the different stages of the disorder,
with the age of the patient, and with the presence of other complicating
factors such as syphilis. If the vascular lesion is in the cortex, the pupils
may be unequal in size, the larger one usually being on the side
opposite the cortical lesion. A homolateral, dilated, and fixed pupil is
occasionally seen when a massive intracerebral hemorrhage has caused
impaction of the temporal lobe into the incisura with compression of
the third cranial nerve. Conjugate deviation of the head and eyes
together, or of the eyes alone, is frequently present in patients with
large cerebral lesions. The deviation is *toward* the lesion in hemispheric abnormalities and *away* from it in brain stem abnormalities if

the lesion is destructive in nature. In irritative lesions the opposite sequence of events occurs. Deviations of the head and eyes tend to disappear as the general condition of the patient improves.

Stiffness of the neck is a common finding in patients with an intracerebral or primary subarachnoid hemorrhage and is related to the presence of blood in the spinal fluid. Because nuchal rigidity also suggests the possibility of impending herniation of the cerebellar tonsils through the foramen magnum, one should seek an expert opinion before performing a lumbar puncture upon such patients.

Changes in the reflexes and the plantar responses can usually be explained on the basis of the focal lesion. All of the tendon reflexes may be lost in the comatose state immediately following the onset of the vascular lesion; more commonly, however, the reflexes are hyperactive on the side opposite the cerebral lesion. In patients with a unilateral lesion the plantar response may be extensor on *both* sides if cerebral edema has caused compression of the midbrain with impaction into the incisura.

Neurovascular Examination

After the general neurologic testing, certain neurovascular tests must be performed on patients whose neurologic symptoms suggest vascular etiology.

Neck Flexion. Both resistance and pain on neck flexion can be indicative of meningeal irritation which might be secondary to blood in the subarachnoid space.

Palpation. The possibility of occlusive disease in a large vessel can be quickly assessed by simultaneous bilateral palpation of the following major arteries: first the superficial temporal arteries, then the carotids at their bifurcations and low in the neck, the subclavian arteries, above and below the clavicles, and finally the brachial and radial arteries, the abdominal aorta, and pulses in the lower extremities. If any pulses are diminished or absent, more detailed evaluation is required.

Diminished pulsation in one *superficial temporal artery* suggests disease of the external or common carotid artery on that side; increased pulsation sometimes indicates stenosis or occlusion of the internal carotid, with development of collateral flow through the external carotid system.

Palpation of the *internal carotid artery* in the pharynx with a gloved finger can sometimes be helpful, since absence of pulsation suggests disease of the internal carotid artery. Pulse delay in one *radial artery* compared with that of the other is almost pathognomonic of subclavian steal.

Auscultation. After auscultation of the heart, the stethoscope should be used to listen for bruits above the aortic and pulmonary areas and along the course of the subclavian arteries below and above the clavicle; then along the course of the vertebral and carotid arteries at various points, particularly at the bifurcation of the carotid artery behind the angle of the mandible, at the subclavian-vertebral junction and over the mastoids. Lastly, the bell of the stethoscope should be applied to the orbit.

There is some debate about the diagnostic value of bruits. Loud intracranial bruits are normal in children and are sometimes heard in adults with no symptoms of cerebral vascular disease, but in others no bruits are heard despite severe stenosis of a vessel. Nevertheless, a bruit is one of the few clinical signs of atherosclerosis. Bruits heard at the carotid bifurcation suggest disease of the common, internal, or external carotid artery; those at the subclavian-vertebral junction suggest abnormality of the vertebral artery.

Ophthalmodynamometry. This test is used to measure pressure in the ophthalmic artery, which is the first sizable branch of the internal carotid artery. Pressure in the ophthalmic artery is usually a reflection of pressure in the carotid system and can give a clue to carotid disease.

The pupils need not be dilated and no anesthetic is needed for the performance of this test. A spring-loaded gauge is placed against the eyelid or sclera. Pressure is increased on the gauge while pulsations in the retinal arterioles are visualized with an ophthalmoscope. The dynamometer pressure at the point where the retinal arterioles cease to pulsate is equal in grams to the systolic pressure of the ophthalmic artery. This pressure is normally about equal in the two eyes and should be a little more than half that in the brachial artery recorded in millimeters of mercury with a sphygmomanometer. Brachial blood pressures must be recorded in both arms so that the interrelationships between brachial and ophthalmic pressure on both sides can be determined.

In patients with subclavian lesions, blood pressures in the two arms, particularly systolic values, differ by more than 20 mm Hg. Disease of the brachiocephalic artery not only produces unequal brachial blood pressures but sometimes lowers ophthalmic pressure on the right. In disease of the carotid artery the ophthalmic pressure is frequently low on the involved side, but the brachial blood pressures are equal and normal. In bilateral carotid disease both ophthalmic pressures may be low in relation to the brachial pressures. Finally, all ophthalmic and brachial blood pressures may be normal in patients with vertebral-basilar artery disease.

Carotid Massage. Patients with disease of the carotid arteries sometimes have hypersensitive carotid sinus reflexes. The sinus may be massaged to ascertain whether it is responsible for the patient's symptoms, if adequate assistance and an EKG monitor are available. Because of a small but definite risk of inducing cerebral vascular insufficiency or of dislodging an embolus from an atheromatous plaque, compression of the carotid should be performed only by an organized team in a setting where extensive monitoring can be done.

Laboratory Data

Albumin and casts are found in the urine of a great many patients with cerebral vascular lesions, regardless of the type. The associated renal disease may also cause an elevation of the blood urea nitrogen.

It is not unusual for stroke patients to have transient hyperglycemia and glycosuria as the result of a temporary disturbance in the sugar metabolism. Although these findings cannot be correlated with the site of the lesion, they are noted more frequently in patients with cerebral hemorrhage than in patients with infarction or embolism.

The white cell count in the peripheral blood is usually normal in patients with an infarction, but leukocyte counts of 12,000 to 20,000 per cu mm are not uncommon following an intracerebral or subarachnoid hemorrhage or a septic embolus.

Focal abnormalities are found in the electroencephalograms of the majority of patients with vascular lesions in the cerebral hemispheres (Fig. 26). These abnormalities tend to lessen with the passage of time, irrespective of improvement in the focal neurologic signs.

The cerebrospinal fluid pressure is usually normal in patients with cerebral embolus or infarction. Pressures between 200 and 300 mm are present in a small percentage of such cases, but readings greater than 300 are rarely seen. In contrast, the pressure is greater than 200 mm in the majority of patients with an intracerebral or primary subarachnoid hemorrhage.

The cerebrospinal fluid is bloody in all cases following primary subarachnoid hemorrhage, in 85% of the cases of cerebral hemorrhage, and in only 15% of those with cerebral embolism. In most cases of infarction the fluid is clear, although there may be a slight xanthochromic tinge and a few red blood cells are seen on microscopic examination.

The white cell count of the fluid is usually normal in patients with cerebral infarction, although occasionally a slight pleocytosis (up to 50 cells) may be seen. The cell count is usually normal in cases of aseptic cerebral embolism; however, when the embolus is from a septic focus a moderate or severe pleocytosis (up to 4,000 cells) is the rule. In most cases this increase in white cells is due to an aseptic meningeal

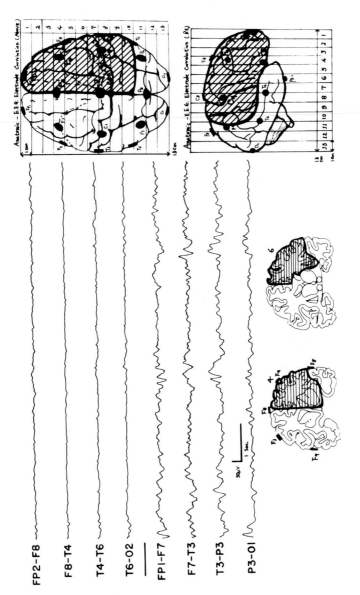

Figure 26.   Virtual absence of the EEG activity over the right hemisphere after infarct from occlusion of middle and anterior cerebral arteries. Diagram shows extent of lesion.

reaction to the septic embolus, as is shown by a normal sugar content of the fluid and the absence of organisms.

In most patients with an intracerebral or subarachnoid hemorrhage, the white cell count of the cerebrospinal fluid is usually in direct proportion to the amount of blood in the fluid. In rare cases of intracerebral hemorrhage the fluid may contain 500 to 4,000 white cells per cu mm and no red cells. We have attributed this to an aseptic meningeal reaction secondary to necrosis of the ventricular wall by hemorrhage which has extended to the ventricles but has not ruptured into them.

When lumbar puncture is performed within twenty-four hours after the onset of a cerebral infarction, the protein content is usually normal if the fluid is clear. A slight elevation (up to 75 mg per 100 ml) is present in about 30% of such cases; but values higher than 100 mg are rare. The protein content of *bloody* fluid is related to the amount of blood present.

When the fluid is clear, the tests for syphilis are negative unless the central nervous system is infected. If the fluid is bloody, the presence of syphilitic reagin in the bloody fluid may cause a false positive reaction. The puncture should be repeated and the fluid tested again after enough time has elapsed for the blood to clear.

The glutamic oxaloacetic transaminase activity is increased in the cerebrospinal fluid in approximately two thirds of the patients with cerebral infarction; the degree of increase is roughly proportional to the size of the lesion.

CHOICE OF NEURORADIOLOGIC PROCEDURES

In cases of suspected vascular episodes, especially when corrective surgery is contemplated, cerebral and aortic arch arteriography should be performed at an appropriate time after the episode. Because arteriography has been known to extend the neurologic deficit during the acute phase, it is important to time this procedure carefully.

Computerized tomography (CT) of the brain is the examination of choice during the acute ictus if the nature of the problem is in doubt. The CT scan will be normal if the patient has ischemia; if infarction, it will remain normal for about twelve hours; and if hemorrhage, it will be abnormal at once. Other information of importance which can be deduced is the presence of edema causing pressure phenomena, hydrocephalus, subdural hematoma, or neoplasm. Several days after onset of infarction, a radiolucency will be easily seen in the area of cerebral edema (Fig. 27). Radiodensity interspersed in the area means that there is hemorrhage. On occasion, the lesion may not be seen without enhancement using *intravenous* injection iodinated contrast material which leaks from the damaged vessels into the parenchyma.

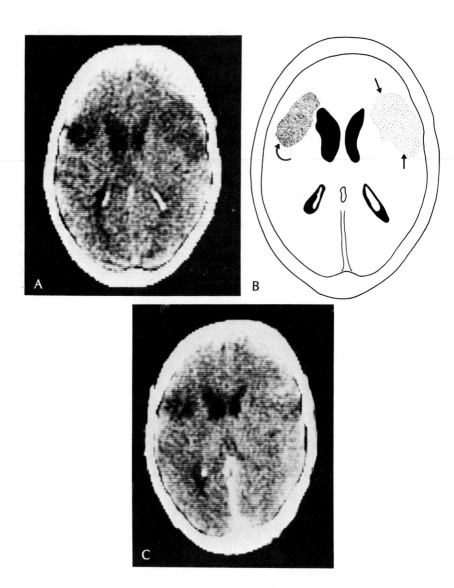

Figure 27. *A, B, C,* Old and recent infarctions. *A* and *B,* Old (curved arrow) and recent (arrows) cerebral infarct in distribution of middle cerebral arteries. There is a shift of the brain to the left because of edema. *C,* Contrast enhancement with Renografin obscures the acute lesion. This emphasizes the necessity for CT scans to be taken both baseline and enhanced with contrast. (Courtesy Dr. Dixon M. Moody.)

In cases of suspected intracranial hemorrhage, CT scan is the procedure of choice (Fig. 28). Location of the blood clot can be identified as an area of increased density. Cerebral angiography can then be performed if an aneurysm or arteriovenous malformation is suspected. Sometimes a large aneurysm can be seen on CT (Fig. 29). The CT scan will be positive even in the earliest intracerebral hemorrhage of appreciable size.

With new generations of fast CT scanners it is probable that regional cerebral blood flow studies will be routinely performed using a readily diffusible gas with high atomic number such as xenon. This has far reaching implications for the diagnosis and treatment of cerebrovascular disease.

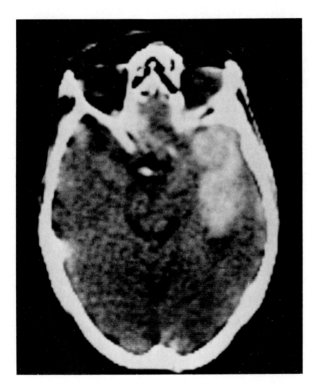

Figure 28. Cerebellar hemorrhage. Homogeneous radiodensity (white area) in central portion of posterior fossa compresses the 4th ventricle (not seen) causing hydrocephalus. Note dilated temporal horns (black densities). (Courtesy Dr. Dixon M. Moody.)

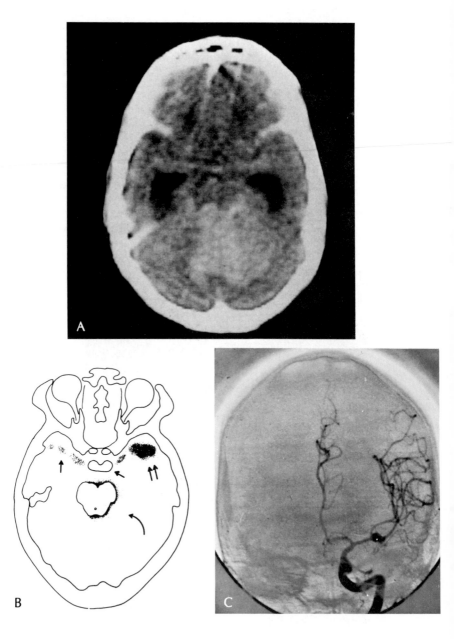

Figure 29. Rupture of a middle cerebral artery aneurysm with subarachnoid hemorrhage. *A*, and *B*, CT scan demonstrates blood in subarachnoid space around brain stem (curved arrow), in sylvian cistern (vertical arrow), and around aneurysm (two arrows). Oblique arrow indicates the dorsum sella. *C*, Angiogram with aneurysm on middle cerebral artery. (Courtesy Dr. Dixon M. Moody.)

DIFFERENTIAL DIAGNOSIS

The diagnosis of a cerebral vascular episode is usually made when focal or general neurologic symptoms suddenly appear in a patient with hypertension, arteriosclerosis, or other evidence of vascular disease.

The logic involved in differential diagnosis is twofold. First, the abnormality must be differentiated from other types of neurologic lesions such as infection, degeneration, or neoplasm; second, an attempt should be made to determine which form of cerebral vascular disorder is present—infarction, hemorrhage, or embolus.

The differential diagnosis is usually not difficult when the history of the patient's illness is known, but is often extremely complicated when the patient is found in a comatose state. For all patients a careful history and examination and the judicious use of laboratory tests are necessary (see page 171).

Although a hemiplegia of sudden onset in a patient with severe hypertension is presumptive evidence of a cerebral vascular lesion, the possibility of uremia or an expanding lesion such as tumor, abscess, or hemorrhage in the cerebrum should not be overlooked. If the patient is comatose and has a normal blood pressure, the diagnostic possibilities include diabetes mellitus, acute alcoholism, extradural or subdural hemorrhage, and drug poisoning.

The odor of acetone on the breath and the presence of sugar in the urine (which may have to be obtained by catheterization) favor a diagnosis of *diabetes*. However, transient glycosuria and even hyperglycemia often occur following cerebral hemorrhage or infarction. The rise in blood sugar which occurs with cerebral vascular episodes is rarely as high as that commonly seen in diabetic coma.

The presence of albumin and casts in the urine favors *uremia*, but this diagnosis cannot be established definitely without a determination of the urea content of the blood. It must also be remembered that cerebral vascular lesions are a common complication of uremia.

An alcoholic odor to the breath, normal blood pressure, no evidence of hemiplegia, and a normal cerebrospinal fluid are characteristic findings in cases of coma due to *acute alcoholism*. The cerebrospinal fluid pressure in some of these cases may be slightly elevated (200 to 300 mm). Since alcoholics are prone to head injuries, the diagnosis of subdural hematoma should always be considered.

Extradural hemorrhage is differentiated from cerebral hemorrhage or infarction by the appearance of symptoms immediately following injury to the head. If the patient is comatose and no history can be obtained, the presence of contusions or lacerations of the scalp which would indicate a head injury is important. Skull radiographs and examination of the cerebrospinal fluid are often helpful. If a fracture of the skull passes through the groove of the middle meningeal artery, the diagnosis of extradural hemorrhage is reasonably certain.

In cases of *subdural hematoma*, it is important that the diagnosis be made promptly because immediate operation may be necessary to save the patient's life. Unfortunately, it is often difficult to differentiate between this condition and other cerebral vascular lesions, especially in cases where the head injury that produced the subdural hemorrhage was relatively minor and occurred several days or weeks before the onset of symptoms. Adding to the difficulty is the fact that hypertension and subdural hematoma frequently occur together.

The diagnosis of subdural hematoma should be considered if there are fluctuations in the patient's state of consciousness and a history of recent head injury. Other clinical findings that favor the diagnosis of subdural hematoma include displacement of a calcified pineal gland on skull radiographs and the presence of blood or xanthochromic cerebrospinal fluid under increased pressure. Occasionally, however, the fluid from a patient with subdural hematoma will be clear, with or without an increase in pressure.

Whenever the diagnosis of subdural hematoma cannot be definitely excluded by the history and examination, a CT brain scan should be performed or small trephine openings made in both temporal regions. False localizing signs are not uncommon in cases of subdural hematomas, nor is it rare to find a clot on both sides.

Neoplasm or *abscess* is usually differentiated from a vascular lesion by the slow and progressive evolution of symptoms. The characteristic findings in patients with brain tumors are "choked discs," normal blood pressure, and clear or slightly yellow cerebrospinal fluid under increased pressure, with a normal cell count and an increased protein content. Exactly the same findings are present in patients with brain abscess, except that the cerebrospinal fluid usually shows mild or moderate pleocytosis.

The history of numerous previous convulsions and the occurrence of a convulsion before the onset of the coma, together with a normal blood pressure and normal cerebrospinal fluid are more likely in the case of epilepsy.

The differential diagnosis between cerebral hemorrhage and cerebral infarction or embolus is important chiefly in regard to the prognosis as to recovery from the "shock" and as to the degree of recovery of the focal neurogic signs. It is also of importance if anticoagulants are to be administered.

The diagnosis of *cerebral embolism* is suggested by the sudden onset of neurologic symptoms in a patient with acute or chronic endocarditis, atrial fibrillation, recent myocardial infarction, septicemia, or a septic focus. In these cases clinical evidence of embolic phenomena is often present elsewhere in the body.

It may be difficult to differentiate between *cerebral hemorrhage* and *infarction*, since both conditions occur in patients of the same age group and in patients with arteriosclerosis and hypertension. The following points favor the diagnosis of intracerebral hemorrhage:

1. Convulsion which is approximately twice as frequent at the onset in such cases as in patients with a cerebral infarction.

2. Severe headache, nausea, or vomiting at the onset.

3. Cheyne-Stokes or labored respirations.

4. Conjugate deviation of the eyes.

5. Stiffness of the neck.

6. Quadriplegia.

7. Bilateral Babinski signs.

8. Bloody cerebrospinal fluid, especially in patients with hemiplegia or aphasia.

In patients with *primary subarachnoid hemorrhage*, headache is a prominent symptom and meningeal irritation, stiffness of the neck, and Kernig's sign develop rapidly. It must be remembered that an aneurysm may be so located that it bleeds into both the subarachnoid space and the cerebrum when it ruptures, in which instance signs suggesting intracerebral hemorrhage will be present.

COURSE

The course of the illness depends on the type and extent of the lesion and the presence or absence of other complicating factors. The mortality is about 80% following an intracerebral hemorrhage of any appreciable size, about 50% following a subarachnoid hemorrhage, and about 30% if a major vessel is occluded by a thrombus. When a small vessel is the site of a thrombus or an embolus, the patient usually survives the insult unless there are serious complicating factors.

In fatal cases the duration of life after the onset of illness varies from a few hours to several months (Table 22). With the exception of rupture of a large aneurysm, cerebral vascular episodes are not a cause of sudden death (within minutes). Death following hemorrhage may occur within three to twelve hours, but as a rule it is delayed for at least one day and often for as long as two weeks. Occasionally a patient with cerebral hemorrhage may live for several months. Death within twenty-four hours is rare in patients with a cerebral infarction or embolus and most commonly occurs several days to several weeks after the onset.

The *focal* neurologic symptoms in cases of cerebral hemorrhage, with few exceptions, are most severe immediately following the onset.

Table 22.   Length of Survival in 243 Cases of Fatal Cerebrovascular
Lesions (in Percentages)

(After Aring and Merritt)

	Hemorrhage		Infarction	
Length of Life after Onset	Intracerebral (115 cases)	Primary Subarachnoid (18 cases)	Athero-thrombosis (89 cases)	Embolism (21 cases)
Less than 12 hours	4	22	0	0
12 to 24 hours	3	11	1	0
1 to 4 days	41	28	30	38
5 to 14 days	39	11	39	38
2 weeks to 2 months	12	22	23	19
2 months to 6 months ...	1	6	7	5
Total	100	100	100	100

In a small percentage of cases an increase in severity or extent over a
period of a few hours may be explained by an increase in the size of the
hemorrhage. Progression of focal neurologic signs is unusual in patients with cerebral infarction or embolism. When it occurs, it can be
explained as due to an independent involvement of other vessels or by
the propagation of thrombus to the point of origin of another branch of
the thrombosed vessel. In patients with thrombosis of the basilar or
posterior inferior cerebellar arteries, however, progression of focal
neurologic signs and symptoms over a period of a few hours or a day or
two is not uncommon.

As a rule, the general symptoms produced by stroke are also most
intense immediately after the onset, but occasionally there will be a
progressive increase in the depth of coma. In fatal cases, the terminal
stage of the disease is characterized by a progressive rise in the
temperature, pulse and respiratory rate, and a decline in the patient's
state of consciousness.

Prognosis

The prognosis for return of function cannot be predicted with any
degree of certainty during the first few days or weeks following a
stroke. In most nonfatal cases there is usually some improvement
which may be dramatic, function being completely restored within a
few hours or a few days. Some attribute the fleeting nature of the
symptoms in such cases to cerebral vascular spasm; but the more
probable explanation is transient cerebral ischemia associated with
microembolism. More commonly, improvement takes place slowly and
usually the patient is left with some permanent residua such as

difficulty in walking, in use of the hand for skilled acts, and in speaking. In some patients there is no improvement.

About half of all patients who survive stroke remain permanently disabled and face the danger of recurrence within weeks, months, or years. About half of the patients suffering cerebral infarction will eventually die of heart disease.

In elderly patients with generalized atherosclerosis, the clinical course may be punctuated by the occurrence of many small cerebrovascular lesions called lacunes. These may produce minimal symptoms and signs such as dizziness, weakness or numbness, and dysarthria.

PREVENTION OF STROKE

An awareness of certain recognizable factors which predispose to stroke—the stroke-prone profile—can be used to identify the person who is at increased risk of stroke and to institute prophylactic measures. First and foremost is the history of hypertension, hyperlipoproteinemia, hyperuricemia, diabetes mellitus, or coronary artery disease in parents and siblings.

In addition to genetic susceptibility, there are various environmental factors such as excessive intake of cholesterol and fat, cigarette smoking, and possibly even chronic psychic stress as exemplified by prolonged emotional upheaval and conflict.

Of the above, sustained hypertension is by far the most important; and it has been determined that if either systolic or diastolic blood pressure is chronically elevated above normal for one's age, the risk of stroke (and also of myocardial infarction) is greatly increased. The higher the blood pressure, the greater the risk. It is essential that families of patients who are known to be hypertensive be screened and those people who are hypertensive be identified early, so that continuous effective reduction of blood pressure to within normal or near normal limits can be achieved. Drugs to decrease platelet adhesiveness are considered by some to be of value in prevention of strokes.

Patients as well as families predisposed to atherosclerosis should be placed on a prudent diet with a relatively low fat and cholesterol intake to maintain them at lean body weight and to reduce the likelihood of development of atherosclerosis and diabetes mellitus. They should be counseled to abstain from using tobacco.

TREATMENT

Therapy can be divided into two phases. The first phase is directed toward saving the life of the patient; the second, toward rehabilitation. A detailed discussion of treatment is contained in the book *Cerebrovascular Disorders* by Toole and Patel.

PHASE I–SAVING LIFE

Medical Treatment of Infarction

Adrenocorticosteroids. Surrounding every cerebral infarction is a zone of edema which, if large enough, can produce complications; some, such as herniation of the uncus through the incisura, can be fatal. In such cases adrenocorticosteroids—for example, dexamethasone 10 mg every six hours—may be life-saving. Their use for patients suffering neurological complications of cranial arteritis can dramatically reverse its process.

Vasodilators. Inhalation of CO_2 and the use of other vasodilators such as papaverine are of no value in arresting or reversing infarction, and may actually do harm by dilating the vascular bed in the normal part of the brain, thus diverting blood away from the ischemic zone.

Anticoagulants. Anticoagulants cannot be expected to produce a resolution of the neurologic signs produced by stroke and should be given only for the purpose of halting their progression or preventing additional episodes. Heparin, coumarin, or warfarin is of value in patients with (1) transient ischemic attacks, (2) arterial emboli usually associated with valvular heart disease, and (3) a predisposition to venous thrombosis.

Anticoagulant therapy should not be given until the possibility of intracranial hemorrhage has been ruled out, or to a patient with hypertension or a tendency to bleeding. Furthermore, in patients suffering with cerebral embolism resulting in sustained neurologic deficit, the prevailing opinion is that anticoagulant therapy should not be used until the possibility of hemorrhagic infarction has subsided—approximately two weeks following the ictus.

Heparin should be given for the first twenty-four to forty-eight hours along with a coumarin drug until the latter has had time to take effect. Then coumarin should be continued alone. There is no agreement as to how long anticoagulant therapy should be continued, but most clinicians administer coumarin for about three months. Patients with recurrent embolic phenomena associated with cardiac disease are an exception and anticoagulants can be continued indefinitely. The appearance of signs of bleeding anywhere in the body is an indication for immediate cessation of anticoagulant therapy and possibly for the administration of vitamin K_1 oxide.

Medications which decrease platelet adhesiveness and aggregation have been advocated for the prevention of transient ischemic attacks which are considered to be the result of fibrin platelet embolism. Of these agents acetyl salicylic acid (aspirin) 600 to 1200 mg daily or dipyridamole appears to be adequate to abolish further episodes.

Nonsurgical Treatment of Hemorrhage

The chief danger to patients with cerebral hemorrhage is death from collapse of the vital centers, which is apt to occur if the bleeding continues. Unfortunately, there is no known method of stopping the hemorrhage unless it is related to a systemic disease such as thrombocytopenic purpura; in such cases transfusions and the administration of vitamin K may be helpful.

Lumbar Puncture. Intracerebral or subarachnoid hemorrhage often leads to increased intracranial pressure, which may be lowered by the removal of cerebrospinal fluid. The procedure seems to be of greatest value in cases of subarachnoid hemorrhage. In patients with primary intracerebral bleeding it may cause transtentorial or foraminal herniation.

Dehydrating Agents. Increased intracranial pressure may also be treated by the rectal administration of 8 ounces of a 25% solution of magnesium sulfate, or by mannitol, glycerol or urea given intravenously. Care should be taken not to cause excessive dehydration.

Surgical Treatment

Operative removal of the hematoma should be considered for all patients who survive the initial hemorrhage and who show evidence of increasing intracranial pressure (papilledema or rising cerebrospinal fluid pressure). Although the results obtained with evacuation of clots deep in the cerebral hemispheres and basal ganglia have been discouraging, removal of clots confined to one lobe of the cerebrum or of the cerebellum have proved life-saving and are often of benefit in decreasing the severity of the neurologic deficit. Unfortunately, the extremely poor general condition of most patients who have had a cerebral hemorrhage is a deterrent to the widespread use of this form of treatment.

Attempts to reestablish the circulation by removal of thrombus from the carotid or vertebral artery or by the reconstruction of arteries stenosed or completely occluded by arteriosclerotic plaques have been effective in preventing the recurrence of symptoms in patients with carotid or vertebral-basilar insufficiency. Operation should be performed during the interval between attacks and not while the patient is in the throes of ischemia or evolving infarction because restoration of high pressure and flow may convert the infarcting area to hemorrhage.

To bypass an occlusive lesion in the internal carotid artery or the middle cerebral artery, anastomosis of the superficial temporal artery, or in some instances, the occipital artery, to a cortical branch of the middle cerebral artery had been advocated.

The indications for microvascular bypass procedures are not yet agreed upon. Initial follow-up of patients undergoing microvascular bypass procedures shows evidence that the procedure may be worthwhile. It is most commonly used for those patients with recurrent transient ischemic attacks who have an inaccessible lesion in the internal carotid artery or the middle cerebral artery with inadequate collateral circulation.

PHASE 2–REHABILITATION

Physical and rehabilitation therapy are of great importance in helping the patient to achieve the maximum recovery of function. The physiatrist should be consulted as soon as possible for advice with regard to the positioning of the patient in bed, and the modes of therapy to be applied in the early and convalescent stages. Therapy directed toward the restoration of function should be begun as soon as the patient has recovered from the initial insult. Massage and passive movements of the affected limbs are useful in preserving circulation and nutrition and help to prevent the development of ankylosis. The slightest voluntary movements should be encouraged. Systematic passive and active exercise of all joints of the affected arm and leg should be done for ten minutes several times a day.

As soon as the patient has regained sufficient strength and his general condition permits, he should be encouraged to sit up in a chair for gradually increasing intervals. Walking should be aided at first by allowing the patient to lean on an attendant. A four-legged walker should be substituted as soon as practicable and discarded only when strength of trunk and leg muscles is sufficient to support the patient. Daily exercise and muscle training should be continued as long as necessary to ensure maximal return of function.

The presence of a sensory defect or hemianopia retards rehabilitation of the hemiplegic patient, but does not make it impossible. In general, it can be said that the results of physical therapy in patients with hemiplegia are directly related to the motivation and diligence of the patient and the therapist.

The treatment of speech disorders requires patience on the part of the therapist and persistent effort on the part of the patient. Best results are obtained when re-education exercises are given by a specialist.

REFERENCES

Austin, G., Laffin, D., and Hayward, W.: Evaluation and Selection of Patients for Microneurosurgical Anastomosis in the Treatment of Cerebral Ischemia. In Current Controversies in Neurosurgery, T. P. Morley, editor, Philadelphia, W. B. Saunders Co., 1976, p. 294–303.

Blaisdell, W. F. et al,: Joint Study of Extracranial Arterial Occlusion: IV. A Review of Surgical Considerations, J.A.M.A., 209, 1889, 1969.

Carter, A. B.: The Immediate Treatment of Non-Embolic Cerebral Infarction, Quart. J. Med., 28, 125, 1959.

Chater, N., Popp, J.: Microsurgical Vascular Bypass for Occlusive Cerebrovascular Disease: Review of 100 Cases, Surg. Neurol. 6, 115, 1976.

Evans, G.: The Clinical Effects on Symptoms of Cerebral Ischemia by Agents Which Affect Platelet Adhesiveness, in Cerebral Vascular Disorders. Proceedings of the Eighth Princeton Conference, New York, Grune & Stratton, 1973.

Graylyl, O., Schmiedek, P., Spetzler, R. et al.: Clinical Experiences with Extra-intracranial Arterial Anastomoses in 65 Cases, J. Neurosurg., 44, 313, 1976.

Hamilton, M., and Kellett, R. J.: The Effect of Antihypertensive Therapy on the Course of Cerebral Vascular Disease, Bull. N.Y. Acad. Med., 45, 933, 1969.

Koos, W. Th., Böck, F. W.: Spetzler, Georg Thieme Verlag, 1976.

Matsumoto, N. et al.: Natural History of Stroke in Rochester, Minnesota, 1955 Through 1969: An Extension of a Previous Study, 1945 Through 1954, Stroke, 4, 20, 1973.

McKissock, W., Richardson, A., and Taylor, J.: Primary Intracerebral Hemorrhage. A Controlled Trial of Surgical and Conservative Treatment of 180 Unselected Cases, Lancet, 2, 221, 1961.

Meyer, J. S.: Modern Concepts of Cerebrovascular Disease, New York, Spectrum Publications Co., 1975.

Millikan, C. H.: Anticoagulant Therapy in Cerebrovascular Disease, in Cerebrovascular Survery Report for Joint Council Subcommittee on Cerebrovascular Disease, National Institute of Neurological Diseases and Stroke and National Heart and Lung Institute. R. G. Sickert, editor, Bethesda, Md., National Institutes of Health, January, 1976.

Moossy, J. et al.: Chairman, Pathology and Laboratory Procedures Study Group, Report of the Joint Committee for Stroke Facilities, III. The Laboratory Evaluation of Neurovascular Disease, Stroke, 3, 505, 1972.

Peszczynski, M. et al.: Chairman, Rehabilitation Study Group, Report of the Joint Committee for Stroke Facilities, II. Stroke Rehabilitation, Stroke, 3, 375, 1972.

Ramey, I. G. et al.: Chairman, Nursing Study Group, report of the Joint Committee for Stroke Facilities, IV. Guidelines for the Nursing Care of Stroke Patients, Stroke, 3, 633, 1972

Sörnäs, R., Ostlund, H., and Müller, R.: Cerebrospinal Fluid Cytology After Stroke, Arch. Neurol., 26, 489, 1972.

Symonds, C., and Mackenzie, L.: Bilateral Loss of Vision from Cerebral Infarction, Brain, 80, 415, 1957.

Thompson, J. E., Austin, D. J., and Patman, R. D.: Carotid Endarterectomy for Cerebrovascular Insufficiency: Long-term Results in 592 Patients Followed up to Thirteen Years, Ann. Surg., 172, 663, 1970.

Whisnant, J. P. et al.: Chairman, Prevention Study Group, Report of the Joint Committee for Stroke Facilities, V. Clinical Prevention of Stroke, Stroke, 3, 806, 1972.

Wylie, E. J., and Ehrenfeld, W. K.: Extracranial Occlusive Cerebrovascular Disease, Diagnosis and Management, Philadelphia, W. B. Saunders Co. 1970.

Yasargil, M. G.: Microsurgery Applied To Neurosurgery, New York, Academic Press, 1969.

SYNDROMES PRODUCED BY VASCULAR LESIONS IN THE BRAIN

Ischemia and Infarction

Thrombosis or embolism of the individual cerebral arteries produces syndromes that are characteristic for each artery. Because a knowledge of these syndromes is important in making the differential diagnosis between cerebrovascular lesions and other diseases of the brain, the clinical pictures produced by occlusion of the more important vessels are described in detail.

Carotid System

Common and Internal Carotid Arteries. Occlusion of the common or internal carotid does not produce any neurologic deficit in persons with normal aortocranial circulation because of the extensive anastomoses between the two carotid systems and between the carotid and the vertebral-basilar systems (see page 150). Because atherosclerosis usually affects more than one artery, asymptomatic atheromatous stenosis or occlusion is not common, although cases have been reported in which 1 to 4 of the arteries supplying the brain have been occluded without producing symptoms. Abnormalities are found in the extracranial arteries in more than one half of the patients with symptomatic cerebral infarction.

The internal carotid supplies the homolateral eye and the frontal lobe, as well as parts of the temporal and parietal lobes. The hallmarks of major disease in this vessel are transient attacks of homolateral blindness, contralateral hemiplegia or hemianesthesia and, if the lesion is in the dominant hemisphere, aphasia. These episodes usually terminate within five to thirty minutes but may last as long as twenty-four hours; they are probably caused by emboli originating from a plaque in the neck and lodging in the intracranial arteries. Isolated or recurrent ischemic episodes of this nature are observed in about one third of patients who eventually have infarction. In about a third of the patients the episodes subside, leaving no residuum.

The onset of symptoms and signs of occlusion of the internal carotid artery may be sudden or may follow one of these transient attacks, leading to hemiplegia or hemiparesis with a cortical type of sensory loss. Aphasia occurs when the dominant hemisphere is infarcted; homonymous hemianopia is present in about 10% of the cases; and rarely homolateral blindness may occur if the ophthalmic artery is occluded. Occasionally coma is one of the initial features of the disease.

Anterior Cerebral Artery. The anterior cerebral artery gives off short ganglionic branches which travel through the anterior perforated space to supply the anterior limb of the internal capsule, the head of the caudate nucleus, and the putamen. Then the trunk courses forward, upward and then backward over the corpus callosum providing blood to it and to the medial surface and superior part of the cerebral hemisphere (paracentral lobule) (Fig. 30). The area of the motor and sensory cortex which controls the legs is within the distribution of this vessel. In the dominant hemisphere, the subcortical white matter beneath Broca's speech area is nourished by ganglionic branches.

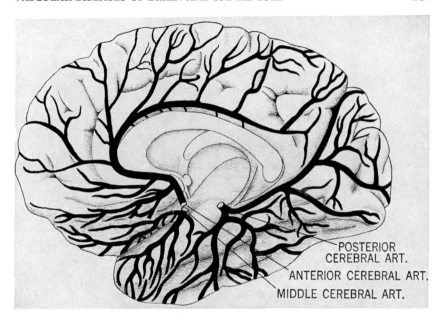

POSTERIOR CEREBRAL ART.
ANTERIOR CEREBRAL ART.
MIDDLE CEREBRAL ART.

Figure 30. Mesial view of cerebral hemispheres showing distribution of anterior and posterior cerebral arteries. (Merritt. H. H., Adams, R. D., and Solomon, H. C.: *Neurosyphilis,* courtesy Oxford University Press.)

Occlusion of the proximal portion of the anterior cerebral artery is uncommon, but obstruction of one or more of its branches is not infrequent and is followed by paralysis and sensory loss affecting chiefly the leg of the opposite side. If the dominant hemisphere is affected, the picture may include mental confusion, clouding of consciousness, and aphasia—symptoms thought to result from infarction of the central white matter of the frontal lobe and the white matter beneath Broca's area.

Middle Cerebral Artery. The middle cerebral artery nourishes the lateral portions of the cerebral hemisphere including the parietal cortex and subcortical white matter of the insula, and the lateral part of the frontal, temporal and parietal lobes (Fig. 31). It also gives off the lenticulo-optic and lenticulostriate arteries which supply the head of the caudate nucleus and the anterior limb of the internal capsule as well as the putamen, external capsule, and claustrum (Fig. 32).

The middle cerebral artery and its branches are occluded more frequently than any other cerebral vessel except possibly the internal carotid artery. Occlusion of the main trunk causes softening of a large portion of the cerebral hemisphere with the resultant contralateral hemiplegia, hemianesthesia, and homonymous hemianopia. If the

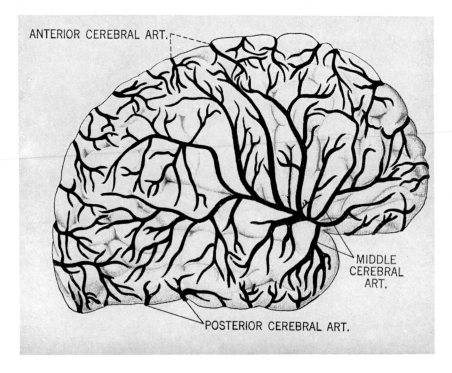

Figure 31. Lateral view of cerebral hemisphere showing distribution of middle cerebral artery. (Merritt, H. H., Adams, R. D., and Solomon, H. C.: Neurosyphilis, courtesy Oxford University Press.)

dominant hemisphere is involved, aphasia is also present. Athero-thrombosis or embolism occurs more commonly in one or more of the branches than in the main trunk itself; as a consequence the entire syndrome of the middle cerebral artery is rare and fragments such as hemiplegia, alexia, agnosia, apraxia, or word deafness appear as isolated phenomena. Unlike the hemiplegia that follows anterior cerebral artery occlusion, the paralysis of the face and arm is often more complete than that of the leg.

Posterior Cerebral Artery. This artery usually arises from the basilar artery but is sometimes a branch of the internal carotid. It conveys blood to the inferior and medial portions of the posterior temporal and occipital lobes (including the area striata), and to the optic thalamus by way of the thalamogeniculate and thalamoperforating branches.

If the main trunk of the artery is thrombosed, both the thalamus and the occipital lobe are damaged and the signs will consist of the thalamic syndrome together with homonymous hemianopia. Should the thalamogeniculate branch alone be involved, only the thalamic

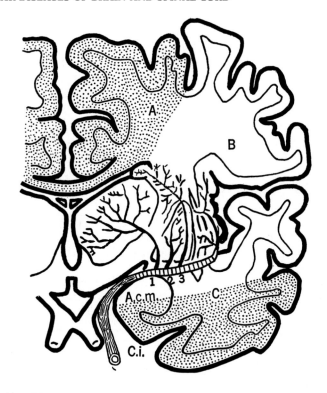

Figure 32.   Sagittal section of cerebral hemisphere showing tissue irrigated by A, anterior cerebral, B, middle cerebral, C, posterior cerebral arteries. (Merritt, H. H., Adams, R. D., and Solomon, H. C.: *Neurosyphilis*, courtesy Oxford University Press.)

syndrome will develop; if just the calcarine branches are thrombosed, contralateral homonymous hemianopia is the only clinical sign. Thrombosis of smaller branches may give rise to parts of these syndromes.

The usual components of the thalamic syndrome are a flaccid type of transient hemiparesis or hemiplegia; permanent impairment of superficial sensation and loss of deep sensation; agonizing, burning pain; and choreoathetoid movements, ataxia or tremor. All these signs and symptoms occur on the side opposite the lesion. In some instances involving the dominant hemisphere, occlusion in the vertebrobasilar distribution results in thalamic infarction with aphasia and at times permanent amnestic syndrome.

Occlusion of the thalamoperforating artery results in softening of the anterior portions of the thalamus and destroys the termination of the dentatorubro-thalamic pathway and subthalamic structures; the ventrolateral nucleus, which is the terminus of the secondary sensory pathways is spared. The chief clinical sign of thrombosis of the thalamoperforating artery is the choreoathetoid movements of the opposite extremities without significant loss of cutaneous sensibility.

Bilateral Multiple Infarctions (Pseudobulbar Palsy). The term *bulbar palsy* is used to describe a syndrome characterized by paralysis or weakness of the muscles supplied by the medulla oblongata (bulb). *Pseudobulbar* palsy may result from bilateral lesions in the cerebral hemisphere due to any cause but is most common in patients with multiple cerebral infarctions. The usual sequence of events is infarction with residual hemiplegia, followed by infarction in the other hemisphere, so that both sides of the body and the bulbar muscles are affected. Pseudobulbar palsy may occur without paralysis of the extremities if the lesions are localized in the corticobulbar fibers. This syndrome ofter includes a loss of emotional control, with unprovoked outbursts of laughing or crying, especially when corticothalamic fibers are interrupted.

The Vertebral-Basilar System

Vertebral Arteries. The two vertebral arteries give off many branches to muscles in the neck through which they anastomose with muscular branches of the external carotid artery. Branches to the spinal cord anastomose at several levels with the anterior median spinal artery, and at the level of the foramen magnum each vertebral artery gives rise to a spinal ramus which joins with that of the opposite side to form the anterior median spinal artery. The posterior spinal artery and the posterior inferior cerebellar arteries are also branches of the vertebral (page 150).

After entering the cranium through the foramen magnum the vertebral arteries travel along the anterior surface of the medulla oblongata until they join together at the pons to form the basilar artery.

Symptoms resulting from occlusion of a vertebral artery are indistinguishable from those caused by occlusion of a posterior inferior cerebellar artery.

Basilar Artery. The basilar artery (Fig. 33) is formed by the junction of the two vertebral arteries and supplies blood to the pons, midbrain, and cerebellum. It terminates by forming the two posterior cerebral arteries.

Occlusion of the basilar artery produces symptoms which vary depending upon the site of the occlusion and the efficiency of the collateral circulation; only rarely is it asymptomatic. Sudden occlusion of the basilar artery produces sudden coma and disastrous neurologic damage (Fig. 34). In many patients, however, infarction is preceded by attacks of focal neurologic symptoms and signs (transient ischemic attacks). These attacks commonly consist of vertigo, difficulty with or

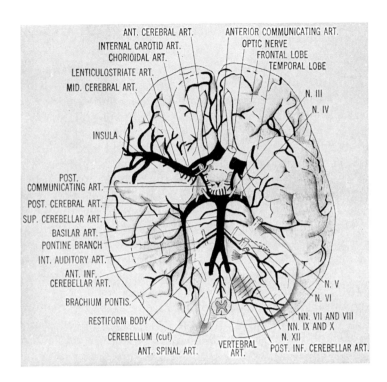

Figure 33.   Arterial circulation of the base of the brain. (Merritt, H. H., Adams, R. D., and Solomon, H. C.: *Neurosyphilis*, courtesy Oxford University Press.)

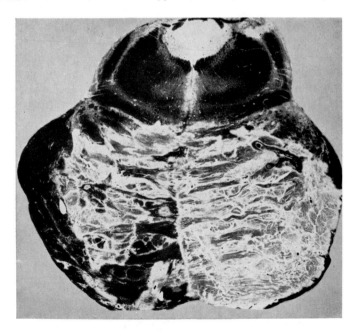

Figure 34.   Necrosis of pons and midbrain due to basilar artery occlusion (not shown). Myelin sheath stain. (Courtesy Dr. Philip Duffy.)

191

slurring of speech, confusion, transient loss of postural tone (drop attacks), hemiplegia or paresthesias on one side of the body. The findings of basilar thrombosis include disorders of the eye movements, blindness and pupillary abnormalities. Unilateral or bilateral paralysis of the third, fourth, or sixth nerves; disorders of gaze; and involvement of the descending sympathetic pathways occur in a small percentage of the cases. The pupils are usually small and fixed to light, but when the nucleus of the third nerve is damaged the pupil is large and fixed to both light and accommodation. Pseudobulbar signs (dysarthria, dysphagia, bilateral facial weakness, and paralysis of the tongue) may be found. A crossed paralysis with involvement of one of the cranial nerves (usually the oculomotor) and paralysis of the opposite side of the body is seen occasionally. The deep reflexes are increased and bilateral extensor plantar responses are common. Sphincter incontinence is almost always present.

The syndromes resulting from insufficiency in the circulation of the individual vessels which supply the brain stem have been named after the authors who first described them, but it is more sensible to refer to these syndromes in terms of the zone of the brain stem which has been damaged. Each side of the brain stem can be divided into two areas: (1) the paramedian and (2) the lateral. The paramedian area is nourished by short perforating arteries which arise from the basilar or vertebral arteries. The lateral area is supplied by surface conducting arteries which travel some distance from their point of origin before entering the brain stem.

1. *Paramedian area.* The structures in the paramedian area which are associated with identifiable deficits are the somatic motor nuclei of the third, fourth, sixth, and twelfth cranial nerves; the medial lemniscus; and the corticospinal tract. Occlusions of vessels in this area result in paralysis of one or more cranial nerves on the same side of the body as the lesion and paralysis of the arm and leg on the contralateral side (alternating hemiplegia).

Midbrain: When the softening is limited to the third nerve nucleus and the cerebral peduncle, there is ophthalmoplegia on the side of the lesion and paralysis of the arm and leg on the opposite side (Weber's syndrome). The ophthalmoplegia is characterized by ptosis of the lid and a dilated pupil fixed to light and accommodation. The eyeball is deviated outward as result of paralysis of the median rectus muscle. Because of the considerable length of the oculomotor nucleus and its emerging fibers, a small lesion may not destroy all the cells and fibers. In such cases some of the muscles innervated by the third nerve may be spared.

If the softening includes the medial lemniscus and red nucleus, contralateral hemianesthesia and involuntary movements of a choreiform nature are also present (Benedikt's syndrome).

Pons: Occlusion of the paramedian arteries in the pons produces a softening in the nucleus of the sixth nerve, the seventh nerve as it hooks around the sixth nucleus, and the corticospinal tract (Millard-Gubler syndrome). The eye on the side of the lesion is deviated inward because of paralysis of the abducens muscle. If the lesion is extensive, there is paralysis of conjugate gaze to the side of the lesion—that is, paralysis of inward movements of the eye opposite the lesion as well as paralysis of outward movements of the homolateral eye. All the muscles on the homolateral side of the face are paralyzed and there is paralysis of the arm and leg on the contralateral side. Rhythmic contractions of the palate (palatal myoclonus) may occur with any vascular lesion of the brain stem which injures the olivo-dentato-rubral connections. This condition most commonly results in lesions involving the paramedian area of the pons.

Medulla oblongata: Occlusion of one of the arteries supplying the paramedian area in the medulla causes softening which involves the pyramid, the nucleus of the twelfth nerve, the medial lemniscus and the medial portion of the olive. The result is paralysis and atrophy of the homolateral half of the tongue, paralysis of the opposite arm and leg and impairment of the tactile sensation in the trunk and extremities on the paralyzed side.

2. *Lateral area.* The circumferential arteries that supply the lateral area of the brain stem also nourish the cerebellum. Thrombosis in one of these vessels will cause dysfunction of the cerebellar hemisphere and of the nuclei and tracts in the lateral portion of the brain stem. The important structures in this area of the brain stem are the visceral motor nuclei of the fifth, seventh, and tenth cranial nerves; the sensory nuclei of the fifth and eighth cranial nerves; the descending sympathetic pathways; and the ascending spinal lemniscus.

Midbrain: The lateral area of the midbrain is supplied by the superior cerebellar artery. Thrombosis of this vessel produces a syndrome with contralateral hemiplegia and hemisensory deficit as well as symptoms of cerebellar dysfunction, including homolateral choreiform movements—the result of damage to the brachium conjunctivum. The impairment of pain and temperature involves the entire contralateral half of the body.

Pons: The anterior inferior cerebellar artery supplies the lateral area of the brain stem in the region of the pons. Thrombosis of this vessel produces a clinical picture which includes homolateral deafness, facial paralysis, Horner's syndrome, and loss of touch sensibility in the face (all on the side of the lesion); and impairment of pain and temperature

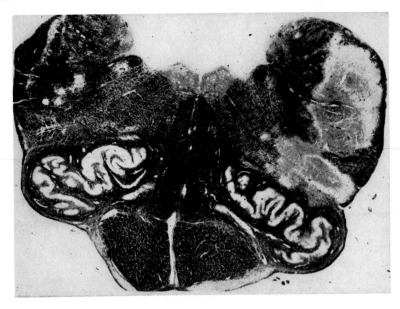

Figure 35. Encephalomalacia in territory of posterior inferior cerebellar artery
resulting from thrombosis of vertebral artery.

in the contralateral arm, leg, trunk, and occasionally face. Nystagmus
and homolateral cerebellar signs are also present. The main sensory
nucleus of the fifth nerve and the nuclei of the seventh and eighth
cranial nerves are involved along with corticobulbar and corticospinal
fibers and the spinothalamic tract.

  Medulla oblongata: The lateral area of the medulla oblongata is
supplied by the posterior inferior cerebellar artery which arises from
the vertebral artery (Fig. 35). The signs and symptoms that result from
occlusion of these arteries (Wallenberg's syndrome) include dysphagia
and dysarthria due to weakness of the homolateral palatal muscles
(innervated by the nucleus ambiguus of the tenth nerve); impairment of
pain and temperature sense on the homolateral side of the face
(descending root and tract of the trigeminal nerve); Horner's syndrome
on the side of the lesion (descending sympathetic fibers); nystagmus
(vestibular nuclei); cerebellar dysfunction in the homolateral arm and
leg (restiform body and cerebellum); and impairment of pain and
temperature on the opposite half of the body (spinal lemniscus).

Intracerebral Hemorrhage

  The signs and symptoms produced by bleeding depend upon its size
and location in the brain. A pea-sized hemorrhage in the centrum

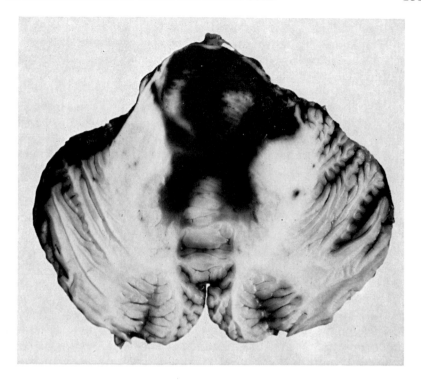

Figure 36. Hypertensive (primary) pontine hemorrhage with extension
into the fourth ventricle.

semiovale causes no detectable signs or symptoms, whereas a similar
lesion strategically located in the brain stem causes widespread abnormalities. Because the basal ganglia and adjacent internal capsule are
affected in more than two thirds of hemorrhages, hemiplegia with or
without a hemianopia or hemianesthesia is common. Hemorrhages into
other locations within the cerebral hemisphere produce signs accompanying destruction of the nervous tissue in those areas first, and then
secondary effects from the mass of blood which acts as a tumor if the
hemorrhage is large. Signs and symptoms of increased intracranial
pressure may develop, and in cases of brain stem or cerebellar hemorrhage there may be signs of an acutely expanding posterior fossa lesion
for which emergency neurosurgical decompression is necessitated.

Lacunar State (État Lacunaire)

Sustained hypertension accelerates atherosclerosis and their dual
effects are doubly dangerous. Small arteries and arterioles already
thickened as a result of hypertension may become occluded with

thrombus, while others may be plugged with emboli from atherosclerotic plaques in larger arteries upstream. The microinfarctions
which result are called "lacunes" (pools). A multiplicity of lacunes is
called the "lacunar state" (état lacunaire).

Lacunes are the most common cerebral vascular lesions found at
autopsy of elderly patients. They appear as irregular cavities from 0.5 to
15.0 mm in size, are usually multiple and distributed through the
putamen, pons, thalamus, caudate nucleus, internal capsule, corona
radiata, and cerebellar white matter, roughly in that order of frequency.
Lacunes result from occlusion of penetrating arteries of the paramedian
group and are not related specifically to disease of the internal carotid
artery or diabetes mellitus. They usually represent the end stage of
hypertensive vascular disease, although at times a small embolus from
an ulcerated atherosclerotic plaque can produce lacunar infarction.

In most patients these lesions apparently do not cause recognizable
symptoms and signs. However, five characteristic syndromes have
been described. Those resulting from single lacunes are:

1. Homolateral cerebellar ataxia and pyramidal tract signs in which
there is weakness involving legs more than arms. The responsible
lesion is thought to lie where the corona radiata funnels into the
internal capsule. The ataxia, which involves the leg more than the arm,
is probably caused by damage to the corticopontine-cerebellar pathways rather than by actual involvement of the cerebellum.

2. Isolated hemiplegia. This syndrome most commonly results from
infarction in the internal capsule (less commonly in the basis pontis),
on the side opposite the hemiplegia. Of course there is no sensory
deficit or aphasia.

3. The "dysarthria-clumsy hand syndrome," characterized by a
sudden onset of moderate to severe dysarthria, accompanied by central
facial weakness, deviation of the tongue on protrusion, slight dysphagia, weakness, clumsiness and awkwardness of the affected hand,
and ataxia demonstrable on the finger-to-nose test. Mild imbalance is
noted on walking, and examination reveals some asymptomatic corticospinal tract signs. The lesion responsible is probably in the pons.

4. Pure sensory stroke involving the face, arm, and leg. The patient
complains of paresthesias described as numbness, tingling, stiffness, a
pressing sensation, or a dead feeling. The affected side may feel
distorted in size or compressed as in a vise. This syndrome is probably
the result of a lacune in the posterolateral nucleus of the thalamus.

5. The clinical picture occurring in association with multiple
lacunes is the same as that found in pseudobulbar palsy (described on
page 190). Because these lesions are located bilaterally in the basal
ganglia and the brain stem, patients are commonly misdiagnosed as
having Parkinson's disease, particularly since they may eventually

become quite rigid and have a small-stepped gait. The patient does not, however, develop tremor at rest.

The practical importance of these lacunar syndromes is that once they are diagnosed, angiography is not needed. The parenchymatous lesions are too small to be seen on CT scan. Furthermore, anticoagulants are potentially harmful because the patients are almost always hypertensive. The treatment of choice then is gradual reduction of systemic arterial blood pressure to levels which are more nearly normotensive for the patient's age.

Fibromuscular Hyperplasia

Fibromuscular hyperplasia is a disease of the intima and media of large arteries which produces hyperplastic changes of a segmental nature along their course. This can result in segmental stenosis of the lumen and occasionally aneurysmal dilatation. The disorder is of unknown etiology and is not the result of atherosclerosis or inflammation. It most commonly occurs in women and it may be found in renal, coronary, and cervicocranial arteries. There are a few reports of intracranial and vertebral artery involvement but most commonly the disease is found in the cervical portion of the internal carotid artery. It is usually asymptomatic in nature and is discovered by a physician who listens to the neck for murmurs. Some patients develop ischemia in the area of distribution of the involved artery, in which case surgical reconstruction of the artery with dilatation of the stenoses is often successful.

In other patients, there may be associated intracranial arterial aneurysms which may need treatment (see section on aneurysm, page 199).

Hypertensive Encephalopathy

Although the term hypertensive encephalopathy is sometimes used loosely to indicate any type of cerebrovascular disease in patients with hypertension, it actually designates an acute or subacute disorder of the nervous system developing as a result of severe hypertension and renal disease (usually malignant nephrosclerosis but occasionally glomerulonephritis or chronic pyelonephritis).

The pathogenesis of the symptoms has not been clearly elucidated; however, edema is the most striking feature observed at autopsy. In addition, numerous small infarcts and petechial hemorrhages are found in the cortex. In occasional cases a massive hemorrhage is the cause of death.

The common symptoms are headache; convulsions; amaurosis; transient periods of confusion, stupor or coma; and in some cases focal neurologic signs such as hemiplegia, aphasia, or hemianopia. Papilledema, hemorrhages and exudates in the retina, severe hypertension, and urinary abnormalities due to concomitant renal disease are present in almost all cases. The cerebrospinal fluid may be under increased pressure, and in some cases contains an increased amount of protein, with values occasionally as high as 200 mg per 100 ml.

Hypertensive encephalopathy is distinguished from uremia because the blood urea nitrogen is normal or only slightly elevated. In cases of malignant nephrosclerosis, however, uremia and hypertensive encephalopathy may occur together as terminal events. Confusion with tumor of the brain is hardly likely in the presence of the severe hypertension with kidney damage. Treatment consists of rapid reduction of systemic arterial pressure to the range of 140/80 mm Hg by whatever means is necessary. Details may be found in *Cerebrovascular Disorders* by Toole and Patel.

Brain Death

Patients with intracranial vascular castastrophes may lose all brain function despite the continuation of heart beat and detectable blood pressure. If the following clinical conditions are met, the diagnosis of brain death can be made and all life-support systems can be stopped: the absence of all neural reflexes; no movement, either spontaneous or reflex; no spontaneous respirations; pupils that are dilated and fixed to light; and no deviations of the eyes in response to caloric testing. In addition the patient must not be hypothermic or show evidence of poisoning and there must be no detectable electrical activity on two successive electroencephalograms made twelve to twenty-four hours apart. If an EEG is not available, the total and persistent absence of all clinically elicitable brain stem reflexes will have the same connotation.

REFERENCES

SYNDROMES PRODUCED BY VASCULAR LESIONS IN THE BRAIN

Becker, D. P., Robert, C. M., Jr., Nelson, J. R., and Stern, W. E.: An Evaluation of the Definition of Cerebral Death, Neurology, *20*, 459, 1970.

Beecher, H. K.: Ethical Problems Created by the Hopelessly Unconscious Patient, N. Engl. J. Med., *278*, 1425, 1968.

Biemond, A.: Thrombosis of the Basilar Artery and the Vascularization of the Brain Stem, Brain, *74*, 300, 1951.

Bradshaw, P., and Casey, E.: Outcome of Medically Treated Stroke Associated with Stenosis or Occlusion of the Internal Carotid Artery, Br. Med. J., *1*, 201, 1967.

Cook, A. W., Plaut, M., and Browder, J.: Spontaneous Intracerebral Hemorrhage, Arch. Neurol., *13*, 25, 1965.

Dustan, H. P. et al.: The Effectiveness of Long-Term Treatment of Malignant Hypertension, Circulation, *18*, 644, 1958.

Fisher, C. M. et al.: Acute Hypertensive Cerebellar Hemorrhage: Diagnosis and Surgical Treatment, J. Nerv. & Ment. Dis., *140*, 38, 1965.

Foley, J. M.: Precipitating Factors in Focal Cerebral Ischemia, in *Modern Neurology: Papers in Tribute to Derek Denny-Brown*, edited by S. Locke, Boston, Little Brown & Co., 1969, pp. 491–496.

Gifford, R. W., Jr., and Richards, N. G.: Hypertensive Encephalopathy. I. Etiology, Pathology, and Clinical Findings, Curr. Concept. Cerebrovas. Dis.—Stroke, *5*, 43, 1974.

Gurdjian, E. S., Darmody, W. R., and Thomas, L. M.: Recurrent Strokes Due to Occlusive Disease of Extracranial Vessels, Arch Neurol., *27*, 447, 1969.

Hunt, T. K., Blaisdell, F. W., and Okimoto, J.: Vascular Injuries of the Base of the Neck, Arch. Surg., *98*, 586, 1969.

Janeway, R. et al.: Vertebral Arterial Obstruction with Basilar Impression: An Intermittent Phenomenon Related to Head Turning, Arch. Neurol., *15*, 211, 1966.

Javid, H. et al.: Natural History of Carotid Bifurcation Atheroma, Surgery, *67*, 80, 1970.

Kubik, C. S., and Adams, R. D.: Occlusion of the Basilar Artery, Brain, *69*, 6, 1946.

Maddison, F. E., and Moore, W. S.: Ulcerated Atheromas of the Carotid Artery, Am. J. Roentgen., *107*, 540, 1969.

Moossy, J.: Cerebral Infarcts and the Lesions of Intracranial and Extracranial Atherosclerosis, Arch. Neurol., *14*, 124, 1966.

Patel, A. and Toole, J. F.: Subclavian Steal Syndrome Reversal of Cephalic Blood Flow, Medicine, *44*, 289, 1965.

Rey-Billett, J.: Cerebellar Hemorrhage, Neurology, *10*, 217, 1960.

Simeone, F. A., and Goldberg, H. I.: Thrombosis of the Vertebral Artery from Hyperextension Injury to the Neck, J. Neurosurg., *29*, 540, 1968.

Sindermann, F., Bechinger, D., and Dichgans, J.: Occlusions of the Internal Carotid Artery Compared with Those of the Middle Cerebral Artery, Brain, *93*, 199, 1970.

Ziegler, D. K., Zosa, A., and Zileli, T.: Hypertensive Encephalopathy, Arch. Neurol., *12*, 472, 1965.

SPONTANEOUS SUBARACHNOID HEMORRHAGE AND INTRACRANIAL ARTERIAL ANEURYSMS

The most common cause of bleeding into the subarachnoid space is trauma to the head. Hemorrhage into the subarachnoid space may also occur in patients with blood dyscrasias, intracranial neoplasms, arteriovenous malformations, certain toxic or infectious diseases of the nervous system, or intracerebral hemorrhages. In this section we will consider only spontaneous subarachnoid hemorrhage and intracranial arterial aneurysm.

Among the 6,368 cases reported in *Intracranial Aneurysms and Subarachnoid Hemorrhage: A Cooperative Study*, 1966, 92% had subarachnoid hemorrhage; 51% resulted from intracranial aneurysm, 8% from arteriovenous malformation, and 0.9% from a combination of these two lesions. In 43% no intracranial vascular lesions could be found on angiography. In 70% of the cases the hemorrhage was presumably related to hypertension, and in about 2% it was due to a blood dyscrasia. In 4% a neoplasm was found, and another 4% had emboli. In 13% no cause could be ascertained. These results will change because of the increased use of CT scans of the cranium which delineate lesions precisely and permit repeated examination to assess changing conditions.

In cases of subarachnoid hemorrhage, the overall mortality was 44%. Nearly a third of these deaths occurred within two days of the onset, another 18% occurred within seven days, and a total of 76% occurred within six weeks. Of those who died, 85% were found at autopsy to have parenchymatous as well as subarachnoid hemorrhage. However, the percentages differ in children because arteriovenous malformation is more common than aneurysm.

Intracranial Aneurysms

Incidence. Intracranial aneurysms are found in approximately 4% of all autopsies performed on adults, and the autopsy statistics from general hospitals show that approximately 10% of all cerebral vascular lesions are due to rupture of an intracranial aneurysm. In patients younger than forty-five, however, intracranial aneurysms are responsible for more than 50% of all fatal cerebral vascular lesions. In the age range from forty-five to sixty-four, the incidence is 14%; after sixty-five years it falls to about 2%.

Symptoms related to an aneurysm in the subarachnoid space may develop at any age, but appear most commonly between forty-five and sixty (Table 19, page 164). In the Cooperative Study, 4,880 patients with first subarachnoid hemorrhage and aneurysms were reported; 2% were under twenty years of age; 16% were between twenty and thirty-nine; 65% were between forty and sixty-four; and 17% were over sixty-five. The two sexes were represented about equally.

Pathologic Considerations. The vast majority of aneurysms in the subarachnoid space are due to a congenital weakness of the involved vessels. In most cases this weakness is the result of maldevelopment of the media, particularly at the point of bifurcation where the muscular coat is incomplete, allowing the intima to bulge through. In some cases the media is weak as a result of a systemic abnormality affecting the connective tissue (Ehlers-Danlos syndrome). Other conditions that may be responsible for intracranial aneurysms include septic emboli (which cause mycotic aneurysms), syphilis and arteriosclerosis. Among the 572 cases reported by McDonald and Korb in 1939, the vessels were normal in 32.7%; arteriosclerotic changes were found in 49.5%, syphilitic changes in 5.6%, and mycotic aneurysms in 12.2%. Most of the mycotic aneurysms were found in young patients and were associated with bacterial endocarditis. Arteriosclerotic changes were most common in patients over forty. The frequenoies of the different types of aneurysms have changed over the years and mycotic and syphilitic aneurysms are now uncommon.

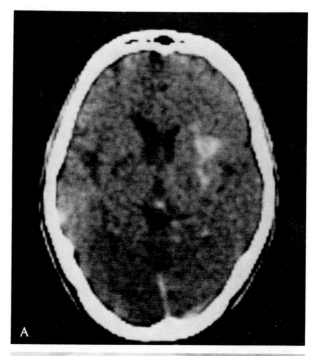

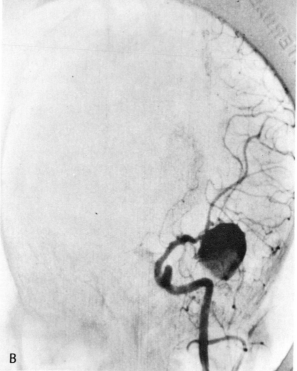

Figure 37. Giant middle cerebral artery aneurysm with hemorrhage into temporal lobe. *A,* On CT scan the round density in the anterior portion of the middle cranial fossa is the aneurysm. The amorphous density posterior to the aneurysm is the hematoma. *B,* Cerebral angiogram demonstrates the aneurysm and elevation of the middle cerebral artery by the hematoma. (Courtesy Dr. Dixon M. Moody.)

Intracranial aneurysms range in size from the microscopic to those as large as an orange (Fig. 37). It is quite likely that an individual aneurysm may vary in size from time to time; for example, a small aneurysm may dilate and later regress somewhat. Small aneurysms do not cause any pathologic changes in the nervous system unless their location is such that they compress one of the cranial nerves. The larger aneurysms may erode the sella turcica and base of the skull and compress neighboring cerebral tissue, the pituitary gland and cranial nerves. Some aneurysms lie free in the meshes of the subarachnoid space; others are partially buried in the substance of the brain.

Although any of the intracranial arteries may be the site of an aneurysm, over 95% of these lesions occur in the internal carotid distribution (Table 23). The vast majority are located near the basilar surface of the skull, but some are found in the hemispheric fissures— most commonly, the fissure of Sylvius. The larger aneurysms may be partially or completely filled with an organized clot which occasionally may be calcified. Intracranial aneurysms are usually single, but two or more have been found in approximately 20% of the cases.

Symptoms and Signs. Arteriosclerosis and hypertension are common findings in middle-aged or elderly patients with intracranial aneurysms, and in patients with mycotic aneurysms septic foci may be observed.

The symptoms and signs produced by intracranial aneurysms may be divided into those resulting from compression of cranial nerves or cerebral substance, and those due to bleeding. Pressure by an unruptured aneurysm on cranial nerves or on the brain itself may result in focal neurologic deficits and occasionally headaches or seizures. The most common deficits are visual defects and partial or complete paralysis of the muscles supplied by the third or the sixth nerve. Depending upon whether the optic nerve, chiasm, or optic tract is

Table 23.   Site Distribution of Single Aneurysms

	No. of Cases	%
Middle cerebral	529	20.0
Internal carotid	1104	41.2
Anterior cerebral	895	33.5
Posterior cerebral	22	0.8
Basilar	77	2.9
Vertebral	25	0.9
Cerebellar	20	0.7
Total	2672	100

Sahs, Perret, Locksley, and Nishioka, *Intracranial Aneurysms and Subarachnoid Hemorrhage.* Philadelphia, J. B. Lippincott, 1969.

compressed by the aneurysm, the visual defect may consist of amblyopia in one eye, bitemporal hemianopia, or a homonymous field defect. The other focal neurologic signs are usually associated with a large aneurysm involving one of the branches of the middle cerebral artery in the sylvian fissure or one of the branches of the vertebral-basilar arterial system in the posterior fossa.

In more than 90% of the cases intracranial aneurysms are "silent" until they rupture. Symptoms develop in most patients while they are pursuing their normal daily activities, and in approximately a third during sleep. Only occasionally is the rupture related to trauma or to physical exertion. The initial symptom in most cases is pain in the head or headache which is localized to the occipital region or to one side. The headache usually becomes generalized in the later stages and is followed in most cases by the development of confusion, delirium, or lethargy. In about 15% the onset of hemorrhage is marked by convulsions, usually of a generalized nature. Loss of consciousness at the onset is a grave prognostic sign. Stiffness of the neck and Kernig's sign occur in practically all cases within a few hours of the onset.

Cranial nerve palsies, particularly of the third nerve, may develop as a result of sudden compression of the nerves or hemorrhage into their sheaths. Occasionally there are hemorrhages into the eye, commonly subhyaloid in location. The tendon reflexes may be hyperactive on the paralyzed side. The plantar response may be extensor on both sides, even in the absence of any paralysis.

The vital signs may be entirely normal, particularly if the hemorrhage is a small one. More commonly, however, the temperature is moderately elevated (100 to 102° F) for the first few days after the hemorrhage and the pulse and respiratory rates are slightly increased. Hypertension is present in more than 50% of the cases (Tables 22 and 23).

Laboratory Data. Although leukocytosis is often present, the significant laboratory findings are in the cerebrospinal fluid. The pressure is almost always increased, the usual range being from 200 to 600 mm of cerebrospinal fluid. The fluid is uniformly bloody, the amount of blood depending on the size of the hemorrhage. The white cell count and the protein content of the fluid are increased in proportion to the number of red blood cells.

In nonfatal cases, the protein content and the white cell count decrease as the fluid becomes less bloody. However, there may be a relative increase in the white blood cells, presumably caused by the irritating effect of the blood in the meninges.

Diagnosis. The diagnosis of subarachnoid hemorrhage due to ruptured aneurysm is suspected in any patient who has sudden onset of headache followed by stiffness of the neck and one or more of the other symptoms described above. Acute bacterial meningitis and other conditions in which there is bleeding into the subarachnoid space must be considered. The differential diagnosis of subarachnoid hemorrhage from intracerebral hemorrhage, cerebral trauma, cerebral tumors, and vascular malformations is considered on pages 178 and 179. The entire intracranial arterial system must be visualized by arteriography in order to ascertain the cause and location of the bleeding and in addition to determine whether there are multiple vascular abnormalities or anomalies such as an unusual configuration to the circle of Willis or multiple arterial aneurysms.

If a ruptured aneurysm is the cause of hemorrhage, cerebral angiography will demonstrate the aneurysm in approximately 80% of the cases. In the remaining 20% the aneurysm is either too small or technical problems such as vasospasm or poor contrast prevent visualization of the bleeding point.

Course and Prognosis. The mortality is much greater in patients with ruptured aneurysms than in those who have no demonstrable cause for bleeding.

The clinical course of patients who survive the first few hours is subject to considerable variation. In some fatal cases the aneurysm may continue to leak slowly until it finally bursts again after a few days. In others, the aneurysm may seal off completely only to rupture suddenly after a varying interval of time. In patients whose rupture heals, the blood in the subarachnoid space is removed and the symptoms of headache and mental cloudiness gradually improve, The headache becomes intermittent before it disappears entirely in the course of a few weeks. When focal neurologic signs are present, they usually improve to some extent or disappear entirely.

In a few cases, internal hydrocephalus develops as a sequel to spontaneous subarachnoid hemorrhage. It is apparently due to the development of adhesive arachnoiditis in the basal cisterns. In rare cases pituitary insufficiency ensues because of damage to the gland by blood or by a large aneurysm. In other cases, inappropriate secretion of anti-diuretic hormone results in reduced urinary output and fluid retention.

Treatment. Once the definitive diagnosis has been made by four vessel angiography, the patient should be sedated and blood pressure kept in slightly hypotensive ranges with antihypertensive medication if necessary. Analgesics should be prescribed for headache and repeated lumbar punctures to control intractable headache. Epsilon amino caproic acid (EACA) accelerates the clotting process and should be administered in the majority of cases to help prevent repeat hemorrhage.

If the angiogram reveals a large subdural hematoma or intracerebral hematoma, this should be evacuated as an emergency. In those patients who do not exhibit marked arterial spasm and who show little neurological deficit, surgery should be carried out in about seven to fourteen days to prevent recurrent hemorrhage.

More advances have been made in the surgical treatment of intracranial aneurysms than probably any other field of neurosurgery over the past ten years. The present methods of direct exposure of the aneurysm with an operating microscope, adrenocorticosteroids, hypotension, and drainage of CSF for brain relaxation result in an operative mortality and morbidity of less than 5% to 10%. The great majority of aneurysms are surgically accessible and should be clipped. Those which cannot be clipped should be reinforced with plastics. Carotid artery ligation should be reserved for internal carotid artery aneurysms in selected patients.

Arteriovenous Malformations. About half of patients with arteriovenous malformations do well with medical management. About 20% die because of intracerebral hemorrhage and another 20% develop a significant disability over the years with progressive hemiparesis, mental confusion, severe headaches, and uncontrolled seizures.

The larger central arteriovenous malformations which present with seizures should be treated with anticonvulsant therapy alone. Smaller arteriovenous malformations which demonstrate a propensity for bleeding and which are located in an accessible area can be removed. The operating microscope and bipolar coagulation have greatly decreased the morbidity and mortality of surgical treatment. Embolization of arteriovenous malformation with various materials also offers hope for improved surgical management.

The evacuation of large intracerebral hematomas and subdural hematomas secondary to arteriovenous malformations may be life saving.

REFERENCES

SPONTANEOUS SUBARACHNOID HEMORRHAGE AND INTRACRANIAL ANEURYSMS

Drake, C. G.: Intracranial Aneurysms, in The Nervous System, The Clinical Neurosciences, edited by Donald B. Tower, 2, 287, 1975.

Drake, C. G., and Girvin, J. P.: The Surgical Treatment of Subarachnoid Haemorrhage With Multiple Aneurysms. In: Controversies in Neurosurgery, edited by T. P. Morley. Philadelphia, W. B. Saunders Co., 1976, p. 275–278.

du Boulay, G. H.: Some Observations on the Natural History of Intracranial Aneurysms, Br. J. Radiol., 38, 721, 1965.

Duvoisin, R. C., and Yahr, M. D.: Posterior Fossa Aneurysms, Neurology, 15, 231, 1965.

Forster, F. M., and Alpers, B. J.: Anatomical Defects and Pathological Changes in Congenital Cerebral Aneurysms, J. Neuropath. & Exptl. Neurol., 4, 146, 1945.

French, L. A., Chou, S. N.: Conventional Methods of Treating Intracranial Arteriovenous Malformations. In: Progress in Neurological Surgery, Krayenbuhl. H., Maspes, P., Sweet, W., editors, Vol. 3, Basel & New York, S. Kayer, 1967.

Hudson, C. H., and Raaf, J.: Timing of Angiography and Operation in Patients with Ruptured Intracranial Aneurysms, J. Neurosurg., 29, 37, 1968.

Luessenhop, A. J. et al.: Surgical Management of Primary Intracerebral Hemorrhage, J. Neurosurg., 27, 419, 1967.

McCormick, W. F., and Nofzinger, J. D.: Saccular Intracranial Aneurysms. An Autopsy Study, J. Neurosurg., 22, 155, 1965.

McKissock, W., Richardson, A., Walsh, L., and Owen, E.: Multiple Intracranial Aneurysms, Lancet, 1, 623, 1964.

Mount, L. A., and Brisman, R.: Treatment of Multiple Intracranial Aneurysms, J. Neurosurg., 35, 728, 1971.

Nibbelink, D. W., and Sahs, A. L.: Cooperative Study of Intracranial Aneurysms and Subarachnoid Hemorrhage, in Cerebrovascular Survey Report for Joint Council Subcommittee on Cerebrovascular Disease, National Institute of Neurological Diseases and Stroke and National Heart and Lung Institute, R. G. Sickert, editor, Bethesda, Md., National Institutes of Health, 1970, pp. 176–193.

Pool, J. L.: Treatment of Arteriovenous Malformations of the Cerebral Hemispheres, J. Neurosurg., 19, 136, 1962.

Pool, J. L., and Potts, D. G.: Aneurysms and Arteriovenous Anomalies of the Brain: Diagnosis and Treatment, New York, Hoeber Medical Division, Harper & Row, 1965.

Slosberg, P.: Non-operative Management of Ruptured Intracranial Aneurysms. In: Clinical Neurosurgery, Baltimore, Williams & Wilkins, 1944, pp. 90–98.

Svien, H. J. and McRae, J. A.: Arteriovenous Anomalies of the Brain. Fate of Patients not Having Definite Surgery, J. Neurosurg., 23, 23, 1965.

Yarsargil, M. G.: Microneurosurgery Applied to Neurosurgery. Stuttgart, Georg Thieme Verlag, 1969, pp. 119–150.

VASCULAR DISEASES OF THE SPINAL CORD

Anatomic Considerations

The greatest portion of the blood is supplied to the cord by the anterior median spinal artery which arises from paired spinal rami and runs along its entire length on the anterior surface. The pial arteriolar plexus and the paired posterior spinal arteries supply the posterior aspect of the cord. These arteries all originate from the vertebral arteries. The anterior and posterior systems are joined at various levels by other arteries that spring from the aorta and the vertebral, subclavian and iliac arteries (Figure 38).

In the cervical region, the anterior median artery is reinforced at several levels by unpaired medullary arteries arising from the vertebrals and the blood supply is rich.

In the thoracic segment where the anterior median spinal artery is joined by only a few branches of the thoracic aorta, the blood supply is sparse. For this reason and because the midthoracic cord is supplied only by the terminal portions of blood columns that descend from the subclavian-vertebral arteries and ascend from the abdominal aorta, the thoracic cord is particularly predisposed to vascular insufficiency and infarction.

The blood supply to the lumbar and sacral cord is derived from a

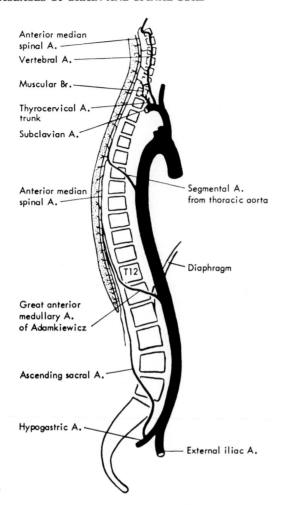

Anterior median spinal A.

Vertebral A.

Muscular Br.

Thyrocervical A. trunk

Subclavian A.

Anterior median spinal A.

Segmental A. from thoracic aorta

Diaphragm

T12

Great anterior medullary A. of Adamkiewicz

Ascending sacral A.

Hypogastric A.

External iliac A.

Figure 38. The anterior median spinal artery is joined at various levels by arteries which arise from the vertebral and subclavian arteries, the aorta, and the iliac arteries.

particularly large artery, the great anterior medullary artery, which is usually found at the level of L_1 or L_2 (occasionally as high as T_{12} or as low as L_4). This artery, which may be paired or single, travels through the appropriate vertebral foramen on the nerve root and anastomoses with the anterior median spinal artery. The conus medullaris and the cauda equina are supplied by sacral branches ascending from the iliac arteries.

The venous system is plexiform and interconnects freely with the radicular veins lying within the subarachnoid space. These radicular veins empty into the epidural venous plexus, which in turn communicates with the inferior vena cava and the azygos system through the perivertebral plexus.

Infarction (Myelomalacia)

Softening or infarction of the spinal cord (myelomalacia) occurs whenever there is an occlusion of the anterior median spinal artery or one of its main collaterals.

Etiology. Although atherosclerosis is the most common cause, spinal infarction may result from syphilis and tuberculosis. When there is a severe inflammatory reaction in the meninges such as acute purulent meningitis, tuberculous meningitis or syphilitic meningitis or after an intraspinal injection, thrombosis may occur without any proliferative changes in the walls of the spinal vessels. The anterior spinal artery or one of its major collaterals may be occluded by an abscess in the epidural space or by extramedullary tumors, especially metastatic tumors or Hodgkin's granuloma. Occlusion of the intercostal or lumbar branches of the aorta may result from a dissecting or arteriosclerotic aneurysm of the aorta. In rare cases, infarction of the cord has followed contrast angiography of the abdominal aorta, or angiography of any major spinal artery tributary. Treatment consists of CSF exchange lavage to remove the iodinated material. This may be due to a direct toxic effect of the contrast material. Compression of the spinal cord by an extradural hemorrhage as a complication of anticoagulant therapy is another possible cause of softening.

Symptoms and Signs. The symptoms and signs produced by thrombosis of the anterior spinal artery or one of its main collaterals depend on the level of the lesion. If the occlusion is in the *cervical* region, there is a sudden onset of tetraplegia, incontinence of urine and feces, and impairment or loss of pain and temperature sensation below that level. The focal atrophy and paralysis of the arms and hands are due to destruction of the anterior horn cells, and paralysis of the trunk and legs is due to corticospinal tract damage. The effects produced by. occlusion of the anterior spinal artery in the *thoracic* region are similar, except that the arms are spared.

If the arterial occlusion is in the *lumbar* region, the clinical signs include paraplegia, disturbances of urination and defecation, and impairment of pain and temperature sensation. The paralysis below the level of the lesion is usually flaccid in the initial stage. The loss of pain and temperature sense is greater than that for other modalities. The deep reflexes may be absent for an indefinite period; when they return, they are brisk. The plantar responses are extensor.

Diagnosis. A vascular lesion of the spinal cord should be suspected whenever the symptoms of transverse myelitis appear suddenly. Since arteriosclerosis so rarely causes thrombosis of spinal vessels, some other etiology should be sought. The possibilities of Hodgkin's disease or a tumor which has metastasized to the spine must always be considered.

Compression of the cord by extramedullary tumors causes a much more gradual onset of paralysis than that produced by vascular lesions. It must be remembered, however, that in Hodgkin's disease or metastatic carcinoma the vascular lesions of the cord sometimes lead to partial or complete subarachnoid block. In these cases, the onset of symptoms may be sudden.

Differentiation between vascular lesions of the spinal cord and acute transverse myelitis or myelopathy of multiple sclerosis can be extremely difficult unless other portions of the nervous system show signs of involvement by these diseases.

Prognosis. The prognosis for return of function is poor in patients with an acute lesion of the spinal cord secondary to occlusion of its blood supply.

Treatment. In patients with infarction of the cord, one must treat not only the symptoms produced by the neurologic lesion but also the underlying disease. Because of the severe degree of sensory loss, excellent nursing care is essential. Unless the skin is kept scrupulously clean and the patient's position is changed frequently, the development of extensive decubiti is almost inevitable. The bladder should be emptied by catheterization, and permanent bladder drainage should be established by means of a suprapubic cystotomy or by an indwelling catheter. The paralyzed limbs should be massaged and exercised passively several times daily.

Treatment of the disease responsible for the thrombosis of the spinal vessels includes chemotherapy for acute purulent meningitis, antisyphilitic treatment for syphilitic meningitis or endarteritis, and x-ray treatment for metastatic carcinoma or Hodgkin's disease. Unfortunately, such treatment cannot be expected to produce any significant degree of improvement, since it is impossible to restore nervous tissue that has been destroyed.

Hematomyelia

Etiology. Hematomyelia, or hemorrhage into or upon the substance of the cord, is practically always due to trauma. Only in rare cases is it the result of a blood dyscrasia or the rupture of an arteriovenous malformation or an arteriosclerotic blood vessel.

Pathologic Findings. In the initial stage the cord is swollen at the site of the hemorrhage, and some blood may extend several segments above and below the level of the hemorrhage. On section a fresh clot is seen filling the central part of the cord. Although the most severe damage to the gray matter of the cord, the white matter may be partially or entirely destroyed at the site of the hemorrhage. If the patient survives, the blood is liquefied and removed by phagocytes. Since glial replacement is usually incomplete, a syrinx or cavity is formed at the site of the lesion and sometimes extends over several segments of the cord.

Symptoms and Signs. The symptoms of hematomyelia develop suddenly, in most cases immediately after an injury to the spine such as occurs in falls or in diving. The severity of the symptoms depends on the size of the hemorrhage. If the hemorrhage is small there may be only spastic weakness associated with hyperactive reflexes in the lower extremities and a transient disturbance of bladder control. If the hemorrhage is large there will be signs of a physiologic transection of the cord: (1) flaccid paralysis of the muscles and a dissociated sensory loss in the segments at the level of the lesion; and (2) flaccid paralysis, complete sensory loss, absent reflexes, and loss of sphincter control below this level. As the blood is absorbed, the deep reflexes return and become hyperactive and the patient's symptoms improve. Mobility of the lower extremities returns, and the sensory loss becomes less severe; but muscles innervated by the segments at the level of the lesion become atrophied.

Differential Diagnosis. Other diseases of the cord cause signs of physiologic transection, but hematomyelia may be differentiated, since the sudden onset that follows severe trauma excludes practically all other conditions except compression of the cord by fracture and dislocation of one or more vertebrae. The diagnosis is made by x-ray films and by lumbar puncture, which gives evidence of complete subarachnoid block.

Treatment. Treatment in the early stages of hematomyelia is similar to that for myelomalacia. In the later stages of hematomyelia, however, physical therapy is more important because of the greater degree of spontaneous recovery and the possibility of partial or complete rehabilitation. In some cases braces to support the trunk and lower extremities may be required to enable the patient to walk.

REFERENCES

VASCULAR DISEASES OF THE SPINAL CORD

Djindjian, R. et al. Angiography of the Spinal Cord, Baltimore, University Park Press, 1970.

Garland, H., Greenberg, J., and Harriman, D. G. F.: Infarction of the Spinal Cord, Brain, 89, 645, 1966.

Gillilan, L. A.: Arterial and Venous Anatomy of the Spinal Cord, in Cerebral Vascular Diseases, Transactions of the Seventh Princeton Conference, J. Moossy and R. Janeway, editors, New York, Grune & Stratton, 1971, pp. 3–9.

Harik, S. I., Raichle, M.D., and Reis, D. J.: Spontaneously Remitting Spinal Epidural Hematoma in a Patient on Anticoagulants, N. Engl. J. Med., *284*, 1355, 1971.

Henson, R. A., and Parsons, M.: Ischaemic Lesions in the Spinal Cord, An Illustrated Review, Quart. J. Med., *36*, 205, 1967.

Herdt, J. R., DiChiro, G., and Doppman, J. L.: Combined Arterial and Arteriovenous Aneurysms of the Spinal Cord, Radiol., *99*, 589, 1971.

Kempinsky, W. H.: Paraparesis Associated with Atherosclerotic Aneurysm of Abdominal Aorta, Neurology, *6*, 368, 1957.

Margolis, G.: Circulatory Dynamics of the Spinal Cord, in *Cerebral Vascular Diseases*, Transactions of the Seventh Princeton Conference, J. Moossy and R. Janeway, editors, New York, Grune & Stratton, 1971, pp. 10–17.

Moersch, F. P., and Sayre, G. P.: Neurologic Manifestations Associated with Dissecting Aneurysm of the Aorta, J.A.M.A., *144*, 1141, 1950.

Toole, J. F.: Some Vascular Disorders Affecting the Spinal Cord, Curr. Concept. Cerebrovas Dis. Stroke, *4*, 11, 1969.

Chapter 3

Tumors

INTRACRANIAL TUMORS

General Considerations

The term *intracranial tumor* includes all neoplasms arising from the skull, meninges, blood vessels, ductless glands, cranial nerves, brain tissue or congenital rests, as well as metastatic tumors, parasitic cysts, granulomas, lymphomas, and vascular malformations.

Classification. Intracranial tumors may be divided into nine subdivisions as follows:

1. Tumors of the skull
   A. Hyperostosis
   B. Osteomas
   C. Hemangiomas
   D. Metastatic
   E. Granulomas
   F. Involvement of the skull in systemic diseases
      a. Xanthomatosis
      b. Osteitis deformans
2. Tumors of the meninges
   A. Meningiomas (arachnoidal fibroblastoma)
   B. Gliomatosis
   C. Sarcomatosis
   D. Metastatic
3. Tumors of the cranial nerves
   A. Gliomas of the optic nerve
   B. Neurofibromas
4. Tumors of the supportive tissue (gliomas)
5. Tumors of the ductless glands
   A. Pituitary
   B. Pineal
6. Congenital tumors
   A. Craniopharyngiomas
   B. Cholesteatomas
   C. Chordomas
   D. Teratomas and dermoids
   E. Cysts
7. Blood vessel tumors
   A. Hemangioblastomas
   B. Angiomas
8. Granulomas and parasitic cysts
   A. Tuberculomas
   B. Syphilomas
   C. Parasitic cysts
   D. Cryptococcal granulomas
9. Metastatic

Pathology. The symptoms which develop with various types of intracranial tumors are related to the nature of the tumor and to its location. These are dependent in part upon the destructive nature of the growth and in part upon the secondary effects of increased intracranial pressure. Details of the pathological changes will be considered in the discussion of the various types of tumors.

Pathogenesis. Almost nothing is known of the cause or mode of growth of primary intracranial tumors. Inheritance plays no significant role except in rare conditions such as von Recklinghausen's disease and tuberous sclerosis. Since our knowledge is so meager, it is not surprising that trauma should be presumed as a causative or precipitating factor. Individual cases have been reported in which, after an interval of months or years, tumors (particularly meningiomas) have developed in the neighborhood of injured intracranial structures. There are no statistics, however, to indicate that intracranial tumors are common sequels of minor or severe injuries to the head.

Brain tumors have been produced in animals by chemical carcinogens, such as anthracine derivatives and N-nitroso compounds, and by viruses. These experiments have not helped in the understanding of the pathogenesis of brain tumors in man.

Incidence. The incidence of intracranial tumors and of the various sub-types in hospital statistics depends not only upon the diagnostic skill of the staff members but also upon the presence on the staff of skilled neurosurgeons and neurologists to whom these cases are referred by the general practitioner. The statistics of the past century indicated that tumors of the brain are present in approximately 2% of all necropsied cases. At the present time, intracranial tumors, of primary or secondary nature, constitute a larger proportion of admission to a neurological service than any other disease of the nervous system with the exception of cerebral vascular disease associated with arteriosclerosis and the acute or subacute infectious diseases of the nervous system.

Frequency of Various Sub-types. The exact frequency of various sub-types of intracranial tumors is not known. For obvious reasons, hospitals with large neurological and neurosurgical clinics (Table 24) show a higher percentage of the slower growing tumors in their statistics than do general hospitals without such services. In the latter

Table 24.   Incidence of the Various Types of Intracranial Tumors

	Number of Cases			
Type of Tumor	Cushing	Grant	Total	%
Gliomas	862	1010	1872	43
Meningiomas	271	407	678	15
Pituitary Adenomas	360	206	566	13
Acoustic Neuromas	176	110	286	6.5
Metastatic	85	196	281	6.5
Congenital	113	70	183	4
Blood Vessel Tumors	41	64	105	3
Miscellaneous	115	263	378	9
Total	2023	2326	4349	100.0

there is a preponderance of the more malignant gliomas and metastatic tumors. Parasitic and granulomatous tumors are rare in the United States and Europe, but are still occasionally found in South America, Asia, and Africa.

Age Incidence. Intracranial tumors of all types may have their initial symptoms at any age. In general, however, they occur predominantly in early adult life or in middle age. They are relatively infrequent before the age of ten and after the age of seventy. While a few general statements may be made concerning the age incidence of the various sub-types of tumors, it must be realized that there are numerous exceptions. The common tumors of childhood and the first two decades of life (Table 25) are gliomas of the cerebellum, brainstem and optic nerve, pinealomas, craniopharyngiomas, teratomas and granulomas. Tumors of adult life and early middle age include meningiomas, neurofibromas, gliomas of the cerebral hemisphere, particularly glioblastoma multiforme, and the pituitary tumors. Metastatic tumors are most frequent in late middle life.

Sex Incidence. Intracranial tumors in general are slightly more common in men. Cerebellar medulloblastomas, cerebral astrocytomas and glioblastomas are more commonly seen in men than in women while the reverse is true of the meningiomas and acoustic neuromas.

Symptomatology. The signs and symptoms of intracranial tumors are customarily divided into two groups. The first or general symptoms include a wide variety of manifestations presumably due to a disturbance of cerebral function resulting from edema, increased intracranial pressure and other unknown factors. The second group is composed of special symptoms and signs which can be attributed to localized destruction or compression of nervous tissue.

Special Symptoms and Signs. Since there is no significant difference between the special symptomatology of intracranial tumors and that of

Table 25.   Tumors of the Brain in Children and Adolescents

Type of Tumor	No. of Cases	%
Gliomas	94	57
Craniopharyngiomas	26	16
Hemangiomas	12	7
Meningeal Tumors	10	6
Tuberous Sclerosis	6	4
Metastatic	4	2
Neurofibromas	3	2
Pituitary Adenomas	2	1
Various or Unclassified	9	5
Total	166	100

other types of lesions, they will not be discussed in detail here. Constellations of symptoms which may occur with a particular type of tumor or with tumors which have a predilection for certain localities are discussed in the appropriate section.

General Symptoms and Signs. It must be stated at the outset that no constellation of symptoms is pathognomonic of an intracranial tumor. Headache, vomiting, and choked disc, the triad of symptoms commonly considered characteristic of brain tumors, may appear early in the course of some cases, in others not until the terminal stages, while in some it may never develop at all. Other general symptoms and signs of intracranial tumors are convulsive seizures, abnormal states of consciousness, mental symptoms, and diplopia or blurred vision. Vasomotor phenomena, cardiac arrhythmias or bradycardia may appear as terminal symptoms.

Headaches. The headaches which occur in patients with intracranial tumors cannot be differentiated either by their nature or their location from headaches due to other causes. Severe recurrent headaches in a person previously free of them should put one on his guard. The headache may be localized, but more commonly it is generalized or more intense in the frontal or occipital region, regardless of the location of the tumor. Localized tenderness of the scalp or the underlying skull is not of absolute localizing value, but it is occasionally found in close relationship to the tumor. The headaches of intracranial tumors are usually intermittent, occurring at irregular intervals and lasting for several minutes or hours. They may be increased by change of posture, coughing or straining. With progress of the growth they tend to become more frequent and of longer duration. The incidence of headaches in patients with brain tumors is high (estimated at 90 per cent by some authors) but its absence, especially when there are few other generalized symptoms, cannot be taken as evidence that a tumor is not present. The cause of the headaches is not known. They are not directly related to the level of intracranial pressure and it is probable that pressure on or traction of pain-producing structures (dura, blood vessels or nerves) plays a role in their appearance.

Nausea and Vomiting. Nausea and vomiting are much less frequent than headache. Projectile vomiting without nausea or headache is rare and it usually occurs as a symptom of a cerebellar tumor in childhood.

Choked Discs. Swelling of the optic nerve head with engorgement of the retinal veins and hemorrhages into the nerve and adjacent retina (choked disc) is a common finding in patients with intracranial tumors, but absence of these changes in the optic nerve cannot be taken as evidence against the diagnosis. The incidence of choked discs is variously estimated as between 50 and 90% of the cases, depending to a great extent upon the stage of the disease at which the examination is made. The nature and location of the tumor are also important factors in the development of choked discs. In general, it may be said that choked discs appear early in all patients with intracranial tumors of whatever nature if they are so located as to interfere with the circulation of the cerebrospinal fluid and produce an internal hydrocephalus. Thus, tumors which occlude the third ventricle, the cerebral aqueduct, fourth ventricle or the foramina of exit of the fluid in the posterior fossa produce a high incidence of choked discs. Examples of such tumors are gliomas of the thalamus, cysts of the third ventricle, pinealomas, and posterior fossa tumors in general (cerebellopontine angle tumors, medulloblastomas, and cerebellar astrocytomas or hemangioblastomas). On the other hand, large tumors can invade and entirely destroy one of the cerebral hemispheres without producing choked discs. Tumors which are confined to the cerebral hemisphere do not cause choked discs until they grow to a size for which the natural elasticity of the intracranial contents cannot compensate. Intracranial tumors with a relatively low incidence of choked discs are pituitary adenomas, slowly growing cerebral astrocytomas, small meningiomas on the convexities of the cerebral hemispheres and gliomas of the brainstem.

The pathological physiology underlying the development of choked discs has never been clearly elucidated. It is generally assumed to be due to an increase in the pressure in the central retinal vein. Its appearance in patients with a brain tumor is practically always accompanied by other evidence of increased intracranial pressure, such as an increase in the cerebrospinal pressure or changes in the bones of the skull (increase in digital markings and erosion of the clinoid process of the sella turcica) in the roentgenograms. On the other hand, even in the presence of a high degree of increased intracranial pressure, the optic discs may be normal. In patients with a tumor compressing the optic chiasm or optic nerve, the optic disc may be atrophied without any evidence of "choking." If a tumor compressing one optic nerve grows to a size sufficient to produce a generalized increase in intracranial pressure, there may be optic atrophy in one eye and choked disc in the other (Foster Kennedy syndrome). In these cases the tumor is on the side opposite to that of the choked disc. With this exception an unequal degree of swelling in the two optic discs has no localizing value and is possibly related to a difference in the intraocular tension in the two eyes. Choking of the discs is rarely seen in patients with a high degree of myopia, or with preexisting optic atrophy.

It is not always possible to differentiate with certainty between the choked discs due to intracranial tumor and swelling of the nerve head associated with multiple sclerosis, other demyelinating diseases or arterial disease of the retina. As a rule in choked disc the swelling of the nerve head is greater than in the optic neuritis of multiple sclerosis. The hemorrhages in the retina in choked disc are usually confined to the nerve head or the adjacent retina, while in arterial disease of the retina, hemorrhagic areas are often found at a distance from the nerve head. Characteristic of the latter condition, also, are changes in the caliber and silver wire appearance of the arteries.

Visual acuity is normal in the early stages of choked disc, but there is an enlargement of the blind spot, proportional to the degree of swelling

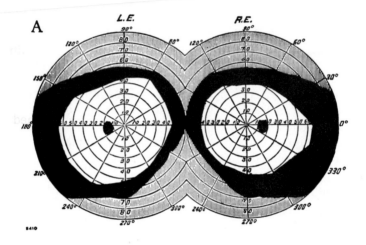

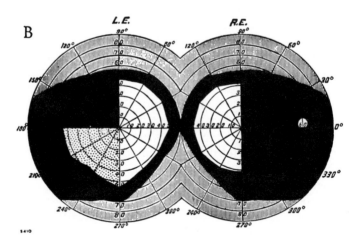

Figure 39.   Visual field defects in intracranial tumors. *A*, Enlargement of blind spots and constriction of peripheral fields with increased intracranial pressure. *B*, Bitemporal hemianopia with pituitary adenoma. (Merritt, H. H., Mettler, F. A., and Putnam, T. J.: Fundamentals of Clinical Neurology, courtesy The Blakiston Co.)

of the nerve head. These findings are so characteristic of choked disc that they serve as a fairly accurate differential between choked disc and optic neuritis. In the latter, visual acuity is usually greatly diminished and there may be central or para-central scotomata, with or without enlargement of the blind spots.

When swelling of the optic disc persists for many weeks or months, a secondary type of atrophy develops in the optic nerve. The peripheral fields are constricted (Fig. 39) and there is a gradual failure of central vision which sometimes progresses to complete amblyopia. As the atrophy of the nerve head advances, there is usually a decrease in the degree of choking of the disc.

Convulsions. Convulsive seizures of a focal or generalized nature are common in patients with tumors in the cerebral hemispheres (Table 26), they are rare with tumors in the brainstem or posterior fossa (Table 27). The focal seizures of brain tumor do not differ in any way from those which occur with organic lesions in the brain from other causes (birth injury, head injury, etc.). Nor do the generalized seizures differ from those of so-called idiopathic epilepsy, except that rarely, if ever, does one find the classical petit mal attacks with their characteristic wave and spike formation in the electroencephalographic tracings. Prolonged coma following a generalized seizure or transient

Table 26. Incidence of Convulsions in Cerebral, Cerebellar and Pituitary Tumors

	No. of	Cases with Seizures	
Location of Tumor	*Cases*	*Number*	*%*
Cerebrum	397	138	35
Cerebellum	247	12	5
Pituitary	79	0	0
Total	723	150	21

Table 27. The Incidence of Convulsive Seizures in 247 Patients with Tumors of the Cerebellum

Type of Seizure	No. of Cases	% (247 cases)
Generalized	6	2.4
Jacksonian	1	0.4
Cerebellar fits	5	2.0
Total	12	4.8

hemiparesis (Todd's paralysis) following a jacksonian, focal or generalized seizure is more common in patients with a tumor than in those having convulsive seizures caused by other conditions.

Seizures are not infrequently the first symptom of an intracranial tumor and this diagnosis must be considered in all patients with seizures, especially if the first attack occurs after the third decade of life. Seizures may be the predominating or only symptom of slowly growing tumors for several or many years.

With tumors of the cerebral hemispheres the incidence of seizures is roughly proportional to the length of time the tumor has been present. They occur in nearly 70% of the vascular tumors of the cortex; in over 50% of the astrocytomas; in approximately 40% of the meningiomas and in about one fourth of the rapidly fatal glioblastomas (Table 28).

Since tumors in any portion of the cerebral hemispheres may cause generalized convulsive seizures, this symptom in itself has no localizing value (Table 29). Jacksonian or focal sensory seizures localize the lesion to the motor-sensory strip of the opposite hemisphere. Seizures preceded by or consisting mainly of olfactory or gustatory hallucinations (uncinate fits) localize the lesion to the temporal lobe, but do not indicate the side of the lesion. Visual phenomena preceding or accompanying a convulsive seizure localize the lesion to either the temporal or occipital lobe, but usually these symptoms have no lateralizing value. As a rule, hallucinations of formed images with or without an auditory accompaniment occur with lesions in the temporal lobe and unformed images (flashes of lights) with lesions in the occipital lobe. Hemianoptic visual field defects indicate that the tumor is in the opposite temporal or occipital lobe. Psychomotor seizures may occur

Table 28. The Relative Frequency of Convulsive Seizures in Various Types of Tumors of the Cerebral Hemisphere
(Modified from Hoefer, Schlesinger and Pennes,
A. Res. Nerv. & Ment. Dis., Proc., 1947)

Type of Tumor	No. of Cases	% with Seizures
Hemangioma and blastoma	13	69
Cysts	5	60
Astrocytoma	85	55
Abscess	12	50
Meningiomas	84	41
Metastatic tumors	34	35
Glioblastomas	149	31
Other gliomas	34	26
Subdural hematoma	17	23

Table 29.   The Frequency of Various Types of Seizures in 47 Patients with Astrocytomas of the Cerebral Hemispheres
(Modified from Hoefer, Schlesinger and Pennes,
A. Res. Nerv. & Ment. Dis., Proc., 1947)

Type of Seizure	Frontal	Temporal	Parietal	Occipital	Two or More Lobes
Generalized	12	5	3	2	4
Jacksonian	2	..	1	..	..
Focal (motor)	9	2	3	..	9
Focal (sensory)	2	..	1	..	2
Aphasia	..	1	1	..	1
Uncinate	..	2	..	..	2
Visual	..	1	..	1	1
Auditory	..	..	1	..	..
Psychic	..	4	..	..	1
Simple faint	6	..	..	..	2
Petit mal	1	1	..	..	..
Other*	3	..	..	..	1

* Includes such symptoms as vertigo, enuresis, sweating and repetitiousness, one such case.

with tumors in any portion of the cerebrum, but they are more commonly associated with lesions in the temporal lobe.

Mental Symptoms. The mental symptoms of intracranial tumors include general hebetude, lethargy, drowsiness, changes in personality, disorders of conduct, impairment of the mental faculties and psychotic episodes. Any or all of these symptoms may occur with any of the intracranial tumors, and although they have no localizing value, they are more common with tumors in the anterior portions of the cerebral hemisphere. Urinary incontinence, or rather an indifference to the propriety of the act of voiding, is a rare symptom and is usually associated with a tumor of the frontal lobe.

Diagnosis of Intracranial Tumors

The diagnosis of an intracranial tumor and its exact location are made from the history, the physical findings and the results of laboratory examinations: roentgenograms of the skull, electroencephalography, examination of the cerebrospinal fluid, echoencephalography, radioactive scanning techniques, visualization of the cerebral ventricles and subarachnoid spaces by ventriculography or pneumoencephalography, the visualization of the cerebral vasculature by angiography and computer assisted tomography.

History. The diagnosis of an intracranial tumor should be entertained whenever focal neurological symptoms develop slowly and gradually increase in severity. Although occasionally symptoms of brain tumor may have a sudden and dramatic onset, they more commonly evolve over a period of weeks, months or years. The occurrence of convulsive seizures, headaches, dizziness, mental symptoms or the slow development of focal neurological symptoms always leads to concern regarding the possibility of an intracranial tumor.

Physical Examination. Significant findings on examination which point to the diagnosis of an intracranial tumor are choked discs and signs of focal damage to the nervous system. Although an intracranial tumor may be present without either of these findings, the diagnosis can rarely be made in the absence of both. It must be kept in mind, however, that these symptoms may also appear in conditions other than intracranial tumors.

When focal neurological signs are present, the localization of intracranial tumors can be made from their nature. A careful examination of the visual fields and speech functions should never be neglected. If the condition of the patient does not permit an accurate perimetric examination, a simple confrontation test may give valuable information. If there are no abnormal findings on neurological examination, localization of the tumor will depend upon the results of other examinations.

False localizing signs may occur when there is a high degree of increased intracranial pressure or distortion of the intracranial structures. Unilateral or bilateral weakness of the external rectus muscles may result from compression of one or both sixth cranial nerves against the floor of the skull. Less common false localizing signs include: Hemiplegia on the same side as the tumor, presumably caused by distortion of the brain and compression of the opposite cerebral peduncle against the incisura of the tentorium; homonymous hemianopia on the same side as the tumor due to distortion of the brain and compression of the opposite posterior cerebral artery; third nerve paralysis accompanied by a fixed dilated pupil on the same side as the tumor, resulting from a downward herniation of the hippocampus through the tentorium; changes in the visual fields due to compression of the optic chiasm or tracts by a dilated third ventricle.

Laboratory Examination. ROENTGENOGRAPHY. Examination of the skull with conventional radiological techniques contributes information of value in the diagnosis of a brain tumor in two thirds and has localizing value in approximately one third of the cases.

Lateral and anteroposterior stereoscopic views of the skull may give evidence of the presence of an intracranial tumor by showing: Displacement of a calcified pineal gland; absorptive changes in the bones of the skull (increase in the convolution markings on the skull and erosion of the clinoid processes); or, in children, separation of sutures. Localization of the site and even the histological type of the tumors may occasionally be deduced from characteristic abnormalities in the roentgenograms. Calcification within the substance of gliomas occurs in approximately 12% of the cases. Approximately 50% of the meningiomas can be diagnosed from atrophic or hypertrophic changes in the bone overlying the tumor or from the presence of abnormal vascular channels in the skull adjacent to the tumor. Seventy to 80% of the craniopharyngiomas can be diagnosed by the presence of calcium in the tumor. Pituitary tumors are accompanied by an enlargement and erosion of the sella turcica, except when the growth is still too small to produce a deformity of the sella or is almost entirely extrasellar. The histological type of the pituitary tumor also can be inferred from the presence or absence of the characteristic changes of acromegaly in the skull and other bones of the body. Acoustic neuromas may cause erosion of the petrous ridge and dilatation of the internal acoustic meatus. Gliomas of the optic nerve are often accompanied by an enlargement of the optic foramen. In a high percentage of cases, angiomas and other vascular anomalies will show calcification of a curvilinear nature. The sarcomas, hemangiomas, myelomas and other tumors involving the skull are manifested by defects in the bones. Metastatic carcinomas may be accompanied by a combination of absorptive and proliferative changes in the bone which may simulate Paget's disease.

ELECTROENCEPHALOGRAPHY. Electroencephalography is of particular value in localizing tumors of the cerebral hemisphere which are near the surface. Focal abnormalities in the electrical activity (Fig. 40) are helpful in indicating the site of a lesion but their character does not make possible an absolute differential diagnosis between a tumor and other lesions of the cortex. An increase in the degree of abnormality on repeated testing is in favor of the diagnosis of a tumor. Deep-seated tumors of the hemispheres or tumors of the posterior fossa may be accompanied by a diffuse slowing of the electrical activity of the cerebral cortex.

EXAMINATION OF THE CEREBROSPINAL FLUID. Although cerebrospinal fluid examination is abnormal in a large percentage of patients with brain tumor, this examination is no longer of prime importance, as noninvasive diagnostic tests are readily available. In a large percentage of cases examination of the cerebrospinal fluid gives valuable information in the diagnosis of intracranial tumors. When there is a high degree of choked disc, the performance of a lumbar puncture is accompanied by definite danger. If, however, a diagnosis cannot be made without the aid of the cerebrospinal fluid findings, the puncture is justified. It is hardly necessary to state that a lumbar puncture should not be made

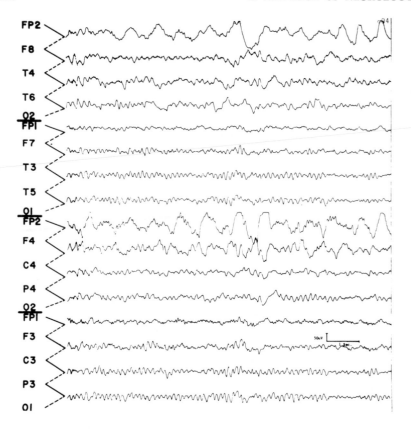

Figure 40. Slow wave focus in a brain tumor. The EEG shows rhythmic and arrhythmic slowing in the frontal area (Fp2) with extension of the irregular slowing into the lateral frontal and temporal areas (P8, T4, and T6).

when the diagnosis is already obvious, nor should it be performed with the patient in the sitting position.

The abnormalities characteristic of an intracranial tumor are an increased pressure and an increased protein content. In 70%, the pressure is greater than 200 mm of water and the protein content is greater than 100 mg. Other changes in the fluid, such as xanthochromia or pleocytosis occur in less than one third of the cases.

The lumbar cerebrospinal fluid is xanthochromic in approximately 30% of the cases. The yellow color of the fluid is usually associated with a high protein content, but occasionally it may be due to a previous extravasation of blood from the tumor.

The cell count in the fluid is greater than 5 per cu mm in approximately 30% and greater than 10 in 17%. Cell counts greater than 100 are uncommon and greater than 1,000 distinctly rare, although a number of such cases are recorded in the literature. A high cell count in the fluid is usually associated with a rapidly growing tumor which is situated close to the ventricular system and has undergone necrosis or is the site of a hemorrhage.

The cells in the spinal fluid are usually lymphocytes, polymorphonuclear leukocytes or other cells normally found in the blood. With the exception of carcinomatous, sarcomatous or diffuse involvements of the meninges by other neoplasms, it is rare to find tumor cells in the fluid. In patients with medulloblastoma, it is common to find these cells on millipore examination of the fluid.

The protein content of the lumbar fluids is greater than 45 mg in 70% and greater than 100 mg in approximately 30% of the cases. A protein content greater than 100 mg in cases with a supratentorial tumor is usually associated with a glioma or a metastatic tumor located near the ventricles or a meningioma which has extended deep into the cerebral substance. A protein content greater than 100 mg is common with neuromas of the acoustic nerve, but is rare with other posterior fossa neoplasms.

The colloidal tests on the fluids are abnormal in about one fourth of the cases, but elevation of the gamma globulin content of the fluids is rare.

Discounting possible laboratory errors, the serological tests for syphilis are negative unless there is a coincidence of syphilis and brain tumor.

ECHOENCEPHALOGRAPHY. Echoencephalography is the term coined by Leksell in 1956 for a technique where the position of the midline structure is determined by passing a beam of pulsed ultrasound through the head in the temporoparietal region and recording the returning echoes. The midline structures, usually the lateral walls of the third ventricle, but also the septum pellucidum, pineal, and interhemispheric fissure send back echoes which can be used to determine the presence or absence of displacement of these structures. A positive test has the same significance as lateral displacement of a calcified pineal gland.

Echoencephalography is an easy, rapid and harmless procedure with greater than 90% accuracy in determining the position of the midline. It is of value in all patients in whom the diagnosis of a brain tumor is considered.

VENTRICULOGRAPHY AND ENCEPHALOGRAPHY. The injection of air into the ventricles and the subarachnoid spaces was formerly one of our most valuable aids in the diagnosis and localization of brain tumors but the introduction of the noninvasive test, computerized x-ray tomography (CT brain scan) has greatly reduced the frequency of its use. It is especially valuable in outlining lesions in the ventricles and in the suprasellar region. It is also of importance in determining the presence and extent of cortical atrophy and enlargement of the ventricles and subarachnoid spaces.

ANGIOGRAPHY. The visualization of cerebral blood vessels by the injection of radiopaque dyes was introduced by Moniz in 1927. Angiography has the advantage over air injection in that it is a less traumatic procedure with a very low mortality rate. Untoward side symptoms—general prostration, increase in focal symptoms, convulsive seizures—occur in less than 10 per cent of the cases. These symptoms are usually transient.

The technique of angiography is not difficult but it requires close cooperation between the operator and technicians. The radiopaque

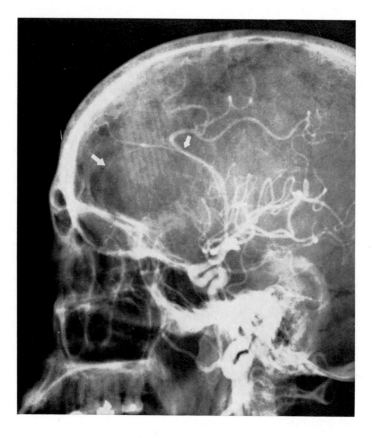

Figure 41.   Olfactory groove meningioma. Angiogram. Elevation and displacement of arteries on inferior surface of the frontal lobe (arrows). The site and location of the tumor are defined by the oval avascular area. (Courtesy Dr. Ernest Wood.)

substance is injected into the cerebral circulation by percutaneous puncture of the femoral artery with subsequent passage of the catheter to the major arteries going to the brain. Serial films in various positions are taken at rapid intervals during the injection (Figs. 41 and 42).

Angiography is of particular value in the differential diagnosis of brain tumor from cerebral vascular lesions, aneurysms and angiomatous malformations.

RADIOACTIVE SCANNING. Extracranial localization of brain tumors by means of their differential uptake of gamma-emitting labeled carriers is a valuable diagnostic aid. Radio-iodinated human serum albumin, radio-mercury-tagged Chlormerodrin (Technetium[99]) or other sub-

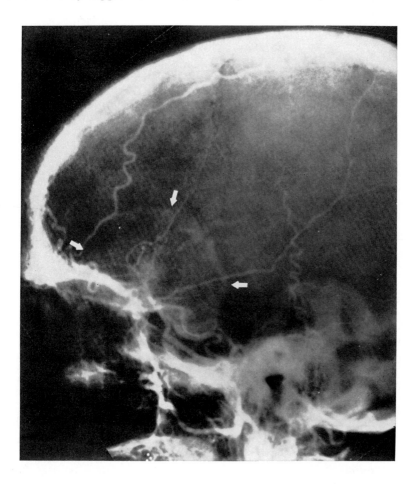

Figure 42.   Meningioma of the sphenoid ridge. External carotid angiogram. Numerous branches near the pterion supply the core of the tumor and a well-defined corona of new vessels (arrows) define the size of the tumor. (Courtesy Dr. Ernest Wood.)

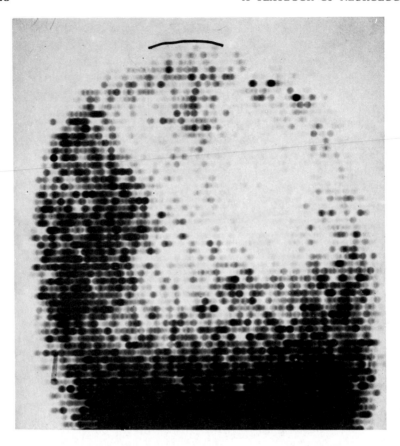

Figure 43.   Radioactive scanning of left temporoparietal glioblastoma.
Lateral view. (Courtesy of Dr. C. Douglas Maynard.)

stances are injected intravenously and isotope scanning is made at times of injection and at intervals of twenty-four, forty-eight and seventy-two hours. Lesions in the cerebral hemispheres can be localized by finding an abnormal concentration of the radioactive substance (Fig. 43) and the nature of the lesion can be conjectured by the rapidity of the appearance and disappearance of the abnormal collection. Lesions which preempt blood supply or are characterized by unique hypervascularity are best seen immediately after injection. Meningiomas generally appear by twenty-four hours after injection. Gliomas appear at twenty-four hours and become more obvious by forty-eight hours. Cystic lesions may appear later. Avascular lesions, third ventricular lesions and cerebellar lesions are not well seen.

It is a harmless procedure and should be used in all patients suspected of having a brain tumor to determine the need for more intensive studies and as a means of analyzing the effects of chemotherapy, radiotherapy or surgery without recourse to repeated angiography or other invasive studies.

COMPUTERIZED X-RAY TOMOGRAPHY (CT BRAIN SCAN). The introduction of computerized tomography of the brain is the greatest advance in diagnosis of brain tumors and other lesions since angiography was first used in 1927 (Figs. 44 and 45).

Computerized tomography has the advantage over pneumoenceph-alography and angiography in that it is a noninvasive technique with little or no mortality or morbidity. There will still be a place for air encephalography and angiography but the CT brain scan will replace to a great extent those techniques in the localization of lesions within the central nervous system and the diagnosis of the nature of the lesion in many of the cases, especially with the aid of intravenously injected contrast media. The technique is especially valuable in the diagnosis of tumors, cerebral hemorrhage, softening and atrophy and in following the course of patients with these lesions. The cost of the equipment and the necessity of an exacting degree of cooperation of the patient limit to some extent its value. The test has not been performed in enough

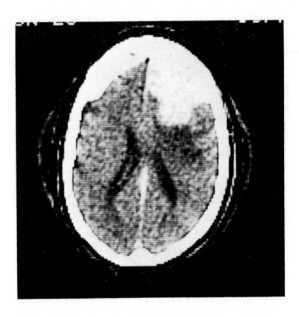

Figure 44.   Falx meningioma in occipital region, CT brain scan.
(Courtesy of Dr. Harry H. White.)

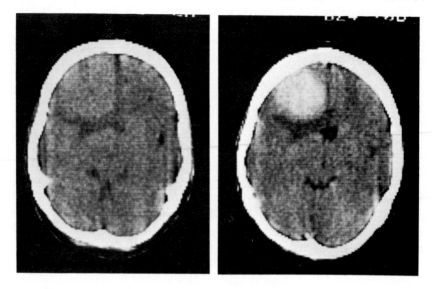

Figure 45.   CT brain scan. Left frontal lobe meningioma, pre and post contrast.
(Courtesy of Dr. Sadek Hillal.)

patients to give an accurate evaluation of its capabilities and limitations but it can be said that there has been a great reduction in the number of air encephalograms and angiograms in all the clinics where CT brain scan is available.

CT brain scan has almost entirely replaced angiography in the routine diagnosis of brain tumor, but angiography is still of importance in determining the vascular supply of tumor, and in the diagnosis of intracranial aneurysms.

Differential Diagnosis. Intracranial tumors must be differentiated from other morbid conditions accompanied by focal neurological signs or signs of increased intracranial pressure. As this obviously encompasses the whole field of neurology, it is necessary to limit discussion to the more common diseases with symptomatology which may mimic that of intracranial tumor. These include cerebral vascular accidents, infections of the nervous system, epilepsy, the demyelinizing diseases, degenerative diseases and subdural hematoma. With all of the diagnostic methods available at the present time, errors in the diagnosis of intracranial tumors are rarely justified.

CEREBRAL VASCULAR ACCIDENTS. Cerebral vascular accidents are differentiated from intracranial tumors by the sudden onset of symptoms and lack of progression of focal signs. Occasionally the symptoms of an intracranial tumor may also have a sudden onset, and in rare instances there may be a progressive increase in the severity of the neurological signs in patients with cerebral vascular lesions. The presence or absence of arteriosclerosis and hypertension is not of absolute diagnostic significance since intracranial tumors are common in the age group that is subject to arteriosclerosis; moreover, cerebral vascular accidents may occur in the absence of hypertension or other signs of arteriosclerosis.

The establishment of the correct diagnosis may be especially difficult in patients with cerebral vascular disease accompanied by changes in the optic disc simulating the choked disc of increased intracranial pressure. Choking of the disc may occur in patients with an intracranial hemorrhage who survive for several days or weeks after its onset. If the cerebrospinal fluid is bloody immediately after the onset of symptoms, the diagnosis of an intracerebral hemorrhage is most probable. If the fluid is clear, it may not be possible to establish the diagnosis without craniotomy. Failure to establish the correct diagnosis before operation is not of serious importance because operative treatment is indicated in this type of cerebral vascular accident.

Cerebral thrombosis or cerebral embolus is differentiated from intracranial tumor by the lack of progression of symptoms. In doubtful cases, examination of the cerebrospinal fluid gives valuable diagnostic aid. In cerebral thrombosis the cerebrospinal fluid pressure is normal even in the cases with changes in the fundi similar to choked disc, unless either cardiac failure or uremia is also present. The latter diagnosis is readily established or excluded by the level of urea in the serum. In addition to the presence or absence of increased cerebrospinal fluid pressure, the level of protein content in the cerebrospinal fluid is also of value in the differential diagnosis. A slight increase in the protein content in the range of 50 to 75 mg is not uncommon in patients with cerebral vascular accidents but values over 100 mg per 100 ml are strongly in favor of the diagnosis of a tumor. Repeat electroencephalograms are of value in the differential diagnosis of occlusive vascular lesions and tumor. The changes in the electroencephalogram persist or increase in severity in patients with tumors, whereas there is a tendency toward reversal to normal in patients with cerebral thromboses.

Echoencephalography and radioactive scanning are also of value in the differential diagnosis. The correct diagnosis can be established in practically all cases by CT brain scan or angiography (Fig. 44).

Intracranial aneurysms which are silent until their rupture do not offer any difficulty in diagnosis. The differential diagnosis in cases with an aneurysm so located as to compress the optic chiasm, cranial nerves or the cerebral substance can be established by angiography.

INFECTIONS OF THE NERVOUS SYSTEM. Patients with acute infections of the meninges with symptoms simulating those of brain tumors are readily diagnosed by the results of an examination of the cerebrospinal fluid. The same is true of the subacute infections of the meninges with tuberculosis, syphilis or the yeast organisms. Localized granulomatous lesions due to these organisms cannot be differentiated from other intracranial tumors unless there is an accompanying meningitis.

Septic thromboses of the intracranial venous sinuses are diagnosed by the presence of a source for the infections and of the cerebrospinal fluid findings characteristic of an aseptic meningeal reaction. This is also true in the majority of the intracranial abscesses, except when they are well encapsulated.

Acute or subacute infections of the central nervous system with the filtrable viruses are diagnosed by their clinical course and by the changes in the cerebrospinal fluid.

DEMYELINIZING DISEASES. Multiple sclerosis is characterized by a multiplicity of symptoms and signs and by a remitting course. Occasionally in multiple sclerosis and more frequently in Schilder's disease, the signs and symptoms may be progressive and localized to one region of the cortex or the brainstem. A normal cerebrospinal fluid pressure and the absence of focal electroencephalographic changes are against the diagnosis of a tumor. Rarely, however, a CT brain scan may be necessary to exclude the diagnosis of tumor.

EPILEPSY. Since convulsive seizures are a common symptom of intracranial tumors, this diagnosis should be considered in every case with seizures. This is true regardless of the age of the patient or the type of the seizure, with the exception of true petit mal. Significant factors in favor of the diagnosis of an intracranial tumor are onset of seizures after the second decade of life, a focal character to the seizures, the presence of transient neurological signs following a seizure, the progressive evolution of focal neurological signs or the presence of focal abnormalities in the electroencephalogram. As a rule, the likelihood of an intracranial tumor as the cause of convulsive seizures in any given patient decreases with the passage of years if choked discs or focal neurological signs do not develop. There are exceptions to this rule because intracranial tumor may be present for many years with convulsive seizures as their only symptoms. A negative CT brain scan or angiogram is of value in excluding an intracranial tumor.

DEGENERATIVE DISEASES. The degenerative diseases which may simulate intracranial tumors by the slow progression of mental symptoms or focal neurological signs, particularly aphasia, are the presenile psychoses, Pick's and Alzheimer's diseases. The diagnosis of tumor is excluded by the normal cerebrospinal fluid pressure, normal roentgenograms of the skull, and absence of focal abnormalities in the electroencephalogram. The diagnosis of tumor can be excluded with certainty by the results of the CT brain scan.

Table 30.   Comparison of the Duration of Symptoms before
Admission to the Hospital in the Various Types of Intracranial Tumors

Type of Tumor	No. of Cases	Duration of Symptoms (in months)				
		Less than 1	1 to 4	4 to 12	12 to 36	Over 36
Glioma	47	13	20	6	4	4
Meningioma	21	1	4	8	5	3
Metastatic	14	2	10	1	..	1
Neurofibroma	7	..	..	..	4	3
Pituitary adenoma	6	..	1	..	..	5
Miscellaneous	5	1	1	1	1	1
Total	100	17	36	16	14	17

SUBDURAL HEMATOMA. Acute subdural hematomas are readily differentiated from intracranial neoplasms by the history of a recent head injury. CT brain scan may be necessary to exclude the diagnosis of a chronic subdural hematoma in cases where the initial head injury was of such a mild nature that it has been forgotten, or in chronic alcoholics who may have injured their head in an alcoholic debauch.

Clinical Course and Treatment

The clinical course of patients with intracranial tumors is closely related to the type of tumor. For this reason it is more appropriate to discuss this subject in more detail in connection with the various types of tumors. In general, it may be said that the symptoms and signs of intracranial tumors are usually of slow onset (Table 30) and they progress in most instances until they cause the death of the patient. Remissions are relatively infrequent but they may occur even in the most malignant tumor.

The treatment of brain tumors is surgical extirpation, when possible, followed by radiation therapy when indicated. If the tumor cannot be removed in toto, partial removal followed by radiation therapy may appreciably lengthen the period of useful life. In general it can be said that patients with meningiomas, acoustic neuromas, cystic astrocytomas of the cerebellum, colloid cysts of the third ventricle, lipomas, angiomatous malformations, and some of the granulomas and congenital tumors can be cured by surgical removal of the tumor. The infiltrating gliomas cannot be entirely extirpated. In these cases, biopsy for the establishment of the diagnosis, partial removal, when clinically feasible, and radiation therapy are the accepted treatment.

There has recently been a tendency in some clinics to administer radiation therapy without operative confirmation of the diagnosis when the presence of a malignant glioma or metastatic tumor seems probable. This course is justified only when the characterisic vascular patterns of such tumors can be demonstrated in the angiograms. The question of radiation therapy versus surgical removal of pituitary adenomas and other tumors is considered in the discussion of these tumors.

Chemotherapy of malignant gliomas is still in the experimental stage.

Hypertonic solutions formerly given to alleviate the symptoms due to increased intracranial pressure have been replaced by the administration of corticosteroids, particularly dexamethasone. Prompt improvement of the symptoms due to increased pressure and partial or occasionally almost complete remission of focal symptoms often result for a limited period of time.

REFERENCES

Bailey, P.: Intracranial Tumors, Springfield, Charles C Thomas, 1933. 475 pp.
Bailey, P., Buchanan, D. N., and Bucy, P. C.: Intracranial Tumors of Infancy and Childhood, Chicago, University of Chicago Press, 1939. 598 pp.
Brinker, R. A., King, D. L., and Taveras, J.: Echoencephalography, Am. J. Roentgen., 93, 781, 1965.
Clifford, J. R., Connolly, F. S., and Vorhees, R. M.: Comparison of Radionuclide Scans with Computerized Tomography in Diagnosis of Intracranial Disease, Neurol., 26, 1119, 1976.
Cushing, H.: Intracranial Tumours: Notes upon a Series of 2000 Verified Cases with Surgical-Mortality Percentages Pertaining Thereto, Springfield, Charles C Thomas, 1932. 150 pp.
Dandy, W. E.: Ventriculography following the Injection of Air into the Cerebral Ventricles, Ann. Surg., 68, 5, 1918.
————: Roentgenography of Brain after Injection of Air into Spinal Canal, Ann. Surg., 70, 397, 1919.
Grant, F. C.: A Study of the Results of Surgical Treatment of 2,326 Consecutive Patients with Brain Tumors, J. Neurosurg., 13, 479, 1956.
Hoefer, P. F. A., Schlesinger, E. B., and Pennes, H. H.: Seizures in Patients with Brain Tumors, A. Res. Nerv. & Ment. Dis., Proc., 26, 50, 1947.
Jacobs, L., Kinkel, W. B., and Hefner, R. L.: Autopsy Control of Computerized Tomography. Experience with 6,000 Cases, Neurol., 26, 1111, 1976.
Liebner, E. J., Pretto, J. I., Hochhauser, M., and Kassaraba, W.: Tumors of the Posterior Fossa in Childhood and Adolescence. Their Diagnostic and Radiotherapeutic Patterns, Radiology, 82, 193, 1964.
Low, N. L., Correll, J. W., and Hammill, J. F.: Tumors of the Cerebral Hemispheres in Children, Arch, Neurol., 13, 547, 1965.
McMenemy, W. H., and Cumings, J. N.: The Value of the Examination of the Cerebrospinal Fluid in the Diagnosis of Intracranial Tumors, J. Clin. Path., 12, 400, 1959.
Merritt, H. H.: The Cerebrospinal Fluid in Cases of Tumors of the Brain, Arch. Neurol. & Psychiat., 34, 1175, 1935.
Moniz, E.: L'encéphalographie artérielle, son importance dans la localisation des tumeurs cérébrales, Rev. Neurol., 2, 72, 1927.
Odom, G. L., Davis, C. H., and Woodhall, B.: Brain Tumors in Children; Clinical Analysis of 164 Cases, Pediatrics, 18, 856, 1956.
Rhoton, A. L., Jr., Carlsson, A. M., and Ter-Pogossian, M. M.: Brain Scanning with Chlormerodrin Hg[197] and Chlormerodrin Hg[203], Arch. Neurol., 10, 369, 1964.

Robbins, L. L.: *Golden's Diagnostic Roentgenology*, Baltimore, Williams & Wilkins, 1936–1964, 3388 pp. 3 vols.
Schlesinger, E. B., de Boves, S., and Taveras, J.: Localization of Brain Tumors Using Radioiodinated Human Serum Albumin, Am. J. Roent., Radium Ther. & Nuclear Med., *87*, 449, 1962.
Taveras, J. M., and Wood, E. H.: *Diagnostic Neuroradiology*, 2nd Ed., Baltimore, Williams & Wilkins. 1976, 1250 pp.

TUMORS OF THE SKULL

Hyperostoses. Local overgrowth of the bones of the skull may be secondary to intracranial tumors, particularly meningiomas, or it may occur independent of the presence of such tumors. The present discussion will be confined to the latter group.

Hyperostoses may involve either the outer or inner tables of the skull. Those involving the outer table are of no importance except for the disfigurement they produce when they grow to a large size. Those involving the inner table rarely grow to sufficient size to compress the intracranial content. Hyperostosis of the inner table of the frontal bone is a common incidental finding in routine roentgenograms of the skull, especially in middle-aged or elderly women. Attempts have been made to associate these changes in the skull with headaches and other somatic symptoms common at the time of the menopause. The frequency of hyperostosis of the frontal bone in patients without symptoms makes it unlikely, however, that overgrowth of the inner table of the frontal bone (hyperostosis frontalis interna) is related to dysfunction of the endocrine glands or that it is the cause of various symptoms which may be present in these patients.

Osteomas. Osteomas of the skull may arise in the paranasal sinuses, particularly the frontal and ethmoid sinuses, or from the cortex of the calvarium.

Osteomas of the nasal sinuses cause an enlargement of the sinus and localized pain or headache. As the tumor grows, it extends into the orbit or into the anterior fossa of the skull. Extension into the orbit may cause displacement of the eyeball; orbital cellulitis may also develop. Symptoms of frontal lobe damage are uncommon, but erosion of the dura may cause cerebrospinal fluid rhinorrhea, pneumatocele, meningitis or abscess formation. The diagnosis of osteomas of the nasal sinuses with intraorbital or intracranial extension can be made from the roentgenograms. The treatment is surgical removal.

Osteomas of the calvarium may arise from either the outer or inner table. Those of the outer table frequently follow trauma. Osteomas of the inner table rarely reach sufficient size to compress the underlying brain tissue. Treatment includes complete removal of the osteoma together with the repair of any dural defect. The defect in the bone is replaced by a tantalum plate.

Hemiangiomas. Hemangiomas are congenital vascular anomalies which may involve the bones of the skull or the spinal column. In the skull they vary from small solitary lesions remaining stationary in size to huge masses or multiple lesions which grow progressively larger and communicate with large masses of vessels in the scalp or on the surface of the brain.

Small hemangiomas of the skull may produce no symptoms. When the inner table of the skull is penetrated, however, headaches, jacksonian or generalized seizures and focal neurological signs may result. Hemangiomas are diagnosed by the characteristic roentgenographic findings of areas of decreased density with linear trabeculations or by angiography. Solitary lesions may be removed surgically. Multiple or large lesions are treated by radiation therapy which may retard the growth or even diminish the size of the lesions.

Metastatic Tumors. Metastatic tumors of the bones of the skull may be secondary to malignant tumors in any portion of the body. Carcinoma is the most common type and the breast is the most frequent site of the primary lesion. Since metastases to the skull are usually blood-borne, the lesions are commonly multiple and accompanied by pulmonary metastases.

Metastatic tumors in the skull are seldom of sufficient size to produce neurological symptoms unless they are located at the base where they may produce single or multiple cranial nerve palsies. The presence of metastatic lesions in the skull is of importance mainly as evidence of generalized carcinomatosis and as an indication that they or other metastatic lesions are the cause of focal neurological signs which may be present. Metastatic lesions of the skull are diagnosed by the appearance in the roentgenograms of irregular areas of complete or incomplete destruction, giving a moth-eaten appearance to the involved bone. Occasionally there may be a mixture of bone destruction and new bone proliferation, with a picture suggesting that of Paget's disease of bone. When the diagnosis of metastatic carcinoma of the skull is established, operative treatment is contraindicated. Radiation therapy is sometimes of value in retarding the rate of growth of the tumors.

Involvement of the skull by carcinoma of the nasal sinuses (Schmincke's tumor) is by direct extension rather than by metastasis. These tumors may occur at any age and characteristically produce single or multiple cranial nerve palsies. Erosion of the base of the skull may be seen in the roentgenogram. The cervical lymph nodes may be involved but the diagnosis can be established with certainty before operation only by finding the primary growth on examination of the nasopharynx.

Tumors of the glomus jugulare (chemodectoma, nonchromaffin

paraganglioma or carotid body tumor) arise from nonchromaffin tissue in the region of the jugular bulb and invade the neighboring temporal and occipital bones. Progressive deafness and a bloody aural discharge are the common presenting symptoms. With growth of the tumor into the posterior fossa there may be paralysis of the lower cranial nerves, and signs of pressure on the brainstem and cerebellum.

Involvement of the Skull in Systemic Diseases. The bones of the skull may be involved in xanthomatosis (Hand-Schüller-Christian disease), multiple myeloma, osteitis deformans (Paget's disease) and osteitis fibrosa cystica. The symptomatology and signs of these conditions are considered in detail elsewhere.

Other Tumors of the Skull. The skull may be affected by tuberculous or syphilic infection, benign giant-cell tumors, cholesteatomas or extension of primary carcinomas of the scalp. A rare tumor of bone, composed of a large number of eosinophils, is known as an eosinophilic granuloma. This is considered to be a benign expression of Hand-Schüller-Christian disease. The treatment is surgical removal or radiation therapy. Steroid therapy has been reported to be effective in the treatment of eosinophilic granuloma of bones.

REFERENCES

Avery, M. E., McAfee, J. G., and Guild, H. G.: The Course and Prognosis of Reticuloen-dotheliosis (Eosinophilic Granuloma, Schüller-Christian Disease, and Letterer-Siwe Disease), Am. J. Med., 22, 636, 1957.

Flosi, A. Z. et al.: Treatment of Eosinophilic Granuloma by Corticotropin: Report of 4 Cases with Disappearance of the Bone Lesions, J. Clin. Endocrin. Metabol., 17, 994, 1957.

Godtfredsen, E.: Neurologische Symptome bei Maligen Rhinopharynxtumoren, Acta Psychiat. et Neurol., 16, 47, 1941.

Lederer, F. L. et al.: Nonchromaffin Paraganglioma of the Head and Neck. Ann. Otol., Rhinol., & Laryng., 67, 305, 1958.

Needles, W.: Malignant Tumors of the Nasopharynx, J. Nerv. & Ment. Dis., 86, 373, 1937.

Pool, J. L., Potanos, J. N., and Krueger, E. G.: Osteomas and Mucoceles of the Frontal Paranasal Sinuses, J. Neurosurg., 19, 130, 1962.

Rice, R. P., and Holman, C. B.: Roentgenographic Manifestations of Tumors of the Glomus Jugulare (Chemodectoma), Am. J. Roentgen., 89, 1201, 1963.

Sbarbaro, J. L., and Francis, K. C.: Eosinophilic Granuloma of Bone, J.A.M.A., 178, 706, 1961.

Session, R. T. et al.: Surgical Experiences with Tumors of the Carotid Body, Glomus jugulare and Retroperitoneal Nonchromaffin Paraganglia. Ann. Surg., 150, 808, 1959.

Tumors of the Meninges

Meningiomas. It is generally accepted that meningiomas (meningeal fibroblastomas, leptomeningiomas, arachnoidal fibroblastoma, dural endothelioma) are tumors which arise from cell clusters principally associated with the arachnoidal villi. They are as a rule discrete nodules which vary in size from that of a small pea to a grapefruit. They

produce symptoms by compression of the underlying nervous parenchyma. Not infrequently they invade the bones of the skull but only
rarely do they break through the pial membrane and grow within the
substance of the nervous system.

Pathology. Grossly these tumors are commonly round or nodular
masses which compress and excavate the underlying portion of the
nervous system. Occasionally they occur in diffuse sheets (meningioma
en plaques). The meningiomas are firm in consistency and rarely
undergo cystic degeneration. The following characteristics are of
clinical and surgical importance: They are sharply circumscribed; they
invade the adjacent dura and frequently the bones as well; they have a
rich vasculature which is derived mainly from the meningeal branches
of the external carotid artery; they stimulate growth in the adjacent
bone and occasionally erode it; they have a tendency to recur.

The microscopic pathology of meningiomas is quite variable. Bailey
and Bucy divided them into nine types. Cushing and Eisenhardt gave
the same number of sub-types but used a slightly different terminology.
According to the latter authors the most common types are the
meningothelial without reticulin or collagen formation, the psam-
momatous type and the fibroblastic. Less common forms are the
angioblastic, epithelioid, sarcomatous, osteoblastic, chondroblastic
and lipoblastic types.

Incidence. Meningiomas constitute 10 to 15% of all the intracranial
tumors admitted to large neurosurgical clinics. Meningiomas may
occur at any age but they are predominantly tumors of adult or early
middle life. The average age at onset of symptoms in Cushing and
Eisenhardt's series was thirty-eight years, which was eight years
younger than the average age on admission. Meningiomas are rare in
childhood. The youngest patient in Cushing's series was five years old,
while Frazier and Alpers reported a patient of three.

Meningiomas are more common in women than in men in the ratio of
3 to 2. Race incidence is not remarkable except for their rarity in the
Negroes of the United States.

Factors cited as important in the causation of meningiomas or the
precipitation of symptoms include trauma and pregnancy. Cushing and
Eisenhardt found a history of trauma in nearly one third of their cases.
In some, the direct relation of the blow to the locus of the ensuing
growth was so precise that the conclusion was inescapable that the
trauma was an etiological factor. The onset of symptoms of a meningioma as well as of other types of intracranial tumors is frequent in the
late months of pregnancy. This can possibly be explained on the basis
of an increased hydration of the brain.

SYMPTOMS AND SIGNS. The symptoms of meningiomas are similar to
those of other intracranial tumors, but owing to their predilection for

certain regions and their tendency to produce proliferation of the bones, they present special features which may make it possible to diagnose their presence before operation. Another feature of meningiomas, which is characteristic but by no means pathognomonic, is the long duration of symptoms. Since meningiomas grow very slowly, it is not uncommon for symptoms of a generalized nature (headache, vomiting, mental changes) or focal symptoms (convulsions, hemiplegia) to be present for several or many years before the patient is admitted to a hospital for diagnosis and treatment. The average duration of symptoms before operation in Cushing and Eisenhardt's series was eight years, but cases have been reported in which local bony swelling or focal convulsive seizures indicating the presence of a meningioma have extended over a period of from twenty to thirty years. On the other hand, a short duration of symptoms does not exclude the diagnosis of meningioma. Even though symptoms may have been evident for only a few weeks or even a few days, it is not unusual to find a large meningioma which must have been present for many months or years.

The vast majority of intracranial meningiomas are located (Table 31) in the parasagittal region (Figs. 46 and 47) on the convexity of the cerebral hemispheres, on the sphenoidal ridge or on the floor of the anterior fossa either in the olfactory groove or above the sella turcica. Less common sites include the posterior fossa, the peritorcular region, the temporal fossa and the falx. Contrary to general opinion, meningiomas arising from the cranial base are as common as those underlying the vault. Multiple meningiomas occur in less than 1 per cent of the cases and occasionally there is the combination of a meningioma and a tumor of another type (neurofibroma or glioma), particularly in von Recklinghausen's syndrome.

Table 31. The Anatomical Distribution of Meningiomas

Site of Tumor	No. of Cases	%
Parasagittal	65	21
Convexity of hemispheres	54	17
Sphenoidal ridge	53	17
Floor of anterior fossa	57	18
Posterior fossa	23	7
Peritorcular	12	4
Temporal fossa	8	3
Falx, gasserian and other	23	7
Spinal	18	6
Total	313	100

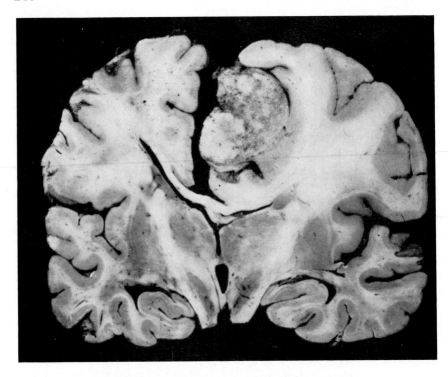

Figure 46. Parasagittal meningioma. (Courtesy Dr. Philip Duffy.)

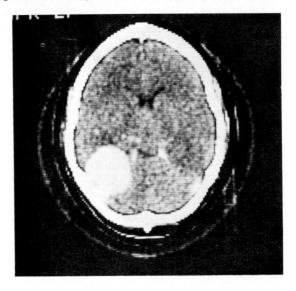

Figure 47. Meningioma, left parietal lobe, CT brain scan.
(Courtesy of Dr. Harry H. White.)

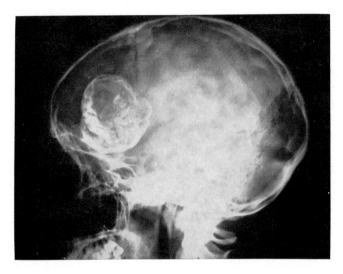

Figure 48.   Meningioma of olfactory groove with extensive calcification.

Parasagittal and Convexity. The symptoms and signs of menin-giomas located in the parasagittal region or on the convexity of the hemisphere (Fig. 48) are those appropriate to tumors in these regions and the diagnosis of a meningioma can be made with certainty only when characteristic changes are noted in the bones of the skull.

Sphenoid Ridge. The meningiomas of the sphenoid ridge are charac-terized by exophthalmos, as result of orbital hyperostosis, by visual defects and by extra-ocular palsies. Cushing and Eisenhardt divide the meningiomas of the sphenoid ridge into three groups. The first in-volves the deep or clinoidal third of the ridge and the presenting symptom is usually unilateral failure of vision associated with a primary optic atrophy. Other symptoms and signs include unilateral exophthalmos, homonymous visual field defects, homolateral oculomotor palsies, contralateral choked discs, numbness of the brow due to involvement of the ophthalmic branch of the trigeminal nerve and olfactory or gustatory hallucinations with or without convulsive seizures. Late symptoms are polyuria, adiposity, changes in personality and other mental symptoms, and contralateral hemiparesis; these are attributed to compression and dislocation of the tuber cinereum, and the frontal lobes.

In the second group, the tumor arises in the middle portion of the sphenoid ridge and differs in symptomatology from the first mainly in the fact that bilateral choking of the disc rather than unilateral optic atrophy is a common early finding. As the tumor grows toward the midline, the signs and symptoms are similar to those of tumors of the inner third of the sphenoid ridge.

The third group—meningiomas of the outer third of the greater wing of the sphenoid bone—is subdivided into two types. The first is a flat tumor (meningioma en plaque) characterized by unilateral non-pulsating irreducible exophthalmos, enlargement of the temporal bone and the roentgenographic finding of thickening of the orbital roof and of the floor of the middle fossa. The second sub-type of meningioma of the greater wing of the sphenoid bone is the large round or globoid tumor which grows into the sylvian fissure. The symptoms and signs of this tumor are those due to intracranial pressure and convulsive seizures, which are more frequently generalized than jacksonian in nature. Olfactory and gustatory hallucinations as well as visual hallucinations are common. The latter are apt to be so vivid that the patient can describe in detail the people and objects in his hallucinations.

Anterior Fossa. Meningiomas on the floor of the anterior fossa are divided into two groups. The first, those arising from the tuberculum sellae, compress the optic chiasm and produce a syndrome similar to that of a pituitary adenoma. There may be absorptive changes in the sella or hyperostosis of the planum sphenoidale. Suprasellar meningiomas can be visualized in the CT brain scan or pneumoencephalograms but they cannot be differentiated from aneurysms except by the results of angiography.

The second group of anterior fossa meningiomas arise from the olfactory groove. These tumors usually grow to a very large size and spread to the other half of the anterior fossa. For this reason the symptoms are quite variable. Unilateral anosmia is a common early finding. The Foster Kennedy syndrome, *i.e.,* homolateral optic atrophy and contralateral choked disc, is a frequent finding when the tumor remains localized to one side. Headaches, progressive failure of vision and mental deterioration are the symptoms characteristic of tumors which compress or distort both optic nerves and frontal lobes.

Posterior Fossa. Meningiomas of the posterior fossa are relatively uncommon, representing approximately 5% of the intracranial meningiomas. They may compress the cerebellar hemisphere and produce signs and symptoms of increased intracranial pressure with or without indications of cerebellar dysfunction. Meningiomas arising from the tentorium of the cerebellum may extend above the tentorium to involve the occipital or temporal lobes. Those on the lower surface of the tentorium compress the trigeminal nerve and grow into the cerebellum. Meningiomas in the cerebellopontine angle produce a syndrome similar to that of an acoustic neurinoma. They can usually be differentiated from the latter by preservation of vestibular responses. A favorite site of origin for posterior fossa meningiomas is the basilar groove. These tumors may grow downward through the foramen magnum, compressing the cervical portion of the spinal cord and producing a complex symptomatology. Paralysis of one or several of the lower cranial nerves on the side of the tumor may be the presenting symptom. Occasionally it may be weakness and paresthesias of the homolateral upper extremity. Extension of the growth may produce signs of increased intracranial pressure, progressive involvement of the cranial nerves and signs of compression of the lower medulla and upper cervical cord. The mode of progress of the symptoms of cord compression is quite characteristic. The motor weakness in the upper extremity extends to the ipsilateral leg and then to the contralateral leg and arm. There may be atrophy of the muscles of the ipsilateral upper extremity and stereoanesthesia in the hand. The degree of cutaneous sensory loss is quite variable. There may be a loss of pain and temperature sense on the opposite or even on both sides of the body. Pain in the occipital region and stiffness of the neck are almost always present. The diagnosis of meningiomas in the region of the foramen magnum can usually be made from the typical progression of symptoms. Roentgenographs of the base of the skull may show changes in the bones or enlargement of the foramen magnum. Partial or complete subarachnoid block is usually present on lumbar puncture. The diagnosis can be established or excluded by myelography.

Peritorcular. The meningiomas which arise in the region of torcula compress the occipital lobe and commonly produce homonymous field defects as one of the early symptoms.

Falx. Meningiomas which arise from the inner surface of the falx may invade one or both hemispheres. Their symptomatology is similar to that of other tumors of the cerebral hemispheres. The chief difference between the parasagittal and falx meningiomas is that the latter are entirely hidden by the overlying cortex.

DIAGNOSIS. The location of intracranial meningiomas is made by the presence of symptoms characteristic of the region affected. In addition plain roentgenograms of the skull may show calcification in the tumor, proliferative changes in the neighboring skull, or enlargement of the vascular channels of the meningeal arteries supplying the tumor. Meningiomas can be demonstrated clearly in the angiograms of the external carotid artery. They can also be clearly demonstrated in the CT brain scan and isotope brain scan.

CLINICAL COURSE AND TREATMENT. The meningiomas grow more slowly than any of the other intracranial tumors and their clinical course usually extends over many years. Small tumors are not an unusual finding in routine necropsies but as a rule, if untreated, meningiomas will almost always lead to death.

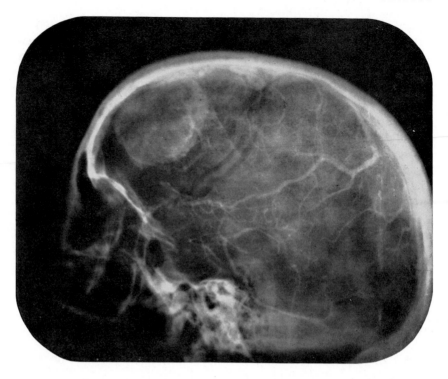

Figure 49. Meningioma of convexity. Persistence of dye in tumor in venous phase of angiography indicating extreme degree of vascularity of tumor. (Courtesy Dr. Juan Taveras.)

The preferred treatment of meningiomas is surgical extirpation. They respond poorly to radiation therapy. The discrete nature of the meningiomas makes them especially suitable for removal in *toto* and complete cures are common, although surgical treatment is by no means always successful. Their large size, extreme vascularity (Fig. 49) and tendency to occur in regions where access to them is difficult make the operative mortality rate between 5 and 10%. Moreover, there is a tendency for the tumor to recur if any portion of the involved dura or bone is not removed, so that in a sizable percentage of cases, the symptoms will return after a few or many years. On the whole, however, the results of the surgical treatment of meningomas by a skilled neurosurgeon are gratifying.

Other Tumors of the Meninges. The dura mater may be the site of single or multiple metastases from carcinomatous or sarcomatous tumors in any portion of the body. The leptomeninges and subarachnoid spaces may be invaded in a diffuse manner by gliomas, particularly the medulloblastomas, sarcomas, melanomas, carcinomas, lymphomas, reticulum cell sarcomas, and in the course of the leukemias. The symptoms resulting from a diffuse involvement of the meninges by tumor are extremely variable. The diagnosis is usually made from the finding of the primary site of the tumor or from the presence of tumor cells in the cerebrospinal fluid. The finding of a low glucose content in the cerebrospinal fluid in the absence of bacteria or yeast organisms is a point in favor of the diagnosis of diffuse neoplastic involvement of the meninges.

REFERENCES

Barrows, H. S., and Harter, D. H.: Tentorial Meningiomas, J. Neurol. Neurosurg, & Psychiat., 25, 40, 1962.
Cherington, M., and Schneck, S. A.: Clivus Meningiomas, Neurology, 16, 86, 1966.
Cushing, H.: The Meningiomas Arising from the Olfactory Groove and Their Removal by the Aid of Electro-surgery, Lancet, 1, 1329, 1927.
Cushing, H., and Eisenhardt, L.: Meningiomas Arising from the Tuberculum Sellae, with Syndrome, Arch. Ophthal., 1, 1 and 168, 1929.
————: Meningiomas: Their Classification, Regional Behavior, Life History, and Surgical End Results, Springfield, Charles C Thomas, 1938, 785 pp.
DeBusscher, J., van Renynghe de Voxvrie, G., and Hoffman, G.: Meningiomas of the Lateral Recess, Act. Neurol. et Pschiat, Belg., 57, 67, 1957.
Ellenberger, C., Jr.: Preoptic Meningiomas. Syndrome of Long-standing Visual Loss, Pale Disk Edema, and Optociliary Veins, Arch. Neurol., 33, 671, 1976.
Gassel, M. M., and Davies, H.: Meningiomas in the Lateral Ventricles, Brain, 84, 605, 1961.
Grant, F. C.: Clinical Experience with Meningiomas of the Brain, J. Neurosurg., 11, 479, 1954.
Hoessly, G. F., and Olivecrona, H.: Report on 280 Cases of Verified Parasagittal Meningioma, J. Neurosurg., 12, 614, 1955.
Hughes, I. E., Adams, J. H., and Ilbert, R. C.: Invasion of the Leptomeninges by Tumour: The Differential Diagnosis from Tuberculous Meningitis, J. Neurol., Neurosurg., & Psychiat., 26, 83, 1963.
Onofrio, B. M., Kernohan, J. W., and Uihlein, A.: Primary Meningeal Sarcomatosis, Cancer, 15, 1197, 1962.
Sachs, E., Jr., Avman, N., and Fisher, R. G.: Meningiomas of Pineal Region and Posterior Part of 3rd Ventricle, J. Neurosurg., 19, 325, 1962.
Stein, B. M., Leeds, N. E., Taveras, J. M., and Pool, J. L.: Meningiomas of the Foramen Magnum, J. Neurosurg., 20, 740, 1963.
Tucker, R. I., Holman, C. B., McCarthy, C. S., and Dockerty, M. B.: The Roentgenological Manifestations of Meningiomas of the Tuberculum Sellae, Radiology, 72, 348, 1959.
Tveten, L.: Primary Meningeal Melanosis, Acta Path. et Microbiol. Scandinav., 63, 1, 1965.
White, J. C., Schwab, R. S., and Sahinalp, L.: Parasagittal Meningiomas of the Longitudinal Sinus and Falx, J. Neurosurg., 17, 197, 1960.

Tumors of the Cranial Nerves

Compression or invasion of the cranial nerves by benign or malignant tumors is discussed elsewhere. This section will be limited to the consideration of the tumors which develop within these nerves. Any of the cranial nerves may be the site of origin of a neurofibroma, particularly in von Recklinghausen's disease, but those most commonly affected are the optic nerve (by glioma) and the eighth nerve, and to a less extent the fifth nerve (by neurofibroma).

Gliomas of the Optic Nerve. Gliomas of the optic nerve may arise in the intraorbital division of the optic nerve, the post-ocular portion or in the chiasm. Most of these tumors are in the intraorbital division. The rarity of gliomas of the optic nerve and chiasm is shown by the fact that Martin and Cushing found only 7 gliomas in 233 cases with tumors involving the region of the chiasm. Davis collected from the literature 380 cases of glioma of the optic nerve and reported 5 cases in which the glioma was found in association with von Recklinghausen's disease. Although the tumor may be composed of any type of gliogenous cells, most commonly it is made up of piloid astrocytes.

Gliomas of the optic nerve occur predominantly in childhood. Progressive loss of vision, unilateral amblyopia or hemianoptic field defects are the characteristic presenting symptoms. These tumors grow slowly and lead to complete blindness in the course of several months or years. Proptosis, unilateral loss of vision, strabismus and swelling of the optic disc are the common signs of tumor in the nerve. Bilateral visual loss with various types of field defects and optic atrophy are characteristic of involvement of the chiasm by the tumor. The diagnosis of glioma of the optic nerve can usually be made on basis of clinical findings. Roentgenograms may show enlargement of the optic foramen (Fig. 50) or an anterior extension of the supraseller fossa (J-shaped

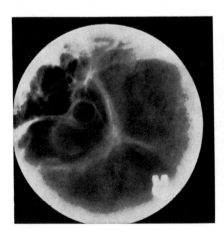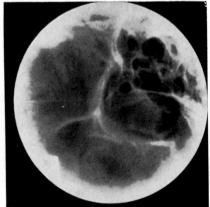

Figure 50. Optic nerve glioma. Symmetrical enlargement of the optic foramen on right. Compare with normal on left. (Chutorian, A. M., Schwarz, J. F., Evans, A., and Carter, S.: Courtesy Neurology.)

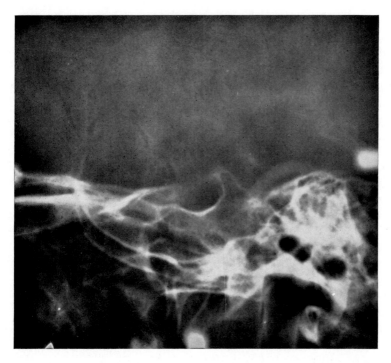

Figure 51. Optic nerve glioma. Anterior extension of the suprasellar fossa—J-shaped sella. (Chutorian, A. M., Schwarz, J. F., Evans, A., and Carter, S.: Courtesy Neurology.)

sella) (Fig. 51) and the tumor can be demonstrated in the C. T. brain scan. Gliomas of the nerve may be removed surgically. When the chiasm is involved, radiation therapy delays or arrests the progressive course of the disease. A malignant form of the tumor occurs occasionally in adult life. These tumors composed of rapidly growing glia cells destroy the optic nerves and chiasm and spread to involve the hypothalamus and neighboring portions of the brain.

REFERENCES

Chutorian, A. M., Schwarz, J. F., Evans, R. A., and Carter, S.: Optic Gliomas in Children, Neurology, 14, 83, 1964.
Davis, F. A.: Primary Tumors of the Optic Nerve (Phenomenon of Recklinghausen's Disease), A.M.A. Arch. Ophth., 23, 735 and 957, 1940.
Dodge, H. W., Jr., et al.: Gliomas of the Optic Nerves, Arch. Neurol. & Psychiat., 79, 607, 1958.
Hoyt, W. F., Meshel, L. G., et al.: Malignant Optic Gliomas of Adulthood, Brain, 96, 121, 1973.
Jackson, H.: Orbital Tumours, J. Neurosurg., 19, 551, 1962.
MacCarty, C. S., et al.: Tumors of the Optic Nerve and Optic Chiasm, J. Neurosurg., 33, 439, 1970.

Martin, P., and Cushing, H.: Primary Gliomas of the Chiasm and Optic Nerves in their
Intracranial Portion, Arch. Ophthal., 52, 209, 1923.
Taveras, J. M., Mount, L. A., and Wood, E. H.: Value of Radiation Therapy in the
Management of Glioma of the Optic Nerves and Chiasm, Radiology, 66, 518, 1956.

Neurofibromas of the Eighth Cranial Nerve. Acoustic Neuroma
(Acoustic Neurinoma, Perineural Fibroblastoma of the Eighth Nerve, Cerebellopontine Angle Tumor). There has been considerable discussion as
to the exact embryological origin of tumors involving the eighth nerve
but the opinion most widely accepted at present is that they arise from
the sheath of Schwann cells and that the appearance of nerve fibers
within the tumor is due to the fortuitous inclusion of normal fibers of
the nerve.

Pathology. According to the best evidence, acoustic neuromas originate in the peripheral portion of the vestibular division of the eighth
nerve in the porus acousticus. Small tumors in this location are
occasionally a chance finding at necropsy. By the time the tumor is
recognized clinically, it is mainly intracranial and of a large size. It is
oval or nodular in shape and is sharply circumscribed (Fig. 52). Fresh
specimens vary considerably in appearance and consistency. As a rule,
they are grayish yellow in color and firm in consistency. Cystic
degeneration occurs occasionally. The shape of the larger tumors is
irregular in order to conform to the walls of the posterior fossa. The
surface of the tumor is covered with numerous vascular attachments.

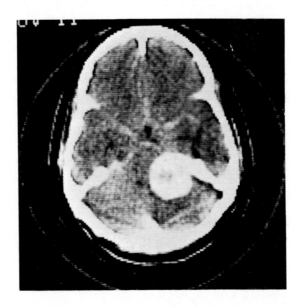

Figure 52.   CT brain scan, acoustic neuroma. (Courtesy of Dr. Harry H. White.)

The eighth nerve and usually also the seventh nerve are surrounded by the tumor, the neighboring cranial nerves are stretched and the adjacent brainstem is compressed and excavated.

Microscopically the tumor is composed of dense interlacing fibrous bands and a loose reticular tissue, in varying proportions. The fibrous appearing portions of the tumor are composed of elongated cells with oval nuclei. The nuclei have a tendency to be arranged in parallel rows or palisades. The reticular tissue is composed of round cells of varying size and lying in a loose tissue network. Collagen, elastic fibrils, fibrogen fibrils and reticulin can be demonstrated by appropriate stains.

Incidence. Tumors of the acoustic nerve constitute 5 to 10% of all intracranial tumors. In the majority of cases the onset of symptoms is in the third to sixth decade of life (Table 32). Onset of symptoms before the age of twenty is so rare that the occurrence of posterior fossa symptoms before that age should lead to a consideration of another type of tumor (usually a glioma). Approximately 60% of the cases are women. The isolated occurrence of bilateral acoustic neuroma on a familial basis is considered to be an oligosymptomatic form of neurofibromatosis.

Symptoms and Signs. Acoustic neuromas grow slowly and symptoms are usually present for many months or several years before the diagnosis is established. In the 42 cases reported by Olsen and Horrax the duration of symptoms before operation varied from six months to ten years with average of two years. In 1 case impairment of hearing had been present for thirty-two years. Loss of hearing, with or without tinnitus, is the first symptom in practically all cases and may precede the development of other symptoms by a period of many years. A careful inquiry may be necessary to establish these symptoms since partial or complete loss of hearing in one ear may not be noticed by the patient. With growth of the tumor there are symptoms and signs of

Table 32.   Age Incidence of Acoustic Neuroma

(Modified from Pool and Pava, *Acoustic Nerve Tumors*, Charles C Thomas, 1957)

Age	No. of Cases	%
0–10	3	1
11–20	29	6
21–30	78	17
31–40	114	24
41–50	135	29
51–60	77	17
61–70	27	6
	463	100

involvement of other cranial nerves, the brainstem, cerebellum or of increased intracranial pressure (Tables 33 and 34).

The *eighth cranial nerve* is involved in all of the cases. Tests made with an audiometer will show that loss of hearing of the nerve type is present in practically all cases.

Symptoms of involvement of vestibular portion of the eighth nerve may be entirely lacking but a sensation of giddiness or unsteadiness of gait is present in a large percentage of cases. Recurrent attacks of severe vertigo, similar to those of Ménière's syndrome, are rare. Complete or partial loss of response of the vestibular apparatus to caloric stimulation is such a constant finding that if a normal response is obtained on stimulation of the affected ear, the diagnosis is doubtful. Horizontal nystagmus is present in almost all cases. Occasionally there is vertical nystagmus.

Involvement of one or more of the *other cranial nerves* is practically always present. This is usually limited to the same side as the tumor but rarely the nerves on the opposite side may be affected. The fifth cranial nerve is involved in nearly 50% of the cases. Paresthesias in the

Table 33. The Incidence of Various Symptoms in 122 Patients with Acoustic Neuroma

(After Pool and Pava, *Acoustic Nerve Tumors*, Charles C Thomas, 1957)

Symptoms	No. of Cases	%
Deafness	107	88
Headache	80	65
Ataxia of Gait	80	65
Tinnitus	67	55
Hypesthesias or Paresthesia of Face	57	47
Diplopia or Blurred Vision	18	15

Table 34. The Frequency of Neurological Signs in 122 Patients with Acoustic Neuroma

(After Pool and Pava, *Acoustic Nerve Tumors*, Charles C Thomas, 1957)

Sign	%
Deafness	97
Nystagmus	80
Impairment of Caloric Reaction	98
Choked Disc	59
Fifth Cranial Nerve Palsy	47
Sixth Cranial Nerve Palsy	6
Seventh Cranial Nerve Palsy	65
Tenth Cranial Nerve Palsy	23
Cerebellar Ataxia	65

face are not uncommon, but severe neuralgical pains of the type of *tic douloureux* are rare. Loss of the corneal reflex is the most common sign of trigeminal involvement. Cutaneous hypesthesia in the distribution of the fifth nerve is present in two thirds of the cases and weakness of the muscles of mastication in one third.

Diplopia due to involvement of the sixth cranial nerve is present in less than 10% of the cases. Injury to the sixth cranial nerve is often associated with an increase in intracranial pressure and is not necessarily due to direct pressure on the nerve by the tumor.

Paralysis, or more usually, a partial weakness of the facial muscles on the homolateral side, is present in about 65% of the cases. Conjunctivitis or corneal ulcers are not uncommon complications when there is complete facial paralysis and corneal anesthesia.

Paresis or weakness of the muscles of the palate, tongue and neck occurs in a small percentage of the cases.

Signs and symptoms of pressure on the *brainstem and cerebellum* are present in practically all cases in the later stages of the disease. These usually take the form of ataxia of the gait and incoordination in the use of one or both upper extremities. Loss of cutaneous sensation or spastic weakness of one side of the body is rare. The sensory involvement and motor weakness may be on the same side or on the opposite side to that of the tumor. The presence of a homolateral sensory loss or motor weakness is explained as result of distortion of the brainstem. The reflexes are usually normal. They are occasionally less active than normal. In the patients with a spastic weakness they are increased and an extensor plantar response is present.

General Symptoms and Signs. Suboccipital discomfort and stiffness of the neck are common. Headaches, nausea and vomiting, dullness of the mental faculties, choked discs and secondary optic atrophy are an indication of internal hydrocephalus. These are usually late symptoms and, although they were almost constant in the cases recorded in the older literature, the diagnosis is usually established at the present time before these symptoms appear.

Laboratory Findings. The cerebrospinal fluid is usually under increased pressure, but the pressure may be normal in the early stage. The chief characteristic of the cerebrospinal fluid in patients with an acoustic neuroma is an increase in the protein content. This is almost constant and values over 150 mg per 100 ml are common. Appropriate x-ray examination of the skull may show an enlargement of the porus acousticus internus or an erosion of the petrous ridge. The pneumoencephalogram may show absence of air in the cerebellopontine angle and displacement and rotation of the fourth ventricle. The electroencephalogram may show the changes which are characteristic of increased intracranial pressure, with sometimes an exaggeration of the abnormalities in the posterior portion of the cerebral hemispheres.

Diagnosis and Differential Diagnosis. The diagnosis of an acoustic neuroma is made on the appearance of symptoms and signs of involvement of the eighth cranial nerve, followed by signs and symptoms of involvement of the neighboring cranial nerves, cerebellum and brainstem. Tomography, polytome studies and CT brain scan (Fig. 52) help to confirm the diagnosis. A posterior fossa myelogram is sometimes necessary if the tumor is small.

The syndrome of an acoustic neuroma may be simulated by any tumor in the cerebellopontine angle. These include neuromas of the fifth or other cranial nerves, meningiomas, papillomas, gliomas and cysts in the lateral recess, aneurysms and inflammatory processes. The diagnosis can be established in most cases from the history and the neurological findings, the results of the labyrinthine tests and the examination of the cerebrospinal fluid. If the initial symptoms are not referable to the eighth nerve, if the vestibular response to the caloric test is preserved or if the cerebrospinal fluid protein content is normal, the diagnosis of an acoustic neuroma is hazardous.

Course and Treatment. Untreated, the course of an acoustic neuroma is always progressive. There may be some fluctuation in the severity of symptoms but death is almost inevitable. The average duration of life of untreated cases is three and one-half to five years after the diagnosis is established. Fatal cases with symptoms of only a few months or many years' duration are not rare, however. Acoustic neuromas do not respond to radiation therapy and the only treatment is surgical removal.

Total removal of the tumor is the goal today. Seventh cranial nerve paralysis can frequently be avoided by meticulous microdissection of the tumor off of the nerve, particularly in small or medium sized lesions. Elderly patients with large tumors are best treated with intracapsular removal. Preoperative ventricular shunting in patients with large tumors is often helpful. Reoperation, if necessary, can be done quite safely.

REFERENCES

Cook, A. W., and Browder, E. J.: Total Removal of Acoustic Neuroma, Arch. Neurol., *21*, 7, 1969.
Cushing, H.: *Tumors of the Nervus Acusticus and the Syndrome of the Cerebellopontile Angle*, Philadelphia, W. B. Saunders Co., 1917, 296 pp.
Glasscock, N. E., Hays, J. M., and Murphy, J. P.: Complications in Acoustic Neuroma Surgery, Ann. Otol. Rhinol. Laryngol., *84*, 530, 1975.
Olivecrona, H.: Analysis of Results of Complete and Partial Removal of Acoustic Neuromas, J. Neurol., Neurosurg. & Psychiat., *13*, 271, 1950.
Olsen, A., and Horrax, G.: Symptomatology of Acoustic Tumors with Special Reference to Atypical Features, J. Neurosurg., *1*, 371, 1944.
Pennybacker, J. B., and Cairns, H.: Results in 130 Cases of Acoustic Neurinoma, J. Neurol., Neurosurg. & Psychiat., *13*, 272, 1950.

Pool, J. L., Pava, A., and Greenfield, E.: *Acoustic Nerve Tumors, Early Diagnosis and Treatment*, 2nd Ed. Springfield, Charles C Thomas, 1970, 232 pp.

Thomsen, J.: Suboccipital Removal of Acoustic Neuromas. Results of 125 Operations, Acta Otolaryngol.: *81*, 466, 1976.

————: Cerebellopontine Angle Tumors other Than Acoustic Neuromas, a Report of 34 Cases, A Presentation of Bilateral Acoustic Neuromas, Acta Otolaryngol., *82*, 106, 1976.

Young, D. F., Eldridge, R., and Gardner, W. J.: Bilateral Acoustic Neuroma in a Large Kindred, J.A.M.A., *214*, 347, 1970.

Neurofibromas of the Fifth Cranial Nerve. Neurofibromas of the gasserian ganglion or of the fifth nerve in the middle or posterior fossa are quite rare. Only a small number of cases are reported in the literature. When the tumor is confined to the gasserian ganglion and middle fossa, the signs are usually limited to sensory loss (with or without spontaneous pain) in the face, and paralysis and atrophy of the muscles of mastication. With growth of the tumor into the posterior fossa there are signs and symptoms of involvement of the lower cranial nerves, medulla and cerebellum. Roentgenograms of the base may show erosion of the foramen ovale or foramen rotundum.

Acoustic neuromas and involvement of the fifth nerve by metastatic tumor or carcinoma of the nasopharynx should be considered in the differential diagnosis. Treatment is by surgical removal.

REFERENCES

Gordy, P. D.: Neurinoma of the Gasserian Ganglion, J. Neurosurg., *22*, 90, 1965.

Olive, I., and Svien, H. J.: Neurofibromas of the Fifth Cranial Nerve, J. Neurosurg., *14*, 484, 1957.

Schisano, G., and Olivecrona, H.: Neurinomas of the Gasserian Ganglion and Trigeminal Root, J. Neurosurg., *17*, 306, 1960.

Gliomas

Gliomas are neoplasms which arise from primitive forms of the glial cells. They constitute nearly 50% of all intracranial tumors. Several attempts have been made to subdivide the gliomas into groups according to the embryological origin of the tumor cells. For various reasons no one of these classifications is entirely satisfactory but the one introduced by Bailey and Cushing is most widely used. The value of their classification lies in the fact that the various types of glial tumors have a different life history (Table 35), and although any of them may occur at any age or in any portion of the central nervous system, there is a tendency for some to occur at certain ages and to have a predilection for special regions of the nervous system.

Table 35.   The Average Survival Period for the Various Types of Gliomas

Type of Tumor	Survival* (in months)
Spongioblastoma multiforme	12
Medulloblastoma	17
Ependyblastoma	19
Astroblastoma	28
Ependymoma	32
Spongioblastoma unipolare	46
Oligodendroglioma	66
Astrocytoma—protoplasmic	67
Astrocytoma—fibrillary	86

* From earliest known symptoms.

Table 36.   The Incidence of the Various Types of Gliomas

Type	No. of Cases	%
Astrocytoma	255	38
Spongioblastoma multiforme	208	31
Medulloblastoma	86	11
Astroblastoma	35	5
Spongioblastoma polare	32	5
Oligodendroglioma	27	4
Ependymoma	25	4
Pinealoma	14	2
Ganglioneuroma	3	..
Neuroepithelioma	2	..
Total	687	100

The relative incidence of the various types of gliomas is given in Table 36, which is taken from Cushing's monograph. Included in this table are the pinealomas, which will be considered elsewhere, and the ganglioneuromas and neuroepitheliomas which are so rare as to cast some doubt upon their existence as separate entities.

There is considerable difference in the gross appearance of the various forms of gliomas. The slowly growing astrocytomas may appear firmer than the surrounding brain tissue, while the rapidly growing glioblastoma is soft and necrotic in appearance. In all forms of gliomas there is, as a rule, no sharp dividing line between the tumor and the neighboring brain tissue. The tumor growth tends to follow fiber pathways and may spread through one entire hemisphere or across the corpus callosum into the other hemisphere. Necrosis with cyst formation is not rare. Small hemorrhages are common in the more malignant types but large hemorrhages are infrequent.

A brief discussion of the more common forms of gliomas is given below. It must be remembered that these tumors do not always occur in pure culture and that mixed or transitional forms are not rare.

Astrocytomas. The astrocytomas, which constitute approximately 40% of the gliomas, are tumors composed almost entirely of astrocytes. These tumors tend to infiltrate large areas and may undergo cystic degeneration. Occasionally there may be a large cyst with only a small nodule of tumor in the cyst wall. Astrocytomas grow much more slowly than other gliomas but they can hardly be called benign since complete surgical removal is only occasionally possible.

Astrocytomas may occur in any portion of the brain, cerebellum or spinal cord. They may occur at any age but astrocytomas of the cerebellum, particularly the cysts with a mural nodule, occur predominantly in children or young adults and are rare after the age of thirty. Astrocytomas are treated by surgical excision and radiation therapy. Complete cure is possible when the tumor is cystic with a mural nodule, as sometimes occurs in the cerebellum, and survival with several to many years of useful life is sometimes possible even in the diffuse astrocytomas of the cerebral hemispheres.

A distinctive syndrome is produced by astrocytomas in the hypothalamic region in infants. The syndrome, first described by Russell in 1951, is characterized by emaciation and failure of the infant to thrive normally in spite of adequate caloric intake, unusual alertness, hyperactivity, euphoria and evidences of autonomic dysfunction. Only a small number of cases have been reported, but there are probably a much larger number of cases that have not been reported or have not been diagnosed.

Astrocytomas are also common in optic nerve and brainstem. In these sites the nuclei of the cells are apt to be elongated and arranged in parallel lines giving a palisade-like appearance (piloid astrocytoma). These tumors have been described in the older literature by terms such as central neurons and spongioblastoma polare. Involvement of the optic nerve and chiasm is discussed on page 246.

Brain Stem Glioma. Infiltration of the brainstem by astrocytomas or other forms of glioma is most commonly seen in children or young adults, although it is not rare in middle-aged adults. Multiple cranial nerve palsies and signs of involvement of the long tracts in the brainstem are the characteristic clinical features. Increased intracranial pressure and choked disc develop when the aqueduct of Sylvius is occluded by the tumor or when the brainstem enlarges to a size sufficient to interfere with the drainage of cerebrospinal fluid. This is usually a late development and it is not rare for death to ensue before choked discs develop.

Any of the cranial nerve nuclei may be affected, but unilateral or bilateral sixth nerve paralysis is the most common sign. Paralysis of the facial nerve, deafness and palatal weakness, all usually unilateral, are the next most common symptoms. With growth of the tumor, there may be signs of involvement of the cerebellar peduncles, corticospinal tract and spinal lemniscus. A glioma may infiltrate the pons and destroy some nuclei and fiber paths but leave others relatively unaffected.

It is important to differentiate between gliomas of the brainstem and extramedullary tumors in the posterior fossa (neurofibromas, meningiomas and cysts) which are amenable to therapy. The differential is not always possible before operation. Some points which are of value in the localizing of the lesion within the brainstem are: (1) The young age of the patient; (2) the presence of paralysis of conjugate gaze rather than a simple paralysis of one external rectus muscle; (3) the development of signs of injury to the long tracts before the appearance of choked discs; and (4) the appearance of signs and symptoms which rarely result from compression of the brainstem, i.e., Horner's syndrome, vertical nystagmus and singultus. Frequently, the diagnosis of an intrapontine glioma can be established by the demonstration of enlargement of the pons in the CT brain scan.

If the diagnosis of an intramedullary tumor can be established by the presence of the characteristic clinical findings, treatment should be with radiation therapy. Reduction in the severity of symptoms and prolongation of the course often result. When there is any reasonable doubt as to whether the tumor is extra- or intramedullary, exploratory operation is justified.

Oligodendroglioma. Oligodendrogliomas are tumors which are derived from primitive forms of the oligodendroglia. They constitute less than 5% of all gliomas and are found chiefly in the cerebral hemispheres of young adults. They are firm in consistency and are more often circumscribed than the more rapidly growing gliomas. Hemorrhagic areas and cystic degeneration are uncommon. Microscopically the appearance is quite characteristic. The tumor is quite cellular with the cells uniform in size and shape, fairly evenly spaced in a loose meshwork. The nuclei of the cells are round with a large amount of chromatin and are surrounded by a faint halo of cytoplasm. Small flecks of calcium are present in about 50% of these tumors.

Oligodendrogliomas occur in the cerebral ventricles (lateral or third) or in the cerebral hemispheres. Those in the cerebral ventricles tend to occur at an earlier age, have a shorter duration than those in the cerebral hemispheres, and are characterized clinically by the presence of signs and symptoms of increased intracranial pressure without convulsive seizures or focal neurological signs.

Increased intracranial pressure is a relatively late sign in the oligodendrogliomas of the hemisphere. Focal neurological signs and convulsive seizures, generalized or jacksonian, are common.

The diagnosis of an oligodendroglioma can sometimes be made by finding the characteristic flecks of calcium in the tumor in the roentgenograms.

Oligodendrogliomas are rarely amenable to complete surgical removal. Partial removal of the tumor with subsequent radiation therapy may give the patient several or many years of useful life.

A more malignant tumor of the oligodendroglia with numerous mitotic figures is known as the oligodendroblastoma.

Glioblastoma Multiforme (Spongioblastoma Multiforme). The glioblastoma multiforme is the most rapidly growing form of glioma. Grossly, these tumors appear soft with numerous small yellow areas of degeneration or petechial hemorrhages. Microscopically, the tumor is cellular and is composed of cells of many sizes and shapes. Mitotic figures and bizarrely shaped giant cells with many nuclei are common.

Glioblastoma multiforme constitutes about one third of all the gliomas. They may occur in any part of the central nervous system but they are most frequently found in the cerebral hemisphere of adults (Figs. 53 and 54). They invade large portions of the hemisphere and

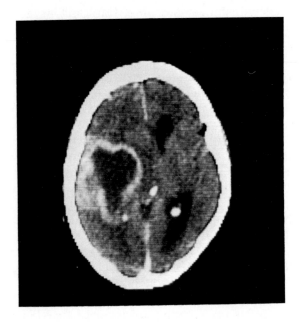

Figure 53.   CT brain scan, Glioblastoma, ring enhancement. (Courtesy of Dr. Sadek Hillal.)

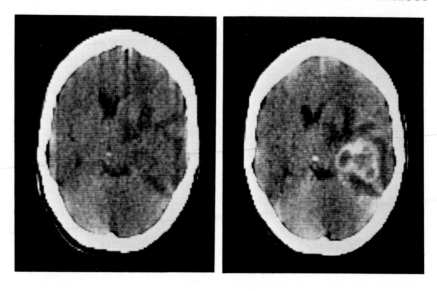

Figure 54. CT brain scan. Glioblastoma. Pre and post enhancement.
(Courtesy of Dr. Sadek Hillal.)

often spread to the opposite hemisphere by way of the corpus callosum. They may seed into the cerebrospinal fluid and produce tumors in remote regions of the nervous system. They are rapidly fatal, leading to death within one year in the vast majority of the cases. The invasive nature of the tumor makes them unsuitable for surgical removal. They respond poorly to radiation therapy, but prolongation of life for months or years is possible with intensive therapy.

Medulloblastomas. The medulloblastomas constitute about 10% of the gliomas. These tumors are derived from the most primitive form of glial cell. They may occur in any part of the nervous system but they are predominantly a tumor of the cerebellum. The tumor is reddish in color and soft in consistency. Commonly it arises in the posterior midline or vermis of the cerebellum and invades the fourth ventricle and the neighboring cerebellar hemispheres. It is a cellular tumor containing numerous mitotic figures. The predominant cell has a round or oval nucleus with abundant chromatin and scanty cytoplasm. There is no characteristic arrangement of the cells but occasionally there may be pseudorosette formations. Other types of cells, such as spongioblasts and neuroblasts, are scattered throughout the tumor.

Although medulloblastomas may occur in adults, they are most frequently seen in infants or young children and are relatively rare after the age of twenty. Increased intracranial pressure as the result of an internal hydrocephalus is an early sign. Headaches, vomiting and unsteadiness of the gait are usually the presenting symptoms. Separation of the cranial sutures, choked discs and nystagmus are common findings. The medulloblastoma is a rapidly growing tumor and is usually fatal within a year although cases are on record with a survival period of many years. The medulloblastoma has a tendency to metastasize through the subarachnoid spaces to the cerebral hemisphere or to the spinal cord and rarely to other parts of the body, particularly when procedures for shunting of the cerebrospinal fluid have been performed. Thus symptoms of involvement of the cranial nerves, cerebral cortex, spinal cord or spinal nerve roots (particularly those of the cauda equina) are not rare in the later stages of the disease. Although they may occasionally appear to be sharply circumscribed, they cannot be removed in their entirety by surgery and recurrence is almost inevitable. They are influenced to a moderate degree by radiation therapy. According to Ingraham, Bailey and Barker the survival period is directly related to the total dosage. The tendency of these tumors to spread to other portions of the nervous system through the cerebrospinal fluid pathways makes it advisable to radiate the entire nervous system as well as the site of the tumor.

Ependymoma. Ependymomas are tumors composed of primitive forms of the ependymal glia. They may occur in relationship to any part of the ventricular system (lateral, third or fourth ventricles or spinal

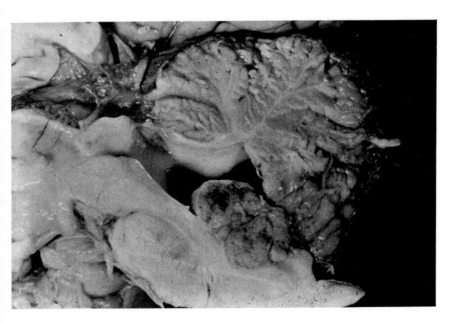

Figure 55. Ependymoma of fourth ventricle. (Courtesy Dr. J. Kepes.)

canal) but they are most common in the fourth ventricle (Fig. 55). The tumors arise from the ventricular walls, fill the ventricular cavity and invade the adjacent tissues. Grossly, they are firm grayish tumors. Occasionally, there are small areas of cystic degeneration and flecks of calcium. Microscopically, they are composed of polyhedral cells with a moderate amount of cytoplasm fitted tightly together in a mosaic pattern and spindle-shaped cells with a rather long, fine process terminating on a blood vessel wall and forming a corona about the vessel. Both of these cells contain small round or rod-shaped bodies within the cytoplasm known as blepharoplasten.

Ependymomas may occur at any age but they are most common in children. Ependymomas arising from the lateral ventricles produce symptoms similar to other tumors of the cerebral hemisphere. Those in the fourth ventricle produce a clinical picture simulating that of the medulloblastomas. Ependymomas of the central canal may involve an extensive longitudinal area of the spinal cord.

Ependymomas are rarely amenable to complete surgical removal and they respond only slightly to radiation therapy. They are relatively malignant, with an average life history of two and one-half to three years.

REFERENCES

Bailey, P. and Cushing, H.: A Classification of the Tumors of the Glioma Group on a Histogenetic Basis with a Correlated Study of Prognosis, Philadelphia, J. B. Lippincott Co., 1926, 175 pp.

Barnett, H. J., and Hyland, H. H.: Tumours Involving the Brain-stem, Quart. J. Med., 21, 265, 1952.

Bucy, P. C., and Thieman, P. W.: Astrocytomas of the Cerebellum, Arch. Neurol., 18, 14, 1968.

Glassauer, F. E., and Yuan, R. H. P.: Intracranial Tumors with Extracranial Metastases, J. Neurosurg., 20, 474, 1963.

Ingraham, F. D., Bailey, O. T., and Barker, W. F.: Medulloblastoma Cerebelli, New Eng. J. Med., 238, 171, 1948.

Jelsman, R., and Bucy, P. C.: Glioblastoma Multiforme, Arch. Neurol., 20, 161, 1969.

Kricheff, I. I., Becker, M., Schneck, S. A., and Taveras, J. M.: Intracranial Ependymomas. A Study of Survival in 65 Cases Treated by Surgery and Irradiation, Am. J. Roentgen., 91, 167, 1964.

Paterson, E.: Distant Metastases from Medulloblastoma of the Cerebellum, Brain, 84, 301, 1961.

Roberts, M., and German, W. J.: A Long-term Study of Patients with Oligodendrogliomas, J. Neurosurg., 24, 697, 1966.

Russell, A.: A Diencephalic Syndrome of Emaciation in Infancy and Childhood, Arch. Dis. Childh., 26, 274, 1951.

Shapiro, W. R., and Young, D. F.: Treatment of Malignant Glioma. A Controlled Study of Chemotherapy and Irradiation, Arch. Neurol., 33, 494, 1976.

Smith, R. A., Lampe, I., and Kahn, E. A.: The Prognosis of Medulloblastoma in Children, J. Neurosurg., 18, 91, 1961.

Torrey, E. F., and Uyeda, C. I.: The Diencephalic Syndrome of Infancy, Am. J. Dis. Child., 110, 689, 1965.

White, H. H.: Brain Stem Tumors Occurring in Adults, Neurology, 13, 292, 1963.

White, P. T., and Ross, A. T.: Inanition Syndrome in Infants with Anterior Hypothalamic Neoplasms, Neurology, 13, 974, 1963.

Tumors of the Ductless Glands

Pinealomas. Pinealomas and pineoblastomas are generally considered as belonging to the class of the gliomas. They are relatively rare, constituting only 2% of the gliomas in Cushing's series. Grossly, they are similar in appearance to the medulloblastoma, and are composed of nests of tumor cells separated by areas of cells with a lymphoid appearance. The tumor cells are large and spherical with large vesicular nuclei and processes which may end in typical bulbs. Pineoblastomas are rarer than pinealomas and are composed of small cells with round nuclei and little or no cytoplasm. Occasionally the pineal gland may be the site of a teratoma or a malignant tumor called germinoma. These tumors are prone to metastasize widely.

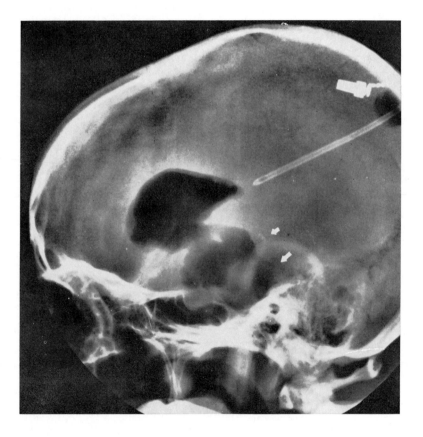

Figure 56. Pinealoma. Ventriculogram. The lateral ventricles and anterior three fourths of the third ventricle are enlarged. The posterior part of the third ventricle is obliterated by a mass which envelops calcified portion of the pineal (upper arrow). The aqueduct is displaced downward and occluded (lower arrow). (Courtesy Dr. Ernest Wood.)

Tumors of the pineal gland occur most commonly between the ages of fifteen and twenty-five years. Nearly 90% of the reported cases have been in the male sex. They vary in size from a few millimeters to several centimeters in diameter. They have a slow rate of growth but, owing to their peculiar location, they have a relatively short life history, usually under two years, although cases with a duration of five or more years are not rare.

Pinealomas compress the anterior quadrigeminal plate and occlude the aqueduct of Sylvius (Fig. 56) causing an internal hydrocephalus and choking of the disc. Characteristic symptoms and signs include paralysis of upward gaze (Parinaud's syndrome), dilatation of the pupils with loss of the pupillary reflexes to light and accommodation, and impairment of hearing. Signs of involvement of the cerebrum or the cerebellum may develop late in the course of the tumor as the result of its extension. Precocious puberty occurs in a small percentage of cases. It is now generally agreed that precocious puberty, diabetes insipidus and other signs and symptoms of involvement of the hypothalamus are due to a secondary involvement of the latter area as result of increased intracranial pressure or the presence of tumor cells in this region. The presence of pineal tumors in the pituitary and hypothalamic region is explained by some as the result of seeding of the tumor through the subarachnoid spaces and by others as due to presence of tumor cells of the germinoma type in this region.

Pineal tumors are not easily accessible to operative approach, and are usually treated by radiation therapy, together with shunting procedures to relieve hydrocephalus. Survival for more than five years can be obtained in about two thirds of the cases.

REFERENCES

Cummins, F. M., Taveras, J. M. and Schlesinger, E. B.: Treatment of Gliomas of the Third Ventricle and Pinealomas, Neurology, 10, 1031, 1960.
Horrax, G.: Further Observations on Tumor of the Pineal Body, Arch. Neurol. & Psychiat., 35, 215, 1936.
Horrax, G., and Bailey, P.: Tumors of the Pineal Body, Arch. Neurol. & Psychiat., 13, 423, 1925.
Kageyama, N. and Belsky, R.: Ectopic Pinealoma in the Chiasma Region, Neurology, 11, 318, 1961.
Russell, D.: Ectopic Pinealoma, Its Kinship to Teratoma of the Pineal Gland, J. Path. & Bact., 68, 125, 1954.

Tumors of the Pituitary Gland

J. Lobo Antunes, M.D.

Tumors of the pituitary gland have been classified in three types, according to their staining characteristics using the classical histological techniques: *chromophobe adenomas*, the most common type, *acidophilic adenomas*, which cause acromegaly and, the least common, *basophilic adenomas*, associated with Cushing's disease. It has become apparent in recent years, particularly since the advent of specific and sensitive techniques for measuring the different pituitary hormones, that such classification is of limited usefulness. Indeed, most pituitary tumors secreting growth hormone, or prolactin are chromophobe adenomas, and therefore the concept that chromophobe tumors are essentially non-functioning had to be revised. With the development of more accurate radiographic techniques it has been found that a number of patients with pituitary dysfunction and a variety of clinical pictures, such as amenorrhea-galactorrhea, are, indeed, harboring small secreting tumors *(microadenomas)*, that can not be detected by the standard radiological procedures. Although it is generally considered that pituitary adenomas represent about 10% of all intracranial tumors, its real incidence is probably considerably higher if one includes these small secreting tumors that are not diagnosed due to the paucity of their neurological manifestations. In fact, small pituitary adenomas are an incidental finding in about 25% of all glands studied in large autopsy series.

A classification more satisfactory, that is, from a clinical point, divides pituitary tumors into *secreting* and *nonsecreting*. The former are subdivided according to which hormone is produced in excess— growth hormone (GH), prolactin (Prol.), adrenocorticotropin (ACTH), thyrotropin (TSH) or gonadotropins, luteinizing hormone (LH) and follicle-stimulating hormone (FSH). From a therapeutic point it is also important to consider the size of the lesion, and the criteria first proposed by Hardy are particularly useful. The term *enclosed adenomas* applies whenever the floor of the sella turcica is intact, whereas in the case of *invasive adenomas* there is erosion of the floor. Further qualification depends on whether the tumor remains *intrasellar* or whether there is an *extrasellar* (more frequently *suprasellar*) extension. The designation of *microadenoma* applies to tumors smaller than 10 mm in diameter.

PATHOLOGY. Pituitary tumors are more frequent in the third and fourth decades and they affect both sexes equally. The great majority are, by standard histological techniques, chromophobe tumors. Macroscopically some of these are well encapsulated, while others behave more like focal hyperplasias. They are usually dark, soft and not infrequently hemorrhagic, necrotic or cystic. Microscopically the cells are arranged in a syncytial or sinusoidal pattern. Eosinophilic and basophilic tumors are usually smaller.

Using specific immunocytochemical techniques it has been demonstrated that a number of chromophobe tumors are actively secreting hormones, particularly prolactin and growth hormone, and occasionally both of them. It has also been noticed that the small secreting adenomas occupy different locations in the gland, which follow closely the normal distribution of the various cell types. Thus tumors that secrete growth hormone are usually lateral and superficial, and prolactin secreting adenomas are also lateral, but deeper. ACTH secreting tumors are deep and centrally placed and the rare TSH producing adenomas, more superficial.

As the adenoma progressively grows, it displaces and eventually destroys the adjacent functioning parenchyma, and enlarges the sella turcica; further expansion depends in part on the size of the aperture of the diaphragma sellae. Frequently they extend upwards filling the suprasellar cisterns, impinging on the recesses of the third ventricle and, rarely, obstructing the foramina of Monro, causing hydrocephalus. They occasionally expand laterally into the cavernous sinus or the temporal fossa, grow forwards under the frontal lobes or caudally into the interpeduncular cistern. Not infrequently they cause erosion of the floor of the sella protruding into the sphenoid sinus.

Intracranial or extracranial metastases from pituitary adenomas are exceptional, and the term pituitary carcinoma is, on histological grounds, rarely justifiable. Some cases may show, however, remarkable invasive characteristics together with rapid growing and anaplastic features.

A number of families have been reported, with a high incidence of hyperplasia or tumors involving multiple endocrine glands including parathyroids, pituitary, pancreatic islets, thyroid and adrenal cortex, many of which are functional. This *multiple endocrine adenomatosis* is inherited as an autosomal dominant trait with high penetrance.

Tumors of the posterior lobe (neurohypophysis) are extremely rare and behave like hypothalamic gliomas. They are of two distinct morphological types: gliomas (infundibulomas), or choristomas (myoblastomas or granular cell tumors).

CLINICAL FEATURES. The clinical manifestations of pituitary adenomas depend on their local expansion with displacement and compression of the adjacent neural and vascular structures, and on the endocrine dysfunctions they produce.

Neurological Symptoms. Headaches, frequently frontal, are a common complaint, and they are usually attributed to pressure upon the diaphragma sellae and adjacent structures. *Visual symptoms* are also frequent, and are practically constant in cases with suprasellar extension. The patients may complain of progressive blurring or dimming of vision. When present, visual field defects involve the temporal fields (bitemporal hemianopsia) (Fig. 57), starting with the upper quadrants. With further growth of the tumor the lower nasal quadrants and finally

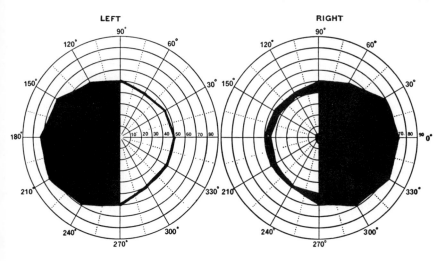

Figure 57. Chromophobe adenoma. Bitemporal hemianopia; visual acuity O.D.
15/200, O.S. 15/30. (Courtesy Max Chamlin.)

the upper nasal quadrants may be also compromised. In some cases the macular fibers of the chiasm are affected first giving rise to a central hemianoptic scotoma, which may be missed unless the central fields are also examined. More rarely, loss of vision in one eye or a homonymous hemianopsia are the presenting visual symptoms. Examination of the optic fundi frequently reveals pallor or atrophy of the optic discs, and only exceptionally, papilledema.

Involvement of other cranial nerves, particularly of III, IV and VI is present in 5 to 15% of the cases, and indicates lateral extension of the tumor. In these cases facial hypesthesia is occasionally noticed.

Other neurological manifestations depend on the direction of growth of the tumor. Thus some patients with large suprasellar extensions may present signs of hypothalamic dysfunction, including diabetes insipidus, and hydrocephalus. Tumors that insinuate under the frontal lobes may cause personality changes or dementia. Seizures and a number of motor and sensory symptoms occasionally occur. Cerebrospinal fluid rhinorrhea is not unusual in cases where the tumor has eroded the base of the skull.

Pituitary tumors occur only rarely in children or adolescents. When present they seem to have a higher incidence of extrasellar extensions, and obesity and extraocular palsies are more frequently seen. Enlargement of adenomas during pregnancy has also been reported. This is of particular importance in women with amenorrhea and infertility in whom pregnancy was induced in the presence of an unrecognized pituitary tumor.

About 5% of patients with pituitary tumors will present with the picture of *pituitary apoplexy*. This frequently simulates a subarachnoid hemorrhage, with a sudden onset of severe headaches, nausea, vomiting, alteration of consciousness, diplopia, and sometimes, rapid and progressive visual loss. More rarely facial paresthesias, seizures or focal signs also occur. A lumbar puncture may show increased pressure, pleocytosis or fresh blood. The diagnosis of pituitary apoplexy is then made by the finding of an enlarged sella turcica in radiographs of the skull, and changes consistent with a sellar tumor in the angiogram. A detailed history will reveal that endocrine changes had been present for a while. Pituitary apoplexy usually results from an hemorrhagic infarction of an adenoma.

Endocrine Symptoms. Hypopituitarism. A variable degree of hypopituitarism is present in the majority of patients with pituitary adenomas, particularly when they have reached a considerable size. It is important to emphasize, however, that a number of patients with microadenomas will have preserved function, and this is why early recognition and treatment of these lesions is imperative. Secretion of gonadotropins is affected first and this will lead in women to irregularities of the menstrual periods and amenorrhea, and in men to loss of libido and decreased potency. In late cases, oligospermia or azoospermia and testicular atrophy may be present. The skin is often thin, smooth, and dry; its peculiar pallor and inability to tan have been related to loss of the melanocyte-stimulating hormone. There is a decrease in axillary and pubic hair, and in the frequency of shaving. Due to decrease in ACTH and TSH production, patients frequently complain of lethargy, weakness, fatigability, intolerance to cold and constipation. Acute adrenal crisis with nausea, vomiting, hypoglycemia, hypotension and even circulatory collapse may also occur, particularly in response to stress. Diabetes insipidus is only rarely seen.

Prolactin Secreting Adenomas. These are the most common of all secreting pituitary adenomas. In fact, hyperprolactinemia is present in about 70 to 75% of all patients with pituitary tumors. Although the increased prolactin may not give rise to any clinical manifestations, a large number of women will complain of amenorrhea, sometimes associated with galactorrhea, which may have started after oral contraceptives were discontinued. In males decreased sexual potency, and, more rarely, galactorrhea, may be present. It is important to emphasize that serum prolactin measurement and radiographic studies of the skull should be obtained in all women in reproductive age, presenting with amenorrhea because a significant number of them will have a pituitary adenoma.

Growth Hormone Secreting Adenomas. Excessive secretion of growth hormone results in the picture of *gigantism*, if it begins before

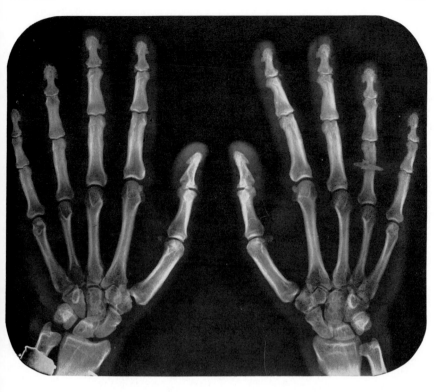

Figure 58. Acromegaly. Tufting of terminal phalanges. (Courtesy Juan Taveras.)

closure of the epiphysis occurs, or *acromegaly* (Figs. 58 to 60) if it starts later. When fully developed, acromegaly is easily recognized, due to excessive skeletal and soft tissue growth. The facial features are coarse, with a large bulbous nose, prominent supraorbital ridges and a protruding mandible, with separated teeth and thick lips. The hands and feet are enlarged, and the patient frequently has a slightly kyphotic posture. The voice is harsh, and increased sweating is frequently noticed. Visceromegaly is also part of the clinical picture. These changes are usually slowly progressive. Patients complain of headaches, fatigue, muscular pain, paresthesias, sometimes manifesting as a carpal tunnel syndrome, visual disturbances and impairment of gonadal function. Generalized arthritis, and diabetes mellitus are a frequent component, and thyroid enlargement and hirsutism may also be present. A number of these patients will show increased prolactin secretion as well. Increased mortality associated with acromegaly is now well documented.

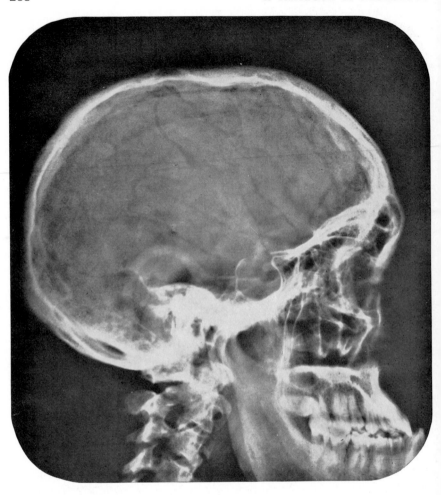

Figure 59. Pituitary tumor. Chromophile adenoma with ballooning of sella turcica, prognathism, and enlargement of bones of skull. (Courtesy of Juan Taveras.)

The facial features of acromegaly are occasionally present with no chemical evidence of an endocrine abnormality. These cases of "inactive" or "burned-out" acromegaly are probably caused by a secreting tumor that has spontaneously regressed.

Cushing's Syndrome. The clinical manifestations known as Cushing's syndrome result from hypercortisolism which is not always due, as originally thought by Cushing to a basophilic pituitary tumor secreting excessive amounts of ACTH. In fact only about 10% of the cases of Cushing's syndrome are caused by pituitary tumors. Others are due to adrenal adenomas or carcinomas, or a variety of malignant

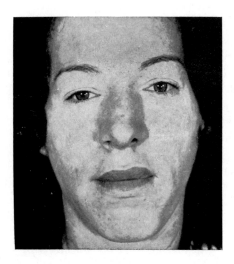

Figure 60.   Chromophile adenoma of pituitary. Prognathism and enlargement of nose in acromegaly. (Courtesy of Dr. E. Herz.)

tumors which produce "ectopic" ACTH. In other cases, one may find an adrenal hyperplasia, and in these patients, although basal ACTH levels may be normal, there is a disturbance of its secretory rhythm, that points to a hypothalamic dysfunction as the primary mechanism.

When fully developed, the clinical syndrome includes a plethoric appearance, with rounding of the face, trunkal obesity, hirsutism, purple striae in the skin of the abdomen, breasts and thighs and there is a tendency for excessive bleeding from scratches. Other manifestations include hypertension, osteoporosis, diabetes, polycythemia, lympho- and eosinopenia, and electrolyte imbalance. Visual symptoms in the cases associated with pituitary adenomas are uncommon, since the tumors are usually small. Chromophobe tumors may develop after adrenalectomy for Cushing's disease *(Nelson's syndrome)*, and many of these cases will show abnormal pigmentation of the skin.

Other Secreting Tumors. Pituitary tumors secreting TSH and causing hyperthyroidism have been reported. Adenomas secreting excessive amounts of gonadotropins are even more exceptional.

Diagnosis. *Radiographic Techniques.* Meticulous radiological evaluation is important in the differential diagnosis of sellar and parasellar lesions, and to determine the extent of the lesion. This is obviously crucial for adequate planning of the treatment. Plain radiographs of the skull associated with polytomography are essential to evaluate the intrasellar growth of the lesion. Most pituitary tumors (Fig. 59) will enlarge the sella and modify its contour—"ballooning"—thinning the dorsum, floor and, sometimes, the clinoid processes. The micro-adenomas do not increase the volume of the sella, but almost always will cause an asymmetrical depression of the floor ("double floor"), detectable only with polytomography. Erosion of the floor of the sella and extension into the sphenoid sinus can also be appreciated.

In patients with acromegaly other abnormal features can be demonstrated with simple radiological techniques. These include enlargement of the paranasal sinus, increase in thickness of the cranial bones, enlargement of the mandible, and separation of the teeth. Hypertrophy of the hands, enlargement of the ungual tufts of the terminal phalanges and hypertrophy of the soft tissues of the pad of the heel are also typical findings. Radiographs of the spine will reveal an increase in antero-posterior diameter of the vertebral bodies and progressive kyphosis.

To determine the degree of extrasellar extension of the tumor contrast studies are necessary. Pneumoencephalography (or in cases with obstruction of the foramina of Monro, ventriculography) with tomography are particularly helpful in delineating the size and shape of a suprasellar extension, which usually presents as a dome-shaped mass just above the diaphragma sellae, filling the suprasellar cisterns and, frequently, blunting the anterior recesses of the third ventricle.

Lateral displacement of the intracavernous portion of the internal carotid artery and elevation of the initial segments of the anterior cerebral arteries are the characteristic angiographic findings. A tumor blush may be visualized with appropriate techniques. Angiography is also important in excluding the presence of an intracranial aneurysm, which may simulate a pituitary adenoma.

Isotopic scanning is of limited value except for tumors with large suprasellar components.

Computerized tomography (Fig. 61) may eventually replace the contrast studies in the evaluation of these lesions, since it demonstrates the presence and size of a pituitary adenoma very nicely. These are better visualized with contrast material. The technique is also helpful in demonstrating the presence of a cyst or an "empty sella."

Endocrine Evaluation. Endocrine evaluation of patients with pituitary tumors depends on the assessment of the function of the target organs, and the direct assay in the blood of the anterior pituitary hormones. Adrenal function can be evaluated by measuring the urinary excretion of 17-hydroxy and 17-ketosteroids, cortisol levels, and the response to stimulation with ACTH or suppression with dexamethasone. These tests as well as direct assay of ACTH are indispensable in the diagnosis of Cushing's disease. Radioimmunoassay of LH, and FSH, and measurement of testosterone levels are good indicators of gonadal function. Prolactin can be measured by radioimmunoassay and values in excess of 20ng/ml in men, and 25ng/ml in

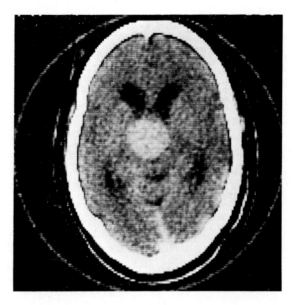

Figure 61.   CT brain scan. Pituitary tumor. (Courtesy Dr. Harry H. White.)

women are considered abnormal; levels above 300ng/ml are practically diagnostic of a pituitary tumor. In these situations the increase in prolactin by chlorpromazine of TRH (TSH-releasing hormone) and its suppression by L-Dopa are usually less pronounced than normally. Hypersecretion of growth hormone can also be documented by radioimmunoassay. Equally important for the diagnosis is the fact that the increased levels cannot be suppressed by hyperglycemia. Finally, thyroid hormone measurements are readily available. Elevation of TSH associated with hyperthyroidism has been found in the rare cases of TSH secreting tumors.

DIFFERENTIAL DIAGNOSIS. The diagnosis of pituitary tumors depends on a thorough radiological and endocrine evaluation. A number of other sellar and parasellar lesions can, however, simulate the clinical and sometimes radiographic features of a pituitary adenoma. These include tumors such as craniopharyngiomas, which usually manifest at an earlier age and are frequently calcified, meningiomas, optic gliomas, chordomas, atypical teratomas, dermoid tumors, metastasis and invasive nasopharyngeal carcinomas. Intrasellar or parasellar aneurysms can be diagnosed by angiography. Mucoceles of the sphenoid sinus may occasionally be difficult to distinguish from an invasive adenoma. Chronically increased intracranial pressure may cause enlargement of the sella turcica and visual symptoms.

In recent years increasing attention is being paid to the so-called *empty-sella* syndrome. In this situation, the subarachnoid space extends into the sella through an incompetent diaphragma flattening the gland against the floor. These cases are sometimes found following the incidental discovery of a large sella, or during a work-up for headaches. A number of cases have been reported, where pseudotumor cerebri was present, and a possible role of increased intracranial pressure in causing the empty sella has been suggested. Cerebrospinal fluid rhinorrhea has also been described in this situation. Endocrine abnormalities, when present, are usually mild. The diagnosis is made by pneumoencephalography with tomographic cuts and, more recently, by the CT brain scan. An *acquired empty sella* has occasionally followed surgical procedures.

TREATMENT. The first steps in the treatment of pituitary adenomas are the correction of any electrolyte imbalance and, if needed, institution of replacement therapy, particularly thyroid and steroid hormones. These should be started if hypopituitarism is suspected, and immediately after blood specimens for the necessary endocrine evaluation, are obtained. Adequate steroid coverage must be provided for both radiographic and surgical procedures.

The goals of treatment are different for the secreting tumors, and in particular the microadenomas, and the non-secreting lesions, usually chromophobe adenomas, presenting with visual compromise. In the first case, a biological cure is to be attained, correcting the hypersecreting status and preserving the normally functioning gland. This can often be achieved by selectively removing the tumor. In the latter cases, a more radical tumor excision, decompression of the optic pathways and prevention of recurrence are the main objectives.

Not all pituitary tumors will require immediate treatment. In some cases an enlarged sella turcica is found in the absence of any neurological or endocrine manifestations. These patients should be closely watched and the treatment deferred, although progression of the lesion may of course occur. The same attitude seems justified in patients who present with acromegalic features but no chemical evidence of active disease.

Radiotherapy and surgery are the two basic and frequently complementary modalities of treatment.

*Radiotherapy.*Conventional irradiation using external beams and total doses of about 5000 r is indicated as the initial form of treatment in patients who constitute poor operative risks, or in the small, non-secreting tumors, with minimal or no visual involvement. If visual deterioration occurs in these cases, surgical decompression is indicated. Radiotherapy should also be given following surgery, in all cases where only a subtotal removal of the tumor was performed, since it has been demonstrated that it significantly reduces the incidence of recurrences. If these occur, surgical decompression through a subfrontal or transsphenoidal approach is usually preferable than a second course of radiotherapy. Radiotherapy is contraindicated in cases of pituitary apoplexy, or when there has been a rapidly progressive visual deficit.

In the case of secreting tumors, conventional radiotherapy effectively decreases the abnormal hormonal levels, although restoration of complete normal values occurs only infrequently. In addition, these results may only be observed several months after the treatment has been completed. One should also notice that radiotherapy is not without complications such as radiation necrosis of the brain, and rarely visual deterioration.

A number of rather sophisticated irradiation techniques have also been proposed in an attempt to achieve a better rate of cure particularly of the hypersecreting adenomas. These include proton beam and heavy particles irradiation and the implantation inside the sella of radioactive isotopes like yttrium (^{90}Y) and gold (^{198}Au). These forms of treatment, although having a better result in reducing abnormal hormonal levels, have also a number of undesirable side effects including a considerably high incidence of post-treatment hypopituitarism.

Surgical Treatment. Surgical approaches to the pituitary gland have changed in recent years due first to introduction of antibiotics and steroids, and lately to the development of microsurgical techniques and the transsphenoidal approach. This technique was actually used extensively by Hirsch and Cushing, but became less popular in favor of the transcranial subfrontal approach. Both methods, however, have their indications, and the choice of one over the other depends on a variety of factors.

Transsphenoidal removal of a pituitary tumor is indicated in the presence of a secreting microadenoma because it allows the selective removal of the tumor, with preservation of the remaining gland. In these cases radiotherapy is usually deferred, except in the cases where a biological cure was not achieved. In general, however, a rapid reduction of the abnormal hormonal levels is obtained. The transsphenoidal approach is also the method of choice for tumors that invade the sphenoid sinus, in cases that are poor surgical risks or in the presence of a picture of pituitary apoplexy.

In cases with suprasellar extensions and an enlarged sella, either functioning or non-functioning, both transsphenoidal or subfrontal approaches can be used. In these situations an intracapsular removal and decompression of the optic pathways are attempted, and radiotherapy should follow surgery.

A transcranial approach is indicated in patients with suprasellar lesions and a small sella, or in the presence of extrasellar extensions into the anterior or temporal fossas. Again, in these cases, radiotherapy should also be given.

Mortality with the transsphenoidal approach is about 1 to 2%, and with the transcranial procedure 3 to 5%. Other, less used forms of treatment include stereotactic radiofrequency lesions and cryohypophysectomy.

Medical Treatment. In recent years attempts have been made to control pituitary hypersecreting states with a variety of drugs. Bromocriptine, an ergot derivative, is effective in reducing hyperprolactinemia, and has also been reported to diminish growth hormone secretion in patients with acromegaly. Cyproheptadine, an anti-serotonin drug, has been employed in Cushing's disease, and seems to cause return to normal of the elevated corticosteroid levels in these patients. Long term results with these drugs are, however, not available, and it seems that when the medication is discontinued there is a prompt return to the previous abnormal states.

REFERENCES

Antunes, J. L. et al.: Prolactin Secreting Pituitary Tumors, Ann, Neurol., 2:148, 1977.
Bonneville, J. F., et al.: Delineation of Pituitary Tumors by Angiotomography, Neuroradiology 11:49, 1976.
Hankinson, J., and Banna, M.: *Pituitary and Parapituitary Tumors.* Philadelphia, W. B. Saunders Co., 1976. 217 pp.
Harris, J., and Levene, M. B.: Visual Complications Following Irradiation for Pituitary Tumors and Craniopharyngiomas, Radiology, 120:171, 1976.
Hirsch, O.: Symptoms and Treatment of Pituitary Tumors, Arch. Otolaryng., 55, 268, 1952.
Jenkins, J. S.: *Pituitary Tumors.* New York, Appleton-Century-Crofts, 1973, 206 pp.
Kleinborg, D. L., Nod, G. L., and Frantz, A. G.: Galactorrhea; a Study of 235 Cases Including 48 with Pituitary Tumors, N. Engl. J. Med., 296, 589, 1977.
Kohler, P. O., and Ross, G. T.: *Diagnosis and Treatment of Pituitary Tumors.* New York, Excerpta Medica, 1973, 343 pp.
Krieger, D. T. et al.: Cyprohepatidine-induced Remission of Cushing's Disease. N. Engl. J. Med., 293: 893, 1975.
Nardich, T. et al.: Evaluation of Sellar and Parasellar Masses by Computerized Tomography, Radiology, 120, 91, 1976.

Congenital Tumors

H. Houston Merritt

Craniopharyngiomas. Craniopharyngiomas (Rathke's pouch tumor, hypophyseal duct tumors, adamantinoma) are tumors which arise from remnants of the hypophyseal duct. They constitute approximately 4% of all intracranial tumors. Owing to their location they produce a syndrome similar to that of pituitary adenomas or other tumors in the

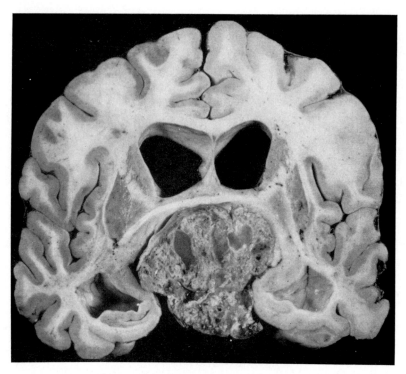

Figure 62.   Craniopharyngioma. Large tumor obstructing third ventricle and causing
hydrocephalus. (Courtesy Dr. Abner Wolf.)

suprasellar region. They vary from small, solid, well-circumscribed
nodules to huge multilocular cysts invading the sella turcica and also
displacing neighboring cerebral structures (Fig. 62). The cysts are filled
with a turbid fluid which may contain cholesterin crystals. There are
three histological types of craniopharyngioma: (1) Mucoid epithelial
cysts lined with ciliated columnar and mucus-secreting cells; (2)
squamous epitheliomas composed of islands of squamous epithelium
with cystic degeneration; and (3) adamantinomas, consisting of epithelial masses forming a reticulum resembling enamel pulp of developing
teeth. Occasionally teratomas may arise from epithelial remnants of the
hypophyseal stalk. Craniopharyngiomas are predominantly a tumor of
infancy or childhood, with onset of symptoms before the age of fifteen
in 50% of the cases, but symptoms may have their onset at any age and
cases with initial symptoms after the age of fifty or sixty are not rare.

The development of symptoms is usually slow but occasionally they
are of rapid or sudden onset. In the majority of cases the initial signs
and symptoms are those of pituitary hypofunction. These are followed

by evidence of involvement of the optic chiasm, optic tract or one of the optic nerves. Diabetes insipidus is not infrequently seen. Owing to the tendency of these tumors to invade the third ventricle, choked disc and other signs of increased intracranial pressure are more common than in pituitary adenomas.

The diagnosis of craniopharyngiomas can usually be made from the age of the patient and the presence of calcification in the suprasellar region in the roentgenograms. The latter is present in about 80% of the cases. Although the sella turcica may be eroded, it is uncommon for it to be ballooned in the same manner as occurs in pituitary adenomas. When the onset of symptoms is delayed until adult life and there is no calcification in the tumor, the diagnosis cannot be established before operation.

The treatment of craniopharyngiomas is total removal of all of the solid tumor, evacuation of the cyst and removal of the cyst wall followed by radiation therapy. This has resulted in a cure in a high percentage of the cases now that adequate endocrine therapy is available.

REFERENCES

Bartlett, J. R.: Craniopharyngiomas, An Analysis of some Aspects of Symptomatology, Radiology and Histology, Brain, 94, 725, 1971.
Bingas, B., and Wolter, M.: Das Kraniopharyngiom, Fortschr. Neurol. Psychiat., 36, 117, 1968.
Katz, E. U.: Late Results of Radical Excision of Craniopharyngiomas in Children, J. Neurosurg., 42, 86, 1975.
Russell, R. W. R., and Pennybacker, J. B.: Craniopharyngioma in the Elderly, J. Neurol., Neurosurg. & Psychiat., 24, 1, 1961.
Svien, H. J.: Surgical Experiences with Craniopharyngiomas, J. Neurosurg., 23, 148, 1965.

Cholesteatomas. Cholesteatomas (pearly tumors, epidermoids) are a rare type of intracranial tumor which may arise within the tables of the skull or in relationship to the dura. They may occur in any portion of the cranial cavity. The most common sites are (Table 37) the cerebellopontine angle, the suprasellar region, the fourth ventricle, the pineal recess and over the convexity of the hemispheres. Cholesteatomas vary

Table 37.   The Location of Intracranial Cholesteatomas

Site of Tumor	No. of Cases	%
Suprasellar	44	39
Parapontine	53	47
Fourth ventricle	15	14

in size from small nodules to large masses which cover almost an entire hemisphere. They are usually sharply demarcated and completely encapsulated and have a pearly appearance. Occasionally they may burrow into the cerebrum or brainstem. Microscopically the tumor is divided into four layers: Stratum durum, granulosum, fibrosum, and cellulosum.

Cholesteatomas may occur at any age but they are more common in young adults. The signs and symptoms are related to the site of the tumor. Large cholesteatomas may overlie the cerebral hemisphere without producing any significant symptoms. The diagnosis of chole-steatomas in the suprasellar region or in the posterior fossa is rarely made before operation. Those which underlie the cranial vault can be recognized from the characteristic shadow in the roentgenograms, a large evenly calcified area with sharp margins.

Cholesteatomas grow relatively slowly and the rate of progression of symptoms is related to the site of the tumor. Rapid advancement of symptoms is the rule when the tumor is in the fourth ventricle or cerebellopontine angle. Those over the cerebral hemisphere may be present for ten, twenty or more years without any symptoms.

Treatment consists of surgical removal of the entire tumor with its capsule.

REFERENCES

Fawcitt, R. A. and Isherwood, I. R.: Radiodiagnosis of Intracranial Pearly Tumors with Particular Reference to the Value of Computer Tomography, Neuroradiology, 11, 235, 1976.
Keville, F. J., and Wise, B. L.: Intracranial Epidermoid and Dermoid Tumors, J. Neurosurg., 16, 564, 1959.
Toglia, J. U., Netsky, M. G., and Alexander, E., Jr.: Epithelial (Epidermoid) Tumors of the Cranium. Their Common Nature and Pathogenesis, J. Neurosurg., 23, 384, 1965.
Tytus, J. S., and Pennybacker, J.: Pearly Tumours in Relation to the Central Nervous System, J. Neurol. Neurosurg. & Psychiat., 19, 241, 1956.

Chordomas. Chordomas are tumors which develop from remnants of the notochord. Approximately 60% arise at the upper end of the notochord at the clivus Blumenbachii, or at the junction of the sphenoid and occipital bones, about 30 per cent are in the sacrococcygeal region and 10% elsewhere along the spine. These tumors have a smooth nodular surface of a milky-white color. The cut surface resembles cartilage but is softer and often of jelly-like consistency. There may be cystic areas filled with slimy mucus. The characteristic feature of the histological structure is the presence of large masses of spherical, oval or polygonal cells, arranged in groups or cords, with large vacuoles in the cytoplasm containing mucin (physaliferous cells).

The intracranial chordomas are highly invasive. They spread along the floor of the posterior fossa, damaging cranial nerves and compressing the brainstem. They may grow forward and produce a bitemporal hemianopia as a result of involvement of the optic chiasm. They also invade the nasopharynx or the intracranial sinuses and may extend into the neck.

Chordomas which arise from the lower end of the notochord compress the roots of the cauda equina. Those which arise along other portions of the spinal cord compress and sometimes invade the substance of the spinal cord.

The diagnosis of an intracranial chordoma cannot be made with certainty before operation except when the tumor invades the nasopharynx or neck and histological identification is possible. It should be suspected whenever there are multiple cranial nerve palsies or when erosion of the floor of the skull in the region of the clivus Blumenbachii can be demonstrated in the roentgenograms. Treatment is by operation followed by radiation therapy. Complete removal is rarely possible, but growth of the tumor is inhibited by radiation.

REFERENCES

Adson, A. W., Kernohan, J. W., and Woltman, H. W.: Cranial and Cervical Chordomas, Arch. Neurol. & Psychiat., 33, 247, 1935.
Chutorian, A.: Intracranial Chordoma in Children, Arch. Neurol., 17, 89, 1967.
Furlow, L. T.: Intracranial Chordoma, Arch. Neurol. & Psychiat., 34, 839, 1935.
Kamrin, R. P., Potanos, J. N., and Pool, J. L.: An Evaluation of the Diagnosis and Treatment of Chordoma, J. Neurol., Neurosurg., & Psychiat., 27, 157, 1964.
Schechter, M. M., et al.: Intracranial Chordomas, Neuroradiology, 8, 67, 1974.

Dermoids and Teratomas. Dermoids and teratomas which involve the central nervous system do not differ from similar tumors found in other portions of the body. They tend to occur along the central axis, involving the regions of the pituitary and pineal glands, the fourth ventricle or the distal end of the spinal cord. Dermoids and teratomas vary greatly in size and are composed of a wide variety of tissue, including elements of any of the three germ layers. Cystic degeneration is common. Although these tumors are present from birth, the onset of symptoms may be delayed for many years. More commonly, however, symptoms develop in the first decade of life. Ingraham and Bailey report that teratomas constitute 4% of all intracranial tumors and 18% of all spinal tumors in childhood.

The signs and symptoms which occur with teratomas are similar to those of other tumors. Varying degrees of calcification in the tumor may be seen in roentgenograms but the diagnosis can rarely be made before operative exposure of the tumor.

The end result of the surgical removal of teratomas depends on the degree of malignancy and invasiveness of the tumor. The results in 15 cases reported by Ingraham and Bailey were as follows: Two living more than five years after the operation without evidence of recurrence; 5 living less than five years after operation without recurrence; recurrence of the tumor in 2; 6 dead.

REFERENCES

Arseni, C. et al.: Cerebral Dermoid Tumors, Neurochirurgie, 19, 114, 1976.
Herrschaff, H.: Die Teratome des Zentralnervensystems, Deutsche Zeitschrift für Nervenheilkunde, 194, 344, 1968.
Higashi, K. and Wakuta, Y.: Epidermoid Tumor of the Lateral Ventricle, Surg. Neurol., 5, 363, 1976.
Spiegel, A. M. et al.: Diagnosis of Radiosensitive Hypothalamic Tumors without Craniotomy, Endocrine and Neuroradiological Studies of Intracranial Atypical Teratomas, Ann. Int. Med., 85, 290, 1976.
Tomlinson, B. E., and Walton, J. N.: Granulomatous Meningitis and Diffuse Degeneration of the Nervous System due to an Intracranial Epidermoid Cyst, J. Neurol. Neurosurg. and Psychiat., 30, 341, 1967.

Cysts (Colloid Cysts of the Third Ventricle). Cystic degeneration may occur in many of the various types of intracranial tumors previously described. A large cyst with a mural nodule is most frequently seen in association with astrocytomas, particularly those in the cerebellar

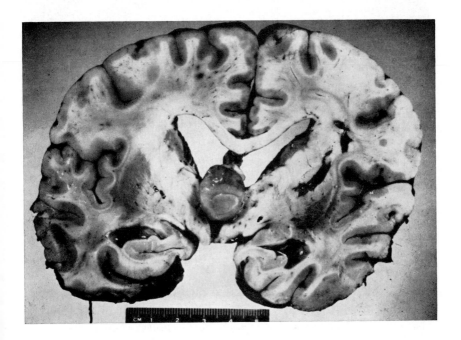

Figure 63.   Colloid cyst of third ventricle. (Courtesy Dr. Philip Duffy.)

hemispheres, and in hemangioblastomas. A rare type of cystic tumor which occurs within the cavity of the third ventricle is known as a colloid cyst. Presumably this tumor arises from the anlage of the paraphysis. It is located in the anterior superior part of the third ventricle (Fig. 63) and has the gross appearance of a small white ball. The cyst wall is composed of a layer of cuboidal and columnar ciliated cells and a layer of connective tissue. The cyst is filled with a homogeneous gelatinous material which becomes rubbery on fixation with formalin. In 1933, Dandy collected 16 cases from the literature and reported 5 additional cases. The age of the patients at the time of onset of symptoms varied between ten and sixty, with the majority being in the third to fifth decades. Mental symptoms are common. Intermittent attacks of headache, dizziness, and weakness and numbness of the extremities, sometimes related to changes in posture, are characteristic symptoms. They are presumed to be due to an acute hydrocephalus produced by a shift of the tumor so that it blocks the foramina of Monro. This train of symptoms may occur, however, on change of posture with

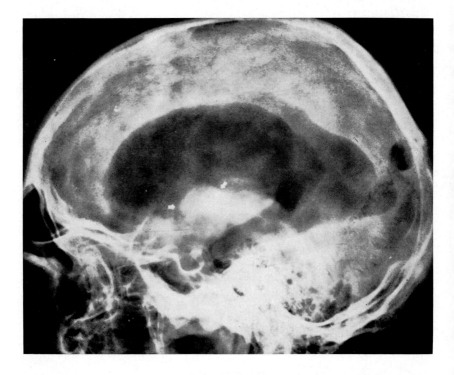

Figure 64. Colloid cyst of third ventricle. Ventriculogram. Oval mass in the third ventricle projects into the lateral ventricle producing severe degree of hydrocephalus. (Courtesy Dr. Ernest Wood.)

a tumor anywhere in the cranial cavity. The diagnosis of a colloid cyst of the third ventricle can be made from the appearance of the characteristic defect in the third ventricle in the ventriculogram (Fig. 64). Colloid cysts must be differentiated from other tumors which invade the third ventricle, such as gliomas, papillomas of the choroid plexus, craniopharyngiomas, pineal tumors and pituitary adenomas. The differential diagnosis between a colloid cyst and other tumors in the third ventricle cannot always be made before operation, unless signs and symptoms characteristic of the various other types of tumors are present or unless the colloid cyst can be clearly visualized by ventriculography or CT brain scan. The treatment of colloid cysts is complete surgical removal through the foramen of Monro after frontal craniotomy.

REFERENCES

Brunette, J. R., and Walsh, F. B.: Neurophthalmological Aspects of Tumors of the Third Ventricle, Canadian Med. Assoc. J., 98, 1184, 1968.
Cairns, H., and Mosberg, W. H., Jr.: Colloid Cyst of Third Ventricle, Surg., Gynec. & Obst., 92, 545, 1951.
Dandy, W. E.: Benign Tumors in the Third Ventricle of the Brain, Springfield, Charles C Thomas, 1933, 171 pp.
Netsky, M.: Neuroepithelial Colloid Cysts of the Nervous System, Neurol., 16, 887, 1966.

Papillomas of the Choroid Plexus. Papillomas of the choroid plexus may be found in the lateral or third ventricles, but they are more commonly found in the fourth ventricle. Grossly they are tufted, reddened mulberry growths which may grow to a large size and may undergo cystic degeneration. Microscopically, the tumor is composed of papillae which have a central core of connective tissue and are covered by cuboidal choroidal epithelium. Papilloma of the choroid plexus is a rare tumor. Matson and Crofton collected 83 cases from the literature and Cushing found 12 instances in his series of 2000 cases of verified intracranial tumors. They may occur at any age but are common in children or young adults. Papillomas of the choroid plexus located in the lateral recess of the medulla may be accompanied by an excessive formation of cerebrospinal fluid. There are no signs or symptoms which are characteristic of papillomas of the choroid plexus. The diagnosis of an intraventricular tumor, but not the histological type, can be made by the result of air injection or CT brain scan.

REFERENCES

Laurence, K. M., Hoare, R. D., and Till, K.: The Diagnosis of the Choroid Plexus Papilloma of the Lateral Ventricle, Brain, 84, 628, 1961.

Matson, D. D., and Crofton, F. D. L.: Papilloma of the Choroid Plexus in Childhood, J. Neurosurg., 17, 1002, 1960.
Nassar, S. I., and Mount, L. A.: Papillomas of the Choroid Plexus, J. Neurosurg., 29, 73, 1968.

Blood Vessel Tumors and Malformations. Vascular tumors of the nervous system are divided into two main groups generally referred to as angiomas and angioblastomas. An angioma is a malformation composed of blood vessels of adult structure, whereas the angioblastoma is a tumor comprised of embryonic vascular channels and blood vessel-forming cells. There have been a number of different classifications of the vascular anomalies and malformations of the nervous system. The most comprehensive is that of Noran. The various types of vascular anomalies or malformations are shown in Table 38, separated according to the site of the lesion.

SINUS PERICRANII. This is a vascular tumor composed of thin-walled vascular spaces interconnected by numerous anastomoses which protrude from the skull and communicate with the superior longitudinal sinus. The tumor appears early in life and may enlarge slowly over a period of many years. The tumor is soft and compressible and increases in size when the venous pressure in the head is raised by coughing, straining or lowering the head. The external tumor may occur at any portion of midline of the skull, including the occiput, but it is most commonly found in the midportion of the forehead. Except for the external swelling there are usually no symptoms. Rarely there may be a pulsating tinnitus, increased intracranial pressure or variable cerebral symptoms. In roentgenograms there is a defect in the underlying bone,

Table 38. Pathological Classification of Intracranial Vascular Tumors and Malformations

(Modified from Noran, Arch. Path., 1945)

I.   Angiomatous lesions (comprised of adult vascular elements)
    A.   Sinus pericranii
    B.   Meningeal angioma
        1. Angioma of the meninges
        2. Meningeal varix or varicosity
        3. Sturge-Weber disease
    C.   Parenchymatous angioma
        1. Telangiectasis (capillary); Rendu-Osler disease
        2. Parenchymal varix or varicosity
        3. Cavernous angioma or cavernoma
        4. Racemose angioma
II. Angioblastic lesions (embryonic vascular tumors)
    A.   Angioblastic meningiomas
    B.   Parenchymal angioblastomas (von Hippel-Lindau disease)

through which the external lesion communicates with the longitudinal sinus.

MENINGEAL ANGIOMA. Angiomas of the meninges are vascular malformations composed of various combinations of adult arteries, veins, capillaries and cavernous spaces. These tumors are rare and only a small number are recorded in the literature. They may be confined to one region of the brain or they may cover both hemispheres (Fig. 65). They may be found on the surface of the cerebrum, cerebellum, brainstem or spinal cord. There is no characteristic clinical picture for angiomas of the meninges. Convulsive seizures, various focal symptoms and signs and symptoms of subarachnoid bleeding may occur.

STURGE-WEBER DISEASE (KRABBE-WEBER-DIMITRI DISEASE). The two cardinal features of Sturge-Weber disease are a localized atrophy and calcification of the cerebral cortex associated with an ipsilateral port-wine colored facial nevus usually in the distribution of the first division of

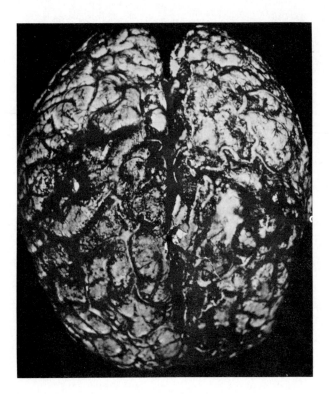

Figure 65. Meningeal angiomatosis. Extensive cerebral angiomatous malformation. (Yakovlev, P. I., and Guthrie, R. H., courtesy Arch. Neurol. & Psychiat.)

the trigeminal nerve. Angiomatous malformation in the meninges, ipsilateral exophthalmos, glaucoma, buphthalmos, angiomas of the retina, optic atrophy and dilated vessels in the sclera may also be present. Any portion of the cerebral cortex may be affected by the atrophic process but the occipital and parietal regions are most commonly involved.

In the atrophic cortical areas there is a loss of nerve cells and axons and a proliferation of the fibrous glia. The small vessels are thickened and calcified, particularly in the second and third cortical layers. Small calcium deposits are also present in the cerebral substance (Fig. 66), and rarely there are large calcified nodules. When an angioma is present, it is limited to the meninges overlying the area of shrunken

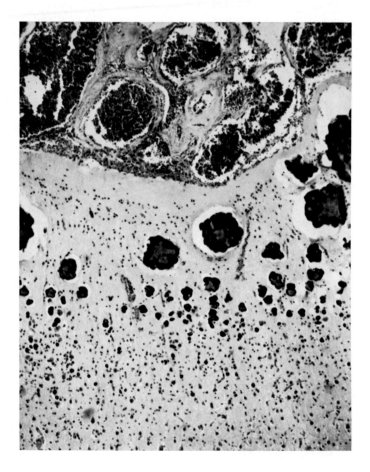

Figure 66.   Sturge-Weber syndrome. Angiomatous malformation in meninges and calcification in cortex. H & E. stain. (Courtesy Dr. Philip Duffy.)

cortex. It is now generally agreed that the atrophy and calcification of the cortex are not secondary to the angiomatous malformations of the leptomeninges.

Sturge-Weber syndrome is probably more common than would be concluded from the relatively small number of cases that are recorded in the literature. Yakovlev and Guthrie, for example, found 6 cases in the clinical material of the Epileptic Colony at Monson, Massachusetts. It is possible for the combination of a port-wine facial nevus and localized cortical atrophy to exist without clinical symptoms, but in the majority of cases convulsive seizures are present from infancy. Mental retardation, contralateral hemiplegia (Fig. 67) or hemianopia are also present in a high percentage of cases.

The diagnosis of Sturge-Weber disease can be made without difficulty from the clinical syndrome. The presence of the cortical lesion can be demonstrated in the majority of cases by the appearance of

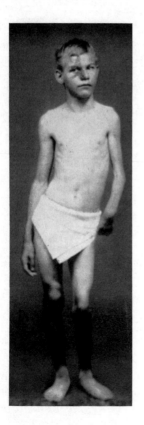

Figure 67.   Sturge-Weber disease. Right facial nevus in patient with convulsions and left hemiparesis. (Courtesy Dr. P. I. Yakovlev.)

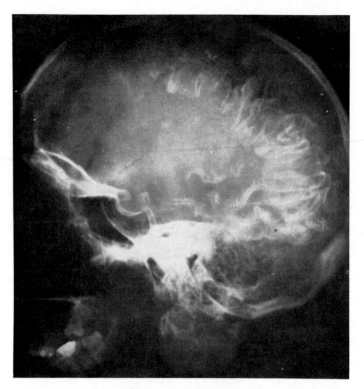

Figure 68.   Sturge-Weber disease. Intracerebral calcification.
(Courtesy Dr. P. I. Yakovlev.)

characteristic shadows in the roentgenograms (Fig. 68). The calcified area in the cortex appears as a sinuous shadow with a double contour, showing both the gyri and sulci of the affected cerebral convolutions. The lesions in the occipital or parietal lobes are usually more definitely calcified than those which occur in the frontal lobe.

The treatment of patients with Sturge-Weber disease is essentially symptomatic. Anticonvulsive drugs should be given for the seizures. Radiation therapy has been recommended but there is no evidence that it is of any benefit. Hemispherectomy may be of benefit in the control of the convulsive seizures.

PARENCHYMATOUS ANGIOMAS. Vascular malformations of the parenchyma of the nervous system are variously classified as telangiectases, varices and angiomas (cavernous, venous, arterial and arteriovenous).

Telangiectases are a collection of engorged capillaries or cavernous spaces which are separated by relatively normal brain tissue. They are usually small and poorly circumscribed and may be found in any portion of the nervous system. Multiple lesions in the nervous system may be present in association with telangiectasis in the skin, mucous membranes, respiratory, gastrointestinal and genitourinary tracts (Rendu-Osler syndrome).

Varices consist of abnormal, dilated thin-walled vessels situated either within the nervous substance or on its surface.

Angiomas are composed of closely packed vascular channels which may simulate cavernous spaces, veins, arteries or a mixture of these elements. These tumors may be located in any part of the nervous system. They are usually single but multiple lesions may occur. While angiomas are congenital malformations and are relatively fixed lesions, there is considerable variation as to the time of onset of symptoms of their presence. In many cases this is in childhood but occasionally it is delayed to late middle life. Convulsive seizures and intermittent headaches, similar in character to that of migraine, are the most common presenting symptoms. Focal neurological signs, such as hemiplegia or hemianopia may develop when there is rupture of the abnormal vascular channels. Increased intracranial pressure may occur when there is extensive hemorrhage into the cerebral substance or subarachnoid space or when there is congestion of the cerebral substance as result of thrombosis of the large tortuous vessels. Recurrent attacks of bleeding into the subarachnoid space are common in patients with cerebral angiomas.

The diagnosis of a cerebral angioma can sometimes be made from the roentgenograms when there is calcification in the vessels (Fig. 69). In the absence of calcification the diagnosis can be established by CT brain scan or angiography (Fig. 70).

The mortality rate is less than 20%. Death is usually the result of an extensive intracerebral or subarachnoid hemorrhage. The life span of the remaining 80% is not significantly affected although one half of them may have minor or major neurological deficits as the result of bleeding from the lesion or suffer from recurrent convulsive seizures. Small superficially located angiomas can be removed surgically but excision of large deep-seated lesions is not advised. Embolization of large malformations has reduced symptoms in a number of patients with reduction of frequency of seizures, decreased headache and reversal of progressive neurological deficit. It has also allowed surgeons to remove malformations that were previously considered inoperable.

HEMANGIOBLASTOMAS. Hemangioblastomas are tumors composed of embryonic vascular elements. They were formerly considered to be exclusively tumors of the cerebellum, but they may also occur in the cerebral hemispheres. Hemangioblastomas in the cerebellar hemispheres are often associated with angiomatosis of the retina, cysts of the

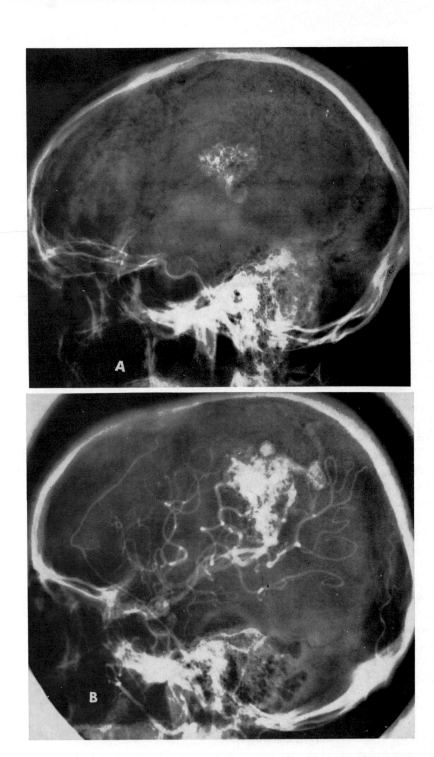

Figure 69. Arteriovenous malformation. Angiogram showing enlargement of branches of middle cerebral artery abruptly terminating in a plexus of abnormal arterioles and venules. (Courtesy Dr. Ernest Wood.)

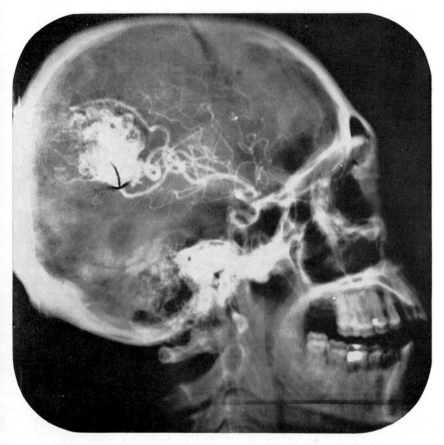

Figure 70.   Arteriovenous malformation of parieto-occipital region as
demonstrated by angiography. (Courtesy of Dr. Juan Taveras.)

kidney and pancreas and there is a tendency to a familial occurrence
(von Hippel-Lindau syndrome). The tumors in the cerebellum may be
solid, but more commonly they consist of a large cyst filled with yellow
fluid which may be dark as result of hemorrhage, and a small mural
nodule of tumor tissue. The tumor consists of many capillaries and a
variable amount of cellular tissue.

Symptoms of hemangioblastoma of the cerebellum may develop at
any age, but they most commonly appear in the fourth to sixth decades.
Headache and choked discs are the most common clinical features.
Signs and symptoms of cerebellar dysfunction may or may not be
present. There may be associated angioblastic tumors in the brainstem
or spinal cord. A syringomyelic cavitation of the cervical cord and
medulla is also occasionally present. Polycythemia and pheo-

chromocytomas are not infrequently associated with a hemangioblastoma of the cerebellum.

The diagnosis of hemangioblastoma of the cerebellum can be made without difficulty when there is an associated tumor in the retina. In the absence of the latter, the diagnosis should be considered in all middle-aged patients with signs and symptoms of a cerebellar tumor, especially if there is no obvious source for a metastatic lesion. The diagnosis of a tumor of the cerebellum is established by ventriculography, angiography or CT brain scan. Treatment is evacuation of the cyst and removal of the mural nodule. Complete cure can be effected in the cases with a single tumor.

REFERENCES

Chao, D. H.: Congenital Neurocutaneous Syndromes of Childhood. III. Sturge-Weber Disease, J. Ped., 55, 635, 1959.
Cramer, F., and Kimsey, W.: The Cerebellar Hemangioblastomas, Arch. Neurol. & Psychiat., 67, 237, 1952.
Henderson, W. R., and Gomez, R. de R. L.: Natural History of Cerebral Angiomas, British Med. J., 4, 571, 1967.
Hilal, S. K., and Michelson, J. W.: Therapeutic Embolization for Extra-axial Vascular Lesions of the Head, Neck, and Spine, J. Neurosurg., 43, 275, 1975.
Illingworth, R. D.: Pheochromocytoma and Cerebellar Hemangioblastoma, J. Neurol. Neurosurg. and Psychiat., 30, 443, 1967.
McCormick, W. F., Hardman, J. M., and Boulter, T. R.: Vascular Malformations ("Angiomas") of the Brain with Special Reference to Those Occurring in the Posterior Fossa, J. Neurosurg., 28, 241, 1968.
Melmon, K. L., and Rosen, S. W.: Lindau's Disease, Review of the Literature and Study of a Large Kindred, Am. J. Med., 36, 595, 1964.
Mohan, J., Brownell, B., and Oppenheimer, D. R.: Malignant Spread of Hemangioblastomas. Report of Two Cases, J. Neurol., Neurosurg, and Psychiatry, 39, 515, 1976.
Noran, H. H.: Intracranial Vascular Tumors and Malformations, Arch. Path., 39, 393, 1945.
Olivecrona, H.: The Cerebellar Angioreticulomas, J. Neurosurg., 9, 317, 1952.
Paterson, J. H., and McKissock, W.: A Clinical Survey of Intracranial Angiomas with Special Reference to their Mode of Progression and Surgical Treatment. A Report of 110 Cases, Brain, 79, 233, 1956.
Pia, H. W., et al.: Cerebral Angiomas, Advances in Diagnosis and Therapy. New York, Springer, 1975, 285 pp.
Pool, J. L., and Potts, D. G.: Aneurysms and Arteriovenous Anomalies of the Brain, New York, Hoeber Medical Division of Harper & Row, 1965.
Svien, H. J., and McRae, J. A.: Arteriovenous Anomalies of the Brain. Fate of Patients not Having Definitive Surgery, J. Neurosurg., 23, 23, 1965.
Wohlwill, F. J., and Yakovlev, P. I.: Histopathology of Meningo-Facial Angiomatosis (Sturge-Weber's Disease). Report of Four Cases, J. Neuropath. & Exper. Neurol., 16, 341, 1957.
Yakovlev, P. I., and Guthrie, R. H.: Congenital Ectodermoses (Neurocutaneous Syndromes) in Epileptic Patients, Arch. Neurol. & Psychiat., 26, 1145, 1931.

ARTERIOVENOUS ANEURYSMS. Direct connection between an artery and a vein in the brain, with the exception of carotid-cavernous sinus fistula, is practically always the result of a congenital defect in the development of these vessels. Although any vessel may be affected, the vein of

Galen is most frequently involved. Only a small number of patients have been reported. The symptoms and signs, which usually develop in infancy or early childhood, include headache, convulsive seizures, hydrocephalus, and cardiac failure. Death usually results from cardiac failure or cerebral decompensation. A few patients have been cured by surgical ligation of the arterial feeders from the posterior and middle cerebral arteries and plication of the aneurysm.

Embolization of the malformation with elastic spheres has symptomatically improved a number of these patients with reduction of headache, risk of hemorrhage and reversal of cardiac failure.

REFERENCES

Gold, A. P., Ransohoff, J., and Carter, S.: Vein of Galen Malformation, Acta Neurol. Scand., 40, Suppl. 11, 1, 1964.
Gomez, M. R., et al.: Aneurysmal Malformation of the Great Vein of Galen Causing Heart Failure in Early Infancy. Report of Five Cases, Pediatrics, 31, 400, 1963.

Granulomas

Granuloma formation may occur in the nervous system as a result of infections with syphilis, tuberculosis, fungi, sarcoidosis, and the larvae of various intestinal parasites.

Tuberculomas. Tuberculomas of the brain are always secondary to tuberculosis elsewhere in the body, which, however, need not be clinically active. Small or microscopic tuberculomas are a frequent finding in patients with tuberculous meningitis but in the majority of cases there is no clinical evidence of the presence of these small tuberculomas. Tuberculomas of sufficient size to produce focal neurological signs or an increase in intracranial pressure are a rarity in the United States at the present time. This is in contrast to their frequency before 1900 when Starr (Table 39) found that they constituted approximately one third of all intracranial tumors. The incidence of tuberculomas of the brain continues to be high in Spain, Portugal, South America and India. In the latter country Dastur and Desai report that tuberculomas constituted 30.5% of 373 verified intracranial tumors in the years 1957 to 1963.

Solitary tuberculomas have been found in all portions of the nervous system. They may involve the dura, arachnoid or substance of the nervous system and have a histological appearance similar to tuberculomas elsewhere in the body. Although they may be found in patients of any age, they are most common in children or young adults.

The symptoms produced by tuberculomas are similar to those of any tumor and it is rarely possible to make an etiological diagnosis before

Table 39.   The Relative Incidence of Various Types of Intracranial Tumors Before 1900

Type of Tumor	Children	Adults
Tuberculomas	152	41
Sarcoma	34	86
Glioma	37	54
Gliosarcoma	5	25
Cystic	30	2
Carcinoma	10	31
Gummata	2	20
Other	30	41
Total	300	300

operation in the absence of a frank tuberculous meningitis. The clinical course is usually short, but there may be remissions. Complete healing with calcification may rarely occur.

A presumptive diagnosis of tuberculoma can be made before operation when there is evidence of active tuberculosis elsewhere in the body or in the presence of a positive tuberculin reaction in a child. The laboratory studies are not conclusive. The cerebrospinal fluid is under increased pressure and may contain cells. The latter finding is not, however, rare in other types of intracranial tumors. The cerebrospinal fluid sugar content is normal and tubercle bacilli are not found unless there is diffuse tuberculous meningitis.

It was formerly thought that tuberculomas were not amenable to operation but with the use of electrocautery and the administration of streptomycin and isoniazid, it is now possible to remove solitary tuberculomas of the cerebral meninges and cortex without the subsequent development of tuberculous meningitis. Diffuse meningeal tuberculomas of the cerebral cortex or cerebellum as well as solitary tuberculomas in the substance of the brainstem cannot, for obvious reasons, be treated surgically. Chemotherapy is the only, although not very promising, form of treatment in such cases.

REFERENCES

Asenjo, A., Valladares, H., and Fierro, J.: Tuberculomas of the Brain, Arch. Neurol. & Psychiat., 65, 146, 1951.

Dastur, H. M., and Desai, A. D.: A Comparative Study of Brain Tuberculomas and Gliomas Based Upon 107 Case Records of Each, Brain, 88, 375, 1965.

Obrador, S.: Intracranial Tuberculomas. A Review of 47 Cases, Neurochirurgia, Fortschr. d. Neurol. und Psychiat., 1, 150, 1959.

Sibley, W. A., and O'Brien, J. L.: Intracranial Tuberculomas. A Review of Clinical Features and Treatment, Neurology, 6, 157, 1956.

Starr, M. A.: Organic Nervous Diseases, Philadelphia, Lea Brothers & Co., 1903, 751 pp.

Cryptococcal Granulomas. The central nervous system is involved in practically all patients in whom the meninges are affected by cryptococci. Usually, however, this takes the form of microscopic foci of necrosis filled with the organisms. Occasionally, however, large fibrous nodules may be present within the substance of the nervous system or invading it from the meninges. These granulomatous nodules may be present in the cerebral hemispheres, brainstem, cerebellum, or rarely in the spinal cord. The diagnosis cannot be established unless the accompanying meningitis is of sufficient degree to produce a cellular reaction in the cerebrospinal fluid, and the organism can be cultured from the fluid. Surgical excision is rarely successful.

REFERENCES

Cox, L. B., and Tolhurst, J. C.: Human Torulosis, London, Oxford University Press, 1946, 149 pp.
Daniel, P. M., Schiller, F., and Vollum, R. L.: Torulosis of Central Nervous System, Lancet, 1, 53, 1949.
Krainer, L., Small, J. M., Hewlitt, A. B., and Deness, T.: A Case of Systemic Torula Infection with Tumor Formation in the Meninges, J. Neurol., Neurosurg. & Psychiat., 9, 158, 1946.

Metastatic Tumors

Metastatic tumors constitute 10 to 20% of all intracranial tumors. The figures from large neurosurgical clinics such as that of Cushing (4.2%) and Dandy (10%) are unduly low because patients with metastatic tumors of the brain are, for obvious reasons, rarely referred to the neurosurgeon. Globus and Meltzer found that 13.5% of all the brain tumors at the Mt. Sinai Hospital were of metastatic origin. The reported incidence of autopsy-proven metastases to the brain from carcinoma elsewhere in the body varies according to whether the study is made in a general hospital or in a hospital for the care of the chronically ill. Chason and his associates report a 12% incidence in 525 cases autopsied at the Detroit Receiving Hospital and 24% of 571 cases at the Dearborn Veterans Administration Hospital.

Metastatic tumors in the brain are usually a manifestation of generalized dissemination of the tumors. Histological examination of the lung shows evidence of a primary tumor or secondary metastases in approximately 80% of the cases. Signs and symptoms of intracranial metastases, however, may precede any clinical evidence indicative of the presence of a primary lesion. In approximately one half of the 57 cases reported by Globus and Meltzer the primary site of the metastatic lesion was not apparent on clinical study. On the other hand, it is not

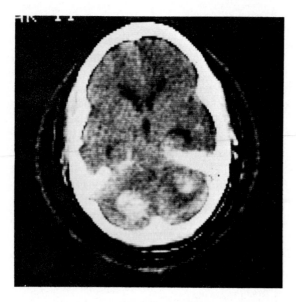

Figure 71.   CT brain scan. Cerebral metastases.
(Courtesy Dr. Harry H. White.)

uncommon to find at necropsy small metastatic lesions in the brain
which have caused no symptoms. Practically any malignant tumor may
metastasize to the brain but in approximately 60% of the cases the
primary tumor is a carcinoma of the breast or lung (Table 40).
Metastatic tumors of the brain may occur at any age but they are most
common in the fourth to seventh decades of life, paralleling the age
incidence of malignant tumors in general. There is no significant
difference in the incidence in the two sexes.

Multiple lesions in the brain are the rule but in some series the
incidence of solitary nodules is as high as 25%. It is probable, however,
that if a careful histological examination were made of the entire
nervous system, the figure would be much lower. Metastatic tumor may
be found in any portion of the central nervous system. They are most
common in the hemisphere of the cerebrum or cerebellum. Nodules in
the dura mater are not uncommon and rarely there may be a diffuse
infiltration of the leptomeninges (carcinomatosis, melanosis or sarcomatosis of the meninges).

Metastatic tumors vary in size from microscopic collections of
neoplastic cells to lesions which involve an entire hemisphere. They
vary in gross appearance from hard, pale nodules, sharply circumscribed from the surrounding tissue, to soft, hemorrhagic-
appearing lesions. Areas of cystic degeneration filled with a gelatinous

Table 40.   Primary Sites of Metastatic Tumors of the Brain
(Modified from Aronson, Garcia and Aronson, Cancer, 1964)

Type and Site of Primary Tumor	No. of Cases	%
Carcinoma		
Lung	184	46
Upper respiratory tract	14	3
Breast	51	13
Gastrointestinal tract	34	9
Pancreas	8	2
Liver and gallbladder	5	1
Endocrine organs	7	2
Urinary tract	10	3
Reproductive organs	15	4
Melanoma	13	3
Other and unknown	17	4
Non-epithelial		
Leukemia	27	7
Sarcoma	12	3
Total	397	100

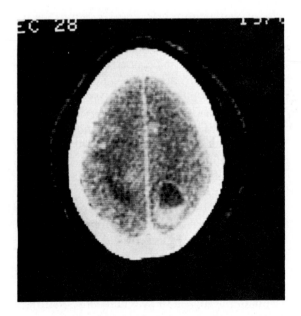

Figure 72.   CT brain scan. Cerebral metastases.
(Courtesy Dr. Harry H. White.)

fluid are not uncommon. Although the histological appearance of the metastatic tumor is similar to that of the primary lesion, it is not always possible to determine the site of the primary tumor from the appearance of the metastasis.

The clinical signs and symptoms of metastatic tumor are similar to those of other tumors and are dependent on the site of the lesion. In the majority of the cases, the signs and symptoms are predominantly those of a single lesion even though several or many tumors may be found at autopsy. Characteristic of metastatic tumors is the rapid onset and progression of symptoms. The duration of life after the appearance of signs of intracranial metastases is usually only a matter of a few months. The extremes vary from a few days to several years. Survival for one year after the onset of neurological signs and symptoms is rare, except in patients with metastatic hypernephromas.

Carcinomatosis of the Meninges. Diffuse involvement of the leptomeninges is a rare complication of metastatic tumors to the nervous system. Headaches, dementia and multiple cranial nerve palsies are the most common manifestations. The cerebrospinal fluid is usually under increased pressure with a lymphocytic pleocytosis and a decreased sugar content. Tumor cells may be found in the fluid. The course is rapidly progressive with death within a few weeks or months from the onset of the symptoms.

The diagnosis of metastatic intracranial tumor as the cause of neurological signs and symptoms can be made without difficulty in patients with a known malignant primary tumor or with evidence of metastases in other portions of the body. The possibility of a metastatic tumor should be considered in all middle-aged or elderly individuals in whom the neurological symptoms have developed in the course of a few weeks or months. Metastatic tumors are sufficiently common to make it mandatory to have a roentgenogram made of the chest of all patients in whom the diagnosis of an intracranial tumor is considered.

If the diagnosis of a metastatic intracranial tumor is definitely established, operation is rarely advisable. It must be remembered, however, that the finding of a malignant tumor, such as carcinoma of the colon, or the history of a previous operation for the removal of a carcinoma of the breast cannot be taken as prima facie evidence that the lesion in the nervous system is metastatic unless there is evidence of generalized metastases. The coincidence of a malignant tumor of the breast or the abdominal viscera and a benign tumor of the brain is occasionally encountered.

If there is reasonable doubt as to the metastatic nature of the lesion, an exploratory craniotomy is justified. In some instances, the removal of a large single metastatic tumor may relieve the symptoms and give the patient several or many months of useful life. Radiation therapy may be given to retard the rate of growth of the intracranial metastases.

REFERENCES

Aronson, S. M., Garcia, J. H., and Aronson, B. E.: Metastatic Neoplasms of the Brain: Their Frequency in Relation to Age, Cancer, 17, 558, 1964.
Fischer-Williams, M., Bosanquet, F. D., and Daniel, P. M.: Carcinomatosis of the Meninges, Brain, 78, 42, 1955.
Fox, H. J., et al.: Neurocutaneous Melanosis, Arch. Dis. Childhood, 39, 508, 1964.
Globus, J. H., and Meltzer, T.: Metastatic Tumors of the Brain, Arch. Neurol. & Psychiat., 48, 163, 1942.
Hazra, J., Mullins, C. M., and Lott, S.: Management of Cerebral Metastases from Bronchiogenic Carcinoma, Johns Hopkins Med. Bull., 130, 377, 1972.
Hoffman, H. J., and Freeman, A.: Primary Leptomeningeal Melanoma in Association with Giant Hairy Nevi, J. Neurosurg., 26, 62, 1967.
Moersch, F. P., Love, J. G., and Kernohan, J. W.: Melanoma of the Central Nervous System, J.A.M.A., 115, 2148, 1940.
Vieth, R. G., and Odom, G. L.: Intracranial Metastases and Their Neurosurgical Treatment, J. Neurosurg., 23, 375, 1965.

Pseudotumor Cerebri
(Benign Intracranial Hypertension)

Headache, choked discs and diminution of visual acuity may occur in patients who do not have any of the usual causes of increased intracranial pressure (intracranial mass lesions, obstruction of the flow of the cerebrospinal fluid, intracranial infections, hypertensive encephalopathy or chronic retention of carbon dioxide in pulmonary disease). This condition has been described by the terms pseudotumor cerebri, serous meningitis and otitic hydrocephalus. It is also called benign intracranial hypertension because spontaneous recovery generally occurs but visual acuity may be severely damaged.

The increased intracranial pressure is associated with a wide variety of conditions, but the mechanism of the increase in pressure is obvious in only a few of them. Increased venous pressure with a disproportion in the rate of formation and absorption of cerebrospinal fluid can explain the situation in the patients with thrombosis of the intracranial sinuses or veins, but the mechanism of the increased pressure is not evident in most of the remaining patients. The fact that the ventricles and subarachnoid spaces are smaller than normal raises the possibility that edema of the cerebral substances is the cause of the increased pressure.

The conditions commonly associated with benign increased intracranial pressure can be divided into five groups. New causes are being constantly added, including adrenal hyperplasia, vitamin A, vitamin B or iron deficiency and allergic reactions to penicillin and other drugs.

With the diagnostic methods now available it is rare for an intracranial tumor to be present and not detected as the cause of the increased intracranial pressure. This mistake, however, can be and still is made.

Treatment. Thrombosis of the lateral sinus can be treated surgically and the patients in whom the condition is associated with endocrine

Table 41. Presumed Causes of Benign Increased Intracranial Pressure (Pseudotumor Cerebri)

1. Intracranial venous thromboses (sagittal, straight or lateral sinuses, vein of Galen)
2. Disorders of endocrine glands
   A. Adrenal (Addison's disease, Cushing's syndrome, with steroid therapy)
   B. Ovarian (menstrual dysfunction with obesity, pregnancy, menarche, administration of contraceptive hormones)
   C. Parathyroid (hypoparathyroidism)
   D. Thyroid, hyper- and hypothyroidism
3. Vitamin and drug therapy
   A. Excessive dosage of vitamin A in children and adolescents
   B. Tetracycline, penicillin and other drugs in infants
4. High protein content in the cerebrospinal fluid in patients with polyneuritis or tumors of the cauda equina
5. Unknown

disorders can be treated by replacement therapy. When the symptoms are due to treatment with adrenal steroids, ovarian hormones (contraceptive pills) and overdosage of vitamin A, withdrawal of therapy is indicated. Reduction in weight is indicated in the obese females with menstrual dysfunction. Lumbar puncture with removal of fluid at intervals of one to seven days is often of value in relieving the pressure until spontaneous stabilization occurs. Subtemporal decompression or lumbo-peritoneal shunts may be necessary to prevent severe damage to the optic nerve.

REFERENCES

Bradshaw, P.: Benign Intracranial Hypertension, J. Neurol., Neurosurg. & Psychiat., 19, 28, 1956.
Greer, M.: Benign Intracranial Hypertension,
   1. Mastoiditis and Lateral Sinus Obstruction, Neurology, 12, 472, 1962.
   2. Following Corticosteroid Therapy, Neurology, 13, 439, 1963.
   3. Pregnancy, Neurology, 13, 670, 1963.
   4. Menarche, Neurology, 14, 569, 1964.
   5. Menstrual Dysfunction, Neurology, 14, 668, 1964.
   6. Obesity, Neurology, 15, 382, 1965.
Hagberg, B., and Sillinpää, M.: Benign Intracranial Hypertension (Pseudotumor Cerebri), Acta Paediat. Scand., 59, 328, 1970.
Lysak, W. R., and Svien, H. J.: Long-Term Follow-Up on Patients with Diagnosis of Pseudotumor Cerebri, J. Neurosurg., 25, 284, 1966.
Walker, A. E., and Adamkiewcz, J. J.: Pseudotumor Cerebri Associated with Prolonged Corticosteroid Therapy, J.A.M.A., 188, 779, 1964.
Walsh, F. B., Clark, D. B., Thompson, R. S., and Nicholson, D. H.: Oral Contraceptives and Neuro-ophthalmologic Interest, Arch. Ophth., 74, 628, 1965.

NORMAL PRESSURE HYDROCEPHALUS IN ADULTS

In recent years the term *normal pressure hydrocephalus* has been given to a syndrome which develops in middle-aged or elderly adults characterized clinically by dementia, a spastic-ataxic or -apraxic gait, and urinary incontinence with a normal cerebrospinal fluid pressure. There is enlargement of the ventricles and the basal cisterns on pneumoencephalography, but the injected air does not pass over the surface of the cerebral cortex.

This rare syndrome is apparently due to an obstruction in the passage of fluid from the ventricular system into the subarachnoid spaces or to a failure of absorption of the fluid in the cerebral venous sinuses. In a number of patients there was a previous history of subarachnoid hemorrhage, an inflammatory process in the meninges, or a tumor which interfered with the absorption or circulation of the cerebrospinal fluid. In a number, but not all of the cases, the symptoms have been alleviated by ventriculo-atrial or ventriculo-peritoneal shunt.

The dementia is differentiated from that associated with cortical atrophy due to cerebral arteriosclerosis, presenile dementia or other degenerative disease by the typical findings on pneumoencephalography and by the pattern of distribution of radionuclide following subarachnoid injection. The isotope remains concentrated in the ventricles and basal cisterns and does not pass over the convexities of the cerebral hemispheres.

The findings on neurological examination have varied. The dementia and gait disturbance are constant. There may be also spasticity of the lower extremities with hyperactive knee jerks and extensor plantar responses. The cerebrospinal fluid is usually entirely normal, but in occasional cases there has been a slight increase in pressure and in the cellular and protein content. The results of subarachnoid air injection and isotope cisternography establish the diagnosis and are an indication for the performance of shunting procedures.

REFERENCES

Adams, R. D.: Further Observation on Normal Pressure Hydrocephalus, Proceed. Royal Society Med., 59, 1135, 1966.
Adams, R. D., et al.: Symptomatic Occult Hydrocephalus with Normal Cerebrospinal Fluid Pressure, N. Engl. J. Med., 273, 117, 1965.
Benson, D. F., et al.: Diagnosis of Normal Pressure Hydrocephalus, N. Engl. J. Med., 283, 609, 1970.
Geschwind, N.: The Mechanism of Normal Pressure Hydrocephalus, J. Neurol. Sci., 7, 481, 1968.
Hogan, P. A., and Woolsey, R. M.: Hydrocephalus in the Adult, J.A.M.A., 198, 524, 1966.
James, A. E., et al.: Normal-Pressure Hydrocephalus, Role of Cisternography in Diagnosis, J.A.M.A., 213, 1615, 1970.
Michelsen, W. J., et al.: Factors Involved in Surgical Management of Normal Pressure Hydrocephalus, Acta Radiologica, 13, 570, 1972.

SPINAL TUMORS

Tumors which involve the spinal cord or its roots are similar in their nature and origin to intracranial tumors. They may arise from the

parenchyma of the cord, its roots, the meningeal coverings, the intraspinal vascular network or the vertebral column. In addition there may
be metastases from tumors elsewhere in the body.

Spinal tumors are divided according to their location into two large
groups: the intramedullary and extramedullary. Extramedullary tumors
may be intradural, extradural or extravertebral. Occasionally, an extradural tumor may extend through the intravertebral foramina and lie
partially within and partially outside of the spinal canal (dumbbell or
hourglass tumors).

Table 42.   Relative Frequency of Various Types of Spinal Tumor

	Elsberg	Sloof, et al.	Total	%
Neurofibromas	70	383	453	29
Meningiomas	73	338	411	26
Gliomas	33	291	324	21
Sarcomas	31	157	188	12
Angiomas	9	82	91	6
Metastatic & others ..	32	71	103	6
Total	248	1322	1570	100

**Table 43.   The Location of Spinal Tumor with Reference to the Spinal
Cord and Its Covering**

(567 Cases Collected from the Literature)

	No. of Cases	%
Extradural	141	25
Extramedullary	334	59
Intramedullary	62	11
Cauda equina	30	5
Total	567	100

**Table 44.   The Relative Frequency of Benign and Malignant Spinal
Tumors**

	Elsberg	Sloof, et al.	Total	%
Benign	149	721	870	56
Malignant	74	501	575	37
Metastatic, Vascular & others ..	17	100	117	7
Total	240	1322	1562	100

Pathology. The histology (Table 42) of the various types of primary and secondary tumors is, with minor modifications, exactly the same as that of the intracranial tumors and need not be repeated in detail here. It should be emphasized that tumors of the substance of the spinal cord are relatively rare and represent only a little more than 10% (Table 43) of all spinal tumors. On the other hand the benign encapsulated tumors (Figs. 73 and 74) (meningiomas and neurofibromas) are common and constitute approximately two thirds of all of the primary spinal tumors and over one half of all spinal tumors of primary or metastatic origin (Table 44). Vascular malformations are not infrequent (Fig. 75).

Incidence. Tumors of the spinal cord are much less frequent than intracranial tumors, the ratio being about 1 to 4. The incidence in the two sexes is approximately equal with the exception that meningiomas

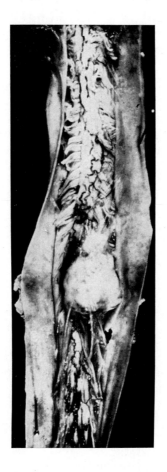

Figure 73.   Meningioma of lower cervical spinal cord. (Courtesy Dr. Abner Wolf.)

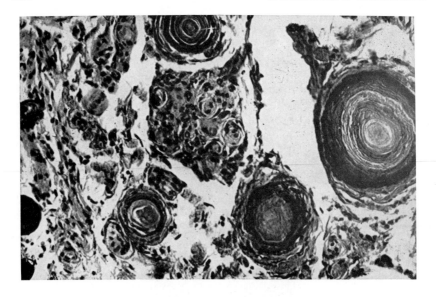

Figure 74.   Meningioma of spinal cord with whirls.

Table 45.   Age Incidence of Spinal Tumors of all Types
(Data Compiled from the Literature)

Age in Years	No. of Cases	%
0–9	19	2
10–19	98	10
20–29	156	16
30–39	177	18
40–49	238	25
50–59	186	19
Over 60	101	10
Total	975	100

are more common in women. Spinal tumors occur predominantly in young or middle aged adults, and are relatively rare in childhood or in old age (Table 45). Hamby was able to collect from the literature only 214 cases in children (Table 46). Spinal tumors are more common in the thoracic region, but when the actual length of the various portions of the spinal cord is taken into consideration, the distribution is relatively equal.

Symptomatology. Extramedullary tumors produce symptoms by pressure on the nerve roots, compression of the spinal cord and

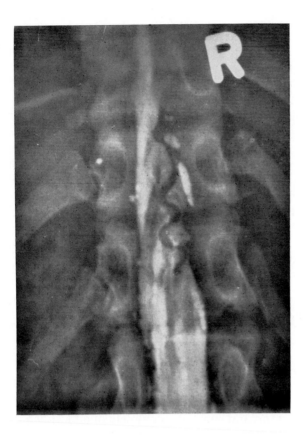

Figure 75. Vascular malformation. Myelography demonstrating large tortuous vessels on the surface of the lower thoracic cord. (Courtesy Dr. Gordon Potts and Dr. Juan Taveras.)

Table 46.   The Incidence of Tumors of the Spinal Cord in Childhood
(After Hamby, J. Neuropath. & Exper. Neurol., 1944)

Type of Tumor	No. of Cases	%
Gliomas	44	21
Sarcomas	42	19
Dermoids	37	17
Neurinomas	23	11
Lipomas	10	5
Meningiomas	10	5
Chloromas	9	4
Blood vessel tumors	7	3
Sympathetic tumors	6	3
Miscellaneous tumors	26	12
Total	214	100

occlusion of the spinal vessels. The symptoms of intramedullary tumors are the result of destruction of parenchyma by the tumor and compression of adjacent areas.

EXTRAMEDULLARY TUMORS. Extramedullary tumors are usually limited to several segments of the spinal cord and commonly produce signs and symptoms of a partial or complete transverse myelitis. The first symptoms are pains and paresthesias as result of compression of nerve roots. This is soon followed by sensory loss, weakness and muscular wasting in the distribution of the affected root or roots. Compression of the spinal cord of a mild or moderate degree interrupts the function of the fibers in the peripheral portion of the cord. The early signs of cord compression are: (1) Spastic weakness of the muscles below the level of the lesion; (2) impairment of cutaneous and proprioceptive sensation below the level of the lesion; (3) impairment of the control of the bladder and to less extent of the rectum; and (4) increase in the reflexes with extensor plantar responses and loss of appropriate abdominal skin reflexes.

There may be considerable variation in the severity and distribution of the motor weakness and sensory loss depending to some degree on the location of the tumor in relation to the anterior, lateral or posterior portion of the spinal cord. Laterally placed tumor may produce a typical Brown-Séquard syndrome.

Severe compression of the spinal cord is followed by necrosis of the parenchyma with destruction of gray as well as white matter, producing the symptoms and signs of a complete or almost complete transection of the cord. There is wasting and atrophy of the muscles at the level of the lesion, and below the level of the lesion there is: Paraplegia in flexion; complete loss of all forms of sensation; loss of the appropriate abdominal skin reflexes and the presence of reflexes of defense.

Symptoms and signs of compression of the conus or cauda equina are considered later.

Occlusion of the spinal vessels not infrequently occurs with extraspinal tumors, particularly metastatic carcinoma, lymphogranulomas (Hodgkin's disease) or epidural infections. When the spinal vessels are occluded, there is myelomalacia of the cord with symptoms and signs similar to those which are seen with severe compression necrosis of the cord. Occlusion of spinal vessels may also occur in combination with cord compression.

INTRAMEDULLARY TUMORS. Intramedullary tumors may be confined to a few segments of the cord but not uncommonly they extend over many segments. For this reason the signs and symptoms of intramedullary tumors are much more variable than those of extramedullary tumors. If the tumor is localized to one segment of the cord, the syndrome is similar to that of extramedullary tumors. When they extend over many segments, the clinical picture may simulate that of syringomyelia.

REGIONAL SYNDROMES. *Foramen Magnum Tumors*. Tumors in the high cervical region may extend through the foramen magnum and lie partially intracranially and partially intraspinally. The syndrome produced by such tumors is quite variable with a mixture of signs and symptoms due to paralysis of one or more of the cranial nerves on one side and signs and symptoms of cord compression. The syndrome produced by these tumors (usually meningiomas) is described on page 242.

Cervical Tumors. Involvement of the upper segments of the cervical cord is accompanied by pain or paresthesias in the occipital or cervical region and stiffness of the neck. There is weakness and wasting of the neck muscles. Below the level of the lesion there is a spastic tetraplegia. Occasionally there may be a hemiplegia on one side and a paralysis of the lower extremity on the opposite side. Impairment of sensation extends to the level of the area supplied by the trigeminal nerve. Pain and temperature sense in the distribution of the trigeminal nerve may be affected in patients with intramedullary tumors extending upward to involve the descending root of the nerve. The characteristic findings which make it possible to localize the upper level of spinal tumors in the middle and lower cervical segments are given in outline form below.

Fourth Cervical. Paralysis of the diaphragm.

Fifth Cervical. Atrophic paralysis of the deltoid, biceps, supinator longus, rhomboids and spinatus muscles. The upper arms hang limp at the side. The sensory level extends to the outer surface of the arm. The biceps and supinator reflexes are lost.

Sixth Cervical. Paralysis of triceps and wrist extensor. The forearm is held semi-flexed and there is a partial wrist drop. The triceps reflex is lost. Sensory impairment extends to a line running down the middle of the arm slightly to the radial side.

Seventh Cervical. Paralysis of the flexors of the wrist and of the flexors and extensors of the fingers. Efforts to close the hands result in extension of the wrist and slight flexion of the fingers ("preacher's hand"). The sensory level is similar to that of the sixth cervical segment but slightly more to the ulnar side of the arm.

Eighth Cervical. Atrophic paralysis of the small muscles of the hand with resulting "clawhand" ("*main-en-griffe*"). Horner's syndrome, unilateral or bilateral, is characteristic of lesions at this level. Sensory loss extends to the inner aspect of the arm and involves the little, ring, and ulnar aspect of the middle finger.

Other signs of cervical tumors include nystagmus which is most commonly seen with intramedullary tumors in the upper segments. This is presumably due to damage to the median longitudinal fasciculus. Horner's syndrome may be found with intramedullary lesions in any portion of the cervical cord as result of injury to the descending sympathetic pathways.

Thoracic. Localization of tumors in the thoracic region of the cord is usually made on basis of the sensory level. It is difficult to determine the location of lesions in the upper half of the thoracic cord by testing the strength of the intercostal muscles. Lesions which affect the lower abdominal muscles but spare the upper ones can be localized by the observation that the umbilicus moves upward when the patient attempts to flex the head on the chest against resistance (Beevor's sign). The abdominal skin reflexes are absent below the level of the lesion.

Lumbar. Lesions in the lumbar region can be localized by the level of the sensory loss and motor weakness. Tumors which compress only the first and second lumbar segments cause a loss of the cremasteric reflexes. The abdominal reflexes are preserved and the patellar and achilles reflexes are increased.

If the tumor affects the third and fourth segments of the lumbar cord and does not involve the roots of the cauda equina, there is weakness of the quadriceps muscles and loss of the patellar reflexes with hyperactive achilles reflexes. More commonly lesions at this level also involve the cauda equina and there is a flaccid paralysis of the lower extremities with loss of both knee and ankle reflexes. There may be, however, a spastic paralysis of one lower extremity with increased ankle reflex on that side and a flaccid paralysis and loss of reflexes on the other side as result of compression of the roots of the cauda equina.

Conus and Cauda Equina. The initial symptom of tumors which involve the conus or cauda equina is pain in the back or in the lower extremities often leading to a diagnosis of "sciatica." Bladder symptoms and impotence are also commonly seen early in the course. With extension of the growth there are a flaccid paralysis of the lower extremities, atrophy of the leg muscles and foot drop. Fibrillary twitchings may be seen in the atrophied muscles. Sensory loss is usually present in the lower lumbar and in the sacral dermatomes. This may be very slight or it may be so severe that trophic ulcer develops over the lumbosacral region, the buttocks, the hips or heels. Headache, diplopia and choked discs may occur in patients with tumors in the low thoracic or lumbosacral regions. These symptoms are due to hydrocephalus, which is presumably the result of interference of drainage of cerebrospinal fluid by the high protein content.

Diagnosis of Spinal Tumors. Tumors compressing the spinal cord or the cauda equina are characterized by radicular pains and the slow evolution of signs of an incomplete transverse lesion of the cord or signs of compression of the roots of the cauda equina. Extramedullary tumors which do not compress the spinal cord may produce symptoms as the result of interfering with the blood supply of the cord. In the majority of such cases, the symptoms are of sudden onset and the tumor is of metastatic origin or is of granulomatous nature. A careful study should be made for evidence of a primary tumor or for evidence of Hodgkin's or other granulomatous lesions elsewhere in the body.

The diagnosis of an intraspinal tumor can be established before operation with almost absolute certainty with the help of certain diagnostic aids. These include roentgenograms of the spine and visualization of the subarachnoid space with Pantopaque or air. Tumors and vascular malformations can be visualized by spinal angiography.

Roentgenograms. Tumors within the spinal cord may be visualized by roentgenogram when they produce any of the following: (1) Localized destruction of the vertebrae or their processes. (2) Changes in the contour of or separation of the pedicles. The interpedicular distance should be measured and compared with the normal. Localized enlargement of the spinal canal is usually diagnostic of an intraspinal tumor but an enlargement over many segments may be due to a developmental anomaly. (3) Distortion of paraspinal tissues by tumors (frequently a neurofibroma) which extend through the intervertebral foramen. (4) Proliferation of bone. This is rare except in osteomas and sarcomas, but is also occasionally seen in hemangiomas affecting the bone and meninges. (5) The presence of calcifications. Calcium deposits are occasionally present in meningiomas or congenital tumors.

The Cerebrospinal Fluid. The characteristic cerebrospinal fluid findings of intraspinal tumors are incomplete or complete subarachnoid block and an increased protein content. Complete or incomplete subarachnoid block is present in practically every patient with a spinal tumor that is large enough to compress the spinal cord and produce signs and symptoms of a partial or complete transverse lesion. The cerebrospinal fluid dynamics are normal with tumors of the cauda equina which lie below the level of the puncture and with extradural tumors which do not compress the cord. Normal or nearly normal dynamics may be present with small tumors, particularly those in the cervical region, which lie intradurally or intramedullary and have not blocked the subarachnoid space. In the latter cases neurological signs and symptoms of a complete transverse myelitis are rarely, if ever, found.

When there is complete subarachnoid block, the fluid is usually yellowish in color as result of the high protein content. The fluid may be slightly yellow or clear and colorless when the subarachnoid block is incomplete. The fluid removed from above the level of cauda equina tumors usually has a slight yellow tinge. The cell count is usually normal but a slight pleocytosis is found in approximately 30% of the cases. Cell counts between 25 and 100 per cu mm are found in about 15%. The protein content is increased in over 95%. Values over 100 mg are present in 60% and over 1000 mg in 5% (Table 47). The sugar content is normal and the chloride content is normal except in the fluids with a high protein content when it is moderately reduced.

Myelography. Myelography (Figs. 76, 77 and 78) with radiopaque oils (preferably Pantopaque) or air is of value in localizing the level of lesions which compress the spinal cord and in establishing the diagnosis of tumors of the cauda equina. The opaque oil should be removed after the completion of the fluoroscopic examination and the taking of roentgenograms. An extradural tumor will displace the dura towards the subarachnoid space and deform the dye column on its outer aspect (Fig. 76). A subdural extramedullary lesion lying within the subarachnoid space displaces the spinal cord away from the tumor, and the tumor may be outlined by Pantopaque (Fig. 77). An intramedullary tumor will cause enlargement on the dye column from its inner aspect (Fig. 78).

Differential Diagnosis. Spinal tumors must be differentiated from other conditions with progressive signs of disease of the spinal cord, including syphilis, multiple sclerosis, syringomyelia, combined system disease, amyotrophic lateral sclerosis, anomalies of the cervical spine and base of the skull, adhesive arachnoiditis, radiculitis of the cauda equina, hypertrophic arthritis and ruptured intervertebral discs.

Syphilis may produce signs and symptoms of a transverse lesion of the cord. The diagnosis of syphilis is established by the serological findings in the cerebrospinal fluid. In addition, subarachnoid block rarely occurs as result of syphilitic involvement of the meninges. When it is found and does not clear up with antisyphilitic treatment, exploration is justified because the treatment of a syphilitic granuloma is by operation.

Multiple sclerosis with a complete or incomplete transverse lesion of the cord can be differentiated from spinal cord tumors by the remitting course, the presence of signs and symptoms of injury to other parts of the nervous system and by the normal cerebrospinal fluid dynamics. Complete subarachnoid block may occur occasionally with swelling of the cord when there is an acute lesion as result of multiple sclerosis or other demyelinizing processes. The acute onset of the symptoms is of value in differentiating these cases from tumors of the spinal cord.

The differential diagnosis between syringomyelia and intramedullary tumors is complicated by the fact that the coincidence of the two is not uncommon. Extramedullary tumors in the cervical region may give localized pains and muscular atrophy together with a Brown-Séquard syndrome, producing a clinical picture similar to that of syringomyelia.

Table 47. **The Protein Content of the Cerebrospinal Fluid in 36 Cases with Spinal Tumors**

Protein Content (mg per 100 ml)	No. of Cases	%
Less than 45	5	14
45–100	7	19
100–1000	22	61
More than 1000	2	6
Total	36	100

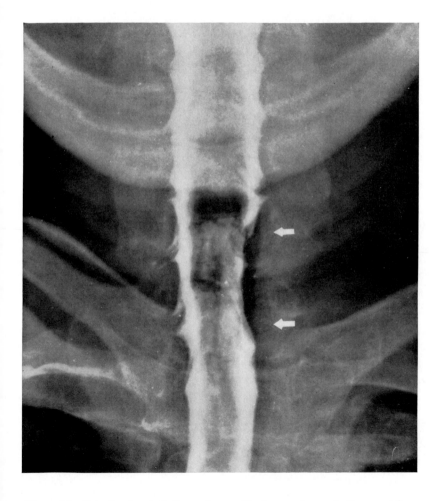

Figure 76. Extradural metastatic carcinoma. Myelogram demonstrating smooth even impression upon the lower cervical subarachnoid outline (arrows), obliteration of nerve root shadows and slight displacement of spinal cord. (Courtesy Dr. Ernest Wood.)

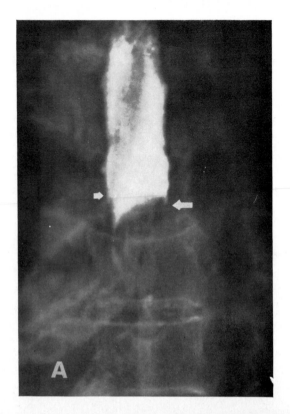

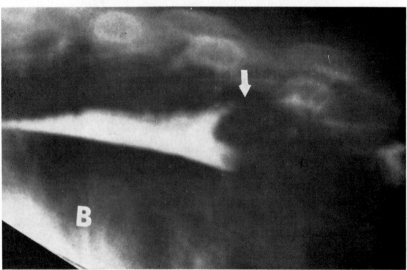

Figure 77. Spinal meningioma. Myelogram. *A*, Frontal view shows sharply margi-nated edge of an intradural tumor (large arrow) displacing the spinal cord and compressing it (small arrow) to a narrow band. *B*, Lateral view shows tumor outline (arrow) with the compressed cord shadow situated ventrally. (Courtesy Dr. Ernest Wood.)

310

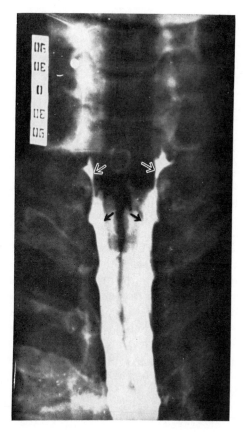

Figure 78.   Intramedullary tumor. Myelogram showing widening of the cervical cord
shadow by the tumor. (Courtesy Dr. Gordon Potts and Dr. Juan Taveras.)

The diagnosis of syringomyelia is likely when trophic disturbances are
present and the cerebrospinal fluid dynamics are normal. The differential can be made with certainty only by exploratory operation in the
rare cases of syringomyelia with complete subarachnoid block.

Combined system disease is diagnosed by the neurological findings,
the normal cerebrospinal fluid dynamics and the characteristic changes
in the blood.

The combination of atrophy of the muscles of the upper extremity
and a spastic weakness in the lower extremities which are common
findings in patients with amyotrophic lateral sclerosis may suggest the
diagnosis of a cervical cord tumor. The latter is excluded by the normal
sensory examination, the presence of fibrillation or atrophy in muscles
in the lower extremities, and normal cerebrospinal fluid dynamics.

Osteoarthritis of the cervical spine with or without rupture of the intervertebral discs may produce symptoms and signs of root irritation and compression of the spinal cord. The osteoarthritis can be diagnosed by the roentgen-ray findings. Myelography may be necessary to determine whether there is concomitant disease of the disc or whether an extramedullary tumor is also present.

Anomalies in the cervical region or at the base of the skull, such as platybasia or Klippel-Feil syndrome, are diagnosed by the characteristic roentgenographic findings.

The arachnoid may be thickened in patients with primary disease of the spinal cord such as syringomyelia, syphilis or multiple sclerosis. In these cases the thickening of the arachnoid does not play any significant role in the production of the cord symptoms. The pia-arachnoid may be thickened in the absence of intrinsic spinal cord disease following infections of the spinal meninges or hemorrhage into the meninges secondary to trauma, following the injection of serum, Lipiodol, spinal anesthetics and other substances into the subarachnoid space, and following the removal of extramedullary tumors. Occasionally the meninges may become so thickened as to interfere with the circulation in the cord and produce signs and symptoms of a transverse lesion. Spinal subarachnoid block may be present. The cerebrospinal fluid protein content is moderately elevated. There may be a complete arrest of the oil on Pantopaque myelography or a separation of the oil column into globules at the site of the lesion. Operative separation of the adhesions and removal of the thickened arachnoid are not followed by any significant improvement in the symptoms, especially when they are due to myelomalacia secondary to vascular damage.

The signs and symptoms of ruptured intervertebral disc in the lumbar region may be similar to those of a cauda equina tumor. Extensive sensory or motor loss is much more common in the latter. In addition, the protein content of the cerebrospinal fluid is usually greater than 100 mg per 100 ml, whereas such values are rare with ruptured intervertebral disc. The differential diagnosis can usually be established by the size and position of the defect in the myelograms.

Course and Prognosis. Benign tumors of the spinal cord are characterized by a slowly progressive course extending over several or many years. The paraplegia is of the spastic type and sensory loss is incomplete until there is a complete transverse necrosis of the cord. The paralysis is of the flaccid type and the sensory loss is complete when there is complete myelomalacia.

Although the symptoms are usually inexorably progressive, occasionally there may be partial or complete remission in symptoms in the patients with extramedullary tumors, particularly extradural cysts.

Sudden onset of signs and symptoms of a complete transverse myelitis may occur with spinal tumors which compress the spinal vessels. This most commonly occurs with metastatic tumors or Hodgkin's disease.

Treatment. The treatment of spinal tumors is by operation or radiation. Surgical therapy of cord tumors is indicated whenever there is evidence of compression of the spinal cord or the roots of the cauda equina. Surgical therapy is of little or no value in the patients with signs and symptoms of a transverse myelitis which result from compression of the spinal vessels by extramedullary tumors such as lymphogranulomas or metastatic tumors. In general the best results are obtained when the signs and symptoms are due solely to compression of nervous tissue by meningiomas, neurofibromas, lipomas and other benign encapsulated tumors. Complete restoration may occur even in patients in whom a severe spastic paraplegia has been present for several or many years. Very little or no improvement can be expected when there is a flaccid paraplegia as result of complete necrosis of the cord substance secondary to compression of or interference with its circulation.

Complete removal of the tumor is only rarely possible in patients with intramedullary gliomas, gliomas of the conus and cauda equina, chordomas, dermoids, angiomas and metastatic tumors. Partial removal followed by radiation therapy may result in improvement in the signs and symptoms.

REFERENCES

Auld, A. W., and Buerman, A.: Metastatic Spinal Epidural Tumors, Arch. Neurol., 15, 100, 1966.

Austin, G.: The Spinal Cord; Basic Aspects and Surgical Considerations, 2nd Ed., Springfield, Charles C Thomas, 1972, 762 pp.

Benson, D. F.: Intramedullary Spinal Cord Metastases, Neurology, 10, 281, 1960.

Bergstand, A., Höök, O., and Lidvall, H.: Vascular Malformations of the Spinal Cord, Acta Neurol. Scand., 40, 169, 1964.

Blockey, N. J., and Schorstein, J.: Intraspinal Epidermoid Tumors in the Lumbar Region of Children, J. Bone & Joint Surg., 43B, 556, 1961.

Elsberg, C. A.: Surgical Diseases of the Spinal Cord, Membranes and Nerve Roots, New York, Paul B. Hoeber, Inc., 1941, 598 pp.

Frazier, C. H., and Allen, A. R.: Surgery of the Spine and Spinal Cord, New York, D. Appleton, 1918, 971 pp.

Glassauer, F. E.: Thoracic and Lumbar Intraspinal Tumors Associated with Increased Intracranial Pressure, J. Neurol., Neurosurg. & Psychiat., 27, 451, 1964.

Krueger, E. G., Sobel, G. L., and Weinstein, C.: Vertebral Hemangioma with Compression of Spinal Cord, J. Neurosurg., 18, 331, 1961.

Lin, T. H.: Intramedullary Tuberculoma of the Spinal Cord, J. Neurosurg., 17, 497, 1960.

Lombardi, G., and Passerini, A.: Spinal Cord Tumors, Radiology, 76, 381, 1961.

McKissock, W., Bloom, W. H., and Chynn, K. Y.: Spinal Cord Compression Caused by Plasma-Cell Tumors, J. Neurosurg., 18, 68, 1961.

Norstrom, C. W., Kernohan, J. W., and Love, J. G.: One Hundred Primary Caudal Tumors, J.A.M.A., 178, 1071, 1961.

Otenasek, F. J., and Silver, M. L.: Spinal Hemangioma (Hemangioblastoma) in Lindau's Disease, J. Neurosurg., 18, 295, 1961.

Patterson, R. H., Jr., Campbell, W. G., Jr., and Parsons, H.: Ependymoma of the Cauda Equina with Multiple Visceral Metastases, J. Neurosurg., 18, 145, 1961.

Pickens, J. M. et al.: Teratoma of the Spinal Cord. Report of a Case and Review of the Literature, Arch. Path., 94, 448, 1975.

Rosenquist, H., and Saltzman, G. F.: Sacrococcygeal and Vertebral Chordomas and Their Treatment, Acta Radiol., 52, 177, 1959.

Shapiro, J. H., and Jacobson, H. G.: Differential Diagnosis of Intradural (Extramedullary) and Extradural Spinal Canal Tumors, Radiology, 76, 718, 1961.

Smith, R.: An Evaluation of Surgical Treatment for Spinal Cord Compression Due to Metastatic Carcinoma, J. Neurol., Neurosurg. & Psychiat., 28, 152, 1965.

Taveras, J. M., and Wood, E. H.: Diagnostic Neuroradiology, 2nd Edition, Baltimore, The Williams & Wilkins Co., 1976, 1250 pp.

Vieth, R. G., and Odom, G. L.: Extradural Spinal Metastases and Their Neurosurgical Treatment, J. Neurosurg., 23, 501, 1965.

Webb, J. H., Craig, W. M., and Kernohan, J. W.: Intraspinal Neoplasms in the Cervical Region, J. Neurosurg., 10, 360, 1953.

Wood, E. H., Jr.: An Atlas of Myelography, Washington, D. C., Registry Press, 1948, 111 pp.

TUMORS OF THE PERIPHERAL NERVES

Solitary tumors (usually neurofibromas) may develop on any of the peripheral nerves, but more commonly these tumors are multiple and are a part of the syndrome of neurofibromatosis. The symptoms which are produced by tumors of peripheral nerves are similar to those produced by other lesions. They are discussed in Chapter 4. This section will be limited to the consideration of the cases with multiple tumors of the nerves.

Neurofibromatosis

Neurofibromatosis (von Recklinghausen's disease) is an inherited disorder characterized by the development of multiple tumors of the spinal or cranial nerves, tumors of the skin and cutaneous pigmentation. The disease has a great variety of other manifestations too numerous to be included in a short description.

Etiology and Pathology. It is generally agreed that the manifestations of the disease are due to an abnormality in germ plasm which results in localized overgrowth of various mesodermal and ectodermal elements in the skin, peripheral nerves, central nervous system and at times in other organs of the body.

The pathological manifestations of the disease are variable and widespread. Most characteristic are the tumors of the peripheral nerve. These may occur as nodules scattered along the course of the nerve in their peripheral or in their intracranial or intraspinal portions or they may occur on the terminal distribution of the fibers in a widespread fashion (plexiform neuroma). Coincidental with the neuromas there may be tumors of the meninges (meningiomas), tumors of the glia cells (astrocytomas, ependymomas, glioblastomas and the like), as well as small nodules of gliosis or glial proliferation within the central nervous system.

Changes in the skin, in addition to the plexiform neurofibromas, include pedunculated or sessile polypi, café-au-lait spots and port-wine or anemic nevi.

Other lesions include changes in the bones (osteitis fibrosa cystica), local overgrowth of tissue causing hemihypertrophy of tongue, face, extremities or viscera. Associated maldevelopments are not uncommon and the coincidence of neurofibromatosis and syringomyelia is not rare. Dysfunctions of the various endocrine glands may also be conjoined. The occurrence of pheochromocytoma or cystic lung disease has been reported in a number of cases.

Premature puberty, gynecomastia, and disorders of growth are uncommon features of the disease. Glaucoma, buphthalamos, glioma of the optic nerve and involvement of the uveal coat are occasionally seen.

Incidence. Neurofibromatosis is relatively rare in the fully developed form, but abortive forms with only selected features of the disease are more common. It may be transmitted as a Mendelian dominant, appearing usually in the same form in successive generations. Skipping of one or more generations may occur or there may be abortive or partial forms. The disease is more common in men and may be transmitted by either parent.

The lesions in the nerves and skin may be present at birth but more commonly they do not appear until puberty and grow slowly or rapidly after this time.

Symptoms and Signs. For purposes of description the symptoms and signs of neurofibromatosis are divided into those which pertain to the nervous system and those of other systems. Serious disability is usually due to the presence of tumors on the nerves in the cranium or spinal cord or to the coincidence of meningeal or gliogenous tumors of the nervous system.

Patients with von Recklinghausen's disease may be divided into three groups according to whether the tumor formation occurs only on the peripheral portion of the nerve (peripheral type), nerve root (central type) or on both (mixed type). In the peripheral form of the disease nodules of various size appear on the nerves of the somatic or autonomic nervous system. These are most common on the nerve trunks of the extremities, but they may also be found on the nerves of the head, neck and body (Fig. 79). The various trunks and plexuses of the autonomic system are not infrequently affected. The number of nodules in individual cases vary from a few to many thousands and

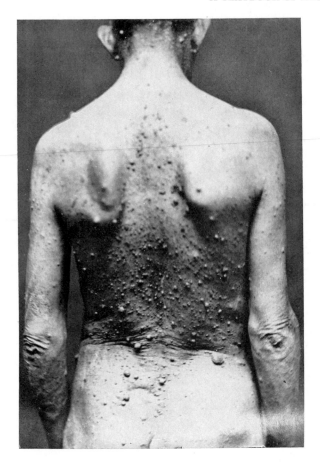

Figure 79. von Recklinghausen's disease. Multiple subcutaneous nodules
(neurofibromas) on trunk and extremities. (Courtesy Dr. P. I. Yakovlev.)

their size from that of a small seed to that of an orange. The tumors
often do not give rise to any symptoms except that they may be painful
to pressure or be the cause of neuralgic or paresthetic pains. Only rarely
is there any weakness, atrophy or sensory loss in the distribution of the
affected nerve.

Neuroma formation in the terminal distribution of the nerve fibers
(plexiform neuroma) may be accompanied by a diffuse proliferation
and fibrosis of the affected parts. The resulting picture has been
described by the term elephantiasis neuromatosa. There may be overgrowth of all tissues of one extremity or localized overgrowth of the
tissues of the head or trunk. As a result there may be elephantiasis of
one extremity or hypertrophy of one half of the face, lips or tongue.

Table 48. The Frequency of Involvement of the Cranial Nerves in 45 Necropsy-Studied Cases of Neurofibromatosis

Nerve	No. of Cases
Vagus	29
Trigeminal	12
Hypoglossal	7
Spinal accessory	6
Oculomotor	6
Glossopharyngeal	4
Optic	4
Auditory	3
Abducens	3
Trochlear	3
Olfactory	1

Overgrowth of the skin of the skull, neck or other portions of the body may be of such an extent that the excess tissue falls in loose folds of enormous size, over the eyes, shoulders or trunk. Hypertrophy of the viscera has been reported in association with the plexiform neuromas of the autonomic nervous system.

In the central or mixed form of neurofibromatosis, the symptoms and signs are those which are appropriate to tumors in the spinal cord or cranium. Small neurofibromas may be present on the spinal roots or larger ones on the cauda equina without any clinical symptoms. Large fibromas in the cervical or thoracic portion of the cord compress the spinal cord and produce a Brown-Séquard syndrome or the signs and symptoms of a transverse lesion of the spinal cord.

Large fibromas on the roots of the cranial nerves may be accompanied by symptoms and signs of increased intracranial pressure and those due to compression of the brainstem. A form of central neurofibromatosis has been reported by Gardner and Frazier in which bilateral involvement of the eighth cranial nerve is the only manifestation. According to Thomson, however, the tenth and the fifth cranial nerves are much more frequently involved than the eighth nerve (Table 48) in the usual form of neurofibromatosis.

Neurological symptoms may also appear in patients with von Recklinghausen's disease as the result of the presence of meningiomas, gliomas of the optic nerve, cerebrum or spinal cord or the coincidence of syringomyelia or other congenital defects.

The cutaneous manifestations of the disease are of little importance in regard to the production of signs and symptoms. These, together with the overgrowth of skin and other tissues associated with the plexiform neuromas, are, however, the source of considerable suffering because of the unsightly deformities and disfigurements they produce.

Subperiosteal fibromas may cause rarefaction of any of the bones with the formation of bone cysts (osteitis fibrosa cystica). Spontaneous fractures of the spine or long bones may occur.

Laboratory Data. There are no significant laboratory findings in patients with neurofibromatosis, except the changes in the cerebrospinal fluid and roentgenograms which may accompany the presence of large tumor masses in the skull or spinal cavity, and the changes in the bone which are associated with subperiosteal neurofibromas.

Diagnosis. The diagnosis is made without difficulty from the characteristic lesions in the skin and peripheral nerves. The diagnosis in the pure central form can be made only from the family history and the finding of neurofibromata at operation. The changes in the bone can be differentiated from those of hyperparathyroidism by determination of the blood calcium content.

Course and Prognosis. The course is often relatively benign with no shortening of the life span. The lesions, when fully developed, may remain stationary for many years. Occasionally there may be, without any adequate explanation, periods of rapid growth of the lesions. The prognosis in the patients with lesions on the cranial nerves or spinal roots is poor because of the disabling nature of the symptoms they produce and because they are usually multiple. Sarcomatous degeneration sometimes occurs in the peripheral tumors and leads to a fatal outcome.

Treatment. There is no adequate treatment for the disease. The peripheral tumors and hypertrophic folds of skin should be removed only when they interfere with normal activity or are disfiguring. Their removal, however, may lead to an increase in the malignancy of the growths. Intraspinal and intracranial tumors should be removed when possible.

REFERENCES

Canale, D., Bebin, J. and Knighton, R. S.: Neurologic Manifestations of von Reckling-hausen's Disease of the Nervous System, Confin. Neurol., 24, 359, 1964.
Chao, D. H.-C.: Congenital Neurocutaneous Syndromes in Childhood, J. Ped., 55, 189, 1959.
Crowe, F. W., Schull, W. J., and Neel, J. V.: *A Clinical, Pathological and Genetic Study of Multiple Neurofibromatosis*, Springfield, Charles C Thomas, 1956, 181 pp.
D'Agostino, A. N., Soule, E. H., and Miller, R. H.: Sarcomas of the Peripheral Nerves and Somatic Soft Tissues Associated with Multiple Neurofibromatosis (von Reckling-hausen's Disease), Cancer, 16, 1015, 1963.
Fienman, N. J., and Yakovac, W. C.: Neurofibromatosis in Childhood, J. Pediatrics, 76, 339, 1970.
Gardner, W. J., and Frazier, C. H.: Bilateral Acoustic Neurofibromas, Arch. Neurol. & Psychiat., 23, 266, 1930.
Martin, J. J.: Les Lesions Cérébelleuses de la Neurofibromatose de von Recklinghausen, Acta Neurol. et Psychiat., Belg., 61, 1117, 1961.
Massaro, D., Katz, S., Matthews, M. J., and Higgins, G.: Von Recklinghausen's Neurofibromatosis Associated with Cystic Lung Disease, Am. J. Med., 38, 233, 1965.

Penfield, W., and Young, A. W.: The Nature of von Recklinghausen's Disease and the Tumors Associated with It, Arch. Neurol. & Psychiat., 23, 320, 1930.

Rosendahl, T.: Some Cranial Changes in Recklinghausen's Neurofibromatosis, Acta Radiol., 19, 373, 1938.

Saxena, K. M.: Endocrine Manifestations of Neurofibromatosis in Children, Am. J. Dis. Child., 120, 265, 1970.

Thomson, A.: On Neuroma and Neurofibromatosis, Edinburgh, Turnbull & Spears, 1900, 168 pp.

von Recklinghausen, F.: Ueber die multiplen Fibrome der Haut und ihre Beziehung zu den multiplen Neuromen, Berlin, A. Hirschwald, 1882, 144 pp.

Chapter 4

Trauma

CRANIOCEREBRAL TRAUMA

Types of Head Injuries

Craniocerebral trauma may be divided according to the nature of injury to the skull into three groups: (1) Closed head injuries; (2) depressed fracture of the skull; and (3) compound fracture of the skull. This division is mainly of importance with regard to whether operative therapy will be necessary or not in the management of the patient. The prognosis for life and recovery of function is dependent more on the nature and severity of the damage to the brain than to the injury to the skull.

Closed head injuries are those in which there is no injury to or only a linear fracture of the skull. These cases can be subdivided according to the severity of damage to the cerebral substance into two main groups: patients with no significant degree of structural damage to the brain, usually designated by the term *simple concussion*; and those with destruction of brain tissue related to edema, contusion, laceration and hemorrhage.

Simple depressed fractures of the skull are those cases in which the pericranium is intact but a fragment of fractured bone is depressed inward to compress or injure the underlying brain substance.

The term *compound fracture* of the skull indicates that the pericranial tissues have been torn and that there is direct communication between the lacerated scalp and the cerebral substance through the depressed or comminuted fragments of bone and lacerated dura.

The complications of head injury include vascular lesions (hemorrhage, thrombosis or aneurysms), infections (osteomyelitis, meningitis or abscess), rhinorrhea, otorrhea, pneumocele, leptomeningeal cysts, injury to the cranial nerves and focal cerebral lesions. The sequelae of head injury are convulsive seizures, psychoses and mental disturbances, and the so-called post-traumatic syndrome, which has no established pathologic basis.

Pathology. There is some disagreement with regard to the term *concussion.* Some authors limit its use to those cases where there is only brief loss of consciousness and in whom there is no permanent damage to neural tissue.

Others include under concussion all patients with head injury who do not have objective evidence of cerebral damage regardless of the duration of the coma. In the patients with prolonged coma there may be dissolutions of neurons or other damage to brain tissue. The loss of consciousness characteristic of concussion is presumably due to a physiological disturbance, the exact nature of which has not been fully elucidated. Experimental studies indicate that it is a specific type of reaction to neural trauma related to the displacement of the brain caused by sudden movement of the head.

The experimental and pathologic evidence regarding cerebral edema following head injury is conflicting. The presence of swelling of the brain after trauma is supported by the work of some authors but denied by others. Clinical experience as well as the appearance of brains at operation strongly indicate that edema of the brain following head injury is a real entity.

The cerebral substance may be contused or lacerated even when

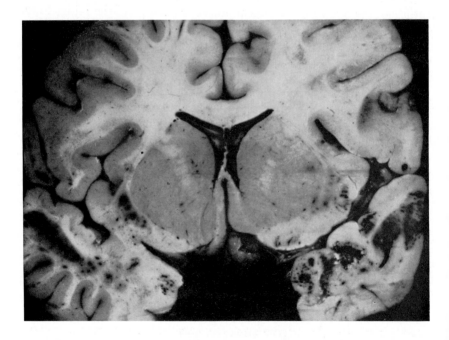

Figure 80.   Cerebral trauma. Contusion of temporal poles with fresh hemorrhages in temporal lobes. (Courtesy Dr. Philip Duffy.)

there is no injury to or only a linear fracture of the skull as well as when there is a compound or depressed fracture of the skull. The injury to the brain may be directly beneath the site of the blow to the skull, it may be in the opposite hemisphere when the injury is to the lateral surface of the skull or at the opposite pole of the hemisphere when the injury is in the occipital or frontal regions (contrecoup injury). Owing to the frequency of injuries to the occipital region, the frontal and temporal poles (Fig. 80) are commonly the sites of contusion and laceration.

The degree of damage to the meninges and cerebral substance is related to the force of the blow. With minor injuries there are petechial hemorrhages in the surface of the cortex and a mild degree of meningeal hemorrhage. With more severe injuries the meninges and cortical substances are torn and there may be an extensive hemorrhagic necrosis of the cortex and the subcortical white matter. In addition there may be small or large hemorrhages into the basal ganglia, brainstem or other portions of the brain (Fig. 81) far removed from the actual site of injury. Laceration of the middle meningeal artery or the dural sinuses is followed by bleeding into the extradural spaces, except in older patients where the bleeding may be in the subdural space.

Rupture of arachnoidal vessels produces hemorrhage into the subarachnoid space which may extend also into the subdural space. It is probable, however, that subdural hemorrhage is more commonly due to

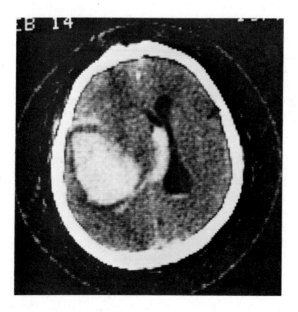

Figure 81.   Large hemorrhage in substance, brain trauma.
(Courtesy of Dr. Harry H. White.)

rupture of the vessels which bridge the space between the arachnoid and the dura mater.

Depressed fractures of the skull may not be accompanied by any injury to the brain or the cerebral substance beneath the depressed fragment may be compressed or contused. The superior longitudinal sinus may be torn or compressed and thrombosed by depressed fractures of the vertex.

Penetration of the skull and cerebral substance by bullets, bomb fragments and other missiles causes necrosis and hemorrhage into the tissue around the track of the missile.

The evolution of the pathological changes in the patient who recovers is related to the nature of the injury. Superficial lacerations of the meninges and cortex heal by gliosis, with the formation of small punched-out areas, denuded of their meningeal covering. These areas usually retain a yellowish color due to the presence of blood pigment (plaques jaunes). Larger areas of necrosis which extend deep into the cerebral substance heal by the formation of scar tissue which is composed of glia, fibroblasts and meninges (meningocerebral cicatrix). The introduction of scalp or other infected tissues into the cranium may be followed by the development of an abscess or meningitis.

Incidence. Injuries to the head are frequent in both civil and military practice. Craniocerebral trauma is the cause of death in a high percentage of the fatalities in battle and it is one of the more common causes of accidental deaths in civil life. Head injury may occur at any age, but adult men are most frequently affected. It is a common complication of delivery and is frequent in infancy and childhood as a result of falls. Automobile and motorcycle accidents are the most common cause of head injury in civil life. Kehlberg estimates that approximately three million persons sustain head injury in motor vehicle accidents each year in the United States resulting in 30,000 deaths.

Perforating wounds with compound fractures are common in military practice. In civil life, however, "closed head" injuries predominate. In the 7,031 cases reported by the Mocks, there was no fracture of the skull in 58%. In Munro's series of 1,203 cases (Table 49), nonoperative cases comprised 63%; compound fracture of the skull was present in 11.3% and depressed fracture in 4.5%.

Symptoms and Signs. Disturbance of consciousness is the most common symptom of head injury. Coma or loss of contact with the environment of short duration is a characteristic feature of simple concussion. Coma may be more prolonged, lasting for several hours or days, when there is edema, hemorrhage, dissolution of cortical neurons, contusion or laceration of the cortex. The duration of the coma is dependent on the site and severity of the injury. Coma prolonged over several days or many weeks is not uncommon when the brain or

Table 49. Ratio of Occurrence and Mortality Rate of Various Types of Head Injury and Complications in 1,203 Cases

	Total		% Mortality
	Number	%	
Nonoperative cases	758	63.0	13.9
Operative cases	444	37.0	32.4
Depressed fractures	55	4.5	5.4
Compound fractures	136	11.3	30.8
Extradural hemorrhages	38	3.1	55.2
Subdural hemorrhages	215	17.8	36.2

brainstem has been severely contused or lacerated. Loss of consciousness in patients with perforating wounds of the skull and brain is related to the size of the missile and to the region of the brain injured. Penetration of the frontal or parietal lobes by small missiles may not cause loss of consciousness, while those which pass through the petrous bone into the cerebellum and posterior fossa commonly produce coma of several or many days' duration.

On recovering consciousness, the severity and nature of the symptoms are related to the degree of brain damage. Patients with a minor degree of concussion may be normal within a few minutes. Others may be slightly dazed for a few minutes and complain of headaches for twelve to twenty-four hours. The period of mental confusion is prolonged, roughly proportional to the degree of brain injury, whenever there is contusion or laceration of the cortex. Surgical shock may be present, particularly if there is injury to the other portions of the body. Headaches and dizziness may be present after a head injury regardless of the severity of brain damage. The presence of hemiplegia, aphasia, cranial nerve palsies and other focal neurological signs is dependent on the extent and site of the damage to intracranial structures. These will be considered in detail later.

Laboratory Data. The laboratory studies which are of most importance in patients with craniocerebral injuries are roentgenograms or the skull, echoencephalograms, CT brain scan, electroencephalograms and examination of the cerebrospinal fluid.

Roentgenograms of the skull are important to determine the degree of injury to the skull and whether there is displacement of the pineal gland or other midline structures. The latter can be more accurately determined by echoencephalography and CT brain scan which will also reveal the presence of hemorrhages into the brain substance, or into the subdural or epidural spaces.

The cerebrospinal fluid is entirely normal when there has been only

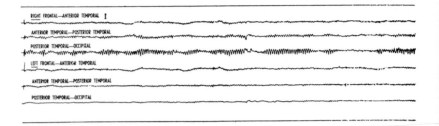

Figure 82. Cerebral trauma. Electroencephalogram showing depression of cortical activity on left side in patient with fracture of occipital bone. (Courtesy Dr. P. F. A. Hoefer.)

a cerebral concussion. The fluid is clear and colorless and under increased pressure when the injury is complicated by cerebral edema. The fluid is bloody and under increased pressure when there is contusion or laceration of the cerebral substance. The cerebrospinal fluid findings in the various complications of head injuries are considered under the appropriate headings.

With head injury of any type there is usually a suppression of the electrical activity of the cerebral cortex at the time of injury (Fig. 82). With recovery, the activity returns to normal, often going through a phase in which there is generalized slowing and an increase in voltage. Areas of focal damage to the cortex may show evidence of abnormal activity (slowing and spike activity) for many weeks or months after the injury. These abnormalities are of importance with regard to the possibility of later development of convulsive seizures. A common feature of the electroencephalograms of all patients with head injuries is an undue susceptibility of the cortical activity to overventilation. This may persist for many weeks.

Course and Prognosis. The prognosis in patients with head injury is related to the site and severity of the injury. The mortality rate is nil in the patients with simple concussion and is less than 2% when there is a mild degree of cerebral edema and congestion. The mortality rate increases greatly when the cortex is contused (5%) or lacerated (41%). Death may result in the period immediately following the injury or it may be delayed for several weeks. Death may be due to the direct effect of the injury or the complications which ensue.

With concussion or with minor degrees of cerebral edema or contusion, the patients recover from the coma with no residuals. There may be loss of memory for the events which occurred in the immediate period following the recovery of consciousness (post-traumatic amnesia) and a similar amnesia for the events immediately preceding the injury (pre-traumatic amnesia). The length of both pre- and post-traumatic amnesia is related to the severity of the brain damage. With a minor degree of concussion they may both be entirely absent, but when there has been severe contusion and laceration or other injury of the brain, periods of amnesia may extend over days or weeks. In the weeks following recovery from the injury there is a partial return of memory for events which occurred before and after the accident and a reduction of the period of absolute memory loss.

Headaches, dizziness or vertigo may be present in the immediate post-traumatic period. These usually disappear within a few weeks, but they may be prolonged for many months. With severe injuries to the brain and prolonged coma, there is usually a period of mental cloudiness and confusion before full consciousness is restored. Headaches, dizziness, vertigo and the other features of the post-traumatic syndrome may be present as well as signs of cranial nerve injuries or focal damage to the brain. With the passage of time there is usually a considerable degree of improvement in the signs and symptoms of brain damage but permanent sequelae are not uncommon when there has been extensive damage to the brain.

Treatment. Treatment of patients with craniocerebral injuries is operative and nonoperative. The operative therapy of the complications of head injuries is discussed below. Simple wounds of the scalp should be thoroughly cleaned and sutured. Compound fractures of the skull should be completely debrided with removal of all fragments of bone and necrotic tissue. Operative treatment of compound fractures should be performed as soon as possible, but it can be delayed for twenty-four hours until the patient is transported to a hospital equipped for this purpose, or until the patient has recovered from surgical shock if this complication is present. Elevation of small depressed fractures need not be performed immediately, but the depressed fragments should be elevated before the patient is discharged from the hospital.

The nonoperative therapy is concerned chiefly with the general care of the patient and the control of increased intracranial pressure. Placement of extradural pressure monitors may be of aid in the management of increased intercranial pressure. The patient should be kept in a quiet room and disturbed as little as possible. Roentgenograms of the skull, echoencephalography and CT brain scans are important for diagnosis and for medicolegal purposes. These can be deferred until the condition of the patient permits his removal to the x-ray room, except when the diagnosis of an extradural or subdural hematoma is considered. The position of a comatose patient should be changed frequently. The bladder should be emptied by catheter and the bowels by enema. The bed should be kept clean. Clots of blood on the nares or external ear can be removed by gentle wiping but these orifices should not be probed.

The patient should be carefully examined to determine the state of awareness and the presence or absence of signs of injury to the cerebral substance or the cranial nerves. Variations in the level of consciousness while the patient is under observation or the development of a hemiplegia or other focal neurological signs should lead to the consideration of the diagnosis of an extradural or subdural hematoma. The vital signs should be recorded at two- to four-hour intervals. Fluids and a soft liquid diet can be administered by mouth if the patient is conscious and able to swallow.

If the patient remains in coma for more than twelve hours, nutrition can be administered by nasal tube or parenterally. The administration of sedative drugs should be avoided if possible. Restlessness may be combatted by small doses of paraldehyde or other sedatives. The use of morphine is contraindicated because it depresses respiration. Excessive sedation with barbiturates and other sedative drugs may prolong the period of mental confusion and restlessness. Meticulous attention should be given to pulmonary care. Serial determinations of blood gas values are necessary to properly assess pulmonary function in the comatose or confused patient.

Lumbar puncture should be performed for diagnostic purposes. Increased intracranial pressure can be combatted by the administration of steroids, particularly Decadron (dexamethasone) or by the intravenous administration of hypertonic solutions of sucrose. Care should be taken to see that the patient is not dehydrated by such measures, and fluid intake should be kept at an adequate level by parenteral injections if necessary.

Patients with simple concussion should be kept under observation for twenty-four hours and allowed to return to their usual activities after another twenty-four to forty-eight hours. The period of bed rest and convalscence of patients with more severe head injuries must be determined by the response of the patient to the treatment administered. Care should be taken not to overemphasize the severity of the injury or prolong the period of invalidism unnecessarily. The patient should be allowed out of bed as soon as his condition permits. Activity should be gradually increased during the hospital stay. Convalscence should be continued at home with graduated exercises. Return to active work should be deferred for two to three months after discharge from the hospital whenever there has been a severe degree of brain injury. The use of alcohol is interdicted because of the decrease in the tolerance which occurs in patients with head injury.

REFERENCES

Brock, S.: *Injuries of the Brain and Spinal Cord and Their Coverings*, 5th Ed., New York, Springer Publishing Co., 1974, 962 pp.

Caveness, W. F., and Walker, A. E.: *Head Injury. Conference Proceedings*, Philadelphia, J. B. Lippincott Co., 1966, 589 pp.

Crompton, M. R.: Brainstem Lesions due to Closed Head Injuries, Lancet, *1*, 669, 1971.

Hoefer, P. F. A.: The Electroencephalogram in Cases of Head Injury, in *Injuries of the Brain and Spinal Cord and Their Coverings*, 4th Ed., S. Brock, Editor, Chapter 25, pp. 707–732, Baltimore, Williams & Wilkins, 1960.

Kehlberg, J. K.: Head Injury in Automobile Accidents, in *Head Injury. Conference Proceedings*, W. F. Caveness, and A. E. Walker, Editors, Philadelphia, J. B. Lippincott Co., 1966, 589 pp.

Merritt, H. H.: Head Injury, War Medicine, *4*, 61, 187, 1943.

Miller, J. D. and Jennett, W. B.: Complications of Depressed Skull Fractures, Lancet, *2*, 991, 1968.

Mock, H. E.: *Skull Fractures and Brain Injuries*, Baltimore, Williams & Wilkins, 1950, 806 pp.

Mock, H. E., and Mock, H. E., Jr.: Management of Skull Fractures and Brain Injuries, J.A.M.A., *120*, 498, 1942.

Munro, D.: *Cranio-cerebral Injuries*, New York, Oxford University Press, 1938, 412 pp.

Munro, D.: *The Treatment of Injuries to the Nervous System*, Philadelphia, W. B. Saunders Co., 1952, 284 pp.

Rowbotham, G. F.: *Acute Injuries of the Head*, Baltimore, Williams & Wilkins, 4th Ed. 1964, 584 pp.

Russell, W. R.: *The Traumatic Amnesias*, London, Oxford University Press, 1971.

Shenkin, H. A., and Bouzarth, W. F.: Clinical Methods of Reducing Intracranial Pressure, N. Engl. J. Med., *282*, 465, 1970.

Symonds, C.: Concussion and Its Sequelae, Lancet, *1*, 1, 1962.

Walker, A. E., Caveness, W. F., and Critchley, M.: *The Late Effects of Head Injury*, Springfield, Charles C Thomas, 1969, 560 pp.

Complications of Head Injuries

Vascular Lesions

The vascular complications of head injury include subarachnoid hemorrhage, extradural hemorrhage, subdural hemorrhage, subdural hygroma, intracerebral hemorrhage, cerebral thrombosis and arteriovenous aneurysms.

Subarachnoid Hemorrhage. Some extravasation of blood into the subarachnoid spaces is to be expected in any patient with an injury to the head. In most cases it is of little clinical importance except to indicate that the brain has been injured and to warn the physician that serious damage to the brain or its coverings may have occurred. No specific treatment for simple subarachnoid bleeding is needed.

Extradural Hemorrhage. Hemorrhage into the extradural space is generally due to a tear in the wall of one of the meningeal arteries, usually the middle meningeal artery, but in approximately 15% of the cases the bleeding is from one of the dural sinuses. The dura is separated from the skull by the extravasated blood. The size of the clot increases until the ruptured vessel is occluded by the formation of a clot in its torn walls. Usually the hematoma is quite large and is located over the convexity of the hemisphere in the middle fossa but occasionally the hemorrhage may be confined to the anterior fossa, possibly as result of tearing of an anterior meningeal artery. Extradural hemorrhage in the posterior fossa may occur when the torcular Herophili is torn. Bilateral extradural hemorrhages are extremely rare. In the vast majority of cases, the hematoma is on the side of the head injury. Since the body has no mechanism for the absorption of an extradural hemorrhage, the clotted blood remains in the epidural space as a tumor until removed by operation. Organization of the clot by the dura does not occur because hemorrhage into the epidural space usually causes death within a few days.

Incidence. Extradural hemorrhage is a relatively rare complication of head injury. It was found in 0.4% of 46,574 unselected cases treated by Lin, Cook and Browder. This figure is probably more representative of the incidence than the figure of 3% given by McKissock and his associates, by Munro and Maltby and by Woodhall, Devine and Hart because the cases studied by these authors were mainly those with relatively severe injuries. The pathological studies of Vance and of Le Count and Apfelbach, who report extradural hemorrhage in over 20% of fatal head injuries, are not an indication of its frequency but attest to the seriousness of this complication.

Symptoms and Signs. The typical sequence of events in a patient with an extradural hemorrhage is as follows: Loss of consciousness at the time of the injury, a lucid interval of several hours' duration, and a subsequent relapse into coma accompanied by the development of a hemiplegia. The initial coma is due to concussion or cerebral trauma. The secondary loss of consciousness and hemiplegia is the result of compression of the brain by expansion of the hemorrhage. The relatively slow development of the symptoms of cerebral compression is explained by the close adherence of the dura to the skull.

The typical sequence of events described above is not present in as high a percentage of the cases as is commonly assumed. In some series of cases the lucid interval was absent in over 50%. This is due to the fact that the degree of damage to the brain at the time of the injury was sufficient to cause the coma produced by it to merge with that resulting from compression of the brain by the hematoma. The hemiplegia is usually contralateral to the hematoma, but occasionally it is on the same side. The mechanism of the production of homolateral hemiplegia has not been clearly demonstrated but is generally assumed to be due to compression of the opposite cerebral peduncle against the tentorium.

In the usual case the signs of brain compression, coma and hemiplegia develop within a few hours after the accident. Occasionally, they may be delayed for several days or as long as two to three weeks. The optic discs are usually normal in the patients who develop signs of cerebral compression within a few hours of the injury, but choked discs may develop in the patients who live for two to three weeks after the injury. Convulsive seizures are rarely seen, but jacksonian or generalized seizures have been reported in a few cases. The presence of cerebellar signs, nuchal rigidity and drowsiness, together with a fracture of the occipital bone should lead to the suspicion of a clot in the posterior fossa.

A finding of value in the diagnosis and localization of an extradural hemorrhage is a dilated pupil which does not react to light or accommodation. This dilated, fixed pupil, usually accompanied by other signs of paralysis of the third nerve, is always on the same side as the clot and is due to compression of the third nerve by the hippocampal gyrus when herniated over the free edge of the tentorium.

Laboratory Data. The results of examination of the cerebrospinal fluid, while not diagnostic, are of value. However, with current diagnostic techniques, CSF examination is most often unnecessary. The pressure is over 200 mm of water in approximately two thirds of the cases. The fluid is usually clear, but it may be bloody if there has been contusion or laceration of the brain in addition to the extradural hemorrhage.

The results of the x-ray examination of the skull are of great diagnostic aid. The presence of a fracture line which crosses the groove of one of the meningeal arteries, displacement of the pineal gland or an abnormal echoencephalogram are strong supporting evidence for the diagnosis of a hematoma. The diagnosis of an extradural clot can be made by angiography (Fig. 83) and CT brain scan (Figs. 84 and 85).

The electroencephalogram may also give information which will be of value in the establishment of the diagnosis. Abnormalities in the electrical activity of the cerebral cortex are commonly present. These abnormalities may be generalized or more intense on one side of the head. The electroencephalogram is of value in localizing the site of the lesion when the abnormalities are limited to one side of the head, but the site of the lesion cannot be determined with certainty when abnormalities are generalized, even though they are more intense on one side. A normal electroencephalogram does not exclude the diagnosis of an extradural hemorrhage.

Diagnosis. The diagnosis of extradural hemorrhage can be made without difficulty in patients with the typical clinical history and x-ray evidence of a fracture through one of the meningeal arteries or large sinuses. The remainder should be diagnosed if the variations in the clinical picture are kept in mind and diagnostic exploratory trephine openings in the skull are made if indicated by CT brain scan or angiography. The anterior fossa should be explored if a clot is not found in the usual site.

Course and Prognosis. Extradural hemorrhage is the most fatal

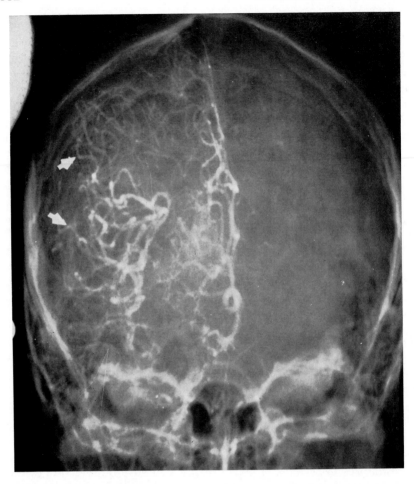

Figure 83. Extradural hematoma. A clear avascular area is present between the inner table of the skull and the surface vessels of the brain in the angiogram. The vessels are displaced inward (arrows) but there is relatively little contralateral displacement of the anterior cerebral artery owing to the rigidity of the dura mater between the hematoma and the brain. Compare with Figure 112. (Courtesy Dr. Ernest Wood.)

complication of head injury. The mortality rate is nearly 100 per cent in untreated cases and it is over 50% in the treated cases. The high mortality rate in treated cases is due in part to delay in establishing diagnosis and in part to the severity of concomitant brain damage. In untreated cases death usually occurs within twelve to seventy-two hours after the injury, but rarely the patient may live for two to three weeks. The clinical course in fatal cases is a gradual increase in the depth of the coma with death ensuing as a result of failure of the cardiac and respiratory centers.

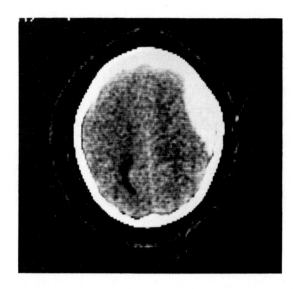

Figure 84.   Epidural hematoma, CT brain scan.
(Courtesy of Dr. Harry H. White.)

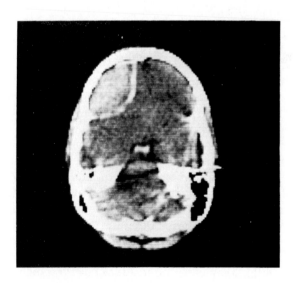

Figure 85.   Epidural hematoma, CT brain scan.
(Courtesy of Dr. Sadek Hillal.)

Treatment. The treatment of extradural hemorrhage is removal of the clot through an enlargement of trephine openings in the skull. The bleeding point should be identified and either ligated or clipped if arterial, or closed with muscle if venous. Postoperative treatment includes transfusions and other methods to combat shock, and treatment of the cerebral edema. The operative results are dependent to a great extent upon the degree of associated brain damage. If this is slight, complete recovery is the rule, with disappearance of the hemiplegia or other focal neurological signs. Occasionally, a very large clot may dislocate the brain so greatly that secondary hemorrhages occur in the brainstem. In such cases recovery may not be possible even though the original head injury had not produced any other serious change.

REFERENCES

Coleman, C. C., and Thomson, J. L.: Extradural Hemorrhage in the Posterior Fossa, Surgery, *10*, 985, 1941
Hawkes, C. D., and Ogle, W. S.: Atypical Features of Epidural Hematoma in Infants, Children and Adolescents, J. Neurosurg., *19*, 971, 1962.
Ingraham, F. D., Campbell, J. B., and Cohen, J.: Extradural Hematoma in Infancy and Childhood, J.A.M.A., *140*, 101, 1949.
Le Count, E. R., and Apfelbach, C. W.: Pathologic Anatomy of Traumatic Fractures of Cranial Bones and Concomitant Brain Injuries, J.A.M.A., *74*, 501, 1920.
McKissock, W., Taylor, J. C., Bloom, W. H., and Till, T.: Extradural Hematoma, Observations on 125 Cases, Lancet, *2*, 167, 1960.
McLaurin, R. L., and Ford, L. E.: Extradural Hematoma. Statistical Survey of Forty-seven Cases, J. Neurosurg., *21*, 364, 1964.
Munro, D., and Maltby, G. L.: Extradural Hemorrhage, Ann. Surg., *113*, 192, 1941.
Vance, B. M.: Fractures of the Skull, Arch. Surg., *14*, 1023, 1927
Whittaker, K.: Extradural Hematoma of the Anterior Fossa, J. Neurosurg., *17*, 1089, 1960.
Woodhall, B., Devine, J. W., Jr., and Hart, D.: Homolateral Dilatation of the Pupil, Homolateral Paresis and Bilateral Muscular Rigidity in the Diagnosis of Extradural Hemorrhage, Surg., Gynec. & Obst., *72*, 391, 1941.

Subdural Hemorrhage. A collection of blood between the dura and arachnoid in the subdural space is known as a subdural hematoma. It is practically always secondary to a severe or minor injury to the head but may occur in connection with blood dyscrasias or cachexia in the absence of trauma. Subdural hematoma has been reported as the result of blast injury and has been found in the newborn and infants as a complication of delivery and postnatal trauma. Organized subdural hemorrhages were formerly a common finding at necropsy in psychotic patients, especially those suffering with dementia paralytica. Such hematomas were described in the literature as pachymeningitis hemorrhagica interna and were considered to be of syphilitic origin. It is now recognized that syphilis played no role in the production of these hematomas and that they were the result of head trauma in convulsive seizures or other blows to the head.

Pathology. The bleeding in the subdural space is practically always of venous origin except when the branches of the middle meningeal artery are lacerated by a fracture of the skull. In older patients the dura does not strip and the acute hemorrhage occurs in the subdural space with clinical symptoms of an epidural hematoma. The fluid in the subdural space may be admixed with cerebrospinal fluid if the arachnoid is torn. When the fluid collection is composed mainly of cerebrospinal fluid, it is known as a subdural hygroma. The hemorrhage is usually over the convexity of the hemisphere in the region of the frontal and parietal lobes. Occasionally it may be confined to the anterior or temporal fossa and rarely, to the posterior fossa. The hematoma is bilateral in approximately 15% of the cases.

Blood which is extravasated into the subdural space is not absorbed but is organized or encapsulated by the dura. Fibroblasts proliferate from the inner surface of the dura and invade the clot at all points where it is in contact with the dura. Newly formed capillaries enter the clot and gradually absorb the liquefied blood. If the clot is small, it is completely organized by fibroblasts. When the clot is large, fibroblasts not only invade the clot directly, but they also grow along the undersurface of the clot to form new membranes on the inner surface of the clot, as well as on the surface adjacent to the dura (Fig. 86). Thus the incompletely liquefied clot is encapsulated.

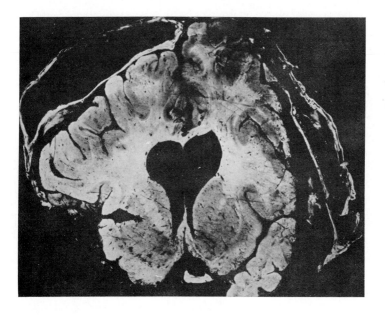

Figure 86.   Bilateral chronic subdural hematoma. (Munro, D., and Merritt, H. H., courtesy Arch. Neurol. & Psychiat.)

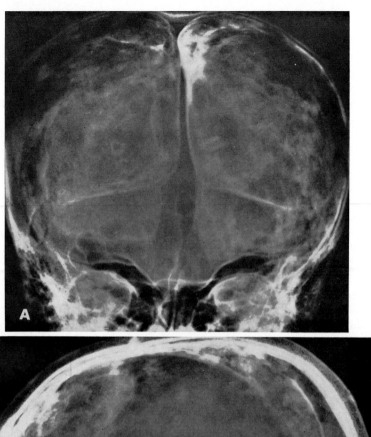

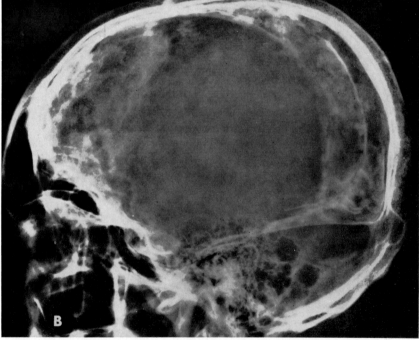

Figure 87. Calcified subdural hematomas. In the frontal view (A) bilateral shell-like calcifications form a cast of the cerebral hemispheres. In the lateral view (B) two calcified shells related to each hematoma are seen—the outer calcified membranes near the bony skull and the inner membranes separated from the outer by relatively clear zones—between which there are irregular calcified deposits. (Courtesy Dr. Ernest Wood.)

336

If death does not occur, the end result of a small subdural hematoma is a thickening of the dura by the addition of the organized membrane. When the clot is large, a subdural cyst with inner and outer membranes is formed and in some cases it may become calcified (Fig. 87).

The cerebral cortex is compressed and molded by the clot. The compression of the cortex may result in the herniation of the cerebral substance through the tentorium and damage to remote portions of the nervous system, producing false localizing signs. The opposite posterior cerebral artery may be compressed producing a homolateral hemianopia, or the opposite cerebral peduncle may be caught against the tentorium and cause a homolateral hemiplegia. Paralysis of the oculomotor nerves or disorganization of gaze may result from hemorrhages in the brainstem as a result of compression of its vessels. Since subdural hematoma is due to venous bleeding, the increase in intracranial pressure develops slowly. Herniation of the hippocampus through the free edge of the tentorium and compression of the third nerve with a dilated fixed pupil are not often seen as an early sign, but may occur as a late sign.

Incidence. The incidence of subdural hematoma following injury to the head is variously estimated at 1 to 10% depending upon the severity of the injury. The figure of 17% given by Munro is representative of the experience of a neurosurgeon whose service received a high percentage of severe head injuries. The figure of 1% given by Laudig and his associates is in agreement with our experience and that of Lin, Cook and Browder (2%) with unselected head injuries. Subdural hematoma in adults occurs predominantly in men, because of the greater incidence of head injury in that sex. The high incidence of subdural hematoma in chronic alcoholics is mainly due to the frequency of injury to such patients.

Subdural hemorrhage was found in 245 (8%) of 3,100 consecutive autopsies of psychotic patients by Allen, Moore and Daly. Subdural hematoma was found in all types of psychotics but was more common in the senile, epileptics, alcoholics and paretics, who are all more prone to head injury. Men predominated in this series by a ratio of 1:5 to 1. The figures of these authors are for the years 1914 to 1934, and are much higher than those of today.

The incidence of subdural hematoma in infancy has never been accurately determined. The frequency of all types of intracranial hemorrhage in the newborn is estimated as 2 to 3%. This figure is obviously too low. Subdural hematoma constitutes only a small portion of these, but the experience of pediatric neurosurgeons would indicate that subdural hematoma is more frequent in infants than is commonly supposed. Ingraham and Matson report an average of 17 cases per year at the Children's Hospital in Boston and the Hospital for Sick Children in Toronto reports an incidence of 5.2% in a series of 4,465 cases admitted after injury to the head.

Symptoms. Subdural hematomas are commonly divided into acute or chronic types according to whether the symptoms of the hematoma develop at the time of the injury or whether they appear after a latent interval of several weeks or months. In some of the latter cases the head injury may have been so slight that it has been forgotten.

There are no characteristic symptoms which will serve to differentiate an acute subdural hematoma from cerebral contusion or laceration or a chronic hematoma from an intracranial neoplasm. The symptoms of an acute subdural hematoma usually develop within the first few days after the injury. Headache is almost invariably present. The state of consciousness is variable and is dependent to some extent on the degree of concomitant cerebral damage. After recovery from the coma due to the injury, the development of irritability, mental confusion or varying degrees of coma is a common occurrence in patients with a subdural hematoma. Similarly there may be fluctuations in the level of consciousness from day to day or during one day. Hemiplegia or central facial weakness is present in approximately 50% of the cases. The paralysis is usually on the side opposite to the hematoma, but it may be on the same side. Convulsive seizures, usually generalized, occur in less than 5% of the cases. Aphasia is uncommon and hemianopia does not occur unless the optic radiations have been contused or the opposite posterior cerebral artery has been compressed by dislocation of the cerebrum. In the latter case, the hemianopia is homolateral to the hematoma.

The symptoms of a chronic subdural hematoma are similar to those of an acute hematoma. The symptoms usually date from the time of the injury. Intermittent headache, slight or severe impairment of the intellectual faculties and a hemiparesis are the most characteristic symptoms. In patients in whom the initial trauma was so slight that it is not remembered, the symptoms are identical with those of any expanding intracranial lesion and are indistinguishable from those of a neoplasm.

Signs. The common signs of an acute subdural hematoma are fluctuations in the level of consciousness and hemiplegia. The hemiplegia, which may be present on recovery of consciousness or develop in the next few days, is most commonly of the spastic type with increase in the deep reflexes and Babinski sign. Changes in the vital signs are not present unless there is associated cerebral injury. Choked discs are rarely seen. Inequality in the size of the pupils is frequent. The size of the pupils has no value in localizing the hematoma unless one pupil is large and does not react to light. This large, non-reacting pupil, which is on the same side as the hematoma, is much less common in patients with a subdural hematoma than in patients with extradural hemorrhages. Weakness of the extraocular muscles or disorganization of gaze may rarely be seen as a result of hemorrhages into the brainstem.

The signs of a chronic subdural hematoma are similar to those of an acute hematoma except that convulsive seizures and choked discs are more frequently seen.

Laboratory Data. The cerebrospinal fluid is usually bloody due to concomitant brain damage. Occasionally the fluid will be entirely clear and under normal pressure. Roentgenograms of the skull may or may not show evidence of a linear fracture. Displacement of a calcified pineal gland, if present, or shift of the mid-line in the echoencephalogram is of value in establishing the diagnosis of a hematoma. The electroencephalogram may show a difference in the electrical activity of the two hemispheres (Fig. 86). Carotid angiograms demonstrate inward displacement of the terminal branches of the middle cerebral artery (Fig. 87). The diagnosis can be established by CT brain scan or angiography (Figs. 88 and 89).

Diagnosis. Since there is no characteristic symptomatology for either an acute or chronic subdural hematoma, the diagnosis of subdural hemorrhage is difficult. The hematoma is commonly accompanied by cerebral contusion and laceration, and the situation is further complicated by the fact that subdural hemorrhage is frequent in patients addicted to the use of alcohol who are admitted to a hospital in coma or semicoma and are unable to give a history of an accident. In these cases, the erroneous diagnosis of spontaneous intracerebral or subarachnoid hemorrhage may be made. The results of neurological examination are not conclusive because focal neurological signs are absent in approximately half of the cases, and when present they do not serve to differentiate between hematoma and cerebral contusion or laceration.

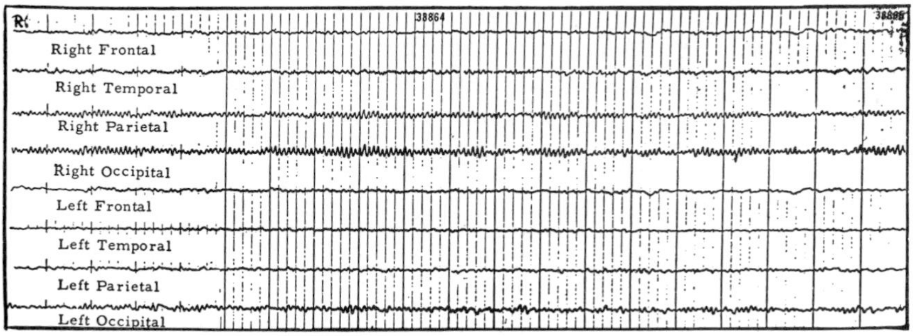

Figure 88. Subdural hematoma. Electroencephalogram showing depression of activity on the side of the hematoma—lower four tracings. (Courtesy Dr. Paul F. A. Hoefer.)

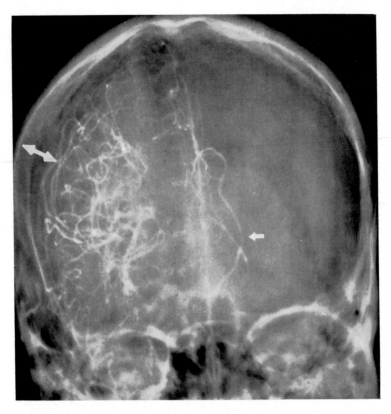

Figure 89. Subdural hematoma. Carotid angiogram. The pial vessels are separated from the inner table of the skull (double arrow). The anterior cerebral artery (single arrow) is displaced beneath the falx. Compare with Fig. 83. (Courtesy Dr. Ernest Wood.)

Roentgenograms of the skull, echoencephalography, examination of the cerebrospinal fluid, electroencephalogram, angiogram, CT brain scan (Figs. 90 and 91) and ventriculogram or pneumoencephalogram are of diagnostic value, but the diagnosis of a subdural hematoma can be excluded or established with certainty only by the placing of burr holes on both sides of the skull. The diagnosis should be considered in any patient who has suffered a head injury if there are fluctuations in level of consciousness, if focal neurological signs develop or if the patient does not respond satisfactorily to adequate treatment of a head injury.

Treatment. The treatment of subdural hematoma is evacuation of the clot and neomembrane through trephine openings or craniotomy. Since subdural hematoma is frequently bilateral, both sides should be explored. There have been reports in the literature of cases in which the

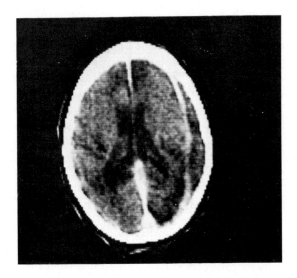

Figure 90.   Subdural hematoma, CT brain scan.
(Courtesy of Dr. Harry H. White.)

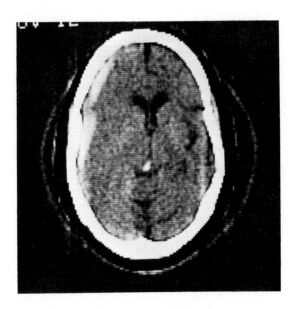

Figure 91.   Subdural hematoma, CT brain scan.
(Courtesy of Dr. Harry H. White.)

diagnosis of subdural hematoma has been established by angiography and in which spontaneous resorption of the hematoma has occurred. Clinical experience would indicate that this sequence of events is rare and that, unless a subdural hematoma of any appreciable size is removed, most patients will die or suffer serious sequelae.

SUBDURAL HEMORRHAGE IN INFANTS. As previously noted, the incidence of subdural hematoma in infancy is more frequent than commonly supposed. According to Ingraham and Matson pre- or postnatal trauma is practically a constant etiologic factor. In malnourished and diseased infants it may take less injury to produce this lesion, and in poor economic surroundings the exposure rate to trauma is high. The absence of the history of an injury should not militate against the diagnosis of hematoma. The pathology of subdural hematoma in infancy is similar to that in adults. Bilateral hematomas are much more common. The pathological findings in the cases of Ingraham and Matson are given in Table 50.

Symptoms of subdural hematoma in infants usually appear within a few days of the trauma, but they may be delayed for several weeks and months. Convulsive seizures, jacksonian or generalized, are the most common presenting symptoms, occurring in over one half of the cases. Other symptoms include irritability, excessive crying, restlessness and various degrees of depression of consciousness. The signs in order of frequency of occurrence are: fever, hyperactive reflexes, bulging fontanelle, enlargement of the head (hydrocephalus), papilledema, paralyses, and fracture of the skull. The diagnosis of subdural hematoma in infants can be established by tapping the subdural space on both sides.

The treatment of subdural hematoma in infants differs from that in adults. The sudden removal of large bilateral hematomas may be followed by an acute cerebral edema. Ingraham and Matson, therefore,

Table 50.   Summary of Pathologic Findings in 98 Cases of Subdural Hematoma in Infants

(After Ingraham and Matson, J. Ped., 1944)

	Unilateral	Bilateral	Total
Grossly bloody or xanthochromic fluid found on subdural puncture	18	70	88
Excessive clear fluid with elevated protein found on subdural puncture	3	7	10
Subdural membrane established by trephination and removal at craniotomy	30	32	62
Solid blood cot in addition to fluid still present in sac at time of craniotomy	7	13	20

advise that only 10 to 15 ml of fluid be removed from each side at the first tapping and that the tap be repeated daily on alternate sides for a period of one to two weeks. With adequate fluid and food intake the patient improves steadily, gains weight, becomes normally hydrated and is ready for the second stage, the placing of bilateral burr holes. The purpose of the procedure is to evacuate all remaining fluid and clots. If these are found after repeated taps, subdural peritoneal shunts are performed. The membrane then resorbs.

Subdural Hygroma. An excessive collection of fluid in the subdural space is known as subdural hygroma. Dandy lists three causes. The first and by far the most common is cranial trauma with tearing of the arachnoid and escape of cerebrospinal fluid into the subdural space. In these cases the fluid is usually admixed with blood due to coincident rupture of meningeal vessels. The second is a subdural effusion secondary to an infection of the meninges or the skull. This is most commonly seen in connection with influenzal meningitis and mastoiditis. The third cause of a subdural hygroma is the rupture of the arachnoid at the basal cistern in cases of communicating hydrocephalus.

The signs and symptoms of subdural hygroma (Table 51) following head injury are similar in character and in evolution to those of a subdural hematoma. The diagnosis, as with subdural hematoma, can be made with certainty only by trephine openings in the skull. Drainage of the fluid will result in relief of the symptoms in these cases when there is a large collection of fluid and there is no other associated pathologic condition. If satisfactory resorption does not occur, shunting of the subdural space may be necessary.

Table 51.   Symptoms in 33 Cases of Subdural Hygroma
(After Wycis, J. Neurosurg., 1945)

Symptoms	No. of Times Recorded
Headache	12
Dizziness	5
Nervousness and irritability	7
Loss of memory and confusion	6
Restlessness	4
Aphasia	5
Hemiparesis or hemiplegia	6
Drowsiness	4
Semicoma	3
Stupor	7

REFERENCES

Abbott, W. D., Due, F. O., and Nosik, W. A.: Subdural Hematoma and Effusion as a Result of Blast Injuries, J.A.M.A., *121*, 739, 1943.

Allen, A. M., Moore, M., and Daly, B. B.: Subdural Hemorrhage in Patients with Mental Disease, N. Engl. J. Med., *223*, 324, 1940.

Aring, C. D., and Evans, J. P.: Aberrant Location of Subdural Hematoma, Arch. Neurol. & Psychiat., *44*, 1296, 1940.

Bender, M. B.: Recovery from Subdural Hematoma without Surgery, J. Mt. Sinai Hosp., *27*, 52, 1960.

Cole, M., and Spatz, E.: Seizures in Chronic Subdural Hematoma, N. Engl. J. Med., *265*, 628, 1961.

Hendrick, E. B., Harwood-Hash, D. C. F., and Hudson, A. R.: Head Injuries in Children. A Survey of 4465 Consecutive Cases at the Hospital for Sick Children, Toronto, Canada, Chir. Neurosurg., *11*, 46, 1963.

Ingraham, F. D., and Matson, D. D.: Subdural Hematoma in Infancy, J. Ped., *24*, 221, 1944.

Laudig, G. H., Browder, J., and Watson, R. A.: Subdural Hematoma, Ann. Surg., *113*, 170, 1941.

Leary, T.: Subdural Hemorrhages, J.A.M.A., *103*, 897, 1934.

Maltby, G. L.: Visual Field Changes and Subdural Hematomas, Surg., Gynec., & Obst., *74*, 496, 1942.

McLaurin, R. L., and McLaurin, K. S.: Calcified Subdural Hematomas in Childhood, J. Neurosurg., *24*, 648, 1966.

McLaurin, R. L., and Tutor, F. T.: Acute Subdural Hematoma, Review of Ninety Cases, J. Neurosurg., *18*, 61, 1961.

Munro, D., and Merritt, H. H.: Surgical Pathology of Subdural Hematoma, Arch. Neurol. & Psychiat., *35*, 64, 1936.

Nelson, J.: Involvement of the Brain Stem in the Presence of Subdural Hematoma, J.A.M.A., *119*, 864, 1942.

Yashon, D. et al.: Traumatic Subdural Hematoma of Infancy. Long-term Follow-up of 92 Patients, Arch. Neurol., *18*, 370, 1968.

Intracerebral Hemorrhage. Intracerebral hemorrhages accompanying head injury are usually multiple and small in size. They are most commonly found in the neighborhood of the contused or lacerated brain but may be in areas far removed from the original injury. Occasionally there may be a large solitary subcortical hematoma. Solitary hematomas of sufficient size to require surgical removal were found in 0.3% of unselected head injuries by Lin, Cook, and Browder. The symptomatology of a solitary hematoma is indistinguishable from that of extradural or subdural hemorrhage. Increased intracranial pressure and focal neurological signs, usually a hemiplegia, develop within a few hours or a few days of the accident. The diagnosis is established by CT brain scan (Fig. 92). Operative removal of the intracortical clot is feasible and may be followed by improvement in the general condition of the patient and a decrease in focal signs. The occurrence of intracerebral hemorrhage weeks or months after a trauma, so-called late apoplexy, has a doubtful relationship to the injury.

Cerebral Thrombosis. Thrombosis of the contralateral posterior cerebral artery is a rare complication of distortion of the brain by an

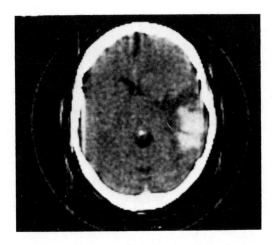

Figure 92.   CT brain scan, intracerebral hemorrhage.
(Courtesy of Sadek Hillal.)

extradural or subdural hematoma. Injury to the wall of the carotid or
other arteries may be followed by thrombosis of these vessels. Thrombosis of branches of the cerebral arteries occasionally develops several
days or weeks following a head injury in elderly patients with cerebral
arteriosclerosis. It is difficult if not impossible, to assess on clinical
evidence the role of the cerebral trauma in the production of the
thrombosis in these cases.

Arteriovenous Fistulas. Trauma is a common cause of arteriovenous
fistulas. These fistulas are usually due to laceration of the internal
carotid artery as it passes through the cavernous sinus by penetrating
missiles or fracture of the sphenoid bone. Immediately following the
injury the patient may become aware of a bruit, which is synchronous
with the pulse. The other symptoms are similar to those of cavernous
sinus obstruction from other causes. Exophthalmos, distended orbital
and periorbital veins, and paralysis of cranial nerves, most commonly
the sixth, can all be traced to increased tension in the cavernous sinus
due to direct infusion of arterial blood (Fig. 93). The bruit and the
exophthalmos may be reduced by manual occlusion of the carotid
artery in the neck. If spontaneous regression does not occur, ligation of
the internal or common carotid artery may be necessary. If there is total
diversion of the flow from the carotid artery into the fistula, more
extensive procedures may be necessary, with ligation of the internal
carotid in the neck and the internal carotid and ophthalmic artery
intracranially. More recently, intravascular techniques have been developed to occlude these lesions.

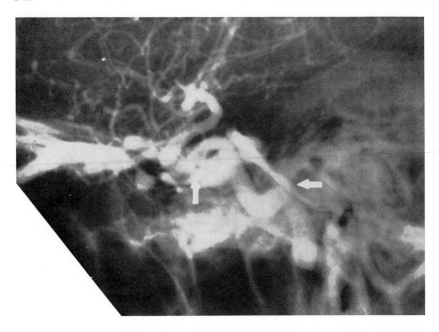

Figure 93. Carotid cavernous sinus fistula. Carotid angiogram. Large communication (vertical arrow) between the carotid artery (above) and the cavernous sinus. In addition to the enlarged orbital veins which drain forward from the cavernous sinus, there is backward drainage through the petrosal sinus (transverse arrow). (Courtesy Dr. Ernest Wood.)

REFERENCES

Dott, N. M.: *Carotid-Cavernous Arteriovenous Fistula, in Clinical Neurosurgery,* Volume 16, Baltimore, Williams & Wilkins, 1969, 513 pp.
Echols, D. H., and Jackson, J. D.: Carotid-Cavernous Fistula, J. Neurosurg., *16,* 619, 1959.
Hayes, G. J.: Carotid Cavernous Fistulas: Diagnosis and Surgical Management, Am. Surgeon, *24,* 837, 1958.
Lin, T. H., Cook, A. W., and Browder, E. J.: Intracranial Hemorrhage of Traumatic Origin, Med. Clin. North Am., *42,* 603, 1958.

Infections

Infections within the intracranial cavity following injury to the head may be extradural, subdural, subarachnoid (meningitis) or intracerebral (abscess).

Extradural Infections. These are usually accompanied by infection of the external wound and osteomyelitis of the skull and can be diagnosed by inspection of the wound and by roentgenograms. Treatment includes debridement of infected bone, evacuation of the abscess and administration of antibiotics.

Subdural Abscess. This is one of the rarest suppurative lesions following head injury. It may be a complication of subdural hematoma. Symptomatology is similar to that of subdural abscess from other causes and includes localized headache, fever, stiffness of the neck, jacksonian seizures and focal neurological signs. The cerebrospinal fluid is under increased pressure and shows signs of an aseptic meningeal reaction, i.e., a pleocytosis and increased protein content with a normal sugar content and a negative culture. Treatment of subdural abscess secondary to head injury is similar to that for subdural abscess due to other causes.

Meningitis. Meningitis may develop following compound fractures, penetrating missiles, or linear fractures which extend into the nasal sinuses or the middle ear. Any of the pathogenic organisms may be the cause of the meningitis but the staphylococcus, streptococcus, pneumococcus and the influenza bacillus are most frequently found. The incidence of meningitis in civilian practice was estimated by Munro as less than 1% in patients with "closed head" injuries and approximately 6% in patients with compound fracture of the skull. The incidence of meningitis is affected by the degree of care in the treatment of the scalp and skull wound.

Meningitis commonly develops two to eight days following the injury but the onset may be delayed for several or many months, particularly in patients with fractures through the mastoid or nasal sinuses. Recurrence of the meningitis with as many as 7 or 8 attacks has been reported. The presence of a cerebrospinal fluid fistula with rhinorrhea favors the recurrence of meningitis. Treatment in such cases must include the closure of this fistula after the patient has recovered from the meningitis.

The treatment of post-traumatic meningitis follows the same principles as those outlined for the treatment of meningitis from other sources.

Brain Abscess. Intracerebral abscess may follow compound fractures of the skull and the entrance of penetrating missiles. This is a rare complication of head injury and is usually related to infection in the scalp wound. The symptoms of the abscess commonly develop in the first few weeks after the injury but they may be delayed for several months. The symptomatology, course and treatment of cerebral abscess following head injury are the same as those of abscess due to other causes.

Rhinorrhea

Cerebrospinal fluid may drain from the nose when there has been a fracture of the cribriform plate with herniation of a fragment of the dura and arachnoid through the fracture. Drainage of cerebrospinal fluid is usually preceded by bleeding from the nose and is not recognized until the bleeding has ceased. Isotope cisternography is of value in diagnosing and localizing the site of the leak. Drainage of the cerebrospinal fluid is not of itself of great importance but meningitis will almost invariably result unless the fistula closes spontaneously or is closed by an operation.

Otorrhea

Drainage of cerebrospinal fluid from the ear associated with fracture of the temporal bone is an uncommon complication of head injury, occurring in about 2 or 3% of the cases. The drainage is usually of transient duration. If it persists, the rent in the dura should be repaired surgically.

Pneumocele

The presence of air in the cranial cavity is a rare complication of head injury. The air is usually in the frontal region in association with a fracture of one of the frontal sinuses, but cases have been reported with an occipital pneumocele following fracture through the mastoid. The air may not appear for several days after the injury and then only after the patient sneezes or blows his nose.

The pneumocele may be asymptomatic but headaches or mental symptoms may be present. Signs of increased intracranial pressure do not develop unless the pneumocele becomes infected or filled with fluid. The diagnosis of pneumocele is made by the roentgenograms. If spontaneous absorption of the air does not occur, the opening in the frontal sinus should be covered with a strip of fascia lata through a transfrontal craniotomy in order to relieve whatever symptoms may be present and to prevent the development of an intracranial infection.

Leptomeningeal Cysts

A rare complication of head injuries is the formation of a cyst in the space between the pia mater and the arachnoidal membrane. This complication may develop when there is a linear fracture of the skull with separation of the edges of the fracture and laceration of the dura. In such cases, the arachnoid may be caught between the edges of the fracture. Pulsation of the brain forces fluid into the cyst and produces erosion of the skull. This complication is most commonly seen following fracture of the skull in infants and young children. Convulsive seizures, mental retardation and increased intracranial pressure are the common signs and symptoms. The diagnosis is made from roentgeno-graph of a circular or oval area of erosion of the skull in a patient who has had a previous fracture of the skull. Treatment consists of excision of the cyst and repair of the dural defect.

Cranial Nerve Palsies

Injury to the cranial nerves is a frequent complication of fracture at the base of the skull. In addition, the cranial nerves, especially the olfactory, may be torn or bruised by the movement of the brain within the skull.

The incidence of cranial nerve injury and the frequency of involvement of the individual nerves in civil practice vary considerably from that in war casualties. This difference is mainly due to the frequency of involvement of the peripheral branches of these nerves by explosive missiles in war injuries.

Foerster reported cranial nerve injuries in 423 of 3,907 (11%) cases of head injury in World War I, with a preponderance of involvement of the fifth and seventh nerves.

In civil life, the frequency of damage to cranial nerves was reported by Russell as 7% and by Friedman and Merritt as 4%. A considerably higher incidence of cranial nerve damage is reported by some authors who include all visual complaints and vertigo or dizziness as an indication of damage to the optic or auditory nerves.

Cranial nerve palsies, when present, can usually be detected as soon as the patient recovers from the coma of the injury. Occasionally, the paralysis may not be evident for several days. Facial paralysis, for example, may have its onset several days after a severe head injury. Partial or complete recovery of function is the rule with traumatic injuries to the cranial nerves, with the exception of the first or second nerves.

Focal Cerebral Lesions

Focal brain lesions are much less common in the injuries of civil life than in those of war. Hemiplegia and speech disturbance are the most common symptoms of focal brain damage in both civil and war injuries. Symptoms of damage to the occipital lobe or cerebellum are found almost exclusively in war casualties.

Hemiplegia was found in 9% and disturbance of speech, aphasia or dysphasia, in 6% of the 255 cases reported by Glaser and Shafter. Complete or almost complete return of motor power and speech function is the rule when the deficit is the result of compression of the brain by a hematoma, but a severe residual defect may be expected when there has been extensive laceration of the brain substance.

Injury to the hypothalamus or the pituitary gland is a rare complication of head injury. Transient or permanent diabetes insipidus has been reported in a few cases, probably as result of injury to the supraoptic-hypophyseal tract. Anosmia is usually also present in these cases as a result of injury to the olfactory bulb.

Acromegaly and other pituitary disorders have been reported as sequelae of head injury. Traumatic hemorrhage into the pituitary gland may be followed by the development of pituitary cachexia, Simmonds' disease, but it is unlikely that acromegaly and other evidence of pituitary hyperfunction could result from trauma. Some cases of narcolepsy have been attributed to cerebral trauma, but since there is no known anatomical basis for narcolepsy it is difficult to prove or disprove the claims that it may be caused by a head injury.

Parkinsonism and other basal ganglia syndromes have been reported following head trauma. In some of these cases the temporal relationship between the injury and the development of symptoms is such that there may be a possible relationship between the symptoms and the trauma. In the majority of the cases, however, it is quite doubtful whether the trauma played even a contributing role in the onset of the symptoms.

Sequelae of Head Injuries

Epilepsy

Convulsive seizures are an infrequent symptom of the acute phase of a head injury. Rarely, they may occur immediately following or within the first few days of the injury. In these cases the seizures are related to the acute brain damage or to the presence of hematomas or meningitis. In the majority of the cases, however, seizures do not develop until several months after the injury, six to eighteen months being the most common interval. Seizures which follow head injury may be of any type except the classic petit mal, and contrary to the usual impression, they are more often generalized than focal in nature.

The exact incidence of seizures following head injury is unknown. The figures given in the literature vary from 2.5 to 40%. The lower figure is probably correct if all types of head injury are included. As a rule, the more severe the injury, the greater the likelihood that seizures will develop. The incidence is as high as 50% when there has been penetration of the dura and laceration of the underlying cortex with formation of a cerebromeningeal scar. There is no evidence that the retention of a deeply situated foreign body predisposes to the development of seizures.

Little is known about the prophylaxis of seizures in patients with head injuries. A thorough debridement of a compound fracture, removal of all foreign material and necrotic cerebral tissue, and suturing of the dura should decrease the amount of scar formation and thus the tendency toward seizures. Some evidence has been accumulated with regard to the prediction of the subsequent occurrence of seizures. The persistence in the electroencephalogram of a focus of abnormal cortical activity beyond several months after the injury is suggestive evidence that seizures will ultimately develop. It has been recommended that all patients with severe head injuries receive anticonvulsant medication for a year or two after the injury. The value of such treatment is unproven, but the idea has merit and anticonvulsant medication should be given to those patients with a persistent focus of abnormal electrical activity in the electroencephalogram.

The prognosis for remission of seizures is good in patients in whom they occur in the first few days or weeks after the injury. If the seizures are a manifestation of an acute injury to the brain, they are rarely a persistent sequel. There may be a remission of the seizures at any time. Recent studies by Caveness, Walker and Ascroft indicate that the prognosis for the cessation of the seizures is not as poor as was formerly thought.

The treatment of post-traumatic epilepsy is both medical and surgical. As a rule these patients do not respond as well to medical therapy as patients with so-called idiopathic epilepsy, but surprisingly good results can be obtained in a large percentage of the cases. Medical treatment, as outlined in Chapter 9, should be given a trial in all cases and operation reserved for the few who are not benefited by this form of therapy. Operative treatment should be carried out only in neurosurgical clinics where there are adequate facilities for localizing the abnormal cortex which is presumably responsible for the seizures. This area may be removed with or without excision of the neighboring scar. Medical treatment should be given to the patients for two to three years following the operation even if there are no seizures. The results of surgery are not universally good, but about 50% of the cases so treated are relieved of their attacks.

Psychoses and Mental Disturbances

Transient psychotic episodes and some permanent impairment of the mental faculties are not uncommon after injuries to the head but long-continued psychotic episodes are rare. Karnosh stated that reports from mental hospitals in this country indicate that traumatic insanity is responsible for only 0.6% of the annual admissions to mental hospitals. Vyner and Swire in England found that insanity had followed a head injury in 0.8% of the patients in a mental hospital.

Serious residual mental defects are found only after a severe injury. Practically every patient with severe brain injury shows mental changes immediately after recovery of consciousness, and frequently the steps to complete recovery are semi-stupor, bewilderment, a Korsakow-like phase, and euphoria. In the patients who do not recover fully, the clinical syndromes are usually classified as traumatic delirium, mental deterioration, and post-traumatic personality disorders. Focal neurological signs and convulsive seizures are common in these patients. Less severe disturbances of the mental faculties, such as impairment of memory and minor changes in personality, which do not make confinement in an institution necessary are frequent and can be expected in a high percentage of elderly patients. The relationship of head injury to the subsequent development of other types of psychoses is a medicolegal problem which has not been solved. It is reasonable to assume that a severe head injury may adversely influence preexisting pathological processes in the brain and accelerate the progress of organic disease such as cerebral arteriosclerosis. The problem is not so simple in connection with dementia praecox, manic-depressive and other psychoses which do not have any known pathology. It seems unlikely that head trauma could have any causal relationship to these conditions.

Post-traumatic Syndrome

Approximately 35 to 40% of patients who sustain minor or severe injuries to the head complain of headache, dizziness, insomnia, irritability, restlessness, inability to concentrate, hyperhidrosis, depression and other personality changes. This group of symptoms, which may be present for only a few weeks or persist for years, has been described by the terms post-concussional state and post-traumatic neurosis. Neither of these terms is satisfactory since they imply that the symptoms manifested by the patient are either directly the result of injury to the brain or that they are due to the psychological reaction of the patient to the injury. Extensive physiological and psychological studies of these patients have not yielded any criteria which make it possible to clearly define the role of either physiological or psychological factors in the production of the symptoms. In some patients the symptoms appear to be related to the brain damage and in others, they seem to be entirely psychological in origin, but in the majority both factors play a contributing role.

There is no direct correlation between the severity of the injury and the development of post-traumatic symptoms. The symptoms may develop in patients who were only dazed by the injury, but they do occur in a higher percentage of the patients who were rendered unconscious. In such patients, however, the incidence of the post-traumatic symptoms is not related to the duration of either the retrograde amnesia, the coma or the post-traumatic amnesia. The symptoms which are commonly present in adults after head injury are relatively rare in children but behavioral disorders and personality changes are not infrequent.

Post-traumatic symptoms may develop in patients who had previously shown a normal adjustment to life, but they are more apt to occur in patients who had manifested neurotic symptoms before the injury. Factors such as hazardous occupations, domestic or financial difficulties and the desire to obtain compensation, financial or otherwise, tend to produce and prolong the symptoms once they have developed.

Symptoms. The headaches usually have their onset coincidental with the return of consciousness but occasionally they may not appear until the patient is ambulatory. At first, the headache is severe and more or less constant. As the days go by, it decreases in severity and there are periods of relative freedom. As a rule, the periods in which the patient is free of headache become longer and after a week or two, the headaches are paroxysmal. Usually, the headache is described as a dull aching, throbbing, or pressure sensation. Sometimes they are described as quite severe, "a bursting feeling." Occasionally the headaches develop without any apparent reason, waking the patient out of a sound sleep. More frequently they occur with excitement or when the patient tries to concentrate. Such headaches are reported by many patients as recurring daily over a period of years. In others, and this represents the majority, their severity and frequency diminish with the passage of time, usually disappearing entirely within six to twelve months.

Dizziness is a fairly constant symptom of the post-traumatic syndrome. Again, as with the headaches, it usually makes its appearance quite early after return of consciousness. Many patients report that the least movement in bed will produce severe vertiginous attacks. In other instances, the dizziness first appears when the patient begins to get on his feet. The dizziness, like headaches, after a time becomes paroxysmal in character, produced by quick movements, turning about or attempting to rise from a recumbent position; not infrequently the attacks of dizziness are associated with headache. Some patients will find that putting the head in certain positions will precipitate vertigo. Rarely, indeed, is the dizziness associated with any nystagmus. At times, nausea and even vomiting accompany a dizzy attack, but this effect is rarely long-continued. Labyrinthine tests, as a rule, throw little light on the mechanism, although in some instances these tests will indicate disturbance of the vestibular connections.

Insomnia is usually a bothersome symptom and obviously real enough. Patients have difficulty in getting to sleep, and when they do fall asleep, they complain that it is a restless sleep in which they feel half awake, that it is broken by periods of wakefulness and interspersed with terrifying dreams, frequently in relation to the events of the accident. Disturbance of sleep continues, as a rule, as long as the other symptoms are relatively severe.

Irritability, restlessness, lack of ability to concentrate, change of personality and depression all fall into one group of symptoms. The patients state that they cannot stand noises, are bothered by children, cannot enjoy themselves, find even the television unpleasant, have little control of their temper or emotions, and, in general, are a burden to themselves and a great trial to the family. The reality of these changes is borne out by the accounts of family and friends, and very frequently is obvious to the examiner.

Hyperhidrosis, while not as frequent as the other symptoms, may be present to such an extent that it leaves no doubt in the observer's mind that there is a marked vasomotor instability.

Prognosis. The prognosis in cases of so-called post-traumatic syndrome is uncertain. In general, progressive improvement may be expected with the passage of time. The duration of symptoms is not directly related to the severity of the injury. In some patients with only a mild injury, symptoms continue for a long period, whereas patients with severe injuries may have only mild or transient symptoms following their convalescence. By and large, however, it is a matter of two to six months in the majority of cases, before the headache and dizziness as well as the more definite mental changes will show much improvement. Slight residuals are to be expected over a much longer period, and in those patients who develop convulsive seizures, it is often six to eighteen months before the first attacks occur, so that there is no definite assurance that things are going to go entirely well until at least a year or two have transpired. Definitely functional or psychoneurotic symptoms are added to the picture quite often and the prognosis must then be modified by taking into account the individual patient and the circumstances surrounding his life and activities.

Treatment. The general medical, surgical and psychological treatment of the patient immediately after the injury is of great importance in the prevention of post-traumatic syndrome. To many patients the idea of an injury to the head is bound up with the fear of all sorts of disasters, such as that injury to the brain often leads to the development of insanity or brain tumor. Not infrequently, the physician and lawyer add to the worry by making too much of the injury, telling the patient how near to death he may have been, being unduly concerned about later symptoms, keeping the patient from reasonable activity, and intensifying whatever worrries he may have. As the weeks and months pass with continuance of symptoms, the patient's worst fears seem to be materializing. If, in addition, the patient finds himself economically handicapped and in dire financial straits, another cause for the development and continuance of symptoms is present. Legal activity induces a real complication in almost every case and prolongs the period of disability.

With the exception of surgical operation for the rare case of subdural hematoma, physiotherapy and re-education of neurological defects and the administration of anticonvulsive drugs in the patients with seizures, treatment is largely in the field of psychotherapy. *Reassurance is important at all times.* An adept examination and evaluation followed by relatively long talks with the patient, in which the whole matter is explained to him in detail, are the first essentials. Constant attention must be given to relieve fears of serious outcome, always remembering that patients reflect the attitudes and anxieties of their physicians. While it is wise to keep a patient quiet for a number of days after any moderately severe head injury, when he gets about, it is important to see that there is enough activity to keep his mind engaged, and his hands occupied. The patient should be induced to take regular exercise, to enter into various simple pastimes, such as playing cards, going to the theater, dances, and engaging in other forms of diversion. This not only occupies his time, but also tends to convince him that he does not need to have undue concern about his condition. He should be allowed to return to part-time work as soon as possible and to full-time work after an interval of another one to two weeks.

Sedatives, tranquilizers and analgesic drugs in moderation are helpful. *Phenobarbital* and *antihistamines* for dizziness and *aspirin* for headache usually are helpful. Relief of financial difficulties, settlement of insurance or liability claims are also important. Most of the cases that are seen today have insurance, industrial accident or liability claims, and it is perfectly obvious that when difficulty arises about the settlement of such claims, the functional and even the organic symptoms are prolonged.

REFERENCES

Appelbaum, E.: Meningitis Following Trauma to the Head and Face, J.A.M.A., *173*, 1818, 1960.

Brenner, C., Friedman, A. P., Merritt, H. H., and Denny-Brown, D. E.: Post-traumatic Headache, J. Neurosurg., *1*, 379, 1944.

Brisman, R., et al.: Cerebrospinal Fluid Rhinorrhea, Arch. Neurol., *22*, 245, 1970.

Caveness, W. F., Walker, A. E., and Ascroft, P. B.: Incidences of Post-traumatic Epilepsy in Korean Veterans as Compared with Those from World War I and World War II, J. Neurosurg., *19*, 122, 1962.

Corsellis, J. A., and Brierley, J. B.: Observations on the Pathology of Insidious Dementia Following Head Injury, J. Ment. Sci., *105*, 714, 1959.

Courville, C. B., and Blomquist, O. A.: Traumatic Pachymeningitis Interna and Subdural Abscess, Arch. Surg., *42*, 890, 1941.

Dillon, H., and Leopold, R. L.: Children and the Post-Concussion Syndrome, J.A.M.A., 175, 86, 1961.

Frable, M. A., Oppenheimer, P., and Harrison, W.: Cerebrospinal Otorrhea, Arch. Otol., 75,, 208, 1962.

Friedman, A. P., Brenner, C., and Denny-Brown, D. E.: Post-traumatic Vertigo and Dizziness, J. Neurosurg., 2, 36, 1945.

Friedman, A. P., and Merritt, H. H.: Damage to Cranial Nerves Resulting from Head Injury, Bull. Los Angeles Neurol. Soc., 9, 135, 1944.

Glaser, M. A., and Shafter, F. P.: Skull and Brain Traumas, J.A.M.A., 98, 271, 1932.

Jennett, W. B., and Lewin, W.: Traumatic Epilepsy after Closed Head Injuries, J. Neurol., Neurosurg., & Psychiat., 23, 295, 1960.

Karnosh, L. J.: Traumatic Neuroses and Psychoses, West J. Surg., 49, 606, 1941.

Kaufman, H. H.: Nontraumatic Cerebrospinal Fluid Rhinorrhea, Arch. Neurol., 21, 59, 1969.

Leigh, A. D.: Defects of Smell after Head Injury, Lancet, 1, 38, 1943.

Miller, H.: Mental Sequelae of Head Injury, Proceed. Royal Soc. Med., 59, 257, 1966.

Miller, H., and Stern, G.: The Long-term Prognosis of Severe Head Injury, Lancet, 1, 225, 1965.

Russell, W. R.: The Anatomy of Traumatic Epilepsy, Brain, 70, 225, 1947.

Strich, S. J.: Shearing of Nerve Fibers as a Cause of Brain Damage Due to Head Injury, Lancet, 2, 443, 1961.

Vyner, H. L., and Swire, H.: Sequelae in Posttraumatic Psychoses, Psychiatric Quart., 15, 343, 1941.

Walker, A. E.: *Posttraumatic Epilepsy,* Springfield, Charles C Thomas, 1949, 86 pp.

Walker, A. E., and Jablon, S.: Follow-up of Head-Injured Men of World War II, J. Neurosurg., 16, 600, 1959.

Walker, A. E., Caveness, W. F., and Critchley, M. (Eds.): *The Late Effect of Head Injury,* Springfield, Charles C Thomas, 1969.

Walker, A. E., et al.: Life Expectancy of Head-Injured Men With and Without Epilepsy, Arch. Neurol., 24, 95, 1971.

TRAUMA TO THE SPINAL CORD

Trauma to the spine may produce symptoms and signs as result of injury to the nerve roots or substance of the spinal cord.

Etiology. The spinal cord and the nerve roots may be injured by stab wound, gun shots, shrapnel and other penetrating missiles and by fracture or fracture dislocation of the vertebral bodies or their processes. At birth the spinal cord may be torn in delivery, especially with breech presentations. Injuries to the vertebrae may occur as result of direct violence but more commonly they are the result of excessive flexion or extension of the spine in falls, diving, and automobile accidents.

Damage to the cord from trauma may result from: (1) Simple concussion without direct trauma to the cord; (2) compression, contusion or laceration of the cord substance by penetrating missiles or by fracture dislocation; (3) hemorrhage into its substance (hematomyelia); and (4) by compression of its vascular supply. Any level of the spinal column may be injured but in civil life the most common sites of injury are at the level of the fifth and sixth cervical and the eleventh and twelfth thoracic vertebrae.

Pathology. It should be emphasized that the injury to the bony spine is of little practical importance except when this injury also affects the spinal cord or its roots.

The pathology of spinal concussion has not been clearly elucidated. The term is used to describe those patients in whom there are transient neurological symptoms as a sequel to blast injuries or direct injuries. Presumably there is swelling, edema and congestion of the cord as result of transmission of pressure waves to the substance of the cord.

Direct injury to the cord by penetrating missiles or by compression fractures or fracture dislocations, produces a variable degree of damage to the cord substance (Fig. 94). There may be a complete or incomplete transverse section of the cord at the affected segments, or hemorrhage into the cord at the site of the injury and into the neighboring segments.

The appearance of the cord at the level of the injury is subject to variations dependent on the nature of the injury. The cord may appear edematous and swollen if it is not compressed by the fractured vertebrae or bony spicules. When the cord has been damaged by penetrating missiles or crushed by the vertebrae, the affected segments are soft and mushy or the cord may be completely severed. Serious injury to the white matter or segments of the cord is followed by secondary degeneration in the fiber tracts. Segments above the level of the injury will show a loss of the fibers in the posterior and to a less extent in the lateral funiculi, while the degeneration in the segments below the level of the lesion will be confined to the lateral and anterior funiculi.

Chronic adhesive arachnoiditis may occur as a sequel of injury to the spinal cord. This is due to a progressive proliferation of the arachnoid membrane. This complication is relatively infrequent and is most common after minor injuries to the cord. Amyloidosis of the liver,

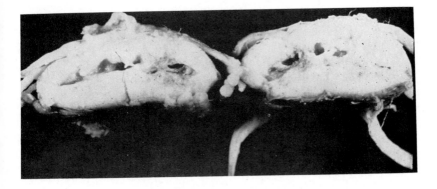

Figure 94.   Spinal cord trauma. Myelomalacia of cord following trauma.
(Courtesy Dr. Abner Wolf.)

spleen, kidneys, and adrenal cortex may follow chronic infections of the genitourinary tracts or decubitis ulcers. An ossifying fibro-myopathy not infrequently develops around the major joints in the lower extremities of the patients who have suffered a complete transection of the cord. Cystitis, pyelitis and urolithiasis are not uncommon complications in patients with disturbance of the innervation of the bladder.

Symptoms and Signs. The symptoms and signs of injury to the spinal cord are related to the level of the injury. Damage to the roots of the cauda equina causes a flaccid paralysis and sensory loss in the area supplied by the affected roots together with paralysis of the bladder and rectum. Injury to the spinal cord by fracture or fracture dislocation of the spine results in a complete motor, sensory and sphincter paralysis and absence of reflexes below the level of the lesion. The severity of the symptoms at the onset is not an accurate index of the degree of cord injury because of the development of so-called cord shock. The duration of this period of cord shock is quite variable. In severe injuries to the cord it may persist for several weeks and it is prolonged by the presence of bed sores or any infection. When the injury is of a minor degree, there may be rapid improvement within a few hours or days.

A complete transection of the cord results in a permanent motor and sensory paralysis below the level of the lesion and a temporary paralysis of the bladder and rectum and loss of tendon and cutaneous reflexes.

Incomplete transverse section of the cord is followed by a variable degree of motor and sensory loss below the level of the lesion depending on the severity of the damage. Unless complicated by spinal shock, the reflexes are exaggerated and there is an extensor plantar response. Bladder and rectal paralysis may also be present.

Hemorrhage into the substance of the cord (hematomyelia) may accompany compression of the cord by dislocation of the spine or it may occur as result of trauma independently of any fracture or dislocation of the spine. The symptoms of hemorrhage into the cord usually appear immediately following the injury (fall or dive), but in rare cases they may be delayed for a few hours. The most common site for hemorrhage into the cord is in the lower cervical region. There is a flaccid paralysis of the muscles at the level of the hemorrhage as result of injury to the ventral horn cells and a spastic weakness, partial sensory loss and sphincter disturbances below the level of the lesion. The severity of the latter symptoms depends upon the extent of the damage to the tracts in the cord by the hemorrhage.

Diagnosis. The diagnosis of injury to the spinal cord is made from the history of trauma and the clinical findings. The level of the injury is determined by the results of the neurological examination and the findings on roentgenographic examinations of the spine. The diagnosis as to whether the spinal cord is compressed by the dislocated or fractured vertebrae is made from the x-ray findings and from the presence of subarchnoid block on the lumbar puncture. The cerebrospinal fluid is bloody when the vessels in the meninges or cord are ruptured. The protein content is increased when there is subarachnoid block or when the fluid is bloody. Subarachnoid block may rarely be present as the result of edema or swelling of the cord without cord compression.

Course and Prognosis. The mortality rate with spine injuries in military life is estimated at about 80%. The rate is lower with injuries in civil life. The immediate prognosis for life is especially poor when the lesion is in the upper cervical cord because of the development of respiratory paralysis. Fatalities in patients with lesions below the fifth cervical segment are uncommon in the period immediately following the injury in absence of damage to other viscera. Death may follow after a period of weeks or months as the result of bed sores, urinary sepsis or septicemia.

In the patients who survive, some degree of improvement of the neurological signs is to be expected in all cases except when the cord is transected. Considerable improvement is the rule when the symptoms are due mainly to hemorrhage into the cord (hematomyelia). With resorption of the hemorrhage there is an improvement in the spastic weakness of the lower extremities, as well as a decrease in the sensory defect, which in some cases amounts to an almost complete disappearance of these symptoms. There is, however, usually some atrophy of the muscles supplied by the anterior horn cells at the level of the lesion.

In incomplete transverse lesions of the cord, there is usually a considerable degree of return of motor and sensory function. Bladder and rectal control usually returns to normal. The deep reflexes in the lower extremities remain exaggerated and it is common for an extensor plantar response to persist.

When the cord has been completely severed, the motor paralysis and sensory loss will be permanent. The further evolution of the symptoms and signs in these cases depends upon the restoration of function in the isolated segment of the cord. In the period immediately following the injury, the function of the isolated segment is in complete abeyance, due to the development of the state of spinal shock. During this stage there is absence of the deep and superficial reflexes and atonic paralysis of the bladder and rectum. Recovery from the stage of spinal shock occurs in the majority of the patients within the space of a few weeks or months. Recovery is prevented or retarded by the presence of bed sores or urinary sepsis.

With recovery from spinal shock there is a return of the tendon reflexes, which frequently become quite brisk, although the arc of the movement and the duration of the reflex are less than those which occur with incomplete lesions of the cord. Concomitant with the return of the reflexes, there are signs of other reflex activity in the isolated cord. In the majority of the cases the return of reflex activity is accompanied by the development of reflex spasms of the paralyzed limbs. These spasms, of a flexor or extensor nature involving many or all of the paralyzed muscles, may be evoked by a variety of stimuli to the anesthetic area. They are the result of heightened sensitivity of the isolated segment of the cord which is released from the control of higher centers. The classical reflex spasm is the withdrawal reflex, or so-called defense reflex. This can be obtained by the application of any noxious stimulus to the foot or to the lower leg. There is dorsiflexion of the great toe and ankle, flexion of the knee on the thigh and the thigh on the abdomen. In some cases, a noxious stimulus is necessary to evoke these reflex spasms. In others, the reflex may be so sensitive that it is aroused by the touch of the bedclothes or a slight draft of air. It was formerly thought that flexor spasms were characteristic of a complete transection of the cord and that the occurrence of extensor spasms indicated that the lesion was incomplete. The error of this concept was shown by Macht and Kuhn who found that extensor spasms predomi-nated over flexor spasms in 19 of 28 patients with verified transection of the cord. In 5 patients the muscles remained flaccid without the occurrence of any spasms.

Bladder and rectal function improves and with proper training automatic control of these functions can be developed in almost all of the patients except those with injury to the sacral outflow.

The loss of vasomotor control to the extremities and the splanchnic area results in a number of disturbances of the autonomic nervous system including orthostatic hypotension, paroxysmal hypertension on filling of the bladder or rectum and disturbances of sweating and heat regulation.

The late complications which may develop in patients with trau-matic, as well as other forms of paraplegia, include amyloidosis, testicular atrophy, pyelonephritis, cystitis and nephrolithiasis.

Treatment. Patients with injury to the spine should be handled with great care immediately after the injury in order to prevent further dislocation of fractured or dislocated bone and added injury to the cord. The patient should be moved only on a rigid stretcher or frame. The neck should be held extended and all flexion of the spine prevented. If surgical shock is present or there are severe injuries to other parts of the body, these should be treated immediately.

In the past it was customary to operate on most patients with acute spinal cord injury in order to "decompress" the damaged cord. It has become apparent that such operations are not of much value and operations are now done only to remove foreign material and damaged soft tissue in cases with compound fractures of the vertebrae.

The care of patients with trauma to the spinal cord includes the treatment of the complications as outlined below and general measures directed toward obtaining the maximum degree of functional activity. Surgical shock, if present, should be treated by transfusions. The bladder should be evacuated by catheterization. The development of bed sores should be prevented, if possible, by keeping the bed clean, by the use of air or water mattresses and by frequent changing of the position of the patient. In the convalescent stage, treatment includes massage, muscle training and the application of suitable braces. With extensive training, ambulation can be obtained in practically all patients with lesions below the cervical segments of the cord.

Treatment of Complications: BLADDER. The ultimate objective in the treatment of the bladder dysfunction in patients with a transected cord is an automatic bladder with twenty-four hour control. There is some disagreement as to the best method of obtaining this objective. Constant tidal drainage is preferred by some while suprapubic cystotomy is preferred by others. The purpose of both of these methods is to prevent the development of infection and to increase gradually the bladder capacity to normal. Once this has been obtained the catheter is removed for increasing lengths of time until it is evident that the patient can reflexly empty the bladder at intervals of three to five hours. This result can be obtained by proper training in all patients with injury to the spinal cord except when the bladder is completely denervated by destruction of the sacral cord. Control of the interval between voidings can be obtained in these patients but the constant use of a catheter is required.

BED SORES. Decubitus ulcers will develop in practically all of the patients with complete transection of the cord unless measures to prevent their occurrence are vigorously pursued. These ulcers develop wherever bony prominences are covered by skin: The sacrum, trochanters, heels, ischium, knees and anterior superior iliac spine are the most common sites. Every effort should be made to prevent the development of bed sores by the use of air mattresses, the elimination of pressure points by padding, frequent changing of position of patient, and by keeping the bed scrupulously clean. A small percentage of bed sores will heal with conservative therapy. Others will need operative intervention. Primary closure of the wound, if possible, gives the highest percentage of cures.

NUTRITIONAL DEFICIENCY. Paramount in the treatment of the patient is attention to the general nutrition. Early loss of weight occurs in many of the patients as result of anorexia. A high caloric, high vitamin diet should be given. In addition, loss of protein through the decubiti must be combatted by giving an excess of protein in the diet and the parenteral administration of protein hydrolysates, plasma and whole blood. The latter is also of value in combatting the anemia which often develops.

MUSCULAR SPASMS. In many cases the flexor or extensor spasms are painful and interfere with the rehabilitation of the patient. Occasionally conservative methods, warm tub baths, the administration of curare or minor operations on nerves or muscles which eliminate "trigger action" are successful. In other cases more radical measures are necessary. Munro recommends laminectomy with anterior rhizotomy from the tenth dorsal to the second sacral segments. The operation is performed while cystometry is in progresss. The roots are stimulated electrically before sectioning in order to preserve the outflow to the bladder. This operation abolishes all reflex activity in the lower extremity and improves the function of the bladder by eliminating spread of reflex activity from the legs to the abdominal musculature.

Reflex activity of the isolated segment of the cord can also be abolished by the intrathecal injection of 10 to 15 ml of absolute alcohol. Some workers object to this form of therapy on the grounds that the treatment of the bladder dysfunction is complicated by the destruction of the sacral outflow to that organ.

PAIN. Various types of pain in the anesthetic areas are reported by approximately 25% of the patients with a complete transverse lesion of the cord. These may be in the form of sharp shooting pains in the distribution of one or more roots, burning pain which is poorly localized, or deep pain localized in the viscera. Numerous forms of therapy have been recommended for the relief of these pains, including placebos, spinal anesthesia, posterior rhizotomy, sympathectomy, chordotomy and posterior column tractotomy. None of these forms of therapy has been uniformly successful. The best results were obtained by Freeman and Heimburger who obtained complete relief of the pain in 34 and improvement in 9 of 45 patients by chordotomy at level of the first dorsal segment.

REHABILITATION. The ultimate aim in all patients with spinal cord injuries is ambulation and economic independence. This can be accomplished in practically all patients with injuries below the cervical cord. This is best done in a rehabilitation center which has trained personnel and adequate equipment. Diligent cooperation of the patient with the physiatrist and the application of supportive braces are of paramount importance. When the upper extremities are paralyzed as result of damage to the cervical cord, the therapeutic goal is more limited, but pneumatic devices controlled by intact muscles which permit useful motion of paralyzed upper extremities are being introduced.

REFERENCES

Bors, E., and French, J. D.: Management of Paroxysmal Hypertension Following Injuries to Cervical and Upper Thoracic Segments of the Spinal Cord, Arch. Surg., 64, 803, 1952.
Bosch, A., Stauffer, S., and Nickel, V. L.: Incomplete Traumatic Quadriplegia. A Ten Year Review, J.A.M.A., 216, 473, 1971.
Brock, S.: Injuries to the Brain and Spinal Cord and Their Coverings, 5th Ed., Baltimore, Williams & Wilkins, 1974.
Bucy, Paul C., and Perot, P. L., Jr.: Injury to the Spinal Cord. In The Nervous System, E. B. Tower, Editor-in-Chief, Volume 2, 421, 1975. New York, Raven Press.
Dietrick, R. B., and Russi, S.: Tabulation and Review of Autopsy Findings in Fifty-five Paraplegics, J.A.M.A., 166, 41, 1958.
Hardy, A. G., Rossier, A. B.,: Spinal Cord Injuries. Orthopedic and Neurologic Aspects, Stuttgart, Thieme, 1975.
Kuhn, R. A.: Functional Capacity of the Isolated Human Spinal Cord, Brain, 73, 1, 1950.
Leventhal, H. R.: Birth Injuries of the Spinal Cord, J. Ped., 56, 447, 1960.
Martin, J., and Davis, L.: Studies Upon Spinal Cord Injuries: Altered Reflex Activity, Surg., Gynec. & Obst., 86, 535, 1948.
Munro, D.: The Rehabilitation of Patients Totally Paralyzed below the Waist, with Special Reference to Making Them Ambulatory and Capable of Earning Their Own Living: An End-result Study of 445 Cases, N. Engl. J. Med., 250, 4, 1954.
———: Treatment of Fractures and Dislocations of the Cervical Spine, Complicated by Cervical-Cord and Root Injuries, N. Engl. J. Med., 264, 573, 1961.
Prather, G. C., and Mayfield, F. H.: Injuries of the Spinal Cord, Springfield, Charles C Thomas, 1953, 396 pp.
Schneider, R. C., and Schemm, G. W.: Vertebral Artery Insufficiency in Acute and Chronic Spinal Trauma, J. Neurosurg., 18, 348,1961.
Towbin, A.: Spinal Cord and Brain Stem Injury at Birth, Arch. Path., 77, 620, 1964.

RUPTURE OF THE INTERVERTEBRAL DISCS

Rupture of the intervertebral disc into the body of the vertebrae was noted by Schmorl in 1927 and fragments of material described as chondromas had been removed from the spinal canal by neurosurgeons before Mixter and Barr in 1934 clearly demonstrated that these chondromas were, in reality, fragments of a degenerated and extruded intervertebral disc. The extruded material may herniate beneath the annulus fibrosus or it may rupture through the degenerated annulus and lie within the spinal canal.

Rupture of the nucleus pulposus of the intervertebral disc can produce pain by pressure on nerve roots. The dislocated disc material may also produce sensory loss and paralysis by pressure on the roots or on the spinal cord. Although rupture of the intervertebral disc may occur at any level of the spine, the prolapse is usually at the lower lumbar or lower cervical levels.

Pathogenesis. Trauma of a minor or severe degree is the cause of the rupture of the disc in the majority of the cases. Lifting in the bent-forward position and sudden straining with the back in an unusual position are the commonly reported types of injuries. The symptoms may appear immediately or after an interval of several months or years. Since rupture of the disc occurs predominantly in the fourth to sixth decades of life, it is probable that degenerative changes which begin in the prime of life predispose to herniation of the nucleus pulposus.

Incidence. The frequency of rupture of the intervertebral disc is attested to by the fact that most neurosurgeons and many orthopedic surgeons have been able to collect a large number of cases since the report of Mixter and Barr. It is now generally agreed that in the vast majority of the cases, symptoms which were formerly diagnosed as "sciatica" are due to rupture of the intervertebral disc.

Rupture of the intervertebral disc is most common in the fourth to sixth decades of life. It is rare before the age of twenty-five and uncommon after the age of sixty. Approximately 70 to 80% of the reported cases have been in men.

Symptoms and Signs. The signs and symptoms of herniation of the intervertebral discs are related to the size and location of the extruded material. Laterally placed protrusions confined to one interspace produce signs of injury to a single nerve root. Midline protrusion of the disc in the lumbar region may cause compression of one root, the roots on both sides of one segment or all of the roots of the cauda equina. Small laterally placed extrusions in the thoracic region rarely produce any symptoms, owing to the lack of relationship of the root to the extruded material. Larger lesions may compress the cord and produce signs commonly associated with extramedullary lesions at that level. Laterally placed extrusions in the cervical region (usually at the sixth or seventh cervical vertebrae) may compress a single nerve root, but owing to the relatively small size of the spinal canal at this level, signs of compression of the cervical cord are also apt to be present.

A characteristic, but not constant feature, of the symptoms of ruptured intervertebral disc is their remitting nature. It is common for the patient to give a history of two or more previous attacks of symptoms which disappeared after a period of several weeks or months.

Rupture of the Lumbar Intervertebral Discs. In over 90% of the cases the rupture occurs at the level of the fourth or fifth lumbar interspace. Pain in the lower part of the back radiating down the posterior surface of one, or occasionally both, legs produces the syndrome which has been known for many years as sciatica. In the first few years after the discovery of the role of rupture of the intervertebral disc in the production of pain in the back and the leg, it was claimed that rupture of the disc accounted for almost 100% of the cases of sciatica. It is obvious that these claims are exaggerated, but it is probable that rupture of the intervertebral disc is the cause of the symptoms in the vast majority (probably more than 80%) of patients with recurrent attacks of sciatica.

Pain in the lower back and buttocks, radiating down the posterior surface of the thigh and calf is the most constant and characteristic symptom of protrusion of the fourth or fifth lumbar disc. Paresthesias in the foot or leg are common, but motor weakness and sensory loss are not conspicuous features. The severity of the pain is subject to considerable variation but it is often of such a degree that it prevents the afflicted individuals from any productive work. The pain is often relieved or decreased in severity when the patient lies on a firm bed. It is usually worse when the patient is sitting or bending than when standing. Some patients may assume bizarre postures which they have found to produce amelioration of their pains. The pains may be increased by coughing, sneezing or straining.

On examination there is straightening of the normal lumbar curve and a scoliosis, which is usually away from the side of the sciatic pain. Movements of the lumbar spine are limited and there may be spasm of the erector spinae muscles. Palpation along the course of the sciatic nerve causes a mild or moderate degree of pain. Straight leg raising is limited (Lasègue's test) in the majority of the cases. Objective motor weakness is present in only a small percentage of the cases. This is usually confined to a slight paresis of the extensor of the great toe, the tibialis anterior or the gastrocnemius muscle. A mild degree of hypesthesia to touch or pinprick is present in over 50 per cent of the cases. This impairment is usually in the distribution of the fifth lumbar or first sacral segment and, rarely, in the fourth lumbar segment when the rupture is at the level of the third interspace. Decrease or loss of the ankle reflex is the rule with herniation of the lumbosacral disc.

The characteristic findings in patients with ruptured intervertebral disc at the common lumbar levels are given below.

Third lumbar space: Tenderness to percussion of third lumbar spinous process, normal ankle jerk, but reduced or absent knee jerk, weakness of the quadriceps femoris muscles, and hyperesthesia on the medial aspect of the leg and foot.

Fourth lumbar space: Tenderness to percussion of fourth lumbar spinous process, a normal knee and ankle jerk, but the latter may be diminished if there is multiple root involvement, absent or diminished posterior tibial reflex, weakness of extension of the great toe and ankle, and hypesthesia on the anterior aspect of the leg and great toe.

Fifth lumbar space: Tenderness on percussion of fifth lumbar spinous process, diminished or absent ankle jerk, weakness of the gastrocnemius and soleus muscles, and hypesthesia on the lateral aspect of the leg and foot and the third, fourth and fifth toes.

Rupture of the Thoracic Discs. Rupture of the thoracic discs is relatively rare. Arseni and Nash found 12 in 2544 patients (0.5%) who were subjected to operation in their clinic. Ruptured discs in the upper and middle thoracic segments produce pain in the back at the appropriate level and may compress the cord with resulting paraparesis or paraplegia. Lesions at the level of the eleventh and twelfth segments compress the conus and cauda equina with pain in the thoracolumbar region which may be referred to the legs, impairment of the anal and vesical sphincters and a complete or incomplete motor and sensory syndrome of injury to the conus and cauda equina.

Rupture of the Cervical Discs. Herniation in the cervical region accounts for approximately 5 to 10% of all cases with extrusion of the intervertebral disc. The discs between the fifth and sixth and between the sixth and seventh cervical vertebrae are most commonly involved. The frequency of rupture at the various levels is shown in Table 52.

Small laterally placed extrusions of the disc cause stiffness of the neck, pain in the shoulder and down the arm into the hand. With involvement of the sixth cervical root there are paresthesias and sensory impairment in the dorsum of the hand, slight paresis of the biceps brachii and diminution of the biceps reflex. Involvement of the seventh cervical root is characterized by paresthesias and sensory loss in the index finger and often in the middle and ring fingers, slight weakness of the triceps muscle and impairment or loss of its reflex.

A midline or large laterally placed disc in the cervical region may compress the spinal cord and produce the signs and symptoms of an incomplete transverse lesion of the cord or a Brown-Séquard syndrome.

Diagnosis. The diagnosis of a ruptured intervertebral disc is made from the appearance of the characteristic symptoms and signs of sciatica when the lesion is in the lumbar region and from the signs and symptoms of root or cord compression when the rupture is in the thoracic or cervical region. History of previous trauma is found in over one half of the cases and there is a tendency for remission and relapse of symptoms over a course of several or many years. The findings on

Table 52.   Frequency of Compression of the Cervical Roots by Ruptured Intervertebral Disc

(After Yoss, Corbin, MacCarty and Love, Neurology, 1957)

Cervical Root	%
Fifth	2
Sixth	19
Seventh	69
Eighth	10
	100

radiological examination of the spine are of value but are not always diagnostic. There may be loss of the normal curvatures, scoliosis, arthritic changes, narrowing of the intervertebral spaces and in the cervical region, narrowing of the intervertebral foramina in the oblique views. The protein content of the cerebrospinal fluid is usually elevated but it may be normal. Values in the range of 50 to 75 mg per 100 ml are common with lumbar herniations. Values over 100 mg are rare except in the cases with subarachnoid block. Subarachnoid block is not found when the rupture is in the lumbar region below the level of the puncture, but partial or complete subarachnoid block is frequently present with extrusions in the thoracic or cervical regions. The diagnosis of an extruded disc can be established with almost absolute certainty with the intraspinal injection of contrast media. By the injection of Pantopaque (which should be removed after the study is completed), the outlines of the subarachnoid space can be demonstrated in its entire extent. Defects in filling of the root sleeves indicate a laterally placed disc. Defects in the outline of the subarachnoid space (Fig. 95) or complete interruption of flow of the dye may be found with larger or centrally placed lesions.

Electromyography or electrical testing of the peripheral nerves is of value in localizing the site of the ruptured disc.

Rupture of the intervertebral disc must be differentiated from other lesions which cause root or spinal cord compression. These include primary and metastatic tumors, spinal injuries and anomalies, hypertrophic arthritis of the spine, other diseases of the spine and pelvic bones and tumors in the pelvis. In the cervical region, cervical rib and compression of brachial plexus by the scalene muscles must be considered also in the differential diagnosis. Little difficulty in the differential diagnosis of these various conditions should be encountered if the results of the neurological examination and the x-ray examination of the spine and other bones are carefully evaluated.

Treatment. When signs of cord compression are present, surgical treatment is indicated immediately. Otherwise more conservative methods of therapy should be tried. Limitation of activity, the wearing of a brace or corset or complete rest in bed on a hard mattress supported by a firm board may result in a complete remission of symptoms. Traction on the leg or extension of the neck may also be of value. Conservative treatment should be tried for several weeks or months before decision for surgical therapy is reached. The relapsing nature of the syndrome and the frequency of relief of symptoms from simple therapeutic measures have led to a great reduction in the number of patients who are treated by operative measures. Failure of conservative measures, undue severity of the pain, the development of signs of cord compression or severe weakness of muscles are indications for surgical

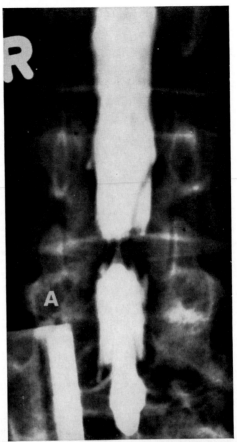

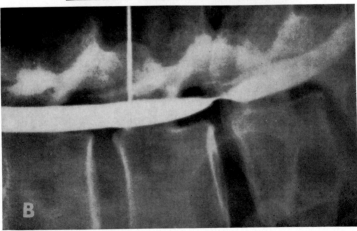

Figure 95. Ruptured intervertebral disc. In the frontal myelogram (A) there is a transverse defect in the opaque column at the L 4–5 level. In lateral view (B) the defect is ventral to the subarachnoid contrast medium and directly behind the intervertebral space at L 4–5. (Courtesy Dr. Ernest Wood.)

therapy. The operative mortality is negligible, the relief of symptoms is dramatic in many of the cases, and postoperative sequelae are uncommon. The question as to whether spinal fusion should be performed at the same time as the removal of the ruptured disc has not been settled. It is now generally agreed, however, that when there is no other abnormality of the spine, simple removal of the disc is sufficient. Failures in the surgical treatment have resulted chiefly from faulty diagnosis, improper localization of the lesion, failure to remove completely all of the extruded disc and the presence of multiple herniations. The results of operative therapy in several large series of cases indicate that complete relief of the severe pain is obtained in approximately 60% of the cases and partial relief of the pain in another 20 to 30%. Some pain in the back may be a constant sequel and return to occupations which require the lifting of heavy weights is inadvisable. Results of thoracic disc removal are often poor. Ligation or operative injury of vessels important for nutrition of the cord may produce myelomalacia.

REFERENCES

Abbott, K. H.: Anterior Cervical Disc Removal and Interbody Fusion. A Preliminary Review of 101 Patients Followed for One to Three Years, Bull. Los Angeles Neurol. Society, 28, 251, 1963.
Arseni, C., and Nash, F.: Thoracic Intervertebral Disc Protrusion, J. Neurosurg., 17, 418, 1960.
De Palma, A. F., and Rothman, R. H.: The Intervertebral Disc, Philadelphia, W. B. Saunders Co., 1970.
Gurdjian, E. S., et al.: Results of Operative Treatment of Protruded and Ruptured Lumbar Discs, J. Neurosurg., 18, 783, 1961.
Love, J. G., and Schorn, V. G.: Thoracic Disk Protrusions, J.A.M.A., 191, 627, 1965.
Mixter, W. J., and Barr, J. S.: Rupture of the Intervertebral Disc with Involvement of the Spinal Canal, N. Engl. J. Med., 211, 210, 1934.
Schmorl, G.: Die pathologische Anatomie der Wirbelsäule, Verhandl. d. deutsch. orthop. Gesellsch., 21, 3, 1927.
Semmes, R. E.: Ruptures of the Lumbar Intervertebral Disc: Their Mechanism, Diagnosis and Treatment, Springfield, Charles C Thomas, 1964.
Sullivan, C. R., Bickel, W. H., and Svien, H. J.: Infection of Vertebral Interspaces after Operations on Intervertebral Disks, J.A.M.A., 166, 1973, 1958.
Yoss, R. E., Corbin, K. B., MacCarty, C. S., and Love, J. G.: Significance of Symptoms and Signs in Localization of Involved Root in Cervical Disk Protrusion, Neurology, 7, 673, 1957.

INJURY TO CRANIAL AND PERIPHERAL NERVES

Neuritis

The term neuritis is generally used to denote damage to the nerves from any cause whatsoever. In the majority of instances dysfunction of the nerve is not due to an infectious process and the term neuropathy is preferred by some authors.

Etiology. The peripheral nerve and the cranial nerves are subject to injury by a variety of processes, including trauma, infections, tumors, toxic agents, vascular and metabolic disturbances. Trauma is the most common cause of localized injury to a single nerve (mononeuritis) whereas toxic agents and metabolic disturbances usually produce a diffuse involvement of many nerves (polyneuritis).

Pathology. The pathological changes which develop in a damaged nerve depend on the severity of the injury. Temporary interruption of function may occur when the nerve is subjected to a moderate degree of pressure or when it is only slightly damaged by some other process. In such cases, with the exception of a mild edema of the nerve at the site of injury, there are no pathological changes. When the injury is severe enough to damage the axis cylinder and myelin sheath, the nerve undergoes degeneration and subsequent regeneration (Wallerian degeneration). When there is a severe injury to a peripheral nerve at any one point, the sheath at the point of injury is destroyed. Subsequently there is a degeneration of the axon and myelin sheaths in the entire length of the nerves distal to the point of injury and a similar degeneration proximally to the next node of Ranvier. This process starts within twenty-four hours but takes many days for its completion. The axons become enlarged, fragmented and then disappear. The myelin sheaths swell and break up into globules of fatty material. If the continuity of the nerve has not been interrupted, the subsequent regeneration usually proceeds in an orderly fashion. In the degenerated portion of the nerve, the Schwann cells in the sheath undergo changes in form and increase in number. There is also an increase in the endoneural cells. These, together with other phagocytic cells, clear away the debris resulting from the breakdown of the myelin and axon. This process is well advanced within two weeks of the injury and usually complete at the end of one to two months. After all of the debris has been removed, the nuclei of the Schwann cells are arranged in orderly rows, which apparently serve to guide the course of the axon from its point of regeneration to its end organ in the muscle, skin, blood vessels or glands. The rate of regrowth of the axon is variable but it is roughly figured as 1 mm per day. Deposition of myelin around the axon follows its regeneration. Thus it can be seen that the time between injury and restoration of function is measured in months when a nerve is injured at some distance from its ending.

If the nerve has been completely severed, the orderly process described above is interfered with in proportion to the width of the separation of continuity of the proximal and distal ends. If this distance is great, regeneration will not be possible unless the ends are apposed at operation. When the distance is small, the fibrillary process of the axon penetrates the fibrin and connective tissue in the scar and enters the distal end of the nerve. Some of these may be deflected from their course by the scar and turn on themselves to form a neuroma.

There is usually no significant change in the spinal cord with injury to the peripheral nerves. The ventral horn cells which are the origin of the damaged peripheral nerve fibers undergo changes which are described by the term axonal reaction. The cell loses its pyramidal shape, the Nissl granules are displaced to the periphery and the nucleus is eccentric. This is a reversible reaction and the cell soon returns to normal except when the damage to the axon is close to the spinal cord or brainstem. When there is a severe degeneration of sensory or mixed nerves of long standing, there may be degeneration of the axons and myelin sheaths in the posterior funiculi.

General Symptomatology. The symptoms and signs which develop after injury to a nerve are related to the type of nerve affected. If the nerve subserves mainly a motor function, the defect will be manifest by flaccid paralysis, wasting and loss of the reflex of the muscle innervated by the nerve. If the affected nerve contains sensory fibers, there is loss of sensation in an area which is usually slightly less than that of the anatomical distribution of the nerve. Vasomotor disorders and so-called trophic disturbances are more common when a sensory or mixed type of nerve is injured than when a motor nerve is damaged.

Partial injury or incomplete division of a nerve may be accompanied by pains which may be stabbing in character, dysesthesias in the form of pins and needles sensation and rarely severe, burning pains described by the term causalgia.

Complete or incomplete interruption of the nerve may be followed by a variety of changes in the skin, mucous membranes, bones and nails classified as vasomotor or trophic disturbances.

Injury to motor nerve is followed by an alteration of the reaction of the nerve and the muscle to electrical stimulation. Electrical tests are of value in determining whether an injury to the nerve or lower motor neuron is present and in following the course of recovery in a patient with a damaged nerve. Injuries to the peripheral nerves are accompanied by changes in the skin resistance and by changes in the electromyogram.

Diagnosis and Differential Diagnosis. The diagnosis of injury to one or more peripheral nerves can usually be made by the distribution of the motor and sensory deficits. These are considered in connection with the description of isolated peripheral nerve lesions. The differential between lesions of the spinal roots and one or more peripheral nerves can usually be made by the fact that the muscular weakness and sensory loss are of a segmental rather than of a nerve distribution.

The differential diagnosis between polyneuritis and other causes of generalized weakness is discussed in the consideration of the various forms of polyneuritis.

Prognosis. The prognosis with injury to the peripheral nerves is related to the severity of the injury and to some extent to the site of the injury.

As a rule the nearer the site of the injury to the nervous system, the less is the probability of regeneration of a completely severed nerve. This is particularly true of the cranial nerves. It should be noted that regeneration does not occur in the first or second cranial nerves, which are in reality a part of the central nervous system.

When the injury to a peripheral nerve is of a minor nature and there is no degeneration, complete recovery may take place in a few days or weeks. Recovery will be slow and not entirely complete when the nerve is severely injured and permanent loss of function is the rule when the nerve is severed and the gap between the two ends or the severity of the scar formation is such that the regenerating axon cannot reach the distal end of the nerve.

Treatment. When a peripheral nerve is severed by trauma, the ends should be anastomosed at operation. There is no agreement as to the best time to explore and treat by surgical methods lesions of the peripheral nerves, when it cannot be determined whether there has been anatomical or physiological interruption of the nerve. The opinion, at the present time, is that operation should be performed as soon as possible whenever there is any doubt as to the state of the nerve.

After surgical therapy or in patients who do not need operative therapy, there should be immediate cooperation with the rehabilitation service. Paralyzed muscles should be given passive movements and weak muscles given reeducative exercises. If the hand is affected the patient should be given a soft or semisolid ball to hold to hasten the return of strength and dexterity to the fingers. There is disagreement as to whether electrical stimulation is of value. Some authors claim that muscular wasting is less when electrotherapy is given.

Splints, braces and other corrective appliances should be used when the lesion produces a deformity. These should be removable for the regular application of physiotherapy.

REFERENCES

Benisty, A., and Buzzard, E. F.: *The Clinical Forms of Nerve Lesions,* London, University of London Press, 1918. 235 pp.
————: *The Treatment and Repair of Nerve Lesions,* London, University of London Press, 1918. 181 pp.
Denny-Brown, D., and Brenner, C.: Paralysis of Nerve Induced by Direct Pressure and by Tourniquet, Arch. Neurol. & Psychiat., 51, 1, 1944.

Dyck, P. J., Thomas, P. K., and Lambert, E. H.: Peripheral Neuropathy. (Two volumes). Philadelphia, W. B. Saunders Co., 1975, 1438 pp.

Harris, W.: Neuritis and Neuralgia, London, Oxford University Press, 1926, 418 pp.

Haymaker, W., and Woodhall, B.: Peripheral Nerve Injuries, 2nd ed., Philadelphia, W. B. Saunders Co., 1953. 333 pp.

Lyons, W. R., and Woodhall, B.: Atlas of Peripheral Nerve Injuries, Philadelphia, W. B. Saunders Co., 1949. 339 pp.

Pollack, L. J., and Davis, L.: Peripheral Nerve Injuries, New York, Paul B. Hoeber, Inc., 1933. 678 pp.

Seddon, H. J.: Peripheral Nerve Injuries, Medical Research Council Special Report Series No. 282, London, Her Majesty's Stationery Office, 1954.

Stookey, B.: Surgical and Mechanical Treatment of Peripheral Nerves, Philadelphia , W. B. Saunders Co., 1922. 475 pp.

Sunderland, S.: Nerves and Nerve Injuries, Edinburgh, E. and S. Livingstone Ltd., 1968.

Tinel, J.: Nerve Wounds. Symptomatology of Peripheral Nerve Lesions Caused by War Wounds, London, Balliere, Tindall and Cox, 1917. 317 pp.

Woodhall, B., and Beebe, G. W.: Peripheral Nerve Regeneration. A Follow-up Study of 3,656 World War II Injuries. Veterans Administration Monographs, Washington, 1956.

Cranial Nerves

Olfactory Nerve and Tract. Disturbances of the sense of smell may occur as a result of injury to the nasal mucosa, the olfactory bulb, its filaments, or its central connections. Lesions of the nerve cause a diminution or loss of the sense of smell. Injury to the central connections is not usually accompanied by any detectable loss of olfactory sense. Occasionally, however, olfactory hallucinations of a transient and paroxysmal nature occur in patients with lesions in the temporal lobe. Loss of the sense of smell is often accompanied by an impairment of taste, since the latter is dependent to a great extent upon volatile substances in foods and beverages.

Temporary impairment of the sense of smell is seen frequently in connection with the common cold. Inflammatory or neuritic lesions of the bulb or tract are uncommon, although these structures may be involved in meningitis or in multiple peripheral neuritis. The olfactory bulb or tract may be compressed by meningiomas, metastatic tumors or aneurysms in the anterior fossa or by infiltrating tumors of the frontal lobe. The filaments of the olfactory nerve may be torn from the cribriform plate or the olfactory bulb may be contused or lacerated in injuries to the head. Leigh reported disturbances of olfactory sense in 7.2% of 1,000 cases of head injury observed at a military hospital. The loss was complete in 4.1% and partial in 3.1%. Recovery of the sense of smell occurred in only 6 of the 72 cases. Parosmia (perversion of sense of smell) was present in 12 cases. In the study of head injuries in the civilian population, Friedman and Merritt found that the olfactory nerve was damaged in 11 of 430 cases or 2.6%. In all cases the anosmia was bilateral. In three cases the loss was transient and disappeared within two weeks of the injury.

Parosmia, or perversion of the sense of smell, is not accompanied by impairment of olfactory acuity, and is most commonly due to lesions of the temporal lobe, but it has been reported when the injury was probably in the bulb or tract. Hallucinations of smell may occur in psychotics, or they may be an aura of the seizures in patients with convulsive seizures (hippocampal or uncinate gyrus fits). The aura in such cases is usually an unpleasant odor which is described with difficulty

Increased sensitivity to olfactory stimuli is rare, but cases have been reported in which the sense of smell is so acute that it is a source of discomfort. This symptom is usually an accompaniment of a neurosis.

Optic Nerve and Tract. The retina, optic nerve and tract are subject to injury from a great variety of causes with resulting loss of vision, impairment of the pupillary light reflexes and abnormalities in the size of the pupil (see Table 53).

Changes in the retina or optic nerve occur as the result of direct trauma, damage by various toxins, or: (1) systemic diseases such as chronic nephritis, diabetes mellitus, leukemia, anemia, polycythemia, nutritional deficiencies, syphilis, tuberculosis, the lipodystrophies, giant cell arteritis and generalized arteriosclerosis; (2) in demyelinizing disease and in heredodegenerative diseases of the nervous system; (3) as a result of local conditions such as chorioretinitis, glaucoma, tumors, congenital anomalies and thrombosis or embolism of the veins or arteries of the retina; (4) infiltration or compression of the nerve by gliomas, meningiomas, pituitary tumors, craniopharyngiomas, metastatic tumors or aneurysms; and (5) in increased intracranial pressure of whatever cause. Most of the conditions enumerated above are considered elsewhere, and discussion here will be limited to optic neuritis and atrophy.

Optic Neuritis and Atrophy. Optic neuritis is a term which is loosely used to describe lesions of the optic nerves accompanied by a diminution in visual acuity, with or without changes in the peripheral fields of vision, due to inflammatory, degenerative, or demyelinizing processes and to toxic agents. On ophthalmoscopic examination in the early stage of optic neuritis, the disk may appear normal or there may be swelling and congestion of the nerve. In the late stage, the disk is pale and smaller than normal.

Toxic Optic Neuritis. The optic nerve or retina may be injured by a great variety of toxic substances, including methyl alcohol, ethyl alcohol and tobacco, quinine, pentavalent arsenicals, thallium, lead, mercury and other metals.

Alcohol-Tobacco Amblyopia. This term is used to describe the optic neuritis which develops as the result of long-continued use of both tobacco and ethyl alcohol. It has been postulated that the lesion is

Table 53. Effects Produced by Lesions of the Eye, Optic, Oculomotor and Sympathetic Pathways on the Pupils

Site of Lesion on Right Side	Size of Pupil		Reaction of Homolateral Pupil to Stimulation by Light Directed into		Consensual Reaction of Contralateral Pupil to Stimulation by Light Directed into		Accommodation Convergence Reaction
	Right	Left	Right	Left	Right	Left	
Retina	Dilated	Normal	Impaired	Normal	Impaired	Normal	Normal
Optic nerve	Dilated	Normal	Lost	Normal	Lost	Normal	Normal
Optic chiasm	Normal	Normal	Normal*	Normal*	Normal*	Normal*	Normal
Optic tract	Normal	Normal	Normal*	Normal*	Normal*	Normal*	Normal
Optic radiation	Normal	Normal	Normal	Normal	Normal	Normal	Normal
Periaqueductal region†	Contracted	Normal	Lost	Normal	Normal	Lost	Normal
Oculomotor nuclear complex or nerve	Dilated	Normal	Lost	Normal	Normal	Lost	Lost on right
Sympathetic pathways	Contracted	Normal	Normal	Normal	Normal	Normal	Normal

*No reaction of the pupils if the beam of light is focused sharply on the amblyopic portions of the retina.
†Argyll Robertson pupil.

primarily an interstitial neuritis with destruction of the papillomacular bundle. A more reasonable hypothesis, however, is that the ganglion cells in the macular region of the retina are damaged. The neuritis, which is most commonly seen in middle-aged or elderly males who smoke a pipe and drink alcohol in moderate or large quantities, affects both eyes. At the onset there is a central or para-central scotoma for colors which progresses to a complete central scotoma. The peripheral fields of vision are normal. The occurrence of alcohol-tobacco amblyopia in association with pernicious anemia has been noted by several authors, and it has been suggested that malabsorption of vitamin B_{12} may be a factor in the cause of alcohol-tobacco amblyopia. Absolute withdrawal of all forms of alcohol and tobacco will result in an improvement in vision unless the disease has progressed to the point of complete atrophy of the retinal cells or of the optic nerve.

RETROBULBAR NEURITIS. The term retrobulbar neuritis is used to indicate an acute affection of the optic nerve accompanied by loss of visual acuity, with or without objective changes in the fundus. In the majority of the cases, retrobulbar neuritis is an episode in the course of one of the demyelinizing diseases, such as multiple sclerosis, and is readily diagnosed as such. When optic neuritis occurs alone, it has been the common practice to search for foci of infection, especially in the accessory nasal sinuses. Spontaneous improvement, which is the rule in retrobulbar neuritis, is often attributed to whatever treatment is given. Since the first attack of multiple sclerosis may not be followed by a further onslaught until many years later, it is not always possible to establish or exclude this diagnosis in a case showing only retrobulbar neuritis. Indeed, cases have been observed over a period of many years in which a single or recurrent attacks of retrobulbar neuritis have not been followed by any other evidence of central nervous system disease.

The symptoms of retrobulbar neuritis are a rapid loss of vision in one (Fig. 96) or both eyes, often accompanied by slight pain, especially on movements of the eyeball. The pupillary reactions are usually preserved. Presence or absence of changes in the optic disk is presumably related to the distance of the lesions from the nerve head. If the lesion is near the chiasm, the fundus appears normal or there is only slight congestion. When the lesion is in the distal portion of the nerve, the optic disk is swollen or frankly choked, with hemorrhages in the nerve head or adjacent retina. The visual acuity is usually reduced due to the presence of a central scotoma. Various types of visual field defects are found, depending on whether the lesion is in the proximal portion of the nerve, the chiasm or optic tract.

In the majority of cases of retrobulbar neuritis, the course is one of gradual improvement with return of vision to or near to normal. With

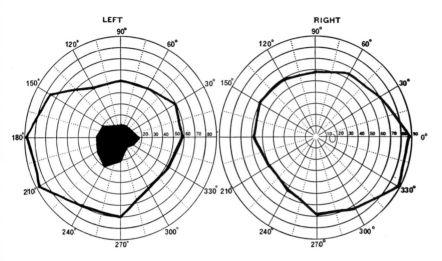

Figure 96. Retrobulbar neuritis. Large central scotoma in left eye. Visual acuity, O.D. 15/15, O.S. 1/400. (Courtesy Dr. Max Chamlin.)

recurrent attacks the degree of permanent visual loss is greater, and atrophy of the nerve is apparent, especially in the temporal half of the disk (temporal pallor). Total loss of vision is rare, however.

Recognition of multiple sclerosis as the cause of retrobulbar neuritis is not difficult when other signs of the disease are present. In the absence of these signs, retrobulbar neuritis must be differentiated from choked disk or optic neuritis from other causes. The severe degree of visual loss and the tenderness of the eyeballs to pressure serve to distinguish the swelling of the optic disk which occurs in retrobulbar neuritis from the choking resulting from increased intracranial pressure. The improvement in the degree of visual loss as well as the results of x-ray examination of the skull serve to differentiate the optic atrophy secondary to retrobulbar neuritis from that which occurs with aneurysms, pituitary adenomas and other tumors in the anterior fossa, or as the end-result of long-sustained increased intracranial pressure.

OPTIC CHIASM AND TRACT. Lesions of the optic chiasm are usually due to aneurysms, pituitary and other tumors and are considered in detail elsewhere. Diminution of visual acuity and visual field defects have been reported as the result of damage to the optic nerve, chiasm or tracts by thickening of the meninges surrounding them. This so-called chiasmal arachnoiditis has been found at operation in patients who have suffered minor or severe cerebral trauma or who have had a previous meningeal infection, particularly syphilitic meningitis. Improvement in vision sometimes occurs when the thickened adherent meninges are separated from the optic chiasm. Necropsy examinations of such cases are rare and at the present time there is not sufficient evidence to enable us clearly to delineate the syndrome.

Oculomotor, Trochlear and Abducens Nerves. Injury to the nerves or nuclei which innervate the ocular muscles produces diplopia, deviation of the eyeball and impairment of ocular movements.

Complete lesions of the third nerve, or its nucleus, produce paralysis of the extrinsic muscles of the eye supplied by this nerve (medial rectus, superior rectus, inferior rectus, inferior oblique, and levator palpebrae superior) as well as the constrictor of the ciliary muscles. There is ptosis of the lid, with loss of the ability to open the eye; the eyeball is deviated outward and slightly downward; the pupil is dilated, does not react to light and the power of accommodation is lost. Partial lesions of the third nerve or its nucleus produce fragments of the above picture, according to the extent of involvement of the nerve fibers or neurons.

Lesions of the fourth nerve or nucleus produce a paralysis of the superior oblique muscle and cause an impairment of the ability to turn the eye downward and outward. This defect is in part compensated by the actions of the external and inferior rectus muscles. Deviation of the eyeball is slight and diplopia is prevented by inclining the head forward and to the side of the normal eye.

Injury to the sixth nerve causes a paralysis of the external rectus muscle. The eyeball is deviated inward and diplopia is present in practically all ranges of movement of the eye, except on gazing to the side opposite the lesions. Lesions in the brainstem which involve the sixth nerve nucleus are accompanied by a paralysis of lateral gaze. On attempting to look toward the affected side, neither eyeball will move beyond the midline. The intactness of the third nerve on the opposite side can be demonstrated by the ability of the patient to innervate the internal rectus muscle of that eye in accommodation-convergence movements.

Paralysis of the ocular muscles may result from injury to the corresponding motor nerves or their cells of origin by a great variety of conditions, including trauma, neurosyphilis, multiple sclerosis and other demyelinizing diseases, tumors or aneurysms at the base of the skull, acute or subacute meningitides, thrombosis of intracranial venous sinuses, encephalitides, acute anterior poliomyelitis, diphtheria, diabetes mellitus, syringobulbia, vascular accidents in the brainstem, lead poisoning, botulism, alcoholic polioencephalitis (Wernicke's encephalitis), osteomyelitis of the skull, and following spinal anesthesia or simple lumbar puncture. Ocular palsies are frequently seen in the course of myasthenia gravis, ocular myopathy and rarely in progressive bulbar palsy, polyneuritis, or progressive muscular dystrophy. The ocular manifestations of the majority of the above conditions are considered elsewhere. Discussion in this chapter will be restricted to the disturbance of eye movement found in patients with increased intracranial pressure.

PARALYSIS OF EYE MUSCLES ASSOCIATED WITH INCREASED INTRACRANIAL PRESSURE. The sixth nerve has a long course from its point of emergence from the brainstem to the external rectus muscle in the orbit. Although it lies in a fluid-cushioned channel for a portion of this course, the nerve is peculiarly subject to injury by compression against the floor of the skull when intracranial pressure is increased from any cause. Thus a unilateral or bilateral paralysis of the external rectus muscle may develop in patients with increased intracranial pressure. In these cases the paralysis is of no value in localizing the site of the lesion.

The third nerve is only rarely injured by increased intracranial pressure. The nerve may be damaged when the increase in pressure develops slowly as is the case with tumors of the brain, but is more apt to be injured when the increased pressure is of sudden onset, with herniation of the uncinate gyrus through the tentorial notch and compression of the nerve. It is most commonly seen in patients with massive intracerebral or with extradural or subdural hematomas. These patients are usually comatose, making it impossible to test the movements of the eyes, but paralysis of the third nerve is manifest by dilatation of the pupil and absence of its reaction to light. The presence of a dilated pupil which does not react to light in a comatose patient is of localizing value in that it indicates that the lesion is on the same side as the abnormal pupil. Mere inequality of pupils is of no localizing value.

Fifth (Trigeminal) Nerve. Injury to the fifth cranial nerve causes: Paralysis of the muscles of mastication with deviation of the jaw toward the side of the lesion; loss of the ability to appreciate light tactile, thermal, and painful sensations in the face; and loss of the corneal and sneezing reflexes.

Lesions in the pons usually involve the motor and main sensory nuclei producing a paralysis of the muscles of mastication and a loss of sensation of light touch in the face. Lesions in the medulla affect only the descending root and produce a loss of the sensations of pain and temperature together with a loss of the corneal reflex.

The fifth nerve may be injured by trauma, neoplasms, aneurysms, or meningeal infections. Occasionally it may be involved in poliomyelitis and generalized polyneuritides. The sensory and motor nuclei in the pons and medulla may be destroyed by intramedullary tumors or vascular lesions. In addition, the descending root is frequently damaged in syringobulbia and multiple sclerosis. The fifth nerve is the site of a neuralgic disturbance, trigeminal neuralgia.

TRIGEMINAL NEURALGIA (TIC DOULOUREUX). Tic douloureux is a disorder of the sensory division of the trigeminal nerve, characterized by recurrent paroxysms of sharp, stabbing pains in the distribution of one or more branches of the nerve.

Etiology and Pathology. The etiology of this neuralgia is unknown. Various contributing factors are cited, such as trauma and infections in the teeth, jaw or accessory nasal sinuses. In the vast majority of cases, there is no organic disease of the fifth nerve or central nervous system. Degenerative or fibrotic changes in the gasserian ganglion have been reported but are too inconstant to be considered as having any causal relationship to the symptoms. In some cases the trigeminal nerve has been found to be compressed by tumors or anomalous blood vessels, and rarely pains typical of trigeminal neuralgia have occurred in patients with lesions in the brainstem as result of multiple sclerosis or vascular lesions which involve the descending root of the fifth nerve. It has been suggested that the attacks of facial pain in trigeminal neuralgia are due to a paroxysmal discharge in the descending nucleus of the nerve. The discharge is presumed to be related to an excessive inflow of impulses to the nucleus. This hypothesis is supported by the facts that typical attacks of trigeminal neuralgia have been relieved occasionally by section of the greater auricular or occipital nerves and that an episode of trigeminal neuralgia can be interrupted by the intravenous injection of Dilantin Sodium.

Incidence. Trigeminal neuralgia is the most frequent of all neuralgias. The onset is usually in middle or late life, but it may occur at any age. Typical trigeminal neuralgia has been reported in children under the age of ten years but it is distinctly uncommon before the age of thirty-five. The incidence is slightly greater in the female than the male.

Symptoms. The pains of trigeminal neuralgia occur in paroxysms. In the interval between the attacks, the patient is free of symptoms except for fear of an impending attack. The pains are described by the patients as searing or burning in nature, coming in lightning-like jabs in the distribution of one or more branches of the nerve. A paroxysm may last only a minute or two or it may be prolonged for fifteen or more minutes. The frequency of attacks varies from many times daily to several times a month. The patients cease to talk when the pains strike. Rarely the affected individual may rub or pinch the face or make violent convulsive movements of the face and jaw (tic convulsif). Watering of the eye on the involved side may occur. There is no objective loss of cutaneous sensation during or following the paroxysms but the patient may complain of hyperesthesia of the face. A characteristic feature of many cases is the presence of a trigger zone, stimulation of which sets off one of the typical paroxysms. This is often a small area on the cheek, lip or nose. The trigger zone may be stimulated by facial movements or by chewing. The patient may attempt to keep his face immobile during conversation or go without nourishment for days in order to prevent an attack of pain.

The pain is strictly limited to one or more branches of the fifth nerve and does not spread beyond the distribution of this nerve. The second or third division is more frequently involved, the latter slightly less frequently than the former. The first division is primarily affected in less than 5%. Pain originally confined to one division may spread to one or both of the other divisions. In cases of long duration, all three divisions are affected in approximately 15%. The affection is occasionally bilateral (5%) but paroxysms on both sides at one time are rare.

Signs. The physical findings in patients with trigeminal neuralgia are normal. The patients may be undernourished or emaciated due to the fear of provoking an attack by eating. There is no objective sensory loss and motor function of the nerve is normal. The results of laboratory examinations are normal.

Diagnosis. The diagnosis of trigeminal neuralgia can usually be made without difficulty from the description of the pains. Also characteristic is the method used by many patients to demonstrate the site of origin and mode of spread of the pain. They will not touch the area but with the tip of the index finger held a short distance from the face indicate the site of origin and spread of the painful spasm.

Differential Diagnosis. Trigeminal neuralgia must be differentiated from other types of pain which occur in the face or head, particularly infections of the teeth and nasal sinus. Although the pains of dental and nasal sinus disease differ from those of trigeminal neuralgia in that they are usually steady and throbbing and persist for many hours, most patients with trigeminal neuralgia have numerous operations on the sinuses and most of the teeth are removed before the diagnosis is established. Conversely, it is also remarkable that many patients with diseased teeth are referred to neurologists with the diagnosis of trigeminal neuralgia. In these cases, the role of the diseased tooth in the production of pain can be demonstrated by syringing it and the surrounding gum tissue with ice water.

The pain of herpes zoster may simulate that of trigeminal neuralgia but the appearance of the vesicles establishes the correct diagnosis. Post-herpetic neuralgia in the face is practically always in the distribution of the first division and differs from trigeminal neuralgia in its continuous nature.

Glossopharyngeal neuralgia may be confused with neuralgia of the third division of the trigeminal nerve. The diagnosis of glossopharyngeal neuralgia can be established by spraying the tonsillar region with local anesthetics.

Tumors of the gasserian ganglion, as well as tumors and other lesions in the cerebellopontine angle, may produce pain in the face. The facial pain which results from lesions of the nerve differs from that of trigeminal neuralgia in that it is steady and lasts for many hours or days, but occasionally it is paroxysmal. Areas of anesthesia in the face, loss of the corneal reflex, atrophy and weakness of the masticatory muscles, together with evidence of involvement of other cranial nerves exclude the diagnosis of trigeminal neuralgia.

Persistent or remitting neuralgic pains in the head, face and neck, which differ from trigeminal neuralgia in that they are not confined to the distribution of the trigeminal nerve, have been classified under the term of atypical facial neuralgia. It is thought by some that they are due to a disturbance of the sympathetic nervous system or that they represent a variant of migraine. Relief of symptoms has been reported following operations on the cervical and dorsal sympathetic ganglia, sectioning of the greater petrosal nerve and by cutting the periarterial sympathetics. The area adjacent to the temporal artery is most frequently the site of this type of pain. In some cases these pains are a manifestation of conversion hysteria.

Pains in the face may occur in patients who have degenerative changes in the temporomandibular joint as result of malocclusion of the teeth. Evidence of changes in the joint in the roentgenograms helps to establish this diagnosis. The symptoms are relieved by the correction of the malocclusion.

Course. The course of trigeminal neuralgia is characterized by remissions. In the majority of cases the paroxysms of pain are present for several weeks or months and then cease spontaneously. The remission may be of short duration or the pains may be entirely absent for months or even years. There is a tendency for the attack-free intervals to become shorter as the patient grows older, and a permanent disappearance of the symptoms is rare. The affection is never fatal in itself, but frequent paroxysms may incapacitate the patient, or even the fear of an impending attack may prevent productive work. Some authors comment on the fact that most of the patients bear their pains stoically and that suicide or morphine addiction is rare.

Treatment. Many unsuccessful forms of medical therapy have been recommended in the past for the treatment of trigeminal neuralgia. The pains are so severe that they are not relieved by analgesic drugs except morphia, the use of which is contraindicated. It has been shown that diphenyl hydantoin (Dilantin) injected intravenously will abort an acute attack and that the daily administration of the drug will prevent recurrence of the pain in many of the patients. The dosage needed, 0.4 to .07 gm daily, is greater than that tolerated by most patients. Another anticonvulsant has been found to be more effective than diphenyl hydantoin with less toxic side effect. This drug, 5-carbamyldibenz (b, f) azepin (Carbamazepine, Tegretol) produces a complete remission of symptoms in a high percentage of cases when used alone or in combination with diphenyl hydantoin. The dose is 200 mg two to five times daily.

The operative procedures which have been devised for the control of trigeminal neuralgia include alcohol injection of the nerve or ganglion, partial section of the nerve in the middle or posterior fossa, decompression of the root, and medullary tractotomy. The number of these operations is an indication that no one of them has been entirely satisfactory either because of the complications of the procedure, failure to obtain satisfactory relief, or the development of numbness and paresthesias in the anesthetic areas. At the present time percutaneous thermal destruction of the affected branch extracranially is the preferred treatment when medical therapy is ineffective.

Seventh (Facial) Nerve. The facial nerve, as it leaves the brainstem, has two divisions: the motor root and the nervus intermedius. These two divisions have little in common from a physiologic point of view. The functions of the intermedius are much like those of the glossopharyngeal. It conducts taste sensation from the anterior two thirds of the tongue, and supplies autonomic fibers to the submaxillary and sphenopalatine ganglia which innervate the salivary and lacrimal glands. There is disagreement as to whether the seventh nerve has any somatic sensory function. It is supposed to carry proprioceptive impulses from the facial muscles and cutaneous sensation from a small strip of skin on the posteromedial surface of the pinna and around the external auditory canal. In fact, however, sensory loss can rarely be detected in patients with lesions of the seventh nerve. Similarly impairment of hearing is seldom found, although the ear is supposed to become more sensitive to low tones when the stapedius is paralyzed.

Injuries to the facial nerve produce a paralysis of the facial muscles with or without loss of taste on the anterior two thirds of the tongue and a disturbance in the secretion of the lacrimal and salivary glands depending upon the portion of the nerve which is involved. Lesions of the nerve near its point of origin or in the region of the geniculate ganglion are accompanied by a paralysis of the motor, gustatory and autonomic functions of the nerve. Lesions of the nerve between the geniculate ganglion and the point of separation of the chorda tympani produce the same dysfunction as that of injury in the region of the geniculate ganglion except that the lacrimal secretion is not affected. Involvement of the nerve at the region of the stylomastoid foramen results only in paralysis of the facial muscles.

Lesions of the facial nucleus in the brainstem cause a paralysis of all facial muscles. Lesions of the motor cortex or the connections between the cortex and the facial nucleus are accompanied by a partial paralysis which is usually most severe in the muscles of the lower half of the face (supranuclear palsy). There may also be an inequality of the movement of the facial muscles to voluntary and emotional stimuli.

Etiology of Facial Paralysis. Owing to their superficial site the peripheral branches of the seventh nerve are subject to injury by stab wounds, cuts, gunshot wounds, and the pressure of forceps at birth. Rarely, the nerve may be injured by pressure against a hard object in sleep. It may be injured in operations on the mastoid, in the operative treatment of acoustic neuromas or trigeminal neuralgia and in operations on the parotid gland. Foerster reported facial nerve injury in 120 of 3,907 cases (3%) of head injury in World War I. Comparable figures were reported by Russell in World War II. In a series of civilian head injuries, Friedman and Merritt found that the seventh nerve was injured in 7 of 430 cases (1.6%). Damage to the seventh nerve which accompanies head injury is commonly associated with fracture of the temporal bone and usually is present immediately after the injury. Occasionally, however, the onset of the facial paralysis may not be manifested for several days after the accident. The mechanism of this delayed paralysis is not clear. Improvement is the rule when damage to the nerve is associated with head trauma, but recovery may not be complete.

Within the skull the nerve may be damaged by tumors, aneurysms, infections of the meninges, leukemias, osteomyelitis, herpes zoster, Paget's disease, sarcomas and other tumors of the bone. The nerve is occasionally affected in the course of a generalized polyneuritis. It is involved in a large percentage of the patients with the so-called Guillain-Barré syndrome and in diphtheritic polyneuritis but only seldom in the diabetic or alcoholic forms. Involvement of the facial nerve is common in leprosy. The peripheral portion of the nerve may be compressed by tumors of the parotid gland. A few cases with recurrent facial palsy in association with facial edema, cheilitis, lingua plicata and migraine have been reported in the literature (Melkersson's syndrome). Facial palsy is rare in mumps but is common in uveoparotid fever or meningeal forms of sarcoidosis.

Bilateral facial palsy may be caused by many of the conditions which produce a unilateral paralysis. It is most frequently seen in polyneuritis, leprosy, leukemia, and meningococcal meningitis.

The facial nucleus may be damaged by tumors, inflammatory lesions, vascular lesions, acute poliomyelitis, and demyelinizing processes.

Bell's Palsy. Not infrequently, paralysis of the seventh nerve may occur without any known cause. This so-called Bell's palsy often follows exposure to cold as in riding in an open car, and is thought to be due to swelling of the nerve within the fallopian canal. Bell's palsy occurs at all ages, but is slightly more common in the third to fifth decades. The frequency of involvement on the two sides is approximately equal. Occasionally the paralysis may recur, either on the same or opposite side.

Alter reports that there is a tendency for the familial occurrence of Bell's palsy.

Symptoms. The onset of facial paralysis may be accompanied by a feeling of stiffness of the muscles but pain is rarely present, except when the paralysis is the result of herpes zoster.

Signs. The signs of complete paralysis of the seventh nerve can be divided into motor, secretory and sensory. When the damage to the nerve is severe, the facial paralysis is obvious even when the face is at rest. There is sagging of the muscles of the lower half of the face and occasionally of the lower lid. The normal folds and lines around the lips, nose and forehead are ironed out and the palpebral fissure is wider than normal. There is complete absence of all voluntary and associated movements of the facial and platysmal muscles. On attempting to smile, the lower facial muscles are pulled to the opposite side. This distortion of the facial muscles may give the false appearance of deviation of the protruded tongue or the open jaw. Saliva and food are apt to collect on the paralyzed side. The patient is unable to close the eye and on attempting to do so the eyeball can be seen to be diverted upward and slightly inward (Bell's phenomenon). When the lesion is peripheral to the ganglion, the lacrimal fibers are spared and there is excessive collection of tears in the conjunctival sac due to the failure of the tears to be expressed into the lacrimal duct by movements of the lids. The corneal reflex is absent due to paralysis of the upper lid. Preservation of corneal sensation is manifested by blinking of the other lid. Secretion of tears is diminished only when the lesion is proximal to the geniculate ganglion. Decrease in salivary secretion and loss of the sense of taste in the anterior two thirds of the tongue are present when the chorda tympani is affected.

Although the seventh nerve presumably transmits proprioceptive sense from the facial muscles and cutaneous sensation from a small area of the pinna and the external auditory canal, loss of these sensations is rarely detected.

Partial injury to the facial nerve produces a weakness of the upper and lower halves of the face. Occasionally, however, the lower half may be more affected than the upper. More rarely, the opposite occurs.

Course. Recovery from facial paralysis depends upon the severity of the lesion. If the nerve is anatomically sectioned, the chances of complete or even partial recovery are remote. In the vast majority of cases and especially in so-called Bell's palsy, partial or complete recovery occurs. With complete recovery there is no apparent difference between the two sides of the face either at rest or on motion. When recovery is partial, there is a tendency for contractures to develop on the paralyzed side, so that on superficial inspection it appears that there is a weakness of the muscles on the normal side. The falsity of this impression will be obvious as soon as the patient smiles or attempts to move the facial muscles. Abnormal movements of the facial muscles and a disturbance in the secretion of the lacrimal gland are not infrequent sequelae of a facial palsy. There may be a slight twitch of the labial muscles whenever the patient blinks, or an excess secretion of tears when the salivary glands are activated in eating (syndrome of crocodile tears). In addition to the twitching movements of the labial muscles synchronous with blinking, there may be paroxysmal clonic contractions of all facial muscles which simulate focal jacksonian seizures. These spasms are occasionally seen in patients who have never had any obvious lesion of the facial nerve. The cause of these sequelae is not known. They are attributed by some to misdirection of the regenerated fibers. Others state that they are the result of spread of impulses in the fibers of the nerve.

Diagnosis. The differential diagnosis between a paralysis due to a cortical lesion and that from a lesion of the nucleus or nerve can be made without difficulty except when only a minor degree of weakness is present. The presence of other signs of cortical involvement, sparing of the muscles of the forehead and upper lid and the preservation of electrical reactions, all indicate a supranuclear lesion. In addition, the weakness of a peripheral lesion is equal for all movements, whereas in supranuclear lesions there may be a discrepancy between the extent of volitional and emotional movements. Volitional contractions may be greater or less than those which occur when the patient smiles or laughs.

The differentiation between lesions of the nucleus and the nerve is made by the presence of associated findings. Lesions in the tegmentum of the brainstem are accompanied by a paralysis of lateral gaze due to concomitant injury to the sixth nucleus. Lesions in the basal part of the brainstem will be accompanied by signs of involvement of the corticospinal tract. Lesions of the nerve at the point of emergence from the brainstem by tumors, meningitis and the like are signalized by the association of paralysis of the facial nerve with paralysis of the eighth, sixth and possibly the fifth nerves.

Occasionally, it may be necessary to distinguish between palsy of the facial muscles due to a lesion of the nerve and unilateral involvement of the facial muscles in myasthenia gravis. The differential diagnosis is made from the associated findings in the latter condition and by the response of the muscular weakness to the parenteral injection of neostigmine or edrophonium.

Treatment. It is obvious that attempts should be made to remove the lesion which is causing the facial paralysis when such is found. In all such cases, as well as in the cases of unknown cause, local treatment of the facial muscles is necessary. The purpose of this treatment is to relieve the strain on the relaxed muscles, and to preserve their "tonus." A simple method of splinting the paralyzed muscles is to anchor a piece of adhesive plaster on the side of the forehead, splitting the distal end to form an inverted "Y" and attaching these ends to upper and lower lip in such a manner as to keep them elevated. The patient should massage the facial muscles for five minutes twice daily. The massaging movements should start from the chin and lower lip and be directed upward. Electrical stimulation with a weak galvanic current is also of value. Goggles or plain glasses should be worn to protect the cornea. With return of function the patient should practice movements of the various muscles of the face while standing before a mirror.

Surgical procedures are often of value when spontaneous recovery does not occur. Neurolysis or end-to-end suture may be indicated in extracranial lesions of the nerve or its branches. When the nerve damage is proximal to the stylomastoid foramen, end-to-end suture is not possible and restoration of innervation of the facial muscle can only be obtained by suturing the distal portion of the seventh nerve with the central portion of one of the other cranial nerves. Either the eleventh or twelfth cranial nerve can be used. When the eleventh nerve is used there is permanent paralysis of the sternomastoid and the upper fibers of the trapezius. This results in slight deformity, but contractions of the facial muscles occur whenever the patient attempts to turn the head or elevate the shoulder. Sooner or later a new motor pattern is developed in the cerebral cortex and the movements of the facial muscles are dissociated from those of the shoulder. Anastomosis of the twelfth with the seventh is followed by atrophy and paralysis of one half of the tongue. This causes little discomfort and control of the facial muscles is developed without any apparent adventitious movement of other muscles.

Anastomosis of the facial nerve with either the eleventh or twelfth nerve should be performed as soon as possible when the nerve is cut in mastoid operation or in the removal of acoustic neuromas. In other types of peripheral facial paralysis it should be delayed for six months or more to determine whether spontaneous regeneration will occur.

Steroids have been recommended for Bell's palsy on the basis of relieving edema. Reports of this form of therapy have not been convincing.

Decompression of the nerve in the canal is recommended by some otologists to expedite and enhance return of function in patients with Bell's palsy. The operation is usually performed six weeks after the onset of the paralysis.

Surgery may be necessary to alleviate facial spasm which occurs spontaneously or after partial regeneration of the injured nerve. The nerve or one of its branches, when the spasms are localized, can be injected with alcohol or partially sectioned. These operations occasionally give permanent relief from the spasms but more often the spasms recur when the nerve regenerates. Permanent relief can be obtained by anastomosing the seventh nerve with the eleventh or twelfth cranial nerve.

Eighth (Acoustic) Nerve. Symptoms of involvement of the cochlear branch of the eighth nerve are tinnitus and loss of hearing; those of involvement of the vestibular portion are vertigo, disturbance of equilibrium and impairment of ocular movements.

The loss of hearing which follows infections in the middle ear or changes in the ossicles without injury to the nerve is only for air conduction. Bone conduction is normal although it may appear to be more acute than normal in the Weber test. Loss of hearing is total and permanent when the cochlear branch is anatomically severed. Partial lesions of the nerve or the nuclei in the brainstem produce a diminution of auditory acuity which is greatest for high tones and is frequently accompanied by tinnitus; bone conduction and air conduction are equally diminished. Unilateral lesions of the secondary connections in the brainstem or thalamus are not accompanied by any loss of hearing because of the bilateral nature of these connections. Bilateral loss of hearing is possible with destructive lesions of the trapezoid body in the pons. There is no unilateral degradation in auditory acuity nor differential tonal discrimination when one insulotemporal region of the cortex is destroyed because each cochlea has a physiological representation of equal value in both medial geniculate bodies and in both cerebral hemispheres. There is, however, a slight reduction in acuity of bilateral audition without any loss in differential tonal discrimination. Bilateral destruction of the primary auditory receptive cortex produces a serious loss of auditory acuity. The threshold rises about 70 decibels which means that all but the very loudest scunds of daily life become psychically inaudible. In addition there is complete loss of ability to distinguish between tones and configurations of sound.

Lesions in the secondary auditory centers in the superior temporal convolution of the dominant cortex impair the understanding of spoken words. This is often accompanied by the loss of the ability to understand writing, because of the association of the printed image with the sound of the word.

Acquired (unbalanced) disturbance of the function of the vestibular nerves or nuclei gives rise to vertigo, disturbance of equilibrium and nystagmus. These symptoms are most prominent in acute unilateral lesions which do not completely destroy the nerve or the nucleus, and are minimal when the nerve is sectioned or completely destroyed. Lesions of the vestibular connections with the cerebellum produce a less severe disturbance of equilibrium. Injury to the medial longitudinal fasciculus, one of the main connections of the vestibular nuclei with other nuclei in the brainstem, causes nystagmus when the lesion is in the medulla or the upper part of the cervical cord. If the medial longitudinal fasciculus is damaged in the pons, there is a peculiar dissociation of eye movements known as ophthalmoplegia internuclearis. Attempts to deviate the eyes to the side of lesion result in an incomplete outward movement of the homolateral eye accompanied by nystagmoid movements of this eye and a failure of the opposite eye to move beyond the position of central fixation.

The nuclei of the eighth nerve may be involved in inflammatory processes, tumors, vascular lesions, and demyelinizing processes. The peripheral portion of the nerve may be damaged by inflammatory processes in the meninges, especially acute purulent tuberculous, or mumps meningitis, tumors in the cerebellopontine angle, infections in the ear and mastoid, or by degenerative or toxic processes in the middle or inner ear. The auditory portion of the nerve is occasionally involved in heredodegenerative disease of the nervous system.

The eighth nerve can be damaged by a great variety of toxic substances, including drugs. The most common of the latter are acetylsalicylic acid, quinine and streptomycin. The site of the damage caused by these substances is not known, but it is presumed to be labyrinthine or retrolabyrinthine. A high incidence of vestibular disturbance and a sizable number of cases of deafness, either transient or permanent, will occur with the use of streptomycin if large doses of the drug are given over prolonged periods. As a rule the otitic symptoms develop between the seventeenth and twentieth day if dosage as high as 3 gm a day is given.

Impairment of hearing in one or both ears occurs in approximately 8% of craniocerebral injuries. Fracture of the middle fossa of the skull is the usual cause. The fracture generally involves the middle ear and the resulting loss of hearing is partial and of the middle ear type. When the inner ear or the nerve is damaged, the hearing loss is apt to be total and there is a loss of vestibular reactions. Traumatic lesions of the eighth nerve are often associated with injury to the facial nerve. Tinnitus usually develops when there has been damage to the inner or middle ear. True vertigo in patients with head injury is usually due to concussion of or hemorrhage into the labyrinth. Some authors attribute the dizziness on change of posture, which is a prominent feature of the post-traumatic syndrome, to a minor degree of damage to the labyrinth.

Impairment of hearing is a common accompaniment of the aging process, occurring in over 60% of patients over eighty years of age.

Dizziness and vertigo are also present in a high percentage of elderly patients, especially women.

Damage to the eighth nerve from whatever cause is apt to produce permanent residuals. Improvement in hearing occurs in a fair percentage of the patients with traumatic injury to the nerve. Loss of hearing as result of damage to the nerve by inflammatory processes in the meninges or by toxic substances is usually permanent, probably due to destruction of the inner ear.

Complete destruction of one labyrinth or the vestibular portion of the eighth nerve is not usually accompanied by any disturbance of equilibrium. Ataxia of a moderate or severe degree occurs when both labyrinths or vestibular nerves are affected. The degree of ataxia decreases when the patient learns to compensate for this defect, but difficulty will always be present on attempts to walk in the dark. Functional disturbance of the labyrinth may occur as an isolated event (acute labyrinthitis) or there may be recurrent attacks (Ménière's syndrome).

ACUTE LABYRINTHITIS. The acute onset of symptoms of dysfunction of the labyrinth—vertigo, disturbance of equilibrium, nausea and vomiting—are described by the term "acute labyrinthitis." These symptoms are the same as those which occur in Ménière's syndrome, although in acute labyrinthitis the symptoms are not recurrent and their duration is much longer than is usual in the attacks of Ménière's syndrome.

The etiology of acute labyrinthitis is unknown. It often follows a mild or severe head cold and it is presumed that the inflammatory process may have spread to the inner ear. Against this hypothesis, however, is the fact that the symptoms may occur without any antecedent infection of the nasopharynx. Acute labyrinthitis may occur at any age and affects the sexes equally. The signs and symptoms, severe vertigo, nausea, disturbance of equilibrium and nystagmus, are of sudden onset and may last for several days or weeks. Tinnitus and loss of hearing are usually absent or are inconspicuous features. During the attack there is photophobia and headache and the gait is ataxic. The patient prefers a darkened room and lies quietly in bed without turning the head. Food may be refused because of the nausea and vomiting. After a period of several days or weeks the vertigo diminishes and the nystagmus disappears. There is no specific treatment. Antihistamines or small doses of tranquilizer may be of value.

Acute labyrinthitis must be distinguished from vascular lesions of the hind brain and multiple sclerosis. The former can usually be diagnosed by the presence of signs and symptoms of involvement of other structures in the brainstem, and the latter by the history of previous attacks of the disease or evidence of injury to other parts of the nervous system. Occasionally involvement of the vestibular nuclei may be the first manifestation of multiple sclerosis. A definite diagnosis cannot be made until further evidence of the disease develops. The persistence of nystagmus after complete subsidence of the vertigo is in favor of the diagnosis of multiple sclerosis.

Ninth (Glossopharyngeal) Nerve. The ninth nerve contains both motor and sensory fibers. The motor fibers supply the stylopharyngeus muscle and the constrictors of the pharynx. The sensory fibers carry general sensation from the upper part of the pharynx and the special sensation of taste from the posterior third of the tongue.

Isolated lesions of the peripheral nerve or its nuclei are rare and are not accompanied by any significant disability. Taste is lost on the posterior third of the tongue and the gag reflex is absent on the side of the lesion. Injuries of the ninth nerve by inflammatory or neoplastic processes are usually accompanied by signs of involvement of the neighboring nerves. The tractus solitarius which receives the taste fibers from both the seventh and ninth nerves may be destroyed by vascular or neoplastic lesions in the brainstem.

The ninth nerve is occasionally the seat of a neuralgic disturbance known as glossopharyngeal neuralgia.

GLOSSOPHARYNGEAL NEURALGIA. Glossopharyngeal neuralgia or tic douloureux of the ninth nerve is characterized by paroxysms of excruciating pain in the region of the tonsils, posterior pharynx, back of the tongue and middle ear.

Etiology and Pathology. The etiology of glossopharyngeal neuralgia is unknown and there are no significant pathological changes in the majority of the cases. Occasionally pains in the distribution of the nerve may be associated with injury to the nerve in the neck by tumors.

Incidence. Glossopharyngeal neuralgia is relatively rare, occurring about one twentieth as often as trigeminal neuralgia. Males are more frequently affected than females. The symptoms may develop at any age but the onset is most frequently in the fourth and fifth decades.

Symptoms. The pain of glossopharyngeal neuralgia, except for its distribution, is exactly like that of trigeminal neuralgia. The pains occur in paroxysms, are burning or stabbing in nature, and are localized to the region of the tonsils, posterior pharynx, back of the tongue and the middle ear. They may occur spontaneously but are often precipitated by swallowing, talking or by touching the tonsils or posterior pharynx. The attacks usually last only a few seconds but occasionally they may be prolonged for several minutes. The frequency of attacks varies from many times daily to once in several weeks. Long remissions are common.

Diagnosis. The diagnosis of glossopharyngeal neuralgia can be made from the description of the pain. The only differential diagnosis of any importance is neuralgia of the mandibular branch of the fifth nerve. The diagnosis of glossopharyngeal neuralgia is established when an attack of pain can be precipitated by stimulation of the tonsils, posterior pharynx or base of the tongue or when the pains are relieved by anesthetizing the affected area with 1% Pontocaine. When the membrane becomes anesthetic, the pains disappear and they cannot be precipitated by stimulation with an applicator. During this period the patient is able to swallow food and talk without discomfort.

Course. The paroxysms of pain occur at irregular intervals and there may be long remissions. During a remission the trigger zone disappears. The pains almost always recur sooner or later unless they are prevented by medical therapy or the nerve is sectioned surgically. The disease does not shorten the life of the affected individuals, but they may become emaciated because of the fear that each morsel of food will precipitate a pain paroxysm.

Treatment. Carbamazepine (Tegretol), alone or in combination with Dilantin, is effective in producing a remission of the symptoms in a high percentage of patients. If medical therapy is not effective, the nerve can be sectioned intracranially. The results of the operation are satisfactory. The patient is relieved of the pains and there are no serious sequelae. The mucous membrane supplied by the ninth nerve is permanently anesthetized with loss of the gag reflex of this side. Taste is lost on the posterior third of the tongue. There are no motor difficulties, such as dysphagia or dysarthria, unless the tenth nerve is injured at the operation.

Tenth (Vagus) Nerve. The fibers of the tenth nerve from the nucleus ambiguus innervate the muscles of the pharynx and larynx and those from the dorsal motor nucleus supply the autonomic innervation of the heart, lungs, esophagus and stomach.

Unilateral lesions of the nucleus ambiguus in the medulla produce dysarthria and dysphagia. Since the nucleus has a considerable longitudinal extent in the medulla, it is possible for lesions in the brainstem to produce dysarthria without dysphagia, or *vice versa*, according to the site of the lesion. Lesions confined to the lower portion of the nucleus cause dysphagia, while lesions of its upper portion produce dysarthria.

The dysphagia or dysarthria which accompanies unilateral lesions of the nucleus ambiguus is rarely of a severe degree. The voice may be hoarse but speech is intelligible. Usually there is only slight difficulty in swallowing solid food, but occasionally there is a transient aphagia which will necessitate the administration of food by tube for a few days or weeks. On examination, the palate on the affected side is lax and the uvula deviates to the opposite side on phonation. The palatal reflex is absent on the affected side. Lesions of the nucleus ambiguus on both sides cause a complete aphonia and aphagia. Bilateral destruction of this nucleus is rare except in the terminal stages of amyotrophic lateral sclerosis.

Selective destruction of certain cells in the nucleus ambiguus may occur in the course of syringobulbia or intramedullary tumors and produce paralysis of the vocal cords in adduction. In such cases the patient can talk and swallow without difficulty, but there is inspiratory stridor and dyspnea which may be severe enough to require tracheotomy.

Unilateral lesions of the dorsal motor nucleus are not accompanied by any symptoms of autonomic dysfunction. Bilateral lesions are not compatible with life.

The nuclei of the tenth nerve may be damaged by inflammatory processes (especially acute anterior poliomyelitis), intramedullary tumors, syringobulbia, vascular lesions, demyelinizing diseases, and degenerative processes such as amyotrophic lateral sclerosis.

The nerve or its branches may be involved in polyneuritis, especially in the diphtheritic and so-called "infectious" forms, or compressed by tumors or aneurysms.

Injury to the pharyngeal branches of the nerve results in difficulty in swallowing. Lesions of the superior laryngeal nerve produce anesthesia of the upper part of the larynx and paralysis of the cricothyroid muscle. The voice is weak and soon tires. Involvement of the recurrent laryngeal nerve, which is frequent with aneurysms of the aorta and which occasionally occurs after operations in the neck, causes hoarseness and dysphonia as a result of paralysis of the vocal cords in the cadaveric position. Complete paralysis of both recurrent laryngeal nerves produces aphonia and inspiratory stridor. Partial bilateral paralysis may produce a paralysis of both abductors with severe dyspnea and inspiratory stridor but without any alteration in the voice.

Unilateral lesions of the vagus nerve do not produce any constant disturbance of the autonomic functions of the nerve. The heart rate may be unchanged, slowed or accelerated. The respiratory rhythm is not affected and there is no significant disturbance in the action of the gastrointestinal tract.

Eleventh (Spinal Accessory) Nerve. The spinal portion of the eleventh nerve innervates the sternomastoid and part or all of the trapezius muscles. The fibers from the accessory portion of the nerve have their origin in the nucleus ambiguus and join with the tenth to innervate the larynx. Paralysis of the spinal portion causes an atrophy of the sternomastoid muscle, and a partial atrophy of the trapezius muscles. There is weakness of the rotary movements of the head to the opposite side, and weakness of shrugging movements of the shoulder.

The nucleus of the eleventh nerve may be destroyed by inflammatory degenerative (syringobulbia, amyotrophic lateral sclerosis) and demyelinizing processes in the medulla. The peripheral portion of the nerve may be involved in general neuritides, by inflammatory processes in the meninges, extramedullary tumors, or by necrotic processes in the occipital bone. The muscles supplied by this nerve are frequently involved in the muscular dystrophies, especially in myotonia atrophica.

Twelfth (Hypoglossal) Nerve. The hypoglossal nerve is the motor nerve to the muscles of the tongue.

The nucleus in the medulla or the peripheral nerve may be injured by all the processes mentioned in connection with the tenth and eleventh nuclei. Occlusion of the short branches of the basilar artery which nourish the paramedian area of the medulla produces a paralysis of the tongue on one side and the arm and leg on the opposite side (alternating hemiplegia).

Unilateral injury to the nucleus or nerve results in atrophy and paralysis of the muscles of one half of the tongue. When the tongue is protruded it deviates toward the paralyzed side and while protruded movements toward the normal side are absent or weakly performed. When the tongue lies on the floor of the mouth it deviates slightly toward the healthy side and movement of the tongue toward the back of the mouth on this side are impaired. Fibrillation of the muscles is seen in chronic processes involving the hypoglossal nucleus (syringobulbia, amyotrophic lateral sclerosis).

Bilateral paralysis of the nucleus or nerve produces atrophy of both sides of the tongue and paralysis of all movements, with resultant difficulty in manipulating food in the process of eating and severe dysarthria, especially in the pronunciation of "linguals."

The tongue is only rarely affected with lesions in the cerebral hemispheres or the corticobulbar connections. Occasionally a homolateral weakness of the tongue may accompany severe hemiplegia. This is manifest by a slight deviation of the tongue to the paralyzed side when it is protruded. Moderate weakness of the tongue may accompany pseudobulbar paralysis but this is never as severe as that which occurs with destruction of both medullary nuclei.

Tremors of the tongue are seen in patients with chronic alcoholism. Apraxia of tongue, i.e., inability to protrude the tongue on command, but preservation of the associated movements in eating or licking the lips, is a frequent accompaniment of motor aphasia.

REFERENCES

Alter, M.: Familial Aggregation of Bell's Palsy, Arch. Neurol., 8, 557, 1963.
Amols, W.: A New Drug for Trigeminal Neuralgia (Clinical Experience with Carbamazepine in a Large Series of Patients over Two Years), Trans. Am. Neurol. Assoc., 91, 163, 1966.

Blau, J. N. et al.: Trigeminal Sensory Neuropathy, N. Engl. J. Med., *281*, 873, 1969.

Blom, S.: Tic Douloureux Treated with New Anticonvulsant, Arch. Neurol., *9*, 285, 1963.

Bohm, E., and Strang, R.R.: Glossopharyngeal Neuralgia, Brain, *85*, 371, 1962.

Boone, P. C.: Bell's Palsy, Acta Neurochirurgia, *7*, 16, 1959.

Braham, J., and Saia, A.: Phenytoin in the Treatment of Trigeminal and Other Neuralgias, Lancet, *2*, 892, 1960.

Cheek, C. W., et al.: Acquired Cranial Nerve Lesions Affecting the Ocular System, Am. J. Ophth., *59*, 13, 1965.

Cogan, D. G.: Neurology of the Ocular Muscles, 2nd ed., Springfield, Charles C Thomas, 1956, 295 pp.

———: Neurology of the Visual System, Springfield, Charles C Thomas, 1966, 413 pp.

Dunphy, E. B.: Alcohol-Tobacco Ambylopia; A Historical Survey, Am. J. Ophth., *68*, 569, 1969.

Earl, C. J. and Martin, B.: Progress in Optic Neuritis Related to Age, Lancet, *1*, 74, 1967.

Ekbom, K. A., and Westerberg, C.E.: Carbamazepine in Glossopharyngeal Neuralgia, Arch. Neurol., *14*, 595, 1966.

Ellenberg, C., and Netsky, M. C.: Infarction in the Optic Nerve, J. Neurol. Neurosurg. and Psychiat., *31*. 606, 1968.

Friedman, A. P., and Merritt, H. H.: Damage to Cranial Nerves Resulting from Head Injury, Bull. Los Angeles Neurol. Soc., *9*, 135, 1944.

Green, W. R., Hackett, E. R., and Schlezinger, N. S.: Neuro-Ophthalmologic Evaluation of Oculomotor Nerve Paralysis, Arch. Ophth., *72*, 154, 1964.

Hierons, R., and Lyle, T. K.: Bilateral Retrobulbar Optic Neuritis, Brain, *82*, 56, 1959.

Hassler, R., and Walker, A. E.: Trigeminal Neuralgia, Philadelphia, W. B. Saunders Co., 1970.

Killiam, J. M., and Fromm, G. H.: Carbamazepine in the Treatment of Neuralgia, Arch. Neurol., *19*, 129, 1968.

Konigsmark, B. G.: Hereditary Deafness in Man, N. Engl. J. Med., *281*, 713, 714 and 827, 1969.

Korczyn, A. D.: Bell's Palsy and Diabetes Mellitus, Lancet, *1*, 108, 1971.

Lerman, S., and Feldmahn, A. L.: Centrocecal Scotomata as the Presenting Sign in Pernicious Anemia, Arch. Ophth., *65*, 381, 1961.

Miller, G. R. and Smith, J. L.: Ischemic Optic Neuritis, Am. J. Ophth., *62*, 103, 1966.

Miller, H.: Facial Paralysis, Br. Med. J., *3*, 815, 1967.

Nosik, W. A., and Weil, A. A.: Selective Partial Neurectomy in Hemifacial Spasm and the Electrophysiologic Selection of Patients, J. Neurosurg., *13*, 596, 1956.

Robertson, D. M., Hines, J. D. and Rucker, C. W.: Acquired Sixth Nerve Paresis in Children, Arch. Ophth., *83*, 574, 1970.

Schwartz, J. F., Chutorian, A. M., Evans, R. A., and Carter, S.: Optic Atrophy in Childhood, Pediatrics, *34*, 670, 1964.

Spillane, J. D., and Wells, C. E. C.: Isolated Trigeminal Neuropathy, Brain, *82*, 391, 1959.

Stevens, H.: Melkersson's Syndrome, Neurology, *15*, 263, 1965.

Symonds, C.: Recurrent Multiple Cranial Nerve Palsies, J. Neurol., Neurosurg. & Psychiat., *21*, 95, 1958.

Victor, M., and Dreyfus, P. M.: Tobacco-Alcohol Amblyopia. Further Comments on its Pathology, Arch. Ophth., *74*, 649, 1965.

Walsh, F. B., and Gass, J. D.: Concerning the Optic Chiasm, Am. J. Ophth., *50*, 1031, 1960.

Weber, R. B., Daroff, R. B. and Mackey, E. A.: Pathology of Oculomotor Nerve Palsy in Diabetics, Neurology, *20*, 835, 1970.

Peripheral Nerves

The peripheral nerves are subject to injury by pressure, constriction by fascial bands, and by trauma associated with injection of drugs, perforating wounds, fractures of the bones and stretching of the nerves. Isolated or multiple nerve paralyses may also be associated with a reaction to the injection of sera or with certain toxic or metabolic disturbances.

The radial, common peroneal, ulnar and the long thoracic are the nerves most commonly subject to damage by external pressure. The median nerve is most frequently affected by constriction by fascial bands. The axillary nerve is commonly affected in an allergic reaction to injections of serum, and the sciatic by direct injection of drugs. Any of the peripheral nerves may be damaged by perforating wounds or fractures of the bones. The frequency of the involvement of the peripheral nerves by trauma is shown in Table 54.

Radial Nerve. The radial nerve arises from the posterior secondary trunk of the brachial plexus (C5 to C8). It is predominantly a motor nerve and innervates the chief extensors of the forearm, wrist and fingers (Table 55).

The radial nerve may be injured by cuts or gunshot wounds, by callus formation after fracture of the humerus, by the pressure of crutches or by pressure against some hard surface especially in sleep ("Saturday night palsy").

Table 54.   The Incidence of Peripheral Nerve Lesions by Trauma

(After Woodhall and Beebe, *Peripheral Nerve Regeneration, A Follow-Up Study of 3,656 World War II Injuries,* Veterans Administration Medical Monographs, Washington, 1956)

Nerve	No. of Cases	%
Median	707	19.3
Radial	516	14.1
Ulnar	1000	27.4
Musculocutaneous	44	1.2
Axillary	9	.2
Sciatic-Peroneal	404	11.1
Sciatic-Tibial	394	10.8
Peroneal	341	9.3
Tibial	235	6.4
Femoral	6	0.2
	3656	100.0

Table 55.   Muscles Innervated by the Radial Nerve

In the Arm	In the Forearm
Triceps	Extensor digitorum
Anconeus	Extensor digiti minimi
Extensor carpi radialis longus	Extensor carpi ulnaris
Extensor carpi radialis brevis	Abductor pollicis longus
Brachioradialis	Extensor pollicis brevis
	Extensor indicis

A complete lesion of the nerve in the axilla is characterized by paralysis of the triceps and abolition of the triceps reflex in addition to the other signs of radial nerve palsy which are discussed below. Lesions of the radial nerve in the axilla are usually accompanied by evidence of injury to other nerves in this region. When the nerve is injured in the posteromedial surface of the arm, one or more of its branches to the triceps may be spared so that weakness of extension of the forearm is minimal.

The most common site of injury to the radial nerve is in the middle third of the arm proximal to the branch to the brachioradialis muscle. Lesions of the nerve at this level result in: Weakness of flexion of the forearm due to the paralysis of the brachioradialis muscle, which is a stronger flexor of the forearm than the biceps; and a paralysis of extension of the wrist, the thumb and of the fingers at the proximal joints. Extension at the distal phalanges is performed by the interossei. There is weakness of adduction of the hand as a result of loss of action of the extensor carpi ulnaris and a loss of supination when the forearm is extended since the supinating action of the biceps is evident only when the forearm is flexed. In addition, there is an apparent weakness of flexion of the fingers. This weakness is not real and is due to the faulty posture of the hand. If the wrist is passively extended, it will be seen that the fingers have normal power of flexion.

Sensory loss associated with lesions of the radial nerve is slight and is confined in most cases to a small area on the posterior radial surface of the hand and the first and second metacarpals of the thumb, index and middle fingers.

Lesions of the nerve or its branches in the forearm or wrist are accompanied by fragments of the syndrome described above, according to the site of the lesion.

Complete lesions of the radial nerve are followed by atrophy of the paralyzed muscles. Vasomotor or trophic disturbances are rare unless there is an associated vascular lesion. Causalgia may rarely follow partial injury to the nerve.

Median Nerve. The median nerve is composed of fibers from the sixth, seventh and eighth cervical and first thoracic roots. It arises in two heads, an outer and inner, which are derived from the upper and lower secondary trunks of the brachial plexus. It has important motor and sensory functions. The movements controlled by this nerve are: Pronation of the forearm by the pronator quadratus and the pronator radii teres; flexion of the hand by the flexor carpi radialis and palmaris longus; flexion of the thumb, index and middle fingers by the superficial and deep flexors; and opposition of the thumb (Table 56).

The sensory region of the median nerve comprises the radial side of the palm of the hand, the palmar surface of the thumb, index, middle

Table 56.   Muscles Innervated by the Median Nerve

In the Forearm	Forearm (continued)
Pronator teres	Pronatus quadratus
Flexor carpi radialis	
Palmaris longus	In the Hand
Flexor digitorum sublimis	Abductor pollicis brevis
Flexor digitorum profundus	Flexor pollicis brevis
(radial half)	Opponens pollicis
Flexor pollicis longus	First and second lumbricales

and neighboring half of the ring finger, the dorsal surface of the middle and terminal phalanges of the index fingers, and the radial half of the ring finger.

The median nerve may be injured by dislocation of the shoulder, perforating wounds of the arm or pressure by a tourniquet. It may be cut at the wrist by glass or by attempts at suicide, and by constriction in the carpal tunnel.

Injury to the median nerve in the arm is characterized by: Loss of ability to pronate the forearm; weakness of flexion of the wrist; paralysis of flexion of the thumb and index finger; weakness of flexion of the middle finger; paralysis of opposition of the thumb; atrophy of the muscles of the thenar eminence; and loss of sensation in an area somewhat smaller than that of the anatomical distribution of the nerve.

Lesions of the nerve at the wrist cause a paralysis and atrophy of the thenar muscles and sensory loss in the characteristic distribution.

There is absolute paralysis of very few movements of the wrist or fingers in isolated lesions of the median nerve because of the compensatory action of unparalyzed muscles. Pronation can be accomplished by the action of the deltoid in holding the arm outward when the forearm is flexed and by rotation of the arm inward by the subscapularis when the arm is extended. Flexion of the wrist can be performed by the action of the flexor carpi ulnaris, with deviation of the hand toward the ulnar side of the arm. There is absence of flexion in the index finger and the middle finger although the latter finger is usually influenced by movements of the ring finger and its deep flexor may be supplied by the ulnar nerve. In addition, flexion of the proximal phalanx of the fingers, including the index in association with extension of the distal phalanges, is possible through the action of the interossei. Although the opponens pollicis is paralyzed, feeble movements of opposition can be made by energetic contraction of the adductors which cause the thumb to move to the ulnar edge of the hand by pressing against the base of the fingers.

Partial lesions of the median nerve are more frequent than complete interruption, with dissociation in the degree of involvement of the various muscles supplied by the nerve and with little or no sensory loss. Flexion of the index finger and opposition of the thumb are the movements which are usually most affected in partial lesions.

Vasomotor disturbances are common with median nerve lesions, probably due to associated lesions of blood vessels. The syndrome of causalgia is most commonly associated with lesions of the median nerve.

A slowly developing atrophy limited to the muscles of the outer radial side of the thenar eminence has been described by the term *partial thenar atrophy.* The atrophy is often bilateral and is in excess of the motor weakness. Pain, paresthesia, and a mild degree of impairment of sensation in the distribution of the nerves, with or without motor weakness are fairly common as result of compression of the nerve by the transverse carpal segment. The pains are quite severe awaking the patients from sleep and causing them to shake the hand vigorously to relieve the pain. The pain is usually in the thumb and index finger, but may at times spread to the other fingers of the hand or up the arm to the axilla. These symptoms, described by the term carpal tunnel syndrome, occur most commonly in middle age and are often associated with arthritis or other inflammatory changes in the tendons and connective tissues of wrists and with amyloid disease, myxedema, gout and acromegaly. Surgical division of the transverse ligament results in relief of the pains and paresthesia and gradual decrease in the motor loss if this has developed.

Ulnar Nerve. The ulnar nerve is the main branch of the lower secondary trunk of the brachial plexus. The fibers arise from the eighth cervical and first thoracic segments. The motor fibers innervate the muscles shown in Table 57. The sensory portion of the nerve supplies the skin on the palmar and dorsal surfaces of the little, inner half of the ring finger, and the ulnar side of the hand.

The ulnar nerve is frequently injured by gunshot wounds, direct stabs, fractures of the lower end of the humerus, olecranon or head of the radius. The nerve may be compressed in the axilla by a cervical rib.

Table 57. Muscles Innervated by the Ulnar Nerve

In the Forearm	Hand (continued)
Flexor carpi ulnaris	Interossei
Flexor digitorum profundus	Third and fourth lumbricales
(ulnar half)	Palmaris brevis
	Abductor digiti minimi
In the Hand	Opponens digiti minimi
Adductor pollicis	Flexor digiti minimi
Flexor pollicis brevis	Lumbricalis (ulnar half)

More frequently it is compressed at the elbow in sleep or as an occupational neuritis in workers who rest their elbows on hard surfaces for prolonged periods.

Complete lesions of the ulnar nerve are characterized by: Weakness of flexion and adduction of the wrist and of flexion of the ring and little fingers; paralysis of abduction and opposition of the little finger; paralysis of adduction of the thumb; and paralysis of adduction and abduction of the fingers. There is atrophy of the hypothenar muscles and the interossei. The latter is especially obvious between the thumb and index finger on the dorsal surface of the hand. Sensory loss is greatest in the little finger and to a lesser extent on the inner side of the ring finger. There is clawing of the hand.

Dissociated paralysis of the muscles supplied by the ulnar nerve may occur with partial lesions of the nerve in the arm or forearm.

Trophic and vasomotor symptoms are not a prominent feature of complete lesions of the nerve. There may be some hyperkeratosis or changes in the palmar fascia. "Irritative" lesions may be accompanied by pain but injuries to the ulnar nerve are only rarely accompanied by causalgia.

The diagnosis of ulnar palsy can usually be made without difficulty from the posture of the hand which is always clawed to a more or less degree, the atrophy of the hypothenar eminence and the first dorsal interosseous space, and the characteristic muscular paralysis. One of the diagnostic signs of ulnar palsy, known as Froment's sign, is flexion of the terminal phalanx of the thumb when the patient attempts to hold a paper between the thumb and index finger.

Musculocutaneous Nerve. The musculocutaneous nerve is the main branch of the upper secondary trunk of the brachial plexus. Its fibers arise in the fifth, sixth and seventh cervical segments. The musculocutaneous nerve is a mixed nerve, innervating the coracobrachialis, biceps brachii and brachialis anticus muscles and transmitting cutaneous sensation from the anterior outer part and a small area on the posterior outer surface of the forearm. Isolated injuries of the nerve are rare. It may be involved in traumatic lesions of the brachial plexus.

Lesions of the musculocutaneous nerve produce: Weakness of flexion and supination of the forearm; a small area of hypesthesia or anesthesia on the anterior outer surface of the forearm; atrophy of the muscles on the anterior surface of the arm; and loss of biceps reflex.

Flexor movements of the forearm can still be vigorously performed by the brachioradialis muscle, which is innervated by the radial nerve. If flexion is performed against resistance, it can be noted by palpation that the biceps muscle is inactive. If the forearm is kept in supination, forearm flexion is impossible. Since the biceps is the chief supinator of the forearm, this movement is paralyzed. Loss of function of the coracobrachialis muscle is compensated for by the action of other adductor muscles of the arm.

Axillary Nerve. The axillary nerve, a branch of the posterior secondary cord of the plexus with fibers from the fifth and sixth cervical segments innervates the deltoid muscle and transmits cutaneous sensation from a small area on the lateral surface of the shoulder.

Lesions of the axillary nerve by trauma or by fractures or dislocation of the head of the humerus are usually associated with injury to the brachial plexus. The axillary nerve may be involved alone or in combination with other nerves in the neuritis which follows serum (especially anti-tetanus) therapy.

Lesions of the axillary nerve are characterized by a loss of power in outward, backward and forward movements of the arm due to paralysis of the deltoid muscle. The area of hypesthesia or anesthesia is inconstant and is much smaller than the anatomical distribution of the nerve.

Long Thoracic Nerve. The long thoracic nerve arising from the fifth, sixth and seventh cervical roots is the motor nerve to the serratus magnus muscle.

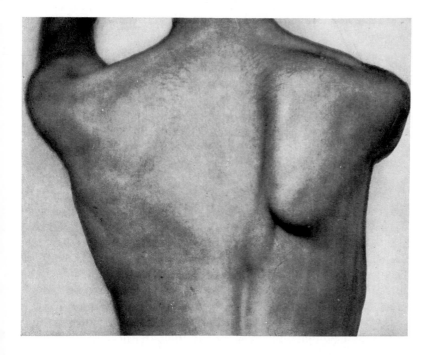

Figure 97. Paralysis of serratus magnus muscle with winging of the scapula.

Lesions of the nerve are most common in men who do heavy labor. It may be injured by continued muscular effort with the arm extended or by carrying heavy, sharp cornered objects on the shoulder (hod carrier's palsy).

Injury to the nerve following acute or chronic trauma is characterized by weakness in elevation of the arm above the horizontal plane. Winging of the scapula is a constant sign when the arm is fully abducted or elevated anteriorly (Fig. 97). Winging is usually absent when the arm is held at the side.

Brachial Cutaneous and Antebrachial Cutaneous Nerves. The brachial and antebrachial cutaneous nerves, branches of the lower secondary trunk of the plexus (C8 T1), are purely sensory in function. They transmit cutaneous sensation from the inner surface of the arm and upper two thirds of the forearm.

These nerves are rarely affected except in injuries of the lower secondary trunk of the brachial plexus. Lesions of these nerves produce hypesthesia on the inner surface of the arm and forearm.

Suprascapular Nerve. The suprascapular nerve arises from the posterior surface of the outer trunk of the brachial plexus, most of its fibers coming from the fifth and sixth cervical roots. It is primarily motor and innervates the supraspinatus and infraspinatus muscles.

Isolated lesions of the nerve are rare. It may be wounded directly, injured in falls or stretched by muscular overaction. It may be involved in association with the axillary nerve in serum reactions or it may be injured in traumatic lesions of the brachial plexus.

Lesions of the nerve produce an atrophic paralysis of the supra- and infraspinatus muscles. Weakness of movements performed by these muscles, i.e., abduction of the shoulder and external rotation of the shoulder, is masked by the action of the deltoid and teres minor muscles.

Lesions of the Brachial Plexus. The fourth, fifth, sixth, seventh and eighth cervical and the first dorsal root contribute to the formation of the brachial plexus (Fig. 98). These roots intermingle to form three primary trunks (upper, middle and lower). The upper primary trunk is composed of fibers from the fourth, fifth and sixth cervical roots; the middle primary trunk from the seventh cervical; and the lower primary trunk from the eighth cervical and first thoracic roots. From the primary trunks there is further redistribution of the fibers which results in the formation of secondary trunks or cords (upper, posterior and lower). The secondary trunks contribute to the formation of the peripheral nerves of the upper extremity as follows: Upper secondary trunk—the musculocutaneous nerve and the outer head of the median; posterior trunk—the axillary and radial nerves; lower secondary—the brachial and antebrachial cutaneous nerves, the ulnar and the inner head of the median.

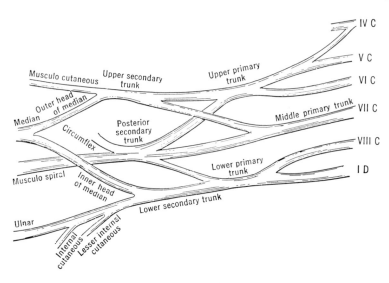

Figure 98. Brachial plexus. (Tinel, J.: *Nerve Wounds*, courtesy Baillière, Tindall & Cox.)

In addition to these major nerves which are formed by fibers in the secondary trunks, collateral branches from the roots and trunks form nerves which innervate the shoulder and scapular muscles, as well as supplying fibers to the inferior cervical ganglion.

From the arrangement of the plexus it is obvious that trauma will affect different groups of nerve fibers according to the site of the lesion. Lesions in the axilla, where all the fibers converge, will affect several trunks. Isolated trunk lesions are more apt to occur when the injury is in the supraclavicular fossa.

The roots or trunks of the brachial plexus may be damaged by cuts, gunshot wounds, or direct trauma. They may be compressed by tumors or aneurysms or stretched and torn by violent movements of the shoulder in falls, dislocations of the shoulder, the carrying of heavy packs on the shoulder (rucksack paralysis) and by traction in delivery in birth.

Various and complex syndromes result from injuries to the plexus. The number of combinations of motor paralysis and sensory loss are great, but several root and trunk syndromes are relatively frequent. Only the latter will be discussed. A minute examination of muscular and sensory disability must be made and studied in connection with anatomic charts of the plexus to determine the site of the lesion and whether the fibers have been injured at their point of emergence from the spinal cord or after the formation of the primary or secondary trunks (Tables 58, 59, 60).

RADICULAR SYNDROMES (ROOTS AND PRIMARY TRUNKS). The syndromes of the roots and primary trunks are essentially those of the roots involved, but partial paralysis and incomplete sensory loss are common since many muscles of the upper extremity receive innervation from two or more roots, and there are extensive substitutions between the various roots.

Table 58.   Innervation of the Important Muscles of the Shoulder Girdle

Muscle	Nerve	Roots
Sternocleidomastoid	Spinal accessory	XI, C2, C3
Trapezius	Spinal accessory	C3, C4
Deltoid	Axillary	C5, C6
Pectoralis major	Ext. and int. ant. thoracic	C5-T2
Pectoralis minor	Ext. and int. ant. thoracic	C7-T2
Serratus magnus	Long thoracic	C5-C7
Levator anguli scapulae	Dorsal scapular	C5
Rhomboideus major	Dorsal scapular	C5
Rhomboideus minor	Dorsal scapular	C5
Latissimus dorsi	Long subscapular	C7, C8
Coracobrachialis	Musculocutaneous	C7
Supraspinatus	Suprascapular	C5, C6
Infraspinatus	Suprascapular	C5, C6
Teres major	Lower subscapular	C5, C6
Teres minor	Axillary	C5, C6
Subscapularis	Upper and lower subscapular	C5, C6

Table 59.   Innervation of the Important Muscles of the Arm and Forearm

Muscle	Nerve	Root
Biceps	Musculocutaneous	C5, C6
Brachialis anticus	{ Musculocutaneous	C5, C6
	{ Radial	C5, C6
Triceps	Radial	C6-C8
Anconeus	Radial	C7, C8
Pronator radii teres	Median	C6
Flexor carpi radialis	Median	C6
Palmaris longus	Median	C6
Flexor carpi ulnaris	Ulnar	C8
Flexor sublimis digitorum	Median	C7-T1
Flexor profundus digitorum	Median, Ulnar	C7-T1
Pronator quadratus	Median	C8, T1
Brachioradialis	Radial	C5, C6
Extensor carpi radialis	Radial	C6, C7
Extensor communis digitorum	Radial	C6-C8
Extensor digiti minimi	Radial	C6-C8
Extensor carpi ulnaris	Radial	C6-C8
Extensor longus pollicis	Radial	C6-C8
Extensor brevis pollicis	Radial	C6-C8
Extensor indicis	Radial	C7, C8

Table 60. Innervation of the Muscles of the Hand

Muscle	Nerve	Root
Palmaris brevis	Ulnar	T1
Abductor pollicis	Median	C6, C7
Opponens pollicis	Median	C6, C7
Flexor brevis pollicis	Median	C6, C7
Abductor digiti minimi	Ulnar	C8, T1
Opponens digiti minimi	Ulnar	C8, T1
Flexor brevis digiti minimi	Ulnar	C8, T1
Lumbricales	Median, Ulnar	C6-T1
Abductor pollicis	Ulnar	C8, T1
Interossei palmaris	Ulnar	C8, T1
Interossei dorsales	Ulnar	C8, T1

Upper Radicular (Erb-Duchenne) Syndrome. Lesions of the upper roots (fourth, fifth and sixth cervical roots or upper primary trunk) are characterized by paralysis of the deltoid, biceps, brachialis anticus, brachioradialis, pectoralis major, supraspinatus, infraspinatus, subscapularis and teres major muscles. If the lesion is near the roots, the serratus magnus, rhomboids and levator anguli scapulae are also paralyzed. In addition, there is partial paralysis of the muscles supplied by the radial nerve because the upper primary trunk contributes to the formation of this nerve.

The motor disability resulting from lesions of the upper radicular group is essentially a paralysis of flexion of the forearm, abduction, internal and external rotation of the arm, as well as weakness or paralysis of apposition of the shoulder blade and backward-inward movements of the arm. The sensory loss is incomplete and consists of a hypesthesia on the outer surface of the arm and forearm. The biceps reflex is absent and percussion of the styloid process of the radius produces a flexion of the fingers instead of the normal flexion of the forearm.

Middle Radicular Syndrome. Injury to the seventh cervical root or the middle primary trunk produces a paralysis of the muscles supplied by the radial nerve with the exception of the brachioradialis, which is spared entirely, and the triceps, which is only partially paralyzed since it receives partial innervation from the upper primary trunk.

The motor weakness is essentially similar to that seen in paralysis of the radial nerve below the origin of the fibers to the brachioradialis or in lead palsy. Sensory loss is inconstant and when present is limited to hypesthesia over the dorsal surface of the forearm and the external part of the dorsal surface of the hand.

Lower Radicular (Klumpke) Syndrome. Injury to the lower primary trunk or eighth cervical and first thoracic root is characterized by paralysis of the flexor carpi ulnaris, the flexor digitorum, the interossei, the thenar and hypothenar muscles. The motor disability is similar to that of a combined lesion of the median and ulnar nerves with a flattened hand or simian griffe.

The sensory disturbance is a hypesthesia on the inner side of the arm, forearm and the ulnar side of the hand. The triceps reflex is abolished. If the communicating branch to the inferior cervical ganglion is injured, there will be paralysis of the sympathetics, with resulting Horner's syndrome.

SECONDARY TRUNK SYNDROMES. Lesions of the secondary trunks of the brachial plexus produce motor and sensory disturbances which closely resemble those which are seen with injuries to two or more peripheral nerves.

The syndrome of the upper secondary trunk is a combination of the signs and symptoms which result from injury to the musculocutaneous nerve and the outer head of the median. Injuries to the latter are accompanied by a paralysis of the pronator radii teres, almost complete paralysis of the flexor carpi radialis and weakness of the flexor pollicis and opponens.

Injury to the posterior secondary trunk produces a paralysis similar to that which results from injury to the radial and axillary nerves.

The syndrome of the lower secondary trunk is the same as that of the ulnar nerve combined with a paralysis of flexion of the fingers as a result of injury to the inner head of the median nerve.

Ischemic Paralysis of the Upper Limb. Paralysis of the muscles of upper extremity may follow injury to the large arteries of the arm. Ischemic paralysis may follow ligation of the major vessels when the collateral circulation is inadequate or it may follow prolonged constriction of the upper extremity by plaster casts.

In the initial stages of ischemic paralysis the distal part of the extremity is cyanotic and edematous. Active movements of the finger and wrist muscles are possible but are of a limited range. There is a diminution in the cutaneous sensibility and all stimuli are poorly localized and have a painful quality. With the passage of time, the cyanosis and edema disappear, the skin becomes smooth and shiny, and the muscles undergo fibrotic changes, and there is an anesthesia which extends in a glove-like distribution to the wrist or middle of the forearm. The hand is held extended and the fingers slightly flexed except when there are associated nerve lesions.

Ischemic paralysis can be differentiated from that due to lesions of the nerves by the absence of pulsations in the radial artery, the glove-like distribution of sensory loss, which does not correspond to that of any peripheral nerve, the fibrous consistency of the tissues and in some cases, by the persistence of feeble, imperfect movements of some of the muscles.

Ischemic paralysis is frequently permanent. Improvement in some cases can be obtained by hot baths, massage, passive movements and electrical stimulation.

Obturator Nerve. The obturator nerve is a mixed nerve which originates in the lumbar plexus from the second, third and fourth lumbar roots. It transmits cutaneous sensation from a small area on the inner surface of the middle side of hip, thigh and knee joint. It innervates the obturator externus muscle, the adductor longus, adductor brevis, gracilis and adductor magnus muscles.

Lesions of the obturator nerve are uncommon. It may be injured by pressure within the pelvis by tumors, obturator hernias or by the fetal head in difficult labor.

Injuries to the obturator nerve results in a severe weakness of adduction and, to a lesser extent, of internal and external rotation of the thigh. Pain in the knee joint is sometimes caused by pelvic involvement of the geniculate branch of the obturator.

Iliohypogastric Nerve. The iliohypogastric nerve is a mixed nerve which originates from the uppermost part of the lumbar plexus and is derived from the twelfth thoracic and first lumbar root. It transmits cutaneous sensation from the outer and upper part of the buttocks and the lower part of the abdomen and supplies partial innervation to the internal oblique and transversalis muscles. Lesions of the iliohypogastric nerve are rare. It may be divided by incisions in kidney operations or together with the iliolingual nerve in operations in the inguinal region. Lesions of these nerves do not produce any significant motor loss and there is only a small area of cutaneous anesthesia.

Ilioinguinal Nerve. The ilioinguinal nerve, a branch of the lumbar plexus, arises from the twelfth thoracic and first lumbar roots. It transmits cutaneous sensation from the upper inner portion of the thigh, the pubic region and the external genitalia. Motor filaments are given off to the transversalis, internal oblique and external oblique muscles. The ilioinguinal is usually injured in connection with the iliohypogastric.

Genitofemoral Nerve. This nerve, which originates from the second lumbar root, is primarily a sensory nerve. It transmits cutaneous sensation from an oval area on the thigh in the region of Scarpa's triangle and from the scrotum and the contiguous area of the inner surface of the thigh. Lesions of the genitofemoral nerve are rare. Irritative lesions of the nerve in the abdominal wall are accompanied by painful hyperesthesia at the root of the thigh and the scrotum.

Lateral Cutaneous Nerve of Thigh. This nerve is formed by fibers from the second and third lumbar roots. It crosses beneath the fascia iliaca to emerge at the anterior superior iliac spine, descends in the thigh beneath the fascia lata and divides into two branches. The posterior branch passes obliquely backward through the fascia lata and transmits cutaneous sensation from the superior external part of the buttocks. The anterior branch, which is more important clinically, pierces the fascia lata through a small fibrous canal about 4 inches below the ligament and transmits cutaneous fibrous sensation from the outer surface of the thigh.

The anterior portion of the nerve is occasionally the site of a sensory mononeuritis, known as *meralgia paresthetica*, with dysesthesias in the nature of tingling, burning, prickling, or pins and needles sensations, with or without sensory loss, in the cutaneous distribution of the nerve. Its long superficial course exposes it to various forms of trauma, but in the majority of the cases there is no history of trauma to explain the onset of symptoms. Various factors which are said to play a contributing role include pressure of tight belts or corsets and intermittent stretching by extensor movements of the thigh in walking. The involvement is unilateral in the vast majority of cases. Men are affected approximately three times as frequently as women.

The diagnosis is not difficult when the dysesthesias are limited to the distribution of the anterior division of the nerve. Pains in the lateral surface of the thigh due to spinal lesions or tumors in the pelvis must be excluded by appropriate diagnostic studies.

The course of meralgia paresthetica is quite variable. Occasionally the symptoms disappear spontaneously after a few weeks. In the vast majority of cases, they will clear up by the removal of tight belts and avoidance of excessive walking. Rarely, it may be necessary to split the fascia lata at the point of emergence of the nerve or correct the angulation of the nerve at the iliac spine.

Femoral Nerve. The femoral nerve arises from the second, third and fourth lumbar nerves. It innervates the iliacus, the psoas magnus, the pectineus, adductor longus, sartorius and quadriceps femoris muscles. It also transmits cutaneous sensation from the anterior surface of the thigh, and by its internal saphenous branch, from the entire inner surface of the leg and the anterior internal surface of the knee.

Traumatic lesions of the femoral nerve are relatively uncommon. It may be compressed by tumors and other lesions in the pelvis or it may be injured by fractures of the pubic ramus or femur. Not infrequently there is no adequate explanation for the occurrence of an isolated femoral nerve palsy. In such cases it is presumed that the lesion of the nerve is due to some toxic factor: diabetes, typhoid, gout, and the like.

Injury to the femoral nerve produces a paralysis of extension of the leg and weakness of flexion of the thigh. When the patient stands erect the leg is held stiffly extended by contraction of the tensor fasciae femoris and the gracilis. Walking on level ground is possible as long as the leg can be kept extended, but if the slightest flexion occurs, the patient sinks down on the suddenly flexed knee. Climbing stairs or walking uphill is difficult or impossible. The quadriceps reflex is lost on the affected side and cutaneous sensation is impaired in an area somewhat smaller than the anatomical distribution of the nerve.

Paralysis of the femoral nerve must be distinguished from hysterical paralysis and reflex muscular atrophies which follow fractures of the femur or lesions of the knee joint. Hysterical paralysis can be diagnosed by the presence of the knee jerk and by special tests. In hysterical paralysis, when the patient is in the recumbent position and attempts to elevate the "paralyzed" limb, there is an absence of the normal fixing movements (downward pressure of the heel) of the opposite extremity.

Orthopedic appliances, which fix the knee joint in extension, are of value in the treatment of femoral nerve paralysis. Transplantation of tendons should be considered when the paralysis persists.

Sciatic Nerve. The sciatic nerve is the largest nerve in the body. Its terminal branches consist of two distinct nerves, antagonists of each other: the common peroneal (external popliteal) and the tibial (internal popliteal) nerves. The former nerve arises from the posterior and the latter from the anterior portion of the sacral plexus (segments L4 to S3). The main trunk of the sciatic nerve innervates the semitendinosus, the long and short heads of the biceps, the adductor magnus and the semimembranosus. The terminal branches of the nerve are considered separately below.

Total paralysis of the sciatic nerve is rare; even with lesion in the thigh the common peroneal nerve is often more severely damaged than the tibial nerve. The sciatic nerve is frequently injured by gunshot, shrapnel or stab wounds. It is only rarely injured in civil life. Partial rupture may result from violent muscular contractions, or the nerve may be injured by fractures of the pelvis or femur, dislocations of the hip, pressure of the fetal head on the plexus in the pelvis, or by tumors in the pelvis. The nerve is occasionally inadvertently injured by intramuscular injection of drugs especially in infants.

Total involvement of the sciatic nerve produces complete paralysis of all movements of the ankle and toes, and weakness or paralysis of flexion of the leg. The patient can stand, but in walking the leg must be raised unduly high to correct for the foot drop. The ankle jerk is lost and cutaneous sensation is lost on the outer surface of the leg, on the instep and sole of the foot and over the toes. Vasomotor and trophic disturbances may also be present.

Sciatica. The sciatic nerve is the seat of a neuralgic disturbance known as *sciatica*. This term is loosely used to describe pains which occur in the lower back and in the leg along the course of the nerve. The term merely describes a set of symptoms which may be due to involvement of any portion of the nerve, including its intraspinal roots.

The concept of the etiology of sciatica has changed with the elucidation of the syndrome of the ruptured intervertebral disc. In the older literature the list of causes of sciatica was long and included: So-called toxic infectious processes, such as alcohol, arsenic, lead, diabetes, gout, syphilis, gonorrhea, phlebitis, and tuberculosis; arthritis of sacroiliac joint; arthritis of the hip; fibrositis; gluteal bursitis; osteitis deformans; sacralization of the fifth lumbar vertebra; pelvic tumors; and an inflammatory neuritis of the nerve. While pains in the lower back which extend down the posterior surface of the leg may be associated with various pathological processes in the pelvis and lower portion of the spine, in the majority of cases the pains are due to a ruptured intervertebral disc. In a lesser number the symptoms are due to arthritis of the sacroiliac joint or spine. The general symptoms and signs of sciatica are discussed below. The distinctive features of ruptured intervertebral discs are considered more fully elsewhere.

Sciatica is most common in the third to sixth decade and occurs about three times as frequently in the male as in the female sex. The pain of sciatica varies greatly in severity. In some cases, it consists of a feeling of discomfort in the lower back and down the posterior surface of the leg. In others, the pain may be so intense as to totally incapacitate the afflicted individual. The pain may be limited to the buttocks and sacroiliac region; it may extend only to the knee; or it may involve the calf and outer surface of the foot. There is usually no weakness, but the patient may keep the knee slightly flexed in walking to prevent stretching of the nerve. On examination the nerve may be sensitive to pressure at any point along its course. Any movement of the lower extremity which stretches the nerve is accompanied by pain and involuntary resistance to the movement. There is limitation of straight leg raising on the affected side and complete extension of the leg is not possible when the thigh is flexed on the abdomen. Similar movements of the unaffected limb can be more fully performed but may produce slight pain on the opposite side. Sensory loss and diminution or loss of the Achilles reflex are rarely found in the sciatica associated with osteoarthritis of the spine or sacroiliac joint and suggest involvement of the nerve roots in the spinal canal.

The clinical course of sciatica is dependent on the nature of the underlying pathological process. In the majority of cases, the symptoms last for several weeks or months and disappear, to recur after a remission of several months or years.

The diagnosis of the cause of pain in the lower back and along the course of the sciatic nerve presents one of the most difficult problems in neurology. A thorough study is usually necessary. This must include an x-ray examination of the hips, pelvis, sacroiliac joint and the lumbosacral spine, examination of the cerebrospinal fluid and in selected cases, myelography. Only by the results of these studies can it be determined with any degree of accuracy whether the symptoms are due to a ruptured intervertebral disc, to a primary or metastatic tumor of the spine, to osteoarthritic changes or other causes.

The treatment of sciatica is essentially that of the underlying cause. The criteria for the operative removal of ruptured intervertebral discs are discussed elsewhere. Sciatica associated with osteoarthritis of the spine or sacroiliac joint is treated by complete rest in bed for a period of several weeks. Traction on the affected leg often lessens the pain and speeds recovery, but occasionally this cannot be tolerated. Radiant heat can be applied by means of electric light bulbs in a cradle over the legs. Analgesic drugs such as aspirin or codeine may be used. With subsidence of pain the patient should be allowed out of bed and to assume gradually usual activities. A back brace can be worn during the waking hours and the bed should have a firm mattress. Injection of the nerve or the epidural space with anesthetic solutions which were quite widely used in the past is rarely necessary at the present time. The treatment of causalgic pains following trauma to the sciatic nerve is discussed on page 414.

COMMON PERONEAL (EXTERNAL POPLITEAL) NERVE. The common peroneal is a mixed nerve which innervates the extensor muscles of the ankle and toes, and the evertors (abductors) of the foot. It transmits cutaneous sensation from the outer side of the leg, the front of its lower third, the instep and the dorsal surface of the four inner toes over their proximal phalanges.

The common peroneal nerve is more frequently subject to trauma than any other nerve of the body. It may be damaged by gunshot wounds in the region of the knee or in the trunk of the sciatic nerve in the thigh.Owing to its superficial position in close relation to the head and neck of the fibula it is injured readily by pressure against hard objects while the patient is asleep, intoxicated or under an anesthetic. It may be stretched by prolonged squatting, compressed in crossing the knees while sitting or by a hard or uneven mattress during sleep, especially in acutely or chronically ill patients. Many cases of simple pressure neuritis of the common peroneal nerve are falsely recorded in literature as being due to such conditions as malarial, typhoid or tuberculous neuritis. The nerve may be injured by ganglion cysts. The cysts, which can usually be palpated at the head of the fibula, compress the nerve and produce foot drop accompanied by burning pains on lateral aspect of the leg, and in the ankle or foot. Relief of symptoms can be obtained by excision of the cyst.

Paralysis of the common peroneal nerve results in a foot drop and inversion of the foot. The patient is unable to dorsiflex the ankle, straighten or extend the toes or evert the foot. The gait is characterized by overflexion of the knee and the slapping of the foot on the floor (steppage gait). Sensory loss is present in an area less extensive than that of the anatomical distribution of the nerve or it may be entirely absent when the injury is due to pressure. Vasomotor and trophic disturbances consisting of swelling, local cyanosis and anhidrosis may also be present.

Complete or partial recovery is the rule when the paralysis is due to transient pressure. Treatment consists of physiotherapy and the use of a foot brace to overcome the foot drop.

TIBIAL (INTERNAL POPLITEAL) NERVE. The tibial branch of the sciatic nerve innervates the muscles on the posterior surface of the leg and the plantar muscles. It transmits sensation from the entire planta, the back and lower part of the leg to the middle third, the outer dorsal surface of the foot and the terminal phalanges of the toes.

Lesions of the tibial nerve are infrequent. It may be injured by gunshot wounds or fractures of the legs. A complete lesion of the nerve is characterized by paralysis of plantar flexion and adduction of the foot, flexion and separation of the toes and a sensory loss in an area less extensive than the anatomical distribution of the nerve. The ankle jerk and plantar reflex are abolished. Causalgia is occasionally seen.

Compression of the posterior tibial branch at the medial malleolus produces pain and paresthesias in the sole of the feet in a manner similar to compression of the medial nerve at the wrist. Decompression results in relief of the symptoms.

Causalgia. Neuralgic pains in the extremities secondary to injury of the nerves were first described by Weir Mitchell. It was formerly considered that this type of neuralgia was found only after injury to the median nerve, but it is now known that it may develop after an injury to any of the sensory or mixed nerves or damage to the plexuses, with or without damage to the major arteries of the extremities.

The pain is usually described as burning in nature (hence the name causalgia) and is constantly present. There is considerable variation in the severity of the pain. In some cases, it is so extreme that the patient is completely incapacitated. The affected limb is constantly protected from movement or external stimuli; and examination of this extremity is strenuously resisted. In others, the pain is severe but the affected extremity can be used (minor causalgia).

Causalgia is usually associated with an incomplete lesion of a nerve. Partial or complete continuity of the nerve may be preserved even though functional loss is complete. The pain is usually limited to the skin distribution of the affected nerve but it may spread to involve the distal part of the extremity or the entire extremity. When more than one nerve is injured, the pain is often in the distribution of only one of the affected nerves. In injuries to the plexus the pain is present in the palm, fingertips, entire hand or arm, rather than in a nerve or root distribution.

Causalgia is a relatively uncommon complication of nerve injuries. It is most frequently seen in military practice. The time of the onset of pain varies from immediately after the injury to an interval of several weeks. Most commonly it appears within a few days of the injury. In the majority of the cases the injury is to the median or sciatic nerves either alone or in combination with other nerves (Table 61).

The pathogenesis of the pains is not known, but it is thought that they are due to an injury of the sympathetic fibers in the nerve trunks. This concept is supported by the fact that relief of symptoms follows the interruption of sympathetic pathways, whereas such operations as neurolysis, removal of neuromas, sectioning and resuturing the nerve usually are of no value.

Examination of motor and sensory function in the affected extremities is made with difficulty in severe cases because any stimulation causes an exacerbation of the pain. In the majority of cases, there is extreme vasodilatation and the extremity is pink, warm and velvety to touch. Perspiration may be increased or decreased. When the pains are severe enough to prevent use of the extremity, there is a rapid development of trophic changes in the skin and nails and periarticular fibrosis.

The course of the condition is quite variable. In mild cases the pain may disappear spontaneously after a few weeks or months without the development of any trophic changes in the affected extremity. Spontaneous remission is less common in severe cases and permanent contactures may result unless the condition is relieved by therapy.

Table 61.   Types of Lesions Producing Causalgia in 100 Cases
(After Rasmussen and Freedman, J. Neurosurg., 1946)

Type of Lesions	Upper Extremity	Lower Extremity
Median nerve	17	
Multiple nerve injuries	28	
Brachial plexus	10	
Ulnar nerve	9	
Radial	6	
Cutaneous nerves of forearm	2	
Digital nerve	2	
Sciatic nerve		8
Tibial nerve		2
Injury to soft tissues	4	1
Fracture of bone or injury to joint	4	6
	82	17

Table 62. Results of Treatment of Causalgia of the Arms and Legs

(After Rasmussen and Freedman, J. Neurosurg., 1946)

	No. of Cases	Relief of Pain				
		Immediate	Within 1 Month	Within Few Mos.	Adequate but Incomplete	Inadequate
Paravertebral block with Novocain	91	6	7	..	32	46
Sympathectomy						
Postganglionic	21	5	5	4	..	7
Preganglionic	14	13	1	0	..	0

Operative procedures on the nerve are rarely followed by relief of the symptoms. The most successful form of therapy is sympathectomy or sympathetic block (Table 62). Preganglionic denervation of the extremity is more effective than postganglionic denervation or paravertebral sympathetic block. In a few cases, a remission is induced by hyperpyrexia produced by the injection of typhoid vaccine intravenously or by means of the fever cabinet.

REFERENCES

Ashenhurst, E. M.: Anatomic Factors in the Etiology of Ulnar Neuropathy, Canadian Med. Asso. J., 87, 159, 1962.

Babbage, N. F.: Burning Foot Syndrome: Bilateral Occurrence with Radical Cure , Med. J. Australia, 1, 764, 1965.

Barrett, R., and Cramer, F.: Tumors of the Peripheral Nerves and So-called "Ganglia" of the Peroneal Nerve, Clinical Orthopaedics, 27, 135. 1963.

Craig, W. S., and Clark, J. M. P.: Obturator Palsy in the Newly Born, Arch. Dis. Childh., 37, 661, 1962.

Curtiss, P. H., Jr., and Tucker, H. J.: Sciatic Palsy in Premature Infants, J.A.M.A., 174, 1586, 1960.

Garland, H., Langworth, E. P., Taverner, D., and Clark, J. M. P.: Surgical Treatment for the Carpal Tunnel Syndrome, Lancet, 1, 1129, 1964.

Hunt, G. M., Abbott, K. H., and Roberts, W. H.: The Median Nerve and Carpal Tunnel Syndrome, Bull. Los Angeles Neurol. Soc., 25, 211, 1960.

Lishman, W. A., and Russell, W. R.: The Brachial Neuropathies, Lancet, 2, 941, 1961.

Mayfield, F. H.: Causalgia, Springfield, Charles C Thomas, 1951, 65 pp.

Nagler, S. H., and Rangell, L.: Peroneal Palsy Caused by Crossing Legs, J.A.M.A., 133, 755, 1947.

Richards, R. L.: Traumatic Ulnar Neuritis: The Results of Anterior Transposition of the Ulnar Nerve, Edinburgh M. J., 52, 14, 1945.

Seddon, H. J.: Peripheral Nerve Injuries, Medical Research Council Special Report, Series No. 282, London, Her Majesty's Stationery Office, 1954.

Stack, R. E., et al.: Compression of the Common Peroneal Nerve by Ganglion Cysts, J. Bone & Joint Surg., 47-A, 773, 1965.

White, H. H.: Pack Paralysis, a Neurological Complication of Scouting, Pediatrics, 41, 1001, 1968.

Wilson, G., and Hadden, S. B.: Neuritis and Multiple Neuritis following Serum Therapy, J.A.M.A., 98, 123, 1932.

Woodhall, B., and Beebe, G. W.: Peripheral Nerve Regeneration. A Follow-up Study of 3,656 World War II Injuries, Veterans Administration Monographs, Washington, 1956.

LUMBAR PUNCTURE AND INTRASPINAL INJECTIONS

Untoward symptoms of a mild nature develop in approximately one third of the patients subjected to a spinal puncture. These symptoms, in the form of headaches and stiffness of the neck, usually develop within eight to forty-eight hours after the puncture. Occasionally they may be accompanied by nausea, vomiting and a rise of body temperature to 101° to 103° F. The headache usually develops a few minutes or several hours after the patient assumes the erect position and is presumably due to traction on the vessels and other pain sensitive structures at the base of the brain as result of intracranial hypotension. The hypotension is due to leakage of fluid into the tissues of the back through the puncture hole in the arachnoid and dura. The symptoms are more apt to develop in patients whose cerebrospinal fluid is normal. If the puncture is repeated at the time of headache, the fluid is unchanged from the original examination with the exception that the pressure may be low. Post-lumbar puncture symptoms commonly last for twenty-four to forty-eight hours, but occasionally they may persist for several weeks. They may be relieved temporarily by the intravenous injection of caffeine in dose of .05 gm, but the most satisfactory treatment is rest in bed for twenty-four to forty-eight hours with the feet elevated slightly above the head.

Rarely these conservative measures will not result in relief of symptoms.

The epidural injection of autologous blood by Di Giovanni and others has resulted in prompt relief.

Rare complications of spinal puncture include: Trauma to the nerve roots by the needle; septic meningitis as result of the introduction of bacteria into the subarachnoid space; herniation of the medulla and cerebellum into the foramen magnum in patients with increased intracranial pressure; and transient paralysis of the sixth cranial nerve. Theoretically it is possible to injure the intervertebral cartilage and produce a herniation of the disc.

Headache may follow puncture of the subarachnoid space for the introduction of anesthetics, air, radiopaque dyes, serum or other substances. In addition, the introduction of foreign substances into the subarachnoid spaces is accompanied by a mild or moderately severe meningeal reaction. The fluid removed four to twenty-four hours afterwards may be slightly cloudy or turbid and contain a few hundred or several thousand leukocytes. The protein content of the fluid may be slightly or moderately elevated, but the sugar content is normal and cultures are sterile excluding the possibility of a bacterial infection.

Other complications of the introduction of foreign substances into the subarachnoid space include arachnoiditis, radiculitis and myelitis as result of injury to the membranes, roots, blood vessels and substance of the cord. These structures are inevitably damaged to a minor degree whenever foreign substances are introduced into a subarachnoid space, but only occasionally is the injury severe enough to be of any significance. Serious damage to the roots and the cord may be produced by the inadvertent injection of solutions contaminated by sterilizing agents. It is also possible that individual sensitivity plays a role in the reactions which occasionally develop after the introduction of anesthetics or other substance, but it is now commonly accepted that the severe degree of adhesive arachnoiditis with ensuing paraplegia, which was reported as the result of spinal anesthesia, was due to contamination of the syringes and tubing by detergent agents used in their cleansing.

In addition to local injury described above, the central nervous system may be damaged during spinal anesthesia as well as with general anesthesia as result of anoxia associated with respiratory or cardiac arrest. If the anoxia is severe and prolonged and if death does not ensue immediately, there is an ischemic necrosis of the neurons in the middle layers of the cortex accompanied by proliferation of the glia. Complete or almost complete recovery is possible but when the brain is severely damaged, serious sequelae are inevitable. Several such cases have been reported in which the patient survived for a number of months in a state of complete decerebrate rigidity and amentia.

REFERENCES

Di Giovanni, A. J., and Dumbar, D. S.: Epidural Injection of Autologous Blood for Postlumbar Puncture Headache, Anesth. and Analg., 49, 268, 1970.

Hoff, E. C., Grenell, R. G., and Fulton, J. F.: Histopathology of the Central Nervous System after Exposure to High Altitudes, Hypoglycemia and Other Conditions Associated with Central Anoxia, Medicine, 24, 161, 1945.

MacRobert, R. G.: The Cause of Lumbar Puncture Headache, J.A.M.A., 70, 1350, 1918.

Merritt, H. H., and Fremonth-Smith, F.: The Cerebrospinal Fluid, Philadelphia, W. B. Saunders Co., 1937, 333 pp.

Paddison, R. M., and Alpers, B. J.: Role of Intrathecal Detergents in Pathogenesis of Adhesive Arachnoiditis, Arch. Neurol. & Psychiat., 71, 87, 1954.

Thorsen, G.: Neurological Complications after Spinal Anesthesia and Results from 2,493 Follow-up Cases, Acta chir. Scandinav. (supp. 121), 95, 1, 1947.

Vandam, L. D., and Dripps, R. D.: Long-term Follow-up of Patients Who Received 10,098 Spinal Anesthetics. Syndrome of Decreased Intracranial Pressure (Headache and Ocular and Auditory Difficulties), J.A.M.A., 161, 586, 1956.

———: Exacerbation of Pre-Existing Neurologic Disease After Spinal Anesthesia, N. Engl. J. Med., 255, 843, 1956.

IONIZING RADIATION

The adult nervous system is relatively resistant to ionizing radiation, but the embryonic nervous system may be damaged by comparatively small dosages.

Experimental work in various species of animal life has shown that the embryonic nervous system is readily injured by radiation, and it is now commonly accepted that microcephaly, hydrocephalus and other development anomalies may occur in the human fetus as result of pelvic irradiation of the pregnant mother. This is particularly true if the radiation is given during the early stage of the development of the fetus.

Little is known with regard to acute damage to the adult nervous system as result of excessively large dosages of ionizing radiations. Fatalities which resulted from explosion of an atom bomb were usually related to blast injury and to the systemic effects of the radiation. The adult nervous system may be damaged occasionally by accidental application of overdosage of radium or other forms of radiation energy or from apparently safe dosages of these agents for the treatment of tumors of the skin or other structures overlying the brain or spinal cord. Unless the dose is excessively high damage to the nervous tissue usually does not become evident until six months or more after the course of therapy. There are thickening and proliferation of the blood vessels and necrosis of the parenchyma in the affected areas. Radiation injury to the brain may produce slowly progressive symptoms suggesting the presence of an intracranial tumor. Injury to the cord is followed by the development of the syndrome of transverse myelitis. Root, plexuses and nerves may be damaged by radiation with resultant motor and sensory defects which have a tendency to progress. Occasionally evidence of damage to the nervous system may appear within three months as result of demyelinating lesions similar to those of multiple sclerosis, without evidence of damage to the blood vessels. Remission of symptoms has been reported in a few such cases.

REFERENCES

Boden, G.: Radiation Myelitis of the Brain-stem, J. Fac. Radiologists, 2, 79, 1950.
Coy, P., et al.: Progressive Myelopathy Due to Radiation, Canad. Med. J., 100, 1129, 1969.
Crompton, M. R., and Layton, D. D.: Delayed Radionecrosis of the Brain Following Therapeutic X-radiation of the Pituitary, Brain, 84, 85, 1961.
Eyster, E. F., and Wilson, C. B.: Radiation Myelopathy, J. Neurosurg., 32, 414, 1970.
Haymaker, W., et al.: Effects of Atomic Radiation of the Brain in Man. A Study of the Brains of Forty-nine Hiroshima and Nagasaki Casualties. J. Neuropath. & Exper. Neurol., 17, 79, 1958.
Hicks, S. P.: Effects of Ionizing Radiations on the Adult and Embryonic Nervous System, A. Res. Nerv. & Ment. Dis., Proc., 32, 439, 1953.
Innes, J. R. M., and Carsten, A.: Demyelinating or Malacic Myelopathy, Arch. Neurol., 4, 190, 1961.
Lampert, P. W., and Davis, R. L.: Delayed Effects of Radiation on the Human Central Nervous System. "Early" and "Late" Delayed Reactions, Neurology, 14, 912, 1964.
Lampert, P., Tom, M. I., and Rider, W. D.: Disseminated Demyelination of the Brain Following Co[60] (Gamma) Radiation, Arch. Path., 68, 322, 1959.
Murphy, D. P.: Outcome of 625 Pregnancies in Women Subjected to Pelvic Radium or Roentgen Irradiation. Am. J. Obst. & Gynec., 18, 179, 1929.

Regan, T. J., Thomas, J. E., and Colby, M. Y., Jr.: Chronic Progressive Radiation Myelopathy, J.A.M.A., *203*, 106, 1968.
Rottenberg, D. A., et al.: Cerebral Necrosis Following Radiotherapy of Extracranial Neoplasms, Ann. Neurol., 1, 339, 1977.
Stoll, B. A., and Andrews, J. T.: Radiation-Induced Peripheral Neuropathy, Br. Med. J., 1, 834, 1966.

ELECTRICAL INJURIES

Injury to the central nervous system or the peripheral nerves may result from the passage of electric currents through the body. As a rule, the passage of a current sufficient to damage the nervous system is fatal. Rarely, however, the patient may survive and shows evidence of damage to the brain, spinal cord or the cranial or spinal nerves.

Accidental contact with high tension currents in the home or industry is the most common cause of electrical injury. Other less common causes of serious electrical injury to the nervous system are lightning-strokes and electric shock therapy of psychoses.

Pathology. Respiratory arrest or ventricular fibrillation is the cause of death in the fatal cases. Injury to the peripheral nerves may be caused by the direct effect of the current, but the lesions in the central nervous system are more probably due to damage to the blood vessels or to cerebral anoxemia secondary to the temporary cardiac and respiratory failure. These include edema, perivascular hemorrhages and areas of cellular loss or demyelinization secondary to vascular damage.

Signs and Symptoms. The symptoms of severe electrical injury are divided into two groups: The acute symptoms and the late manifestations. In the acute state, there is loss of consciousness accompanied in many instances by convulsive seizures. Death results if ventricular fibrillation occurs or if there is a prolonged arrest of respiration.

Late manifestations of electrical injury are extremely rare. Atrophic paralyses as a result of injury to the peripheral nerves or spinal cord are the most common signs. Hemiplegia and other focal cerebral symptoms as well as chorea, dystonia and other signs of injury to the basal ganglia and mental disturbances have been reported as a result of injury to the brain. In some of these cases there was no doubt about the relationship of the shock to the symptoms. In others, it is probable that cerebral arteriosclerosis was a contributing factor in the production of the symptoms.

Treatment. Artificial respiration and the intravenous or intracardiac injection of adrenalin are essential in the acute stage in order to save the patient's life and to prevent further damage to the nervous system by anoxia. The treatment of neurological residuals is the same as for similar defects due to other causes.

REFERENCES

Alexander, L.: Clinical and Neuropathological Aspects of Electrical Injuries, J. Indust. Hyg., 20, 191, 1938.
Langworthy, O. R.: Neurological Abnormalities Produced by Electricity, J. Nerv. & Ment. Dis., 84, 13, 1936.
Morrison, L. R., Weeks, A., and Cobb, S.: Histopathology of Different Types of Electric Shock on Mammalian Brains, J. Indust. Hyg., 12, 324, 1930.
Silversides, J.: The Neurological Sequelae of Electrical Injury, Can. Med. Asso. J., 91, 195, 1964,

DECOMPRESSION SICKNESS

In scuba diving, deep sea diving, caisson work, flying and simulated altitude ascents, rapid reductions in the barometric pressure may occur. These changes can produce lesions involving extremities (bends), cardiorespiratory system (chokes), the skin (itches), and central nervous system. The most serious complication is paralysis of spinal cord origin.

Pathology. Ischemic areas, particularly in the white matter of the thoracic cord, are produced by gas bubbles which may occlude capillaries or veins in the spino-vertebral plexus. Hypoxic changes, edema and ischemic changes secondary to air emboli may develop in the brain.

Signs and Symptoms. Soon after rapid decompression, knife-like chest and abdominal pains may be followed by the onset of paraplegia with motor and sensory levels in the thoracic region. Unless rapid recompression treatment is given, the symptoms may be permanent. Even with prolonged treatment some sequelae may still be noted. Vertigo, deafness, visual disturbances, convulsive seizures and manifestations of focal cerebral involvement have been reported, but permanent lesions of the brain are rare.

Treatment. Recompression in the chamber must be started as soon as possible. This therapy is directed specifically at maintaining pressure over long periods of time so that residual gas bubbles can be recompressed and absorbed and oxygen supplied at increased partial pressure to the damaged tissues. Inadequate recompression may lead to sudden relapse of symptoms and necessitate retreatment to prevent residual damage.

REFERENCES

Behnke, A. R.: Decompression Sickness, Mil. Med., 117, 257, 1955.
Dewey, A. W., Jr.: Decompression Sickness, An Emerging Recreational Hazard, N. Engl. J. Med., 267, 759 and 812, 1962.
Haymaker, W., and Johnston, A. D.: Pathology of Decompression Sickness; Comparison of Lesions in Airmen with those in Caisson Workers and Divers, Mil. Med., 177, 285, 1955.
Richter, R. W., and Behnke, A. R.: Spinal Cord Injury Following a Scuba Dive to a Depth of 350 Feet, U.S. Armed Forces Med. J., 10, 1227, 1959.

Chapter 5

Developmental Defects

Harry H. White, M.D.

A great variety of defects of the brain (Figs. 99 and 100) or spinal cord may be present at birth. The damage may be limited to the nervous system or it may include the bone, skin, or other organs. These defects

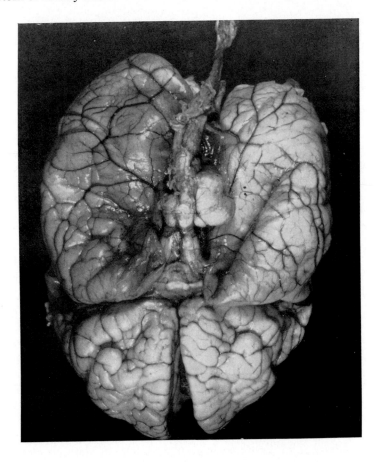

Figure 99. Developmental defect. Microgyria and almost complete agenesis of cerebellum and pons. (Courtesy Dr. Abner Wolf.)

421

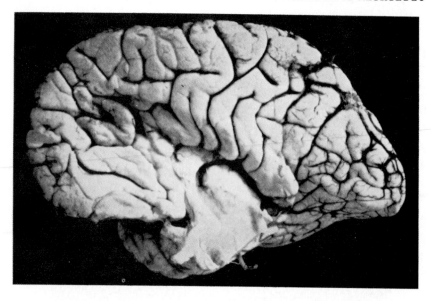

Figure 100. Developmental defect. Abnormal pattern of gyri on mesial aspect of hemisphere and agenesis of the corpus callosum. (Courtesy Dr. Leon Roizin.)

may be extensive, with absence of the cerebral hemispheres (anencephaly), or they may be restricted to the absence of a part or the whole of one structure such as the cerebellum or corpus callosum. Other types of defects which may be found include: Macrogyria; microgyria; heterotopia; porencephaly; hydrocephalus; and failures in the development of or closure of the cranial or spinal bones with or without accompanying damage to the brain or spinal cord.

The causes of these maldevelopments are not known. It is probable that genetic factors play a significant role in most cases, while others are known to be caused by environmental teratogens. The central nervous system of the developing fetus is especially vulnerable to anoxia, ionizing radiation, and certain infectious and metabolic diseases in the mother. The maternal use of alcohol as well as certain drugs including phenytoin and trimethadone may produce mental and somatic deficiencies in the offspring. The central nervous system of the fetus may be severely damaged by maternal infections such as syphilis, toxoplasmosis, cytomegalic inclusion disease, herpes simplex, equine encephalomyelitis, and the bacterial meningitides. In addition, infections and vascular lesions in the early postnatal period may cause extensive damage to the nervous system which simulate developmental defects both clinically and pathologically.

Serious defects in the development of the nervous system usually result in death *in utero* or shortly after birth. Minor defects may be accompanied by no symptoms. Moderately severe defects are usually accompanied by a degree of disability related to the extent and location of the damage. The more common forms of developmental defects, which are compatible with life, are considered here in some detail.

REFERENCES

Bergsma, D. (Ed.): *Birth Defects. Atlas and Compendium.* Baltimore, Williams & Wilkins, 1972, 1006 pp.
Courville, C. B.: *Birth and Brain Damage,* Pasadena, California, Margaret F. Courville, 1971, 408 pp.
Crome, L., and Stern, J.: *The Pathology of Mental Retardation,* 2nd ed., Edinburgh, Churchill Livingstone, 1972, 544 pp.
Dekaban, A. S.: Brain Dysfunction in Congenital Malformations of the Nervous System, in *Biology of Brain Dysfunction,* Vol. 3, ed. by G. E. Gaull, New York, Plenum Press, 1975, pp. 381–423.
Ferrier, P. E.: Editorial: Des Tératogènes, Helv. paediat. Acta, *30,* 5, 1975.
Fraser, F. C., and McKusick, V. A. (Eds.): *Congenital Malformations,* Procds. 3rd Internat. Conf., The Hague, The Netherlands, Amsterdam-New York, Excerpta Medica, 1970, 450 pp.
Hicks, S. P.: Developmental Malformations Produced by Radiation, Am. J. Roent., *69,* 272, 1953.
Holmes, L. B.: Inborn Errors of Morphogenesis, N. Engl. J. Med., *291,* 763, 1974.
———: Congenital Malformations, N. Engl. J. Med., *295,* 204, 1976.
Jellinger, K., and Gross, H.: Congenital Telencephalic Midline Defects, Neuropädiatrie, *4,* 446, 1973.
Jellinger, K., and Rett, A.: Agyria-Pachygyria (Lissencephaly Syndrome), Neuropädiatrie, *7,* 66, 1973.
Monif, G. R. G., and Sever, J. L.: Chronic Infection of the Central Nervous System with Rubella Virus, Neurology, *16,* 111, 1966.
Muir, C. S.: Hydranencephaly and Allied Disorders, Arch. Dis. Child., *34,* 231, 1959.
Page, L. K., Brown, S. B., Gargano, F. P., and Stortz, R. W.: Schizencephaly: a Clinical Study and Review, Child's Brain, *1,* 348, 1975.
Rorke, l. B., and Spiro, A. J.: Cerebral Lesions in Congenital Rubella Syndrome, J. Ped., *70,* 243, 1967.
Smith, D. W.: *Recognizable Patterns of Human Malformation,* 2nd ed., Philadelphia, W. B. Saunders Co., 1976, 504 pp.

CONGENITAL ABNORMALITIES ASSOCIATED WITH CHROMOSOMAL DEFECTS

Some degree and often profound impairments of mental and neurological functions are present in virtually all of the chromosome abnormality syndromes. Down's syndrome (Trisomy 21 Syndrome) is the most common pattern of malformation in man.

The 18 Trisomy Syndrome. The presence of an extra 18 chromosome is characterized by mental retardation, growth deficiency, congenital heart defects, hypoplasia of skeletal muscles, anomalies of the development of the hands and feet, small mandibles, deformed ears and other defects. Failure to thrive is quite common in these babies and only 10% survive the first year of life.

The 13 Trisomy Syndrome. Severe defects in the development of the forebrain are characteristic of this chromosomal syndrome. Failure of separation of the hemispheres (holoprosencephaly), varying degrees of incomplete development of the forebrain and olfactory nerves (arhinencephaly) or absence of the frontal lobes results in severe mental deficiency. Other associated anomalies include cleft lip and palate, defective development of the eyes, malformations of hands and feet and congenital defects of the heart. Death occurs in the first year of life in the majority of cases.

REFERENCES

DeMyer, W., Zeman, W., and Palmer, C. G.: The Face Predicts the Brain: Diagnostic Significance of Median Facial Anomalies for Holoprosencephaly (Arhinencephaly), Pediatrics, *34,* 256, 1964.
DeMyer, W.: The Median Cleft Face Syndrome, Neurology, *17,* 961, 1967.
Gellis, S. S., and Feingold, M.: *Atlas of Mental Retardation Syndromes,* Washington, D.C., U.S. Govt. Printing Office, 1968, 188 pp.
Kakulas, B. A., and Rosman, N. P.: 13–15 Trisomy in Eight Cases of Arhinencephaly, Lancet, *2,* 717, 1965.
Smith, D. W.: *Recognizable Patterns of Human Malformation,* 2nd ed., Philadelphia, W. B. Saunders Co., 1976, 504 pp.
Taylor, A.: Review article. Austosomal Trisomy Syndromes. A Detailed Study of 27 Cases of Edward's Syndrome and 27 Cases of Patau's Syndrome, J. Med. Genet., *5,* 227, 1968.

Down's Syndrome

Down's syndrome (Mongolian idiocy, mongolism) is the term applied to a group of mentally defective patients who have facial and bodily features which have a superficial resemblance to those normally present in the Mongolian race.

Etiology. Down's syndrome is caused by trisomy of chromosome number 21 of the Denver system ("regular" Down's syndrome). Occasionally the extra chromosome is not free, but is translated on another autosome ("translocation" Down's syndrome). The translocation may occur between a chromosome number 21 and one of the 13–15 group or between two numbers 21, or between a number 21 and a number 22. In the majority of the cases the mother is over 35 years of age when the affected individual is born.

Pathology. The brain is small and of abnormal shape possibly related in part to molding by the brachycephalic skull. The frontal and temporal poles are shortened and the occiput is steep. The brain is softer than normal, the convolutions appear simple and broad with fusions of the fissures in some portions of the hemisphere. On microscopic examination the cortical ribbon is narrowed, and there is lack of differentiation of the various cortical areas. There is a decrease in the number of cortical cells, particularly the medium-sized and large pyramidal cells and an increase in the glial elements. There is a reduction in the degree of myelination particularly in the tangential and U-fibers. Pathological changes are present throughout the nervous system and they may be more severe in the cerebellum and brainstem than in the cortex. The morphological changes of Alzheimer's disease are commonly found in patients beyond forty years of age. Regressive changes have been reported in the endocrine glands.

Incidence. Down's syndrome occurs in about 1.5 to 2.0 per thousand births. It accounts for approximately 5% of severe mental defectives of all ages. The incidence rate rises sharply with increasing maternal age, reaching a level of 18 cases per thousand births by age of forty-five years.

The disease has been reported in all races including the Negroes, Indians, Chinese and Japanese. There is a slightly greater incidence in the male than in the female sex. Usually only one child is affected but two or more cases have occurred in one family. The risk of recurrence is about 1% unless the child is a translocation case with a parent who is a translocation-carrier. Under these circumstances there is a relatively high risk for recurrence.

Symptoms and Signs. The two characteristics of the disease are the amentia and various deformities in the configuration of the skull, trunk and extremities. The presence of short ears and small white spots on the iris are also frequent findings.

Physical and mental development is retarded. The affected infants are hypotonic, slow in learning to sit up, walk and talk. The degree of mental defect is subject to some variation. In the majority the intelligence is in the I.Q. range of 25 to 50, but in a few there is a higher degree of mental development, but this rarely reaches a level above an I.Q. of 50. The children are usually docile, of a fairly even disposition and easily managed. Temper tantrums or violent behavior may occur but are exceptional.

Anomalies of the physical structure of the affected infants include: Brachycephalic configuration of the skull; flattening of the face, narrowing and slanting of the palpebral fissures, with epicanthus in about 25% of the cases; shortening of the nose with depression of the bridge; flattening of the ears with deformation of the lobes; broadening and coarsening of the tongue; shortening of the stature; widening and flabbiness of the hands with simian crease on palms (Fig. 101); flattening of the feet with often a large cleft between the first and second toes. In addition, there may be other congenital anomalies such as spina bifida, syndactylism, supernumerary digits and maldevelopment of various organs of the body, particularly the heart.

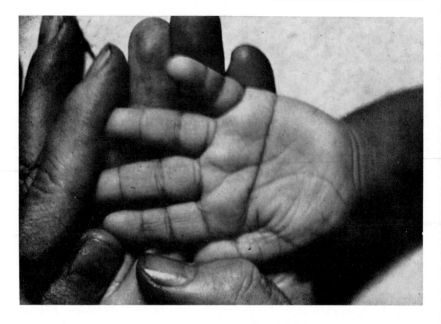

Figure 101.   Down's syndrome. Simian crease on palm. (Courtesy Dr. Arnold Gold.)

Laboratory Data. With the exception of the abnormalities in the roentgenograms of the skull, spine and other bones, the only significant finding in the laboratory examination is a decrease in serotonin and ATPase levels in platelets.

Diagnosis. The diagnosis is usually made without difficulty when feeblemindedness and characteristic bodily defects are present in an infant or child. The diagnosis may be obvious at birth from the appearance of the infant, but these as well as the mental defect may not be obvious until the latter months of the first year of life. The conditions to be considered in differential diagnosis are achondroplasia and cretinism. Achondroplasia is characterized by shortening of the body stature, but the characteristic mongolian features and amentia are not a part of this syndrome. Cretinism is diagnosed by the elevated serum cholesterol and the low uptake of radioiodine.

Prognosis. The prognosis for life is poor. Many of the affected individuals die in infancy. Only a few live beyond the first or second decade. The chief causes of death are congenital heart disease and acute infectious diseases. Chromosome studies of the patient and both parents are necessary for predicting the risk of recurrence in future pregnancies.

Treatment.   There is no effective therapy. Attempts can be made to educate those with a lesser degree of amentia. Institutionalization will be necessary for most cases. Amniocentesis for chromosome studies on any future pregnancy will permit a decision on termination of the pregnancy.

REFERENCES

Aase, J. M., Wilson, A. C., and Smith, D. W.: Small Ears in Down's Syndrome: A Helpful Diagnostic Aid, J. Pediat., 82, 845, 1973.
Breg, W. R., Miller, O. J., and Schmickel, R. D.: Chromosomal Translocations in Patients with Mongolism and in Their Normal Relatives, N. Engl. J. Med., 266, 845, 1962.
Ellis, W. G., McCulloch, J. R., and Corley, C. L.: Presenile Dementia in Down's Syndrome, Neurology, 24, 101, 1974.
Lott, L. T., et al.: Down's Syndrome, Transport Storage and Metabolism of Serotonin in Blood Platelets, Pediat. Res., 6, 730, 1972.
McCoy, E. E., Segal, D. J., Bayer, S. M., and Strynadka, K. D.: Decreased ATPase and Increased Sodium Content of Platelets in Down's Syndrome, N. Engl. J. Med., 291, 950, 1974.
Penrose, L. S.: Mongolism, in Clinical Aspects of Genetics, F. A. Jones, Editor, pp. 8697, London, Pitman Medical Publishing Co. Ltd., 1961.
Polani, P. E.: Cytogenetics of Down's Syndrome (Mongolism), Pediat. Clin. N. Am., 10, 423, 1963.
Solomon, G., et al.: Four Common Eye Signs in Mongolism, Amer. J. Dis. Child., 110, 46, 1965.

AGENESIS OF THE CORPUS CALLOSUM

Defective embryogenesis of the midline telencephalic structures may result in total or partial absence of the corpus callosum. The hippocampal and anterior commissures are likewise absent in many cases. This anomaly may be present without producing signs or symptoms of neurological dysfunction although it is most commonly associated with seizures and varying degrees of mental retardation. The occurrence of clinical symptoms is usually related to other cranial or spinal abnormalities which are present in the majority of patients (hydrocephalus, microgyri, heterotopias, arachnoid cysts, cerebellar dysgenesis, spina bifida and meningomyelocele). Partial or complete agenesis is frequently present with lipomas or cysts in the region of the corpus callosum.

The diagnosis of agenesis of the corpus callosum is made by cranial computerized tomography or air contrast roentgenograms. The anomaly produces marked separation of the lateral ventricles, a concave configuration of the medial walls and dilatation of the caudal portions of the lateral ventricles and a dorsal extension and dilatation of the third ventricle.

REFERENCES

Cooper, W. C., and Van Hagen, K. O.: Lipoma of the Corpus Callosum, Bull. Los Ang. Neurol. Soc., 27, 39, 1962.

de Jong, J. G. Y., Delleman, J. W., et al.: Agenesis of the Corpus Callosum, Infantile
    Spasms, Ocular Anomalies (Aicardi's Syndrome), Neurology, 26, 1152, 1976.
Kazner, E., Lanksch, W., and Steinhoff, H.: Cranial Computerized Tomography in the
    Diagnosis of Brain Disorders in Infants and Children, Neuropädiatrie, 7, 136, 1976.
Loeser, J. D., and Alvord, E. C.: Agenesis of the Corpus Callosum, Brain, 91, 553, 1968.
———: Clinicopathological Correlations in Agenesis of the Corpus Callosum, Neurology,
    18, 745, 1968.
Sadowsky, C., and Reeves, A. G.: Agenesis of the Corpus Callosum with Hypothermia,
    Arch. Neurol., 32, 774, 1975.
Wollschlaeger, G., Wollschlaeger, P. B., Brannan, D. D., and Segal, A. J.: Lipoma of the
    Corpus Callosum, Am. J. Roentgen., 86, 142, 1961.

CONGENITAL HYDROCEPHALUS

Hydrocephalus is a term loosely used to describe a variety of conditions in which there is excess of fluid in the cranial cavity. In a more restricted sense it is reserved for those cases in which there is an accumulation of fluid in the cranial cavity under increased pressure. An excess of fluid may be found in one or both ventricles of patients with atrophic or degenerative lesions. The fluid in these cases is not under increased pressure and is present to fill up the defect occasioned by the lack of cerebral substance (hydrocephalus ex vacuo).

Hydrocephalus may develop in infants or adults as the result of occlusion of the cerebrospinal fluid pathways by tumors in the third ventricle, brainstem or posterior fossa. These are considered elsewhere, and this chapter is concerned only with the type of hydrocephalus which results from obstruction to the normal flow of cerebrospinal fluid by congenital maldevelopment of the brain or intra-uterine infections of the nervous system.

It is customary to divide the cases of congenital hydrocephalus into two groups, communicating and non-communicating, depending on whether there is free communication between the fluid in the ventricles and the basal subarachnoid cisterns. This is determined by ventriculography or pneumoencephalography and more recently by radioisotope encephalograms and CT brain scan. In a strict sense all types of hydrocephalus are "non-communicating" since spinal fluid circulation is obstructed to normal flow and reabsorption at some point in the natural pathway. This classification is useful, however, in planning diversionary routes of circulation by surgical shunts.

Pathogenesis and Pathology. Passage of fluid from the third to fourth ventricle may be prevented by several types of lesions. There may be a complete absence of the aqueduct of Sylvius, but more commonly the canal is narrowed by overgrowth of ependymal cells and glial tissues. The existence of a thin membrane occluding the aqueduct has been reported in a few cases. Obstruction of the outflow from the fourth ventricle may occur as the result of absence or incomplete formation of the foramina of exit (Magendie and Luschka) or the obstruction of these exits by meningeal adhesions secondary to intra-uterine meningitis. In these cases the lateral and third ventricles, the aqueduct and fourth ventricle are all dilated. Communicating hydrocephalus may develop as result of adhesions in the meningeal space of the basal cisterns which prevents flow of spinal fluid over the convexity of the cerebral hemispheres to the pacchionian villae. Theoretically it can result from failure of development or of occlusion of the absorptive mechanism.

In the majority of the cases with congenital hydrocephalus, the defects which produce an interference in the circulation are only one manifestation of a generalized disturbance in the development of the nervous system. Other anomalies include micro- and macrogyria, porencephaly, absence of the corpus callosum, fusion of the cerebral hemispheres, absence of the vermis of the cerebellum, spina bifida, cranium bifidum, meningocele, encephalocele, syringomyelia, hydromyelia and the Arnold-Chiari malformation of the cerebellum and brainstem.

At necropsy the skull is greatly enlarged and the bones are thinned. The sutures are widely separated. The ventricles of the brain are greatly dilated filling almost the entire cranial cavity. The cortical gyri are flattened and narrowed in many cases to the thickness of a ribbon. The basal ganglia appear atrophic. The septum pellucidum is stretched and torn. Various developmental defects may also be present in the brain or spinal cord.

Incidence. Congenital hydrocephalus is a relatively rare condition. The enlargement of the head may develop *in utero* necessitating craniotomy at delivery. More commonly, however, the head is relatively normal in size at birth and the enlargement is first noted in the early months of life. Rarely onset of symptoms may be delayed until adult life, particularly in patients with partial atresia of the aqueduct of Sylvius. Familial incidence of hydrocephalus has been reported.

Symptoms and Signs. In the usual case there is a progressive enlargement of the head in the first few months of life. The cranial bones are thin, the sutures widened and the fontanelles bulge. The roof of the orbit is depressed with downward and outward protrusion of the eyeballs. The sclera is visible beneath the upper lids. Various neurological signs may develop as result of the hydrocephalus or other congenital malformations. Choked discs rarely develop because of the ability of the head to expand. Optic atrophy, deafness, spastic weakness of the legs or arms and cerebellar ataxia are the more common neurological signs. Dandy states that the spastic weakness of the extremities is due to pressure of the dilated fourth ventricle on the brainstem. According to Yakovlev, this sign is due to stretching of corticospinal fibers in the internal capsule by the enlargement of the lateral ventricles.

Mental development is usually retarded. The infants are slow in learning to walk and talk. Occasionally, however, normal mental development may occur in the presence of a severe degree of hydrocephalus.

The roentgenogram shows uniform enlargement of the head, thinning of the calvarium and convolutional markings on the skull bones. The cerebrospinal fluid pressure is increased. The fluid may be normal or there may be a moderate increase in the protein content.

Diagnosis. The diagnosis of congenital hydrocephalus is usually made by the characteristic appearance of the head, and the increase beyond the normal in its measurements in each successive month of life. Subdural hematoma, hydranencephaly, megalencephaly and intracranial tumor are the chief differential diagnoses. Subdural hematoma is excluded by needle puncture of the subdural space. Transillumination of the skull and air encephalography are useful in excluding the latter possibilities. CT brain scan alone will establish an accurate diagnosis in some cases.

Course. The course of congenital hydrocephalus is unpredictable. Some of the severe cases die in the first two years of life but in a number of cases, the obstruction may not be complete and there is a relatively satisfactory adjustment between the rate of formation and absorption of the fluid. The child may develop to adult life with no signs except the enlargement of the head, or there may be some spastic weakness of the extremities and mental retardation. Occasionally this compensation may break down in later life with the development of choked discs and other signs of increased intracranial pressure. Symptoms may develop *de novo* in adult life in patients with partial atresia of the aqueduct of Sylvius.

There have been a number of studies of the course of treated and untreated hydrocephalus. Yashon, Jane and Sugar studied the course of 47 untreated patients. Twenty-three had died. Only 3 of these had survived beyond the fifth year of life. Thirteen of the 24 patients living were nine or more years old at the time of final evaluation. There was no correlation between circumference of the head, the thickness of the cerebral mantle and the final neurological state of the patient.

Laurence and Coates reported on 182 untreated patients. Eighty-one were living with apparent arrest of the hydrocephalus. The vast majority of the fatalities were in the first two years of life. Seventy-three % of the survivors had an I.Q. greater than 50 and 38% an I.Q. greater than 85. During the same period 27 of 56 patients who were subjected to operation were living. They conclude that surgery should be undertaken in rapidly progressing cases in order to prevent further brain damage, but caution must be exercised in arresting or arrested cases.

Foltz and Shurtleff concluded from a five-year study of 113 hydro-cephalic children (65 operated with ventriculo-atrial shunt, 48 unoper-ated) that the survival rate and the mental state of the living children were much better in the operated than in the non-operated cases.

Treatment. In spite of the optimistic figures quoted above for the survival rate of untreated patients, most pediatricians and neurosur-geons are in favor of operative therapy, particularly when there is a progressive increase in the size of the head in the first few months of life. Several neurosurgeons state, however, that arrest or recovery from the hydrocephalus-producing process does not occur in the patients treated by shunting process, thus implying that there would probably be a life-long need for the shunt. Numerous operations have been devised for the relief of congenital hydrocephalus, the most satisfactory of which are excision or coagulation of the choroid plexus, puncture of the third ventricle, and various shunting procedures (ventriculo-cisternal, ventriculo-peritoneal, ventriculo-cardiac, etc.). The ultimate outcome depends on the success of the operation and on whether other serious congenital malformations of the nervous system are present.

REFERENCES

Epstein, F., et al.: Role of Computerized Axial Tomography in Diagnosis and Treatment of Common Neurosurgical Problems of Infancy and Childhood, Child's Brain, 2, 111, 1976.

Foltz, E. L., and Shurtleff, D. B.: Five-year Comparative Study of Hydrocephalus in Children with and without Operation (113 cases), J. Neurosurg., 20, 1064, 1963.

Gomez, M. R., and Reese, D. F.: Computed Tomography of the Head in Infants and Children, Pediat. Clin. N. A., 23, 473, 1976.

Hallar, J. S., Wolpert, S. M., Rabe, E. F., and Hills, J. R.: Cystic Lesions of the Posterior Fossa in Infants: A Comparison of the Clinical, Radiological, and Pathological Findings in Dandy-Walker Syndrome and Extra-Axial Cysts, Neurology, 21, 494, 1971.

Harrison, M. J. G., Robert, C. M., and Uttley, D.: Benign Aqueduct Stenosis in Adults, J. Neurol. Neurosurg. Psychiat., 37, 1322, 1974.

Johnson, R. T.: Hydrocephalus and Viral Infections, Devel. Med. Child Neurol., 17, 807, 1975.

Laurence, K. M.: Neurological and Intellectual Sequelae of Hydrocephalus, Arch. Neurol., 20, 73, 1969.

Laurence, K. M., and Coates, S.: The Natural History of Hydrocephalus, Arch. Dis. Child., 37, 345, 1962.

Lorber, J., and Bhat, U. S.: Posthaemorrhagic Hydrocephalus, Arch. Dis. Child., 49, 751, 1974.

Russell, D. S.: *Observations on the Pathology of Hydrocephalus*, Medical Research Council, Special Report. Series No. 265, London, His Majesty's Stat. Office, 1949.

Shurtleff, D. B., Foltz, E. L., and Loeser, J. D.: Hydrocephalus, Amer. J. Dis. Child., 125, 688, 1973.

Weller, R. O., and Shulman, K.: Infantile Hydrocephalus: Clinical, Histological, and Ultrastructural Study of Brain Damage, J. Neurosurg., 36, 255, 1972.

Yashon, D., Jane, J. A., and Sugar, O.: The Course of Severe Untreated Infantile Hydro-cephalus, J. Neurosurg., 23, 509, 1965.

Young, H. F., et al.: The Relationship of Intelligence and Cerebral Mantle in Treated Infantile Hydrocephalus, Pediatrics, 52, 54, 1973.

MEGALENCEPHALY

Megalencephaly is a rare condition in which the brain is abnormally large and heavy in the absence of other factors such as hydrocephalus, severe edema or hematoma which may produce increased weight of the brain. Structural abnormalities and various malformations are found in the majority of megalencephalic brains. Clinical signs and symptoms are variable and dependent upon the extent and severity of the malformations. Mental deficiency and seizures, evident from early childhood or infancy, are the most common neurological symptoms. Certain progressive encephalopathies of infancy (Tay-Sachs disease, and the spongy degeneration and fibrinoid types of leukodystrophies) may also result in excessively large brains.

The differential diagnosis includes other diseases which produce excessive enlargement of the head in infants. Hydrocephalus is excluded by the presence of normal size ventricles following CT brain scan.

REFERENCES

Crome, L., and Stern, J.: The Pathology of Mental Retardation, 2nd ed. Edinburgh, Churchill Livingstone, 1972, 544 pp.
DeMeyer, W.: Megalencephaly in Children, Neurology, 22, 634, 1972.
Zonana, J., Rimoin, D. L., and Davis, D. C.: Macrocephaly with Multiple Lipomas and Hemangiomas, J. Pediat., 89, 600, 1976.

Table 63.   Site of Lesions in Spina Bifida and Cranium Bifidum

(After Ingraham et al., Spina Bifida and Cranium Bifidum, Harvard University Press, 1944)

Site of Lesion		No. of Cases
Cranial		84
Nasal	5	
Nasopharyngeal	1	
Frontal	6	
Parietal	9	
Occipital	63	
Cervical		23
Thoracic		39
Thoracolumbar		43
Lumbar		205
Lumbosacral		87
Sacral		46
Thoracolumbosacral		10
Pelvic		1
Undesignated		8
Total		546

SPINA BIFIDA AND CRANIUM BIFIDUM

Failure of closure of the bony spine or cranium is known as spina bifida or cranium bifidum. This failure of closure may occur at any level but it is most common in the lumbosacral region of the spine (Table 63).

The defect may be a simple failure of bony union or portions of the nervous system may protrude through the bony defect (Table 64).

Spina Bifida

Spina bifida is defined as a failure in the closure of the spinal column due to a defect in the development of vertebrae. It may be associated with defects in the development of the spinal cord, brainstem, cerebellum or cerebrum, meningoceles, meningomyeloceles, congenital tumors, hydrocephalus or developmental defects in other portions of the body.

Pathology and Pathogenesis. The spinal canal closes by the fourth week and the bony canal by the twelfth week of intrauterine life. The combination of genetic and environmental factors (multifactorial inheritance) is postulated to be the underlying mechanism in the etiology of neural tube defects. The patients with spina bifida can be classified into two large groups: (1) Spina bifida occulta in which there is a simple defect in the closure of the vertebrae; (2) spina bifida with meningocele or meningomyelocele, where the defect in the spinal column is associated with a sac-like protrusion of the skin and meninges overlying the vertebral defect. This sac may contain meninges or portions of the spinal cord.

Incidence. The exact incidence of spina bifida is unknown. Simple

Table 64. The Incidence of Various Types of Lesions in Patients with
Spina Bifida and Cranium Bifidum
(After Ingraham *et al.*, *Spina Bifida and Cranium Bifidum*,
Harvard University Press, 1944)

Type of Lesion	No. of Cases
Spina bifida occulta (13 with lipomas) ...	65
Meningocele	98
Lipomeningocele	14
Myelomeningocele	279
Lipomyelomeningocele	18
Encephalocele	84
Total	558

failure of closure of one or more vertebral arches in the lumbar or sacral region without any other anomaly in the nervous system is a relatively common finding (estimated at 25% by Ingraham and Lowrey) in routine examination of the spine at autopsy or by roentgenogram. Spinal defects of clinical importance are much more rare, occurring in approximately 1 in 4,000 cases admitted to the Children's Hospital in Boston (Ingraham). The incidence is slightly greater in the female sex. There was a history of similar defects in the spinal column in other members of the family in 6% of Ingraham's 546 cases. This figure is consistent with subsequent reports which indicate a recurrence risk of 5% after one affected offspring.

The coincidence of spina bifida and other developmental defects is quite common. Ingraham and his associates found 570 developmental anomalies in 232 of their 546 patients (Table 65). Hydrocephalus was present in 208 cases, clubfoot in 102 and other defects in the vertebrae in 49 cases, including 7 cases of the Klippel-Feil anomaly. Defects in the nervous system were noted in 58 cases, with the Arnold-Chiari malformation in 20.

Although the defect is present before birth, there may be a delay of several or many years before sufficient symptoms develop for the patient to seek medical aid. This fact is of importance, because all

Table 65.   Developmental Anomalies Associated with Spina Bifida and Cranium Bifidum in 546 Cases
(After Ingraham et al., Spina Bifida and Cranium Bifidum, Harvard University Press, 1944)

Anomaly		No. of Cases
Hydrocephalus		208
Clubfoot		102
Bone defects		94
Vertebrae (including 7 cases of Klippel-Feil's syndrome)	49	
Skull	16	
Other bones	29	
Central nervous system defects		58
Cerebrum	20	
Cerebellum and brainstem (including 20 cases of Arnold-Chiari malformation)	26	
Other portions	12	
Hernia		27
Dislocated hip		23
Genitourinary anomaly		11
Congenital heart disease		4
Other		43
Total		570

patients with this developmental defect are not seen in pediatric clinics.

Symptoms and Signs. Spina bifida occulta may be present without any neurological symptoms. Symptoms and signs, when they occur, are related to a concomitant defect in the development of the spinal cord (diastematomyelia, ectopic nerve roots) or the presence of lipomas, dermoids, or other tumors. The symptoms and signs in these cases include: weakness and atrophy of the muscles of the legs, disturbances of the gait, urinary incontinence, impairment of cutaneous and proprioceptive sensations in the lumbar and sacral segments, and loss of tendon reflexes in the legs. Maldevelopment of the feet with valgus, varus or cavus deformities, usually unilateral, and scoliosis are the most common associated structural deformities.

Not infrequently the defect in the spine can be detected by palpation or is evident by the presence of a localized overgrowth of hair or a hard lump in the skin at the site of the defect. A lipoma was present at the site of the defect in 13 of the 65 cases of Ingraham and Lowrey. These lipomas consist of lobules of gritty firm fat bound together by fibrous septa, and may extend from any tissue level of the back of the spinal cord binding the various tissues together and preventing the normal rostral movements of the lower end of the cord with growth. The lipomatous masses may extend into the epidural and subdural spaces and compress the roots of the cauda equina or the lower end of the cord.

Simple meningoceles may occur without any symptoms, but when elements of the spinal cord are present in the sac (myelomeningocele) (Fig. 102), some disability is almost invariably present. The nature of the symptoms is related to the level of the lesion. In the lumbar region they are similar to those which may occur in association with spina bifida occulta, previously enumerated. At higher levels there may be

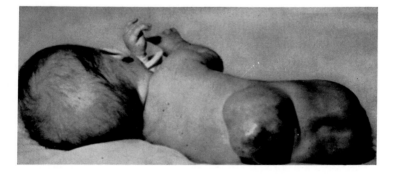

Figure 102.   Spina bifida in lumbosacral region with meningomyelocele and hydrocephalus.

symptoms and signs of complete or incomplete transection of the cord, or combined root and cord symptoms of a syringomyelic character.

Diagnosis. The diagnosis of spina bifida is obvious when the defect is associated with a mass protruding from the spine. In other cases it can be readily diagnosed by the roentgen examination. The finding of a spinal defect in the roentgenogram does not always indicate that the symptoms are due to this defect. It should lead, however, to the consideration of the possibility of the presence of a congenital tumor or some other developmental defect. Recently developed techniques of biochemical analysis of amniotic fluid component (alpha-fetoprotein) and ultrasonography now permit an antenatal diagnosis of some neural tube defects.

Course. The course of patients with defects in the closure of the spine depends on the extent of the lesion and the nature of other congenital defects. Death may occur in infancy as a result of infection of the nervous system secondary to rupture of the sac or as the result of the associated hydrocephalus. Spina bifida occulta with minor defects in the development of the nervous system is compatible with a relatively normal span of life. Neurological signs may increase, however, in severity or develop *de novo* at any time.

Treatment. The treatment of spina bifida and its complications is by surgery. Lipomatous or other types of intraspinal tumors should be removed. Simple meningoceles can be excised when hydrocephalus is not present, or after the latter has been stabilized spontaneously or following surgical treatment. The excision of spinal sacs which contain neural elements is usually attended with poor results, due in part to the frequency of coincidental spinal or cerebral defects. Reduction in the incidence of severe defects may be possible by antenatal diagnosis and termination of pregnancy.

Cranium Bifidum

Defects in the fusion of the cranial bone are known as cranium bifidum. These defects occur in the midline and are most common in the occipital region. The skull defects are usually accompanied by sac-like protrusions of the overlying skin. This sac contains meninges (meningocele) or meninges and cerebral tissue (encephalocele). Other congenital malformations of the nervous system may be present. Hydrocephalus is common when the defect in the skull is in the occipital region.

The occurrence of clinical symptoms and signs in patients with cranial meningoceles or encephaloceles is usually related to the presence or absence of hydrocephalus or other congenital malformations of the nervous system. The actual size of the sac is of importance only in that rupture of the skin and infection of the meninges is more apt to occur when the sac is large.

The treatment of cranial meningoceles or encephaloceles is excision of the sac with its contents and firm closure of the dura. The prognosis is good when only meninges and spinal fluid are contained in the sac. It is poor if large amounts of cerebral tissue are present, if the ventricular system extends into the mass, if hydrocephalus is present, or if there are other serious defects in the nervous system.

REFERENCES

Anderson, F. M.: Occult Spinal Dysraphism, Pediatrics, 55, 826, 1975.
Fishman, M. A.: Recent Advances in the Treatment of Dysraphic States, Pediat. Clin. N. Amer., 23, 517, 1976.
Guthkelch, A. N.: Diastematomyelia with Median Septum, Brain, 97, 729, 1974.
———: Occipital Cranium Bifidum, Arch. Dis. Child., 45, 104, 1970.
Hilal, S. K., Marton, D., and Pollack, E.: Diastematomyelia in Children, Radiology, 112, 609, 1974.
Hoffman, H. J., Hendrick, E. B., and Humphreys, R. P.: The Tethered Spinal Cord: Its Protean Manifestations, Diagnosis and Surgical Correction, Child's Brain, 2, 145, 1976.
Holmes, L. B., Driscoll, S. G., and Atkins, L.: Etiologic Heterogeneity of Neural-tube Defects, N. Engl. J. Med., 294, 365, 1976.
Ingraham, F. D., et al.: Spina Bifida and Cranium Bifidum, Cambridge, Mass., Harvard University Press, 1944, 215 pp.
Karch, S. B., and Urich, H.: Occipital Encephalocele: A Morphological Study, J. Neurol. Sci., 15, 89, 1972.
Lorber, J.: Spina Bifida Cystica. Results of Treatment of 270 Consecutive Cases with Criteria for Selection for the Future, Arch. Dis. Child., 47, 854, 1972.
Laurence, K. M.: The Natural History of Spina Bifida Cystica, Arch. Dis. Child., 39, 41, 1964.
Milunsky, A., and Alpert, E.: Antenatal Diagnosis, Alpha Fetoprotein and the FDA, N. Engl. J. Med., 295, 168, 1976.
Nadler, H.: Present Status of the Prevention of Neural Tube Defects, Pediatrics, 55, 751, 1975.
Thompson, M. W., and Rudd, N. L.: The Genetics of Spinal Dysraphism, in Current Controversies in Neurosurgery, ed. by T. P. Morley, Philadelphia, W. B. Saunders Co., 1976, p. 126.
Shurtleff, D. B., et al.: Myelodysplasia: Decision for Death or Disability, N. Engl. J. Med., 291, 1005, 1974.

ARNOLD-CHIARI MALFORMATION

A congenital anomaly of the hindbrain characterized by a downward elongation of the brainstem and cerebellum into the cervical portion of the spinal cord was originally described by Arnold in 1894 and Chiari in 1895.

Pathology. The cause of this defect is not entirely clear. Because of its common association with spina bifida occulta or the presence of a meningocele or myelomeningocele in the lumbosacral region, it is thought that the downward displacement of the brainstem and cerebellum is due to the fixation of the cord at the site of the spinal defect early in fetal life. With the growth of the spine in the later months of intrauterine life, the adhesions in the lumbar or sacral region prevent the cord from ascending in a normal manner and pull the brainstem and cerebellum downward into the cervical canal. This hypothesis is not applicable to the cases in which there is no defect in the lower spine and fails to account for the other anomalies commonly associated with the hindbrain malformation (absence of the septum pellucidum, fusion of the thalami, hypoplasia of the falx cerebri, fusion of the corporea quadrigemina and microgyri). Some type of developmental arrest and overgrowth of the neural tube in embryonic life is a more plausible explanation of the anomaly.

The gross description of the abnormality has been remarkably similar in all the reported cases. The inferior poles of the cerebellar hemispheres extend downward through the foramen magnum in two tongue-like processes and are often adherent to the adjacent medulla, more than one half of which is usually below the level of the foramen magnum (Fig. 103). The medulla is elongated and flattened anteroposteriorly and the lower cranial nerves are stretched.

Incidence. The Arnold-Chiari malformation is not as rare as would be expected from the small number of cases reported in the literature. Ingraham and Swan found 20 instances of this abnormality in their 290 cases with myelomeningoceles (Table 65). The defect is almost always but not invariably associated with a meningomyelocele or spina bifida occulta in the lumbosacral region. Hydrocephalus is present in the majority of the cases. Other associated defects of development include rounded defect in the bones of the skull (craniolacunia, Lückenschädel), defects in the spinal cord (hydromyelia, double cord), and defects in the spinal column (basilar impression).

Symptoms and Signs. The neurologic signs and symptoms of the Arnold-Chiari malformation which appear in the first few months of life are usually due to hydrocephalus and other developmental defects in the nervous system. The prognosis is poor in these cases. Rarely the onset of symptoms may be delayed until adult life. There may be signs and symptoms of injury to the cerebellum, medulla and the lower cranial nerves, with or without evidence of increased intracranial pressure. The increased intracranial pressure is attributed to occlusion of the basal cisterns by the defect, and the neurological symptoms to compression of the brainstem and stretching of the cranial nerves. Other congenital anomalies, except spina bifida occulta, are rare in the cases with late onset of symptoms.

Diagnosis. The presence of the Arnold-Chiari malformation is quite probable when there is the coincidence of a meningomyelocele, hydrocephalus and craniolacunia in infancy. The diagnosis in adults is usually not made before surgical exploration or necropsy. It should be considered whenever signs and symptoms of damage to the cerebellum, medulla and the lower cranial nerves appear in association with spina bifida. The clinical signs and symptoms of the Arnold-Chiari malformation which occur in adult life may simulate the syndromes produced by tumors of the posterior fossa, multiple sclerosis, syringomyelia and basilar impression. The diagnosis can be established by myelography.

Treatment. The treatment of the condition in infants includes excision of the sac in the spinal region and decompression of the posterior fossa to relieve the hydrocephalus. In adults the posterior fossa should be decompressed. The best results are obtained when few neurological symptoms are present as result of the spinal defect or other congenital anomalies.

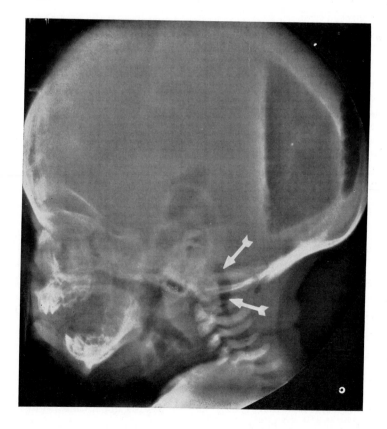

Figure 103. Arnold-Chiari malformation. Ventriculogram showing enlargement of the lateral ventricles. The fourth ventricle is at level of the foramen magnum (arrows). A small quantity of air is seen behind the cerebellar tonsils below the level of the foramen magnum. (Courtesy Dr. Gordon Potts.)

REFERENCES

Arnold, J.: Myelocyste, Transposition von Gewebskeimen und Sympodie, Beitr. path. Anat., 16, 1, 1894.

Banerji, N. K., and Millar, J. H. D.: Chiari Malformation Presenting in Adult Life. Its Relationship to Syringomyelia, Brain, 97, 157, 1974.

Bokinsky, G. E., Hudson, L. D., and Weil, J. U.: Impaired Peripheral Chemosensitivity in Arnold-Chiari Malformation and Syringomyelia, N. Engl. J. Med., 288, 947, 1973.

Caviness, V. S., Jr.: The Chiari Malformations of the Posterior Fossa and their Relation to Hydrocephalus, Devel. Med. Child Neurol., 18, 103, 1976.

Chiari, H.: Ueber Veränderungen des Kleinhirns, des Pons und der Medulla Oblongata in Folge von congenitaler Hydrocephalie des Grosshirns, Denkschr. Akad. Wiss. Wien, 63, 71, 1896.

Emery, J. L., and MacKenzie, N.: Medullo-cervical Dislocation Deformity (Chiari II Deformity) Related to Neurospinal Dysraphism (Meningomyelocele), Brain, 96, 155, 1973.

Gardner, E., O'Rahilly, R., and Prolo, D.: The Dandy-Walker and Arnold-Chiari Malformations, Arch. Neurol., 32, 393, 1975.

Saez, R. J., Onofrio, B. M., and Yanagihara, T.: Experience with Arnold-Chiari Malformation, J. Neurosurg., 45, 416, 1976.

Sieben, R. L. Hamida, M. B., and Shulman, K.: Multiple Cranial Nerve Defects Associated with the Arnold-Chiari Malformation, Neurology, 21, 673, 1971.

Venes, J. L.: Multiple Cranial Nerve Palsies in an Infant with Arnold-Chiari Malformation, Devel. Med. Child Neurol., 16, 817, 1974.

MALFORMATIONS OF OCCIPITAL BONE AND CERVICAL SPINE

The defects in the development of the cervical spine and base of the skull may be divided into the following groups:

1. Basilar impression
2. Malformation of the atlas and axis
3. Malformation or fusion of other cervical vertebrae (Klippel-Feil anomaly)

Any of these malformations may occur singly or together, and in addition they may be associated with developmental defects in the skull, spine, central nervous system or other organs of the body. These deformities can be present without any clinical symptoms, but symptoms may appear as the result of mechanical compression of the neuraxis or the occurrence of an associated malformation of the nervous system.

Basilar Impression

Platybasia, basilar impression and basilar invagination are names frequently used interchangeably for the skeletal malformation in which the base of the skull is flattened on the cervical spine. *Platybasia* (flat base skull) is present if the angle formed by a line connecting the nasion, tuberculum sella and anterior margin of the foramen magnum is greater than 143 degrees (Fig. 104). *Basilar invagination* refers to an

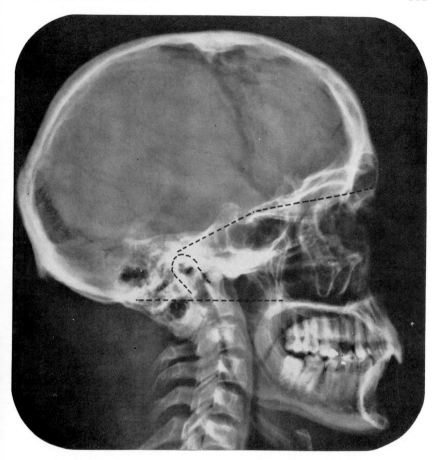

Figure 104. Basilar impression with platybasia. The odontoid process is entirely above Chamberlain's line (hard palate to base of skull). Basal angle is very flat. (Courtesy Dr. Juan Taveras.)

upward indentation of the base of the skull which may be present in Paget's disease, osteomalacia or other forms of bone disease associated with softening of the bones of the skull. An upward displacement of the occipital bone and cervical spine with protrusion of the odontoid process into the foramen magnum constitutes *basilar impression*. Compression of the pons, medulla, cerebellum and cervical cord and stretching of the cranial nerves may result from the upward ascent of the occipital bone and cervical spine and from narrowing of the foramen magnum.

Pathology and Pathogenesis. Minor degrees of platybasia and basilar invagination may produce no symptoms. In the majority of symptomatic cases the deformity is due to a congenital maldevelopment or hypoplasia of the basiocciput resulting in basilar impression, platybasia, partial or complete atlanto-occipital fusion and a narrowed foramen magnum (Fig. 104). An autosomal dominant mode of inheritance has been suggested by some authors. The pons, medulla and cerebellum may be distorted and the cranial nerves stretched. Janeway and Toole have suggested that vertebral artery obstruction during head turning may be significant in the production of brainstem symptoms in basilar impression.

Symptoms and Signs. Basilar impression is a relatively rare condition. Neurological symptoms, when present, usually develop in childhood or early adult life. The head may appear to be elongated and its vertical diameter reduced. The neck appears shortened and its movements may be limited by anomalies of the upper cervical vertebrae. Neurological symptoms include spastic weakness of the extremities, unsteadiness of gait, cerebellar ataxia, nystagmus and paralyses of the lower cranial nerves. Choked discs and other signs of increased pressure may occur when the deformity produces an interference with the circulation of the cerebrospinal fluid. A syringomyelic syndrome may occur, when there is a cavitation of the cervical cord and lower medulla. It is not clear whether this cavitation is the result of the deformation of the nervous structures or whether it is an independent anomaly. Partial or complete subarachnoid block is present at lumbar puncture in the majority of the cases.

Diagnosis. The diagnosis of basilar impression is obvious in the majority of the cases from the general appearance of the patient. It can be established with certainty by the characteristic appearance of the base of the skull in the roentgenograms. The clinical syndromes produced by the anomaly can simulate those produced by multiple sclerosis, syringomyelia, the Arnold-Chiari malformation and posterior fossa tumors. These diagnoses are readily excluded by the roentgenograms.

Treatment. The treatment is surgical decompression of the posterior fossa and the upper cervical cord.

Malformations of the Atlas and Axis

Maldevelopments of the atlas and axis may be found in connection with basilar impression or they may occur independently. Congenital defects resulting in weakness or absence of the structures maintaining stability of the atlanto-axial joints predispose to subluxation and dislocation. Neurological symptoms may be produced by anterior dislocation of the atlas and compression of the cord between the protruding odontoid process and the posterior rim of the foramen magnum. There may be a mild or severe degree of spastic quadriplegia, with or without evidence of damage to the lower cranial nerves. Sensory loss may be absent or of only mild degree. Transitory signs or symptoms of a progressive myelopathy may occur, often following exaggerated movements of the neck or mild trauma. Respiratory embarrassment is prominent when the thoracic muscles are affected. The diagnosis is made by the finding of anterior dislocation of the atlas in the roentgenograms. When the bony changes are slight, and especially when there is little or no posterior dislocation of the odontoid process, the symptoms may be due to other congenital defects, such as syringomyelia or the Arnold-Chiari malformation.

Fusion of the Cervical Vertebrae

Fusion of the upper thoracic vertebrae and the entire cervical spine into a single bony mass was reported by Klippel and Feil in 1912. Since that time a number of cases have been reported in which variations of this deformity were present. In the majority of the cases the abnormality consists of the fusion of the cervical vertebrae into one or more separate masses (Fig. 105). The fusion of the vertebrae is the result of maldevelopment *in utero* and there is evidence of both autosomal dominant and recessive transmission. This anomaly is associated with a short neck, low hairline and limitations of neck movements, especially in the lateral direction. The fusion of the vertebrae is not in itself of any great clinical importance except for the resulting deformity in the appearance of the neck. Clinical symptoms are usually due to the presence of syringomyelia or other developmental defects of the spinal cord, brainstem or cerebellum. Congenital cardiovascular defects have been reported in 4% and genitourinary anomalies in 2% of patients. Congenital deafness due to faulty development of the osseous inner ear has been recorded and estimated to occur in up to 30% of patients by Palant and Carter.

Gunderson and Greenspan have emphasized the much more frequent occurrence of fusion of only two adjacent cervical vertebrae. These patients have a normal morphological appearance, the limited anomaly causing only accentuation of symptoms in the presence of cervical osteoarthritis.

A curious neurological symptom, *i.e.*, the presence of mirror movements in the upper extremities, has been reported to occur in conjunction with the anomaly of the cervical spine. Voluntary movements of one upper extremity are involuntarily imitated to a more or less degree by the other upper extremity. The pathophysiology of these mirror movements is not known. In the reported cases they were present from birth but became less evident as the child grew older.

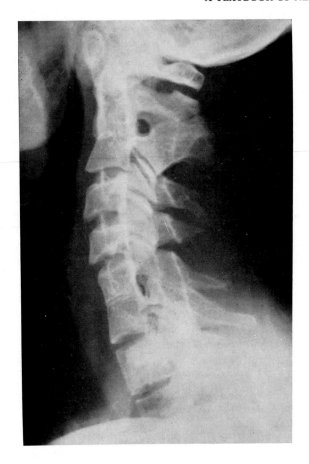

Figure 105.   Fusion of cervical vertebrae. (Klippel-Feil syndrome.)

REFERENCES

Bareš, L.; Basilar Impression and the So-called "Associated Anomalies," Eur. Neurol., 13, 92, 1975.
Bharucha, E. P., and Dastur, H. M.: Craniovertebral Anomalies, Brain, 87, 469, 1964.
DeBarros, M. C., et al.: Basilar Impression and Arnold-Chiari Malformation, J. Neurol., Neurosurg., & Psychiat., 31, 596, 1968.
Dehaene, I., Pattyn, G., and Calliauw, L.: Megadoicho-basilar Anomaly, Basilar Impression and Occipitovertebral Anastomosis, Clin. Neurol. Neurosurg., 78, 131, 1975.
Greenberg, A. D.: Atlanto-Axial Dislocations, Brain, 91, 655, 1968.
Gunderson, C. H., Greenspan, R. H., and Glaser, G. H.: The Klippel-Feil Syndrome: Genetic and Clinical Reevaluation of Cervical Fusion, Medicine, 46, 491, 1967.
Gunderson, C. H., and Solitare, G. B.: Mirror Movements in Patients with Klippel-Feil Syndrome, Arch. Neurol., 18, 675, 1968.
Janeway, R., Toole, J. F., Leinbach, L. B., and Miller, H. S.: Vertebral Artery Obstruction with Basilar Impression, Arch. Neurol., 15, 211, 1966.
Juberg. R. C., and Gershanik, J. J.: Cervical Vertebral Fusion (Klippel-Feil) Syndrome with Consanguineous Parents, J. Med. Genet., 13, 246, 1976.

Klippel, M., and Feil, A.: Un cas d'absence des vertebres cervicales, avec cage thoracique remontant jusqu'a la base due crâne (cage thoracique cervicale), Nouv. Iconog, de la Salpetriere, 25, 223, 1912.

Konigsmark, B. W., and Gorlin, R. J.: Genetic and Metabolic Deafness, Philadelphia, W. B. Saunders Co., 1976, p. 188.

McRae, D. L.: The Significance of Abnormalities of the Cervical Spine, Am. J. Roentgen., 84, 3, 1960.

Mecklenburg, R. S., and Krueger, P. M.: Extensive Genitourinary Anomalies Associated with Klippel-Feil Syndrome, Am. J. Dis. Child., 128, 92, 1974.

Michie, I., and Clark, M.: Neurological Syndromes Associated with Cervical and Craniocervical Anomalies, Arch. Neurol., 18, 241, 1968.

Morrison, S. G., Perry, L. W., and Scott, L. P.: Congenital Brevicollis (Klippel-Feil Syndrome) and Cardiovascular Anomalies, Amer. J. Dis. Child., 115, 614, 1968.

Palant, D. I., and Carter, B. L. : Klippel-Feil Syndrome with Deafness, Am. J. Dis. Child., 123, 218, 1972.

Paradis, R. W., and Sax, D. S.: Familial Basilar Impression, Neurology, 22, 554, 1972.

Taveras, J. M., and Wood, E. H. : Diagnostic Neuroradiology, Baltimore, Williams & Wilkins, 1964, 1960 pp.

Taylor, A. R., and Chakravorty, B. C.: Clinical Syndromes Associated with Basilar Impression, Arch. Neurol., 10, 475, 1964.

Wadia, N. H.: Myelopathy Complicating Congenital Atlanto-Axial Dislocation, Brain, 90, 449, 1967.

PREMATURE CLOSURE OF THE CRANIAL SUTURES

Premature closure of the bones of the skull (craniostenosis) results in a variety of malformations of the skull, described under the terms oxycephaly, brachycephaly, scaphocephaly, plagiocephaly, and trigonocephaly. The chief clinical feature of all of these conditions is the abnormal shape of the skull. Exophthalmos, papilledema or optic atrophy, and the presence of digital markings in the roentgenograms of the skull may also be present. Minor degrees of these abnormalities in the skull may exist without the development of any clinical symptoms. The frequency of involvement of the various sutures is given in Table 66. The defects in the skull may be accompanied by cleft palate, cardiac anomalies, polydactylism, syndactylism and various ocular defects (coloboma, cataracts, retinal detachment, etc.). Convulsive seizures may occur and mental development may be retarded by associated defects in the brain or limitation of its growth by the skull.

According to Park and Powers, these conditions are dependent upon defects in the germ plasm. Familial incidence is not uncommon and defects in the development of other bones, particularly those of the hands and feet (syndactylism) may also be present. There is some disagreement as to the exact mechanism of the production of the cranial deformity. Virchow advanced the hypothesis that when there is a premature synostosis of two cranial bones, normal growth of the brain is inhibited in the direction perpendicular to the obliterated suture line and there is compensatory growth in other directions. Park and Powers explain the premature synostosis on the basis of a defective growth of

Table 66.   The Frequency of Involvement of the Various Sutures in
525 Patients with Craniostenosis
(After Shillito and Matson, Pediatrics, 1968)

Suture Involved	Number of Patients	%
Sagittal alone	289	55
Coronal	127	24.1
Bilateral 61		
Unilateral 66		
Metopic	21	4
Any three sutures	36	6.8
Four or more sutures	30	6.0
Any two unpaired sutures	10	1.8
Lambdoid	12	2.3
Unilateral 7		
Bilateral 5		
Total	525	100

the mesenchyme in which the bone is formed. The bones formed in this defective tissue are smaller than normal and fuse as soon as they approximate. In support of this theory, Reilly found craniostenosis in 30% of his patients with active rickets resulting from various metabolic bone diseases.

Oxycephaly. The characteristic feature of this form of premature closure of the sutures is the great height of the skull, which slopes up to a point at the vertex (tower skull). The forehead is receding, the superciliary and frontal ridges are inconspicuous and the face is narrowed and elongated. The eyeballs are prominent and protruding. The palate is high arched and narrow. The cranial deformity may be present at birth but more commonly it becomes manifest in the first few years of life. Headaches and papilledema may result from increased intracranial pressure. Optic atrophy may occur, secondary to the papilledema or stretching of the optic nerves by the deformity. Other ocular symptoms include divergent strabismus, myopia and nystagmus. The latter is especially common when vision is completely destroyed. Mental retardation, deafness or convulsive seizures are found in a small percentage of the cases.

The roentgenograms of the skull show the characteristic deformity in the shape of the skull. The coronal and sagittal sutures are fused. The orbits are shallow and the accessory nasal sinuses are poorly developed. Digital markings on the inner surface of the skull are prominent.

Brachycephaly. In this form of craniostenosis the head is flattened in the anterior plane, the frontal fossa is shallow and the vault is abnormally high. The defect is due to a premature closure of the coronal sutures. The clinical features are: Prominent forehead with a broad skull, eyes widely separated, short broad nose, bulging eyes, and a prominent jaw.

Scaphocephaly. Premature closure of the sagittal suture results in a deformation of the shape of the skull in which the head is elongated and flattened laterally (Fig. 106). The forehead bulges and the occiput is round and full. This is the most common form of craniostenosis.

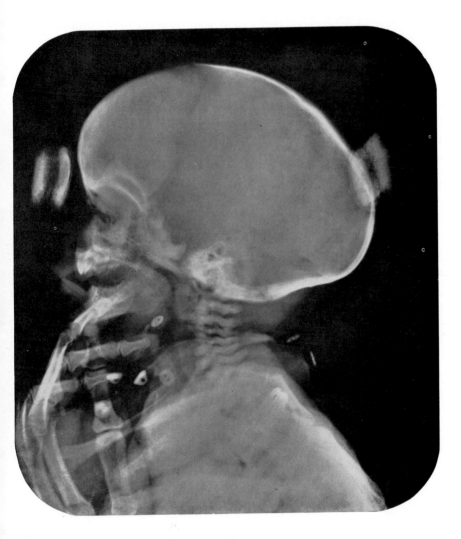

Figure 106. Craniostenosis. Elongation of anterior-posterior diameter of skull due to premature synostosis of sagittal suture. (Courtesy Dr. Juan Taveras.)

Trigonocephaly. The deformity of the skull which results from premature closure of the metopic suture is characterized by triangular appearance of the head when viewed from above, narrow pointed ("keel") forehead with midline ridging and close approximation of the eyes.

Plagiocephaly. An oblique-shaped head results from the premature closure on one side of either the coronal or lambdoid suture. The head appears flat over the involved suture and unusually prominent on the corresponding unaffected side.

Craniofacial Dysostosis (Crouzon's Syndrome). The deformity of the skull and the clinical symptomatology in this form of craniostenosis is similar to that of oxycephaly. The distinguishing features are maxillary hypoplasia with shortness of the upper lip, prognathism and a peculiar "parrot-beak" shape to the nose. The eyes are widely separated.

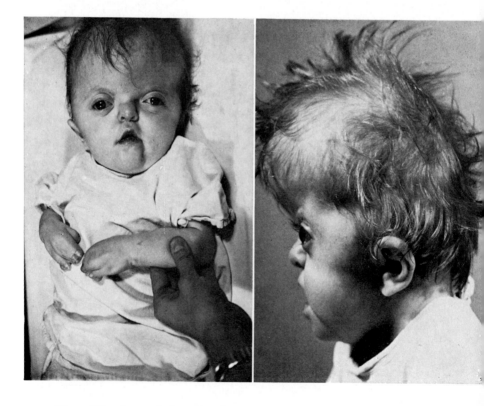

Figure 107.   Acrocephalosyndactyly (Apert's syndrome). The head is shortened in the anterior posterior dimension, the forehead is prominent and the occiput flat. Typical facies showing shallow orbits and proptosis of the eyes, downward slanting palpebral fissures, small nose and low set ears. Osseous and cutaneous syndactyly of the hands and feet.

Exophthalmos and divergent strabismus are characteristic features. The disease is transmitted by an autosomal dominant gene.

Acrocephalosyndactyly (Apert's Syndrome). The deformity of the skull, facial appearance and mode of inheritance is similar to that in Crouzon's syndrome. The distinguishing feature of this anomaly is the presence of syndactyly of the hands and feet. Several phenotypically similar inherited disorders have been reviewed by Smith.

Diagnosis. The diagnosis of premature fusion of the. cranial sutures can be made in most instances by the characteristic appearance of the head. The differentiation between the various forms may not be possible without roentgenograms of the skull. The diagnosis of hydrocephalus should be excluded by the appearance of the skull or by computerized axial tomography.

Treatment. Surgical therapy may be indicated in order to conserve vision and to improve the cosmetic appearance of the head.

REFERENCES

Anderson, F. M., and Geiger, L.: Craniosynostosis. A Survey of 204 Cases, J. Neurosurg., *22*, 229, 1965.

Anderson, F. M., Gwinn, J. L., and Todt, J. C.: Trigonocephaly. Identity and Surgical Treatment, J. Neurosurg., *19*, 723, 1962.

Anderson, H., and Gomes, S. P.: Craniosynostosis, Acta Paed. Scand., *57*, 47, 1968.

Crouzon, M. O.: Dysostose cranio-faciale héréditaire, Soc. med hôp., Paris, *33*, 545, 1912.

Dunn, F. H.: Apert's Acrocephalosyndactylism, Radiology, *78*, 738, 1962.

Foltz, E. L., and Loeser, J. D.: Craniosynostosis, J. Neurosurg., *43*, 48, 1975.

Greitzer, L. J., et al.: Craniosynostosis—Radial Aplasia Syndrome, J. Pediat., *84*, 723, 1974.

Kushner, J., et al.: Crouzon's Disease (Craniofacial Dysostosis). Modern Diagnosis and Treatment, J. Neurosurg., *37*, 434, 1972.

Norwood, C. W., et al.: Recurrent and Multiple Suture Closures after Craniectomy for Craniosynostosis, J. Neurosurg., *41*, 715, 1974.

Park, E. A., and Powers, G. F.: Acrocephaly and Scaphocephaly with Symmetrically Distributed Malformations of the Extremities: a Study of the So-called "Acrocephalosyndactylism," Am. Dis. Child., *20*, 235, 1920.

Reilly, B. J., Leeming, J. M., and Fraser, D.: Craniosynostosis in the Rachitic Spectrum, J. Ped., *64*, 396, 1964.

Shillito, J., and Matson, D. D.: Craniosynostosis. A Review of 519 Surgical Patients, Pediatrics, *41*, 829, 1968.

Smith, D. W.: *Recognizable Patterns of Human Malformation*, 2nd ed., Philadelphia, W. B. Saunders Co., 1976, pp. 234–243.

CERVICAL RIB

The roots of the brachial plexus and the subclavian artery may be compressed by a variety of anomalous or normal structures in the neck and give rise to sensory, motor or vasomotor symptoms in one or both upper extremities. The nerves and the artery may be compressed by a rudimentary cervical rib, a fibrous band, the first thoracic rib or an unusually tight scalene muscle. The onset of symptoms is often related to loss of tonus in the muscles of the shoulder girdle and the descent of the shoulder which normally occurs between childhood and adult life. Traction due to carrying heavy weight and trauma have been cited as precipitous causes.

Incidence. Rudimentary or fully developed cervical ribs are not an infrequent incidental finding at necropsy or in routine roentgenograms of the cervical spine. They do not give rise, however, to any symptoms except in a small percentage of the cases (estimated at 5 to 10%). The

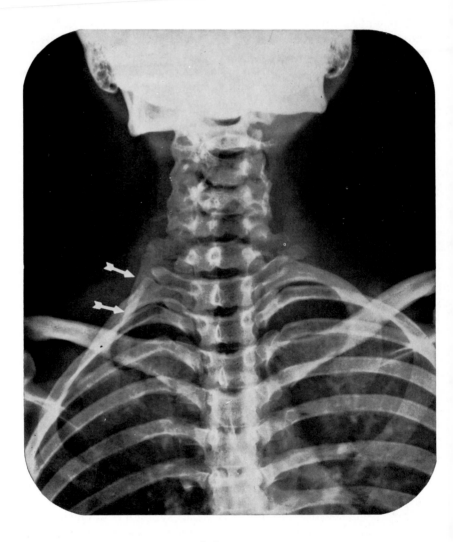

Figure 108.   Cervical rib. (Courtesy Dr. Juan Taveras.)

older literature contains many articles dealing with the symptomatology and treatment of cervical ribs. In recent years the subject has
received less consideration and more attention has been directed
toward the role of herniation of the nucleus pulposus in the production
of pain in the upper extremity. Cases are still seen, however, in which
the symptoms are due to compression of the brachial plexus and the
subclavian artery by cervical ribs, but they are relatively rare. The
syndrome is most apt to develop in the female because of the greater
tendency of the shoulder to sag in this sex.

Symptoms and Signs. The most common sensory symptoms are
pains and paresthesias in the hand and forearm. These may involve the
entire hand, but most frequently they are confined to the ulnar half and
the corresponding portion of the forearm. Complete loss of sensation is
rare. There may be a diminution of the appreciation of pain and light
touch in the hand or forearm which does not necessarily conform to
any root or nerve distribution. Muscular weakness and atrophy are
much less common. When present, they are usually confined to the
small muscles of the hand innervated by the ulnar or median nerves.
There may be a partial atrophy of the thenar muscles and the interossei.

Diagnosis. The diagnosis is made without difficulty when the typical
motor and sensory findings are combined with prominence in the
cervical region above the clavicle and roentgenographic evidence of a
cervical rib (Fig. 108). The diagnosis is more difficult when only one or
two of the clinical features are present. It must be remembered that the
roentgen ray findings are not conclusive because cervical ribs are
frequently present without causing symptoms and, on the other hand,
the roentgenograms cannot show the presence of a fibrous band or a
tight scalene muscle.

In the differential diagnosis, other conditions which give rise to pain
or muscular atrophy in the upper extremity must be considered. These
include syringomyelia, amyotrophic lateral sclerosis, spinal tumors,
osteoarthritis of the spine, herniation of the nucleus pulposus and
compression of the median nerve within the carpal tunnel. In a number
of cases it will be necessary to perform myelography to exclude these
diagnoses. Electromyography and determination of nerve conduction
velocities may prove helpful in the diagnosis in selected cases.

Course. The course is subject to considerable variation. The
symptoms may be subject to frequent remission or they may progress
slowly. The limb may be incapacitated by the pains and paresthesia but
only rarely does an extensive degree of atrophy occur.

Treatment. Temporary relief of the symptoms may be obtained by the
wearing of a sling to support the affected extremities. Exercise which
develops the shoulder muscles and leads to the assumption of a better
posture may be of value. Rest in bed, traction on the neck and the use of

pillows to support the shoulders have all been advocated for the relief of symptoms. Good results have been reported following surgical removal of anomalous ribs, division of fibrous bands or sectioning of the scalene anticus muscles.

REFERENCES

Bergquist, E., Hugosson, R., and Westerberg, C. E.: A Wasted Hand, J. Neurol. Neurosurg. Psychiat., *38*, 100, 1975.
Britt, L. P.: Nonoperative Treatment of the Thoracic Outlet Syndrome, Clin. Orthopaed., *51*, 45, 1967.
Gilroy, J., and Meyer, J. S.: Compression of the Subclavian Artery as a Cause of Ischaemic Brachial Neuropathy, Brain, *86*, 733, 1964.
Kremer. R. M., and Ahlquist, R. E., Jr.: Thoracic Outlet Compression Syndrome, Amer. J. Surg., *130*, 612, 1975.
London, G. W.: Normal Ulnar Nerve Conduction Velocity Across the Thoracic Outlet; Comparison of Two Measuring Techniques, J. Neurol. Neurosurg. Psychiat., *38*, 756, 1975.
Sargent, P.: Lesions of the Brachial Plexus Associated with Rudimentary Ribs, Brain, *44*, 95, 1921.
Urschel, H. C., Jr., and Razzuk, M. A.: Management of the Thoracic-Outlet Syndrome, N. Engl. J. Med., *286*, 1140, 1972.

Chapter 6

Degenerative and Heredodegenerative Diseases

Robert Katzman

There are a wide variety of diseases of the central nervous system of unknown cause, many of which have a hereditary or familial occurrence. In the present state of our knowledge they are grouped under the heading of degenerative or heredodegenerative diseases. It has been the tendency in the past to attribute these diseases to an inherent lack of ability of certain tissues to survive (abiotrophy). This explanation is obviously inadequate and it is quite probable that with the advance of our knowledge, it will be shown that most, if not all, of these morbid conditions are the result of genetically conditioned metabolic defects or damage by exogenous or endogenous toxins.

It should be kept in mind that any portion of the central and peripheral nervous system may be affected in the heredodegenerative disease, and that the different portions may be involved in various combinations. In some families there is a remarkable consistency with regard to the location and extent of the pathological changes. In other families, there may be great discrepancies in the manifestation of the disease between individual members of the family and also between them and members of other families apparently affected with the same disease. Abortive forms (formes frustes) of all of the heredodegenerative diseases are also quite common.

For the sake of convenience in discussion, these diseases have been grouped according to the site of principal damage as follows: (1) Cerebrum and cranial nerves; (2) basal ganglia; (3) cerebellum; (4) spinal cord; (5) peripheral nerves; and (6) muscles.

CEREBRUM AND CRANIAL NERVES

Tuberous Sclerosis

Tuberous sclerosis (Bourneville's disease) is a disease characterized by the development in early life of congenital tumors, or malformations in the nervous system, skin and occasionally in other organs of the body. Prominent clinical features include: (1) Facial nevi ("sebaceous adenoma"); (2) recurrent convulsive seizures; and (3) retardation of mental development.

Pathology and Pathogenesis. The pathological changes are widespread and include lesions in the nervous system, skin, bones, retina, kidney and other viscera.

Nervous System. The brain is usually normal in size, but there are several or many hard nodules on the surface of the cortex. These nodules are smooth, rounded or polygonal and project slightly above the surface of the neighboring cortex. They are whitish in color and firm to the touch. The nodules are of various sizes. Some involve only a small portion of one convolution. Others may encompass the convolutions of one whole lobe or a major portion of a hemisphere. In addition, there may be developmental anomalies of the cortical convolutions in the form of pachygyria or microgyria. On sectioning the hemispheres, sclerotic nodules may be found in the subcortical gray matter, the white matter and the basal ganglia. The lining of the lateral ventricles is frequently the site of numerous small nodules which project into the ventricular cavity ("candle gutterings") (Fig. 109). Sclerotic nodules are less frequently found in the cerebellum, brainstem and spinal cord.

Histologically the nodules are characterized by the presence of a cluster of atypical glial cells in the center and giant cells in the periphery. Calcifications are relatively frequent. Other features include

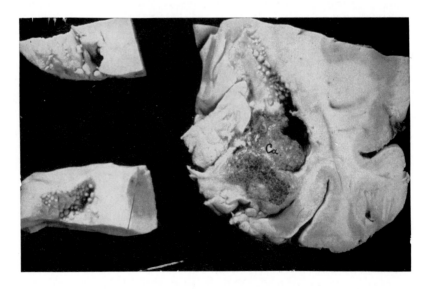

Figure 109.   Tuberous sclerosis. Nodules, "candle gutterings," on surface of ventricles. (Courtesy Dr. Leon Roizin.)

heterotopia, vascular hyperplasia (sometimes with actual angiomatous malformations), disturbances in the cortical architecture and the occasional development of subependymal giant cell astrocytomas.

Skin. The lesions in the skin are multiform and include the characteristic facial nevi (fibroma molluscum) and patches of skin fibrosis. The facial lesions (Fig. 110) are not adenomas of the sebaceous glands but are small hamartomas arising from nerve elements of the skin, combined with hyperplasia of the connective tissue and blood vessels. Lesions similar in composition to those on the face are occasionally found between the nails and the digits of the hands and feet. Circumscribed areas of hypomelanosis or white nevi are common in tuberous sclerosis and are often found during infancy. Although these are less specific than the sebaceous adenoma, they are of importance in suspecting the diagnosis in infants with seizures. Histologically, the skin appears normal, except for the loss of melanin, but ultrastructural studies have shown that the melanosomes are small in size and have reduced content of melanin.

Retina. The retinal lesions are small congenital tumors (phakomas) which may be composed of glia, ganglion cells or fibroblasts. Glioma of the optic nerve has been reported. The occurrence of congenital tumors in the central nervous system and retina in tuberous sclerosis links this condition with the syndrome of von Hippel and Lindau.

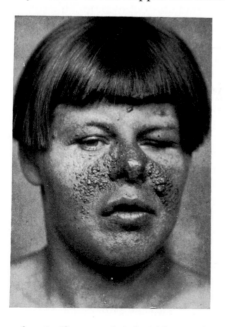

Figure 110.   Tuberous sclerosis. Chararacteristic facial lesions (facial nevi or "sebaceous adenoma"). (Yakovlev, P. I., and Guthrie, R. H., courtesy Arch. Neurol. & Psychiat.)

Other Visceral Lesions. Other lesions include rhabdomyomata of the heart, renal tumors and tumors or cysts in the liver, pancreas, ovary, thyroid or other viscera. The tumors in the kidney involve the cortex and are mixed growths, variously classified as sarcomas, adenomas, fibromas and angiomas.

Incidence. The disease in the well-developed form is rare, accounting for less than one half of 1% of the admissions to colonies for the epileptic or mentally retarded. The incidence of abortive forms with only one or two of the characteristic features of the disease is greater than that of the fully developed syndrome.

The disease occurs sporadically and on a heredofamilial basis. Inheritance appears to involve an autosomal gene with variable penetrance such that the occurrence of one or more of the individual features of the disease is not uncommon. The coincidence of tuberous sclerosis and von Recklinghausen's disease in the same family has been recorded.

Although all races are affected, the disease is uncommon in colored races. There is a greater incidence in the male sex. There is some variation in regard to the age of onset of the characteristic features. The facial nevi (sebaceous adenoma) may be present at birth but more commonly they do not become apparent until the third to sixth years of life. The onset of convulsive seizures is usually in the first or second years of life, but it may be delayed to puberty. A combination of infantile spasms and white nevi frequently herald the disease in infancy. It has been reported that as many as 25% of infants with infantile spasms later develop manifestations of tuberous sclerosis. The mental retardation is usually noted in the early years of life but may be delayed to childhood. In abortive forms, there may be no evidence of mental deficiency.

Symptoms and Signs. The classical features of the disease are the skin lesions, recurrent convulsive seizures, and mental retardation (Table 67). The convulsive seizures may be generalized or focal in nature. There may not be any symptoms to indicate focal damage to the nervous system, but hemiplegia, diplegia, athetosis and other focal signs occur in a small percentage of cases. With the exception of the changes in the retina, lesions in the cranial nerves are rare.

The degree of mental impairment varies from idiocy to a mild degree of mental retardation. In most cases, the onset is early and the deterioration of mental faculties progressive. Stereotyped motor performances and psychotic episodes are not infrequent.

The characteristic facial lesion (Fig. 110) is composed of multiple warty nodules, yellowish pink or brownish red in color, varying in size from that of a millet seed to that of a small pea. These lesions are symmetrically distributed on the side of the nose, the nasolabial fold

Table 67. Frequency of Findings in Tuberous Sclerosis *

	No. of Patients	%
Mental retardation	88	62
Epilepsy	132	93
Adenoma sebaceum	121	85
White nevi	58	41
Other skin lesions	100	70
Retinal tumors	53	37
Intracranial calcifications	68	48

*Based upon 142 patients in the series of Bundey and Evans (1969) and Lagos and Gomez (1967).

and the cheeks in the shape of a butterfly. Occasionally they may spread to involve the forehead and chin. Other skin lesions which may also be present and which link this condition with that of von Recklinghausen's disease are: Pedunculated skin polypi scattered over the head, back, shoulders and pelvic region; raised, but not pedunculated nodules varying in size from that of a pinhead to that of a walnut; areas of fibrous hyperplasia varying in size from that of a half dollar to that of a small saucer (shagreen patches); pigmented nevi and warts; café-au-lait spots; and sharply outlined depigmented patches of skin representing circumscribed hypomelanosis or white nevi which are clinically similar in appearance to the depigmented areas seen in patients with nevus depigmentosus. These can be distinguished from vitiligo by their presence at birth.

Renal tumors are present in over two thirds of the cases; but they are only infrequently detected during life. Tumors of the heart occur in about 5% of the cases. These are small and usually give rise to no symptoms except rarely when they may be the cause of death in infancy. Tumors in the other viscera are usually incidental necropsy findings.

Laboratory Data. The cerebrospinal fluid findings are normal except in the cases with a large intracerebral tumor. Abnormalities in the urine may be present in the patients with renal tumors.

Focal or diffuse abnormalities may be found in the electroencephalogram of patients with convulsive seizures. Infantile myoclonic epilepsy with hypsarrhythmia has been reported in a number of the patients. Small or moderate-sized areas of calcification within the substance of the cerebrum or cerebellum are found in the roentgenograms of the skull in about half of the cases. In addition there may be islands of increased density in the skull overlying cortical nodules. Punched-out, cyst-like foci in the terminal phalanges of the hands and feet are occasionally found.

Diagnosis. The diagnosis is made without difficulty when all three features of the disease are present, or when the characteristic facial lesions are combined with feeblemindedness or epilepsy. The diagnosis is not justified by the occurrence of epilepsy in association with pedunculated tumors, fibromas or café-au-lait spots in the skin in the absence of the typical facial nevi. Other findings in favor of the diagnosis of tuberous sclerosis are tumors in the retina, small scattered areas of calcification in the brain in the roentgenograms (Fig. 111) of the skull and "candle-gutterings" in the walls of the lateral ventricles in the pneumoencephalograms. Computerized tomography (CT) has proved to be especially helpful in the diagnosis of tuberous sclerosis. The scan may show multiple small punctate to nodular lesions in the periventricular area as well as nodules in the cortex, white matter, and basal ganglia (Fig. 112). The CT may also show ventricular dilatation when one of the nodules obstructs the foramen of Monro or other cerebrospinal fluid pathways.

Tuberous sclerosis must be differentiated from other diseases with congenital tumors in the skin, nervous system and retina, including von Recklinghausen's disease, von Hippel-Lindau disease and angiomatosis of the brain with vascular nevi on the face. The differential

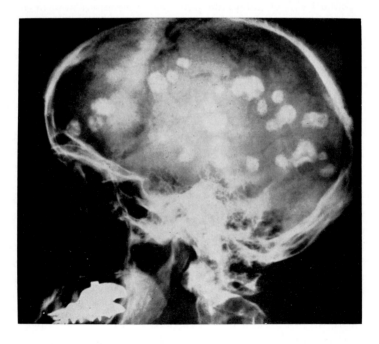

Figure 111.   Tuberous sclerosis. Calcified nodules in the cerebrum.
(Courtesy Dr. P. I. Yakovlev.)

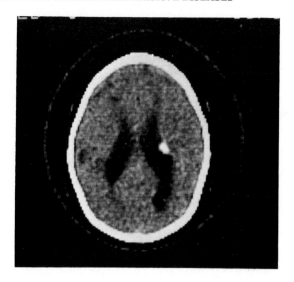

Figure 112. CT brain scan. Tuberous sclerosis. Dilatation of ventricles with nodule in wall of one ventricle. (Courtesy Dr. Harry H. White.)

can usually be made from the presence of the typical features of these three conditions.

The symptomatology of toxoplasmosis may occasionally have a superficial resemblance to that of tuberous sclerosis. The differential is made by the absence of the facial lesions in the former as well as by the specific skin test.

Course and Prognosis. The prognosis is poor and the course is progressive in the full-blown syndrome. The seizures increase in frequency and the severity of the mental defect is progressive. Death usually occurs before the thirtieth year of life. The average duration of life is less than fifteen years. Approximately 30% die before the fifth year and nearly 75% before the twentieth year of life. Death may be due to marasmus, brain tumor, intercurrent infection, status epilepticus or renal failure. In the abortive form there may be a relatively normal life span, particularly if there is no serious degree of mental retardation and the seizures are infrequent or absent.

Treatment. There is no specific treatment. Seizures should be treated by anticonvulsant drugs and patients with severe degrees of mental defect should be institutionalized.

REFERENCES

Babonneix, L.: A propos de l'épiloia, Arch. de méd. d. enf., *31*, 133, 1928.
Berland, H. I.: Roentgenological Findings in Tuberous Sclerosis, Arch. Neurol. & Psychiat., *69*, 669, 1953.

Bielschowsky, M., and Gallus, M.: Ueber Tuberoese Sklerose, J. f. Psych. u. Neurol., 20, 1, 1913.
Bundey, S., and Evans, K.: Tuberous Sclerosis, A Genetic Study, J. Neurol., Neurosurg., and Psychiatry, 32, 591, 1969.
Cares, R. M.: The Tuberous Sclerosis Complex, J. Neuropath. & Exper. Neurol., 17, 247, 1958.
Gomez, M. R., Mellinger, J. F., and Reese, D. F.: The Use of Computerized Transaxial Tomography in the Diagnosis of Tuberous Sclerosis, Mayo Clin. Proc., 50, 553, 1975.
Jimbow, K., Fitzpatrick, T. B., Szabo, G., and Hori, Y.: Congenital Circumscribed Hypomelanosis: A Characterization Based on Electron Microscopic Study of Tuberous Sclerosis, Nevus Depigmentosus, and Piebaldism, J. Inv. Dermatol., 64, 50, 1975.
Martin, G. I., et al.: Computer-Assisted Cranial Tomography in Early Diagnosis of Tuberous Sclerosis, J.A.M.A., 235, 2323, 1976.
Pampiglioni, G., and Pugh, E.: Infantile Spasms and Subsequent Appearance of Tuberous Sclerosis Syndrome, Lancet, 2, 1046, 1975.
Rizzuto, N., and Ferrari, G.: Familial Infantile Myoclonus Epilepsy in a Family Suffering from Tuberous Sclerosis, Epilepsia, 9, 117, 1968.
Scheig, R. L., and Bornstein, P.: Tuberous Sclerosis in the Adult, Arch. Int. Med., 108, 789, 1961.
Yakovlev, P. I., and Guthrie, R. H.: Congenital Ectodermoses (Neurocutaneous Syndromes) in Epileptic Patients, Arch. Neurol. & Psychiat., 26, 1145, 1931.

Menkes Kinky Hair Disease
(X-Chromosome Linked Malabsorption)

In 1962, Menkes and his colleagues described a family with a sex-linked recessive disorder characterized by abnormality of scalp hair, failure to grow, seizures and early death. Pathologically, there is widespread degeneration of the cerebral cortex and cerebellar atrophy. Over 35 cases have now been reported. Only males are affected. The scalp hair is sparse, wiry, kinky and colorless; on microscopic examination, there is longitudinal twisting of the hair (pili torti), periodic variations of hair diameter (monilethrix) and ragged fracture of the end of the hair (trichorrhexis nodosa). Micrognathia is often present. The infant fails to gain weight or achieve developmental milestones and develops a seizure disorder. Later, hyperactive reflexes and rigidity may develop. Death usually occurs in the first three years. This disease is due to a copper deficiency, tissue analyses showing a low level of copper and of copper-containing enzymes. Danks and co-workers have demonstrated a primary defect in copper transport, particularly affecting intestinal absorption of copper. Antenatal diagnosis has been made by demonstration of reduced uptake of copper into cell cultures of amniotic fluid. Feeding of large doses of copper has not helped, but treatment with intravenously administered copper has been reported successful in one case.

REFERENCES

Danks, D. M. et al.: Menkes' Kinky-Hair Syndrome, Lancet, 1, 1100, 1972.
Horn, N.: Copper Incorporation Studies on Cultured Cells for Prenatal Diagnosis of Menkes' Disease, Lancet, 1, 1156, 1976.

Menkes, J. H. et al.: A Sex-Linked Recessive Disorder with Retardation of Growth, Peculiar Hair and Focal Cerebral and Cerebellar Degeneration, Pediatrics, *29*, 764, 1962.

Linear Nevus Sebaceous with Convulsions and Mental Deterioration

In recent years there have been reports on small number of patients with a syndrome similar to that of tuberous sclerosis or Sturge-Weber disease. These patients have all been infants with a linear nevus on the face or head combined with ocular lesions, convulsive seizures and mental retardation. The cutaneous and ocular lesions are present at birth. There have not been any reports on the pathological changes in the nervous system. The convulsive seizures and mental retardation are indicative of cerebral involvement.

REFERENCES

Blanchine, J. W.: Nevus Sebaceous of Jadassohn, Amer. J. Dis. Child., *120*, 223, 1970.
Feuerstein, R. C., and Mims, L. C.: Linear Nevus Sebaceous with Convulsions and Mental Retardation, Amer. J. Dis. Child., *104*, 675, 1962.
Monahan, R. H., and Hill, C. W.: Multiple Choristomas, Convulsions and Mental Retardation as a New Neurocutaneous Syndrome, Amer. J. Ophth., *64*, 529, 1967.

Primary Degeneration of the Corpus Callosum
(Marchiafava-Bignami Disease)

Primary degeneration of the corpus callosum is a disease which occurs almost exclusively in middle-aged or elderly Italian men addicted to the use of wine and is characterized by mental symptoms and signs of focal or diffuse disease of the brain. The disease was first described by Marchiafava and Bignami in 1903.

Etiology. The cause of the degenerative changes in the corpus callosum is not known. The relative specificity of the disease for the Italian male suggests that constitutional liability is a factor in its occurrence. It is possible, that in addition to constitutional factors, the type of alcohol may be of importance because addiction to crude Italian wine (dago-red) is recorded in some of the isolated cases of non-Italian stock.

Pathology. The *sine qua non* of Marchiafava-Bignami disease is necrosis of the medial zone of the corpus callosum. The dorsal and ventral rims are spared. The necrosis varies from softening and discoloration (Fig. 113) to cavitation and cyst formation. Usually all stages of degeneration are found in any given case. In the majority of cases, the rostral portion of the corpus callosum is affected first. The lesions arise

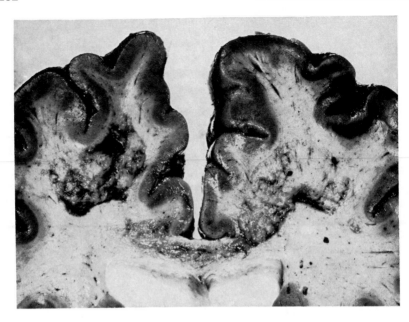

Figure 113. Marchiafava's disease. Acute necrosis of corpus callosum and neighboring white matter of the frontal lobes. (Merritt, H. H., and Weisman, A. D., courtesy J. Neuropath. & Exper. Neurol.)

as small symmetrical foci which extend and become confluent. Although medial necrosis of the corpus callosum is the principal pathological finding, there may be, in addition, degeneration of the anterior commissure (Fig. 114), the posterior commissure, the centrum semiovale and subcortical white matter, the long association bundles and the middle cerebellar peduncles. All these lesions, wherever situated, have a constant bilateral symmetry. Usually spared are the internal capsule, corona radiata and subgyral arcuate fibers. The gray matter is not grossly affected.

Few diseases have such a well-defined pathological picture. The corpus callosum may be infarcted as a result of occlusion of the anterior cerebral artery, but the symmetry of the lesions, the sparing of the gray matter and the occurrence of similar lesions in the anterior commissure, long association bundles and cerebellar peduncles are found only in Marchiafava's disease.

The microscopic alterations are the result of a sharply defined necrotic process with loss of myelin but relative persistence of axis cylinders in the periphery of the lesions. No evidence of inflammation is found as a rule, aside from a few perivascular lymphocytes. In most cases fat-filled phagocytes are common. Gliosis is usually not well

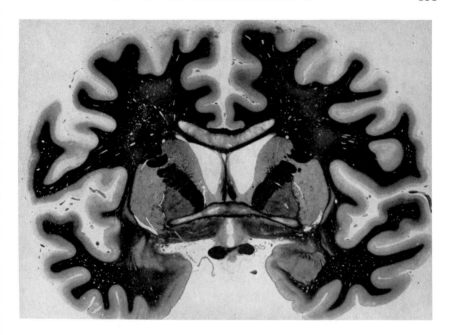

Figure 114. Marchiafava-Bignami disease. Medial necrosis of the corpus callosum and anterior commissure with sparing of the margins. (Courtesy Dr. P. I. Yakovlev.)

advanced. Capillary endothelial proliferation may be present in the affected area but no thrombi are seen in the vessels.

Incidence. More than 100 cases have been recorded in the literature since the original report in 1903. Almost all of the cases have been in the male sex and with a few exceptions of Italian stock. The onset of symptoms is in middle or late life.

Symptoms and Signs. The onset is usually insidious and the initial symptomatology so nonspecific that an accurate estimation of the exact time is difficult. The clinical picture is quite variable with a mixture of focal and diffuse signs of cerebral disease.

Mental symptoms are almost always present and are variously characterized by manic, paranoid and delusional states, depression, extreme apathy or dementia. Convulsions are common. Tremors, aphasia, apraxia, transitory hemiparesis and other motor disabilities may be found.

Diagnosis. The diagnosis of Marchiafava-Bignami disease can rarely be made with certainty during life. It can be suspected, however, when an elderly Italian man with a history of alcoholism develops an organic psychosis or dementia together with convulsions, aphasia or other focal cerebral symptoms. The differential diagnosis under these circumstances lies between senile and presenile dementias and frontal lobe tumor.

Course. The disease is usually slowly progressive and results in death within three to six years. In an occasional case there is a temporary remission.

Treatment. There is no adequate therapy.

REFERENCES

Fittipaldi, C.: Sul morbo di Marchiafava (degenerazione primitiva sistematizzata delle vie commessurali dell'encefalo), Riv. di pat. nerv., *50*, 427, 1937.
Ironside, R., Bosanquet, F. D., and McMenemey, W. H.: Central Demyelination of the Corpus Callosum (Marchiafava-Bignami Disease). With Report of a Second Case in Great Britian, Brain, *84*, 212, 1961.
King, L. S., and Meehan, M. C.: Primary Degeneration of Corpus Callosum (Marchiafava's Disease), Arch. Neurol. & Psychiat., *36*, 547, 1936.
Marchiafava, E.: The Degeneration of the Brain in Chronic Alcoholism, Proc. Roy. Soc. Med., *26*, 1151, 1933.
Marchiafava, E., and Bignami, A.: Sopra un' alferazione del corpo calloso osservata in soggetti alcoolisti, Riv. di pat. nerv., *8*, 544, 1903.
Merritt, H. H., and Weisman, A. D.: Primary Degeneration of the Corpus Callosum (Marchiafava-Bignami's Disease), J. Neuropath. & Exper. Neurol., *4*, 155, 1945.
Nielsen, J., and Courville, C.: Central Necrosis of Corpus Callosum (Marchiafava-Bignami's Disease), Bull. Los Angeles Neurol. Soc., *8*, 81, 1943.

Central Pontine Myelinolysis

In 1959, Adams, Victor and Mancall described a distinct and previously unrecognized entity characterized by the destruction of myelin localized to the base of the pons. Since that time over 100 cases have been reported in the literature. In most of these, there was a history of chronic alcoholism or other conditions associated with malnutrition. The lesion may involve the entire base of the pons (Fig. 115) or only a small portion of this structure. There is destruction of the myelin with relative preservation of the axis cylinders and the pontine nuclei in the affected area.

The majority of the cases reported are young or middle-aged, although the disease can occur in children and in elderly individuals. Typically, there is a history of alcoholism and associated malnutrition, but other systemic disorders may be present. Central pontine myelinolysis is often associated with diseases of other organs: liver (cirrhosis, Wilson's disease); kidney (vascular nephropathy, kidney transplant); and brain (Wernicke's disease, tumors). Occasional cases have been associated with diabetes, amyloidosis, leukemia and various infections.

Initially, the diagnosis was made solely at necropsy. The first case of central pontine myelinolysis diagnosed in life was presented by

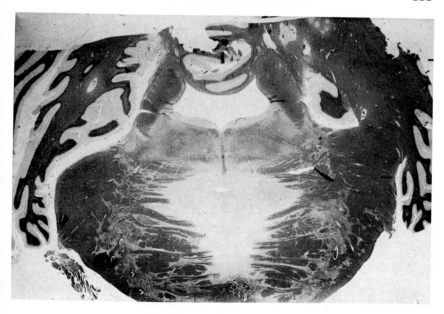

Figure 115.   Central pontine myelinolysis. Section through rostral pons showing characteristic lesion. (Courtesy Dr. J. Kepes.)

Paguirigan and Lefken (1969). Their diagnosis was made in a forty-seven-year-old man with a history of chronic alcoholism who had an acute illness associated with severe electrolyte disturbance, convulsions, and lethargy. Following successful treatment of the electrolyte disturbance, there was progressive corticospinal and corticobulbar disease resulting in quadriplegia and facial, glossal, and pharyngeal paralysis with mutism. The patient was able to move his eyelids. This clinical syndrome is found in about half the patients reported since 1969, and it has become relatively easy to recognize during life. The patients, although mute, are not necessarily comatose, since a response of blinking eyelids can often be elicited. The disease runs a rapid course, with death usually occurring within a few days or weeks after onset of symptoms. The principal pathological change, that is, demyelination, is potentially reversible, and some patients have now been carried through the acute illness.

The electrolyte changes present in a portion of the cases include marked hyponatremia, hypokalemia, and hypochloremia. The serum osmolality is reduced, but the urine osmolality is normal. Thus, these changes are consistent with inappropriate secretion of antidiuretic hormone and should be treated with fluid restrictions. In some instances, there is pulmonary hypoventilation with marked buildup of

pCO_2. An increase in cerebrospinal fluid pressure has been reported in a few cases, but the fluid is usually normal.

The etiology of the disease remains obscure. Pathological evidence has been interpreted to support both a vascular etiology and a toxic-metabolic etiology, the latter being favored by many authors.

REFERENCES

Adams, R. D., Victor, M., and Mancall, E. L.: Central Pontine Myelinolysis, Arch. Neurol. & Psychiat., 81, 154, 1959.

Aleu, F. P., and Terry, R. D.: Central Pontine Myelinolysis, Arch. Path., 76, 140, 1963.

Burcar, P. J., Norenberg, M. D., and Yarnell, P. R.: Hyponatremia and Central Pontine Myelinolysis, Neurology, 27, 223, 1977.

Chason, J. L., Landers, J. W., and Gonzalez, J. E.: Central Pontine Myelinolysis, J. Neurol., Neurosurg., & Psychiat., 27, 317, 1964.

Cole, M., Richardson, E. P., Jr., and Segarra, J. M.: Central Pontine Myelinolysis, Neurology, 14, 165, 1964.

Finlayson, M. H., Snider, S., Oliva, L. A. and Gault, M. H.: Central Pontine Myelinolysis. Two Cases with Fluid and Electrolyte Imbalance and Hypotension, J. Neurol. Sci., 18, 399, 1973.

Paguirigan, A. and Lefken, E. B.: Central Pontine Myelinolysis, Neurology, 19, 1007, 1969.

Powers, J. M. and McKeever, P. E.: Central Pontine Myelinolysis. An Ultrastructural and Elemental Study, J. Neurol. Sci., 29, 65, 1976.

Tomlinson, B. E., Pierides, A. M. and Bradley, W. G.: Central Pontine Myelinolysis. Two Cases with Associated Electrolyte Disturbance, Quart. J. Med., New Series, 45, 373, 1976.

Wiederholt, W. C., Kobayashi, R. M., Stockard, J. J., and Rossiter, V. S.: Central Pontine Myelinolysis. A Clinical Reappraisal, Arch. Neurol., 34, 220 , 1977.

Hereditary Optic Atrophy

(Leber's Disease)

A hereditary disease of the optic nerve, characterized by loss of central vision with relatively normal peripheral fields, was described by von Graefe in 1858. The disease was named after Leber who reported 15 cases in 4 different families in 1871. The disease usually affects young men. The onset is often acute, simulating an optic neuritis.

The mode of inheritance of Leber's disease is not fully understood. It is usually transmitted from mother to son, it occasionally occurs in females who may then transmit it to their sons. The characteristic findings at autopsy are a primary neuronal degeneration of the retina and optic nerve with marked demyelination of the geniculocalcarine fibers, but with preservation of the calcarine cortex. Rarely are other signs of disease of the nervous system, including nystagmus, ataxia, intention tremor, convulsive seizures and increased reflexes found; demyelination of other parts of the brain and the dorsal columns of the spinal cord may occur in such instances. The visual loss usually develops suddenly without any obvious cause, but occasionally it may be preceded by some acute infection. There is a cloudiness of central vision which progresses to a central or paracentral scotoma. Both eyes are affected simultaneously in most cases. The fundi are usually normal at the onset. Occasionally there may be hyperemia, edema or blurring of the disc margins. In the late stages of the disease the disc is atrophic, particularly on the temporal side. The visual acuity is reduced and there is a central or rarely a paracentral scotoma for both form and color. Occasionally only color vision may be affected. The peripheral fields are normal in most cases but may be moderately constricted. The progress of the disease is usually rapid, commonly reaching its maximum extent within a few weeks. It rarely progresses to complete blindness. With arrest of the progression there is a tendency for slight improvement in vision; this is probably explained as the result of the patient learning to accommodate for the central scotoma and to use the periphery of the retina to better advantage.

The diagnosis of hereditary optic atrophy is usually made when the typical visual disturbance is found in a patient with a similar type of visual loss in other members of the family. It is distinguished from tobacco-alcohol amblyopia by the difference in the age of onset and clinical course of the two conditions, the latter generally coming on late in life and improving with abstinence from tobacco and alcohol. Tabetic optic atrophy is readily recognized by its progressive course and the serological findings.

Several other related syndromes of inherited optic atrophy distinct from Leber's have been described. These include a congenital or infantile form of optic atrophy with insidious onset and a dominant mode of inheritance. A sex-linked form of hereditary optic atrophy with onset at ages five to seven has been reported. A recessive inheritance of optic atrophy in association with diabetes insipidus and diabetes mellitus with gradual loss of visual acuity beginning in early childhood has been described in several families. Patients with retrobulbar neuritis do not have the family history nor is the pattern of visual loss the same. Rarely, tumors involving the optic chiasm may simulate Leber's disease; these should be ruled out by roentgenograms of the skull and CT brain scan.

No treatment is of any value. Since the degree of visual loss remains stationary after reaching a certain point, the patient should be encouraged to adjust his life to the amount of vision preserved.

REFERENCES

Adams, J. H., Blackwood, W., and Wilson, J.: Further Clinical and Pathological Observations on Leber's Optic Atrophy, Brain, 89, 15, 1966.

Brodrick, J. D.: Hereditary Optic Atrophy with Onset in Early Childhood, Brit. J. Ophthal, 58, 817, 1974.

Flynn, J. T., and Cullen, R. F.: Disc Oedema in Congenital Amaurosis of Leber, Brit. J. Ophthal., 59, 497, 1975.

Kjer, P.: Infantile Optic Atrophy with Dominant Mode of Inheritance. In: *Handbook of Clinical Neurology*, Vol. 13, Neuroretinal Degenerations, P. J. Vinken and G. W. Bruyn, Eds. North-Holland Publishing Co., Amsterdam, 1972, pp. 111–123.

Leber, T.: Ueber hereditäre und congenital angelegte Sehnervenleiden, Arch. f. Ophth. 17, 249, 1871.

Page, M. McB., Asmal, A. C., and Edwards, C. R. W.: Recessive Inheritance of Diabetes. The Syndrome of Diabetes Insipidus, Diabetes Mellitus, Optic Atrophy and Deafness, Quart. J. Med., 45, 505, 1976.

Pilley, S. F. J., and Thompson, H. S.: Familial Syndrome of Diabetes Insipidus, Diabetes Mellitus, Optic Atrophy, and Deafness (Dismoad) in Childhood, Brit. J. Ophthal., 60, 294, 1976.

Von Graefe: Ein ungewöhnlicher Fall von hereditäre Amaurose, Arch. f. Ophth., 4, 266, 1858.

Went, L. N., De Vries-De Mol, E. C., and Volker-Deiben, H. J.: A Family with Apparent Sex-Linked Optic Atrophy, J. Med. Genetics, 12, 94, 1975.

Progressive Ophthalmoplegia

Progressive ophthalmoplegia, a disease of familial or sporadic incidence, is characterized by a progressive paralysis of the external muscles of the eye. The onset is usually in early childhood, but may be delayed to late middle life. Frequently, the condition starts with a slight ptosis of the lids and progresses over a number of years to complete paralysis of all of the external muscles of the eye. Only rarely are the intrinsic muscles affected. Occasionally, the paralysis of the muscles of one eye may precede that of the other eye by several or many years.

Ophthalmoplegia may occur in association with a wide variety of symptoms and signs of involvement of the nervous system including retinitis pigmentosa, cerebellar ataxia, spastic paraplegia, dystonia, motor neuron disease, peripheral neuropathy, congenital paralysis of the facial muscles and other conditions. Many of the patients with this "ophthalmoplegia-plus" may be more appropriately classified as having the Kearns-Sayre syndrome. The Kearns-Sayre syndrome consists of the association of progressive external ophthalmoplegia with pigmentary degeneration of the retina, heart block, and elevated cerebrospinal protein. The syndrome is not inherited, and onset is usually before age twenty. There is often involvement of various neurological structures and limb weakness. Abnormal mitochondria containing paracrystalline inclusions are seen on ultrastructural examination of muscle biopsies. The involvement of the heart may lead to early death. It is especially important to identify patients with the Kearns-Sayre syndrome, since the associated cardiopathy may require treatment with a pacemaker.

The course of the disease in patients with ophthalmoplegia is progressive for a number of years. There may be a spontaneous arrest before there is complete paralysis of all of the extrinsic eye muscles, but the latter is the rule. In the absence of more widespread involvement of the nervous system or other organs, the length of life is not affected by the disease.

The diagnosis of ocular myopathy is not difficult when the onset is in infancy or early childhood. Refsum's syndrome should be excluded by determination of phytanic acid. Cases with late onset must be differentiated from myasthenia gravis, exophthalmic ophthalmoplegia associated with Graves' disease and diseases which destroy the nuclei in the brainstem.

REFERENCES

Beckett, R. S., and Netsky, M. G.: Familial Ocular Myopathy and External Ophthalmoplegia, Arch. Neurol. & Psychiat., 69, 64, 1953.

Berenberg, R. A. et al.: Lumping or Splitting? "Ophthalmoplegia-Plus" or Kearns-Sayre Syndrome? Ann. Neurol., 1, 37, 1977.

Butler, I. J., and Gadoth, N.: Kearns-Sayre Syndrome. A Review of a Multisystem Disorder of Children and Young Adults, Arch. Intern. Med., 136, 1290, 1976.

Danta, G., Hilton, R. C., and Lynch, P. G.: Chronic Progressive External Ophthalmoplegia, Brain, 98, 473, 1975.

Davidson, S. I.: Abiotrophic Ophthalmoplegia Externa, Brit. J. Ophth., 44, 590, 1960.

Drachman, D. A.: Ophthalmoplegia Plus the Neurodegenerative Disorders Associated with Progressive External Ophthalmoplegia, Arch. Neurol., 18, 654, 1968.

Gibbert, F. B.: Ophthalmoplegia in Acute Polyneuritis, Arch. Neurol., 23, 161, 1970.

Kearns, T. P., and Sayre, G. P.: Retinitis Pigmentosa, External Ophthalmoplegia and Complete Heart Block, Arch. Ophth., 60, 280, 1958.

Kiloh, L. G., and Nevin, S.: Progressive Dystrophy of the External Ocular Muscles (Ocular Myopathy), Brain, 74, 115, 1951.

Magora, A., and Zauberman, H.: Ocular Myopathy, Arch. Neurol., 20, 1, 1969.

Mathew, N. I., Jacob, J. C., and Chandy, J.: Familial Ocular Myopathy with Curare Sensitivity, Arch. Neurol., 22, 68, 1970.

Nicolaissen, B., and Brodal, A.: Chronic Progressive External Ophthalmoplegia, Arch. Ophth., 61, 202, 1959.

Rosenberg, R. N., et al.: Progressive Ophthalmoplegia, Arch. Neurol., 19, 362, 1968.

Marcus Gunn Phenomenon

A reflex elevation of the eyelid in association with movements of the jaw was described by Marcus Gunn. The cause and the anatomical pathway of this reflex are unknown. The reflex is unilateral and occurs in patients who have a partial ptosis of one lid. Movements of the jaw, particularly those which involve lateral deviation of the jaw, are accompanied by an elevation of the affected lid and widening of the palpebral fissure. The reflex movement occasions no disability except for the embarrassment it may cause the patient while eating in public places.

REFERENCES

Grant, F. C.: The Marcus Gunn Phenomenon, Arch. Neurol. & Psychiat., 35, 487, 1936.
Lewy, F. H., Groff, R. A., and Grant, F. C.: Autonomic Innervation of the Eyelids and the Marcus Gunn Phenomenon, Arch. Neurol. & Psychiat., 37, 1289, 1937.

Congenital Facial Diplegia

Congenital facial diplegia (Moebius's syndrome) is rare. Henderson in 1939 was able to find only 60 cases in the literature since the first description by von Graefe in 1868. The paralysis of the facial muscles may be complete or partial and may be associated with other congenital defects, including other cranial nerve palsies, mental defect, clubfoot and brachial malformations. The symptoms are usually nonprogressive, but in one case, a progressive peripheral neuropathy developed as reported by Rubenstein and his associates.

There are probably multiple etiologies of this congenital defect. In several instances, hereditary factors apparently played a role, since two or more members of a family were affected. Pathological studies may show a hypoplasia of the nuclei in the brainstem and of the nerves and muscles connected with them. Evidence of in utero necrosis of brainstem nuclei has been reported in several cases. This necrosis may have resulted from an episode of anoxia in utero; the brainstem is known to be susceptible at this age. In other cases, the primary defects appear to have involved facial muscles indirectly. In the case reported by Pitner and his associates there was dysplasia of the facial muscles. Although hypoplastic changes were found in the cerebellum and medulla, the facial nucleus and the facial nerves were normal.

When the paralysis is complete, it is usually evident immediately after birth owing to the difficulty in nursing or failure of the eyes to close during sleep. Partial paralysis may not be detected until it is noted that the child's face does not move normally in crying or laughing. The paralysis is complete in about one third of the cases. In the remainder the muscles of the upper half of the face are more severely affected than those of the lower half, a condition which is different from that usually seen in either supranuclear or peripheral palsies. Facial diplegia occurred as an isolated phenomenon in only about 15% of the reported cases. In the original description of Moebius's syndrome, patients also had abducens paralysis (70%). Other congenital abnormalities include ophthalmoplegia externa (25%), ptosis (10%), lingual palsy, unilateral or bilateral (18%), clubfoot (30%), brachial malformations (22%), pectoral muscle defects (13%) and mental deficiency (10%).

REFERENCES

Hanson, P. A., and Rowland, L. P.: Möbius Syndrome and Facioscapulohumeral Muscular Dystrophy, Arch. Neurol., 24, 31, 1971.

Henderson, J. L.: The Congenital Facial Diplegia Syndrome, Brain, 62, 381, 1939.

Murphy, J. P., and German, W. J.: Congenital Facial Paralysis, Arch. Neurol. & Psychiat., 57, 358, 1947.

Olson, W. H., et al.: Moebius Syndrome, Lower Motor Neurone Involvement and Hypogonadotropic Hypogonadism, Neurology, 20, 1002, 1970.

Pitner, S. E., Edwards, J. E., and McCormick, W. F.: Observations on the Pathology of the Moebius Syndrome, J. Neurol., Neurosurg. & Psychiat., 28, 362, 1965.

Rubenstein, A. E., Lovelace, R. E., Behrens, M. M. and Weisberg, L. A.: Moebius Syndrome in Kallmann Syndrome, Arch. Neurol., 32, 480, 1975.

Sprofkin, B. E., and Hillman, J. W.: Moebius's Syndrome—Congenital Oculofacial Paralysis, Neurology, 6, 50, 1956.

Thakkar, N., et al.: Möbius Syndrome Due to Brain Stem Tegmental Necrosis, Arch. Neurol., 34, 124, 1977.

Laurence-Moon-Biedl Syndrome

A syndrome characterized by the combination of retinitis pigmentosa, mental deficiency, polydactylism and signs of a polyglandular deficiency was described in 1866 by Laurence and Moon.

The syndrome is rare and little is known of the pathogenesis or pathology. It is more common in the male and the mode of inheritance is autosomal recessive. The signs usually appear in childhood and include obesity, retardation of sexual development, polydactylism and

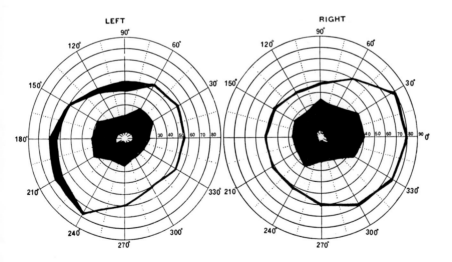

Figure 116.   Retinitis pigmentosa. Annular scotomata. Visual acuity, O.D. 15/15, O.S. 15/40. (Courtesy Dr. Max Chamlin.)

pigmentary degeneration of the retina. Some degree of mental deficiency is almost always present and occasionally it may be severe. There is considerable variation in the degree of retinal degeneration but partial or almost complete blindness (Fig. 116) is the rule. Hypogenitalism is more frequent in males than in females. There is now evidence that this may be due to abnormalities in hypothalamic control of pituitary function. Diabetes insipidus may also occur. The adrenal and thyroid glands are usually spared. Bodily growth may be reduced and some patients may remain dwarfs. The occurrence of retinitis pigmentosa, adiposity and impotence in association with spinocerebellar degeneration was reported by Francois and Descamps suggesting a relationship between Laurence-Moon-Biedl syndrome and the cerebellar ataxias.

The syndrome may occur in an abortive form with absence of one or more of the principal clinical features. The signs and symptoms are stationary except for the visual loss which is usually progressive. Although the condition is compatible with a normal life span, early death often occurs due to coincidental kidney abnormalities or congenital heart disease. The severity of the mental defect and visual loss is the chief factor which determines whether or not the affected individual will make a satisfactory adjustment to life.

REFERENCES

Bauman, M. L. and Hogan, G. R.: Laurence-Moon-Biedl Syndrome. Report of Two Unrelated Children Less Than 3 Years of Age, Am. J. Dis. Child., 126, 119, 1973.
Biedl, A.: Uber das Laurence-Biedlsche Syndrom, Med. Klin., 29, 839, 1933.
Klein, D., and Ammann, F.: The Syndrome of Laurence-Moon-Bardet-Biedl and Allied Diseases in Switzerland, J. Neurol. Sciences, 9, 479, 513, 1969.
Koepp, P.: Laurence-Moon-Biedl Syndrome Associated with Diabetes Insipidus Neurohormonalis, Europ. J. Pediat., 121, 59, 1975.
McLaughlin, T. G., and Shanklin, D. R.: Pathology of Laurence-Moon-Bardet-Biedl Syndrome, J. Path. and Bacteriol., 93, 65, 1967.
Perez-Palacios, G., et al.: Pituitary and Gonadal Function in Patients with the Laurence-Moon-Biedl Syndrome, Acta Endocrinol., 84, 191, 1977.

Myoclonus Epilepsy

Myoclonus epilepsy is a group of heredofamilial diseases characterized by the onset in childhood of myoclonic jerks, convulsive seizures, various neurological signs and mental deterioration.

Myoclonus in patients with primary convulsive disorders occurs only sporadically. Myoclonus, however, is an almost constant feature both in patients with myoclonus epilepsy and in patients with several other diffuse diseases of the nervous system. The myoclonus is often increased.by photic stimulation and by sensory stimulation such as the tapping of a limb, and during the course of voluntary movement, so-called intention myoclonus. A severe from of intention myoclonus occurs in some patients following cerebral anoxia or cardiac arrest. Myoclonus occurs together with signs of cerebellar dysfunction as cardinal features of the Ramsay Hunt syndrome (1921). Myoclonus is a prominent feature of slow virus diseases such as subacute sclerosing panencephalitis and Jakob-Creutzfeldt disease. It is a prominent feature of many of the sphingolipidoses, particularly in the juvenile and adult forms.

Myoclonus epilepsy is a rare disease. Only a small number of cases have been recorded in the literature and it is only rarely seen on the neurological wards of hospitals for acute or chronic diseases of the nervous system.

The incidence of myoclonic epilepsies varies considerably from country to country. Unverricht first described the disease in Estonia. The highest incidence of the Unverricht form occurs in Finland, a country whose population is closely related to Estonians. The prevalence of myoclonus epilepsy in Finland is 1/27,000. Since the onset of dementia may be late, life span is not materially altered. Lafora bodies are not present in this group. Many of the cases are familial, and there appears to be an autosomal recessive inheritance. The Lafora variety of myoclonus epilepsy also has an autosomal recessive inheritance, but the course is malignant with progressive myoclonus, dementia and incapacitation usually by age twenty, with death often in the third decade.

Myoclonus epilepsy was described as a distinct clinical entity by Unverricht in 1891 and in 1903 by Lundborg. Lafora and Glueck in 1911 described a number of cases which were characterized pathologically by the presence of inclusion bodies in the neurons (Fig. 117).

They are most numerous in the neurons of the dentate nucleus, but may be found in the thalamus, basal ganglia and spinal cord. Schwarz and Yanoff report the finding of these bodies in the nerves, retina, liver, heart and striate muscles. Histochemical evidence suggested that the Lafora bodies might represent a type of glycoprotein. Biochemical analyses of Lafora bodies show that they are comprised primarily of a relatively insoluble polyglucosan and, therefore, this disease might be considered as among the inherited disorders of glycogen metabolism.

At the present time, it seems probable that the forms described by Lafora and Glueck represent a different entity with a different symptomatology from those without Lafora bodies but with degenerative changes in Purkinje cells and neurons in the medial part of the thalamus.

The myoclonic jerks may involve any of the muscles of the body. The extremities are most commonly affected but the muscles of the trunk, face, diaphragm and larynx or pharynx may be involved. The move-

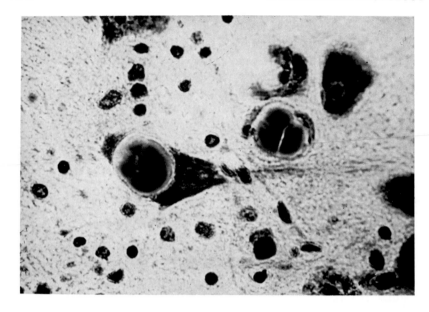

Figure 117. Myoclonus epilepsy. Inclusion body in neurons of substantia nigra. Nissl stain.

ments are quick and forceful. They may be present when the patient is at rest, but they are more numerous when the patient attempts voluntary movements. They may occur so frequently that they interfere with walking or use of the upper extremities. Spontaneous variations in the frequency and severity of the myoclonic jerks are common. The seizures are usually of the grand mal type, but minor seizures often described as petit mal may occur. With progress of the disease, cerebellar incoordination or intention tremor appears. Less commonly signs and symptoms of damage to the basal ganglia, brainstem or retina may develop.

The laboratory findings are normal with the exception of various changes in the electroencephalogram. Wave and spike formations at the rate of three per second are commonly seen in all cortical leads in association with the myoclonic jerks. The abnormalities in the electroencephalogram and myoclonic jerks can be precipitated by stroboscopic light.

The diagnosis is made on basis of the familial or hereditary occurrence of the typical symptom complex. The differential includes Schilder's disease, inclusion body encephalitis and other diseases with myoclonus.

The course of the disease is slowly progressive with incapacitation by the age of twenty in the severe cases. Abortive forms of the disease with only one or two of the classical features may occur.

The convulsive seizures should be treated with anticonvulsant drugs. Several drugs have recently been found to be effective in the treatment of myoclonus. These include the precursor of serotonin, L-5-hydroxytryptophan, and the benzo-diapezine derivative, clonazepam.

REFERENCES

Boghen, D., and Peyronnard, J. -M.: Myoclonus in Familial Restless Legs Syndrome, Arch. Neurol., 33, 368, 1976.

Gambetti, P., Di Mauro, S., Hirt, L., and Blume, R. P.: Myoclonic Epilepsy with Lafora Bodies. Some Ultrastructural, Histochemical, and Biochemical Aspects, Arch. Neurol., 25, 483, 1971.

Goldberg, M. A., and Dorman, J. D.: Intention Myoclonus: Successful Treatment with Clonazepam, Neurology, 26, 24, 1976.

Growdon, J. H., Young, R. R., and Shahani, B. T.: L-5-Hydroxtryptophan in Treatment of Several Different Syndromes in Which Myoclonus is Prominent, Neurology, 26, 1135, 1976.

Hunt, J. R.: Dyssynergia Cerebellaris Myoclonica—Primary Atrophy of the Dentate System: A Contribution to the Pathology and Symptomatology of the Cerebellum, Brain, 44, 490, 1921.

Janeway, R., Ravens, J. R., et al.: Progressive Myoclonus Epilepsy with Lafora Inclusion Bodies. I. Clinical, Genetic, Histopathologic, and Biochemical Aspects, Arch. Neurol., 16, 565, 1967.

Koskiniemi, M., Donner, M., et al.: Progressive Myoclonus Epilepsy. a Clinical and Histopathological Study, Acta Neurol. Scand., 50, 307, 1974.

Lafora, G. R., and Glueck, B.: Contributions to the Histopathology and Pathology of Myoclonic-Epilepsy, Bull. Gov. Hosp. Insane, 3, 96, 1911.

Laitinen, L., and Toivakka, E.: Clonazepam (Ro 5–4023) in the Treatment of Myoclonus Epilepsy. Four Case Reports, Acta Neurol. Scand., 49, Suppl. 53, 72, 1973.

Lundborg, H.: Der Erbgang der progressiven myoklonus-Epilepsie (Myoklonic Epilepsies. Unverrichts familiare Myoklonie), Ztschr. f. d. ges. Neurol. u. Psychiat., 9, 353, 1912.

Schwarz, G. A., and Yanoff, M.: Lafora's Disease. Distinct Clinico-Pathologic Form of Unverricht's Syndrome, Arch. Neurol., 12, 172, 1965.

Swanson, P. D., Luttrell, C. N., and Magladery, J. W.: Myoclonus—A Report of 67 Cases and Review of the Literature, Medicine, 41, 339, 1962.

Unverricht, H.: Ueber familiare Myoclonie, Deutsche Ztschr. f. Nervenh., 7, 32, 1895.

Unverricht, H.: Die Myoclone, Leipzig, Franz Deuticke, 1891, 128 pp.

Ziegler, D. K., Van Speybroech, N. W., and Seitz, E. F.: Myoclonic Epilepsia Partialis Continua and Friedreich Ataxia, Arch. Neurol., 31, 308, 1974.

Progressive Cerebral Degeneration of Infancy
(Progressive Poliodystrophy, Alper's Disease)

The characteristic pathological findings in this type of cerebral degeneration are a severe degree of loss of the nerve cells and glia (status spongiosus) in all layers of the cerebral cortex in all or most of the convolutions of the cerebral hemispheres, with relative preservation of the white matter. The basal ganglia and the cerebellum may also be involved. Clinically the cases have been characterized by the onset of symptoms in early infancy (convulsions, dementia, blindness, deafness and paralysis), a progressive course terminating in death before the age of seven years. There is some question whether this entity constitutes a single disease. Some authors noted that the pathological changes are similar to those that occur with cerebral anoxia and thus attributed them to difficult delivery or repeated convulsions. Several authors have pointed out the similarity of the neuropathological changes to those of Creutzfeldt-Jakob disease and kuru, both "slow-virus" diseases. In some cases familial occurrence suggests an inherited metabolic defect.

In several families the occurrence of hepatic cirrhosis together with progressive degeneration of the cerebral cortex has been noted. The neurological disorder begins between ages one and three with intractable convulsions resulting in a stuporous and demented state, death within ten months of the onset of the symptoms. Evidence of hepatic disease occurs late. In these patients spinal fluid protein was found to be between 90 and 500 mg %. Evidence indicates that the inheritance is recessive in this sub-group.

REFERENCES

Alpers, B. J.: Diffuse Progressive Degeneration of the Gray Matter of the Cerebrum, Arch. Neurol. & Psychiat., 25, 469, 1931.
————: Progressive Cerebral Degeneration of Infancy, J. Nerv. & Ment. Dis., 130, 442, 1961.
Blackwood, W., et al.: Diffuse Cerebral Degeneration in Infancy (Alper's Disease), Arch. Dis. Child., 38, 193, 1963.
Dreifuss, F. E., and Netsky, M. G.: Progressive Poliodystrophy, Am. J. Dis. Child., 107, 649, 1964.
Hopkins, I. J., and Turner, B.: Spongy Glio-Neuronal Dystrophy: A Degenerative Disease of the Nervous System, J. Neurol., Neurosurg., & Psychiat., 36, 50, 1973.
Huttenlocher, P. R., Solitare, G. B., and Adams, G.: Infantile Diffuse Cerebral Degeneration with Hepatic Cirrhosis, Arch. Neurol., 33, 186, 1976.
Janota, I.: Spongy Degeneration of Grey Matter in 3 Children. Neuropathological Report, Arch. Dis. Child., 49, 571, 1974.
Jellinger, K., and Seitelberger, F.: Spongy Glio-Neuronal Dystrophy in Infancy and Childhood, Acta Neuropath., 16, 125, 1970.
Sandbank, U., and Chemke, J.: A Case of Infantile Jakob-Creutzfeldt Disease, Acta Neuropath., 4, 331, 1965.

Leigh's Disease (Wernicke's Encephalomyelopathy in Children)

Leigh in 1951 published the report of his findings in a child with necrotizing lesions in the brainstem somewhat similar to those found in Wernicke's encephalopathy. The necrotic lesions are located in the periaqueductal areas of the midbrain and pons, and the substance of the medulla adjacent to the fourth ventricle (Table 68). The cerebrum,

Table 68. Comparison of Distribution of Brain Lesions in Subacute Necrotizing Encephalomyelopathy and Wernicke's Disease

	SNE (50 cases)	WD (60 cases)
Brainstem	49/50	51/60
Midbrain	44/49	41/57
Tegmentum	39/50	
Substantia nigra	31/50	3/60
Pons	45/49	14/39
Medulla	41/49	34/59
Spinal cord	23/31	1/3
Cerebellum	25/43	11/58
Cerebrum	46/50	57/59
Cortex	5/50	19/57
Basal ganglia	28/43	6/52
Thalamus	20/39	38/56
Hypothalamus	12/44	56/58
Mamillary bodies	7/44	50/52

After: Montpetit et al., 1971.

especially the basal ganglia and the thalamus, cerebellum and the central portion of the spinal cord may also be affected. Pathologically, subacute necrotizing encephalomyelopathy differs from Wernicke's in that the hypothalamus and mamillary bodies are usually spared.

Although approximately 100 cases have been reported, the disease is relatively uncommon. Familial occurrence is frequent, and the disorder appears to be inherited as an autosomal recessive. The onset of symptoms is often insidious. Some infants develop normally for several months or years, others show evidence of damage to the nervous system from early infancy. Respiratory abnormality, a poor cry, and impairment of feeding can be observed in early infancy. Later, impairment of vision and hearing, ataxia, muscular weakness and hypotonia, progressive intellectual deterioration, and seizures appear. Abnormalities of eye movements, including nystagmus, are common, but ophthalmoplegia is rare. Rarely is there muscle involvement. Within a single family, the clinical picture may show significant variation. The affected individuals usually die in the first few years, but a few cases have lived until the first or middle portion of the second decade of life.

Routine laboratory examinations are usually not helpful. Nonspecific changes can appear on the electroencephalogram; the pneumoencephalogram occasionally shows dilatation of ventricles, and the cerebrospinal fluid protein is mildly elevated in about a fourth of the patients. Since the familial incidence suggests an inherited metabolic defect, and since the pathological distribution of lesions partially resembles that of Wernicke's encephalopathy, attention has been given to a possible disorder in intermediary metabolism of lactate or pyruvate. A mild metabolic acidosis frequently associated with a rise in blood lactate and pyruvate and an elevation of plasma alanine is found. In some cases, a decrease in pyruvate carboxylase is reported, and in other cases, a deficiency of pyruvate dehydrogenase has been demonstrated. It has been reported that the level of thiamine triphosphate is decreased in the brain, especially in affected areas, and protein that interferes with the formation of thiamine triphosphate has been reported in the urine of some patients with Leigh's disease. Thus, it seems likely that Leigh's disease represents a common pathological expression of several genetic defects involving pyruvate metabolism.

REFERENCES

Blass, J. P., Cederbaum, S. D. and Dunn, H. G.: Biochemical Abnormalities in Leigh's Disease, Lancet, 1, 1237, 1976.

Crosby, T. W. and Chou, S. M.: "Ragged-Red" Fibers in Leigh's Disease, Neurology, 24, 49, 1974.

Farrell, D. F., Clark, A. F., et al.: Absence of Pyruvate Decarboxylase Activity in Man: A Cause of Congenital Lactic Acidosis, Science, 187, 1082, 1975.

Feigin, I., and Wolf, A.: A Disease in Infants Resembling Chronic Wernicke's Encephalopathy, J. Ped., 45, 243, 1954.

Grover, W. D., Auerbach, V. H., et al.: Biochemical Studies and Therapy in Subacute Necrotizing Encephalomyelopathy (Leigh's Syndrome), J. Ped., 81, 39, 1972.

Leigh, D.: Subacute Necrotizing Encephalomyelopathy in an Infant, J. Neurol., Neurosurg., Psychiat., 14, 216, 1951.

Pincus, J. H., Solitare, G. B. and Cooper, J. R.: Thiamine Triphosphate Levels and Histopathology. Correlation in Leigh Disease, Arch. Neurol., 33, 759, 1976.

Tang, T. T., Good, T. A., et al.: Pathogenesis of Leigh's Encephalomyelopathy, J. Ped., 81, 189, 1972.

Acute Encephalopathy and Fatty Degeneration of the Viscera (Reye's Syndrome)

In 1963 Reye and his co-workers reported clinical and pathological observations in 21 children with encephalopathy and fatty changes in the viscera. Since that time an increasing number of cases have been reported from various parts of the world, and Reye's syndrome is now recognized to be among the ten major causes of deaths in children between one and ten years of age.

Reye's syndrome is usually associated with influenza B or varicella virus infections, although a wide range of viral infections have been reported in individual cases. Outbreaks have occurred following several influenza B epidemics. Often these children (as most children with viral infections) have been treated with antiemetics, aspirin, and acetaminophen; and in some cases, the blood levels of these drugs, especially the salicylates, have been high. However, the etiological role of these drugs has not been established.

Children between the ages of one to eight years are most commonly affected, but the disease occurs from age two months to adolescence. Prodromal symptoms are those of an upper respiratory infection and include fever, rhinorrhea, sore throat, cough, abdominal pain and diarrhea. The onset of the encephalitis is heralded by vomiting followed rapidly by the development of coma and convulsions. Death may occur in one to four days. Neurological symptoms include altered state of consciousness; seizures, either focal or general; and in the terminal stages signs of brainstem dysfunction including decorticate or decerebrate rigidity, and loss of corneal, pupillary and vestibulo-ocular reflexes.

The cerebral symptoms may, in part, be due to the profound hypoglycemia, hyperammonemia and increase in short chain fatty acids in the serum subsequent to the liver involvement. In the liver, there are diffuse deposits of lipid microdroplets and a remarkable absence of any sign of inflammatory reaction or necrosis. Azotemia may also occur as result of fatty degeneration of the kidneys. The most consistent early pathological change in the viscera is in the mitochondria; in fact, the special involvement of the mitochondria, which contain the urea cycle enzymes, may account for the unusual pattern of severe hyperammonemia in the absence of jaundice. The brain is markedly swollen, and there may be cerebellar tonsillar herniation. This cerebral edema is associated with astrocytic swelling and myelin bleb formation, such as is usually seen with cytotoxic edema. There is widespread injury of neuronal mitochondria with swelling and disruption of the mitochondrial matrix similar to that seen in liver mitochondria.

The abnormal laboratory findings include hyperammonemia, hypoglycemia, elevation of blood urea nitrogen, and an elevated glutamic oxalacetic transaminase and lactic dehydrogenase in the serum. There may be protein and red cells in the urine. Serum bilirubin is usually normal. There is an initial metabolic acidosis followed by a respiratory alkalosis. When lumbar punctures are carried out, the opening pressure is greater than 160 mm of water in most cases. There are no polymorphonuclear leukocytes and less than 4 lymphocytes per cu ml. The protein is usually normal. In some patients, the glucose concentration may be markedly reduced in association with hypoglycemia. The electroencephalogram shows diffuse slowing consistent with coma. In most series, the mortality rate is between 80 and 90%; recently, a reduction to 30 to 40% has been achieved with more intensive care, with the use of peritoneal dialysis and exchange transfusions to restore more normal blood levels. The use of orally administered arginine, ornithine, and citrulline to overcome deficiencies in the urea cycle has been suggested.

REFERENCES

Chaves-Carballo, E., Gomez, M. R., and Sharbrough, F. W.: Encephalopathy and Fatty
    Infiltration of the Viscera (Reye-Johnson syndrome). A 17-Year Experience, Mayo
    Clinic Proc., 50, 209, 1975.
Huttenlocher, P. R., Schwartz, A. D., and Klatskin, G.: Reye's Syndrome: Ammonia
    Intoxication as a Possible Factor in the Encephalopathy, Pediatrics, 43, 443, 1969.
Partin, J. C., Partin, J. S., Schubert, W. K., and McLaurin, R. L.: Brain Ultrastructure in
    Reye's Syndrome. (Encephalopathy and Fatty Alteration of the Viscera), J.
    Neuropath. Exp. Neurol., 34, 425, 1975.
Reye, R. D., Morgan, G. and Baral, J.: Encephalopathy and Fatty Degeneration of the
    Viscera, Lancet, 2, 749, 1963.
Rosenfeld, R. G., and Liebhaber, M. I.: Acute Encephalopathy in Siblings. Reye Syndrome
    vs Salicylate Intoxication, Am. J. Dis. Child., 130, 295, 1976.
Snodgrass, P. J., and DeLong, G. R.: Urea-Cycle Enzyme Deficiencies and an Increased
    Nitrogen Load Producing Hyperammonemia in Reye's Syndrome, N. Engl. J. Med.,
    294, 855, 1976.
Thaler, M. M.: Metabolic Mechanisms in Reye Syndrome. End of a Mystery? Am. J. Dis.
    Child., 130, 241, 1976.
Trauner, D. A., Nyhan, W. L., and Sweetman, L.: Short-Chain Organic Acidemia and
    Reye's Syndrome, Neurology, 25, 296, 1975.

Cerebral Palsy

Cerebral palsy (infantile cerebral palsy, Little's disease) is not a disease entity but is the term used to describe a heterogeneous group of cases with damage to the nervous system in utero, at birth, or in early life.

The term cerebral palsy can be broadly used to include all diseases of the nervous system described in this text which are manifested by paralytic symptoms in infancy or childhood. Many of these should properly be excluded because they are progressive diseases which often terminate fatally in the early years of life.

Pathogenesis. It was formerly thought that most of the cases of so-called cerebral palsy were due to injury to the nervous system at birth. It is quite likely that injury to the nervous system during labor and in the period immediately following birth is responsible for the defect in a number of cases, but other factors, many of which are as yet unknown, probably account for many of the cases. All of the factors that play a role are not known, but for convenience they can be divided into five groups: Genetic defects associated with chromosome abnormalities; inherited metabolic defects; prenatal injury to the developing fetus; perinatal damage; and postnatal injury. The pathological findings of Malamud and his associates are shown in Table 69.

Inborn errors of metabolism which can produce damage in the nervous system now number in the hundreds. Most of these are related to the metabolism of the amino acids or glucose. In many of these conditions the damage to the nervous system is diffuse and results mainly in mental retardation, but in some there may be focal damage producing the symptoms of cerebral palsy.

**Table 69.   Classification of Neuropathological Findings in 68 Cases
of Cerebral Palsy**

(After Malamud, Itabashi, Castor and Messinger, J. Ped., 1964)

Type	No. of Cases	%
Malformations	24	35
Destructive processes		
Primary subcortical pathology	25	37
(sequelae of perinatal trauma)		
Primary cortical pathology		
(sequelae of postnatal disorders)	13	19
Status dysmyelinatus		
(sequelae of kernicterus)	6	9
Total	68	100

The developing fetus is susceptible to injury, particularly in the first few months of development, by a large number of factors, including maternal infections, particularly with viruses such as rubella and cytomegalic inclusion and with bacteria and other organisms, particularly toxoplasma. Other factors which may adversely affect the developing fetus include ionizing radiation, malnutrition in the mother and the administration of drugs. Prematurity is also a common cause of mental deficiency and cerebral palsy.

In the perinatal period, the factors of significance are trauma in delivery and anoxia in the immediate period after delivery. Rh incompatibility is often accompanied by hyperbilrubinemia and kernicterus.

In the neonatal period the brain may be injured by trauma, cerebral vascular lesions, infections, and malnutrition. Prolonged convulsive seizures of whatever cause may produce severe brain damage if there is a serious degree of anoxia.

Cerebral palsy is found more frequently in infants who are born prematurely or after difficult labor than in normal infants. The incidence of cerebral palsy is approximately equal in the two sexes.

Symptoms and Signs. Although the symptoms and signs of cerebral palsy are quite variable, the cases are often classified as spastic, athetoid or ataxic. Admixtures are the rule rather than the exception. In addition, there may be signs of damage to the somatic sensory cortex, speech centers, or optic pathways with resultant sensory defects, dysphasia, apraxia or hemianopia. Intellectual defect is not uncommon. Approximately 50% of the cases are definitely mentally retarded. In addition, convulsions, aphasia, apraxia, dysarthria and motor difficulties in the use of the arms and hands may seriously interfere with intellectual performances.

Severe injury to the brain may be obvious at birth by difficulties in feeding, poverty of movements, listlessness and the like. More usually, however, evidence of brain damage may not appear until the age of six months to two years. The infant will fail to hold the head up, sit erect, crawl, walk or talk at the expected time, or abnormal movements may appear. In the less severe cases, the defect may not be manifest for several years, when it is apparent that the child cannot compete physically and intellectually with other children of similar age.

Incidence. An incidence of about 2 per 1,000 live births is widely accepted as a reasonable figure, although variations between 0.6 per 1,000 births in a study in Rochester, Minnesota, and 6 per 1,000 births in a study in Schenectady County, New York, have been reported. Hagberg and co-workers have reported a decrease in the incidence of cerebral palsy in Sweden and Denmark, from 2.2 per 1,000 live births in the mid 1950s to 1.3 per 1,000 live births from 1967 to 1970. This decrease has been attributed to improved prenatal and obstetrical care. However, this trend may be reversed as a consequence of intensive neonatal care units which may salvage babies with brain defects who might previously have died.

In spastic diplegia, there is greater spasticity in the legs than in the arms. In the experience of most pediatric-neurologists, this represents the most common form of cerebral palsy. It is more benign than spastic quadriplegia, with many of the children having normal intelligence. In various series, between 45 and 75% of children with spastic diplegia were premature, and often, there was a history of difficulty in delivery. The pathological finding of periventricular leukomalacia described by Banker and LaRoche is typically associated with this entity, although various malformations also present in this fashion.

Spastic hemiplegia is another common form of cerebral palsy. In a majority of cases, there is a history of difficulty with pregnancy or delivery. The hand is more involved than the leg and may be useless, especially in children with defects of cortical sensory modalities when there may be growth failure of the affected limbs. Convulsions, again, are frequent. Intellect is often normal in children with spastic hemiplegia. Occlusive vascular disease may produce an acute hemiplegia during infancy. Although frequently associated with trauma, infections, congenital heart disease, or sickle cell anemia, the cause of acute infantile hemiplegia is often unknown. The resulting clinical syndrome is similar to that in children with congenital hemiplegia. Occasionally, dystonic posture of the affected limbs may occur.

Some degree of unsteadiness in gait may be associated with many of the forms of cerebral palsy. However, in some children, ataxia appears to predominate. It is important, however, to rule out metabolic disease, cerebellar tumors and malformations which also present as ataxia, and a CT brain scan should be carried out in any infant in whom an ataxic form of cerebral palsy is suspected.

Choreoathetosis is the most common form of the extrapyramidal cerebral palsies. Often the abnormal movements do not manifest themselves until the second year, perhaps because of later maturation of extrapyramidal motor systems. Many cases of choreoathetosis were usually associated with paralysis of upward gaze and a hearing loss, but this variety is now uncommon as Rh incompatibility is routinely determined in pregnant women. Children with athetosis secondary to kernicterus often have normal intelligence. When choreoathetosis occurs as a result of neonatal distress or malformations, the picture is one of marked spasticity and athetosis, and these children are prone to mental retardation. However, even among children with normal intelligence, the impairment of speech and the social problems produced by the movements themselves may make schooling difficult.

The subdivision of children with spastic cerebral palsy into several major syndromes appears to be warranted on pathologic and prognostic bases. Spastic quadriplegia or bilateral hemiplegia was described by Little as "spastic rigidity." In these children, the upper extremities are affected more than the lower extremities, often, with accompanying pseudobulbar signs. Convulsions occur in half the patients. Mental retardation is almost universal. A history of difficulties in delivery or fetal distress, and cystic degeneration of the brain is often found.

Course. The course of these patients is subject to a wide degree of variation. As a rule, the symptoms reach their maximum degree of severity by the age of two to three years. After this there may be some improvement as the patient learns to compensate for his disability. Patients with a mild degree of cerebral damage may develop to normal adult life with only a slight spasticity of the extremities or a mild degree of the athetoid movements. Those with severe damage to the brain may die of intercurrent infection in childhood. When the damage is of a moderately severe degree, and this is not uncommon, the physical handicap is great, requiring special care throughout childhood and special education.

Treatment. Intensive physiotherapy and special education are the main forms of therapy. Orthopedic surgery for the correction of deformities, chiefly of the extremities, is often of great aid in the rehabilitation of the child. With diligent efforts on the part of the therapists and the patient, good results are possible and many of the patients can be rehabilitated to the level where they can compete economically and socially with normal individuals. In some cases, however, the results are discouraging. A disability which was of relatively minor importance in a child may be a serious handicap to an adult.

Drugs with curare-like activity have been used to decrease the spasticity and reduce the severity of the abnormal movements.

Diazepam, dantrolene sodium and baclofen may be of limited value in relieving spasticity. Dextroamphetamine sulfate or methylphenidate hydrochloride may improve the behavior of hyperactive children. Anticonvulsant drugs should be administered to patients with convulsive seizures. Various operative procedures on nerve roots, spinal cord and other parts of the nervous system have been tried in the past with disappointing results. Recently attempts have been made to alleviate the spasticity and abnormal movements by destruction of the globus pallidus or its thalamic connections.

REFERENCES

Banker, B. Q. and LaRoche, J. -C.: Periventricular Leukomalacia of Infancy, A.M.A. Arch. Neurol., 7, 386, 1962.

Hagberg, B., Hagberg, G. and Olow, I.: The Changing Panorama of Cerebral Palsy in Sweden 1954–1970. I. Analysis of the General Changes, Acta Paediatr. Scand., 64, 187, 1975.

Hagberg, B., Hagberg, G. and Olow, I.: The Changing Panorama of Cerebral Palsy in Sweden 1954–1970. II. Analysis of the Various Syndromes, Acta Paediatr. Scand., 64, 193, 1975.

Hsia, Y. E.: Disorders of Amino Acid Metabolism. In: Basic Neurochemistry, 2nd Ed., G. J. Siegel, R. W. Albers, R. Katzman and B. W. Agranoff, Eds., Boston, Little, Brown & Co., 1976, pp. 500–541.

Ingram, T. T. S.: Paediatric Aspects of Cerebral Palsy, Edinburgh, E. and S. Livingstone, Ltd., 1964.

Little, W. J.: The Influence of Abnormal Parturition, Difficult Labours, Premature Birth, and Asphyxia Neonatorum, on the Mental and Physical Condition of the Child, Especially in Relation to Deformities, Trans. Obstet. Soc. London, 3, 293, 1861.

Malamud, N., Itabashi, H. H., et al.: An Etiologic and Diagnostic Study of Cerebral Palsy, J. Ped., 65, 270, 1964.

Menkes, J. H.: Textbook of Child Neurology, Chapter 5: Perinatal Trauma, Philadelphia, Lea & Febiger, 1975, pp. 182–212.

Towbin, A.: Central Nervous System Damage in the Human Fetus and Newborn Infant. Mechanical and Hypoxic Injury Incurred in the Fetal-Neonatal Period, Amer. J. Dis. Child., 119, 529, 1970.

Presenile and Senile Dementia
Alzheimer's Disease and Senile Dementia

One of the most common degenerative diseases of the brain is named after Alois Alzheimer who described the major pathological changes over sixty years ago. For many years, the term "Alzheimer's disease" was limited to the description of cases with an onset in the presenium, that is, before the age of sixty-five or seventy. Clinical, pathological, ultrastructural, and biochemical analyses indicate that Alzheimer's disease and senile dementia are a single process and, therefore, there is now a consensus of opinion to consider them a single disease. Community surveys in Northern Europe and the United States indicate that about 4% of persons over age sixty-five are incapacitated by an organic dementia, and about 10% have progressive mental deterioration but can still function in their community. Pathological studies in the same communities indicate that between 40 and 60% of the brains of patients with organic dementia have Alzheimer's disease. Extrapolating these numbers, there may be as many as 500,000 individuals incapacitated by Alzheimer's disease in the United States today and as many as 1.2 million with an earlier or milder form of this disorder.

Pathology. Alzheimer's disease is characterized by atrophy of the cerebral cortex which is usually diffuse, although it may be more severe in the frontal and temporal lobes (Fig. 118). On microscopic examination, there is loss of both neurons and neuropil in the cortex and, sometimes, secondary demyelination in subcortical white matter. The most characteristic findings are the argentophilic senile plaques and neurofibrillary tangles. The senile plaque (Fig. 119) is found throughout the cerebral cortex, and the number of plaques per microscopic field has been reported by Tomlinson, Blessed, and associates to correlate with the degree of intellectual loss. The senile plaque is composed of enlarged, degenerating axonal endings surrounding a core composed mainly of extracellular amyloid. The degenerating axonal boutons contain lysosomes, degenerating mitochondria, and paired helical filaments. These paired helical filaments, which are about 200 Å wide with a twist every 800 Å along their length, constitute the chief element found in the Alzheimer neurofibrillary tangle. These tangles consist of accumulation of these filaments within

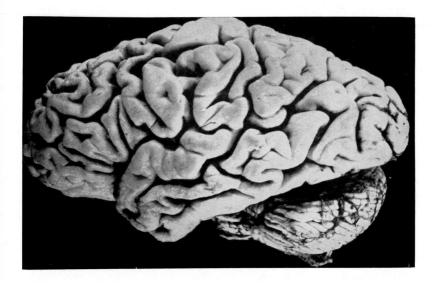

Figure 118.   Presenile dementia. Alzheimer's disease. Diffuse atrophy of brain, especially severe in frontal and temporal lobes. (Courtesy Dr. Leon Roizin.)

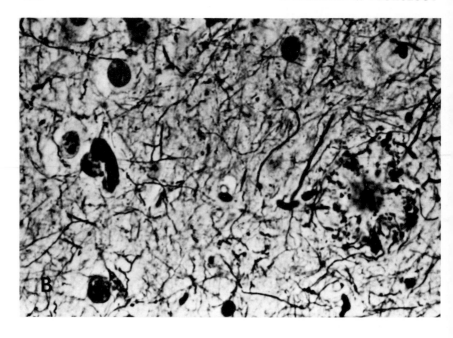

Figure 119.   Alzheimer's disease. Prominent senile plaques on left. Several neurons with neurofibrillary tangles on right. Note also disruption of cortical organization. (Courtesy Dr. Robert Terry.)

the body of a swollen neuron. Neurofibrillary tangles first occur in the hippocampus, but later are found throughout the cerebral cortex. Other less prominent but still common features of Alzheimer's disease include granulovacuolar degeneration of pyramidal cells of the hippocampus and congophilic angiopathy. The Hirano body, a rod-like body containing paracrystalline material, first described in the Guam-Parkinsonism-Dementia complex, is also found in Alzheimer's disease.

Arteriosclerotic changes are absent or are present to only a minor degree in most cases.

Symptoms and Signs. Alzheimer's disease presents as a progressive dementia with increasing loss of memory, intellectual function, and disturbances in speech. In the initial stages, there is a slight dulling of the intellectual faculties. Thought processes are slowed, ability to perform in the social and economic spheres is impaired and memory is defective. Disturbances in the functions of speech are commonly early symptoms; anomia, echolalia, and difficulty in comprehending written and oral speech. To these may be added various apraxias and various types of agnosias.

If the patient has insight into his deterioration, he may become depressed, and signs of a depression are seen in about one-quarter of the patients. Agitation and restlessness also frequently occur. Motor signs are uncommon early in the course, but if the disease progresses, reflex changes may be noted and a slow, shuffling gait will develop. Myoclonus and convulsive seizures occur in some patients late in the course. Rarely, myoclonus has been reported early in the course of the disease. The clinical picture in the terminal stages is strikingly constant. Intellectual activity ceases and the patient becomes meek and reduced to a vegetative condition. Generalized weakness and contractions may develop in the terminal stages. Control of bowel and bladder functions is lost.

Laboratory Data. There are no significant changes in the usual laboratory examinations. The cerebrospinal fluid findings are typically normal. A slight increase in the protein content of the fluid has been noted in a few cases. Generalized slowing is regularly seen in the electroencephalogram. Psychomotor examination is useful in following the progress of the disease. Cerebral blood flow falls as neurons quit functioning and oxygen demand is reduced. Dilatation of the lateral ventricles and widening of the cortical nuclei, particularly in the frontal and temporal regions, are common findings in pneumoencephalograms or CT brain scans in the late stage of the disease. However, a mild degree of cortical atrophy is seen in some older individuals who are functioning normally by clinical and psychological testing.

Differential Diagnosis. The diagnosis of Alzheimer's disease is based upon the development of a progressive dementia with the absence of motor findings in the early stages and the exclusion of other entities that may present with dementia. Documentation of the progression of the dementia by reexamination after several months is useful. Ordinarily, it is easy to differentiate Alzheimer's disease from Korsakoff's psychosis, since in the latter, there is a history of alcoholism, the memory defect is static and other intellectual functions are intact. However, in some cases, confusion arises when a history of progressive memory defect is given and the CT brain scan shows mild atrophy. The condition of "pseudodementia" must be suspected in patients in whom a history of depression preceded the onset of intellectual deterioration. The term "pseudodementia" has been used to describe depressed patients in whom cognitive function is temporarily impaired on a functional basis. Such patients show improvement in intellectual function when their depression is treated. In such instances, reexamination of the patient after several months may clarify the diagnosis.

Rarely, myxedema or pernicious anemia may present with intellectual deterioration as the primary symptom. These diseases can be ruled out by appropriate testing of thyroid function and determination of vitamin B_{12} levels. Dementia paralytica is excluded by the normal cerebrospinal fluid. Huntington's chorea is excluded by the absence of the characteristic choreiform movements and family history of the disease. Brain tumor is excluded by the absence of signs of increased intracranial pressure, focal changes on neurological examination, or focal abnormalities in the electroencephalogram, and the absence of a mass lesion on CT brain scan. Alzheimer's disease is usually differentiated from the subacute progressive dementias such as Jakob-Creutzfeldt disease by the absence of such findings as myoclonus and other motor findings early in the course as well as the absence of the periodic electroencephalogram. The rare occurrence of myoclonus as an early event in Alzheimer's disease may make diagnosis difficult at first, but the differences in progression of the two diseases will clarify the situation in a few months. Cerebral arteriosclerosis usually occurs in the presence of hypertension and other signs of vascular disease and has a step-like progression; particularly in patients with a lacunar state, the early presence of a gait disturbance and later pseudobulbar signs in addition to the dementia help establish the diagnosis.

The differentiation of Alzheimer's disease from normal pressure hydrocephalus is important, since the latter condition may be treated operatively. Most patients with normal pressure hydrocephalus have a preceding history of subarachnoid hemorrhage, head trauma, or meningitis accounting for the development of the hydrocephalus. In cases without an apparent cause, the patients who respond to shunt therapy are those with a history of the onset of progressive unsteadiness of gait together with a psychomotor retardation and a mild intellectual loss and, occasionally, with urinary incontinence. Confirmatory tests for normal pressure hydrocephalus include marked enlargement of the ventricles with minimal cortical atrophy on pneumoencephalogram or CT brain scan and abnormal cerebrospinal fluid flow determined by RISA cisternography or the cerebrospinal fluid infusion test. However, in the absence of a typical clinical history, these laboratory findings by themselves are not sufficient for the diagnosis, since about 10% of patients with Alzheimer's disease have markedly enlarged ventricles together with some evidence of abnormal cerebrospinal fluid flow. If Alzheimer patients are operated upon, they usually show marked postoperative deterioration.

Course. The clinical course is progressive, terminating inevitably in complete incapacity and death. The duration of the disease is usually between four and ten years, with extremes varying from less than one year to more than twenty years. It is customary to separate the cases into two groups according to the rapidity of the progress of the disease: The acute with death commonly between two to five years after onset; and the chronic in which the duration of the disease varies from five to fifteen years.

Treatment. There is no effective therapy. Custodial care is required in the terminal stage of the disease.

REFERENCES

Alzheimer, A.: Uber eine eigenartige Erkrankung der Hirnrinde, Zbl. Nervenheilk., 30, 177, 1907.
Blessed, G., Tomlinson, B. E., and Roth, M.: The Association Between Quantitative Measures of Dementia and of Senile Change in the Cerebral Gray Matter of Elderly Subjects, Br. J. Psychiat., 114, 797, 1968.
Corsellis, J. A. N.: Mental Illness and the Ageing Brain, London, Oxford University Press, 1962.
Delay, J., Brion, S., and Escourolle, R.: L'Opposition Anatomo-clinique des Maladies de Pick et d'Alzheimer; Valeur Diagnostique des Examens Complementaires, Presse med., 65, 1515, 1957.
Faden, A. I., and Townsend, J. J.: Myoclonus in Alzheimer Disease. A Confusing Sign, Arch. Neurol., 33, 278, 1976.
Feldman, R. G.: Myoclonus and Alzheimer Disease, Arch. Neurol., 33, 730, 1976.
Feldman, R. G., Chandler, K. A., Levy, L. L., and Glaser, G. H.: Familial Alzheimer's Disease, Neurology, 13, 811, 1963.
Hirano, A., Dembitzer, H. M., Kurland, L. T., and Zimmerman, H. M.: The Fine Structure of Some Intraganglionic Alterations. Neurofibrillary Tangles, Granulovacuolar Bodies and "Rod-Like" Structures as Seen in Guam Amyotrophic Lateral Sclerosis and Parkinsonism-Dementia Complex, J. Neuropath. Exp. Neurol., 27, 167, 1968.
Katzman, R.: The Prevalence and Malignancy of Alzheimer Disease. A Major Killer, Arch. Neurol., 33, 217, 1976.
Kiloh, L. G.: Pseudo-Dementia, Acta Psychiat. Scand., 37, 336, 1961.
Sim, M., and Sussman, I.: Alzheimer's Disease: Its Natural History and Differential Diagnosis, J. Nerv. Ment. Dis., 135, 489, 1962.
Terry, R. D.: Dementia. A Brief and Selective Review, Arch. Neurol., 33, 1, 1976.
Terry, R. D., Gonatas, N. K., and Weiss, M.: Ultrastructural Studies in Alzheimer's Presenile Dementia, Am. J. Pathol., 44, 269, 1964.
Tomlinson, B. E., Blessed, G., and Roth, M.: Observations of the Brains of Demented Old People, J. Neurol. Sci., 11, 205, 1970.
Wang, H. A., and Whanger, A.: Brain Impairment and Longevity. In: Prediction of Life Span, E. Palmore and F. C. Jeffers, Eds., Lexington, Mass., D.C. Heath & Co., 1971, pp. 95–105.
Wolstenholme, G. E. W., and O'Connor, M.: Alzheimer's Disease and Related Conditions, London, J. & S. Churchill, 1970.

Pick's Disease

Pick's disease is a rare degenerative disease that occurs almost entirely in the presenium. Within this age group, the incidence of Pick's disease is less than one-fiftieth that of Alzheimer's. Pathologically, Pick's disease (Fig. 120) is characterized by severe atrophy of the frontal and temporal poles with sparing of the motor and sensory cortex and the first temporal convolution. On microscopic examination, Pick's disease is characterized by a diffuse loss of neurons, particularly in the outer layer of the cortex. Within remaining neurons, cytoplasmic inclusions called Pick's bodies are found (Fig. 121). Many of the preserved neurons are swollen and have a pale cytoplasm. Glial

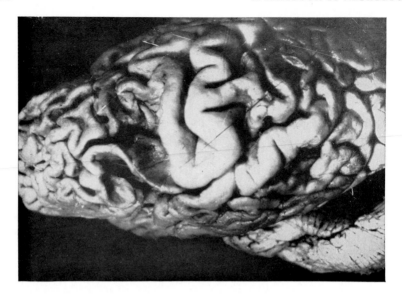

Figure 120.   Presenile dementia. Pick's disease with severe cerebral atrophy. Sparing motor and sensory cortex and first temporal convolution. (Courtesy Dr. P. I. Yakovlev.)

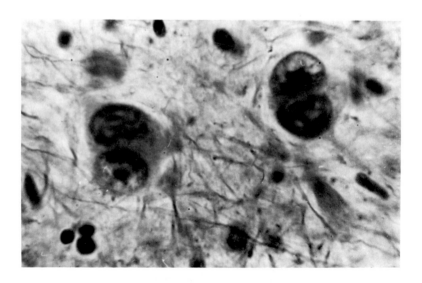

Figure 121.   Intraneuronal inclusions in Pick's disease.
Silver stain. (Courtesy Dr. Asao Hirano.)

proliferation is prominent in both the gray and white matter. The basal ganglia are also involved in high percentage of the cases. Some neurons contain argentophilic intraneuronal inclusions known as Pick's bodies. The inclusions contain many 100 Å neurofilaments, vesicles, and complex lipid bodies. Alzheimer neurofibrillary tangles and senile plaques are not present.

The presentation of Pick's disease is similar to that of Alzheimer's disease. Although in some cases of Pick's disease disturbances in personality, orientation, and attention span are more affected than memory early in the course of this disease as compared to Alzheimer's disease, it is the consensus of opinion that the differential diagnosis can be made only at biopsy and necropsy. Although computerized tomography might be able to demonstrate the localized atrophy in patients with Pick's disease, focal atrophy is also sometimes seen in Alzheimer's disease, and the finding of severe frontal and partial temporal atrophy alone may suggest, but would not prove, the diagnosis in the absence of histological confirmation.

The course is similar to that of Alzheimer's disease. There is no effective treatment.

REFERENCES

Constantinidis, J., Richard, J., and Tissot, R.: Pick's Disease: Histological and Clinical Correlations, Eur. Neurol., 11, 208, 1974.
Pick, A.: Uber die Beziehungen der senilen Hirnatrophie zur Aphasie, Prag. med. Wchnschr., 17, 165, 1892.
Terry, R. D.: Dementia. A Brief and Selective Review, Arch. Neurol., 33, 1, 1976.
Williams, H. W.: The Peculiar Cells of Pick's Disease: Their Pathogenesis and Distribution in Disease, Arch. Neurol. Psychiat., 34, 508, 1935.
Wisniewski, H. M., Coblentz, J. M., and Terry, R. D.: Pick's Disease: A Clinical and Ultrastructural Study, Arch. Neurol., 26, 97, 1972.

BASAL GANGLIA DISEASES

Melvin D. Yahr

The basal ganglia disorders comprise a complex and heterogeneous group of conditions having in common one or more of the following clinical manifestations: abnormal involuntary movements, alterations in muscle tone and changes in body posture. The basis of classifying them into disease entities rests on the nature and degree of severity as well as the combination of this triad of signs and symptoms; the manner of their evolution and progression; the age and mode of onset and the identification of particular etiological or genetic factors. They are described here under the section devoted to degenerative diseases using this term in the broadest sense as many of these disorders may occur as a result of specific infectious processes and toxic agents on the nervous system or secondarily to systemic disease processes such as: vasculitis, metabolic disturbances or endocrine dysfunction.

Although there is little doubt that the basal ganglia are concerned with the control and execution of movement, and much is known about the clinical aspects of the disorders which affect them, our information is far from satisfactory regarding their fundamental, anatomic, physiologic and pathogenetic basis. In fact, basal ganglia disorders are unique among diseases of the nervous system in that in only few instances has it been possible to relate the clinical manifestations to pathological alterations in specific areas of the brain, and even in these the magnitude of the demonstrable morphological changes bears little relationship to the severity of the condition. During the past decade a growing body of evidence has accumulated indicating that the underlying disturbance in these disorders may relate to biochemical changes in the basal ganglia rather than morphological abnormalities.

The most prominent biochemical feature of the basal ganglia is their particularly high content of putative neurotransmitter agents notably acetyl choline (ACH), dopamine (DA) and gamma aminobutyric acid (GABA). The substrates and enzymes necessary for their production and degradation are found within the cellular components of the basal ganglia. In some instances they are produced within the segment in which they have their action, while in others, cellular elements in one area are responsible for their production but they are transported via connecting axons to another, where they are stored and then released to produce their effects. Experimental evidence is available indicating that dopamine for example, is produced in the pars compacta of the substantia nigra and is transported via a neuronal tract, the nigro-striatal pathway to the caudate nucleus and putamen where its action occurs. Normal function in the basal ganglia appears to depend on a homeostatic relationship between these various neurotransmitter agents. Neurophysiologically this balance may be viewed as existing between those whose action is inhibitory in nature (DA and GABA) versus those with excitatory properties (ACH). Disturbances of their homeostasis result in one or another of the symptoms which are generally attributed to this area of the brain. In general, dopamine deficiency allows for cholinergic hyperactivity and can be correlated with the akinetic-rigid disorders such as parkinsonism. Dopamine hyperactivity and/or cholinergic hypoactivity results in the hyperkinetic phenomena encountered in Huntington's chorea. To a considerable extent present approaches to the etiogenesis and treatment of basal ganglia disorders are directed to a better understanding of the role of and reestablishing balance among these neurotransmitter agents.

Chronic Progressive Chorea
(Huntington's Disease, Adult Chorea)

Chronic progressive chorea, more commonly known as Huntington's disease is an hereditary disorder of the central nervous system characterized by the appearance in adult life of choreiform movements and dementia which are progressive in nature. It was first recognized clinically by Waters (1842) but did not become accepted as a clinical entity until the comprehensive description and interpretation of its mode of transmission by George Huntington (1872) after whom the disease was named.

Pathology. At post-mortem examination the brain appears shrunken and atrophic with the cerebral cortex and caudate nucleus being primarily affected (Fig. 122). Histologically, the cerebral cortex shows widespread loss of neurons and diffuse loss of nerve fibers. The caudate nucleus and putamen are severely involved with loss of small neurons and as a result there is atrophy of the strio-pallidal nerve fiber

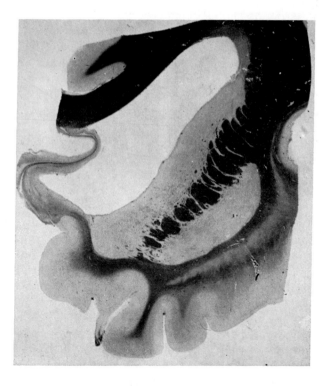

Figure 122.   Huntington's chorea. Atrophy of caudate nucleus and dilatations of lateral ventricle. Myelin sheath stain.

bundles in the lateral segment of the globus pallidus. Less marked changes occur in other structures such as the thalamus and brain stem. A reactive gliosis is apparent in the affected areas. Changes in the cerebral cortex undoubtedly are the cause of the dementia, while the striatal cell loss is held to be responsible for the chorea. In advanced cases the striatum may be completely devoid of cells and replaced by a gliotic process at which time choreic movements abate and are replaced by an akinetic-rigid state terminally. While the etiology and pathogenesis of this disorder remain unknown, some recent findings of selective depletion of neurotransmitter agents in the striatum hold promise of a better understanding of its underlying nature as well as symptomatic control of its manifestations particularly the choreiform movements. A number of investigators utilizing post-mortem material have now shown a selective depletion of GABA and its synthesizing enzyme glutamic acid decarboxylase and a decline in the activity of the acetyl-choline synthesizing enzyme choline-acetyl-transferase in the striatum of patients dying from Huntington's disease. These defects result in a disruption of the homeostatic relationship of these agents and may underlie the choreatic manifestations.

Prevalence and Hereditary Factors. Chronic progressive chorea is not an infrequently encountered disorder. It occurs worldwide and in all ethnic groups. Excluding certain communities where its incidence is particularly high, the prevalence of chronic progressive chorea has been estimated to range from 4 to 7 per 100,000 population. The highest incidence rates have been reported from geographic regions where affected families have resided for many generations. The disease is transmitted from parent to offspring in autosomal dominant fashion with full penetrance. Hence 50% of children of sufferers inevitably will be affected. New mutations are rare and nearly all cases have affected relatives although the familial nature of the disease is often concealed which makes documentation difficult on occasion.

In general, symptoms of the disorder usually appear between thirty-five and forty years of age. However, the range of age of onset spans a considerable number of years with cases recorded as early as five years of age and others at seventy years. Though one cannot generalize about the behavior of the disease in a particular family constellation, in general, considerable similarity exists among sibships; this favors the hypothesis of a single rather than multiple genes as a cause of Huntington's chorea. Considerable effort has been directed toward the development of a test which would permit early detection of the disorder before the appearance of symptoms and prior to childbearing. These have included physiological tests, such as eye movement recordings and H reflex responses; provocative tests with pharmacological agents such as the L-dopa loading test; and the measurement of growth hormone levels particularly in response to insulin induced hypo-glycemia. Though a number of abnormalities in one or another of these parameters have been shown to be abnormal in offspring of Huntington disease patients, none has been validated as being unequivocally predictive. Further, ethical questions have been raised regarding their use in a disease process with as much variability in age of onset and severity and for which no satisfactory treatment exists.

Signs and Symptoms. The two characteristic manifestations of the disease are: choreiform movements and mental deterioration. The two may occur together at onset or one may precede the other by a period of years. In general, the onset of symptoms is insidious beginning with fidgetiness associated with irritability, slovenliness and neglect of duties progressing to frank choreiform movements and dementia. Overt psychotic episodes have been reported to precede or occur during the course of the disease. The disease tends to run its course over a period of fifteen years being more rapid in those with an earlier age of onset.

Choreic Movements. The most striking feature of the disease is the involuntary movements which are purposeless, abrupt and jerky in nature but less rapid and lightning-like than those seen in Sydenham's chorea. Though any of the somatic muscles may be affected those of the trunk and proximal girdle are more frequently involved. In the early stages, or in the less severe form slight grimacing of the face, shrugging of the shoulders and jerking movements of the limbs occur. As the disease progresses twisting and lordotic movements of the trunk especially on walking, associated with more intense arm and leg movements give the individual a dancing, prancing type of gait, which is particularly characteristic of the disorder. The abnormal movements are increased by emotional stimuli, disappear during sleep and become superimposed on voluntary movements to the point that they make volitional activity difficult. With increase in their severity the routine daily activities of living become difficult as does speech in those with oral-facial involvement. At the end stage of the disease previously existing choreic movements may disappear and be replaced by muscu-lar rigidity (see akinetic-rigid form of disease below).

Mental Symptoms. Characteristically these are similar to that of any organic dementia with progressive impairment of memory, loss of intellectual capacity, apathy and inattention to personal hygiene. Early in the disease less profound abnormalities consisting of irritability, impulsive behavior and bouts of depression or fits of violence are not infrequent. In some patients frank psychotic features, schizophrenic in type predominate and the underlying cause is not evident until choreiform movements develop. The dementing and psychotic fea-tures of the disease usually lead to commitment to a mental institution.

Other Neurological Manifestations. Cranial nerves remain intact except for rapid eye movements which are impaired in a large percentage of patients. Sensation is usually unaffected as are the reflexes which are intact and normal in most patients. However, deep tendon reflexes may be found to be hyperactive and the plantar responses abnormal especially in cases with rigidity.

Muscle tone is normal in most patients except for those with the so-called akinetic-rigid variety (Westphal variant). This form usually begins in childhood with proximal muscular rigidity, mental abnormalities and convulsive seizure phenomena. Choreic movements are rare but convulsive seizures are not infrequent. This form of the disease is rapidly progressive with a fatal outcome in less than ten years. During the end stages of the more classical form of Huntington's disorder muscular rigidity and seizure phenomena are not unusual.

Laboratory Data. Routine studies of blood, urine and cerebrospinal fluid show no abnormalities. Growth hormone levels in plasma are elevated and an exaggerated growth hormone response can be shown with insulin induced hypoglycemia. Diffuse abnormalities are seen in the electroencephalogram. Roentgenograms of the skull are normal but computerized axial tomograms show enlarged ventricles with characteristic butterfly appearance of the lateral ventricles, a result of degeneration of the caudate nucleus (Fig. 123). Similar changes can be demonstrated on pneumoencephalography.

Diagnosis and Differential Diagnosis. The diagnosis of Huntington's

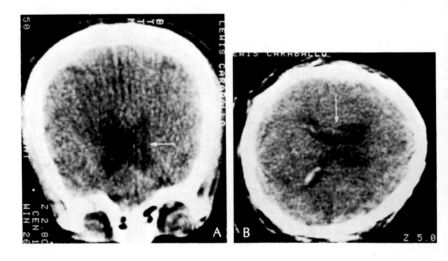

Figure 123.   CT scan showing ventricular enlargement. Note squaring of lateral ventricles. (A) Coronal section, (B) horizontal section.

chorea can be made without difficulty in an adult when the triad of chorea, dementia and a positive family history is present. Difficulties arise when one or another of these may be lacking. Such is the case in individuals whose onset and predominant symptomatology are of psychiatric disturbance as well as those who are reluctant to reveal or have not been apprised of their family background. However, in such instances subsequent developments usually allow for the establishment of a firm diagnosis.

Other conditions in which choreatic movements are a major manifestation can be excluded on clinical grounds. Sydenham's chorea has an earlier age of onset, is self-limited and lacks the characteristic mental disturbances. Chorea and mental disturbances occurring as a manifestation of lupus erythematosus are usually more acute in onset, the choreiform movements more localized and have characteristic serological and serum protein alterations. Involuntary movements occurring in psychiatric patients on long-term treatment with neuroleptic agents, so-called tardive dyskinesia, on occasion pose a problem. However, by and large such movements remain restricted usually to the oral facial musculature and lack the progressive features of Huntington's chorea. The pre-senile dementias, Alzheimer's and Pick's disease, are strikingly similar in their mental disturbances and on occasion exhibit involuntary movements. However, they differ in type and rarely become a prominent feature of the disorder. The peculiarities of the disorder in childhood with rigidity, convulsive seizures and mental retardation require differentiation from other genetically determined disorders such as the leukodystrophies and gangliosidosis. Habit spasms particularly the Gilles de la Tourette's syndrome usually pose little problem in view of the stereotyped nature of the involuntary movements and the characteristic vocalizations.

Treatment. There is at present no known means of altering the underlying disease process or its progressive fatal outcome. Attempts to replace the defect in GABA metabolism by utilizing some of its precursors such as glutamic acid or elevate its level by utilizing inhibitors of GABA catabolism such as dipropyl acetic acid have been unsuccessful. Symptomatic control of the choreiform movements can be accomplished by the use of neuroleptic agents such as haloperidol and chlorpromazine. Recently it has been demonstrated that choline chloride given in dosages of up to 20 gm a day, can ameliorate the choreiform movements to a considerable extent without the attendant rigidity occurring with the use of neuroleptic agents. Utilizing these drugs combined with supervision of the patient's daily activities allows for management at home during the early stages of the disorder. However, as the disease advances confinement to a psychiatric facility becomes necessary.

REFERENCES

Barbeau, A., Chase, T. N. and Paulson, G. W., eds.: Huntington's Chorea 1872-1972, Adv. Neurol., 1, 1973.
Bird, E. D. and Iversen, L. L.: Huntington's Chorea: Post-mortem Measurement of Glutamic Acid Decarboxylase, Choline Acetyl Transferase and Dopamine in Basal Ganglia, Brain, 97, 457, 1974.
Davis, K. L., et al.: Choline in Tardive Dyskinesia and Huntington's Disease, Life Sci., 19, 1507, 1976.
Huntington, G.: On Chorea, Med. & Surg. Reporter, Phila., 26, 317, 1872.
Myrianthopoulos, N. C.: Huntington's Chorea, J. Med. Genet., 3, 298, 1966.
Paulson, G. W.: Predictive Tests in Huntington's Disease. In.: The Basal Ganglia, M.D. Yahr, ed. N.Y., Raven Press, 1976, pp. 317–329.
Perry, T. L., Hansen, S. and Kloster, G.: Huntington's Chorea: Deficiency of δ-aminobutyric Acid in Brain, N. Engl. J. Med., 288, 337, 1973.
Phillipson, O. T. and Bird, E. D.: Plasma Growth Hormone Concentration in Huntington's Chorea, Clin. Sci. Mol. Med., 50, 551, 1976.
Waters, C. O.: Description of Chorea. In: Dunglison, R.: Practice of Medicine. Vol. 2. Philadelphia, Lea & Blanchard, 1842, pp. 312–313.

Gilles de la Tourette's Disease (Maladie de Tic)

This unusual involuntary movement disorder is so distinctive in its clinical characteristics that it warrants separation as a nosological entity. At onset which is during childhood (two to thirteen years of age), facial twitching and grimacing as well as abrupt jerky movements of the muscles of the neck and shoulder occur. Later they spread to involve the limbs and are accompanied by explosive and often foul utterances (coprolalia) with obsessional ideation and hyperactive behavior not infrequently associated. Electroencephalographic abnormalities though non-specific in nature are frequently demonstrated. In patients who have come to necropsy no specific morphological changes in the nervous system have been noted. The disorder increases in severity during childhood but in many cases seems to spontaneously resolve by adult life. Tourette's disease can be differentiated from other dyskinesias of childhood such as simple habit spasms which are more stereotyped and lack coprolalia, Sydenham's chorea which differs in the type of movement disorder and is self limited and Hallervorden-Spatz disease which has other neurological abnormalities in addition to the abnormal movements. The severity of the abnormal involuntary movements and control of the unfortunate verbal outbursts of Tourette's disease can be accomplished with the use of haloperidol in doses from 5 to 20 mg a day.

REFERENCES

Gilles de la Tourette, G.: Étude sur une Affection Nerveuse caracterisée par l'Incoordination Motrice accompagnée d'Echolalie et de Coprolalie (Jumping, Latah, Myriachit), Archives de Neurologie, 9, 19 and 158, 1885.

Sweet, R. D., et al.: Neurological Features of Gilles de la Tourette's Syndrome, J. Neurol.
Neurosurg. Psychiatry, 36, 1, 1973.
Shapiro, A. K., Shapiro, E. and Wayne, H.: Treatment of Tourette's Syndrome with
Haloperidol; Review of 34 Cases, Arch. Gen. Psychiatry, 28, 92, 1973.

Senile Chorea

Choreiform movements may have their initial onset and occur as an isolated symptom in individuals past the sixth decade of life. As a rule they begin insidiously, are mild in nature and usually involve the limbs. However, more complex movements of the lingual-facial-buccal regions are on occasion encountered. Slow progression in intensity as well as extent of the movements may occur over time. There are no associated mental disturbances, nor is a family history of Huntington's chorea obtained. Pathologically, changes are found in the caudate nucleus and putamen, which show cellular loss but not to the degree that is seen in Huntington's chorea. Significantly, there is an absence of degenerative changes in the cerebral cortex. Though some have considered senile chorea to be a variant of Huntington's chorea, it seems more likely that it is a distinctive pathological entity. The etiology of this degenerative process remains unknown but it may well have several underlying causes. In general, the symptoms are mild and there is little need to resort to therapeutic measures. However, in those instances especially where oral-facial and neck muscle involvement occurs, drugs utilized to control chorea as indicated above may prove useful.

Hemichorea

On occasion choreiform movements confined to the arm and leg on one side of the body may develop abruptly in middle-aged or elderly patients. Their sudden onset suggests a vascular basis and indeed they may be preceded by hemiplegia or hemiparesis. In such instances the choreiform movements appear when return of motor function occurs. Though post-mortem examination of such cases are few those reported have shown involvement of the internal capsule with extension to the lateral nuclei of the thalamus, or the sub-thalamic region. By and large they have been of an occlusive or hemorrhagic nature with resultant encephalomalacia.

The severity of the choreiform movements are variable and when severe may be difficult to distinguish from hemiballism (see below). In general the movements tend to diminish over a period of time but they may be persistent and require therapeutic intervention. The agents noted above for the control of choreic movements in general have on occasion proven effective.

Hemiballism

Hemiballism is a rarely encountered symptom which is characterized by continuous uncoordinated activity of the axial and proximal appendicular musculature of such violence that the limbs are forcefully and aimlessly thrown about. Most frequently it develops suddenly involving the arm and leg on one side of the body but may be localized to only one extremity. The terms hemiballism or hemichorea have been used interchangeably by some authors, but the violence of the movements of the former warrants their separate designation.

Hemilballism is the result of a destructive lesion of the contra-lateral sub-thalamic nucleus, corpus luysii, and/or its connections. Vascular lesions, hemorrhagic or occlusive in nature are the most common cause, but hemiballism has been found in association with tumors and has on occasion followed attempted thalamotomy when poor localization of the lesion placement has occurred.

In general, hemiballism occurs in older patients usually after a cerebral vascular accident which has included hemiparesis and/or sensory deficit. As these neurological signs clear, or at a variable interval afterward the ballistic movements begin. They may evolve slowly and increase in intensity or be exceedingly severe at onset. The violent nature of the movements usually completely incapacitates the individual and their persistence may lead to cardiac failure and exhaustion with eventual death. Instances of spontaneous remission after variable periods of time have been reported. More frequently they continue and since they are refractory to drug therapy ventrolateral thalamotomy has been resorted to by some with relief of the movement.

REFERENCES

Alcock, N. S.: A Note on the Pathology of Senile Chorea (Non-Hereditary), Brain, 59, 376, 1936.
Altrocchi, P. H.: Spontaneous Oral-facial Dyskinesia, Arch. Neurol., 16:506–512, 1972.
Martin, J. P. and McCaul, I. R.: Acute Hemiballismus Treated by Ventrolateral Thalamolysis, Brain, 82, 104, 1959.
Weiner, W. J. and Klawans, H. L.: Lingual-facial-buccal Movements in the Elderly. II. Pathogenesis and Relationship to Senile Chorea, J. Am. Ger. Soc., 31, 318, 1973.

Dystonia Musculorum Deformans (Torsion Dystonia)

Torsion dystonia may be viewed as a symptom complex characterized by dystonic movements and postures of varied causation. When a known pathological process is present, the dystonic phenomena usually occur in association with other neurological deficits. Such instances are referred to as a symptomatic torsion dystonia. Separable are cases whose clinical characteristics, genetic background and natural history are so distinctive that they constitute a nosological entity, often referred to as idiopathic torsion dystonia or dystonia musculorum deformans.

Dystonic movements regardless of cause are similar in nature. They evolve slowly and build up to an intense sustained muscular contraction which results in twisting and turning of the bodily part involved. Though intermittent, their repetitive recurring pattern may give the appearance of rhythmicity. Dystonic movements may occur at rest or on action and are often intensified by emotional and physical stress. Though they may affect any or all of the musculature, they have a predilection for the muscles of the trunk, shoulder and pelvic girdles. Involvement of the neck on one side results in torticollis, or if the contraction is backwards, retrocollis; the trunk may be bent back giving rise to a lordosis, or to one side so that scoliosis results. If the pelvis is involved, tortipelvis may be the predominating feature. Associated with these trunk movements are involvement of the limbs with the arm usually extended and hyperpronated and the wrist flexed and fingers extended. The foot becomes plantarflexed and turned inwards. As the disorder progresses the spasms of muscular contraction may become constant so that instead of movement the bodily part remains in a fixed dystonic posture.

Pathology and Pathogenesis. The pathology of dystonia musculorum deformans is unknown. Gross examination of the brain and histological studies by light microscopy have failed to reveal any consistent morphological changes. In view of this, considerable emphasis has been given to the possibility that a biochemical abnormality of the basal ganglia, genetically determined, may underlie the disorder.

That dystonic symptomatology arises from dysfunction within the basal ganglia seems unquestioned since in those instances with symptomatic dystonia such as hepatolenticular degeneration, encephalitis lethargica and Hallervorden-Spatz disease characteristic pathological changes are found in this region. In support of a biochemical abnormality are the well-documented instances of dystonic reactions occurring with the use of pharmacological agents particularly those that affect striatal amine function such as the phenothiazines and levodopa. However, no direct evidence indicating the exact nature of the biochemical disturbance in idiopathic torsion dystonia exists nor have any assays of the monoamines, their enzymes or metabolites in brain been reported.

The hereditary nature of the disorder has long been recognized, but it has only been of recent date that an attempt to clarify its genetic background has been made. Recent reports suggest that the mode of inheritance may be either autosomal recessive or autosomal dominant in type. The autosomal dominant variety has been correlated with elevations of serum dopamine-beta-hydroxylase, an enzyme which catalyzes the conversion of dopamine to noradrenalin. This finding has been interpreted as suggesting overactivity of the sympathetic nervous system. Whether such activity is a result of a disturbance in central regulatory mechanisms or due to secondary changes in peripheral receptors for this neurotransmitter, is not known at present. However, this observation may provide a useful genetic marker in distinguishing certain types of dystonia.

Symptomatic dystonia has occurred with a variety of cerebral disorders including hepatolenticular degeneration, post-encephalitic parkinsonism, perinatal birth injuries, such as kernicterus, brain tumors and has been induced by a variety of pharmacological agents particularly, the phenothiazines, butyrophenones and by levodopa in parkinsonian patients. When a history of any of these known disorders is lacking and the sole manifestation is dystonic movements and/or

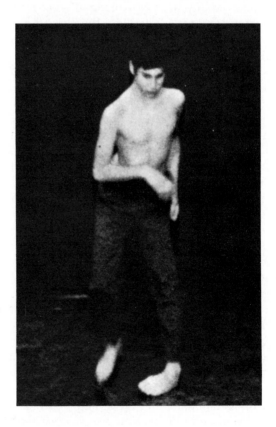

Figure 124. Dystonia.

postures, one can be reasonably certain that the disorder is of idiopathic variety. Two major forms of this type of dystonia have been recognized based on age of onset, clinical characteristics and genetic background.

Signs and Symptoms. The most commonly encountered form of the disease is that which begins in childhood, has an autosomal recessive mode of inheritance and occurs primarily in Ashkenazi Jews. This type generally begins between the ages of five and fifteen years and though its mode of onset may be variable, the most frequent initial symptoms involve the lower extremities with intermittent spasmodic inversion of the foot usually apparent on walking. Bizarre stepping or a bowing gait may be noted when the dystonic movements affect more proximal muscles of the leg or difficulty in placing the heel on the ground when more distal (Fig. 124). As the movements become more intense and the proximal musculature more prominently involved, lordosis and tor-

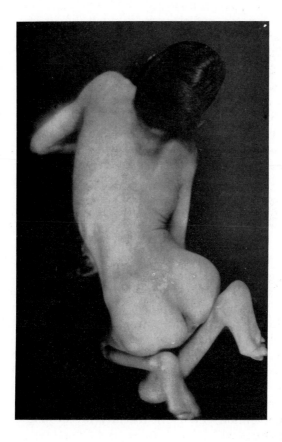

Figure 125.   Dystonia musculorum deformans. Torticollis and tortipelvis.

tipelvis appear (Fig. 125). As the disease progresses neck and shoulder girdle become involved with torticollis becoming apparent. Facial grimacing and difficulties in speech become evident as the muscles subserving these functions become impaired. The continuous spasms over a period of time result in marked distortion of the body to a degree rarely seen in any other disease processes. Although muscle tone and power appear to be normal, the involuntary movements interfere with function to such a degree as to make voluntary activity extremely difficult. In general, mentation remains normal and no alterations in deep tendon reflexes or sensation occur. The rate of progression of this type of dystonia is extremely variable though in most cases it is greatest within the first five to ten years after onset, following which the disease may enter a quiescent, static phase. Periods of remission may occur at any time during the disorder.

The autosomal dominant form is unrelated to ethnic background, tends to have its onset at a later age and runs a more benign course. It frequently begins in adolescence or adult life with upper limb or cervical musculature involvement. Though it tends to remain restricted to the initial bodily area for extended periods of time progression with more generalized symptoms of dystonia usually occurs but of a less disabling nature.

Diagnosis and Differential Diagnosis. The diagnosis of idiopathic torsion dystonia is tenable when typical dystonic movements and postures begin in childhood or young adult life, perinatal and developmental history is normal, there is no antecedent illness or drug ingestion that can be implicated as a cause of the symptoms, no other neurological deficits are found and no abnormalities of copper metabolism are uncovered.

The bizarre nature of the initial symptomatology and their exaggeration under periods of stress, as well as their variability in certain settings not infrequently lead to a diagnosis of "hysteria." This often leads to a long delay in identification of the true nature of the disorder with prolonged periods of needless psychotherapy. Awareness of the capricious nature of the disorder and serial observation of patients can avoid this pitfall. Differentiation from symptomatic forms of dystonia may be difficult during the early phases but by and large the occurrence of additional neurological deficits will resolve the issue.

Treatment. The extreme variability of the natural history of this disorder makes evaluation of the effects of various treatment measures difficult to assess. Dystonic movements have been reported to be effectively controlled for varying periods of time by a variety of drugs, surgical intervention and more recently by the use of bio-feedback techniques. Drugs which have proven useful are those which produce a degree of muscle relaxation such as the diazepams including Valium and clonopin; agents capable of inducing a degree of pseudoparkin-sonism such as the phenothiazines (chlorpromazine), butyrophenones (haloperidol) and carbomazepines (Tegretol) which reputedly depresses neuronal activity in the thalamic nuclei. Stereotactic thalamotomy has been reported to benefit patients for extended periods of time. How-ever, it does require rather extensive bilateral lesions of the ventral lateral nuclei of the thalamus which carries the risk of additional neurological deficit, particularly speech disturbance. Attempts to utilize bio-feedback mechanisms are of too recent origin to fully assess their value in this disorder.

Focal Dystonias

In contrast to the generalized forms of idiopathic torsion dystonia are instances of focal or segmental types of the disorder. It is a matter of controversy as to whether these represent formes frustes of torsion dystonia or are distinctive clinical entities in and of themselves. In favor of the latter are their onset of symptoms in adult life and a tendency for them to remain restricted to specific bodily segments. However, on occasion they may become more generalized. A variety of focal dys-tonias have been identified including writers cramps, some related to muscle groups used in occupational activities, blepharospasm and buccal-mandibular dystonia. However, the most frequently encoun-tered is spasmodic torticollis.

Spasmodic Torticollis (Wry Neck)

The restriction of dyskinetic movements to neck muscles so that abnormal postures of the head result is the distinguishing characteris-tic of this symptom complex. Involuntary activity involves the sterno-cleidomastoids, trapezius, and scalenus muscles in sustained contrac-tions that result in slow, twisting, turning movements of the head (torticollis) (Fig. 126) or less often forward flexion (anterocollis) or forceful extension (retrocollis). In most instances there is bilateral involvement, and the resultant postural deformity is maintained for varying lengths of time. The muscles of the neck appear under tension, and the continual muscular activity may lead to some degree of hypertrophy, especially evident in the sternocleidomastoid. The amount of active motion or static postural deformity is extremely variable. Similar activity may spread to facial and brachial muscula-ture. Some authors have reported that long term observations indicate that two thirds of patients develop additional dystonic features within ten years of onset.

Spasmodic torticollis has variably been described as a psychogenic

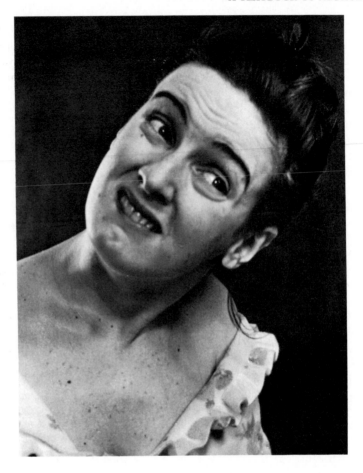

Figure 126.   Spasmodic torticollis.

disorder, a fragment of dystonia musculorum deformans, or a compensatory postural defect in persons with congenital ocular muscle imbalance or defects of the cervical spine or musculature. Hyperthyroidism has been present in a few cases. In some instances it has occurred as part of a wide spectrum of extrapyramidal symptoms that follow encephalitis lethargica. There is no information at present regarding either its pathophysiology or pathology. The disorder has been encountered at all ages, but most frequently makes its appearance during the third to sixth decades of life. The course is extremely variable, being transitory and remitting after a few months in some patients and relentlessly progressive and leading to incapacity in others. Some cases reach a static phase in which movements cease or are minimal, and a minor postural deformity of the head persists.

The evaluation of this condition should include a search for ocular and bony vertebral abnormalities, major psychiatric disturbances, and other neurologic conditions with which it may be associated. Definable conditions account for only a small percentage of cases. In most, no known cause is uncovered.

There is no specific therapy for torticollis except when an underlying correctable disease process is found. Many measures have been recommended to ameliorate the symptoms. Sensory bio-feedback techniques have been utilized with some success. Of the number of pharmacological agents Valium, clonopin and haloperidol have been reported effective in a small series of patients. In those more severely affected a variety of surgical measures have been attempted with inconsistent results. Denervation of the affected muscles by section of the anterior cervical root and/or the spinal accessory nerve has been utilized. Although the movements decrease on the operated side, they frequently recur in the contralateral group of muscles. Bilateral procedures may result in extensive disability. Bilateral thalamotomy has been performed with improvement. However, one is hesitant to recommend a procedure of this magnitude except in extreme situations. A procedure involving iontophoresis of saline into the middle ear, which presumably suppresses labyrinthine function unilaterally, has produced encouraging results in one series.

REFERENCES

Barrett, R. E., Yahr, M. D., and Duvoisin, R. C.: Torsion Dystonia and Spasmodic Torticollis—Results of Treatment with L-Dopa, Neurology, 20, 107, 1970.

Cooper, I. S.: Dystonia: Surgical Approaches to Treatment and Physiologic Implications, Res. Publ. Assoc. Res. Nerv. Ment. Dis., 55, 369, 1976.

Duane, D. D. and Svien, H. J.: Preliminary Evaluation of Labyrinthine Suppression in the Treatment of Spasmodic Torticollis, Neurology, 22, 399, 1972.

Eldridge, R.: The Torsion Dystonias. Literature Review and Genetic and Clinical Studies, Neurology, 20, 1, 1970.

Gilbert, G. J.: The Medical Treatment of Spasmodic Torticollis, Arch. Neurol., 27, 503, 1972.

Herz, E.: Dystonia. I. Historical Review; Analysis of Dystonic Symptoms and Physiologic Mechanisms Involved, Arch. Neurol. Psychiat., 51, 305, 1944.

————: Dystonia. II. Clinical Classification, Arch. Neurol. Psychiat., 51, 319, 1944.

————: Dystonia. III. Pathology and Conclusions, Arch. Neurol. Psychiat., 52, 20, 1944.

Herz, E. and Glaser, G. H.: Spasmodic Torticollis. Clinical Evaluation, Arch. Neurol. Psychiat., 61: 227, 1949.

Korein, J. and Brudny, J.: Integrated EMG Feedback in the Management of Spasmodic Torticollis and Focal Dystonia: A Prospective Study of 80 Patients, Res. Publ. Assoc. Res. Nerv. Ment. Dis., 55, 385, 1976.

Larsson, T., and Sjögren, T.: Dystonia Musculorum Deformans. Genetic and Clinical Population Study of 121 Cases, Acta Neurol. Scan. Supplement 17 (ad Volumen 42), 1966.

Marsden, C. D. and Harrison, M. J. G.: Idiopathic Torsion Dystonia (Dystonia Musculorum Deformans), Brain, 97, 793, 1974.
Marsden, C. D.: Dystonia: The Spectrum of the Disease, Res. Publ. Assoc. Res. Nerv. Ment. Dis., 55, 351, 1976.
Wooten, G. F.: Elevated Plasma Dopamine-β-hydroxylase Activity in Autosomal Dominant Torsion Dystonia, N. Engl. J. Med., 288, 284, 1973.
Zeman, W.: Pathology of the Torsion Dystonias (Dystonia Musculorum Deformans), Neurology, 20, 79, 1970.

The Parkinsonian Syndrome

James Parkinson in 1817, first described the major manifestations of this syndrome which is characterized by tremor, muscular rigidity and loss of postural reflexes. Not only is it one of the most frequently encountered of all the basal ganglia disorders, but parkinsonism is a leading cause of neurological disability in individuals over sixty years of age. Though its exact frequency is unknown, it has been estimated to have a prevalence rate of 100 to 150 per 100,000 population with an incidence of 20 cases per 100,000 annually. As a symptom complex its occurrence has been noted in a number of disease processes either as the sole manifestation or in association with other signs and symptoms. However, in the vast majority of cases no definable cause has as yet been uncovered. Since these latter cases appear to have many features in common, particularly in regard to age of onset and evolution of symptomatology, they have been designated as Parkinson's disease or primary parkinsonism. The cases with definable disease processes are best classified as secondary or symptomatic parkinsonism. This separation into clinical groups cannot be construed as indicative of a difference in pathophysiology or even pathogenetic mechanisms for the underlying basis of symptoms for all parkinsonism may well have a common origin. In fact sufficient evidence now exists that the loss of pigmented neurons particularly in the substantia nigra, locus ceruleus and brain stem nuclei is a common feature in all forms of parkinsonism.

The significance of these morphological changes has become evident since the demonstration that dopamine, a neurotransmitter substance, is found in high concentration in the neostriatum, that is, the caudate nucleus, putamen and pallidum. In parkinsonism, selective depletion of dopamine occurs in these structures and can be correlated with the degree of degeneration of the substantia nigra. Not only has this been shown in man, but it has been experimentally produced in animals. The greater the cell loss in the substantia nigra, the lower the concentration of dopamine in the striatum and the more severe the degree of clinical parkinsonism. The exact mechanism, however, by which selective damage to the substantia nigra occurs is at present unknown.

In the light of these findings parkinsonism may be defined in biochemical terms as a dopamine deficiency state resulting from disease, injury or dysfunction of the dopaminergic neuronal system. The physiologic role of this system appears to be one of inhibitory modulation of the striatum which it produces by counterbalancing the excitatory cholinergic activity in this region. Acetylcholine, the neurotransmitter of this latter system, is in abundant supply in the striatum and its concentration has been shown to be unaltered in parkinsonism. In the normal, healthy state a balance exists between the effects of acetylcholine and dopamine. With loss of the latter the balance is disturbed and cholinergic activity predominates. As yet it is not completely certain as to whether the loss of dopamine is the only defect nor that it is responsible for all of the manifestations of the disorder. Indeed it has been suggested that other neurotransmitters such as noradrenalin, gamma amino butyric acid and serotonin may be either primarily or secondarily involved. It is, however, well established that restoration of striatal dopamine activity results in a beneficial effect on all the symptoms of parkinsonism and is presently the basis for its treatment.

Parkinson's Disease
(Paralysis Agitans, Shaking Palsy)

The largest number of cases of parkinsonism encountered today falls into this category. The disease most frequently has its onset between the ages of fifty and sixty-five years though a rarely encountered juvenile form has also been described. Parkinson's disease affects both sexes, has occurred in all races and throughout the world. Though there is no evidence to indicate a hereditary factor a familial incidence is claimed by some authorities.

The pathological findings are quite striking and characteristic with neuronal loss and depigmentation in the substantia nigra, particularly the zona compacta (Fig. 127). Similarly loss of cells and pigment is noted in the locus ceruleus and in the dorsal vagal nucleus of the brainstem. These areas also show the presence of an intracellular inclusion body—the Lewy body. The exact nature of this inclusion body has not been defined but it is not viral in origin. Though the pathogenesis of Parkinson's disease is unknown, the fact that it makes its appearance in the latter years of life has suggested that it may relate to mechanisms involved in the aging process of neuronal cells particularly in individuals in whom the nigral cells are highly vulnerable to such effects. One of the factors that has been given consideration and for which some evidence exists relates to the enzymes necessary for removing the products of catecholamine metabolism. Hydrogen peroxide is such a by-product and its removal depends on the enzymes

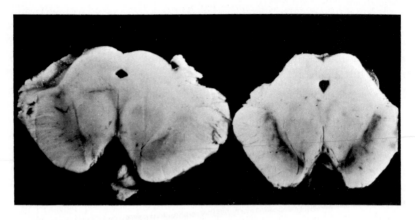

Figure 127.   Parkinson pathology.

peroxidase and catalase both normally in high concentration in the substantia nigra and reduced with aging but more so in Parkinson's brains. Their reduction may allow for the accumulation of hydrogen peroxide and other toxic products which then leads to the destruction of nigral cells and the loss of tyrosine hydroxylase, the enzyme responsible for dopamine production.

The classical triad of symptoms that occur in this disease are tremor, rigidity and akinesia. Of equal frequency and prominence are such abnormalities as disturbances of posture, equilibrium and autonomic function. The early symptomatology more often than not is subtle and indeed elusive as to its exact nature or time of onset. Since Parkinson's disease tends to occur in the middle years of life a sense of slowness or loss of agility of movement, feelings of tremulousness, or even depression with attendant psychomotor retardation may be attributed to advancing years or the involutional state. It is only when one of the cardinal symptoms becomes evident that the situation becomes clear and the appropriate diagnosis is reached. Early valuable signs usually present for years before other more obvious symptoms appear are lack of mobility of facial expression with infrequent blinking of the eyelids, fixed or tilted postures of the trunk, a hesitant rise from a chair in assuming the erect position, associated with an inability to seat oneself with ease. Not infrequently a poverty of movement with tendency to maintain positions for unusually long intervals of time in contrast with the normal tendency to shift and be slightly restless when sitting or standing are other early features. These heralding events all appear to be less well remembered by the patient than the first instance in which tremor or difficulty in the use of the limbs appears and for which

Table 70.   Initial Symptoms in Parkinson's Disease
(After Hoehn and Yahr)

	No. of Cases (183)
Tremor	129
Stiffness or slowness of movement	36
Loss of dexterity and/or handwriting disturbance	23
Gait disturbance	21
Muscle pain, cramps, aching	15
Depression, nervousness, or other psychiatric disturbance	8
Speech disturbance	7
General fatigue, muscle weakness	5
Drooling	3
Loss of arm swing	3
Facial masking	3
Dysphagia	1
Paresthesia	1
Patients with tremor as an initial symptom	70.5%
Average number of initial symptoms per patient	1.4

medical attention is sought. As indicated in Table 70, tremor was the initial complaint in more than 70% of patients. However, it was readily evident on questioning that many could recall one of the above noted ill-defined symptoms being present for years preceding tremor.

The tremor of Parkinson's disease has often been described as having distinctive characteristics. Typically it is referred to as pill-rolling involving the thumb and forefinger, alternatingly evident at rest with a frequency of 4 to 7 per second. However, it can be extremely variable. While its rhythmic alternating nature is a constant characteristic, the rate, amplitude and areas of bodily involvement are not so. Tremor of the so-called action variety, both postural and intentional, of variable frequencies with either minimal or extensive movement of the involved segments of the body both proximal and distal are not infrequently encountered. There is a general tendency for the tremor, once it occurs, to spread and involve other segments, but such is not invariably the case. Instances are encountered where tremor remains localized to the initial site of occurrence, while other features of the disorder may become more widespread. Tremor is an unsettling symptom to patients because it is such a highly visible phenomenon and carries with it undesirable connotations as to the emotional stability of the individual. However, it contributes less to the disability of the parkinsonian than other manifestations of the disease.

Rigidity of the musculature, i.e., resistance to passive movement is present in almost all cases of Parkinson's disease. Initially, it may exist in a mild degree restricted to a few groups of muscles but invariably it progresses to involve more areas of the body. In its early stages when not readily obtainable by passive movements of a limb, it can be induced by having the patient carry out active synkinetic movement of the contralateral limb. Rigidity contributes to the limited range and slowness of movement which characterizes Parkinson's disease but less so than akinesia. It also, to a limited extent, is a cause of the sense of muscle weakness which many patients experience. This latter symptom, however, is usually more apparent than real for in fact the parkinsonian patient can usually carry out an initial forceful contraction but is unable to maintain or do so repetitively. Rigidity has also been implicated as a cause of the postural deformities of limbs and trunk which are so characteristic and frequently encountered. Conceivably the sustained forceful contraction of rigid muscles can produce such abnormalities. However, their early occurrence in parkinsonism when rigidity is barely demonstrable and their experimental production in animals without rigidity in whom the nigrostriatal pathway is interrupted, suggest that it is a symptom in its own right. Indeed accumulated evidence would indicate that striatal imbalance resulting from dopamine deficiency underlies the postural abnormalities.

The body posture of the individual with established Parkinson's disease is characteristic and readily recognizable (Fig. 128). In the erect position the head is bowed, the trunk bent forward, the shoulders drooped, the arms flexed at the elbows with hands held in front of the body and the knees assume a flexed posture. The totality of this appearance is that of an individual whose body is immobilized in an anteriorly shifted overhanging position. Indeed the center of gravity appears to be displaced forward leading to his inability to stand erect without toppling and a tendency to be propulsive when walking. The small-stepped festinating gait is a distinctive feature and results from a combination of akinesia, rigidity and this postural abnormality. Postural abnormalities less profound can be detected in the early stages of parkinsonism. The most common are seen in the upper limbs. A tendency for the hand to assume an ulnar deviated position with flexion of the fingers at the metacarpal phalangeal joints, the so-called "striatal hand" is often encountered. Tilting of the trunk usually to the side opposite to that of initial limb involvement and equinovarus posture of the foot are other postural abnormalities.

One of the most disabling features of Parkinson's disease which bedevils the patient more than any other is the inability to initiate, maintain and perform with rapidity and ease volitional motor activities of the most ordinary sort. This contributes more to the disability of this

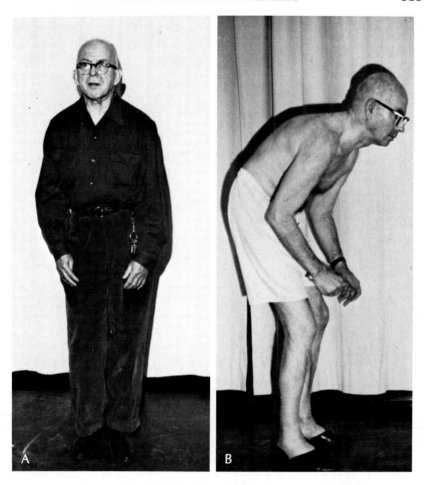

Figure 128. (A) Parkinson patient body posture, front view.
(B) Parkinson patient posture, side view.

disorder than any other symptom. The terms bradykinesia, hypokinesia and akinesia aptly describe the degrees of impaired movement which occur without any disturbance in muscle power, coordination or presence of rigidity. In all the acts of daily living the patient is conscious of delay in execution which at times may reach a total standstill. A meal normally consumed in twenty minutes may be only half eaten in an hour or more. Dressing and washing may require the better part of a morning and walking may be interrupted by the patient coming to a complete halt and being "frozen" in place. The poverty of movement which results from the bradykinetic and akinetic state is apparent in a broad variety of reflex motor activities normally occurring with little or no conscious awareness. Periodic eyeblinking; mimetic facial movements; associated movements of the arms when walking; shifting of weight when standing or sitting; assuming a relaxed posture when sitting are all impaired and rarely occur except with conscious effort. In fact, the patient with Parkinson's disease is under constant stress to voluntarily perform actions which in prior days came naturally and involuntarily. Akinetic mechanisms play a role in the voice-disturbance, namely its reduced amplitude and monotonous quality; the disorder of gait which in addition to its shuffling nature is difficult to start, maintain or alter in tempo on command; and in use of the upper limbs especially in writing. With advancing akinesia patients with Parkinson's disease can rarely maintain the continuous motor activity required in script writing and resort to printing individual letters. The capricious nature of akinesia adds greatly to the misery which the patient experiences. Its intermittent paradoxical nature leads to accusatory remarks by those involved in his daily care regarding the patient's motivation and sense of dependency. The literature on parkinsonism is replete with descriptions of patients who though totally immobile and in need of assistance for any and every act will suddenly rise and move normally for a period of time; the so-called paradoxical akinetic reaction. Family members, nurses and attendants are prone to state "he can do it when he wants to, five minutes ago he couldn't move a muscle now he is able to do anything he wants," as if the phenomenon were willed or strictly a matter of motivational nature. Undoubtedly, psychological factors play a role in chronic illness and Parkinson's disease is no exception, but this profound disturbance in motor activity without question is primarily based on organic neural factors involving the integrative functions of the nervous system at a high level.

A variety of symptoms referable to autonomic dysfunction is encountered in Parkinson's disease. These consist of thermal paresthesias undoubtedly related to alterations in vasomotor control of peripheral blood vessels; hyperhidroses indicating over-activity of sweat gland innervation and a tendency to hypotension with poor baroreceptor mechanisms leading in some instances to orthostatic syncope. Skin changes with eczematous eruption especially over the forehead and sialorrhea are not fully explained as to mechanism and may not be a direct expression of autonomic dysfunction. More likely they relate to the attendant difficulties in personal hygiene.

Considerable comment has been made regarding the intellectual capacity of those with Parkinson's disease. There are some who feel that dementia is an intrinsic characteristic of the disease increasing in severity as it progresses. Others have implied that intellectual deterioration occurs in those with specific manifestations of the disease particularly akinesia. Contrary to these reports are those that contend, as did James Parkinson, that the senses are unaffected. When testing has been carried out so that motor activities play a minor role in their performance and hence akinetic and rigid aspects of the disease are not a factor, it does appear that a number of cognitive, perceptual and memory deficits are present. To some extent the cognitive and perceptual deficits relate to cerebral dominance in that those with minor hemisphere involvement were more seriously affected. These findings suggest that the striatum plays a role in cerebral dominance in addition to the cerebral cortex. Memory deficits encountered in Parkinson's disease are usually not of a major degree. It would appear from these findings that there is an element of intellectual loss but not one of major proportions nor is it an outstanding characteristic of this disease.

Deep tendon reflexes are usually unimpaired in Parkinson's disease though on occasion one may elicit an abnormal extensor plantar response. A hyperactive or exaggerated glabellar reflex (Myerson's sign) is present in most patients and palmomental reflexes are usually positive.

Symptomatic or Secondary Parkinsonism

Parkinsonism has occurred as the predominate manifestation in a variety of diseases and conditions of the nervous system. Included are: poisoning with carbon monoxide, manganese and other heavy metals, brain tumors in the region of the basal ganglia, cerebral trauma, intoxication with neuroleptic agents, infectious processes such as encephalitides, multi-neuronal degenerative disorders of unknown cause and in association with cerebral arteriosclerosis as well as with endocrine dysfunction such as hypoparathyroidism. In most instances the presence of associated neurological deficits, atypical features of the symptomatology and/or other systemic manifestations of the related disease process arouses suspicion that one is not dealing with primary parkinsonism.

Postencephalitic Parkinsonism

One of the most prominent sequelae of the epidemic of encephalitis lethargica (von Economo's disease) that occurred between 1919 and 1926 was the parkinsonian syndrome. The syndrome developed after mild as well as severe encephalitis lethargica, and although in most instances they immediately followed the acute infectious process, in some patients prominent symptoms were not evident for intervals of up to ten years. The causative agent of encephalitis lethargica was never established. However, recent studies suggest that it may have been produced by a virus of the influenza A variety. Parkinsonism appears to have been a unique sequela of this form of encephalitis because it rarely follows any other known viral encephalitides. Pathologically postencephalitic parkinsonism differs from the idiopathic in that cellular loss of the melanin-containing neurons is greater, neuro-fibrillary changes occur in many of the remaining nerve cells and there is an absence of Lewy bodies. Persistent inflammatory changes are occasionally found even years after the initial infectious process. Multi-focal areas of glial scarring may be found throughout the nervous system.

Postencephalitic parkinsonism has a number of distinctive or unique features, including the following: (1) A history of encephalitis lethargica during the epidemic period 1918-1919. Since the pandemic of influenza occurred concurrently with encephalitis, it is essential that careful documentation be undertaken in differentiating these two infectious processes. (2) In addition to any or all of the parkinsonian symptoms indicated above, one or more of the following neurologic deficits may be found: hemiplegia, bulbar or ocular palsies, dystonic phenomena, tics, or behavioral disorders. (3) The parkinsonism itself is as a rule incompletely developed and has been static or slowly progressive over a period of years. (4) Episodes that have been termed oculogyric crises consist of attacks in which spasms of conjugate eye muscles occur so that the eyes are deviated upward, downward, or to one side for minutes or hours at a time.

The response of postencephalitic parkinsonism to treatment with pharmacologic agents differs from that of Parkinson disease. Though improvement of symptoms occurs with levodopa, tolerance is limited. Most must be treated cautiously with less than one half the usual therapeutic dose (2 to 3 gm/day) as they rapidly develop abnormal involuntary movements and are prone to abnormal behavioral reactions. However, most postencephalitics can tolerate large doses of anticholinergic agents.

Arteriosclerotic Parkinsonism
(Pseudo-parkinsonism)

Atherosclerotic involvement of the cerebral vessels has been implicated by some as a cause of parkinsonism. Though the symptoms produced by both disorders appear on superficial examination to resemble each other there are distinctive differences. Indeed, Critchley, who first proposed the term arteriosclerotic parkinsonism in 1929 has more recently re-emphasized the differing nature of the two disorders and has indicated that when there is an underlying substrate of cerebrovascular disease, it be referred to as "pseudo" parkinsonism.

Others have suggested that the nature of the symptomatology warrants abandoning the term arteriosclerotic parkinsonism.

Pathologically, multiple small cerebral infarctions (lacunes) secondary to small vessel occlusion are not infrequently found throughout the brain in these patients. The neuronal cell loss which is diffuse may involve the substantia nigra, but is rarely of an extensive degree when compared to other changes in the central nervous system. In fact, a greater involvement of the globus pallidus is often found as are lesions in the brain stem and cerebral cortex.

Signs and Symptoms. As a rule, the onset of symptoms is insidious with most cases beginning in the seventh decade of life, though on occasion the occurrence has been noted in younger individuals in their fourth decade. Only rarely is there a history of a major stroke preceding onset though symptoms referable to so-called minor strokes may be elicited. Early symptoms usually center around impaired mobility with gait disturbance being the most frequent initial complaint. Other presenting complaints may refer to pseudobulbar phenomena with dysarthria, some degree of dysphasia and emotional incontinence. On occasion, patients will present with progressive intellectual defects in association with poverty of movement. Tremor is a rare finding but alteration in muscle tone does occur. It differs from the cogwheel type, characteristic of Parkinson's disease, in that there is a stiffening of the limb in response to contact and a sense of resistance with attempted change of position. This type of alteration in muscle tone is known as "Gegenhalten." Hyperactive reflexes, abnormal plantar responses, palmomental and snouting reflexes are all usually found.

The course of the disease is progressive usually step wise, and more rapid than Parkinson's disease. Tolerance for the usual anti-parkinson drugs whether anti-cholinergic or dopaminergic is poor.

Striatonigral Degeneration. Striatonigral degeneration is an uncommon form of parkinsonism which was first identified as a separate entity by Adams, et al. in 1961. Clinically, it is difficult to distinguish these patients from those with primary parkinsonism though they have a tendency to show a greater degree of rigidity, a more rapid course and a poor response to pharmacological agents. Pathologically, however, these cases are characterized by neuronal degeneration of the striatum, particularly the putamen, while the substantia nigra is only mildly affected. Neuronal loss occurs in the putamen which is replaced by a dense gliosis with scattered pigment accumulation which may extend into the globus pallidus.

Progressive Supranuclear Palsy. Clincially and pathologically, progressive supranuclear palsy first described by Steele et al. in 1964, can be identified as a distinct disease entity. Pathologically, neuronal loss and the formation of neurofibrillary tangles occur in the pallidum, substantia nigra, superior colliculi and the periaqueductal grey matter as well as the reticular formation and inferior olivary nuclei.

Clinically the condition is characterized by a triad of symptoms referable to parkinsonism, mental disturbance and impairment of eye movements. The onset of the disorder is usually parkinson-like in nature with rigidity, akinesia or disturbances in equilibrium being first noted. The changes in personality and behavior are indicative of an organic dementia usually not of a severe degree. The disturbance of ocular activity is most characteristic with downward gaze being impaired early on, progressing to vertical gaze palsy and finally, to a total ophthalmoplegia. The initial disturbance in downward gaze leads to an abnormal posture of the head in which it is tilted backward to make up for the abnormal position of the eyeballs (Fig. 129). Progressive supranuclear palsy resembles other disorders of the nervous system in which multiple neuronal structures become involved. As a rule such disorders progress rather rapidly and are poorly responsive to treatment. In the case of progressive supranuclear palsy, the Parkinson symptomatology may respond to dopaminergic agents but the rest of the disorder progresses in an unaltered fashion.

Drug-Induced Parkinsonism. The use of neuroleptics as psychotherapeutic or antiemetic agents has resulted in the occurrence of a number of extrapyramidal syndromes. Parkinsonism indistin-

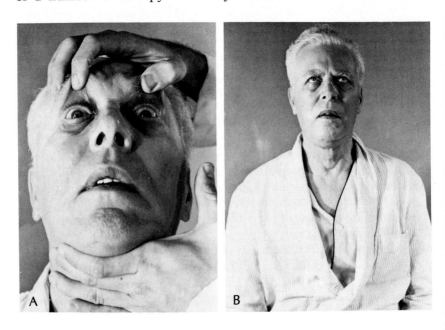

Figure 129.   Progressive supranuclear palsy.

guishable from that previously described, dystonic movements involving the tongue and face, and akathisia, a restless fidgety state with a desire to be in constant motion are those symptoms frequently encountered. Adults are more likely to develop parkinsonism and akathisia, whereas dystonic movements predominate in children. In some instances these reactions are dose-dependent; in others they are related to individual susceptibility. The symptoms usually disappear within a few days when the drugs are withdrawn, but occasionally persist for months. In some subjects permanent remnants of parkinsonian symptoms have been found years after elimination of the drugs. Paradoxically, involuntary movements may make their initial appearance after withdrawal of neuroleptic agents. This condition, termed tardive dyskinesia, tends to occur in older patients who have been on phenothiazine drugs for extended periods of time, during which they have shown signs of parkinsonism. Stereotyped repetitive movements of lips, tongue, and mouth and choreiform movements of limbs and trunk characterize this disorder. It may diminish in intensity or disappear spontaneously after weeks or months, but in some patients it has persisted indefinitely. In most instances the occurrence of basal ganglia symptoms, particularly parkinsonism, can be minimized by the simultaneous administration of one of the centrally active anticholinergic agents, such as Cogentin or Artane. Cautious use of neuroleptics, employing restricted doses and drug holidays in those requiring long-term treatment, may be the best preventive measure.

Parkinson-Dementia Complex of Guam. A syndrome of parkinsonism in association with a severe progressive dementia and motor neuron disease has been described in the indigenous Chamorro population of Guam and the Mariana Islands. The syndrome more commonly affects males and has a typical onset at age fifty to sixty; death usually occurs three to five years after onset. The syndrome is responsible for about 7% of deaths among the adult Chamorro population. The disorder tends to run in families. Motor neuron signs may be upper or lower in nature, resembling amyotrophic lateral sclerosis, which is also extraordinarily common among the Chamorro people (approximately 10% of adult deaths).

Pathologically the syndrome has features of both parkinsonism and Alzheimer's disease. Depigmentation of the substantia nigra and locus ceruleus occurs, as do Alzheimer's neurofibrillary tangles and severe cortical atrophy. Lewy bodies and senile plaques are not present. Motor neuron loss and pyramidal tract degeneration are also seen.

L-dopa therapy alleviates the extrapyramidal symptomatology in this syndrome; the dementia and motor neuron involvements are unaffected. The cause is unknown. It does not appear to be postencephalitic, nor is there evidence to date to suggest a viral etiology.

Laboratory Studies. Routine examination of blood, spinal fluid and urine is normal in all forms of parkinsonism. In primary parkinsonism and the more frequently encountered secondary forms (postencephalitic, progressive supranuclear palsy), the deficiency of dopamine in the striatum has been shown to cause a decrease of its acid metabolite, homovanillic acid (HVA) in the cerebrospinal fluid. The electroencephalogram is usually normal though diffuse slowing may be present. A greater degree of abnormalities usually of a non-specific nature are seen in secondary forms of parkinsonism. Skull roentgenograms and routine isotope brain scanning show no abnormalities. Computerized axial tomography reveals normal findings in parkinsonism but is useful in eliminating disorders whose symptoms are similar such as arteriosclerotic pseudoparkinsonism.

Management. GENERAL PRINCIPLES. Until the etiology and pathogenesis of parkinsonism are defined, its treatment must be considered as symptomatic, supportive and palliative. It is only in the exceptional case of symptomatic parkinsonism resulting from the use of drugs or occurring in association with specific disease processes that treatment of the causative factor may result in eradication of symptoms. The more frequently encountered patient will require lifelong treatment, consisting of the administration of specific medications, supportive psychotherapeutic measures, physical therapy, and, in rare instances, surgical intervention.

As is often the case in a chronic disease of unknown etiology with protean manifestations and no curative therapy, hard and fast rules regarding treatment, when applied indiscriminately to all patients, give less than optimal results. Indeed we have found it wise in Parkinson's disease to highly personalize treatment programs using as a guide not only the patient's symptomatology, but the degree of functional impairment and the expected benefits and risks obtainable from presently available therapeutic agents.

Judiciously employed treatment may control the symptoms of parkinsonism in a large proportion of patients for extended periods of time. In most it allows relatively normal activities of living during most phases of this disorder. The introduction of new pharmacological approaches to its treatment has markedly reduced mortality and forestalled the progressive disabling nature of this disorder.

SUPPORTIVE PSYCHOTHERAPY. The major symptoms of parkinsonism are markedly influenced by psychic factors, and a patient's outlook and motivation will affect the extent to which he can overcome disability. It is important for the physician to provide reassurance, encouragement, and sympathetic understanding to the patient and family so that they may meet the numerous difficulties to be encountered at various stages of the illness. To allay anxieties both should be counseled regarding the meaning of various symptoms, the nature of the disease in terms of its long and variable course, and the potential that most patients can lead active and productive lives for long periods after symptoms begin.

PHYSICAL THERAPY. Simple measures such as heat and massage will alleviate painful muscle cramps and the muscle contraction headache that often accompanies pronounced rigidity of the cervical musculature. Exercises help in preventing flexion contractures. Gait training, walking exercises, and minor rehabilitative measures may enable the patient to maintain his independence with regard to personal hygiene and daily living activities for many more years than his disabilities might otherwise allow. Physical therapy in parkinsonism need not be elaborate, but when indicated should be done frequently and for an indefinite period. The patient should be instructed in simple home exercises and encouraged to develop a program of physical activity. Most patients in the earlier stages like to take long walks and should be encouraged to continue this habit as long as reasonably possible. Every effort should be made to keep them gainfully employed and to adjust their occupations as indicated by their symptoms.

DRUG THERAPY. The drugs now employed in the treatment of parkinsonism are those theoretically capable of restoring normal activity to the striatum. Thus any agent that crosses the blood-brain barrier and enhances the brain's dopaminergic function or that reduces cholinergic activity may be expected to influence parkinsonism favorably. As a general rule a combination of agents with such properties works best.

The dopaminergic system may be functionally enhanced by agents that increase the synthesis of dopamine (this is presumably the modus operandi of levodopa), delay the catabolism of dopamine directly (monoamine oxidase inhibitors), stimulate its release (amphetamine and its analogues), act directly at receptor sites (Piribedil and Bromocriptine), and block the reuptake of monoamines at the synaptic cleft (anticholinergics, amantadine). Of the numerous means for improving dopaminergic function that have been tried to date, the most effective thus far has been the administration of levodopa (3,4-dihydroxyphenyl-L-alanine). Given alone or in combination with a peripheral dopa decarboxylase inhibitor (benserazide, carbidopa), it is appreciably more effective and less toxic than any therapeutic agent previously available for the treatment of Parkinson's disease.

In the selection of patients for treatment with levodopa, the over-all severity of parkinsonism and the degree of functional impairment, as well as the existence of concomitant diseases of other organs, must be carefully considered. As previously stated, patients with minimal signs and symptoms who are able to meet the demands of daily living need not involve themselves in a treatment program that may be rigorous and demanding and carries an implicit risk. The presence of occlusive vascular disease involving the heart or brain warrants careful assessment. Severe angina pectoris or transient cerebral ischemic attacks contraindicate the use of levodopa. A history of episodic cardiac arrhythmia presents an additional hazard. When the arrhythmia is associated with myocardial disease, the use of levodopa must be undertaken with extreme caution. Evidence of prior mental illness, particularly affective disorders or major "psychotic breaks" contravenes the use of levodopa. Although requiring careful monitoring, levodopa has been administered without adverse effects to patients with hepatic, renal, gastrointestinal, and hematopoietic disorders. However, the presence of hemolytic anemia and glucose-6-phosphate dehydrogenase (G-6-PD) deficiency contraindicates its use. L-dopa has been reported to worsen melanotic lesions; its use is contraindicated in such cases.

Clinical experience with levodopa suggests two phases of treatment with which the physician and patient must be familiar. The first or "introduction phase" extends over a period of weeks or months in which the dosage is slowly built up to the therapeutic range. During this phase, tolerance develops to many of the side effects of levodopa; and although improvement of symptoms occurs in most patients, the optimal therapeutic response may not be evident. A "maintenance phase" follows, in which the full benefits of treatment most often occur, and careful patient monitoring with readjustment of dosage and ancillary therapeutic measures may be required to maintain a stable therapeutic response. Each of these phases requires cooperation on the part of the patient and careful management by the physician to achieve the best therapeutic response. Monoamine oxidase inhibitors should be discontinued for at least two weeks prior to the start of levodopa therapy. Pyridoxine (vitamin B_6) is a cofactor for peripheral dopa decarboxylase. Its use in significant amounts will increase peripheral metabolism of dopa to dopamine, which does not cross the blood-brain barrier, and effectively reduce the amount of dopa available to the brain. Therefore patients on levodopa should not receive vitamin preparations containing pyridoxine. Treatment with levodopa may conveniently be initiated with 250 mg given three or four times daily by mouth after meals. If the initial doses are well tolerated, each dose may be increased to 500 mg. Subsequent increments of 125 to 250 mg may be made every two to three days in hospitalized patients or at intervals of one to two weeks in outpatients. It is preferable that no single dose exceed 1.5 to 2.0 gm; hence many patients will be required to take multiple doses throughout a twenty-four-hour period. The dose is gradually increased until either a satisfactory response or a dose-limiting side effect is encountered. The average optimal dose in patients with Parkinson's disease is 5 to 6 gm daily. As a general rule it is often best to settle for a total daily dose that, although failing to control all the symptoms, gives an acceptable degree of improvement and a tolerable level of side reactions. Attempts to eradicate every vestige of the disorder may require doses at which an undue frequency and severity of reactions occur.

It is unusual for patients to enjoy the benefits of levodopa without experiencing some side effects. In most, these effects can be modified to tolerable levels by the judicious use of the drug as well as by ancillary measures. Early in treatment, the major side effects encountered are nausea, vomiting, and anorexia, requiring reduction of dosage and deferral of further increments until such effects subside. Heightened nervous tension and feelings of anxiety necessitate reduction of dosage and a slower build-up to optimal levels. Acute psychotic episodes with delusions, hallucinations, hypomania, or depression are reactions that make it necessary to withdraw the drug. Cardiac dysrhythmia and/or hypotension with syncope is a combination that rarely permits continued use of levodopa. However, patients with orthostatic hypotension may continue treatment, employing commonly used means for its control. Adventitious involuntary movements develop in most patients on long-term levodopa therapy. When they are mild, treatment may be continued at full dosage. In instances in which the movements are excessive or interfere with function, a reduction in dosage is indicated with an attempt to find a level which compromises between a tolerable level of such movements and some degree of improvement of parkinsonian symptoms. No drug has been effective, in our experience, in the treatment of levodopa-induced dyskinesias. Variability in therapeutic response, the so-called "on-off" effect develops in some patients after extended periods of levodopa administration. This apparent loss of "dopa effect" may last for hours or days. Its cause is unknown, and few effective means for relieving it have been found. Laboratory abnormalities with the use of levodopa are few. Occasional transitory alterations in blood chemistry, including elevations of serum glutamic oxaloacetic transaminase (SGOT), alkaline phosphatase, serum glucose, and blood urea nitrogen (BUN) as well as depression of white blood cell count and development of a positive Coombs test have occurred. To date, these have not been associated with symptoms of dysfunction in organ systems, nor has autopsy material shown structural alterations.

The large daily dose of levodopa required, the delayed onset of therapeutic benefits, and some of its side effects can be avoided by the simultaneous administration of a dopa decarboxylase inhibitor. The use of such a combination prevents the peripheral utilization of levodopa, making it more readily and rapidly available for brain metabolism to dopamine. Hence the beneficial effects make their appearance within a matter of days, and side effects such as nausea, vomiting, and anorexia are virtually eliminated. Those side effects originating in the central nervous system, however, are unaffected. A number of such agents have been developed, but not all have been validated for general use in all countries. In the United States and some European and South American countries, Sinemet, as tablets containing carbidopa, 10 or 25 mg, plus levodopa, 100 or 250 mg, is marketed. In general, patients will require carbidopa 100 mg, and levodopa, 1000 mg a day, divided into four equal doses, or approximately one fourth the previous dose of levodopa. Available only in some European countries as Madopar is a combination of benserazide, 25 or 50 mg, and levodopa, 100 or 200 mg. The average required daily dose of this combination is benserazide, 200 mg, and levodopa 800 mg, in four equally divided doses. Aldomet (methyl dopa) in doses of 500 mg (125 mg four times a day) has been used in combination with levodopa, 2 to 4 gm with some effectiveness, but not to the extent of the previously mentioned compounds. A number of other antiparkinsonian agents are useful as adjunctive drugs with levodopa; they are also indicated for those in whom levodopa is contraindicated and are preferred for patients with mild symptoms in the early stages of the disorder. Some are also the drug of choice in drug-induced parkinsonism. Most of these compounds possess central nervous system anticholinergic properties or augment striatal dopaminergic activity. Those most frequently used are trihexyphenidyl (Artane), available in 2 and 5 mg tablets; benztropine (Cogentin), as 1 and 2 mg tablets; cycrimine (Pagitane), as 1.25 and 2.5 mg tablets; and procyclidine (Kemadrin), 2 and 5 mg tablets. All are virtually identical in their therapeutic effectiveness, with little reason except personal preference for choosing one over the other. Treatment should be initiated with small doses such as trihexyphenidyl, 2 mg three times daily, gradually increased until further increases yield no additional benefit or side effects reach an unacceptable degree of severity.

To obtain optimal results with anticholinergic drugs, careful titration of dosage against side effects is required. The goal is to find the dose that yields an optimal compromise between the limited symptomatic improvement of the parkinsonism and the disagreeable symptoms of cholinergic blockage of the central and peripheral nervous systems. Among the latter are blurring of vision, dryness of mouth and throat, anhidrosis, constipation, and urinary urgency, or sometimes, retention. The major symptoms of central anticholinergic intoxication are ataxia, dysarthria, hyperthermia, and a characteristic pattern of mental disturbances, including impairment of recent memory, confusion, delusion thinking, hallucinations, somnolence, and rarely coma.

A number of other agents, not primarily anticholinergics, but with mild central anticholinergic properties, are useful. Diphenhydramine (Benadryl), orphenadrine (Disipal), and chlorphenoxamine (Phenoxene) are all similar in pharmacologic action, and there is no reason except personal preference or individual tolerance in choosing one over the other. In general, diphenhydramine has enjoyed the widest use and can be given in divided dosage up to 150 mg a day. It is particularly useful as an adjunct to levodopa, for in addition to benefiting symptoms of parkinsonism, it allays anxiety and tempers insomnia.

The antidepressants imipramine (Tofranil) and amitriptyline (Elavil) are minimally effective when used alone, but in combination with anticholinergic agents or levodopa they may be beneficial. With administration in limited dosage, one may avoid their adverse effects, which may resemble parkinsonism. Not only are they helpful in improving akinesia and rigidity, but depressive symptoms when present are relieved. Imipramine or amitriptyline, 10 to 25 mg given four times a day, can be safely administered for extended periods.

Introduced as an antiviral agent, amantadine HCl (Symmetrel) was accidentally found to have activity against parkinsonism. Its mechanism of action in this regard is unknown, but it has been postulated that it may augment striatal dopaminergic activity or block cholinergic action. When used alone in doses of 100 mg twice or three times a day, its therapeutic effects are evident within forty-eight to seventy-two hours, consisting of a mild reversal of symptoms of parkinsonism. More effective action can be achieved when it is added to an existing regimen of treatment consisting of anticholinergic agents or levodopa (or both). On occasion amantadine has proved useful during the induction phase of levodopa therapy. Its effects are short lived, tending to diminish after a month and rarely lasting for more than three months. Many of its side effects are similar to those of the anticholinergic agents, particularly the induction of confusional and delusional states. In some patients after long-term use, edema and a form of livedo reticularis develop over the limbs.

Recently clinical trials with a number of new agents designed to overcome the shortcomings of levodopa have been made. In the main, they are directed toward patients who are: unresponsive to levodopa, experience "on-off" response or having an excessive degree of abnormal involuntary movements as a result of its use. Agents that have shown some promise are those having the property of directly activating post-synaptic dopamine receptors in brain—so-called dopaminergic receptor agonists. Some that have received particular attention are Piribedil (Trivastal) and Bromocriptine. Though Piribedil has shown anti-parkinson action, it has offered little advantage over levodopa administered with carbidopa (Sinemet). Indeed, its comparative efficacy is below that achieved with the latter combination. Bromocriptine in rather large doses, 100 to 200 mg a day, has in some patients who have been resistant to treatment produced beneficial effects. However, it does not avoid the side effects of the levodopa-carbidopa combination and additionally carries the risk of increasing behavioral disorders and peripheral vasospastic phenomena. The usefulness of either of these administered as the sole therapeutic agent for the treatment of parkinsonism has not as yet been established. However, when added to an existing therapeutic regimen, in modest doses, they may add additional therapeutic benefit. Though the usual MAO inhibitors have been avoided because of the potential of inducing hypertensive crises, when given with precursors of dopamine, such reactions have not been encountered with the MAOB inhibitor Deprenyl. Given in small doses 10 to 15 mg a day, it has been possible to reduce the required dose of levodopa and produce a more efficacious therapeutic response.

At present there is no doubt that levodopa given in combination with a decarboxylase inhibitor is the best available treatment for the large majority of parkinsonian patients. It is far from ideal but its judicious use benefits a large proportion of those suffering from Parkinson's disease over an extended period of time.

SURGICAL MEASURES. Surgical attempts to alleviate parkinsonism are primarily directed to the interruption of one or more neural pathways, the integrity of which appears essential for the production of symptoms, and at a site where normal sensory and motor functions will not be affected. Lesions produced by electrocoagulation or freezing in the ventrolateral nucleus of the thalamus have relieved contralateral tremor and rigidity in the limbs. However, akinesia and disturbances in gait, posture, and voice are not appreciably improved, and multiple lesions are necessary to relieve cervical, truncal, and bilateral limb symptoms. Since in most cases tremor and rigidity are bilateral, a good result on one side often encourages an attempt to do the same for the other. Most surgeons prefer to wait six months to one year before operating on the second side to minimize the complications that are apt to occur with bilateral procedures. Even so, the bilateral procedure frequently produces adverse effects on speech and, though recovery usually occurs, the patient may retain some degree of dysarthria and hypophonia. Since in most cases the manifestations become bilateral within a year or two of the onset, and disability is eventually due not so much to tremor or rigidity but to akinesia and postural abnormalities, stereotactic surgery benefits only a limited number of patients. The best candidate for surgery is the patient whose chief manifestation is unilateral tremor and rigidity, preferably in the upper extremity, and whose disease seems to progress slowly. These characteristics represent an early stage of the disease, and usually the patient is not yet seriously disabled. Thus, proponents of stereotactic surgery urge that thalamotomy be considered early in the course of Parkinson's disease, although its critics have pointed out that surgery does not benefit the more advanced patients who most need help, nor does it prevent progression of the disease. The introduction of more effective pharmacologic therapy has diminished the enthusiasm for surgical intervention. A balanced judgment would be that thalamotomy be used for cases resistant to other forms of therapy and in which relief of upper limb tremor is desired.

Course. All forms of parkinsonism are progressive disorders of the nervous system leading over variable periods of time to a considerable

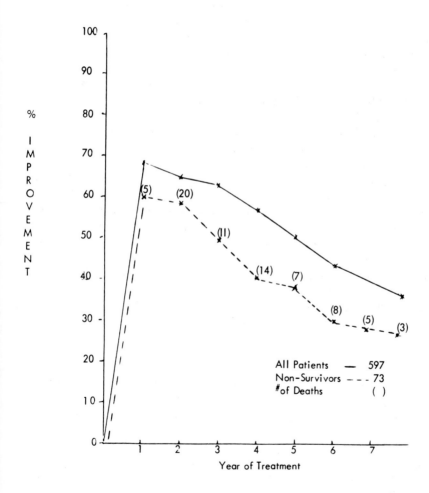

Figure 130. Degree of improvement of Parkinson signs during each year of treatment with levodopa. Non-surviving patients are compared with the total group treated.

degree of motor disability. The most progressive are those in which it is associated with other defects of the nervous system such as progressive supranuclear palsy where a fatal outcome can be expected within five years. Postencephalitic parkinsonism has been unique in that its evaluation has been relatively slow and patients have remained functional for extended periods of time in some instances for thirty years or more. Parkinson's disease or what is now referred to as primary parkinsonism, prior to its treatment with levodopa could be expected to produce severe disability or death in 25% of patients within five years of onset, which rose to 65% in the succeeding five years and to 80% in those surviving for fifteen years. Further it had been estimated that those suffering from Parkinson's disease had a mortality rate three times that of the general population matched for age, sex and racial origin. Though there is no evidence to indicate that levodopa or any other therapeutic agent now in use alters the underlying pathological process or stems the progressive nature of the disease there are indications of a major impact on survival time and functional capacity. Recent studies show that the added risk of mortality from Parkinson's disease has been reduced by one half and that longevity is extended by a number of years. More importantly since the introduction of these newer therapeutic agents the quality of life has been improved for patients with Parkinson's disease in that they do not suffer the degree of incapacity and dependence which previously was characteristic.

However, it must be emphasized that the treatment of parkinsonism is still far from ideal. Long term follow up studies covering periods of time up to eight years during which levodopa has been administered reveal a gradual loss of therapeutic efficacy. Optimal responses are obtained during the first three years of instituting treatment with levodopa regardless of duration of the disease and then diminish (Fig. 130). It is not known at this time whether this relates to intrinsic factors of the disease process itself or to pharmacological properties of the drug.

REFERENCES

American College of Neuropsychopharmacology: Drug Therapy: Neurologic Syndromes Associated with Antipsychotic-drug Use, N. Engl. J. Med., 289, 20, 1973.

Andrews, J. M., Terry, R. D. and Spataro, J.: Striatonigral Degeneration: Clinical-pathological Correlations and Response to Stereotaxic Surgery, Arch. Neurol, 23, 319, 1970.

Behrman, S., et al.: Progressive Supranuclear Palsy. Clinico-pathological Study of Four Cases, Brain, 92, 663, 1969.

Bernheimer, H., et al.: Brain Dopamine and the Syndromes of Parkinson and Huntington: Clinical, Morphological and Neurochemical Correlations, J. Neurol. Sci., 20, 415, 1973.

Blumenthal, H., and Miller, C.: Motor Nuclear Involvement in Progressive Supranuclear Palsy, Arch. Neurol., 20, 362, 1969.

Borit, A., Rubinstein, L. J. and Urich, H.: The Striatonigral Degenerations: Putaminal Pigments and Nosology, Brain, *98*, 101, 1975.

Brody, J. A., Hirano, A., and Scott, R. M.: Recent Neuropathological Observations in Amyotrophic Lateral Sclerosis and Parkinson-Dementia of Guam, Neurology, *21*, 528, 1971.

Costa, E., Cote, L., and Yahr, M. D., eds.: *Biochemistry and Pharmacology of the Basal Ganglia*. Hewlett, N.Y., Raven Press, 1966.

Cotzias, G. C.: Modification of Parkinsonism—Chronic Treatment with L-Dopa, N. Engl. J. Med., *280*, 337, 1969.

Critchley, M.: Arteriosclerotic Parkinsonism, Brain, *52*, 23, 1929.

Dix, M. R., Harrison, M. J. G., Lewis, P. D.: Progressive Supranuclear Palsy (The Steele-Richardson-Olszewski Syndrome), J. Neurol. Sci., *13*, 237, 1971.

Duvoisin, R. C., and Yahr, M. D.: Encephalitis and Parkinsonism, Arch. Neurol., *12*, 227, 1965.

Elizan, T. S., et al.: Amyotrophic Lateral Sclerosis and Parkinsonism-Dementia Complex. A Study in Non-Chamorros of the Mariana and Caroline Islands, Arch. Neurol., *14*, 347, 1966.

————: Amyotrophic Lateral Sclerosis and Parkinsonism-Dementia Complex of Guam, Arch. Neurol., *14*, 356, 1966.

Gamboa, E. T., et al.: Influenza Virus Antigen in Postencephalitic Parkinsonism Brain, Arch. Neurol., *31*, 228, 1974.

Hirano, A., et al.: Parkinsonism-Dementia Complex, An Endemic Disease on the Island of Guam. I. Clinical Features, Brain, *84*, 642, 1961.

Hirano, A., et al.: Amyotrophic Lateral Sclerosis and Parkinsonism-Dementia Complex on Guam, Further Pathologic Studies, Arch. Neurol., *15*, 35, 1966.

Hoehn, M. M. and Yahr, M. D.: Parkinsonism: Onset, Progression and Mortality, Neurology (Minneap.), *17*, 427, 1967.

Hornykiewicz, O.: Dopamine in the Basal Ganglia: Its Role and Therapeutic Implications (Including the Clinical Use of L-Dopa), Br. Med. Bull., *29*, 172, 1973.

————: Neurohumoral Interactions and Basal Ganglia Function and Dysfunction, Res. Publ. Assoc. Res. Nerv. Ment. Dis., *55*, 269, 1976.

Parkinson, J.: *An Essay on the Shaking Palsy*, London, Sherwood, Neely and Jones, 1817.

Sachdev, K. K., et al.: Juvenile Parkinsonism Treated with Levodopa, Arch. Neurol., *34*, 244, 1977.

Sharpe, J. A., et al.: Striatonigral Degeneration: Response to Levodopa Therapy with Pathological and Neurochemical Correlation, J. Neurol. Sci., *19*, 275, 1973.

Steele, J. C., Richardson, J. C., and Olszewski, J.: Progressive Supranuclear Palsy, Arch. Neurol., *10*, 333, 1964.

Yahr, M. D. (ed.): Treatment of Parkinsonism—The Role of Dopa Decarboxylase Inhibitors, Adv. Neurol., New York, Raven Press, 1973.

————: Levodopa, Ann. Intern. Med., *83*, 677, 1975.

————: Evaluation of Long-Term Therapy in Parkinson's Disease: Mortality and Therapeutic Efficacy. In *Advances in Parkinsonism*, W. Birkmayer and O. Hornykiewicz, Eds., Basle, Editiones Roche, 1976, p. 435.

————(ed.): The Basal Ganglia, Res. Publ. Assoc. Res. Nerv. Ment. Dis., *55*, 474, 1976.

Essential Tremor
(Familial Tremor)

This is a monosymptomatic condition in which tremor involving the upper limbs and/or head and face is the primary manifestation. The tremor is rhythmical, regular and is usually more rapid than that encountered in parkinsonism. It is accentuated by emotional factors, more apparent on sustension than rest and may be worsened by volitional movement, especially as it nears completion. The ingestion of alcohol not infrequently suppresses the tremor. The age of onset is variable, but in most cases the disorder begins prior to the age of twenty-five years and tends to persist throughout life. Some progression of the intensity of tremor and spread to other bodily parts usually occur over the years, which may result in significant physical and social disability. There is a strong familial incidence, with occurrence in several successive generations of the same family, though the genetic pattern of inheritance has not been fully established. Its transmission appears to be an autosomal dominant trait. It is also unusually common in males with sex chromosome abnormalities. To date no specific pathologic lesion has been reported in the nervous system of people with this condition. It has been suggested that the condition is an abortive form of parkinsonism and, on occasion, other hallmarks of this disorder have developed after many years. However, such instances are exceptional and in general this concept does not appear justifiable at present. There is no specific effective therapy for controlling the tremor, although beta-adrenergic blocking agents such as propranolol in dosage of 120 to 140 mg a day divided equally into 3 or 4 doses are occasionally effective. Sedatives such as phenobarbital, in dosage of 15 mg 3 times a day, or Valium 10 mg 3 times a day, may reduce the intensity of the tremor. Anxiety tremor and hyperthyroid tremor are quite similar in appearance and may be mistaken for essential tremor. It is of utmost importance to differentiate essential tremor from parkinsonism. By and large, the distinguishing characteristics are earlier age of onset; lack of severe progression, akinesia, rigidity, or postural abnormalities; and the strong family history of tremor.

Senile Tremor

Tremor is a frequent finding in the elderly, most often involving the upper limbs and head. It differs from parkinsonian tremor in that it is finer and more rapid and at first occurs only with voluntary movements. As time goes on it becomes more constant and is also present while the limbs are at rest. There is no associated weakness or alteration in muscle tone. These features differentiate this form of tremor from parkinsonism. The cause is unknown. Since senile tremor has both cerebellar and extrapyramidal features, in that it occurs at rest and with movement, the assumption is that some critical pathway linking these systems has undergone degeneration. There is no effective treatment, although mild benefit may be derived from sedatives or the use of diphenhydramine (Benadryl) given in 25 mg doses 3 times a day. Most patients accept it as another of the many changes that come with advancing years. Occasionally patients have to be reassured that they do not have parkinsonism or some other progressive neurologic disorder.

REFERENCES

Critchley, E.: Clinical Manifestations of Essential Tremor, J. Neurol. Neurosurg. Psychiat., 35, 365, 1972.
Marshall, J.: Observations on Essential Tremor, J. Neurol. Neurosurg. Psychiat., 25, 122, 1962.
Winkler, G. F. and Young, R. R.: Efficacy of Chronic Propranolol Therapy in Action Tremors of the Familial, Senile or Essential Varieties, N. Engl. J. Med., 290, 984, 1974.

Pigmentary Degeneration of the Globus Pallidus (Hallervorden-Spatz disease)

Originally described by Hallervorden-Spatz in 1922, this disorder derives its name from its distinctive pathological changes. These consist of an intense brown pigmentation of the globus pallidus and to a lesser extent of the substantia nigra and red nucleus. The pigment results from the deposition of iron (Fig. 131) which is in granules and amorphous deposits in ganglion cells, the interstitial tissues and walls

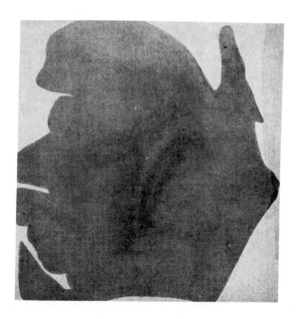

Figure 131. Pigmentary degeneration of globus pallidus, Iron pigment in basal ganglia. Turnbull-blue stain. (Merritt, H. H., Moore, M., and Solomon, H. C., courtesy Am. J. Syph.)

of small blood vessels. In the affected areas one notices a loss of neurons and medulated fibers as well as swollen axon fragments. Some have contended that neuroaxonal degeneration is the basic pathological feature and that the disorder is a juvenile form of this condition. Others contend that it may represent a variant of the lipoidoses.

The disorder is considered to be inherited in an autosomal recessive manner though sporadic cases have also been reported. Its onset is between the ages of seven and twelve, usually with rigidity of the limbs followed by dysarthria, emotional disorders of the pseudobulbar type, dementia and the development of clubfoot deformities. More than 50% of patients show abnormal involuntary movements consisting of either tremor, dystonia or choreoathetosis. Associated findings have included optic atrophy, retinitis pigmentosa, ataxia and myoclonus. In most instances the deep tendon reflexes are hyperactive with abnormal plantar responses. A marked degree of increased muscle tone is present. Recently it has been shown that the diagnosis can be confirmed by determining the uptake of radio-active iron by the basal ganglia. Utilizing the iron isotope ^{59}Fe, one can show increased uptake on scintillation counting in the region of the basal ganglia but in no other regions of the body. These studies in addition to their diagnostic value have suggested that the increased concentration of iron in the pallidum is the result of local storage, rather than any abnormalities of general iron metabolism.

There is no treatment for this disorder at the present time. Chelating agents to reduce iron storage have not proven useful. The disease progresses slowly over a period of five to twenty years with a fatal outcome the result.

REFERENCES

Defendini, R., et al.: Hallervorden-Spatz Disease and Infantile Neuroaxonal Dystrophy. Ultrastructural Observations, Anatomical Pathology and Nosology, J. Neurol. Sci., 20, 7, 1973.

Dooling, E. C., Schoene, W. C. and Richardson, E. P.: Hallervorden-Spatz Syndrome, Arch. Neurol., 30, 70, 1974.

Gilman, S. and Barrett, R. E.: Hallervorden-Spatz Disease and Infantile Neuroaxonal Dystrophy: Clinical Characteristics and Nosological Considerations, J. Neurol. Sci., 19:189, 1973.

Hallervorden, J. and Spatz, H.: Eigenartige Erkrankung im extrapyramidalen system mit besonderer Beteiligung des Globus pallidus und der Substantia nigra., Zentralbl. Gesamte Neurol. Psychiatr., 79, 254, 1922.

Martin, L., Martin, J. J. and Centerick, C.: Forme Infantile de la Maladie de Hallervorden-Spatz. Etude Anatomo-clinique de la Troisième Observation de la Fratrie D. B., Acta Neurol. Belg., 75, 257, 1975.

Szanto, J. and GallYas, F.: A Study of Iron Metabolism in Neuropsychiatric Patients, Hallervorden-Spatz Disease, Arch. Neurol., 14, 438, 1966.

Vakili, S., et al.: Hallervorden-Spatz Syndrome, Arch. Neurol., 34, 729, 1977.

Other Diseases of the Basal Ganglia

In addition to the more common diseases of the basal ganglia previously described, there are a number of rare and less clearly defined diseases which merit only a brief discussion.

Juvenile Paralysis Agitans (Progressive Atrophy of the Globus Pallidus, Progressive Pallidal Degeneration). This is a rare familial disease of the basal ganglia described by Willige and Hunt, characterized by the appearance in childhood or early adult life of symptoms similar to those of paralysis agitans. The condition differs from post-encephalitic parkinsonism in its familial nature, the early age of onset, the slower progress of symptoms and the intensity of the tremor and the rigidity. Although the disease is familial, sporadic cases are reported. Necropsy confirmation of the diagnosis has been obtained in only two cases. In these the changes were limited to a decrease in large nerve cells and an increase in glia in the globus pallidus and to a lesser extent in the putamen, caudate, substantia nigra and the subthalamic nucleus. It is quite probable that some of the cases, which have been reported without necropsy confirmation, represent examples of postencephalitic parkinsonism or progressive hepatolenticular degeneration.

Double Athetosis (Status Marmoratus, Etat Marbré, Congenital Chorea, Infantile Partial Striatal Sclerosis). From the large number of cases classified as Little's disease or birth injury, there has been separated by Anton and the Vogts a small group of cases in which the symptoms are predominantly those of athetosis and dystonia of the trunk, facial and extremity muscles, and in which there is a peculiar marbling or mottling of the basal ganglia. The marbled appearance (Fig. 132) is due to the presence of large bundles of abnormally situated myelin sheaths. The marble appearance is greatest in the caudate and lenticular nucleus, but it may be found in the thalamus, internal capsule and cerebral cortex. The pathogenesis of this overgrowth of myelin is not known. It is thought by some to be the result of excess formation of myelin by the increased number of glial cells which are present in the lesion. The overgrowth of glia is explained by some as the result of anoxia at birth or fetal encephalitis.

The clinical picture is characterized by the appearance in the latter half of the first year of life of choreiform and athetoid movements and rigidity of the muscles. The latter in some instances may assume the character of dystonia. There is some disagreement in regard to the static or progressive nature of the disease. It is Ford's contention that the disease is always static, and that the afflicted child is slow in learning to walk and talk, and that the latter function may be seriously interfered with by the rigidity and abnormal movements of the muscles of phonation. Mental deficiency of a moderate or severe degree may also

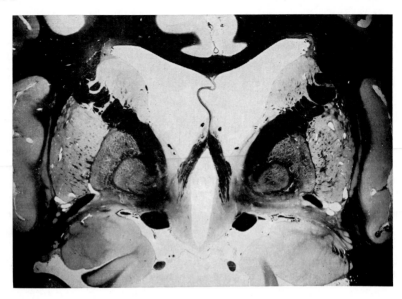

Figure 132.   Status marmoratus of basal ganglia. (Courtesy Dr. P. I. Yakovlev.)

be present. In most cases the mental deficiency appears greater than it actually is due to the motor defects and the defects in vocalization.

Status Dysmyelinatus. An ill-defined pathological syndrome was described by the Vogts in 1919 and 1920 which was characterized by a shrinkage of the caudate nucleus, globus pallidus and subthalamic nucleus and a failure of staining or lack of development of the myelin sheaths in the affected areas. The clinical picture is characterized by the development in the first year of athetoid movements, which are gradually replaced by rigidity before the death of the patient in the second decade of life.

Kernicterus. Severe jaundice of the newborn may occur as the result of erythroblastosis fetalis, associated with Rh and ABO incompatibility of parents. Other causes include prematurity and the use of antibiotic drugs. In this condition the brain may be stained with bile pigment. The staining is most intense in the basal ganglia either as a result of a selective affinity of these regions for the pigment or the result of anoxic degeneration of these nuclei with secondary deposition of the pigments in the destroyed tissues. The mortality rate is high, but it is thought by some pediatricians that at least a portion of the cases of choreoathetosis and mental retardation which are found in the institutions for the feebleminded may be due to the less severe and nonfatal forms of erythroblastosis fetalis.

REFERENCES

Anton, G.: Uber die Beteiligung der grossen basalen Gehirnganglien bei Bewegungsstörungen und insbesondere Chorea, Jahrb. f. Psychiat. u. Neurol., *14*, 141, 1896.
Fitzgerald, G. M., Greenfield, J. G., and Kounine, B.: Neurological Sequelae of "Kernicterus," Brain, *62*, 292, 1939.
Hunt, J. R.: Progressive Atrophy of the Globus Pallidus (Primary Atrophy of the Pallidal System), Brain, *40*, 58, 1917.
Kalinowsky, L.: Familiäre Erkrankung mit besonderer Beteiligung der Stammganglien, Monatsschr. Psychiat., u. Neurol., *66*, 168, 1927.
Lewy, F. H.: Die Histopathalogie der choreatischen Erkrankungen, Ztschr. f. d. ges. Neurol. u. Psychiat., *85*, 622, 1923.
Lowenburg, K., and Malamud, W.: Status Marmoratus, Arch. Neurol. & Psychiat., *29*, 104, 1933.
Margoles, C., et al.: Kernicterus in Japan, World Neurology, *1*, 254, 1960.
Munch-Petersen, C. J.: Studien uber erbliche Erkrankungen des Zentralnervensystems, I. Fälle von heriditärem, striärem Symptomkomplex, Acta Psychiat. et Neurol., *5*, 493, 1930.
Vogt, C.: Quelques Considérations Générales à propos du Syndrôme du Corps Strié, J. f. Psychol. u. Neurol., *18*, 479, 1911.
Vogt, C., and Vogt, O.: Zum Lehre der Erkrankungen des Stirären Systems, J. f. Psychol. u. Neurol., *25*, 627, 1920.
Willige, H.: Ueber Paralysis agitans im jugendlichen Alter, Ztschr. f. d. ges. Neurol. u. Psychiat., *4*, 520, 1911.
Winkelman, N. W.: Progressive Pallidal Degeneration, Arch. Neurol. & Psychiat., *27*, 1, 1932.
Zimmerman, H. M., and Yannet, H.: Cerebral Sequelae of Icterus Gravis Neonatorum and Their Relation to Kernicterus, Am. J. Dis. Child., *49*, 418, 1935.
Zuelzer, W. W.: Neonatal Jaundice and Mental Retardation, Arch. Neurol., *3*, 127, 1960.

CEREBELLUM

The cerebellum and its connections are the primary site of disease in a number of chronic progressive disorders often occurring in a familial or hereditary pattern. There is, as yet no satisfactory means of classifying these disorders due to our limited knowledge of etiologic factors, a considerable variability in the clinical manifestations and the difficulties of correlating clinical signs with changes found in postmortem studies. The salient clinical feature common to these disorders is a chronic slowly progressive ataxia usually beginning in the lower extremities. In addition, signs and symptoms reflecting involvement of the posterior columns, the pyramidal tracts, the pontine nuclei, the basal ganglia and other regions of the brain may occur. As a rule, the clinical picture is fairly constant in a given kindred, but cases of muscular dystrophy, optic atrophy or spastic paraplegia have been found in some affected families.

On histological study there is a selective neuronal system degeneration with reactive gliosis and demyelination. Current nosological concepts of these disorders rest primarily on the distribution of degenerative changes in the nervous system. Indeed, in individual cases, precise diagnosis is often possible only on post-mortem study.

Even then, there may be difficulty in satisfactorily classifying intermediate or mixed cases. For our present descriptive purposes we may somewhat arbitrarily divide the cerebellar system degenerations into several large groups on clinical and pathological grounds as follows:

1. Hereditary spinocerebellar ataxia of Friedreich
2. Hereditary ataxia with muscular atrophy (Levy-Roussy syndrome)
3. Hereditary cerebellar ataxia
   a. resembling olivopontocerebellar atrophy
   b. cerebello-olivary degeneration (Holmes)
4. Olivopontocerebellar atrophy (Dejerine-Thomas)
5. Parenchymatous cerebellar degeneration
6. Other forms of cerebellar ataxia

Hereditary Spinal and Cerebellar Ataxia (Friedreich's Ataxia)

Friedreich's ataxia is a familial and hereditary disease with degenerative changes localized chiefly to the dorsal half of the spinal cord and the cerebellum and characterized clinically by the appearance in the first or second decade of life of ataxia of the extremities and trunk, absence of deep reflexes, loss of proprioceptive sensations in the extremities and extensor plantar responses. Clubfoot and scoliosis are present in a high percentage of the cases. Dysarthria, muscle atrophies and degeneration of the optic nerve may occur in late stages of the disease. Involvement of the heart muscles has been reported in many cases. Diabetes mellitus is present in over 10% of the cases.

Pathology. On gross inspection the spinal cord and cerebellum may appear to be normal. Some authors have noted that the cord appeared to be thinner than normal and the cerebellum somewhat shrunken. The characteristic histological changes in the cord are a degeneration in the posterior funiculi, in the lateral corticospinal tract and the dorsal and ventral spinocerebellar tracts. These degenerative changes are most intense in the dorsal funiculi where there is an extensive degree of gliosis. Degeneration also involves the dorsal roots, the ganglia and the peripheral nerves. There is a loss of cells in Clarke's column and to a lesser extent in the substantia gelatinosa and other cell masses of the posterior horn. Ventral horn cells are usually preserved.

The cerebellum and brainstem are usually normal but shrinkage of the pons and the medulla has been reported. Atrophy of the Purkinje cells and those of the dentate nuclei has been found in some cases. There are no significant changes in the cerebral cortex and the degeneration in the corticospinal tract rarely extends above the level of the medulla.

Recent investigations have shown evidence of defective pyruvate metabolism in some patients with Friedreich's ataxia, but in the majority of cases no consistent biochemical abnormality has been defined.

Incidence. Friedreich's ataxia is one of the more common hereditary diseases of the nervous system. All races are affected and it is slightly more common in the male sex. There is no agreement as to the mode of transmission. It is assumed by some that the presence of both a dominant and recessive gene is necessary for the transmission of the disease. The disease may be inherited directly, but familial incidence is more common. The latter is to be expected from the fact that the early onset of disability in the full-blown disease prevents marriage and the production of offspring. Sporadic or isolated instances of the disease are not uncommon.

The onset is usually in the first or second decade of life. Most commonly it is between the seventh and thirteenth years. Symptoms may be present in infancy and rarely they may not appear until the third decade. Abortive forms, in which only one or two features of the disease are present, *i.e.,* clubfeet, slight ataxia or absent knee jerks, are not uncommon.

Symptoms and Signs. Ataxia, sensory loss, nystagmus, alterations in the reflexes, clubfeet and kyphoscoliosis are the characteristic features of the disease. Optic atrophy, cranial nerve palsies, mental deficiency and deterioration are other less common findings.

Motor System. Ataxia of the gait is the most common symptom and it is usually the first to develop. The difficulty in gait may make its appearance in the latter half of the first decade of life in a child who had apparently been able to walk normally, but more commonly it has been noted that the child was slow in learning to walk, his gait was clumsy and awkward and that he was not as agile as other children. Within a few years after the onset of frank difficulty in locomotion, ataxia appears in the movements of the upper extremities and finally in those of the trunk. The impairment of movements is the result of the combination of cerebellar asynergia with ataxia due to the loss of proprioceptive sense. Movements are jerky, awkward and poorly controlled. Intention tremor, most common in the extremities, may occasionally affect the muscles of the trunk (cerebellar titubation). The muscles of articulation are involved in advanced cases, with explosive or slurred speech or finally a dysarthria of such a severe degree that speech is unintelligible. Pseudoathetoid and choreiform movements of the muscles of the extremities may also be seen.

Weakness of the muscles is common. In some cases this amounts to a complete or almost complete paralysis of the lower extremities with paraplegia in flexion. As a rule the muscles are flabby and disuse atrophy is common in the late stages of the disease. In addition, localized atrophy of the muscles may occur in the late stage. This is most common in the muscles of the distal parts of the extremities but the girdle and trunk muscles are also occasionally involved.

Sensory System. Evidence of involvement of the posterior funiculi is present in almost all cases. Loss of the appreciation of vibration in the extremities is an early sign. Some impairment of position sense in the lower extremities and later in the upper extremities is almost always present. Occasionally, the loss of proprioceptive sense in the trunk muscles confines the patient to bed or makes it necessary that the patient have special support when sitting in a chair. Loss of two-point discrimination and partial or complete astereognosis and some impairment of the appreciation of pain, temperature and tactile sensation are occasionally seen in advanced cases.

Reflexes. The reflexes in the legs are almost invariably absent. Rarely, in otherwise typical cases, they are preserved throughout the course of the disease. The reflexes are usually present in the upper extremities in the initial stages, but they may be absent in the later stages. The plantar responses are extensor in type in practically all cases. Occasionally an extensor response may be found on only one side and rarely the plantar responses may be flexor. The abdominal and cremasteric reflexes are preserved in the majority of cases.

Other Neurological Signs and Symptoms. Nystagmus develops at some stage of the disease in practically all cases. It is commonly of the fixation type, *i.e.,* oscillatory movements of the eyes on movement before coming to rest, but horizontal nystagmus and vertical or rotary nystagmus have been reported. Optic atrophy is an inconstant feature, but its frequency has been emphasized by some authors. Oculomotor paralysis with diplopia, deafness and loss of labyrinthine reactions are rare manifestations. Impairment of the sphincters is uncommon except when the patients are bedridden. It is often difficult to determine whether incontinence in these patients is due to organic damage or to inattention. Mental retardation, progressive deterioration of the mental faculties or psychotic manifestations occur in a small percentage of the cases. The condition is not incompatible with a high degree of intellectual development. The incidence of convulsive seizures is greater than in the general population.

Skeletal Abnormalities. Clubfeet and kyphoscoliosis are the characteristic skeletal deformities. The abnormality in the shape of the foot usually takes the form of a double pes cavus, conjoined with talipes varus or equinovarus. Although not a constant feature of the disease, the foot deformity is present in almost three fourths of the cases, and it is occasionally found in other members of the family as the only sign of the disease. The abnormality of the feet may be present from early infancy or it may not develop until late in the course of the disease. Deformity of the head is a rare finding.

Kyphosis or scoliosis, usually in the upper thoracic regions, is present in over 80% of the cases. The spinal deformity usually develops late and progresses slowly.

Heart. Enlargement of the heart, cardiac murmurs, abnormalities in the electrocardiogram and other signs of heart disease are not uncommon. Boyer and also Hewer found that cardiac involvement in the form of diffuse myocardial fibrosis with coronary thrombosis was a common cause of death.

Laboratory Findings. The laboratory findings are usually normal. Occasionally there is a slight increase in the protein content and rarely a slight pleocytosis in the cerebrospinal fluid. The latter is possibly related to an acute episode in the degenerative process. Abnormalities in the electrocardiogram, related to involvement of the heart muscle, are common.

Diagnosis. The characteristic spinal cord and cerebellar signs in combination with the abnormalities of the feet and spine make the diagnosis a relatively simple matter in classical cases. In sporadic cases with no skeletal deformities, there may be some difficulty in the differential diagnosis between Friedreich's ataxia and multiple sclerosis. The onset of symptoms at an early age and the progressive course of Friedreich's ataxia as well as the relative infrequency of the loss of the deep reflexes in multiple sclerosis are important factors in the differential diagnosis.

Abortive or atypical forms of Friedreich's ataxia are distinguished from other heredodegenerative disease with difficulty unless the typical syndrome is present in other members of the family.

Clinical Course. There are numerous instances in which the disease assumes an abortive form which may be compatible with a relatively normal life span without serious disability. In the majority of the patients, however, in which the onset is in the early years of life, the disease is slowly or rapidly progressive with complete incapacity by the age of twenty. Death usually occurs as the result of intercurrent infections but may result from involvement of the heart muscles.

Treatment. There is no specific treatment which will influence the course of the disease. Tenotomies or other orthopedic operations are indicated for the relief of the foot deformity. Muscle training and re-education are of value in the abortive forms and in the rare cases with spontaneous remissions.

REFERENCES

Blass, J. P., Kark, R. A. and Menon, N. K.: Low Activities of the Pyruvate and Oxoglutarate Dehydrogenase Complexes in 5 Patient with Friedreich's Ataxia, N. Engl. J. Med., *295*, 62, 1976.

Boyer, S. H., Chisholm, A. W., and McKusick, V. A.: Cardiac Aspects of Friedreich's Ataxia, Circulation, *25*, 493, 1962.

Friedreich, N.: Ueber Ataxie mit besonderer Berucksichtigung der hereditaren Formen, Virchows Arch. f. path. Anat., *68*, 145, 1876.

Hewer, R. L.: Study of Fatal Cases of Friedreich's Ataxia, Br. Med. J., *3*, 649, 1968.

Hughes, J. T., Brownell, B. and Hewer, R. L.: The Peripheral Sensory Pathways in Friedreich's Ataxia, Brain, *91*, 803, 1968.

Skre, H., and Loken, A. C.: Myoclonus Epilepsy and Subacute Presenile Dementia in Heredo-Ataxia, Acta Neurol. Scand., *46*, 18, 1970.

Thilenius, O. G. and Grossman, B. J.: Friedreich's Ataxia with Heart Disease in Children, Pediatr., *27*, 246, 1961.

Urich, H., Norman, R. M. and Lloyd, O. C.: Suprasegmental Lesions in Friedreich's Ataxia, Confinia Neurologica, Separatum, *17*, 360, 1957.

Hereditary Ataxia With Muscular Atrophy
(Levy-Roussy Syndrome)

In 1926, Levy and Roussy described a syndrome characterized by impairment of the equilibrium in walking and standing, loss of knee and ankle jerks, wasting of the muscles of the legs and kyphoscoliosis. Typical cerebellar signs and nystagmus are not present. The symptoms develop early in childhood. They progress slowly and in a large percentage of cases arrest before the development of severe disabilities. The disorder is regarded as intermediate between Friedreich's ataxia and Charcot-Marie-Tooth disease. The occurrence of typical Friedreich's ataxia, the syndrome of Levy-Roussy and Charcot-Marie-Tooth disease in different members of the same family has been reported. It is transmitted in a autosomal dominant pattern.

REFERENCES

Oelschlager, R., White, H. H. and Schimke, R. N.: Levy-Roussy Syndrome: Report of a Kindred and Discussion of the Nosology, Acta Neurol. Scand., *47*, 80, 1971.

Roussy, G., and Levy, G.: Sept cas d'une maladie familiale particuliere: Troubles de la marche, pieds bots et areflexie tendineuse generalisee, avec accessoirement, legere maladresse des mains, Rev. Neurol., *33*, 427, 1926.

Rombold, C. R. and Riley, H. A.: The Abortive Type of Friedreich's Ataxia, Arch. Neurol. & Psychiat., *16*, 301, 1926.

Hereditary Cerebellar Ataxia

Marie in 1893 applied the term "hereditary cerebellar ataxia" to a group of cases in which the clinical picture differed from that of Friedreich's ataxia in the late onset of symptoms, more definite hereditary character, exaggeration of reflexes and the frequent occurrence of optic atrophy and oculomotor palsies. Scoliosis, pes cavus, muscle atrophy, Rombergism and other signs of spinal cord involvement were said to be lacking although spasticity was sometimes present. A kindred described by Sanger Brown in 1892 was considered an example of the disorder. The term "Marie's hereditary cerebellar ataxia" was subsequently widely employed to designate such cases.

The original nosological concept has been considerably altered in the light of more recent clinical and pathological observations. Some of the cases on which Marie's concept was based were later found on post-mortem study to have a spinocerebellar degeneration and would now be classified as variants of Friedreich's ataxia. The hereditary cases with a pathologically verified cerebellar degeneration appears to represent a heterogenous group of disorders. Greenfield classified them on the basis of the anatomical distribution of degenerative changes into two major groups: Type A numerically larger, presenting the features of olivopontocerebellar atrophy, and Type B, the relatively rare cerebello-olivary degneration described by Holmes. Konigsmark and Weiner have further subdivided the olivopontocerebellar type into five groups. There is considerable clinical and pathological variability among these cases, even within the same kindred. For example, in the large American family with 53 affected persons described by Schut in 1950 and more recently by Landis, Rosenberg, et al. in 1974, one affected individual had a spinocerebellar degeneration resembling Friedreich's ataxia, one exhibited a spastic paraplegia with minimal ataxia, while the remainder presented a cerebellar ataxia, many with signs of pyramidal tract involvement.

Pathology. In the more common olivopontocerebellar type there is atrophy of the middle cerebellar peduncle, the pontine nuclei, medullary olives, cerebellar cortex and white matter. The cranial motor nerves, especially the oculomotor and hypoglossal nerves and the anterior horn cells are sometimes affected. Degeneration is frequently seen in the long tracts of the spinal cord, but it is not of the severity found in Friedreich's ataxia. Rarely, degenerative changes are found in the dentate nuclei. In the cerebello-olivary type the cortex of the superior surface of the cerebellum and the vermis is particularly affected. The inferior olives are also degenerated. In both types there is profound loss of Purkinje cells and a reduction in the number of cells in the molecular and granular layers and degeneration of the fibers in the folia and white matter of the cerebellum. Ultrastructural studies in members of the Schut family have shown striking proliferation of membranous tubules in some Purkinje cells and aberrant axons in the molecular layer. Vermiform tubules resembling paramyxovirus nucleocapsids were also observed.

Incidence. Hereditary cerebellar ataxia is much less common than Friedreich's ataxia. The age of onset is relatively late, usually in the fourth to sixth decades of life but onset as early as the second and as late as the seventh decade has been recorded. In most of the kindreds studied, autosomal dominant transmission has been observed. Occasional sporadic cases may occur.

Symptoms and Signs. The initial symptom is usually an ataxia of gait. Frequent sudden falls are common. Later, incoordination in the upper extremities, tremor of the hands and dysarthria occur. In advanced stages of the disease, weakness of the legs, rigidity, nystagmus and oculomotor palsies may develop. Optic atrophy occurs frequently in some families but seems to be absent in others. The reflexes may be reduced or hyperactive. Ankle clonus and extensor plantar responses are found in some cases. Mental deterioration may occur late in the course of the disease. Parkinsonism occurs in a proportion of cases of the olivopontocerebellar type.

Diagnosis. The development of a chronic progressive ataxia in an adult known to have affected siblings or antecedents suggests the diagnosis of hereditary cerebellar ataxia. However, the absence of clinical signs of spinal cord involvement does not necessarily exclude a spinocerebellar degeneration. The differential diagnosis between the various forms of cerebellar ataxia and from atypical forms of Friedreich's ataxia is difficult to make on clinical grounds alone. Sporadic cases do not differ in any consistent manner. A biochemical method of identifying affected individuals known to be at risk in a preclinical phase has been reported. If validated, it may enlarge the opportunities for genetic counseling.

Course and Treatment. The course of the disease is progressive, but progress may be so slow that incapacitation does not occur for several or many decades. There is no specific therapy. Cases with rigidity or other features of parkinsonism may benefit from symptomatic treatment with levodopa.

REFERENCES

Brown, S.: Hereditary Ataxy, Brain, *15*, 250, 1892.
Greenfield, J.: *The Spinocerebellar Degenerations.* Springfield, Charles C Thomas, 1954.
Hoffman, P. M., et al.: Hereditary Late-onset Cerebellar Degeneration, Neurology, *21*, 771, 1971.
Holmes, G.: A Form of Familial Degeneration of the Cerebellum, Brain, *30*, 466, 1907.
Konigsmark, B. W., and Weiner, L. P.: The Olivopontocerebellar Atrophies: A Review, Medicine, *49*, 277, 1970.
Landis, D. M. D., Rosenberg, R., et al.: Olivopontocerebellar Degeneration: Clinical and Ultrastructural Abnormaliteis, Arch, Neurol., *31*:295, 1974.
Schut, J. W.: Hereditary Ataxia, Arch. Neurol. & Psychiat., *63*, 535, 1950.

Olivopontocerebellar Atrophy

Dejerine and Thomas in 1900 gave the descriptive name olivopontocerebellar atrophy to a form of chronic progressive ataxia beginning in middle age in which atrophy of the cerebellum, pons and inferior olives are conspicuous findings on post-mortem study. Most cases encountered in clinical practice are sporadic and present a distinctive and generally more consistent clinical picture than the hereditary cases included above among the hereditary cerebellar ataxias. However, Konigsmark and Weiner suggest that many of the sporadic cases probably reflect an unrecognized recessive heredity.

Pathology. Marked shrinkage of the ventral half of the pons, disappearance of the olivary eminence on the ventral surface of the medulla and atrophy of the cerebellum is evident on gross inspection of the brain post mortem. Variable loss of Purkinje cells, a reduction in the number of cells in the molecular and granular layer, demyelination of the middle cerebellar peduncle and the cerebellar hemispheres and a severe loss of cells in the pontine nuclei and olives are found on histological examination. The vermis, the dentate and other cerebellar nuclei, the tegmentum of the pons, the corticospinal tracts and the restiform body are usually well preserved. Degenerative changes in the striatum, especially the putamen, and loss of the pigmented cells of the substantia nigra may be found in cases with extrapyramidal features. More widespread degeneration in the central nervous system including involvement of the posterior columns and the spinocerebellar fibers is often present, especially in the autosomal dominant cases.

Symptoms and Signs. The clinical syndrome of olivopontocerebellar atrophy is characterized by the development in adult or late middle life of a progressive cerebellar ataxia of the trunk and extremities, impairment of the equilibrium and gait, slowness of voluntary movements, scanning speech, nystagmoid jerks and oscillatory tremor of head and trunk. Dysarthria, dysphagia, oculomotor and facial palsies may also occur. Extrapyramidal symptoms occur in a number of cases with rigidity of the muscles, immobile facies and parkinsonian tremor of the extremities. The reflexes are usually normal, but loss of the knee and ankle jerks or extensor responses may occur. Mental deterioration is not rare, but is usually mild. Impairment of sphincter function commonly occurs with urinary and sometimes fecal incontinence.

Diagnosis. Olivopontocerebellar atrophy is differentiated from Friedreich's ataxia by the relatively late onset and the absence of signs and symptoms of spinal cord disease. In familial cases, the differentiation from hereditary cerebellar ataxia is more difficult in view of persisting uncertainties regarding the classification of the hereditary ataxias. The family history is of primary importance. Posterior fossa tumor and cerebellar degeneration occurring as a remote effect of carcinoma should be considered in the differential diagnosis. Some cases with rigidity and tremor may initially be mistaken for Parkinson's disease. Pneumoencephalography or computerized axial tomography usually shows enlargement of the prepontine cistern and fourth ventricle.

Course. The course is slowly progressive with the development of incapacity in five to ten years.

Treatment. There is no specific therapy. Patients with symptoms of parkinsonism may benefit from levodopa therapy.

REFERENCES

Critchley, M. and Greenfield, J. G.: Olivo-Ponto-Cerebellar Atrophy, Brain, *71*, 343, 1948.
Déjerine, J., and Thomas, A.: L'atrophie olivo-ponto-cérébelleuse, N. Iconog. de la Salpêtrière, *13*, 330, 1900.
Francois, J., and Descamps, L.: Hérédo-ataxie par dégénérescence spino-ponto-cérébelleuse avec manifestations tapéto-rétiniennes et cochléo-vestibulaires, Monatsschr. Psychiat. u. Neurol., *121*, 23, 1951.
Geary, J. R., Earle, K. M., and Rose, A. S.: Olivopontocerebellar Atrophy, Neurology, *6*, 218, 1956.
Klawans, H. L. and Zeitlin, E.: L-Dopa in Parkinsonism Associated with Cerebellar Dysfunction (Probable Olivoponto Cerebellar Degeneration), J. Neurol. Neurosurg. and Psychiat., *34*, 14, 1971.

Parenchymatous Cerebellar Degeneration

Intracerebellar atrophy (parenchymatous cerebellar degeneration, lamellar atrophy of Purkinje cells, parenchymatous cortical cerebellar atrophy) is a disease of the cerebellum characterized by the development in middle life of cerebellar symptoms which are limited to or most severe in the lower extremities.

Pathology. On gross inspection there is obvious atrophy of the cerebellum (Fig. 133). Microscopically, there is complete disappear-

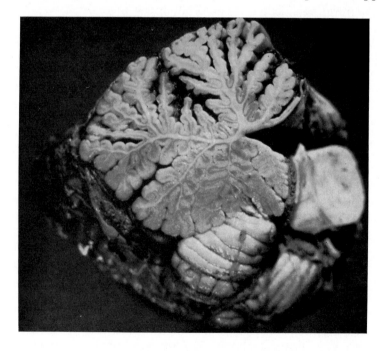

Figure 133. Parenchymatous cerebellar degeneration. Atrophy of cerebellar foliae associated with chronic alcoholism. (Courtesy Dr. Morris Victor.)

ance of the Purkinje cells in the atrophic areas, with preservation of the basket cells and the climbing fibers. The granular and molecular layers are thinned and the white matter of the folia is slightly reduced. The dentate and other nuclei are preserved and there are no changes in the olives, pons or the cerebellar peduncles.

Incidence. Judging from the number of cases in the literature with necropsy examination, the disease is rare, but clinical experiences indicate that it is the most common form of cerebellar ataxia.

Hereditary or familial incidence is denied by most authors. In our experience chronic alcoholism and cancer of the lung or other organs have been the two most common factors of etiological importance.

The onset of symptoms is usually in the fifth to seventh decades of life, but occasionally they may develop in the fourth decade. Males are much more commonly affected than females.

Symptoms and Signs. The initial symptom is difficulty in walking. The gait is wide-based, ataxic and occasionally somewhat spastic. There is intention tremor and ataxia on movements of the legs. With advance of the disease, the ataxia in the lower extremities increases in severity and may spread to involve the upper extremity. Dysarthria may develop. Nystagmus is usually absent but the occurrence of a bizarre movement of the eyes (opsoclonus) has been reported. The reflexes are usually normal but hyperactive reflexes and an extensor plantar response occur in a few cases.

Course and Treatment. The course is slowly progressive and extends over several decades. Occasionally the course may be quite rapid, with death occurring within a few years of the onset. Arrest of the progress is usual in the patients in whom the disease is related to chronic alcoholism, if alcohol is withdrawn. There is no specific therapy.

REFERENCES

Brain, W. R., and Wilkinson, M.: Subacute Cerebellar Degeneration Associated with Neoplasms, Brain, *88*, 465, 1965.
Ellenberger, C., Jr., Campa, J. F., and Netsky, M. C.: Opsoclonus and Parenchymatous Degeneration of Cerebellum, Neurology, *18*, 1041, 1968.
Hagen, P. B., Noad, K. B., and Latham, O.: Syndrome of Lamellar Cerebellar Degeneration Associated with Retinitis Pigmentosa, Heterotopias and Mental Deficiency, Med. J. Australia, *1*, 217, 1951.
McDonald, W. I.: Cortical Cerebellar Degeneration with Ovarian Carcinoma, Neurology, *11*, 328, 1961.
Parker, H. L., and Kernohan, J. W.: Parenchymatous Cortical Cerebellar Atrophy (Chronic Atrophy of Purkinje's Cells), Brain, *55*, 191, 1933.
Romano, J., Michael, M., Jr., and Merritt, H. H.: Alcoholic Cerebellar Degeneration, Arch. Neurol. & Psychiat., *44*, 1230, 1940.
Rossi, I.: Atrophie primitive parenchymateuse du cervelet à localisation corticale, N. Iconog. de al Salpêtrière, *20*, 66, 1907.
Skillicorn, S. A.: Presenile Cerebellar Ataxia in Chronic Alcoholics, Neurology, *5*, 527, 1955.

Victor, M., Adams, R. D., and Mancall, E. L.: A Restricted Form of Cerebellar Cortical Degeneration Occurring in Alcoholic Patients, Arch. Neurol., 1, 579, 1959.

Other Forms of Cerebellar Ataxia

Acute Cerebellar Ataxia in Children. Acute cerebellar ataxia is occasionally seen in young children without any obvious etiology. The neurological symptoms usually have a sudden onset and are preceded in over half of the cases by a nonspecific, undiagnosed illness of the respiratory or gastrointestinal tract. The majority of the children are under the age of five years. Males and females are equally often affected. The usual symptoms are ataxia of the trunk and extremities, disorders of eye movements, tremors of head and trunk, hypotonia and irritability. The disease is usually benign with complete recovery within six months. The etiology is obscure. Multiple sclerosis or other demyelinating disease seems unlikely because of the age of the patients and the lack of recurrences. Infection with poliomyelitis or ECHO viruses has been suggested as the cause.

REFERENCES

Seikert, R. G., et al.: Symposium on Ataxia in Childhood, Proc. Staff Meet. Mayo Clinic, 34, 659, 1959.
Weiss, S. and Carter, S.: Course and Prognosis of Acute Cerebellar Ataxia in Children, Neurology, 9, 711, 1959.

Ataxia Telangiectasia. Hereditary hemorrhagic telangiectasia (Rendu-Osler-Weber disease) has been known for many years. The vascular lesions of this disease can be found in any part of the body including the brain. Hemorrhages may occur in the meninges or parenchyma of the nervous system, but cerebellar ataxia is not part of the clinical picture of the disease.

In recent years a number of cases have been described in which the telangiectases are most prominent in the bulbar conjunctivae (Fig. 134), and they are associated with cerebellar degeneration and sinopulmonary infections. It has been suggested that the syndrome is a fifth form of phakomatosis. The disease was first reported by Madame Louis-Bar in 1941 and since then there have been more than 100 cases reported in the literature. The pathological changes in the neuron system include degeneration of the Purkinje and basket cells and the neurons in the dentate nucleus and inferior olives, granular cells of the cerebellum, demyelination of the posterior columns of the spinal cord, degenerative changes in the ventral horn cells and spinal ganglia.

Other pathological findings include respiratory tract infections, hypoplasia or absence of the thymus, reticuloendothelial malignancies,

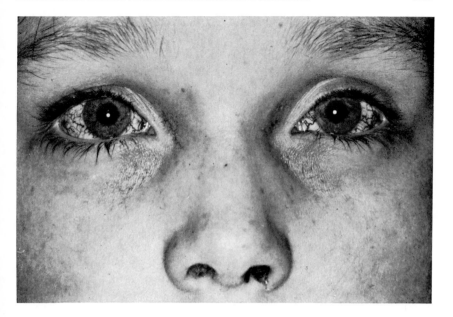

Figure 134. Ataxia telangiectasia. Telangiectases in the bulbar conjunctiva. (Courtesy Dr. G. Gaull.)

hypoplasia of lymphoid tissue and telangiectases in the conjunctivae, skin and nervous system.

There is considerable variation in the clinical symptomatology. Ataxia of gait with onset in infancy is the most common symptom. Other symptoms include nystagmus, dysarthric speech, loss of reflexes, retardation of development and changes in the skin and hair. There is a deficiency of 1A and E globulin in the serum.

The course of the disease is relentlessly progressive with death in childhood, but survival to age of twenty-five years has been reported. Death is usually due to pulmonary infections or malignant tumors of lymphatic or reticuloendothelial origin.

REFERENCES

Aguilar, M. J., et al.: Pathological Observations in Ataxia-Telangiectasia, J. Neuropath. and Exp. Neurol., 27, 659, 1968.

Ammann, M. D., et al.: Immunoglobulin E Deficiency in Ataxia-Telangiectasia, N. Engl. J. Med., 281, 469, 1969.

Harley, R. D., et al.: Ataxia Telangiectasia. Report of Seven Cases, Arch. Ophth., 77, 582, 1967.

Louis-Bar, Madame: Sur un Syndrome Progressif Comprenant des Télangiectasies Capillarres Cutanées et Conjunctivalis Symetriques, a disposition Naevoide et des Troubles cérébelleux, Confinia Neurol., 4, 32, 1941.

Mc Farlin, D. E., Strober, W., and Waldmann, T. A.: Ataxia Telangiectasia, Medicine, 51, 281, 1972.

Bassen-Kornzweig Syndrome. In 1950, Bassen and Kornzweig described a syndrome characterized by thorny appearance of the erythrocytes (acanthosis), steatorrhea, retinitis pigmentosa and a neurological picture resembling Friedreich's ataxia. Since that time less than a dozen cases have been reported. The clinical features of the disease in addition to the abnormality of the erythrocytes include: retinitis pigmentosa, ophthalmoplegia, muscular weakness, cerebellar ataxia, cutaneous sensory loss, disease of the cardiac muscles, and impairment of the absorption of fat from the gastrointestinal tract. There is decrease in the lipid content of the serum, and a complete loss of beta lipoproteins on electrophoretic testing of the serum.

The disease is of special interest because it is the first of the hereditary ataxias in which there is a clue to the metabolic disorder.

REFERENCES

Bassen, F. A., and Kornzweig, A. L.: Malformation of Erythrocytes in a Case of Atypical Retinitis Pigmentosa, Blood, 5, 381, 1950.
Kornzweig, A. L.: Bassen-Kornzweig Syndrome. Present Status, J. Med. Gen., 7, 271, 1970.
Meir, M., et al.: Acanthocytosis, Pigmentary Degeneration of the Retina and Ataxic Neuropathy, a Genetically Determined Syndrome and Associated Metabolic Disorder, Blood, 16, 1586, 1960.
Schwartz, J. F., et al.: Bassen-Kornzweig Syndrome, Trans. Amer. Neurol. Asso., p. 49, 1961.

Marinesco-Sjögren Syndrome. A syndrome characterized by cerebellar ataxia, bilateral cataracts and physical and mental retardation was reported in 1931 by Marinesco, Draganesco and Vasilu. Fourteen cases were reported in 1950 by Sjögren, and since then about 50 cases have appeared in the literature.

The symptoms of cerebellar involvement and the cataracts are evident early in life. Retardation of physical growth of a mild degree is present in most of the patients. The degree of mental retardation is variable, but most of the patients are imbeciles.

The disease does not affect the length of life. The cataracts can be removed by surgery, but the patients may be greatly handicapped by their mental retardation.

REFERENCES

Andersen, B.: Marinesco-Sjögren Syndrome, Spinocerebellar Ataxia, Congenital Cataract, Somatic and Mental Retardation, Develop. Med. Child. Neurol., 7, 249, 1965.
Todorov, A.: Le Syndrome de Marinesco-Sjögren. Première Étude Anatomoclinique, J. Génet. Hum., 14, 197, 1965.

Dyssynergia Cerebellaris Myoclonica (Ramsay Hunt Syndrome). The combination of myoclonus with chronic progressive ataxia first described by Ramsay Hunt and termed dyssynergia cerebellaris myoclonica is a distinctive if rare clinical entity. Atrophy of the dentate nucleus with demyelination of the superior cerebellar peduncles, degeneration of the posterior columns of the spinal cord and to a lesser extent of the spinocerebellar tracts comprise the major pathological alterations. Hunt ascribed the myoclonus to the dentate atrophy, but this may be questioned since dentate lesions are often present in cerebellar degeneration without myoclonus and conversely cases have been described in which the dentate was spared. The clinical manifestations of dyssynergia cerebellaris myoclonica have been described in cases with different pathology, for example, Pallis' case of diffuse lipofucsinosis. Thus the condition must be regarded as a syndrome rather than a specific entity.

REFERENCES

Bonduelle, M., Escourelle, R., Boygues, P., Lormeau, G. and Gray, E.: Atrophie olivo-ponto-cerebellum familiale avec myoclonica, Rev. Neurol., *132*, 113, 1976.
Critchley, M.: Dyssynergia Cerebellaris Progressive, Trans. Am. Neurol. Assoc., *87*, 81, 1962.
Hunt, J. R.: Dyssynergia Cerebellaris Myoclonica, Brain, *44*, 490, 1921.
Pallis, C. A., Duckett, S. and Pearse, A. G. E.: Diffuse Lipofucsinosis of the Central Nervous System, Neurology, *17*, 381, 1967.

MOTOR NEURON DISEASE

Amyotrophic Lateral Sclerosis

ROGER N. ROSENBERG

Amyotrophic lateral sclerosis is a disease of the motor neurons in the brain and spinal cord with atrophy and weakness of the muscles innervated by them and degeneration of the descending motor tracts in the medulla oblongata and spinal cord (Fig. 135).

The disease was first discovered by Charcot and Joffroy in 1869.

All of the motor cells are involved in the terminal stage of the disease but the cases can be divided into three groups in the early stage according to the site of initial involvement: (1) progressive bulbar palsy when the motor cells in the medulla oblongata are involved, (2) progressive muscular atrophy when the muscles of the trunk and extremities are affected first as result of degeneration of the motor neurons in the spinal cord, (3) amyotrophic lateral sclerosis when atrophy of the bulbar and trunk muscles is accompanied by signs of corticospinal tract involvement.

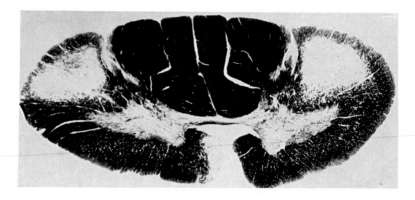

Figure 135.   Amyotrophic lateral sclerosis. Degeneration of lateral and anterior funiculi
of spinal cord. Myelin sheath stain.

Incidence. Amyotrophic lateral sclerosis is a relatively common
disease. The incidence rate recorded by Kurland of 1.4 per 100,000
population has been found in many countries. As many as 10,000
patients may have the disease at any one time in the United States.
Although the disease may occur at any age, it develops mainly in the
fifth, sixth, and seventh decades of life and runs a progressive course
lasting about seven years. The median age of death of patients dying of
amyotrophic lateral sclerosis in the United States is approximately
sixty-two years. The incidence in males is approximately twice that in
females. The familial form of disease has a one-to-one male/female
ratio. There are no well-documented racial differences for ALS with the
exception of foci of the disease on Guam and in Japan.

In the 51 fatal cases reviewed by Vejjajiva, *et al.* in 1969, the clinical
grouping according to presenting symptoms was as follows: 53% of
patients had amyotrophic lateral sclerosis, 27% of patients had progressive muscular atrophy, and 20% of patients had progressive bulbar
palsy. The initial site of involvement was also tabulated and the figures
showed that atrophy begins in the upper extremity in 25% of patients,
in the lower extremity in 25% of patients, in 25% in the head, and about
10% were mixed. The sporadic form of motor neuron disease is
indistinguishable in clinical expression from the hereditary form of
ALS seen in the United States and in the Guamanian and Kii Peninsula
forms, but neuropathological distinguishing features have been reported. Of importance is a recent study by Mulder and Howard in 1976
in which they demonstrated in a prospective study of 100 patients with
this disorder that 20 patients were living at least five years after the
onset of disease. These patients with more benign form of disease did

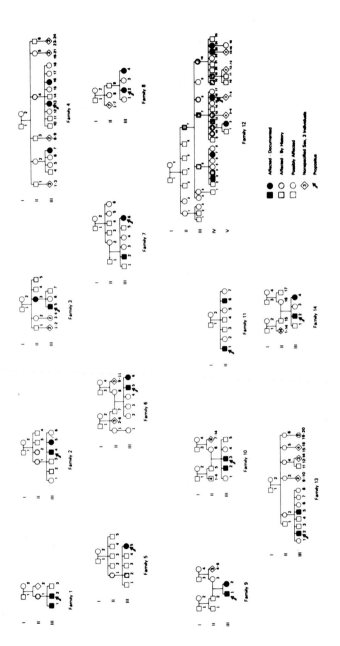

Figure 136. Pedigrees of 14 families in which at least two members have progressive neuron disease.

not have any predictive identifying features and were unique only due to their protracted course.

Etiology. It has been suggested that ALS is the result of a slow viral infection but attempts to isolate a transmissible agent in chimpanzees injected with ALS tissue have not been successful, and attempts to recover virus from neurons fractionated out of ALS spinal cord and fused carrier-helper cells to form heterokaryons have proved negative. Recently Horton, *et al.* in 1976 have identified at least three types of familial motor neuron disease based on clinical, pathologic, and genetic studies of fourteen families (Fig. 136). Most of their families had an inheritance pattern indicative of an autosomal dominant disorder. In a smaller number, an autosomal recessive form of inheritance was suggested. In families with autosomal dominant transmission a spectrum of clinical involvement was recorded from a rapid progressive loss of motor function to a form which was quite benign with some individuals living longer than twenty years (Table 71).

Recently Oldstone and associates have reported finding immune complexes associated with the mesangium of the renal glomerulus and basement membrane in typical patients with motor neuron disease who had a more aggressive form of disease (Fig. 137). This motor neuron disease may be the result in part of an autoimmune disorder and raises speculation as to the primary basis for the break in immunological tolerance in these patients. A slow viral infection such as a mutated polio virus might be pathogenetic. At the present time all that can be said is that the precise mechanism and cause of ALS are not known.

Table 71.   Familial Motor Neuron Disease of Adult Onset

Type 1—short duration
  Clinical: Rapidly progressive loss of motor function with predominantly lower motor neuron manifestations. Pyramidal tract signs may or may not be present.
  Pathology: Limited to anterior horn cells and pyramidal tracts.
  Genetics: Autosomal dominant
              Autosomal recessive?
Type 2—short duration
  Clinical: Identical to type 1
  Pathology: Additional involvement of posterior columns, Clarke's column and spinocerebellar tracts. Surviving anterior horn cells may contain hyaline inclusions.
  Genetics: Autosomal dominant
Type 3—long duration
  Clinical: Slowly progressive loss of motor function with predominantly lower motor neuron manifestations. Pyramidal signs present.
  Pathology: Anterior horn cells, pyramidal tracts, posterior columns, Clarke's column and spinocerebellar tracts. Hyaline inclusions may be found.
  Genetics: Autosomal dominant
              Autosomal recessive?

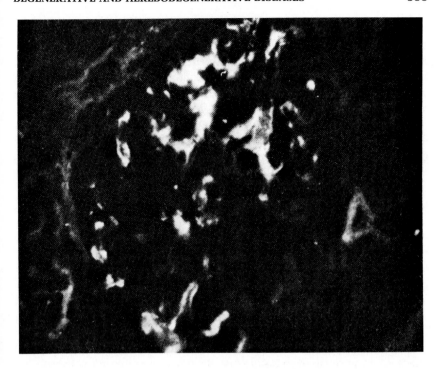

Figure 137. Photomicrograph of a renal glomerulus obtained by biopsy from a patient with ALS. The specimen was stained with a monospecific rabbit antibody to human IgG conjugated to fluorescein isothiocyanate and showed granular deposits of host IgG in the mesangia and along the glomerular basement membrane. Patient died within 2 years of onset of ALS. Reduced to two-thirds from about ×250.

Motor neuron disease has been well studied in recent years on Guam, in the Kepi region of New Guinea, and in the Kii Peninsula of Japan where it occurs with an unusually high incidence. These endemic forms of disease may be the result of environmental factors interacting with multifactorial or polygenetic mechanisms. The incidence of ALS in the Chamorro people on the island of Guam is in the order of 50 to 100 times the rates observed in other nations. The Guamanian form of the disease is clinically indistinguishable from sporadic ALS except patients are younger than those with the sporadic form of ALS and survive somewhat longer. A syndrome consisting of the triad of dementia, parkinsonian rigidity and the findings of ALS has been well documented in these groups.

Pathology. There is degeneration of the motor neurons in the medulla oblongata and in the anterior horns of the spinal cord. Similar degenerative changes with motor neuronal loss are present in the medulla oblongata and in the cortex in Brodman's areas 4 and 6. This results in a secondary atrophy of the musculature innervated by the cranial nuclei and motor anterior horn cells. In the autosomal dominantly inherited form of ALS, in addition to the typical pathological findings of sporadic ALS, there is a degeneration in Clark's column with demyelination of the posterior columns and spinocerebellar tracts of the spinal cord. Bundles of neurofilaments are present in the remaining horn motor neurons of the spinal cord. In the Guamanian form of ALS there are similar widespread neurofibrillary tangles present in remaining cortical motor neurons and in subcortical areas.

Symptoms and Signs. The clinical features of amyotrophic lateral sclerosis are essentially a combination of those which follow destruction of motor cells and those commonly ascribed to degeneration of the corticospinal and corticobulbar pathways. There is, therefore, weakness and atrophy of muscles together with a loss or increase in the deep reflexes, depending upon the degree of muscular wasting and the extent of fiber tract degeneration. Added to these are fibrillations and fasciculations of the muscles.

Muscular weakness is usually the initial symptom. In the majority, weakness is first noted in the extremities, often in the distal portion. Less frequently, the initial symptom is dysphagia. The weakness is usually symmetrical but occasionally only one extremity may be affected at the onset. It usually spreads within a few months to involve the muscles of the other extremities, trunk and those innervated by the brainstem. The mode of extension is quite variable, giving rise to hemiplegic and paraplegic forms. Terminally, there are usually a quadriplegia and bulbar paralysis.

Pains and paresthesias in the extremities occur in approximately one half of the cases. These pains are usually in the nature of an aching sensation in one or more muscle groups. They may precede the onset of obvious weakness and disappear with the advance of paralysis.

Table 72. The Site of Presenting Symptoms in 539 Cases of
Amyotrophic Lateral Sclerosis

| | Site of Initial Involvement (in % of cases) | | | |
| | Medulla | Cervical Cord | Lumbar Cord | Mixed |
Author				
Dana	33	43	18	6
Collins	26	48	13	13
Wechsler et al.	32	38	17	13
Friedman and Freedman	21	31	38	10
Bowman and Meurman	35	44	52	9
Total	147 (27%)	203 (38%)	138 (26%)	51 (9%)

Twitching of the muscle bundles is occasionally a spontaneous complaint of the patient. Muscular fasciculations may be felt or observed by the patient but in many cases they pass unnoticed until attention is called to them by the examining physician.

Urinary frequency, urgency, difficulty in initiating the stream or incontinence occurs in approximately 15 to 20% of the patients. These symptoms usually develop late in the course of the disease.

Mental symptoms are not unusual, occurring in approximately one third of the cases at some stage of the disease. In the majority of cases these so-called mental symptoms are in the nature of uncontrollable outburst of laughing, crying or an admixture of both. If these affective outbursts, which are a characteristic symptom of pseudobulbar palsy, are excluded, mental symptoms are uncommon. In a small percentage of the cases, however, other disturbances in the mental sphere do occur. These include mental deterioration and depressive or other psychotic states. It is felt by some that the mental disturbances are related to the pathology of the disease; others consider them to be an expression of the patient's reaction to the disease.

Muscular Weakness and Atrophy. The weakness of the muscles is usually symmetrical and in the terminal stage of the disease is generalized (Fig. 138). Weakness of the muscles is usually proportional to the degree of atrophy. In the terminal stage there is a severe degree of wasting of all of the affected musculature as well as the overlying fatty and connective tissues.

The muscles of the palate, pharynx and tongue are commonly affected. Weakness of these muscles develops in practically all cases in the terminal stages of the disease and is the initial symptom in approximately 25%. In the initial stages, speech is thick and monotonous due to weakness of the tongue, palate and lips. Mastication is rarely affected, but deglutition is impaired by the inability of the tongue to

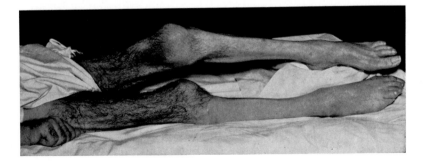

Figure 138. Amyotrophic lateral sclerosis. Atrophy of muscles of thighs and legs with footdrop.

control the movement of food and by weakness of the pharyngeal muscles. In the terminal stages, there may be complete aphasia and tube feeding may be necessary. The tongue is atrophic and the constant fasciculations of the muscles give it the appearance of a bag of worms. Movements of the tongue are weakly performed and the patient may be totally unable to protrude it from the mouth. The muscles of the lower half of the face are weak, giving an expressionless facies, but the muscles of the upper are spared. The extraocular muscles are rarely, if ever, affected.

Fibrillations and Fasciculations. Spontaneous contractions of individual muscle fibers or small muscle bundles are a constant feature of the disease. They are rarely of sufficient magnitude to produce any movements of the joints, except of the fingers. In some cases fibrillations or fasciculations are not a conspicuous feature and careful observations may be necessary to detect them. In other cases, twitchings in the muscles are so numerous that the rapid changes in the contour of the skin are comparable to the movements of the keyboard of a player-piano. The patient should be examined in a warm well-lighted room and the portion of the body under examination should be at rest.

The signification and pathogenesis of fibrillary twitchings and muscular fasciculations are not known. It was thought that they were due to abnormal discharges from ventral horn cells undergoing degenerative changes. This theory is not supported by the electromyographic studies which show that fibrillations continue after blocking the efferent nerves to the muscle.

Sensation. Although impairment of various forms of sensation has been reported in isolated cases, the nature of this sensory loss (often a glove or stocking hypesthesia) has been such that it was of doubtful significance. A slight or moderate diminution of vibratory sensibility is to be expected in patients in the older age groups but the finding of cutaneous anesthesia should cast doubt upon the diagnosis of amyotrophic lateral sclerosis.

Reflexes. There is an increase in the myotatic irritability of the affected muscles which persists until atrophy is complete. The jaw jerk is increased when the corticobulbar tracts are affected. The reflexes in the arms are increased in the early stages of the disease, but they may disappear with progress of the atrophy. The reflexes in the lower extremity are usually hyperactive but they may be decreased or absent when the muscles are atrophied. Ankle clonus is present in a small percentage of the cases. The plantar responses are extensor in type in about three fourths of the cases. The plantar response is absent when there is paralysis of the toe movements. The abdominal skin reflexes are usually absent but they may be preserved even when there is an extensor toe response. The palmomental reflex is present when there is involvement of the medullary tracts.

Laboratory Data. There are no significant findings other than evidence of muscle denervation. Nerve conduction velocity is usually normal but needle electromyography demonstrates muscle denervation, that is, fibrillations and reduced numbers of motor unit potential under voluntary control. It is of value in the early stages, when fasciculations can also be more easily shown by this technique. Giant motor unit potentials on voluntary movement are a feature of anterior horn cell disease.

A slight increase in protein content in the cerebrospinal fluid, with values between 45 and 95 mg per 100 ml, is found in one third of the cases. There is a decrease in the urinary output of creatinine and a slight increase in the output of creatine.

Diagnosis and Differential Diagnosis. The diagnosis of amyotrophic lateral sclerosis is made without difficulty when there is evidence of progressive widespread damage to the ventral horn cells (muscular weakness, atrophy and fasciculations) and injury to the lateral tracts in the spinal cord (hyperactive reflexes and Babinski sign). The diagnosis may be difficult in the early stages of the disease when only one portion of the spinal cord or medulla is affected or when there is no clinical evidence of lateral tract disease.

Among the conditions which may simulate the syndrome of amyotrophic lateral sclerosis are polyneuritis, multiple sclerosis, spinal cord tumor, syringomyelia, osteoarthritis of the spine, cervical ribs and other anomalies in the development of the cervical spine or base of the skull, myasthenia gravis, hyperthyroidism, progressive muscular dystrophy and the Charcot-Marie-Tooth type of muscular atrophy. Differential diagnosis between amyotrophic lateral sclerosis and the conditions listed can be made by a careful study of the patient and the use of the appropriate laboratory examinations. Compression of the spinal cord by neoplasm, ruptured intervertebral disc or bony spicules or intrinsic neoplasm of the cord is excluded by the lack of sensory changes and the normal cerebrospinal fluid dynamics; syringomyelia by the lack of sensory loss or trophic changes; anomalies of the cervical spine and base of the skull by the normal roentgenograms; myasthenia gravis by the failure of the symptoms to improve on test dose of neostigmine; hyperthyroidism by the normal results on testing the functions of the thyroid; progressive muscular dystrophy by the late age of onset and rapid progress of the symptoms; Charcot-Marie-Tooth muscular atrophy by the normal foot, and preservation of cutaneous sensation. The diagnosis of amyotrophic lateral sclerosis should not be accepted when the muscular weakness is limited to one level and does not extend in the course of one or two years. Whenever the diagnosis is questionable, roentgenograms of the spine should be taken at the appropriate level and myelography performed.

Course and Treatment. The course of amyotrophic lateral sclerosis is

Table 73.   The Duration of Life in 77 Cases of Amyotrophic Lateral Sclerosis According to the Site of Onset of Symptoms

(After Friedman and Freedman, J. Nerv. & Ment. Dis., 1950)

Site of Onset	Duration of Life (in months)		
	Minimum	Maximum	Mean
Bulbar..........................	5	41	19
Cervical cord	6	108	34
Lumbar cord	9	120	45
Mixed	12	45	23
Total series	5	120	34

progressive without remission. The average duration of life is approximately three years from the appearance of symptoms. The extremes of duration are from a few months to ten years (Table 73). A duration of life greater than five years after the onset in distinctly uncommon. As would be expected, cases with evidence of involvement of the medulla at the onset have the most rapid course, with a life expectancy of less than three years. Widespread fasciculations are also evidence of a rapidly progressive course. Death in amyotrophic lateral sclerosis may result from inanition, paralysis of the accessory muscles of respiration or aspiration pneumonia.

There is no treatment which will favorably influence the course of the disease.

REFERENCES

Bobowick, A. R., and Brody, J. A.: Epidemiology of Motor Neuron Diseases, N. Engl. J. Med., 288, 1047, 1973.

Brody, J. A., Hirano, A., and Scott, R. M.: Recent Neuropathological Observations in Amyotrophic Lateral Sclerosis and Parkinson-Dementia of Guam, Neurology, 21, 528, 1971.

Charcot, J. M., and Joffroy, A.: Deux cas d'atrophic musculaire progressive avec lesions de la substance grise et des faisceaux anterolateraux de la moelle epinere, Arch. de Physiol. Norm et Path., Par., 2, 354, 629, 744, 1869.

Elizan, T. S., et al.: Amyotrophic Lateral Sclerosis and Parkinsonism-Dementia Complex of Guam, Arch. Neurol., 14, 356, 1966.

Friedman, A. P., and Freedman, D.: Amyotrophic Lateral Sclerosis, J. Nerv. & Ment. Dis., 111, 1, 1950.

Horton, W. A., Eldridge, R., and Brody, J. A.: Familial Motor Neuron Disease, Neurology, 26, 460, 1976.

Mulder, D. W., and Howard, F. M.: Patient Resistance and Prognosis in Amyotrophic Lateral Sclerosis, Mayo Clinic Proc., 51, 537, 1976.

Oldstone, M. B. A., Perrin, L. H., Wilson, C. B., and Norris, F. H.: Evidence for Immune-Complex Formation in Patients with Amyotrophic Lateral Sclerosis, The Lancet, 2, 169, 1976.

Pedreira, F. A., and Long, R. E.: "Arthrogryposis Multiplex Congenita" in One of Congenital Twins, Am. J. Dis. Child., 121, 64, 1971.

Relkin, R.: Arthrogryposis Multiplex Congenita. Report of Two Cases, Review of Literature, Am. J. Med., 39, 871, 1965.
Vestermark, B.: Arthrogryposis Multiplex Congenita. A Case of Neurogenic Origin, Acta Paediatrica Scand., 55, 117, 1966.

Infantile Progressive Spinal Muscular Atrophy (Werdnig-Hoffmann Syndrome)

This syndrome refers to a generalized neurogenic muscular atrophy beginning in the first year of life and progressing to death within the first two years of life. The onset in the first year with a slower progression and prolonged survival into adolesence or early adulthood is known as the Wohlfart-Kugelberg-Welander syndrome and probably represents a benign form of the Werdnig-Hoffmann syndrome. Epidemiologic studies have suggested an autosomal recessive mode of inheritance. Neuropathological findings include loss of anterior horn cell motor neurons and bundles of focal glial hyperplasia in relation to the anterior spinal roots. There is also a predilection for involvement of type 1 muscle fibers. The cause of disease and effective therapy are not known.

REFERENCE

Brandt, S.: Course and Symptoms of Progressive Infantile Muscular Atrophy, Arch. Neurol. & Psychiat., 63, 218, 1950.

Congenital Arthrogryposis

Congenital arthrogryposis is a syndrome associated with fixation of joints at birth with other malformations. It is a rare syndrome due to a diverse etiology. Drachman and Banker have described a spinal form as a result of anterior horn motor neuron injury and loss presumably developing in fetal life. Fibrillations with normal nerve conduction velocities have been found by electromyography indicating the presence of denervation due to neuronal disease. Other patients have a myopathic form of disease. It is presumed the joint fixations result from lack of proper movement in utero due to either neuronal or primary muscle disease. It probably is not etiologically related to Werdnig-Hoffmann syndrome which may also begin in utero and be associated with fixed joints as the syndrome of spinal arthrogryposis is a non-progressive static syndrome and with familial involvement.

REFERENCES

Drachman, D. B., and Banker, B. Q.: Arthrogryposis Multiplex Congenita. Case Due to Disease of the Anterior Horn Cells, Arch. Neurol., 5, 77, 1961.

Byers, R. K., and Banker, B. Q.: Infantile Muscular Atrophy, Arch. Neurol., 5, 140, 1961.
Greenfield, J. G., and Stern, R. O.: The Anatomical Identity of the Werdnig-Hoffmann and
    Oppenheim Forms of Infantile Muscular Atrophy, Brain, 50, 652, 1927.
Norman, R. M.: Cerebellar Hypoplasia in Werdnig-Hoffmann Disease, Arch. Dis. Child.,
    36, 96, 1961.

Juvenile Progressive Spinal Muscular Atrophy (Wohlfart-Kugelberg-Welander Syndrome)

This syndrome has its onset in childhood or adolesence and develops as a progressive, usually proximal neurogenic muscular atrophy which may be confused with Werdnig-Hoffmann disease or limb girdle muscular dystrophy. Since the original descriptions by Wohlfart in 1942 and by Kugelberg and Welander in 1956, over 200 case reports have been published with approximately 100 cases with infantile onset of disease beginning less than two years of age and about 133 cases with onset in the juvenile years between three and eighteen years of age. A family history is positive in most cases inherited in an autosomal recessive manner, but several families have been reported with an autosomal dominant mode of inheritance. Namba, et al. in 1970 reported a sex ratio of about 1 to 1 with infantile onset of disease and Smith and Patel in 1965 found a male/female sex ratio of about 2 to 1. The disease produces weakness and muscular wasting in the proximal muscles of the extremities usually sparing ocular, facial, and other bulbar musculature. Motor and sensory pathways of the spinal cord are not involved. Fasciculations may be present in weak or atrophied muscles. This syndrome is separated from Werdnig-Hoffmann disease by the later onset and benign course and also from amyotrophic lateral sclerosis similarly because of the slow progression of disease and the absence of any involvement of corticospinal tracts. The limb girdle form of muscular dystrophy can be distinguished from this syndrome by findings on electromyography and muscle biopsy. The Charcot-Marie-Tooth form of neuropathy is distinguished as it produces a predominantly distal muscular atrophy and sensory loss which is not characteristic of Wolfhart-Kugelberg-Welander disease.

REFERENCES

Bobowick, A. R., and Brody, J. A.: Epidemiology of Motor Neuron Diseases, N. Engl. J.
    Med., 288, 1047, 1973.
Furukawa, T., et al.: Neurogenic Muscular Atrophy Simulating Fascioscapulohumeral
    Muscular Dystrophy, J. Neurol. Sci., 9, 389, 1969.
Gardner-Medwin, D., et al.: Benign Spinal Muscular Atrophy Arising in Childhood and
    Adolescence, J. Neurol. Sci., 5, 121, 1967.
Kugelberg, F., and Welander, L.: Heredofamilial Juvenile Muscular Atrophy, J. Neurol.
    Sci., 11, 401, 1970.
Magee, K. R., and DeJong, R. N.: Hereditary Distal Myopathy with Onset in Infancy, Arch.
    Neurol., 13, 387, 1965.

Namba, T., Aberfeld, D. C., and Grob, D.: Chronic Proximal Spinal Muscular Atrophy. A Clinical Entity Simulating Muscular Dystrophy, J. Neurol. Sci., 11, 401, 1970.

Peters, H. A., et al.: The Benign Proximal Progressive Muscular Atrophies, Acta Neurol. Scand., 44, 542, 1968.

Wohlfart, G., Fex, J., and Eliason, S.: Heredofamilial Juvenile Muscular Atrophy. A Clinical Entity Simulating Muscular Dystrophy, Acta Psychiat. Neurol. Scand., 30, 395, 1955.

Zellweger, H., et al.: Heritable Spinal Muscular Atrophies, Helv. Paed. Acta, 24, 92, 1969.

Fazio-Londe's Disease

Progressive bulbar paralysis in childhood is the hallmark of Fazio-Londe's disease as emphasized by Gomez in 1962. It is a rare syndrome beginning in childhood resulting in progressive bulbar palsy with minimum involvement of extremity musculature. It may be inherited in an autosomal recessive manner and results in progressive paralysis of the muscles of mastication, facial muscles, pharyngeal and lingual musculature.

REFERENCE

Gomez, M., Clermont, V., Bernstein, J.: Progressive Bulbar Paralysis in Childhood (Fazio-Londe's Disease), Arch. Neurol., 6, 317, 1962.

Familial Spastic Paraplegia

Familial spastic paraplegia is a familial or hereditary disease, characterized by the development in early life of spasticity and weakness of the lower extremities.

Pathology. There are only a small number of necropsy-studied cases reported in the literature. The pathological findings are usually limited to degeneration of the corticospinal tract in the spinal cord. The degeneration is greatest in the lumbar and thoracic segments and is rarely evident above the level of the medulla. Other changes have been reported which indicate that the syndrome of familial spastic paralysis may be akin to Friedreich's ataxia. These include degeneration of the cells in the column of Clarke, in the posterior funiculi and in the spinocerebellar tracts.

Incidence. The disease is rare. The syndrome occurs sporadically as well as on a hereditary or familial basis. Males are more frequently affected than females. The onset of symptoms may be in the first years of life or it may be delayed until puberty. Onset in late adult life has been reported.

Symptoms and Signs. The first symptoms are weakness and stiffness of the legs. The gait is slow, halting and stiff. With progress of the disease, the gait becomes scissored. The patient walks on his toes and talipes varus or equinovarus develops. The knee and ankle jerks are hyperactive with ankle and patellar clonus, extensor plantar response and flexor withdrawal reflexes. There are no sensory defects and the control of the sphincters is normal. Atrophy of the hand muscles has been reported in a few families.

Diagnosis and Course. The diagnosis is made on the familial appearance of spastic weakness of the lower extremities, and the absence of cerebellar symptoms and sensory defects. In sporadic cases, the differential includes multiple sclerosis, tumor and other diseases of the spinal cord. The slowly progressive nature of the disease serves to exclude multiple sclerosis. The normal sensory examination and the absence of spinal subarachnoid block exclude spinal cord tumor.

The course is quite variable. In some cases, the progress of the spasticity and weakness is so slow that the patient reaches adult life or middle age without incapacity. In other cases, the patients become completely paralyzed in the lower extremities and are chair-ridden before the age of fifteen to twenty years. Late symptoms include weakness of the muscles of the trunk and upper extremities and optic atrophy.

Treatment. There is no specific therapy.

Familial Dysautonomia
(Riley-Day Syndrome)

This syndrome presents in early childhood inherited in an autosomal recessive manner and occurring almost entirely in Jewish children. It was first described by Aring and Engel in 1945 and further elucidated in 1949 by Riley, Day, Greely, and Langford. In 1963 Smith, et al. suggested that the disorder was due to a defect in catechol metabolism because increased concentrations of homovanillic acid were excreted in the urine and there was an associated decrease in the concentration of vanillylmandelic acid. These abnormalities in the urinary excretion of these metabolites suggested a defect in the enzyme dopamine-beta-hydroxylase and in 1971 Weinshilboum and Axelrod reported a marked reduction in serum dopamine-beta-hydroxylase activity in some but not all patients with this syndrome. In 1976 Ziegler, Lake, and Kopin reported on the norepinephrine concentration in serum and dopamine-beta-hydroxylase plasma activity in dysautonomic patients when reclining or after standing as compared to normal control subjects. Dysautonomic patients, after standing, did not have a normal increase in their levels of norepinephrine and dopamine-beta-hydroxylase. Further, they became hypotensive. Their data supported the view that hypotension and hypertension in dysautonomia were related to abnormal rates of norepinephrine release. Recently Siggers, et al. have found that a three-fold increase in serum antigen levels of the biologically-active beta subunit of nerve growth factor (NGF) was found for dysautonomic persons as compared with normal subjects. Further, the beta subunit of NGF from dysautonomic persons was functionally abnormal as measured by binding assays and radioimmunoassays. Thus it is suggested that the beta subunit of NGF is qualitatively as well as quantitatively abnormal in dysautonomia. Such abnormalities might provide the molecular explanation for the neuropathologic changes in the peripheral nervous system, autonomic nervous system, and central nervous system. Degeneration has been reported in the dorsal root ganglia, in the thoracic and sacral sympathetic ganglia, in the coeliac plexus, in the reticular formation of the brainstem, and in the preganglionic sympathetic neurons in the lateral horns of the spinal cord, and in the spinothalamic tract, the spinocerebellar tract, and in the posterior columns of the spinal cord. Many of these neuropathologic changes were also recorded in animals immunosympathectomized by raising antibodies to injected NGF during the neonatal period and thus giving pathogenetic relevance to the altered NGF from patient serum.

Children with this disorder develop symptoms in the first five years of life and usually are in the lower ten percentile for height and weight. Manifestations include emotional irritability, insensitivity to painful stimuli, absence of taste discrimination, attacks of severe vomiting and hyperpyrexia, episodes of hyper- and hypotension, episodes of skin blotching alternating with pallor, impaired lacrimation, seizures, absent deep tendon reflexes and dysphagia. Recurrent upper respiratory tract infections with pneumonia may occur. This syndrome is characterized by the occurrence of periodic attacks as mentioned above with death in infancy or early childhood due to pneumonia, hyperpyrexia, severe dehydration with electrolyte abnormalities due to vomiting, upper gastrointestional bleeding, or recurrent generalized major motor seizures.

The important laboratory findings are those of an increased ratio in the urinary excretion of homovanillic acid to vanillylmandelic acid, low serum dopamine-beta-hydroxylase activity and impaired norepinephrine release. Characteristic findings on physical examination include the absence of fungiform and circumvallate papillae of the tongue, absence of the deep tendon reflexes, and impairment in normal lacrimation. There is no satisfactory treatment. The intravenous administration of edrophonium chloride under carefully controlled conditions may result in a transient return of taste, lacrimation, and improvement in dysphagia indicating the disorder in part is related to an alteration in acetylcholine metabolism.

REFERENCES

Brown, W. J., Beauchemin, J. A., and Linde, L. M.: A Neuropathological Study of Familial Dysautonomia (Riley-Day Syndrome) in Siblings, J. Neurol., Neurosurg, & Psychiat., *27*, 131, 1964.

Dancis, J., and Smith, A. A.: Familial Dysautonomia, N. Engl. J. Med., *274*, 207, 1966.

Engel, G. L., and Aring, C. D.: Hypothalamic Attacks with Thalamic Lesions, Arch. Neurol & Psychiat., *54*, 37, 1945.

Goldstein-Nieviazhski, C., and Wallis, K.: Riley-Day Syndrome. Survey of 27 Cases, Ann. Paediat., *206*, 188, 1966.

McKusick, V. A., et al.: The Riley-Day Syndrome—Observations on Genetics and Survivorship, Israel J. Med. Sci., *3*, 372, 1967.

Riley, C. M., Day, R. L., Greely, D. M., and Langford, N. S.: Central Autonomic Dysfunction with Defective Lacrimation. I. Report of Five Cases, Pediatr., *3*, 468, 1949.

Riley, C. M., and Moore, R. H.: Familial Dysautonomia Differentiated from Related Disorders: Case Reports and Discussion of Current Concepts, Ped., *37*, 435, 1966.

Siggers, D. C., et al.: Increased Nerve-Growth-Factor Beta Chain Cross-Reacting Material in Familial Dysautonomia, N. Engl. J. Med., *295*, 629, 1976.

Smith, A. A., and Dancis, J.: Catecholamine Release in Familial Dysautonomia, N. Engl. J. Med., *277*, 61, 1967.

Smith, A. A., Farbman, A., and Dancis, J.: Tongue in Familial Dysautonomia, Am. J. Dis. Child., *110*, 152, 1965.

Smith, A. A., Taylor, T., and Wortis, S. B.: Abnormal Catechol Amine Metabolism in Familial Dysautonomia, N. Engl. J. Med., *268*, 705, 1963.

Weinshilboum, R., and Axelrod, J.: Reduced Plasma Dopamine-Beta-Hydroxylase Activity in Familial Dysautonomia, N. Engl. J. Med., *285*, 938, 1971.

Yatsu, F., and Zussman, W.: Familial Dysautonomia (Riley-Day Syndrome). Case Report with Post-mortem Findings of a Patient at Age 31, Arch. Neurol., *10*, 459, 1964.

Ziegler, M. G., Lake, C. R., and Kopin, I. J.: Deficient Sympathetic Nervous Response in Familial Dysautonomia, N. Engl. J. Med., *294*, 630, 1976.

Syringomyelia

Syringomyelia or cavitation of the spinal cord as it was first known was described by Esteinne in 1546 in his description "La Dissection Du Corps Humain." The precise term syringomyelia referring to a cavitation of the spinal cord is attributed to Charles P. Ollivier D'Angers in 1827. He attributed the abnormal dilatation of the central canal to a developmental anomaly. Syringomyelia since that time has referred to a chronic and progressive disorder with amyotrophy, pain and temperature loss with relatively preserved touch sensation, paraparesis, skeletal defects including scoliosis and associated neurogenic arthropathies. Syringomyelia is quite rare. It occurs more frequently in the male than the female and the first sign of disease begins in the second or third decade of life but rarely it can begin in childhood or late adulthood.

Clinical Manifestations. The presentation and progression of disease depend primarily on the location of the lesions in the spinal cord. The most common location of the syringomyelic cavity is in the lower cervical region (Fig. 139) of the spinal cord near to the central canal

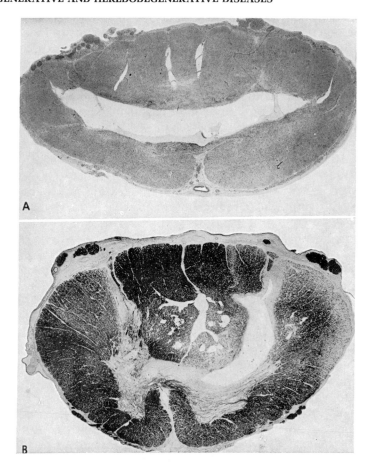

Figure 139. Syringomyelia. Cavitation and gliosis in spinal cord. *(A)* Van Gieson's stain of thoracic cord. *(B)* Myelin sheath stain of cervical cord. (Merritt, H. H., Mettler, F. A., Putnam, T. J., *Fundamentals of Clinical Neurology,* courtesy The Blakiston Co.)

with involvement of anterior horn cells causing amyotrophy beginning in the small muscles of the hands and ascending to the forearms and musculature of the shoulder girdle. Weakness and atrophy develop in the forearms and shoulder girdle muscles with fasciculations and are associated with an early loss of the deep tendon myotatic reflexes in the arms. Scoliosis and kyphosis may occur as a result of atrophy of the dorsomedial and ventrolateral spinal nuclei. The syringomyelic cavity dissects anteriorly and interrupts the decussating spinothalamic fibers mediating pain and temperature and results in loss of these sensations with the relative preservation of light touch. Impairment of pain and temperature with other sensations remaining intact occurs in a shawl distribution across the anterior and posterior upper thorax. Extension of the syringomyelic cavity into the lateral columns of the cord bilaterally results in a paraparesis with spasticity and associated clonus, hyper-reflexia, and extensor plantar responses. Involvement of the posterior column results in loss of position and vibratory sense in the feet and sometimes there is astereognosis in the hands. Impairment of bowel and bladder sphincter functions occur as a late manifestation. The involvement of the secondary order sensory neurons in the spinal cord is associated with deep and severe pain often of a causalgic quality. Horner's syndrome may be seen as a result of damage to the sympathetic neurons in the lateral horn. The presence of dysphagia and pharyngeal weakness and paralysis with weakness and atrophy of the tongue and loss of pain and thermal sensibility in a trigeminal distribution indicates ascent of the syringomyelic process into the medulla producing the syndrome of syringobulbia. Spontaneous fractures and deformities may develop in the knee or shoulder joints (Charcot joints). As re-emphasized recently by Sackellares and Swift in 1976 shoulder enlargement which is painful and associated with complete destruction of the humoral head may develop acutely with cervical syringomyelia early in the course of disease. Angiograms of the shoulder in two adult patients showed hypervascular lesions (Fig. 140). The first clinical manifestation of syringomyelia may be a neuropathic painful shoulder arthropathy.

Pathology. Syringomyelia as defined by Greenfield is a condition with tubular cavitation of the spinal cord extending over many segments. He considered hydromyelia to be a nosologically distinct entity and a cystic expansion of the central canal of the cord. The syringomyelic cavity may be lined by a thick layer of glial tissue and such cavities may be in communication with an enlarged central canal. The syringomyelic cavity is in close relation to the central canal. It may extend almost the entire length of the cord. It varies in transverse diameter but it is usually greatest in the cervical and lumbosacral enlargements. In addition to the cavitation there is proliferation of the glia with gliosis extending into the white matter of the cord. Developmental abnormalities in the cervical spine and base of the skull, namely, platybasia and the Arnold-Chiari malformation with displacement of the cerebellar tonsils into the cervical canal with cord compression are commonly encountered. Associated findings with syringomyelia include ectopic cerebellar tonsils, hydrocephalus, cerebellar hypoplasia, astrocytomas, or ependymomas of the spinal cord.

Gardner has stressed the concept of 'communicating syringomyelia' which refers to a dilated and tense central canal of the spinal cord being in direct communication with the fourth ventricle and developing due

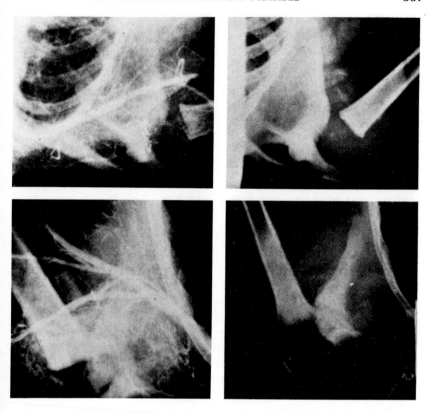

Figure 140. Top left, Case 1, left shoulder shows destruction of humeral head with lesser changes of glenoid fossa, soft-tissue enlargement, and intraarticular calcification. Top right, Case 1, High degree of vascularity present in neuropathic shoulder. Bottom left, Case 2. Right shoulder demonstrates destruction of humeral head, irregularity of glenoid fossa, soft-tissue enlargement, and intraarticular calcification. Bottom right, Case 2. Increased vascularity of shoulder with pooling of contrast in area of proximal humerus and extending into surrounding soft tissue.

to impaired drainage of cerebrospinal fluid from the ventricular system. Impaired drainage from the foramina of Magendie and Luschka resulting in the Dandy-Walker syndrome leads to a communicating syringomyelic cavity which is synonymous in his terms with hydromyelia. The common occurrence of the Arnold-Chiari malformation or ectopic cerebellar tonsils is thus explained on the basis of foraminal herniation of the cerebellar tonsils through the foramen magnum during development. Cavitation in the spinal cord may develop as a sequel of trauma of the spinal cord or be associated with adhesive arachnoiditis.

Lumbar Syringomyelia. The syrinx may develop in the lumbar cord but it is usually occurs in association with a cervical syrinx. A lumbar syrinx results in atrophy in the legs, thigh, and pelvic girdle musculature with a dissociated sensory loss in lumbar and sacral dermatomes. There is a reduction or absence of the deep tendon reflexes in lower extremities and usually the plantar response is flexor. Impairment of bowel and bladder sphincter usually occurs.

Laboratory Data. The cerebrospinal fluid was analyzed by Merritt in 31 cases of syringomyelia with the following findings: 1. The pressure varied between 95 and 285 mm of water pressure; pressure was greater than 200 mm of water pressure in 7 of the 31 patients. A complete subarachnoid block was present in two patients and was confirmed at the time of operation. 2. The cell count varied from 0 to 20 cells, but only one patient had more than 10 cells per cubic millimeter. 3. The protein was greater than 45 mg % in 15 patients and greater than 100 mg % in two patients with subarachnoid block. Dilation of the spinal cord in the cervical region during myelography is of diagnostic value.

Clinical Course. The progression of syringomyelia is usually slow, extending over many years. Rarely it may develop rapidly and usually in those instances where syringobulbia occurs.

Differential Diagnosis. Amyotrophic lateral sclerosis, multiple sclerosis, tumors of the spinal cord, skeletal anomalies of the cervical spine, platybasia, and cervical spondylosis are conditions which must be considered and differentiated from syringomyelia. Myelography is important to determine the presence of a spinal cord tumor and severe spondylosis. Amyotrophic lateral sclerosis can be excluded by the results of the sensory examination. The occurrence of syringomyelia with subarachnoid block can be separated from a spinal cord tumor by myelography.

Cervical ribs may result in progressive weakness and atrophy of shoulder girdle musculature and loss of sensation in dermatomes of a cervical distribution. It should be noted that cervical ribs may be one of the skeletal anomalies associated with true syringomyelia.

Treatment. At the present time there is no specific therapy for syringomyelia. Radiation therapy to reduce glial tissue formation and extension of the syringomyelic cavity is of doubtful benefit. Surgical decompression of a cavity may be helpful in selected patients. Treatment of the associated Arnold-Chiari malformation by widening the foramen magnum has been of significant value. Associated hydrocephalus should be treated with ventricular shunting procedures and the related spinal cord glioma with radiation therapy and surgical decompression.

REFERENCES

Alpers, B. J., and Comroe, B. I.: Syringomyelia with Choked Disc., J. Nerv. & Ment. Dis., *73*, 577, 1931.

Barnett, H. J. M., Foster, J. B., and Hudgson, P.: Syringomyelia, Philadelphia, W. B. Saunders Co., 1973.

Bassoe, P.: The Coincidence of Cervical Ribs and Syringomyelia, Arch. Neurol. & Psychiat., 4, 542, 1920.

Bermann, E. J.: Die Syringomyelic in Kindesalter, Monatschr. f. Kinderh., 37, 1, 1927.

Gardner, W. J.: Hydrodynamic Mechanism of Syringomyelia: Its Relationship to Myelocele, J. Neurol., Neurosurg. & Psychiat., 28, 247, 1965.

Greenfield, J. G.: Syringomyelia and Syringobulbia in Greenfield's Neuropathology, 2nd Ed., (Ed. Blackwood, W., et al.), London, Arnold, 1963.

Hassin, G. B.: Histopathology and Histogenesis of Syringomyelia, Arch. Neurol. & Psychiat., 3, 130, 1920.

Hausman, L.: Macrosoma in a Case of Syringomyelia, Arch. Neurol. & Psychiat., 21, 227, 1929.

Lichtenstein, B. W.: Cervical Syringomyelia and Syringomyelia-like States Associated with Arnold-Chiari Deformity and Platybasia, Arch. Neurol. & Psychiat., 49, 894, 1943.

Love, J. G., and Olafson, R. A.: Syringomyelia: A Look at Surgical Therapy, J. Neurosurg., 24, 714, 1966.

McIlroy, W. J., and Richardson, J. C.: Syringomyelia: A Clinical Review of 75 Cases, Can. Med. Asso. J., 93, 731, 1965.

Netsky, M. G.: Syringomyelia. A Clinicopathologic Study, Arch. Neurol. & Psychiat., 70, 741, 1953.

Poser, C. M.: The Relationship Between Syringomyelia and Neoplasm, Springfield, Charles C Thomas, 1956, 98 pp.

Sackellares, J. C., and Swift, T. R.: Shoulder Enlargement as the Presenting Sign in Syringomyelia, J. A. M. A., 236, 2878, 1976.

Van Epps, C., and Kerr, H. D.: Familial Lumbosacral Syringomyelia, Radiology, 35, 160, 1940.

Wells, C. E. C., Spillane, J. D., and Bligh, A. S.: The Cervical Spinal Canal in Springomyelia, Brain, 82, 23, 1959.

PERIPHERAL NERVES

Peroneal Muscular Atrophy

The Charcot-Marie-Tooth disease or peroneal muscular atrophy is a genetic disorder of the peripheral nervous system primarily involving the peroneal musculature and other distal muscles of both the upper and lower extremities. It is most often inherited as an autosomal dominant disorder and less frequently as an autosomal recessive and sex-linked recessive disease. The specific molecular defect remains unknown.

Pathology. The peripheral nerves in the lower extremities and later in the upper extremities undergo degenerative changes which include demyelination and dissolution of the axon. The occurrence of recurrent demyelination and remyelination with the formation of so-called onion-bulb changes in the peripheral nerve may result in a hypertrophied nerve as a variant and which may be palpated on physical examination. Examination of biopsied skeletal muscle may indicate the occurrence of group atrophy indicative of neurogenic denervation. Pathologic changes have been described in the dorsal root ganglion cells, motor neurons of the spinal cord and the posterior columns of the spinal cord.

Incidence. Peroneal muscular atrophy is a rare disorder most commonly seen as an autosomal dominant inherited genetic disease in large families in which atrophy of the peroneal musculature is the dominant expression. It may also be seen in the spectrum of the spinocerebellar degenerations. It usually begins in the first or second decade of life but delayed onset has been reported. Dyck and Lambert in 1968 and Dyck in more detail in 1975 described an autosomal dominant variant (Type I, dominantly inherited hypertrophic neuropathy) in which slow motor nerve conduction velocities were associated with a hypertrophic form of disease due to recurrent demyelination and remyelination. A second form (Type II, neuronal form of peroneal muscular atrophy) of autosomal dominant disease was not associated with hypertrophy nor with slow conduction velocities but rather with denervation as evidenced by fasciculations and impaired interference patterns on electromyography. A minor variant was a form of peroneal atrophy without sensory involvement.

Clinical Manifestations. The disease beginning in the first decade of life is most characteristic with initial atrophy and weakness of the peroneal musculature of the legs resulting in a steppage gait and obvious footdrop. Skeletal deformities including scoliosis and clubfeet (Fig. 141) are common. Subsequently intrinsic muscle atrophy of the hands and forearms may develop. The occurrence of cerebellar signs and extensor plantar responses indicate a transitional state with the Roussy-Levy or Friedreich's syndromes. Sensory loss is frequent including all forms of sensations in a distal distribution. The deep tendon reflexes are absent at the ankle and reduced at the knee and in the arms.

Laboratory Data. Motor nerve conduction velocities are slowed in the hypertrophic form of disease and denervation on electromyography is present in the neurogenic, non-hypertrophied type. Group atrophy is present upon examination of biopsied skeletal muscle. The cerebrospinal fluid protein is normal in most patients.

Differential Diagnosis. Peroneal muscular atrophy is considered when there is atrophy of the peroneal muscles with scoliosis and foot deformity with a family history. Spinocerebellar disease must be considered with the subsequent development of corticospinal or cerebellar deficits. Optic atrophy and acoustic nerve degeneration may be encountered with hereditary peroneal muscular atrophy as reported by Rosenberg and Chutorian in 1967.

Course and Treatment. The progress of the disease is slow and extends over many decades. Apparent spontaneous arrest is not uncommon. Death does not occur as result of the disease and complete incapacitation is rare. There is no specific treatment. Appliances for

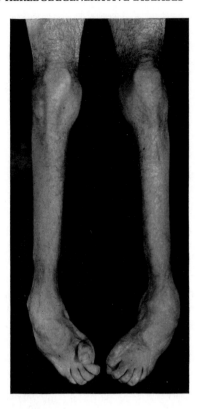

Figure 141. Peroneal muscular atrophy, clubfeet and atrophy of muscles of leg and lower third of the thigh. (Merritt, H. H., Mettler, F. A., and Putnam, T. J.: *Fundamentals of Clinical Neurology*, courtesy The Blakiston Co.)

correction of the footdrop will make it possible for the majority of the patients to remain ambulatory.

REFERENCES

Charcot, J. M., and Marie, P.: Sur une forme particuliere d'atrophie musculaire progressive, souvent familiale debutant per les pieds et les jambes, et atteignant plus tard les mains, Rev. de med., Par., 6, 97, 1886.
Dyck, P. J., and Lambert, E. H.: Lower Motor and Primary Sensory Neuron Disease with Peroneal Muscular Atrophy, I. Neurologic, Genetic, and Electrophysiological Findings in Hereditary Poly-Neuropathies, Arch. Neurol., 18, 603, 1968.
————: II. Neurologic, Genetic and Electrophysiologic Findings in Various Neuronal Degeneration, Arch. Neurol., 18, 619, 1968.
Dyck, P. J.: Inherited Neuronal Degeneration and Atrophy Affecting Peripheral Motor, Sensory, and Autonomic Neurons, Chapt. 41, p. 825, in *Peripheral Neuropathy*, Vol. II., (Ed. by Dyck, P. J., et al.) W. B. Saunders Co., Philadelphia, 1975.
Haase, G. R., and Shy, M.: Pathological Changes in Muscle Biopsies from Patients with Peroneal Muscular Atrophy, Brain, 83, 631, 1960.

Myrianthopoulos, N. C., Lane, M. H., Silberberg, D. H., and Vincent, B. L.: Nerve
    Conduction and Other Studies in Families with Charcot-Marie-Tooth Disease, Brain,
    87, 5; 89, 1964.
Rosenberg, R. N., and Chutorian, A.: Familial Optico-Acoustic Nerve Degeneration and
    Polyneuropathy, Neurol., *17*, 827, 1967.
Schwartz, A. R.: Charcot-Marie-Tooth Disease. A 45-Year Follow-Up, Arch. Neurol., *9*,
    623, 1963.
Tooth, H. H.: *The Peroneal Type of Progressive Muscular Atrophy*, London, H. K. Lewis,
    1886. 43 pp.

Hypertrophic Interstitial Neuropathy
(Dejerine-Sottas Disease)

Dejerine-Sottas disease or hypertrophic interstitial neuropathy is a
recessively inherited disorder producing degeneration of the
peripheral nerves associated with an impressive degree of hypertrophy
of the nerves beginning in infancy or early childhood (Fig. 142). It
usually begins in the lower extremities but gradually extends to the
upper extremities with rare involvement of the cranial nerves. There
may be impairment of sensory functions including vibratory and
position as well as pain and touch sensations with spontaneous
paresthesias and pain. The deep tendon reflexes are absent and the
plantar responses remain flexor. Neuropathologic findings include

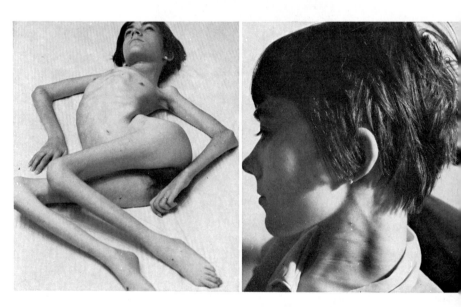

Figure 142. Hypertrophic neuropathy. *(A)* Quadriplegia and severe wasting in
advanced stages. *(B)* Several cervical nerves are visible behind mandible and the greater
auricular nerve can be seen behind the ear.

onion-bulb changes in the peripheral nerve due to redundant numbers of Schwann cells.

Motor nerve conduction velocities are slowed and the cerebrospinal fluid protein may be elevated. This syndrome may be related to peroneal muscular atrophy, but this point can only be precisely determined when the molecular defects are defined in both entities. Dyck has reported a great decrease in the amount of cerebrosides in the presence of a normal amount of sphingomyelin and a moderate increase in sulfatides.

Hypertrophic Neuritis

Course. The disease is usually slowly progressive and is compatible with a relatively normal life span. Some degree of disability is present and complete incapacitation may occur. Occasionally the course of the disease may be punctuated by acute exacerbations and remissions.

Treatment. There is no specific therapy. The usual modes of physical therapy for chronic polyneuritis should be administered. The use of corrective braces will prevent the development of contractures and deformities and prolong the period before the onset of incapacity.

REFERENCES

Austin, J. H.: Observations on the Syndrome of Hypertrophic Neuritis, Medicine, 35, 187, 1956.

Dejerine, J., and Sottas, J.: Sur la nevrite interstitielle, hypertrophique et progressive de Penfance; affection souvent familiale et, a debut infantile caracterisee par une atrophie musculaire des extremities, avec troubles marques de la sensibilite et ataxie des mouvements et relevant d'une nevrite interstitielle hypertrophique a marche ascendante, avec lesions medullaires consecutives, Compt. rend. Soc. de viol., 5, 63, 1893.

Dyck, P. J., and Lambert, E. H.: Lower Motor and Primary Sensory Neuron Disease with Peroneal Muscular Atrophy, Arch. Neurol., 18, 603, and 619, 1968.

Dyck, P. J., et al.: Histological and Lipid Studies of Sural Nerves in Inherited Hypertrophic Neuropathy, Mayo Clin. Proc., 45, 286, 1970.

Dyck, P. J.: Inherited Neuronal Degeneration and Atrophy Affecting Peripheral Motor, Sensory, and Autonomic Neurons, Chapt. 41, p. 825, in *Peripheral Neuropathy,* (Ed. by Dyck, P. J. et al.), Philadelphia, W. B. Saunders Co., 1975.

Gilroy, J., et al.: Chemical, Biochemical and Neurophysiological Studies of Chronic Interstitial Hypertrophic Polyneuropathy, Am. J. Med., 40, 368, 1966.

Symonds, C. P., and Blackwood, W.: Spinal Cord Compression in Hypertrophic Neuritis, Brain, 85, 251, 1962.

Thomas, P. K., and Lascalles, R. G.: Hypertrophic Neuropathy, Quart. J. Med., 36, 323, 1967.

Hereditary Sensory Neuropathy

This disorder is a genetic disease involving the sensory fibers of the peripheral nervous system inherited as an autosomal dominant and producing progressive sensory deficits beginning in the first or second decades of life. There is a progressive loss of pain, thermal sensibility, light touch, and proprioceptive functions with associated absence of the deep tendon reflexes and occasional lightning pains. Characteristic painless ulcerations develop on the feet and the digits of the hands. This disorder seems to be a selective involvement of the sensory neurons in the dorsal root ganglion which undergoes degenerative changes with subsequent neuronal loss. The syndrome must be separated from acute polyneuritis in which there is an exclusive and acute impairment of sensory function devoid of motor impairment. An impairment of pain perception in children must raise the question of the Riley-Day syndrome. With complete absence of cutaneous sensation in children, there may be a complete absence of neurostructures in the skin as reported by Linarelli and Prichard.

The disease is apparently compatible with a long life. The degree of disability is chiefly related to the severity of the trophic changes in the extremities.

REFERENCES

Denny-Brown, D.: Hereditary Sensory Radicular Neuropathy, J. Neurol., Neurosurg. & Psychiat., 14, 237, 1951.
Johnson, R. H., and Spalding, J. M. K.: Progressive Sensory Neuropathy in Children, J. Neurol., Neurosurg., & Psychiat., 27, 125, 1964.
Linarelli, L. G., and Prichard, J. W.: Congenital Sensory Neuropathy, Complete Absence of Superficial Sensations, Am. J. Dis. Child., 119, 513, 1970.
Pallis, C., and Schneeweis, J.: Hereditary Sensory Radicular Neuropathy, Am. J. Med., 32, 110, 1962.
Reimann, H. A., McKechnie, W. G., and Stanisavljevic, S.: Hereditary Sensory Radicular Neuropathy and other Defects in a Large Family, Am. J. Med., 25, 573, 1958.
Schoene, W. C., et al.: Hereditary Sensory Neuropathy, J. Neurol. Sci., 11, 463, 1970.
Turkington, R. W., and Stiefel, J. W.: Sensory Radicular Neuropathy, Arch. Neurol., 12, 19, 1965.

Striatonigral Degeneration
(Joseph's Disease)

Joseph's disease or striatonigral degeneration was described for the first time in 1976 as a form of autosomal dominant striatonigral degeneration occurring in a large family of Portuguese ancestry numbering in excess of 329 persons in eight generations by Rosenberg and Nyhan et al. (Fig. 143). The neuropathologic findings were those of striatonigral degeneration with additional abnormal findings in the dentate nucleus of the cerebellum. The patients described in their report differed clinically from previously described patients with striatonigral degeneration in that the elements of parkinsonian rigidity were minor relative to the marked degree of spasticity. In this variant of

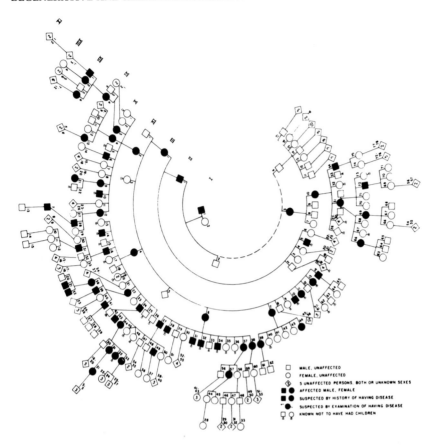

Figure 143. Pedigree of the family showing 329 persons in eight generations with autosomal dominant striatonigral degeneration (Joseph's disease).

striatonigral degeneration, an autosomal dominant mode of inheritance was clearly documented. Subsequently this form of striatonigral degeneration inherited in a dominant manner has been encountered in at least fifteen families most of which are of Portuguese ancestry but which are not known to be directly related. The disease has now been well-described in the inhabitants of the Azores Islands, Portugal, and the United States. The median age of onset of symptoms in affected members was twenty-five years.

Neurologic deficits increased progressively in all affected members and usually resulted in death from pneumonia within fifteen years. An early neurologic symptom is a gait imbalance which is a lurching unsteadiness of gait. Rigidity is present early in the illness and is replaced by progressive spasticity. The lower extremities become progressively stiff and spastic and are held in extension with adductor hypertonicity. Subsequently, speech becomes slow and indistinct. Patients remain ambulatory for ten years after the onset of gait instability. Urinary and bowel incontinence are minimal. Intellectual function remains entirely intact. Upon examination the main findings are weakness of the arms and legs and spasticity especially of the lower extremities. Patellar and ankle clonus were common as were extensor toe responses. The gait was slow with a slight increase in base and lurching from side-to-side due to spasticity. Pharyngeal weakness and spasticity caused difficulty with speech and swallowing. There was a prominence of horizontal and vertical nystagmus with hypermetric and hypometric saccades and impairment of vertical gaze. Facial fasciculations, facial myokymia, and lingual fasciculations without atrophy were common and early manifestations. The cerebrospinal fluid concentration of homovanillic acid was significantly reduced in several affected individuals.

The occurrence of true cerebellar ataxia has been seen in some segments of several affected families establishing a linkage with the spinocerebellar degenerations. Further, significant progressive peripheral neuropathy similar to Machado's disease has also been seen in some family members. Thus a spectrum of involvement with prominent spasticity and pure extrapyramidal signs was seen at one end with some admixture of true cerebellar deficits seen in other segments of the family as an intermediate form and progressive neuropathy seen as a final variant.

There is no specific form of treatment but several patients with prominent spasticity and choking due to pharyngeal involvement have been temporarily improved with Dantrium Sodium. The basic molecular defect remains unknown. The neuropathology is that of a progressive neuronal loss and glial replacement in the striatum and substantia nigra with similar but less intense neuronal loss in the dentate nucleus of the cerebellum.

REFERENCE

Rosenberg, R. N., Nyhan, W. L., Bay, C., and Shore, P.: Autosomal Dominant Striatonigral Degeneration. A Clinical, Pathological and Biochemical Study of New Genetic Disorder, Neurology, 26, 703, 1976.

MUSCLE

H. Houston Merritt, M.D. and Lewis P. Rowland, M.D.

Muscle weakness may result from lesions of the corticospinal tract or the motor unit. Central disorders are accompanied by the distinctive and recognizable signs of upper motor neuron dysfunction. However, lesions of the motor unit, comprising anterior horn cell, peripheral motor nerve, and muscle, are all signified by flaccid weakness, wasting and depression of tendon reflexes and there may be problems identifying disorders that affect one or another of those structures. In recent years, there has been controversy about the classification of individual cases, and debate about some of the criteria used to separate the disorders. Nevertheless, for many reasons, it is still convenient to separate diseases of the motor unit according to the presumed clinical-genetic, electrophysiologic, muscle histology, serum enzymes, and muscle biochemistry, as indicated in Table 74. It is necessary to oversimplify to prepare such a table; the reader must recognize that there are probably exceptions to each of the statements made in the table and individual cases may be impossible to define because of ambiguities or incongruities in clinical or laboratory data. Nevertheless, there is usually consistency between the different sets of data. Moreover, there are syndromes that can be recognized clinically without recourse to any laboratory test, including typical cases of

Table 74. Identification of Disorders of the Motor Unit

	Anterior Horn Cell	Peripheral Nerve	Neuromuscular Junction	Muscle
Clinical				
Symptoms				
Persistent weakness	Yes	Yes	Yes	Yes
Variable weakness	No	No	Yes	No
Painful cramps	Often	Rare	No	Rare
Myoglobinuria	No	No	No	No
Paresthesias	No	Yes	No	No
Bladder disorder	Rare	Occasional	No	No
Signs				
Weakness..............	Yes	Yes	Yes	Yes
Wasting	Yes	Yes	No	Yes
Reflexes lost	Yes	Yes	No (MG)	Yes
Reflexes increased ...... Babinski	Yes (ALS)	No	No	No
Acral sensory loss	No	Yes	No	No
Fasciculation	Common	Rare	No	No
Laboratory				
Serum enzymes ↑	No or mild	No	No	Yes
CSF protein ↑	Yes or mild	Yes	No	No
Motor nerve conduction				
Velocity slow	No, or mild	Often	No	No
↑ or ↓ amplitude ..... (repetitive stimulation)	No	No	Yes	No
EMG "denervation"	Yes	Yes	No	No
"myopathic"	No	No	No	Yes
Biopsy				
Neurogenic features	Yes	Yes	No	No
Myopathic features	No	No	No	Yes

Duchenne dystrophy, Werdnig-Hoffmann disease, peripheral neuropathies, myotonic dystrophy, myotonia congenita, periodic paralysis, dermatomyositis, myasthenia gravis, and the myoglobinurias, to name but a few. Controversies are mostly limited to syndromes of proximal limb weakness without clear signs of motor neuron disease (fasciculation) or peripheral neuropathy (sensory loss, high CSF protein).

Because of the importance given to the laboratory tests, it is appropriate to describe them briefly. In a normal individual, the electromyogram, as recorded with concentric needle electrodes, is silent at rest. With voluntary innervation, motor unit potentials are recorded in numbers roughly proportionate to effort ("interference pattern"); the amplitude and duration of individual potentials have been defined quantitatively. In denervated muscle, fasciculations are seen in resting muscle, the number of motor units under voluntary control is decreased, and both duration and amplitude of individual potentials increase, presumably due to collateral sprouting of nerve fibers, so that the motor unit includes a greater than normal number of muscle fibers. In a typically myopathic disorder, there is no electrical activity at rest, the interference pattern is maintained, and individual potentials are smaller than normal, of reduced amplitude and duration.

In the muscle biopsy, evidence of degeneration and regeneration affects fibers in a random pattern in a myopathy. Some fibers are unusually large and there may be evidence of fiber-splitting. In chronic diseases, there is usually little inflammatory cellular response, or none at all, but in dermatomyositis and polymyositis, infiltration by white blood cells may be prominent. In the dystrophies, there may be infiltration by fat and connective tissue, especially as the disease advances. In denervated muscle, the major fiber change is simple atrophy, and groups of small fibers are typically seen adjacent to groups of fibers of normal size. In histochemical stains, fibers of different types are normally intermixed in a random, checkerboard, pattern but in denervated muscle, fibers of the same staining type are grouped, presumably because of re-innervation of adjacent fibers by one motor neuron. In denervated muscle, angular fibers may be the earliest sign. In other conditions, histochemical stains may give evidence of storage products, such as glycogen or fat, or may signify structurally specific abnormalities, such as nemaline rods, central cores, or other unusual structures.

Serum enzyme determination is another important diagnostic aid. Creatine phosphokinase (CPK) is the most popular enzyme for diagnosis, for it is present in high concentration in muscle, and is not significantly present in liver, lung or erythrocytes. To this extent, it is "specific" and high serum content of CPK is usually indicative of disease of the heart or skeletal muscle. The highest values are seen in Duchenne dystrophy, dermatomyositis, polymyositis, and during attacks of myoglobinuria. In these conditions, other sarcoplasmic enzymes are also found in the serum, including SGOT, SGPT, and lactate dehydrogenase. However, CPK may be increased in neurogenic diseases, too, especially Werdnig-Hoffmann disease, Kugelberg-Welander syndrome, and amyotrophic lateral sclerosis, although not to the same extent as in the myopathies named. For instance, with a CPK test in which the normal maximum is 50 units, values of about 3,000 are common in Duchenne dystrophy or dermatomyositis, may reach 50,000 in myoglobinuria, but in the denervating diseases, CPK values greater than 500 would be unusual. In denervating diseases, the other sarcoplasmic enzymes are not increased in serum. In some individuals, CPK may be increased inexplicably, with no other evidence of any muscle disease. Cardiologists have used isoenzyme analysis of CPK to help differentiate between skeletal muscle and heart as the source of the increased serum activity, but in the differential diagnosis of muscle disease, isoenzyme study has not been helpful, and the appearance of the "cardiac isoenzyme" of CPK does not necessarily implicate the heart when there is limb weakness.

Definitions. Because of the controversies, it is useful to define some terms. *Atrophy* is used in three ways: to denote wasting of muscle in any condition, to denote small muscle fibers under the light microscope, and in the names of some diseases. By historical accident, all the diseases in which the word atrophy has been used in the name proved to be neurogenic (such as peroneal muscular atrophy or spinal muscular atrophy). Therefore, it seems prudent to use the word "wasting" in clinical description of limb muscles, unless it is known that the disorder is neurogenic. *Myopathies* are conditions in which the symptoms are due to dysfunction of muscle and in which there is no clinical evidence of causal emotional disorder or of denervation, on clinical grounds or in laboratory tests. (There is where the controversies arise, because there are arguments about the laboratory tests.) The symptoms of myopathies are almost always due to weakness, but other symptoms include impaired relaxation (myotonia), cramps or contracture (in McArdle disease), or myoglobinuria. *Dystrophies* are myopathies with four special characteristics: 1. They are inherited. 2. All symptoms are due to weakness. 3. The weakness is progressive. 4. There are no abnormalities in muscle other than degeneration and regeneration, or the reaction to these changes in muscle fibers (infiltration by fat and connective tissue), and there is no storage of abnormal metabolic products. In some heritable diseases, weakness is not the dominant symptom (as are familial myoglobinurias) or the syndrome is not usually progressive (as in periodic paralysis or static, presumably congenitive myopathies) and other names are assigned.

Progressive Muscular Dystrophies

Etiology. These inherited diseases are separated from each other on the basis of clinical and genetic criteria, but the inherited biochemical abnormality has not been identified in any of them. Therefore, the pathogenesis of these disorders is not known. Three theories have been advanced in recent years: that there is defective control of muscle function because of a fundamental abnormality in the motor neurons, but one that differs from common denervation; that there is defective nutrition of the fibers because of an abnormality in the microcirculation of muscle; or that there is abnormality of the muscle surface membrane. The neuronal and vascular hypotheses have been contested by contradictory evidence and most investigators now favor the membrane hypothesis, but all the evidence is indirect and the presumed biochemical fault it has is still unknown. Nor, if the genetic fault affects the surface membrane, is it known how this might relate to the characteris-

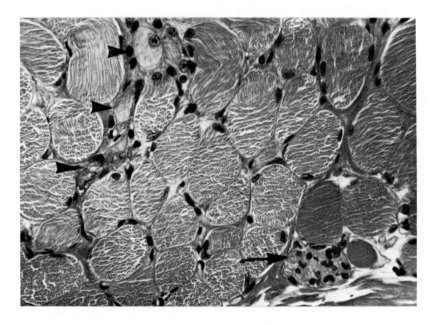

Figure 144. Duchenne's muscular dystrophy. Arrow indicates necrotic muscle fiber undergoing phagocytosis. Several small basophilic, regenerating fibers (arrow heads) form a group. There is also abnormal variation in fiber size and increased dense connective tissue. Magnification, ×400.

tically progressive degeneration of muscle that ultimately leads to its replacement by fat and connective tissue.

Pathology. In the majority of the cases, the significant pathological findings are confined to the muscles. There may be a few degenerative changes in the ventral horn cells or a slight reduction in their number, but as a rule the peripheral and central nervous systems are normal.

In the early stages of the disease, the muscle fibers are rounded and enlarged to more than twice their normal size (Fig. 144). With progress of the disease, there is a longitudinal splitting of some of these large fibers with resulting admixture of fibers of various sizes. This splitting of the fibers is accompanied by hyaline degeneration of the myoplasm, evidence of regeneration, an increase in the number of sarcolemmal nuclei and replacement of the muscle substance by fat and connective tissue.

Classification. Many classifications have been proposed but the one advanced by Walton and Nattrass seems most reasonable. They divide the cases into three groups: Duchenne type; facioscapulohumeral (Landouzy-Déjerine) type; and the limb-girdle type. The major advantage of this classification is one of prognosis, and it also implies a distinct difference between the two most clearly defined types, the Duchenne and facioscapulohumeral. The major drawback is that the category of limb-girdle dystrophy is apt to be a wastebasket and, in addition, transitional and borderline cases are common. The essential features of these three types are shown in Table 75.

Incidence. Progressive muscular dystrophy is a common disease. Herndon reported a prevalence rate of 4 per 100,000 population for North Carolina. This figure is similar to that found for Rochester, Minnesota, by Kurland, and for North Cumberland and Durham Counties in England by Walton and Nattrass. On basis of these figures there are approximately 10,000 cases in the United States at the present time.

The Duchenne type occurs entirely in males and the onset is usually in the first four years of life. The transmission is as a sex-linked recessive trait and the mutation rate is high. The rate of progression is

Table 75. Progressive Muscular Dystrophies

	Duchenne	Facioscapulohumeral	Limb-Girdle
Age at onset	Childhood	Adolescence	Early or late
Sex	Male	Either	Either
Pseudohypertrophy	Common	Rare	Uncommon
Initial distribution	Pelvic girdle	Shoulder girdle	Either
Involvement of face	Rare	Always	Never(?)
Rate of progression	Relatively rapid	Slow (abortive)	Intermediate
Contractures and deformity	Common	Rare	Occasional
Inheritance	Sex-linked recessive	Dominant	Either

relatively rapid, with death in the second or third decade. A milder form of X-linked recessive dystrophy was described by Becker. The clinical features are similar to those of Duchenne dystrophy but the onset is later in childhood or adolescence and the rate of progression is much slower, so that survival into adult years is common.

The facioscapulohumeral type occurs in both sexes. The onset of symptoms may be at any time from early childhood to late adult life. There are many mildly affected abortive cases. Transmission is by an autosomal dominant gene.

The limb-girdle type occurs in either sex and the onset of symptoms is usually in the first three decades of life. There are various modes of inheritance, but it is commonly transmitted as an autosomal recessive trait.

Symptoms. The symptoms are essentially those due to the muscular weakness. In the majority of cases the girdle musculature is more severely affected than that of the distal parts of the extremities. In Duchenne dystrophy the child is clumsy in walking and has difficulty in climbing up and down stairs. Toe walking is a common early symptom. The weakness of the shoulder girdle muscles makes it difficult for the child to raise the arms over the head or lift heavy objects. The weakness of the pelvic girdle muscles gives rise to the characteristic waddling gait and attempts to turn result in much commotion but little progression because the knees cannot be raised properly. The boy may fall frequently and then has trouble rising without assistance.

Signs. There are no cerebral symptoms, but mental retardation seems to be unduly common in the Duchenne type. When the facial muscles are affected in the Landouzy-Déjerine type, the expression is mask-like, the lips are prominent, the eyes are imperfectly closed in sleeping and facial movements are absent in laughing or crying as well as on voluntary efforts in whistling and the like. Involvement of the masticator, palatal and pharyngeal muscles may occur, but is rare. Cardiac failure as the result of involvement of the heart muscles has been reported in a few cases.

In the majority of cases, the dystrophy is limited to the muscles of the trunk and extremities. In Duchenne dystrophy, pseudohypertrophy (Fig. 145) is present in some muscles of the extremities and in others it is entirely absent. More often, there is wasting of some muscle groups and pseudohypertrophy in others. The gastrocnemius, deltoid and triceps are most frequently affected by the pseudohypertrophy. The gait and posture are characteristic. There is an advanced degree of lumbar lordosis (Fig. 146) as a result of weakness of the trunk muscles. There is a steppage, waddling gait. Movements of the arm may be accompanied by winging of the scapula. Weakness of the shoulder girdle muscles

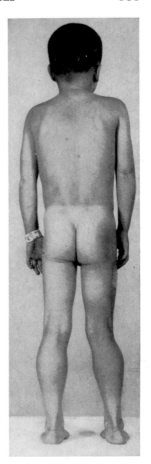

Figure 145. Progressive muscular dystrophy. Pseudohypertrophy of calf muscles.

causes the child to slip through the hands when attempts are made to lift him by placing the hands in the axilla. Another characteristic and diagnostic feature of the disease is the manner in which the patient rises from the supine to the erect position (Gower's sign). The patient first turns over onto the abdomen and raises the trunk to the crawling position. He then places the feet firmly on the floor with the aid of his arms and gradually elevates the upper part of the body by "climbing up his own trunk" with the arms (Fig. 147). With progression of the weakness, the patient is able to rise from the floor only by pulling himself up with his hands on a chair or some other fixed object.

On palpation the hypertrophic muscles feel firm and rubbery. The wasted muscles are often difficult to feel on account of the overlying fat. Pseudohypertrophy may precede the onset of wasting, or it may affect muscles which have never hypertrophied. The involvement of

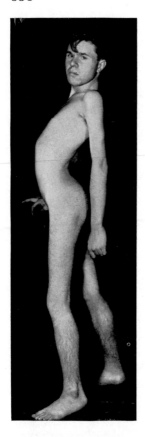

Figure 146. Progressive muscular dystrophy. Lumbar lordosis. (Courtesy Dr. P. I. Yakovlev.)

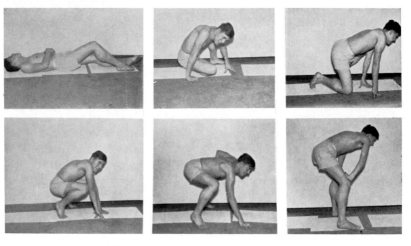

Figure 147. Gowers' sign in patient with Duchenne or Becker variety of muscular dystrophy. Postures assumed in attempting to rise from supine position.

the musculature is usually symmetrical. There are some variations in the degree of weakness on the two sides but involvement limited entirely to one side does not occur. Abnormal movements and fibrillary twitchings of the muscles are not present.

The sensory examination is normal and there are no sphincter disturbances. The deep reflexes may be lost early in the course of the disease or they may persist in wasted muscle. The knee jerks usually disappear before the ankle jerks. Cutaneous reflexes are preserved and the plantar responses are usually flexor.

Laboratory Data. Routine examinations of the blood, urine and cerebrospinal fluid are normal. The excretion of creatinine is decreased in proportion to the amount of loss of muscle substance, in a similar manner to that occurring in other diseases accompanied by muscular wasting. There is an increase in the amount of creatine excreted in the urine, and there is impairment of the ability of the body to store ingested creatine. The significance of the creatinuria is not known. There is no consistent or specific pattern of amino acid excretion.

Increased serum levels of aldolase, lactic dehydrogenase, phosphohexoisomerase, transaminase and creatine phosphokinase have been reported. Serum enzyme levels are most consistently elevated in the early stages of the Duchenne variety of muscular dystrophy. Detection of the disease in the preclinical stage of this form of the dystrophy can be made by determination of the serum enzymes, and detection of the carrier state in unaffected females is manifested by an increase in the serum of creatine phosphokinase. When the serum CPK is definitely increased in a potential carrier of the Duchenne gene, it is likely that the woman is a carrier, but borderline or normal values do not exclude this possibility because even in known carriers (for instance, a woman with both an affected brother and an affected son), CPK is abnormal in only about 80% of the cases. A mild degree of degenerative change in the muscles has also been found in some asymptomatic carriers.

Among the biochemical abnormalities that suggest an abnormality of surface membranes in Duchenne dystrophy are impaired responses of adenyl cyclase to epinephrine and fluoride in muscle, and several abnormalities of erythrocyte membranes, including sodium-potassium ATPase, membrane phosphorylation, osmotic fragility, and some morphological characteristics. Ultrastructural study of muscle has revealed gaps in the plasma membrane of muscle. In contrast to normal surfaces, these gaps seem to be permeable to large molecules such as the protein, horseradish perioxidase, or a dye, procion yellow. Additionally, freeze-fracture studies showed decreased numbers of membrane particles. These abnormalities bear upon theories of pathogenesis, but have not yet had an impact on diagnosis of individual cases.

The electromyogram is of considerable value in diagnosis. The pattern of voluntary effort recorded by means of concentric needle electrodes is characterized by a disintegration of motor unit potentials, many of which become polyphasic and of short duration.

Course. There is considerable variation in the course of these diseases. The prognosis is most favorable when the onset of symptoms occurs after the second decade of life. As a rule, there is a gradual increase in the weakness of the muscles which are first involved and a slwo progress of the wasting to unaffected muscles. The small muscles of the hands and feet are usually last to be affected. Contractures may appear and atrophic changes in the bones have been reported in a few cases. *Formes frustes* with preservation of general good health to old age are not rare in facioscapulohumeral dystrophy, and it is not unusual to find patients who have suffered with the disease for four and five decades but are still able to walk. In the Duchenne form it is common for the disease to progress within a period of five to fifteen years to the stage where the patient is confined to a bed or a wheel-chair. Death may occur from intercurrent infection or from involvement of the respiratory musculature.

Diagnosis. The diagnosis of Duchenne dystrophy can usually be made without difficulty by the onset of muscular weakness in child-hood, the presence of pseudohypertrophy of the muscles, the charac-teristic distribution of the weakness, the family history and the in-creased serum enzyme activity. When the onset is relatively late in life, as in limb-girdle or facioscapulohumeral forms, the diagnosis is made by the distribution of the weakness, the loss of deep reflexes and the absence of evidence of involvement of the spinal cord or peripheral nerves. Determination of the serum enzymes, electromyography and biopsy of the muscles are of value in establishing the diagnosis.

Differential Diagnosis. Progressive muscular dystrophy must be distinguished from the diseases of infancy and childhood which are accompanied by muscular wasting.

Limb-girdle and facioscapulohumeral dystrophy must be distin-guished from diseases of adult life which are accompanied by muscular wasting—myotonic muscular dystrophy, proximal spinal muscular atrophy, peroneal muscular atrophy, amyotrophic lateral sclerosis, atypical forms of polyneuritis, syringomyelia and myositis.

Infantile muscular atrophy is recognized by its onset in infancy, the presence of fibrillations and the rapidly fatal course. Juvenile muscular atrophy (Kugelberg-Welander) may be suspected if fasciculations are seen in a patient who otherwise seems to have limb-girdle or facio-scapulohumeral dystrophy because of proximal limb weakness. In some patients, however, fasciculations are not clinically visible and motor neuron disease is identified only by electromyography and muscle biopsy. This distinction is of some importance because, in general but not always, the prognosis of juvenile neurogenic disease is less serious. Myotonic muscular dystrophy is distinguished from the cases of muscular dystrophy of relatively late onset by the distal weakness, myotonia, and the other characteristic features of the disease, i.e., cataracts, testicular atrophy and early baldness. Peroneal muscular atrophy may be confused with the rare cases of progressive muscular dystrophy with an unusual degree of weakness in the distal portion of the extremities, especially the legs. The presence of cutaneous sensory loss, impairment of the proprioceptive senses and slow motor nerve condition velocity should establish the diagnosis of peroneal muscular atrophy. Amyotrophic lateral sclerosis is distinguished by the extensive degree of atrophy in the distal parts of the extremities, the fibrillary twitchings and hyperactive reflexes. Another feature which is of value in differentiating muscular dystrophy from other diseases of adult life with muscular wasting is the fact that the fat and subcutaneous tissues are usually preserved in muscular dystrophy. In polyneuritis, particularly the Guillain-Barré form, the muscular weakness may occasionally be greatest in the girdle muscles. The acute onset of the symptoms, the increased protein content in the cerebrospinal fluid and the subsequent regression of symptoms should serve to establish the diagnosis. Pseudohypertrophy of the muscles may occasionally be seen in syringomyelia but the other features of the disease should leave no doubt in regard in the diagnosis. The differential diagnosis between polymyositis or dermatomyositis and progressive muscular dystrophy can be made by the lack of family history, much more rapid course, inflammatory response in muscle, and by the characteristic rash of dermatomyositis. Paradoxically, advances in knowledge create new problems in differential diagnosis, for biochemical analysis has shown that some cases formerly classified as limb-girdle dystrophy are due to biochemical disorders, such as lipid storage due to carnitine deficiency or glycogen storage due to acid maltase deficiency, as described below. Genetic analysis has shown that there is an X-linked dystrophy, the Becker type, less severe than the Duchenne type; recognition of Becker cases is facilitated by the recognition of other affected individuals in the same family who are still walking after age twenty, but in sporadic cases, the separation of Becker cases from either Duchenne or limb-girdle cases may be difficult.

Treatment. There is no treatment which has proven to be effective in arresting the course of the disease. Stretching of contractures, bracing and tendon-lengthening operations are advocated with varying degrees of enthusiasm in different centers. When known carriers of the Duchenne gene become pregnant, fetal sex determination permits interruption of pregnancy for boys, but there is no way of identifying affected boys in utero. However, techniques are being developed to sample fetal blood and it is possible that either fetal CPK assay or some other blood test will identify the affected fetus.

REFERENCES

Adams, R. D.: Diseases of Muscle, 3rd Ed. New York, Harper and Row, 1975.
Black, J. T., et al.: Diagnostic Accuracy of Clinical Data, Quantitative Electromyography and Histochemistry in Neuromuscular Disease, J. Neurol. Sci., 21, 59, 1974.
Buchthal, F.: Electrophysiological Signs of Myopathy as related with Muscle Biopsy, Acta Neurol., 32, 1, 1977.
Dubowitz, V., and Brooke, M. H.: Muscle Biopsy: A Modern Approach. Philadelphia, W. B. Saunders Co., 1973.
Duchenne, G.: Note sur l'anatomie pathologique de la paralysie pseudo-hypertrophique dans cinq nouveaux cas, Gaz. d. hôp., Par., 45, 634, 1872.
Emery, A. E. H.: Muscle Histology in Carriers of Duchenne Muscular Dystrophy, J. Med. Genetics, 2, 1, 1965.
————: Genetic Counseling in X-Linked Muscular Dystrophy, J. Neurol. Sci., 8, 579, 1969.
Erb, W. H.: Ueber die "juvenile Form" der progressiven Muskelatrophie and ihre Beziehungen zur sogenannten Pseudohypertrophie der Muskeln, Dtsch. Arch. f. klin. Med., 34, 467, 1884.
Gilroy, J., Cahalan, J. L., Berman, R., and Newman, M.: Cardiac and Pulmonary Complications in Duchenne's Progressive Muscular Dystrophy, Circulation, 27, 484, 1963.
Griggs, R. C., and Moxley, R. T. (Eds): Advances in Neurology. Volume 17. Treatment of Neuromuscular Disease. New York, Raven Press, 1977.
Hanson, P., and Rowland, L. P.: Möbius Syndrome and Facioscapulohumeral Muscular Dystrophy, Arch. Neurol., 24, 31, 1971.
Howells, K. F.: Structural Changes of Erythrocyte Membranes in Muscular Dystrophy, Exp. Res. Med., 168, 213, 1976.
Knight, J. O., and Kakulas, B. A.: The Carrier Problem in Progressive Muscular Dystrophy. Determination of Foetal Sex, Creatine Kinase Studies on Amniotic Fluid, Foetal Blood and Foetal Muscles in Vitro, Proc. Austral. Assoc. Neurol., 7, 85, 1970.
Landouzy, L., and Déjerine, J.: De la myopathie atrophique progressive; myopathie héréditaire, sans neuropathie, débutant d'ordinaire dans l'enfance par la face, Paris, F. Alcan, 1885. 151 pp.
Mabry, C. C., Roeckel, I. E., Munich, R. L., and Robertson, D.: X-Linked Pseudohypertrophic Muscular Dystrophy with a Late Onset and Slow Progression, N. Engl. J. Med., 273, 1062, 1965.
Markand, O. N., North, R. R., D'Agostino, A. N., and Daley, O. D.: Benign Sex-linked Muscular Dystrophy, Neurology, 19, 617, 1969.
McComas, A. J., Sica, R. E. P., Campbell, M. J.: "Sick" Motoneurones. A Unifying Concept of Muscle Disease, Lancet, 1, 321, 1971.
Möbius, P. J.: Progressive Muskelatrophie mit ungewöhnlichem Beginne, Memorabilien, Heilbr., 1, 212, 1881.
Mokri, B., and Engel, A. G.: Duchenne Dystrophy: Electron Microscopic Findings Pointing to a Basic or Early Abnormality in the Plasma Membrane of the Muscle Fiber, Neurology, 25, 1111, 1975.
Moser, H., and Emergy, A. E. H.: The Manifesting Carrier in Duchenne Muscular Dystrophy, Clin. Genet., 5, 271, 1974.
Munsat, T. L., et al.: Serum Enzyme Alterations in Neuromuscular Disorders, J.A.M.A., 226, 1536, 1973.
Panayiotopoulos, C. P., and Scarpalezos, S.: Muscular Dystrophies and Motoneuron Diseases, Neurology, 26, 721, 1976.
Pearce, G. W., Pearce, J. M. S., and Walton, J. N.: The Duchenne Type Muscular Dystrophy: Histopathological Studies of the Carrier State, Brain, 89, 109, 1966.

Penn, A. S., Lisak, R. P., and Rowland, L. P.: Muscular Dystrophy in Young Girls, Neurology, *20*, 147, 1970.

Prosser, E. J., Murphy, E. G., and Thompson, M. W.: Intelligence and the Gene for Duchenne Muscular Dystrophy, Arch. Dis. Child., *44*, 221, 1969.

Roses, A. D., Herbstreith, M., Metcalf, B., and Appel, S. H.: Increased Phosphorylated Components of Erythrocyte Membrane Spectrin Band II with Reference to Duchenne Dystrophy, J. Neurol. Sci., *30*, 167, 1976.

Rowland, L. P. Editor: *Pathogenesis of Human Muscular Dystrophies.* Proceedings of the Fifth International Scientific Conference of the Muscular Dystrophy Association. Amsterdam, Excerpta Medica, 1977.

Roy, L., and Gibson, D. A.: Pseudohypertrophic Muscular Dystrophy and Its Surgical Management: Review of 30 Patients, Canad. J. Surg., *13*, 13, 1970.

Schotland, D. L., Bonilla, E., and Van Meter, M.: Duchenne Dystrophy: Alteration in Muscle Plasma Membrane Structure, Science, *196*, 1005, 1977.

Shaw, R. F., and Dreifuss, E. E.: Mild and Severe Forms of X-linked Muscular Dystrophy, Arch. Neurol., *20*, 451, 1969.

Slucka, C.: The Electrocardiogram in Duchenne Progressive Muscular Dystrophy, Circulation, *38*, 933, 1968.

Thomas, P. K., Schott, G. D., and Morgan-Hughes, J. A.: Adult Onset Scapuloperoneal Myopathy, J. Neurol. Neurosurg. Psychiat., *38*, 1008, 1975.

Walton, J. N.: Carrier Detection in X-linked Muscular Dystrophy, J. Genet. hum., *17*, 497, 1969.

————— (Editor): *Disorders of Voluntary Muscle,* 3rd Ed., Edinburgh, Churchill, Livingstone, 1974.

Walton, J. N., and Nattrass, F. J.: On the Classification, Natural History and Treatment of the Myopathies, Brain, *77*, 169, 1954.

Ocular Muscular Dystrophy. A limited form of muscular dystrophy with restriction of the symptoms to bilateral ptosis and difficulty in swallowing was reported by Taylor in 1915 and in recent years a number of cases have been recorded. The disease is inherited as an autosomal dominant.

The symptoms have their onset in middle or late life and are progressive, but are rarely disabling. Diplopia and difficulty in swallowing are usually the only symptoms, but the face, neck and distal muscles are affected in some cases. Postmortem examination reveals pathological changes in the ocular muscles and no abnormality of oculomotor neurons. The designation "ocular muscular dystrophy" seems appropriate for these cases and the same designation is appropriate for ophthalmoplegic syndromes associated with limb weakness in which electromyographic and histologic study of muscle biopsy provide evidence of myopathy. But there are other cases in which progressive external ophthalmoplegia is associated with peripheral neuropathy, spinocerebellar degeneration, retinopathy or evidence of diffuse cerebral disease. In these cases the ophthalmoplegia may be neurogenic even though the pupil is spared. In one such form, there are distinctive features which warrant specific designation as the Kearns-Sayre syndrome. In this form, never familial and therefore apparently an acquired disease, progressive ophthalmoplegia is accompanied by pigmentary degeneration of the retina before age fifteen. When this combination is recognized, several other abnormalities may be predicted. Almost invariably, there is evidence of heart-block in the ECG, and the CSF protein content is about 100 mg/dl. More than half the patients are affected by short stature, hearing loss, and signs of either cerebellar or corticospinal disorder, or both. In muscle biopsies, there are almost always abnormalities of the mitochondria, and blood lactate may be increased.

REFERENCES

Berenberg, R. A., et al.: Lumping or Splitting? "Ophthalmoplegia Plus" or Kearns-Sayre Syndrome? Ann. Neurol., 1, 37, 1977.
DiMauro, S., et al.: Mitochondrial Myopathies: Which and How Many? In Milhorat A. T., (Ed.). *Exploratory Concepts in Muscular Dystrophy* II., Amsterdam, Excerpta Medica, 1973, pp. 506–515.
Drachman, D. A.: Ophthalmoplegia Plus: The Neurodegenerative Disorders Associated with Progressive External Ophthalmoplegia, Arch. Neurol., 18, 654, 1968.
Karpati, G., et al.: Adult Form of Acid Maltase Deficiency, Ann. Neurol., 1, 276, 1977.
Rowland, L. P.: Progressive External Ophthalmoplegia. I. Vinken, P. J., Bruyn, G. W. (Eds.). *Handbook of Clinical Neurology*, in DeJong, J.M.B.V. (Ed.), *System Disorders and Atrophies*, Part II, New York, American Elsevier Publishing Co., 1975, vol. 22, pp. 177–202.
Victor, M., Hayes, R., and Adams, R. D.: Oculopharyngeal Muscular Dystrophy. A Familial Disease of Late Life Characterized by Dysphagia and Progressive Ptosis of the Eyelids, New Engl. J. Med., 67, 1267, 1962.

Myotonia Congenita

Myotonia congenita, a heredofamilial disease described by Thomsen in 1876, is characterized by the presence of generalized myotonia. Weakness is exceptional and the other stigmata of myotonic dystrophy are lacking: they are not affected by gonadal failure or cataract. According to the classical description the muscles are normal in size or larger than normal. It has been contended that myotonia congenita is merely a monosymptomatic form of myotonic muscular dystrophy and that many of the patients in whom the diagnosis of Thomsen's disease is made in the early years of life later develop the characteristic features of myotonic dystrophy, but in most families the two conditions seem distinct. Myotonia congenita is most frequently inherited in an autosomal dominant pattern, but in some families, recessive transmission seems likely.

Myotonic Muscular Dystrophy

Myotonic muscular dystrophy (myotonia atrophica, dystrophia myotonica) is an inherited disease characterized by myotonia, weakness and wasting of the muscles, especially those of the face and neck, cataracts, early baldness, and testicular atrophy.

Etiology. The disease is inherited as an autosomal dominant trait, but there is no adequate explanation of the pathogenesis of the muscular wasting, cataracts, atrophy of the endocrine glands and other features of the disease. The muscular wasting is similar to that which occurs in progressive muscular dystrophy and is probably related to some, as yet unknown, biochemical defect. The difficulty in relaxation is due to repetitive firing of muscle fibers. The myotonia persists after spinal anesthesia, nerve block or curarization; it is therefore independent of any neural influence but the cause of the repetitive depolarization is not known. Abnormalities of membrane phosphorylation have been reported in both muscle and erythrocytes, again suggesting that the genetic fault affects the muscle surface membrane. In human myotonia congenita and in a genetic myotonia of goats, there is an abnormality of chloride conductance, but the abnormality in myotonic muscular dystrophy seems different and has not been characterized. Myotonia may appear in humans treated with diazacholesterol to block synthesis of cholesterol and this agent has been used to induce experimental myotonia in animals, with results suggesting that altering the lipid composition of muscle surface membranes may be responsible for the tendency to fire repetitively.

Pathology. The changes in the muscles are similar to those which are present in progressive muscular dystrophy and consist of hypertrophy and fragmentation of the muscle fibers, followed by atrophy and replacement by fat and connective tissue. The testes are grossly atrophied and microscopically there is degeneration of the seminiferous tubules with replacement by connective tissue. Changes in the nervous system are absent or of an insignificant nature.

Incidence. Walton and Nattrass estimate that the prevalence rate is about 1 per 100,000 population. On this basis, it is about one fourth as common as Duchenne dystrophy. It is practically always inherited but sporadic cases may occur. Sometimes the disease seems to start at an earlier age and in more severe form in succeeding generations, but this "anticipation" and "potentiation" are regarded by most geneticists as an artifact of observation. Both sexes are affected but the disease is more common in the male. The onset of symptoms is often difficult to determine but it is usually in the second or third decade of life. Myotonia usually precedes the weakness by several or many years. Many patients are unable to date the onset of the myotonia, stating that they have always had difficulty in relaxing the grip, for example. As a rule, myotonia appears in childhood and muscular wasting develops in the late teens or early twenties.

A special form has been recognized when the disease starts in infancy. Although genetic theory would predict that either parent might be affected in an autosomal dominant disease, the affected parent of these infantile cases is almost always the mother. The children have prominent weakness so that difficulty sucking and nursing is common although limb weakness and peripheral myotonia are lacking. Mental retardation is common and may be severe.

Symptoms. The characteristic and diagnostic symptom of the disease is the failure of the muscles to relax promptly after a forceful contraction. The myotonia is most apt to appear when the muscular action is vigorous or when it is made suddenly. Myotonia in the hand muscles, for example, may not be present when the patient fails to make a forceful contraction but it may be most evident when the patient is required to grasp an object firmly. Similarly, myotonia of the leg muscles may appear only when the patient is forced to move his legs suddenly to avoid an obstacle. The distribution of the myotonia is variable. Rarely all of the muscles of the body are affected, but usually it is limited to the muscles of the hands. The patient may become so well adjusted to the difficulty in relaxing the muscles that he or she may not complain of it, and it can be brought out only by direct testing. Myotonia of the leg muscles may cause the patient to fall over curbings or rough places in the ground. With severe myotonic involvement of the trunk muscles the patient may be unable to arise from the ground after falling, and thrash around like a patient in a convulsive seizure.

There is weakness of the muscles which are wasted. When the weakness is confined to the muscles of the neck, it may not be noted by the patient. Vision is lost when cataracts develop.

Signs—Myotonia. The presence of myotonia can be demonstrated by the slow worm-like relaxation of the grip when the patient forcefully grasps the examiner's fingers. It can also be shown by the prolonged contraction and slow relaxation of the thenar muscles when the base of the thumb is struck with a percussion hammer. Myotonia of the tongue muscles is manifested by a sustained localized contraction of the glossal musculature when a tongue depressor is placed under the tongue and the muscle is struck with a percussion hammer. A similar phenomenon can be demonstrated by percussing the muscles of the arm, leg or trunk if they are affected by myotonia. The myotonia may disappear when extensive wasting develops. Most patients with myotonia experience increased stiffness in cold weather, but there is a syndrome in which myotonia, especially of the orbicularis oculi, is characteristically brought out only by cold (paramyotonia). This rare condition, which is inherited in dominant fashion, differs from other myotonic syndromes in that transient attacks of flaccid paralysis may be precipitated by cold. During the paralytic attack the myotonia is abolished.

Weakness and Wasting. Although any of the muscles may be affected in the late stages of the disease, wasting and weakness are commonly confined to the facial and neck muscles in the early stages. Wasting of the facial muscles gives the patient a characteristic long and lean appearance, and an expressionless facies (Fig. 148). Voluntary and emotional movements are weak. The orbicularis oculi are often affected. The sternomastoid and intrinsic muscles of the neck are usually the first muscles to be affected. The patient is unable to lift the head from the bed while in the supine position and rotary movements of the head are weak. The muscles of deglutition are occasionally involved

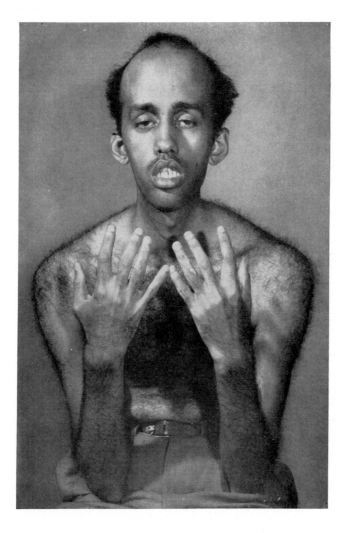

Figure 148.   Myotonic muscular dystrophy. Atrophy of facial, temporal, neck and hand muscles.

and articulation or phonation is frequently impaired. The voice may be weak or nasal in quality. Wasting, with accompanying weakness, may extend to other muscles of the trunk or extremities in late stages of the disease. The muscular wasting is not preceded by hypertrophy and fasciculations do not occur. The heart and the smooth muscles of the gastrointestinal tract are occasionally affected. The sensory examination is normal and deep reflexes are preserved unless the muscles of the extremities are wasted. The cutaneous reflexes are normal.

Other Signs. It is claimed by some that cataracts are present in nearly 100% of the cases. This may be true if the eyes are examined by a slit-lamp, but cataracts which are visible to the naked eye are present in less than one third of the cases in the early stages of the disease. The cataract starts in the posterior portion of the lens and spreads slowly to involve other portions. Senile or pre-senile cataracts are the most common symptom in the parents or grandparents of patients with myotonic dystrophy. Mental retardation is a frequent concomitant of the disease. Many of these patients are found in schools or other institutions for the mentally retarded. Gonadal atrophy appears in the second or third decade. In the male, the testes are small, and there is early impotence. In the female, there is an early menopause and childbearing is rarely possible after the age of thirty. Early baldness commonly occurs in men, but not in women. Endocrine studies afford no basis for allegations of a high frequency of adrenal cortical, thyroidal or pituitary deficiencies.

Laboratory Data. Examinations of the blood, urine and cerebrospinal fluid do not show any significant abnormalities except for a reduction of the gamma globulin content of the serum. There is also a rapid catabolism of 7S gamma globulin. In the myotonic muscles, galvanic stimulation produces a contraction which is sustained as long as the current flows and relaxes slowly after the stimulation is withdrawn (myotonic reaction). The electromyographic concomitant of myotonia is repetitive firing of muscle fibers, induced by movement of the needle, percussion or after voluntary contraction. Reduced duration of individual motor unit potentials is indicative of myopathy as in other dystrophies.

Glycosuria and hyperglycemia are occasionally seen. Disturbance of the creatine and creatinine metabolism, similar to that of progressive muscular dystrophy, occurs when there is a significant degree of muscular wasting. Low basal metabolic rates may occur but remain unexplained. The radioiodine uptake and serum protein-bound iodine are normal. The serum creatine phosphokinase activity may be normal or slightly increased. The ECG is abnormal in most adult cases, with slowed or interrupted atrial-ventricular conduction the most common sign. Sometimes, this is symptomatic, causing syncopal attacks.

Course. Although the disease is progressive, the course is frequently so slow that many patients live to old age without becoming incapacitated. Occasionally they may become bedridden or confined to a bed-chair existence on account of extensive muscular wasting. Limited and oligosymptomatic forms of the disease are not uncommon.

Diagnosis. The diagnosis can be made from the characteristic wasting of the muscles of the neck and face and the myotonia of the extremity musculature. A family history of the disease, alopecia, cataracts and evidences of glandular dysfunction are also present in the majority of the cases. In myotonia congenita, there is ordinarily no weakness, cataracts are lacking and testicular atrophy does not occur. Paramyotonia and hyperkalemic periodic paralysis are distinguished by symptomatic myotonia only on exposure to cold, and by repeated attacks of paralysis. Chondrodystrophic myotonia (or Schwartz-Jampel syndrome) is distinguished by dwarfism, blepharophimosis, kyphoscoliosis and flexion contractures of the limbs (Table 76).

Differential Diagnosis. The unique clinical picture of myotonic dystrophy is not simulated by any other disease of the nervous system. Progressive muscular dystrophy may be considered in the few patients in whom the myotonia is an inconspicuous feature or when it has disappeared. In the latter instance, the history of the previous existence of the myotonia as well as the presence of the other characteristics of the disease should establish the diagnosis.

Treatment. The myotonia can be relieved or alleviated by the oral administration of quinine in the dose of 0.3 to 0.6 gm 3 times a day. Procaine amide (4 to 6 gm daily) is of value in alleviating the myotonia. The drug should be used with caution because a syndrome similar to that of lupus erythematosus has followed its administration. Diphenyl hydantoin (Dilantin) is of value in the control of myotonia. The

Table 76. Conditions Characterized by Myotonia

Inherited Forms
  A. Myotonia congenita
      1. Autosomal dominant form.
      2. Autosomal recessive form.
  B. Myotonic muscular dystrophy.
  C. Hyperkalemic periodic paralysis.
  D. Paramyotonia congenita.
  E. Chondrodystrophic myotonia (Schwartz-Jampel syndrome)
Acquired Forms
  A. Myotonia after diazacholesterol.
  B. Myotonia after 2,4-dichlorophenoxyacetate.
Conditions Resembling Myotonia
  A. Myokymia.
  B. Hypothyroidism.

cataracts can be treated surgically and the endocrine disturbances by
the appropriate substitutive therapy. There is no treatment for the
muscular weakness or wasting.

REFERENCES

Aberfeld, D. C., et al.: Chondrodystrophic Myotonia: Report of Two Cases. Myotonia,
    Dwarfism, Diffuse Bone Disease and Unusual Ocular and Facial Abnormalities,
    Arch. Neurol., 22, 455, 1970.
Barchi, R. L.: Myotonia, An Evaluation of the Chloride Hypothesis, Arch. Neurol., 32,
    175, 1975.
Becker, P. E.: Genetic Approaches to the Nosology of Muscle Disease: Myotonias and
    Similar Diseases, Birth Defects: Orig. Art. Ser., 7, 52, 1971.
Caughey, J. E.: Relationship of Dystrophia Myotonica (Myotonic Dystrophy) and
    Myotonia Congenita (Thomsen's Disease), Neurology, 8, 467, 1958.
Caughey, J. E. and Myrianthopolous, N. C.: Dystrophic Myotonica and Related Disorders,
    Springfield, Charles C Thomas, 1963.
Clark, S. L., Luton, F. H., and Cutler, J. T.: A Form of Congenital Myotonia in Goats, J.
    Nerv. & Ment. Dis., 90, 297, 1939.
Dodge, P. R., Gamstorp, I., Byers, R. K., and Russell, P.: Myotonic Dystrophy in Infancy
    and Childhood, Pediat., 35, 3, 1965.
Drucker, W. D., Rowland, L. P., Sterling, K. and Christy, N. P.: On the Function of the
    Endocrine Glands in Myotonic Muscular Dystrophy, Am. J. Med., 31, 941, 1961.
Dyken, P. R., and Harper, P. S.: Congenital Dystrophia Myotonica, Neurology, 23, 465,
    1973.
Engle, W. K., McFarlin, D. E., Drews, G. A., and Wochner, R. D.: Protein Abnormalities in
    Neuromuscular Diseases—Part I, J.A.M.A., 195, 754, 1966.
Fowler, W. M., Jr., et al.: The Schwartz-Jampel Syndrome. Its Clinical, Physiological and
    Histological Expressions, J. Neurol. Sci., 22, 127, 1974.
Greenhouse, A. H., et al.: Myotonia, Myokymia, Hyperhidrosis and Wasting of Muscle,
    Neurology, 17, 263, 1967.
Griggs, R. C., Davis, R. J., Anderson, D. C., and Dove, J. T.: Cardiac Conduction in
    Myotonic Dystrophy, Am. J. Med., 59, 37, 1975.
Harper, P. S.: Presymptomatic Detection and Genetic Counseling in Myotonic Dystrophy,
    Clin. Genet., 4, 134, 1973.
MacRobbie, D. S., and Friedlander, W. J.: Treatment of Myotonia with Procainamide,
    Arch. Neurol. & Psychiat., 78, 473, 1957.
Munsat, T. L.: Therapy of Myotonia. A Double-blind Evaluation of Diphenylhydantoin,
    Procainamide and Placebo, Neurology, 17, 359, 1967.
Prockop, L. D.: Myotonia, Procaine Amide, and Lupus-Like Syndrome, Arch. Neurol., 14,
    326, 1966.
Pruzanski, W. and Huvos, A. G.: Smooth Muscle Involvement in Primary Muscle
    Diseases: Myotonic Muscular Dystrophy, Arch. Path., 83, 229, 1967.
Roses, A. D., and Appel, S. H.: Phosphorylation of Component A of the Human
    Erythrocyte Membrane in Myotonic Muscular Dystrophy, J. Membrane Biol., 20, 51,
    1975.
Somers, J. E. and Winer, N.: Reversible Myopathy and Myotonia Following the Adminis-
    tration of a Hypercholesterolemic Agent, Neurology, 16, 761, 1966.
Thomsen, J.: Nachträgliche Bemerkungen über Myotonia congenita (Strümpell), Thom-
    sen'sche Krankheit (Westphal), Arch. f. Psychiat., 24, 918, 1892.
Wallis, W. E., Poznak, A. V. and Plum, F.: Generalized Muscular Stiffness, Fasciculation
    and Myokymia of Peripheral Nerve Origin, Arch. Neurol., 22, 429, 1970.
Watters, G. V. and Williams, T. W.: Early Onset Myotonic Dystrophy, Arch. Neurol., 17,
    139, 1967.

Myasthenia Gravis

Myasthenia gravis is a disease due to a defect of neuromuscular transmission caused by the presence of antibodies to the acetyl choline receptor (AChR) and characterized by fluctuating weakness that is improved by inhibitors of cholinesterase.

Etiology and Pathogenesis. The etiology of myasthenia gravis is not known. That is, it is not known how the disease starts. However, the pathogenesis seems clearly related to antibodies to AChR, because an experimental disease has been induced in several different species of animals by immunizing them with AChR purified from the electric organ of eels or torpedo fish, an organ that contains large amounts of AChR. In immunized animals, the weakness has all the essential clinical and physiological characteristics of human myasthenia, and the weakness appears when antibodies to AChR appear in the blood. Antibodies have been localized at the neuromuscular junction in immunocytological studies. Similar antibodies have been demonstrated in virtually all human patients with myasthenia gravis, and in infants of myasthenic mothers, similar symptoms parallel the appearance and disappearance of these antibodies. These facts were established in a series of investigations by the collaboration of workers at the Salk Institute (Lindstrom, Seybold, Lennon) and the Mayo Clinic (Engel, Lambert) and their colleagues and were soon confirmed in several other laboratories in the years between 1973 and 1977. Drachman showed that injection of IgG from human patients can induce features of the disease in mice, and Pinching then found that symptoms were ameliorated by plasmapheresis.

How the antibodies arise is not known, but as in many other autoimmune diseases, a persistent viral infection is suspected. The thymus gland is almost always abnormal, either because of prominent germinal centers or actual tumor formation, and it is presumed that the antibody-forming cells arise there. In the thymus, there are normally epithelioid or "myoid" cells that have histological characteristics of muscle and bear AChR; these cells could present the antigen to thymic lymphocytes. Altered cellular immunity may also play a role, because the experimental disease can be transferred passively by injections of lymph nodes from affected animals, but the role of cellular immunity in the human disease is not clear. There are few familial cases of the disease, but disproportionate frequency of specific transplantation antigen haplotypes in myasthenic patients suggests that genetic predisposition may be important. Other autoimmune diseases also seem to occur with disproportionate frequency in patients with myasthenia, especially hyperthyroidism, other thyroid disorders, systemic lupus erythematosus, rheumatoid arthritis and pemphigus.

Although the antibodies seem to be directed against antigenic determinants on the AChR molecule other than the acetyl choline binding-site, physiological studies indicate impaired responsiveness to the agonist, thereby accounting for the physiological abnormalities, clinical symptoms, and the beneficial effects of drugs that inhibit acetyl cholinesterase.

Pathology. The pathological findings in patients with myasthenia gravis are scant. Examination of other organs of the body with the exception of the muscles and the thymus is usually normal. In approximately 50% of cases there are collections of lymphocytes, or lymphorrhages, in the affected muscles and occasionally in other organs. Usually the muscles bordering the lymphorrhages are normal but occasionally they have undergone degenerative changes. Occasionally there are degenerative changes in the skeletal muscles, or irregular atrophy of fibers, unassociated with cellular accumulations. Round-cell infiltration and necrosis of the cardiac muscle have been reported in a few cases. The thymus contains lymphocytic follicles or is the site of a tumor in most cases. Histologic evidence of thyroiditis is found in about 15% of cases at autopsy.

Incidence. Myasthenia gravis is a common disease. An apparent increase in the incidence of the disease in recent years is probably due to improved diagnosis. According to Kurland the prevalence rate is 3 per 100,000 (or approximately 6,000 cases) in the United States. A similar prevalence rate was given by Garland and Clark for England. Before age forty, the disease is three times more common in women but at older ages both sexes are affected equally.

The onset of symptoms may be at any age, but it is most commonly in the second to fourth decades. It is not rare before ten or after the age of sixty years. Infants born of myasthenic mothers may have a transient myasthenia, which responds to neostigmine and disappears within a few weeks.

Symptoms. The symptoms of myasthenia have three general characteristics which, together, provide a combination that is virtually diagnostic by itself. Formal diagnosis, until recently, depended upon demonstration of the response to cholinergic drugs. In the future, demonstration of circulating antibodies to AChR is likely also to be part of routine diagnosis.

The fluctuating nature of myasthenic weakness is unlike any other disease. The weakness varies in the course of a single day, sometimes within minutes, and it varies from day to day, or for longer periods. Major prolonged variations are termed remissions or exacerbations; when an exacerbation involves respiratory muscles, that is called a crisis. Variations sometimes seem related to exercise; this, and the nature of the physiological abnormality have long been termed "excessive fatigability" but there are practical reasons to de-emphasize fatigability as a central characteristic of myasthenia. Patients with the disease almost never complain of fatigue or symptoms that might be construed as fatigue. Myasthenic symptoms are always due to weakness, not to rapid tiring. In striking contrast, patients who complain of fatigue, if they are not anemic or harboring a malignant tumor, almost always have emotional problems, usually depression.

The second characteristic of myasthenia is the distribution of weakness. Ocular muscles are affected first in about 40% of the cases and they are ultimately involved in about 85%. Ptosis and diplopia are the symptoms that result. Other common symptoms affect facial or oropharyngeal muscles, resulting in dysarthria, dysphagia and limitation of facial movements. Together, oropharyngeal and ocular weakness, or both, cause symptoms in virtually all patients with myasthenia. Limb and neck weakness is also common, but only with cranial weakness, too. Almost never are limbs affected alone.

Respiratory muscles are affected only during crisis. Crisis seems most likely to occur in patients with oropharyngeal weakness, and seems to be provoked by respiratory infection in many cases, or surgical procedures, including thymectomy, although it may occur with no apparent provocation. Systemic illness may aggravate myasthenic weakness for reasons that are not clear; in patients with oropharyngeal weakness, aspiration of secretions may occlude lung passages to cause rather abrupt onset of respiratory difficulty. Major surgery is predictably followed by respiratory weakness without aspiration, however, so this cannot be the entire explanation. "Spontaneous" crisis seems to be less common now than it was a decade or so ago.

The third characteristic of myasthenic weakness is the clinical response to cholinergic drugs. This occurs so uniformly that it has become part of the definition, but it may be difficult to demonstrate in some patients, especially those with purely ocular myasthenia.

Aside from the fluctuating nature of the weakness, myasthenia is not a progressive disease. That is, the general nature of the disease is usually established within weeks or months after the first symptoms. If myasthenia is restricted to ocular muscles for a year, certainly if it is restricted after two years, it is likely to remain restricted, and only in rare cases does it then become generalized. Spontaneous remissions are also most apt to occur in the first two years.

Prior to the advent of respiratory care units and the introduction of positive pressure respirators in the 1960s, crisis was a threatening event, so that the mortality of the disease was about 25%. With improved respiratory care, however, it is now exceptional for patients to die of myasthenia, except when cardiac or renal or other disease complicates the picture.

Signs. The vital signs and general physical examination are usually within normal limits, unless the patient is in crisis. The results of neurological examination depend on the extent of the muscular involvement. The frequency of weakness of the facial and levator palpabrae muscles produces a characteristic expressionless facies with drooping eyelids. When the ocular muscles are involved, there may be ptosis and ocular palsies with diplopia and, rarely, paretic nystagmus. The weakness of the ocular muscles may be a paralysis or weakness of isolated muscles, paralysis of conjugate gaze, complete ophthalmoplegia in one or both eyes, or in a pattern resembling internuclear ophthalmoplegia. Weakness of oropharyngeal or limb muscles, when present, can be shown by appropriate tests. Muscular wasting of variable degree is found in approximately 10% of cases, but this is not focal, and is usually encountered only in patients with malnutrition due to severe dysphagia. Fasciculations do not occur, unless the patient has received excessive amounts of cholinergic drugs. Sensation is normal and the reflexes are preserved, even in muscles that are weak. The sensory examination is normal and the reflexes are preserved even in muscles which are totally unable to perform any voluntary movement.

Laboratory Data. Routine examinations of the blood, urine and cerebrospinal fluid are normal. The characteristic electromyographic abnormality is rapid decline in the height of muscle action potentials evoked by repetitive nerve stimulation at rates less than 15/second. In microelectrode study of intercostal muscle, the amplitude of miniature end-plate potentials is reduced to about 20% of normal and this can be shown to be due to decreased responsiveness of the AChR to agonists applied by microiontophoresis. A new clinical technique, called "single-fiber electromyography" (SFEMG), may become popular in diagnostic evaluation because it is less painful than the traditional form of repetitive stimulation. In this method, a small electrode measures the interval between potentials of the muscle fibers innervated by the same nerve. This interval normally varies, a phenomenon called "jitter," and the temporal limits of jitter have been defined. In myasthenia, the jitter is increased, and when excessively prolonged, an impulse may not appear at all at the expected time; this is called "blocking" and the number of blockings is increased in myasthenic muscle. All of these electrophysiological abnormalities are characteristic of myasthenia, but are occasionally seen in other conditions. The standard EMG is usually normal, occasionally shows a myopathic pattern, and almost never shows signs of denervation unless some other condition supervenes. Similarly, nerve conduction velocities are normal.

Antibodies to AChR may be universally present and a test to demonstrate this would be valuable in diagnosis. Unfortunately, the most sensitive and most specific assay relies upon human AChR as antigen and this is not readily available. Other antigens, such as denervated rat muscle or fish electric organ, can be used but do not give such consistent results.

Other serological abnormalities are encountered with varying frequency but in several studies, antinuclear factor, rheumatoid factor and thyroid antibodies were encountered more often than in control populations. Laboratory (and clinical) evidence of hyperthyroidism occurs at some time in about 5% of patients with myasthenia. Roentgenogram of the chest (including 10° oblique films) provide evidence of thymoma in about 15% of the patients, especially in those older than age forty.

Diagnosis. The diagnosis of myasthenia gravis can be made without difficulty in the majority of cases from the characteristic history and physical examination. The dramatic improvement which follows the injection of neostigmine or edrophonium in a previously untreated case makes the administration of these drugs a valuable diagnostic aid. Return of strength in weak muscles (Fig. 149) occurs so uniformly after the parenteral administration of 1.5 mg of neostigmine that the failure of such a response almost precludes the diagnosis of myasthenia gravis. The excessive response of patients with myasthenia gravis to curare has led to the suggestion that it be used in minute doses to accentuate the symptoms in doubtful cases. The dangers of the use of curare in patients with myasthenia gravis preclude its use as a routine diagnostic test. When the manifestations of the disease are confined entirely to the ocular muscles (ocular myasthenia), the diagnosis may be extremely difficult. The symptoms in these cases respond poorly or not at all to the administration of neostigmine or edrophonium.

In the neostigmine test, 1.5 mg of this drug and 0.6 gm atropine

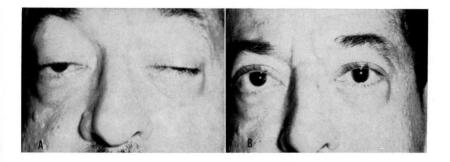

Figure 149. Myasthenia gravis. Severe ptosis of the lids (left). Same patient one minute after intravenous injection of 10 mg of edrophonium (right). (Rowland, L. P., Hoefer, P. F. A., and Aranow, H., Jr.: Res. Publ. Ass. Nerv. & Ment. Dis., courtesy Williams & Wilkins.)

sulfate are given intramuscularly. Objective improvement in muscular power is recorded at intervals from ten minutes to two hours following the injection. Subjective improvement in patients with asthenia due to other causes can be usually detected by the absence of any objective improvement. The effects of the neostigmine are transient and last for only a few hours. It is claimed by some that the weakness following the period of improvement is greater than that present before the injection of the drug. Edrophonium is given intravenously in total dose of 10 mg. The initial dose is 2 mg followed in thirty seconds by an additional 3 mg, and then in another thirty seconds by 5 mg, to maximum of 10 mg. Improvement is observed within thirty seconds and lasts for a few minutes. Because of the immediate and dramatic nature of the response, edrophonium is preferred for evaluation of cranial muscle weakness and neostigmine is now generally reserved for evaluation of limb weakness, which may require more time. Placebo injections are sometimes useful in evaluating limb weakness, but placebos are not necessary in evaluating cranial muscle weakness, which cannot be simulated.

The neostigmine test and the edrophonium tests are seen in patients with myasthenia confined to the ocular muscles. Failure of response to these drugs is sometimes seen in patients with myasthenia confined to the ocular muscles. For all practical purposes a positive response is diagnostic of myasthenia gravis although improvement has been reported in a few cases of other conditions.

Differential Diagnosis. The differential diagnosis includes all diseases which are accompanied by paralysis of the bulbar musculature or by weakness of the muscles of the extremities such as the muscular dystrophies, amyotrophic lateral sclerosis, progressive bulbar palsy, ophthalmoplegias of other cause and the asthenia of psychoneurosis or hyperthyroidism. There is usually no difficulty in differentiating these conditions from myasthenia gravis by the findings on physical and neurological examination and by the failure of symptoms in these conditions to improve following the parenteral injection of neostigmine or edrophonium.

Treatment. The initial management of patients with myasthenia gravis relies mainly on the short-acting anticholinesterase compounds, neostigmine (Prostigmin), pyridostigmine (Mestinon) and ambenonium (Mytelase). Long-acting anticholinesterases, such as tetraethylpyrophosphate and octamethylpyrophosphate have been tried, but the cumulative effects made these compounds too dangerous for use. For long-term management, decisions have to be made about the use of steroids, immunosuppressive drugs, and thymectomy.

Neostigmine. Neostigmine can be given intravenously, intramuscularly and by mouth. For obvious reasons, administration by the oral route is the preferred one. Intramuscular injection is useful as a diagnostic test and as a supplement to oral administration in patients with very severe symptoms. Intravenous administration is rarely necessary and should be used only in extremely severe cases. The amount of neostigmine to be administered should be sufficient to control the symptoms and must be determined for each individual.

Approximately 30 mg of neostigmine when given by the oral route are as effective as 1.5 mg when given intravenously. The response to oral adminstration is slower and is less complete. The tablets for oral administration are 15 mg, and are most effective when taken sublingually. The maintenance dose varies from 1 to 2 tablets in twenty-four hours to 1 to 3 tablets every 2 hours during the day. The first dose in the morning should be given before arising.

For the prevention or alleviation of visceral disturbances, such as salivation, abdominal discomfort, cramps, diarrhea or desire to defecate, which occur in some patients, atropine sulfate 0.3 mg may be taken with the neostigmine. Potassium chloride, ephedrine or amphetamine sulfate may be of use along with the neostigmine. Potassium chloride is given in doses of 1 to 2 gm 3 or 4 times daily, ephedrine in doses of 25 mg or amphetamine sulfate in doses of 10 mg at similar intervals. The benefit of these "adjuvants" has not really been established, but some patients find them useful.

Pyridostigmine (Mestinon). This drug is as effective as neostigmine. Some patients report a longer duration of optimal benefit with a less severe letdown at the end of three or four hours. Average and maximal dosages are about 4 times as great as for neostigmine.

Ambenonium (Mytelase). Ambenonium has an action similar to that of neostigmine or pyridostigmine and is administered in doses of 10 to 40 mg every three or four hours. The drug is also available in solution for parenteral use.

Treatment with neostigmine, pyridostigmine or ambenonium with or without adjuvant therapy should be continued indefinitely. With the onset of a spontaneous remission, the patient may be able to reduce the dosage of the drug or eliminate its use entirely. With relapse of the symptoms, treatment must be reinstituted. Occasionally in the course of therapy the symptoms may become refractory to neostigmine regardless of the size of the dose (myasthenic crisis). Patients with acute paralysis of the respiratory muscles should be intubated, and placed on an artificial respirator. Tracheotomy may be necessary. With complete control of the patient's respirations in the respirator, it is possible to eliminate entirely the use of cholinergic drugs. Reinstitution of therapy with the drug will usually be necessary when the patient is removed from the respirator.

Occasionally it may be necessary to determine whether the so-called myasthenic crisis is due to overdosage of anticholinesterases or refractoriness to their effect. It is thought by some that this differential can be made with edrophonium. If there is no improvement of symptoms with the intravenous administration of 10 mg, it is presumed that the patient has been adequately or perhaps overtreated with anticholinesterases. Temporary improvement following injection of edrophonium is an indication for increased dosage of neostigmine or similar compounds. Many investigators, however, doubt the reliability of this interpretation. If a patient is having respiratory distress, treatment for respiratory failure should be given without awaiting the results of any pharmacological test. For patients who are not in crisis, it has not been demonstrated that decisions based upon the edrophonium test are any more useful than clinical adjustment of dosage.

Thymectomy. In combining the results of thymectomy from several centers about two thirds of the patients with no thymoma improved, with complete remissions in about 25%. When improvement occurs, it may start immediately after the operation or may be delayed for several years. Young patients tend to be selected for surgery and most young patients with myasthenia are women but men also improve. It is not clear whether long duration of symptoms adversely affects the results of operation. In general, patients with thymoma tend to have severe symptoms, but about 25% of these patients also improve after removal of the tumor. Despite these apparently impressive figures, there has been no prospectively controlled study of the operation. Improved surgical and anesthetic techniques, better support for respiratory insufficiency, and antibiotics, however, have so reduced the risks of surgery that most patients who are seriously disabled by myasthenia are selected for surgery. Because these patients are uncommonly encountered in most hospitals, regional centers for thymectomy seem advisable.

Corticosteroids and Immunosuppressive Drugs. The use of prednisone in treating myasthenia is now widespread, although the value of this form of treatment has not been put to controlled trial. Several different regimens are used, depending upon the severity of symptoms. For most patients, 100 mg given on alternate days, is accepted as adequate. But some authorities give the same dose or more daily for patients in crisis. Some start with smaller amounts and gradually increase to the target dosage. Because symptoms may worsen when steroids are first given, it is advisable to have the patient in the hospital when this form of treatment is given. Because of the hazards of chronic steroid therapy, we reserve this treatment for patients with seriously disabling or life-threatening myasthenia who have not responded to thymectomy. Others, however, give prednisone for ocular myasthenia, or in preparation for thymectomy. If there is no response to prednisone, it is not clear how long the trial should continue before it is deemed a failure, but three months of full dosage is probably the minimum. Some investigators report improvement in 80% of patients so treated, but others find the results less impressive. In any case, the significant number of failures has resulted in trials of immunosuppressive drugs, such as azathioprine, methotrexate, or cyclophosphamide. It is not clear whether these drugs are more or less hazardous than steroids, whether prednisone should be continued when they are given, or whether they should be given in arbitrary dosage or with peripheral leukopenia as end-point. It is to be hoped that these questions will be answered by appropriate trials before long.

REFERENCES

Albuquerque, E. X., Rash, J. E., Mayer, R. G., and Satterfield, J. R.; Electrophysiological and Morphological Study of the Neuromuscular Junction in Myasthenia Gravis, Exp. Neurol., 51, 536, 1976.

Alter, M., Talbert, O. R., and Kurland, L. T.: Myasthenia Gravis in a Southern Community, Arch. Neurol., 3, 399, 1960.

Brown, J. C., Charlton, J. E., and Waite, J. K.: A Regional Technique for the Study of Sensitivity to Curare in Human Muscle, J. Neurol. Neurosurg. Psychiat., 38, 18, 1975.

Eaton, L. M., and Lambert, E. H.: Electromyography and Electric Stimulation of Nerves in Diseases of Motor Unit: Observations on the Myasthenic Syndrome Associated with Malignant Tumors, J.A.M.A., 163, 1117, 1957.

Elmqvist, D., and Lambert, E. H.: Detailed Analysis of Neuromuscular Transmission in a Patient with the Myasthenic Syndrome Sometimes Associated with Bronchogenic Carcinoma, Mayo Clin. Proc., 43, 689, 1968.

Engel, A. G.: Immune Complexes at Motor Endplate in Myasthenia Gravis, Mayo Clin. Proc., 52, 273, 1977.

Engel, A. G., Tsujihata, M., Lindstrom, J., and Lennon, V. A.: Endplate Fine Structure in Myasthenia Gravis and in Experimental Autoimmune Myasthenia, Ann. N.Y. Acad. Sci., 274, 60, 1976.

Erb, W.: Zur Casuistik der bulbären Laehmungen: Ueber einem neuen, wahrscheinlich bulbären Symptomencomplex, Arch. f. Psychiat., 9, 336, 1878.

Genkins, G., Papatestas, A. E., Horowitz, S. H., and Kornfeld, P.: Studies in Myasthenia Gravis. Early Thymectomy, Am. J. Med., 58, 517, 1975.

Goldflam, S.: Ueber einen scheinbar heilbaren bulbärparalytischen Symptomencomplex mit Beteiligung der Exteremitäten., Deutsche Zischr. f. Nervenh., 4, 312, 1893.

Greer, M., and Schotland, M.: Myasthenia Gravis in the Newborn, Pediatr., 26, 101, 1960.

Grob, D.: Myasthenia Gravis, Arch. Int. Med., 108, 615, 1961.

Hermann, C., Jr.: Familial Occurrence of Myasthenia Gravis, Ann. N.Y. Acad. Sci., 183, 334, 1971.

Jolly, F.: Pseudoparalysis Myasthenica, Neurol. Centrabl., 14, 34, 1895.

Lindstrom, J., Lennon, V. A., Seybold, M., and Whittingham, S.: Experimental Autoimmune Myasthenia and Myasthenia Gravis: Biochemical and Immunological Aspects, Ann. N.Y. Acad. Sci., 254, 1976.

Lindstrom, J. M., et al.: Antibody to Acetylcholine Receptor in Myasthenia Gravis: Prevalence, Clinical Correlates, and Diagnostic Value, Neurology, 26, 1054, 1976.

Mattell, G., et al.: Effects of Some Immunosuppressive Procedures on Myasthenia Gravis, Ann. N.Y. Acad. Sci., 274, 659, 1976.

McQuillen, M. P., Cantor, H. E. and O'Rourke, J. R.: Myasthenic Syndrome Associated with Antibiotics, Arch. Neurol., 18, 402, 1968.

Osserman, K. E.: Myasthenia Gravis, New York, Grune & Stratton, 1958, 296 pp.

Papatesta, A. E., et al.: Studies in Myasthenia Gravis. Effects of Thymectomy, Am. J. Med., 50, 465, 1971.

Patrick, J., and Lindstrom, J.: Autoimmune Response to Acetylcholine Receptor, Science, *180*, 871, 1973.

Perlo, V. P., et al.: Myasthenia Gravis: Evaluation of Treatment in 1,355 Patients, Neurology, *16*, 431, 1966.

Rowland, L. P.: Immunosuppressive Drugs in Treatment of Myasthenia Gravis, Ann. N.Y. Acad. Sci., *183*, 351, 1971.

Rowland, L. P., Hoefer, P. F. A., Aranow, H., Jr., and Merritt, H. H.: Fatalities in Myasthenia Gravis. A Review of 39 Cases with 26 Autopsies, Neurology, *6*, 307, 1956.

Rowland, L. P., Hoefer, P. F. A. and Aranow, H., Jr.: Myasthenic Syndromes, Res. Publ. Ass. Nerv. Ment. Dis., *38*, 548, 1961.

Santa, T., Engel, A. G., and Lambert, E. H.: Histometric Study of Neuromuscular Junction Ultrastructure. I. Myasthenia Gravis, Neurology, *22*, 71, 1972.

Seybold, M. E., et al.: Experimental Autoimmune Myasthenia: Clinical, Pharmacological, and Neurophysiological Aspects, Ann. N.Y. Acad. Sci., *274*, 275, 1976.

Teng, P., and Osserman, K. E.: Studies in Myasthenia Gravis: Neonatal and Juvenile Types, J. Mt. Sinai Hosp., *23*, 711, 1956.

Toyka, K. V., et al.: Myasthenia Gravis: Passive Transfer from Man to Mouse, Science, *190*, 397, 1975.

Warmolts, J. R., and Engel, W. K.: Benefit from Alternate-day Prednisone in Myasthenia Gravis, N. Engl. J. Med., *286*, 17, 1972.

Familial Periodic Paralysis

Familial periodic paralysis is the name given to a group of familial diseases of unknown etiology characterized by recurrent attacks of

Table 77.   The Clinical Features of Low and High Serum Potassium Periodic Paralysis and Paramyotonia

(Modified from Hudson, Brain, 1963)

	Low Serum Potassium Periodic Paralysis	High Serum Potassium Periodic Paralysis	Paramyotonia Congenita
Age of onset	Usually second or latter part of first decade	First decade	First decade
Sex	Male preponderance	Equal	Equal
Incidence of paralysis	Interval of weeks or months	Interval of hours or days	May not be present; otherwise, interval of weeks or months
Degree of paralysis	Tends to be severe	Tends to be mild but can be severe	Tends to be mild but can be severe
Effect of cold	May induce an attack	May induce an attack	Tends to induce an attack of paralysis
Effect of food (especially glucose)	May induce an attack	Relieves an attack	Relieves an attack of paralysis
Serum potassium	Low	High	Tends to be high
Oral potassium	Prevents an attack	Precipitates an attack	Precipitates an attack

weakness or paralysis of the somatic musculature, accompanied by loss of the deep reflexes and failure of the muscles to respond to electrical stimulation. It was once thought that all cases were associated with a decrease in the potassium content of the serum at the onset of the attacks of weakness. It is now known that three types of the disease can be distinguished on basis of the level of the serum potassium: 1. Hypokalemic, which is by far the most common; 2. hyperkalemic, also called adynamia episodica hereditaria; and 3. normokalemic, the least common of the three forms. Paramyotonia (Eulenburg syndrome) is probably related to the hyperkalemic form of the disease. Although there are clinical distinctions between the three forms (Table 77), these differences are not always demonstrable and identification of the syndromes depends upon the serum potassium content in a spontaneous or induced attack. In all forms there is a strong familial tendency and inheritance is usually an autosomal dominant.

Vacuoles are found in the muscles in the early stages of the disease. These vacuoles seem to arise from both the terminal cisterns of the sarcoplasmic reticulum and from proliferation of the T-tubules. In the later stage there may be degeneration of the muscle fibers, possibly related to a mild degree of weakness in the intervals between.

Hypokalemic Periodic Paralysis

In this form of the disease the potassium content is lowered in a spontaneous attack to values of 3.0 mEq/L or lower. Attacks may be induced by the injection of insulin, epinephrine, flurohydrocortisone or glucose, or they may follow the ingestion of a meal high in carbohydrates. The potassium content of the urine is also decreased in an attack. In the cases described by Conn there was sodium retention and increased aldosterone excretion before the onset of attacks.

Incidence. The disease is rare. There are no large series reported in the literature and only 1 or 2 cases are seen each year in any of the large neurological clinics in this country. Males are affected 2 to 3 times as frequently as females. The first attack usually occurs at about the time of puberty, but it may occur as early as the age of four or be delayed to the sixth decade.

Symptoms and Signs. The attack of muscular weakness usually has its onset after a period of rest. It is common for it to develop during the night or to be present on awakening in the morning. The extent of the paralysis varies from slight weakness of the legs to complete paralysis of all of the muscles of the trunk and extremities. The bulbar musculature and the diaphragm are usually spared, even in the severe attacks, but ptosis of the eyelids may occur. There may be retention of urine and feces during a severe attack. The duration of the individual attack varies from a few hours to as long as twenty-four to forty-eight hours.

According to some patients, there is improvement in the strength of the muscles if they move around and keep active ("walking it off"). The interval between attacks may be as long as a year or one or more attacks of weakness may occur daily. Weakness is especially apt to be present on the morning following the ingestion of a high carbohydrate meal before retiring on the pevious night. There is a frequent association of periodic paralysis with migraine and its coincidence with hyperthyroidism has been noted often. Rarely, the disease may occur in association with heredodegenerative diseases of the nervous system, such as peroneal muscular atrophy.

In the interval between attacks, the patients are usually strong and the potassium content of the serum is normal. In some patients a mild degree of proximal weakness persists. In a mild attack, tendon reflexes and electrical reactions of the muscles are diminished in proportion to the degree of muscular weakness. In severe attacks, the tendon and cutaneous reflexes are absent and the muscles do not respond to electrical stimulation. There is no disturbance of the cutaneous sensibility.

Course. Familial paralysis is not accompanied by any impairment of the general health. As a rule, there is a decrease in the frequency of the paralytic attacks with the passage of the years and it is not uncommon for them to cease altogether after the age of forty or fifty. Fatalities are uncommon but death may occur from respiratory paralysis in severe attacks.

Table 78.   Potassium and Paralysis: Non-inherited Forms

Hypokalemic
- A.   Excessive urinary loss
  1. Hyperaldosteronism.
  2. Drugs: glycyrrhizate (licorice), thiazides, furosemide, chlorthalidone, ethacrynic acid, amphotericin, duogastrone.
  3. Pyelonephritis and renal tubular acidosis.
  4. Recovery from diabetic acidosis.
  5. Ureterocolostomy.
- B.   Excessive gastrointestinal loss
  1. Malabsorption syndromes.
  2. Laxative abuse.
  3. Diarrhea.
  4. Fistulas, vomiting, villous adenoma.
  5. Pancreatic tumor and diarrhea.
- C.   Thyrotoxicosis

Hyperkalemia
- A.   Uremia.
- B.   Addison's disease.
- C.   Spironolactone excess.
- D.   Excessive intake.
  1. Iatrogenic
  2. Geophagia

Diagnosis. The diagnosis can usually be made without difficulty on basis of the familial occurrence of transient attacks of weakness. The diagnosis can usually be confirmed by the finding of a low potassium and high sodium content in the serum during an attack, or by inducing an attack with an infusion of glucose (100 gm) and regular insulin (20 units). In sporadic cases, the first attack has to be differentiated from other courses of hypokalemia (Table 78).

Treatment. Acute attacks, spontaneous or induced, may be safely and rapidly terminated by ingestion of 7 to 10 gm potassium chloride or the equivalent dose of mixed salts of potassium. (Intravenous administration of potassium is usually avoided because of the hazard of inducing hyperkalemia.)

Prophylactic treatment was not satisfactory until recently and numerous regimens were devised in an attempt to reduce the number of attacks; supplementing diet with potassium salts; low-sodium, low-carbohydrate diet; and spironolactone or dexamethasone to promote retention of potassium. The most effective prophylaxis, however, results from oral administration of acetazolamide in doses of 250 to 1000 mg daily. Treatment with acetazolamide may also be followed by improvement of the fixed weakness between attacks that was formerly attributed to "myopathic" changes in the muscles.

The treatment of other forms of hypokalemic paralysis depends upon the nature of the underlying renal disease, diarrhea, drug ingestion, or thyrotoxicosis. Patients with thyrotoxic period paralysis are susceptible to spontaneous or induced attacks during the period of hyperthyroidism; when the patients become euthyroid, spontaneous attacks cease and they are no longer sensitive to infusion of glucose and insulin.

REFERENCES

Conway, M. J., Seibel, J. A., and Eaton, R. P.: Thyrotoxicosis and Periodic Paralysis: Improvement with Beta Blockade, Ann. Intern. Med., *81*, 332, 1974.

Engel, A. G.: Evolution and Content of Vacuoles in Primary Hypokalemic Periodic Paralysis, Mayo Clin. Proc., *45*, 774, 1970.

Engel, A. G. and Lambert, E. H.: Calcium Activation of Electrically Inexcitable Muscle Fibers in Primary Hypokalemic Periodic Paralysis, Neurology, *19*, 851, 1969.

Engel, A. G., Lambert, E. H., Rosevear, J. W., and Tauxe, W. N.: Clinical and Electromyographic Studies in a Patient with Primary Hypokalemic Periodic Paralysis, Am. J. Med., *38*, 626, 1965.

Feldman, D. L. and Goldberg, W. M.: Hyperthyroidism with Periodic Paralysis, Canad. M.A.J., *101*, 667, 1969.

Griggs, R. C., Engel, W. K. and Resnik, J. S.: Acetazolamide Treatment of Hypokalemic Periodic Paralysis. Prevention of Attacks and Improvement of Persistent Weakness, Ann. Intern. Med., *73*, 39, 1970.

Hofmann, W. W. and Smith, R. A.: Hypokalemic Periodic Paralysis Studied *in Vitro*, Brain, *93*, 445, 1970.

Holtzapple, G. E.: Periodic Paralysis, J.A.M.A., *45*, 1224, 1905.

Hudson, A. J.: Progressive Neurological Disorder and Myotonia Congenita Associated with Paramyotonia, Brain, *86*, 811, 1963.

Kao, I., and Gordon, A. M.: Mechanism of Insulin-induced Paralysis of Muscles from Potassium-depleted Rats, Science, 188, 740, 1975.

Layzer, R. B., and Goldfield, E.: Periodic Paralysis Caused by Abuse of Thyroid Hormone, Neurology, 24, 949–952, 1974.

Pearson, C. M. and Kalyanaraman, R.: Periodic Paralysis. In Stanbury, J. B., Wyngaarden, J. B., and Fredrickson, D. S. (Eds.). The Metabolic Basis of Inherited Disease. 3rd Ed., New York, McGraw Hill, 1972, pp. 1180–1203.

Shy, G. M., Wanko, T., Rowley, P. T., and Engel, A. G.: Studies in Familial Periodic Paralysis, Exper. Neurol., 3, 53, 1961.

Van Horn, G., Drosi, J. B. and Schwartz, F. D.: Hypokalemic Myopathy and Elevation of Serum Enzymes, Arch. Neurol., 22, 335, 1970.

Viskopfer, R. J., Licht, A., and Fidel, Chaco, J.: Acetazolamide Treatment in Hypokalemic Periodic Paralysis. A Metabolic and Electromyographic Study, Am. J. Med. Sci., 226, 119, 1973.

Vroom, F. Q., Jarrell, M. A., and Maren, T. H.: Acetazolamide Treatment of Hypokalemic Periodic Paralysis. Probable Mechanism of Action, Arch. Neurol., 32, 385, 1975.

Zierler, K. L.: Speculations on Hypokalemic Periodic Paralysis, Am. J. Med. Sci., 266, 131, 1973.

Hyperkalemic Periodic Paralysis
(Adynamia Episodica Hereditaria)

Tyler, in 1951, recognized a form of familial periodic paralysis in which the attacks were not accompanied by a decrease in the serum potassium content. Gamstorp and Mjönes, in 1956, drew attention to several features of these cases which separated them from the usual cases of periodic paralysis. They proposed the term adynamia episodica hereditaria to describe these cases. The disease is transmitted by a single autosomal dominant gene with almost complete penetrance.

In addition to the absence of hypokalemia in the attacks, the syndrome is characterized by the early age of onset (usually under the age of ten years), the tendency of the attacks to be of shorter duration and less severe, and to occur in the daytime. Myotonia is usually demonstrable by electromyography, but abnormalities of muscular relaxation are rarely symptomatic; myotonic lid-lag (Fig. 150) and lingual myotonia may be the sole clinical evidence of the trait. The serum potassium content and the urinary excretion of potassium may be increased during an attack. It has been suggested that this is due to leakage of potassium from the muscles. The attacks tend to be precipitated by hunger, rest, cold and by the administration of potassium chloride.

The attacks may be terminated by the administration of calcium gluconate, glucose and insulin. Acetazolamide, in oral doses of 250 mg to 1 gm daily, has been effective in reducing the number of attacks or abolishing them altogether. Other diuretics that promote urinary excretion of potassium are also effective.

A variant of adynamia episodica hereditaria has been reported by Poskanzer and Kerr. The disease in their cases (21 members of a family of 45) was characterized by the relative infrequency and the long

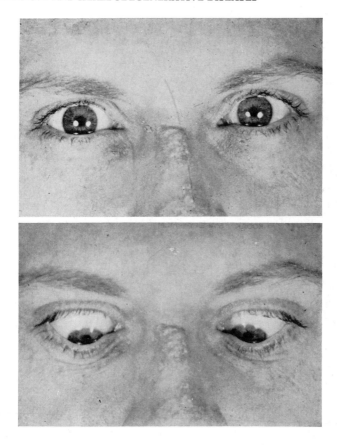

Figure 150.   Paramyotonia congenita. Myotonia of muscles of upper lids on looking downward. (Courtesy Dr. Robert Layzer.)

duration of the attacks. In another form of the disease, cardiac arrhythmias may accompany attacks of paralysis or persist even when the serum potassium content becomes normal.

Paramyotonia Congenita. Whether this is truly a separate genetic entity is now uncertain. All forms of myotonia are aggravated by cold and the attacks of paralysis in Eulenburg's cases suggest that they represented hyperkalemic periodic paralysis. It is possible, however, that there is a disease in which myotonia is detectable or symptomatic only in cold and in which there is no hyperkalemic periodic paralysis.

REFERENCES

Bradley, W. G.: Adynamia Episodica Hereditaria. Clinical, Pathological and Electrophysiological Studies in an Affected Family, Brain, *92*, 345, 1969.

Brillman, J., and Pincus, J. H.: Myotonic Periodic Paralysis Improved by Negative Sodium Balance, Arch. Neurol., 29, 67, 1973.
Danowski, T. S. et al.: Clinical and Ultrastructural Observations in a Kindred with Normohyperkalemic Periodic Paralysis, J. Med. Genet., 12, 20, 1975.
Gamstorp, I., et al.: Adynamia Episodica Hereditaria, Am. J. Med., 23, 385, 1957.
Gamstorp, I.: Adynamia Episodica Hereditaria and Myotonia, Acta. Neurol. Scand., 39, 41, 1963.
Gelfand, M. C., Zarate, A., and Knepshield, J. H.: Geophagia. A Cause of Life-threatening Hyperkalemia, J.A.M.A., 234, 738, 1975.
Layzer, R. B., Lovelace, R. E., and Rowland, L. P.: Hyperkalemic Periodic Paralysis, Arch. Neurol., 16, 455, 1967.
Lisak, R. P., Lebeau, J., Tucker, S. H., and Rowland, L. P.: Hyperkalemic Periodic Paralysis and Cardiac Arrhythmia, Neurology, 22, 810, 1972.
Magee, K. R.: A Study of Paramyotonia Congenita, Arch. Neurol., 8, 461, 1963.
McArdle, B.: Adynamia Episodica Hereditaria and Its Treatment, Brain, 85, 121, 1962.
Perez, G., Siegel, L., and Schreiner, G. E.: Selective Hypoaldosteronism with Hyperkalemia, Ann. Intern. Med., 76, 757, 1972.
Poskanzer, D. C., and Kerr, D. N. S.: A Third Type of Periodic Paralysis with Normokalemia and Favorable Response to Sodium Chloride, Am. J. Med., 31, 328, 1961.
Streeten, D. H. P., Dalakos, T. G., and Fellerman, H.: Studies on Hyperkalemic Periodic Paralysis. Evidence of Changes in Plasma Na and Cl and Induction of Paralysis by Adrenal Glucocorticoids, J. Clin. Invest., 50, 142, 1971.
Van Dellen, R. G., and Purnell, D. C.: Hyperkalemic Paralysis in Addison's Disease, Mayo Clin. Proc., 44, 904, 1969.

Other Diseases of Muscles

Myoglobinuria. When necrosis of muscle occurs acutely, myoglobin escapes into the blood and then into the urine. In the past, the term "myoglobinuria" was reserved for grossly pigmented urine, but modern techniques can detect amounts of this protein so minute that discoloration may not be evident. The clinically important syndromes, however, are associated with gross pigmenturia.

No classification of the myoglobinurias is completely satisfactory, but Table 79 lists the most important causes. Many cases of inherited recurrent myoglobinuria are due to unidentified abnormalities. In three forms, however, the genetic defect has been recognized. In McArdle disease, muscle phosphorylase is lacking. In Tarui disease, the missing enzyme is phosphofructokinase. In DiMauro-Bank disease, the missing enzyme is carnitine palmityl transferase (CPT). The first two enzymes are important enzymes in glycogen metabolism. The third is important in the oxidation of long-chain fatty acids. In all three conditions there is a disorder in the metabolism of a fuel necessary for muscular work, and in all three, exercise is limited by painful cramps after exertion, and myoglobinuria occurs after especially strenuous activity. There may be a subtle difference in the kinds of activity that provoke attacks, more prolonged in CPT deficiency than in the glycogen disorders. The glycogen disorders can be identified by a simple clinical test; a cramp is induced by ischemic exercise of forearm muscles for less than one minute and venous lactate fails to rise as it does in normal individuals or those with CPT deficiency. Specific diagnosis requires histochemical or biochemical analysis of muscle homogenates. All three syndromes are inherited in autosomal recessive pattern.

Another important form of inherited myoglobinuria occurs in "malignant hyperpyrexia" which seems to be due to succinylcholine in some cases and to halothane in others. The characteristic syndrome

Table 79. Classification of Human Myoglobinuria

I. Hereditary Myoglobinuria
  A. Phosphorylase deficiency (McArdle)
  B. Phosphofructokinase deficiency (Tarui)
  C. Carnitine palmityl transferase deficiency (DiMauro)
  D. Incompletely characterized syndromes
    1. Excess lactate production (Larsson)
  E. Uncharacterized
    1. Familial; biochemical defect unknown
      a. Provoked by diarrhea or infection
      b. Provoked by exercise
    2. Familial susceptibility to succinylcholine or general anesthetics ("malignant hyperthermia")
    3. Repeated attacks in an individual; biochemical defect unknown
II. Sporadic Myoglobinuria
  A. Exertion in untrained individuals
    1. "Squat-jump" and related syndromes
    2. Anterior tibial syndrome
    3. Convulsions
    4. High voltage electric shock
  B. Crush syndrome
    1. Compression by fallen weights
    2. Compression by body in prolonged coma
  C. Ischemia
    1. Arterial occlusion
    2. Ischemia in compression and anterior tibial syndromes
  D. Metabolic abnormalities
    1. Metabolic depression
      a. Barbiturate, carbon monoxide, narcotic coma
      b. Diabetic acidosis
      c. General anesthesia
      d. Hypothermia
    2. Exogenous toxins and drugs
      a. Haff disease
      b. Alcoholism
      c. Malayan sea-snake bite poison
      d. Plasmocid
      e. Succinylcholine
      f. Glycyrrhizate, carbenoxolone, amphotericin-B
      g. Heroin
    3. Chronic hypokalemia
    4. Heat stroke
  E. Progressive muscle disease ("polymyositis," "alcoholic myopathy")
  F. Cause unknown

includes widespread muscular rigidity, a rapid rise in body temperature, myoglobinuria and metabolic acidosis. In some cases, muscular rigidity is lacking. The syndrome seems to be transmitted by an autosomal dominant gene with incomplete penetrance in some families. The biochemical abnormality has not been identified and may involve an unusual susceptibility of the sarcoplasmic reticulum to the offending drugs, impairing the ability of the SR to bind calcium.

Most cases of acquired myoglobinuria occur in untrained individuals who are subjected to extremely vigorous exercise, a hazard faced primarily by military recruits. These individuals are otherwise normal. If muscle is compressed, as occurs in the crush syndrome of individuals pinned by fallen timber after bombing raids, or after prolonged coma in one position, myoglobinuria may ensue. Ischemia after occlusion of large arteries may also lead to necrosis of large amounts of muscle. Depression of muscle metabolism, especially after drug ingestion, may also be responsible in some cases. Hypokalemia from any cause may predispose to myoglobinuria, but especially after chronic licorice ingestion. Alcoholics seem especially prone to acute attacks of myoglobinuria, which may punctuate or initiate a syndrome of chronic limb weakness ("alcoholic myopathy").

Whatever the cause, the clinical syndrome is similar: widespread myalgia, weakness, malaise, renal pain, fever. Pigmenturia usually ceases within a few days, but the weakness may persist for weeks, and very high concentrations of serum enzymes may not return to normal for even longer. The main hazard of the syndrome is heme-induced nephropathy with anuria, azotemia and hyperkalemia. Hypercalcemia occurs in a few patients after anuria. Rarely, respiratory muscles may be symptomatically weakened.

Treatment of the acute episode is directed primarily toward the kidneys; promotion of diuresis with mannitol seems desirable whenever there is oliguria. Dialysis and measures to combat hyperkalemia may be necessary. In recurrent cases due to defects of the glycolytic enzymes or to cause unknown, a variety of therapeutic regimens have been tried but the patients usually learn the limits of exercise tolerance. The treatment of malignant hyperthermia is unsatisfactory because the rigidity is not abolished by curare; recent experiments suggest that infusions of procaine may be beneficial.

REFERENCES

Bank, W. J., DiMauro, S., Bonilla, E., Capuzzi, D. M., and Rowland, L. P.: A Disorder of Lipid Metabolism and Myoglobinuria. Absence of Carnitine Palmityl Transferase, N. Engl. J. Med., 292, 443, 1975.
Britt, B. A. and Kalow, W.: Malignant Hyperthermia: A Statistical Review, Can. Anaesth. Soc. J., 17, 239, 1970.

Demos, M. A., Gitlin, E. L., and Kagen, L. G.: Exercise Myoglobinuria and Acute Exertional Rhabdomolysis, Arch. Intern. Med., 134, 669, 1974.
DiMauro, S., and DiMauro, P. M. M.: Muscle Carnitine Palmityl Transferase Deficiency and Myoglobinuria, Science, 182, 929, 1973.
Gordon, R. A., Britt, B. A., and Kalow, W. (Eds.): Malignant Hyperthermia. Springfield, Charles C Thomas, 1973.
Harriman, D. G. F., Summer, D. W., and Ellis, F. R.: Malignant Hyperpyrexia Myopathy, Quart. J. Med., 168, 639, 1873.
Harrison, G. G.: Anaesthetic-induced Malignant Hyperpyrexia: a Suggested Method of Treatment, Br. Med. J., 3, 454, 1971.
Knochel, J. P.: Environmental Heat Illness. An Eclectic Review, Arch. Intern. Med., 133, 841, 1974.
Layzer, R. B., Rowland, L. P. and Ranney, H. M.: Muscle Phosphofructokinase Deficiency, Arch. Neurol., 17, 512, 1967.
McArdle, B.: Myopathy Due to Defect in Muscle Glycogen Breakdown, Clin. Sci., 10, 13, 1951.
Moulds, R. G. W.: Biochemical Basis of Malignant Hyperpyrexia, Br. Med. J., 2, 241, 1974.
Pearson, C. M., Rimer, D. G. and Mommaerts, W. F. H. M.: A Metabolic Myopathy Due to Absence of Muscle Phosphorylase, Am. J. Med., 30, 502, 1961.
Penn, A. S., Rowland, L. P. and Fraser, D. W.: Drugs, Coma and Myoglobinuria, Arch. Neurol., 26, 336, 1972.
Perkoff, G. T.: Alcoholic Myopathy, Ann. Rev. Med., 23, 125, 1971.
Rowland, L. P., and Penn, A. S.: Myoglobinuria, Med. Clin. N. A., 56, 1233, 1972.
Ryan, J. F.: Procaine for Malignant Hyperthermia, N. Engl. J. Med., 291, 210, 1974.

Glycogen Storage Diseases of Muscle. Of the seven major forms of glycogen storage disease in which the enzymatic defect has been identified, muscle is involved in four syndromes.

In Pompe disease, due to acid maltase deficiency, glycogen accumulates in all tissues. The syndrome is evident in the first year of life and all typical cases have been fatal within two years. Quadriparesis is probably due to the combined effects of neuronal dysfunction and myopathy, since glycogen distorts the architecture of both tissues. Cranial muscle function is also disturbed so that the neurological disorder resembles Werdnig-Hoffmann syndrome. This could be fatal in itself, but glycogen accumulation in myocardial fibers leads to cardiomegaly and congestive heart failure. There is no treatment for this autosomal recessive disorder. The disease can be identified in utero because the enzyme is lacking also in amniotic cells and pregnancy can be interrupted.

Glycogen accumulation and lack of the same enzyme may also be found in older children and adults with syndromes that resemble limb-girdle dystrophy or polymyositis. There seems to be unusual propensity to affect respiratory muscles, so that this rare syndrome is probably one of the major myopathic causes of alveolar hypoventilation. Another unusual and unexplained feature is the presence of myotonia in the EMG, although this is not evident clinically. Histologically, there is a vacuolar myopathy and on appropriate stains, the vacuoles are seen to be filled with glycogen. As in the infantile disease, lack of acid maltase can be demonstrated biochemically in muscle biopsies or by measuring the enzyme in urine. The late-onset cases lack the clinical homogeneity of the infantile cases and they probably represent different genetic disorders, because infantile and late-onset cases have not yet been reported in the same family.

In type III glycogen storage disease (limit dextrinosis) due to lack of the debrancher system, the predominant syndrome is hepatomegaly but in some cases there is also a myopathy that resembles limb-girdle dystrophy. Recognition of the disease usually requires biochemical analysis of muscle biopsy.

In type IV storage disease (amylopectinosis or Andersen disease) the dominant syndrome is cirrhosis of the liver in young children, but the abnormal polysaccharide is also stored in muscle and weakness has been a symptom in most of the few reported cases.

The symptoms of McArdle disease and Tarui disease have been discussed above.

REFERENCE

DiMauro, S.: Genetic Heterogeneity in Glycogen Storage Disease. In Rowland, L. P. (Ed.), *Pathogenesis of Human Muscular Dystrophies*. Amsterdam, Excerpta Medica, 1977.

Myopathies Due to Abnormal Metabolism of Fat or Sugar. As histochemical and biochemical methods have been applied to the study of syndromes resembling congenital myopathies, limb-girdle dystrophy, and polymyositis, new abnormalities have been found, although the fundamental disorders are still unknown. Among these are the mitochondrial myopathies, appearing as "ragged red fibers" in the Gomori trichrome stain, and "lipid storage myopathies." The two are linked because lactate acidosis may be found in either and because the histological abnormalities are sometimes found together. Among the lipid storage disorders, some are associated with decreased content of carnitine in muscle alone, some with systemic carnitine deficiency. The clinical disorder of the restricted form is sporadic or familial proximal limb weakness, which may be punctuated by periods of exacerbation but has no other distinctive characteristics. Cramps and myoglobinuria are not found in this syndrome, although they are in the closely related CPT-deficiency. The weakness may improve after oral administration of carnitine. In the systemic disease, there may be similar abnormality in the liver and the disorder is then accompanied by episodic hepatic encephalopathy, which may be fatal. In many cases of lipid-storage myopathy, as defined histologically, carnitine content is normal and the essential abnormality remains to be identified.

Lactic acidosis may accompany lipid storage and is found in a variety of neurological and myopathic syndromes, some including both sets of disorder. Abnormalities of pyruvate dehydrogenase have been found in some of the severe neurological diseases, but elucidation of the myopathic disorders remains a problem. The clinical disorder is one of persistent proximal limb weakness, with or without ophthalmoplegia, or exercise intolerance with excessive rise in serum lactate after exercise.

REFERENCES

Angelini, C.: Lipid Storage Myopathies. A Review of Metabolic Defect and Treatment, J. Neurol., *214*, 1, 1976.
Cornelio, F., et al.: Fatal Cases of Lipid Storage Myopathy with Carnitine Deficiency, J. Neurol. Neurosurg. Psychiat., *40*, 170, 1977.
Engel, A. G., and Angelini, C.: Carnitine Deficiency of Human Skeletal Muscle Associated Lipid Storage Myopathy. A New Syndrome, Science, *179*, 899, 1973.
Jerusalem, F., Spiess, H., and Baumgartner, G.: Lipid Storage Myopathy with Normal Carnitine Levels, J. Neurol. Sci., *24*, 273, 1975.
Sengers, R.C.A., et al.: Cardiomyopathy and Short Stature Associated with Mitochondrial and/or Lipid Storage Myopathy of Skeletal Muscle, Neuropadiatrie, *7*, 196, 1976.

Congenital Myopathies. The increasing use of histochemical techniques has permitted the recognition of unusual structures in the muscles of children with mild forms of myopathic weakness. Although these syndromes are not usually evident in the first year or the second year of life (other than delayed walking), the persistent and relative static weakness suggests that the disorder is congenital. The disorders have been named after the predominant structural abnormality.

In *central core disease,* an amorphous area in the center of the fiber stains blue with Gomori's trichrome stain, in contrast with the red peripheral fibrils. The cores are devoid of enzymatic activity histochemically, and with the electronic microscope the area lacks mitochondria. In *nemaline disease* small rods near the sarcolemma stain bright red with the modified trichrome stain. Ultrastructural and extraction experiments suggest that the rods originate from Z-band material. In *myotubular or centronuclear myopathy,* the nuclei are situated centrally and are surrounded by a pale halo. In *pleoconial myopathy* there are too many mitochondria and in *megaconial myopathy,* the mitochondria are abnormally enlarged, and in some the mitochondria contain abnormal crystalline inclusions. Other less clearly demarcated structural abnormalities have been recognized as well. (Although not a congenital myopathy, non-thyroidal hypermetabolism in adults may be associated with abnormal mitochondria in Luft disease.)

The common clinical syndrome for all of these congenital myopathies is proximal limb weakness. Although usually mild and static, the weakness is occasionally progressive and may even be fatal.

There are other cases of congenital myopathy in which there are nonspecific myopathic changes in the biopsy, with no characteristic structural abnormality. In nemaline disease, the face may be long and lean, with prognathism and other skeletal abnormalities. In myotubular disease, there may be ptosis and ophthalmoplegia. Still another form of congenital myopathy warrants the name arthrogryposis congenita multiplex, because of multiple congenital contractures; most cases of arthrogryposis prove to be neurogenic by electromyography and muscle biopsy, but some are myopathic. In the Prader-Willi syndrome, hypotonia, dysphagia, depressed myotatic reflexes and cryptorchidism may be prominent in infancy but there may be no permanent weakness; the syndrome is later recognized by mental retardation, obesity, short stature, skeletal abnormalities, childhood diabetes and a characteristic facial appearance with a triangular-shaped upper lip.

REFERENCES

Amick, L. D., Johnson, W. W., and Smith, H. L.: Electromyographic and Histopathologic Correlations in Arthrogryposis, Arch. Neurol., 16, 512, 1967.

Bethlem, J., Van Wijngaarden, G. K., Meijer, A. E. F. H. and Fleury, P.: Observations on Central Core Disease, J. Neurol. Sci., 14, 293, 1971.

Dahl, D. S., and Klutzoro, F. W.: Congenital Rod Disease, J. Neurol. Sci., 23, 371, 1976.

Darentl, D. L., et al.: A New Familial Arthrogryposis without Weakness, Neurology, 24, 55, 1974.

DiMauro, S., et al.: Mitochondrial Myopathies: Which and How Many? In Milhorat A. T. (Ed.), Exploratory Concepts in Muscular Dystrophy II. Amsterdam, Excerpta Medica, 1974, pp. 506–515.

Dubowitz, V., and Brooke, M. H.: Muscle Biopsy: A Modern Approach. Philadelphia, W. B. Saunders Co., 1973.

Engel, A. G., Gomez, M. R., and Groover, R. V.: Multicore Disease, Mayo Clin. Proc., 46, 666, 1971.

Engel, W. K., Gold, G. N. and Karpati, G.: Type 1 Fiber Hypotrophy and Central Nuclei, Arch. Neurol., 18, 435, 1968.

Gordon, A. S., et al.: Chronic Benign Congenital Myopathy; Fingerprint Body Type, Canad. J. Neurol. Sci., 1, 106, 1974.

Hall, R. D., and Smith, D. W.: Prader-Willi Syndrome, J. Pediatr., 81, 286, 1972.

Haydar, N. A., et al.: Severe Hypermetabolism with Primary Abnormality of Skeletal Muscle Mitochondria, Functional and Therapeutic Effects of Chloramphenicol Treatment, Ann Intern. Med., 74, 548, 1971.

Kinoshita, M., Satoyashi, E., and Matsuo, N.: Myotubular Myopathy and Type 1 Fiber Atrophy in a Family, J. Neurol. Sci., 26, 575, 1975.

Kinoshita, M., Satoyashi, E., and Suzuki, Y.: Atypical Myopathy with Myofibrillar Aggregates, Arch. Neurol., 32, 417, 1975.

Lenard, H. G., and Goebel, H. H.: Congenital Fiber Type Disproportion, Neuropadiatrie, 6, 220, 1975.

Luft, R., Ikkos, D., et al.: A Case of Severe Hypermetabolism of Nonthyroid Origin with a Defect in the Maintenance of Mitochondrial Respiratory Control: A Correlated Clinical, Biochemical and Morphological Study, J. Clin. Invest., 41, 1776, 1963.

Ortiz de Zarate, J. C. and Maruffo, A.: The Descending Ocular Myopathy of Early Childhood; Myotubular or Centronuclear Myopathy, Europ. Neurol., 3, 1, 1970.

Shy, G. M., et al.: Nemaline Myopathy: A New Congenital Myopathy, Brain, 86, 793, 1963.

Shy, G. M., et al.: Two Childhood Myopathies with Abnormal Mitochondria. I. Megaconial Myopathy. II. Pleoconial Myopathy, Brain, 89, 133, 1966.

Shy, G. M., et al.: New Congenital Non-progressive Myopathy, Brain, *79*, 610, 1956.

Spiro, A. J., Shy, G. M. and Gonatas, N. K.: Myotubular Myopathy, Arch. Neurol., *14*, 1, 1966.

Sugita, H., et al.: Staining of the Nemaline Rod by Fluorescent Antibody Against 10S Actinin, Proc. Japan Acad., *50*, 237, 1974.

Swinyard, C. A.: Multiple Congenital Contractures. Public Health Consideration of Arthrogryposis Multiplex Congenita, J.A.M.A., *183*, 23, 1963.

Zellweger, H., Afifi, A., McCormick, W. F. and Mergner, W.: Benign Congenital Muscular Dystrophy: A Special Form of Congenital Hypotonia, Clin. Pediatr., *6*, 655, 1967.

Zellweger, H., Afifi, A., McCormick, W. F. and Mergner, W.: Severe Congenital Muscular Dystrophy, Am. J. Dis. Child., *114*, 591, 1967.

Tetany

Tetany is a clinical syndrome characterized primarily by convulsions, prolonged spasms of limb muscles (especially distal muscles) and laryngospasm, accompanied by signs of hyperexcitability of peripheral nerves.

Etiology. Although vitamin D deficiency once affected most children in the cities of northern Europe, rickets due to nutritional deficiency is now rare in industrial countries; in the United States, malabsorption syndromes are now responsible for most cases of vitamin D deficiency osteomalacia. This changing pattern has also altered the causes of tetany, which may be induced by any disorder that lowers the serum content of ionized calcium. The relative frequency of causes of tetany due to decreased total serum calcium is now difficult to discern; postoperative hypoparathyroidism is probably most common. Other causes (Table 80) include idiopathic hypoparathyroidism, pseudohypoparathyroidism, intestinal malabsorption and vitamin D deficiency. Another relatively common form of tetany is induced by hyperventilation because the resulting alkalosis decreases the propor-

Table 80.   Causes of Tetany

Hypocalcemia	Hypovitaminosis D
	Resistance to vitamin D
	Intestinal malabsorption
	Renal tubular acidosis
	Hypoparathyroidism
	Pseudohypoparathyroidism
	Infants of hyperparathyroid mothers
	Idiopathic
Alkalosis	Hyperventilation
	Persistent vomiting
	Excessive treatment with alkali
	Hypokalemia (especially aldosteronism)
Hypomagnesemia	
"Spasmophilia"	

tion of ionized calcium in relation to total serum calcium content. Alkalosis induced by persistent vomiting, excessive ingestion of alkali or persistent hypokalemia may also be associated with tetany. In Europe, hyperventilation tetany is also referred to as "spasmophilia," but some authorities reserve this term for tetany that is not associated with any discernible abnormality of calcium metabolism. Hypomagnesemia may also be associated with tetany, but in these cases there is usually also a low serum calcium concentration. Neonatal tetany may be due to the low calcium:phosphorus ratio of cow's milk, maternal hyperparathyroidism or osteomalacia, or due to unknown causes of hypocalcemia.

Symptoms and Signs. The triad of symptoms characteristic of active tetany are carpopedal spasm, laryngospasm and convulsive seizures.

Carpal spasm is an involuntary contraction of the muscles of the upper extremity in which the fingers are flexed at the proximal joint and extended at the distal joints. The wrist and elbow may also be flexed. In pedal spasm there is flexion of the toes at the proximal joint and extension at the distal joints. The plantar surface of the foot is concave. The ankle may be slightly extended and the thighs adducted. Except in severe spasms, voluntary movements of the terminal phalanges of the fingers and toes are preserved. Occasionally, the muscles of the face or other portions of the body may be affected by the spasm. Muscle spasm may last for hours or even days. When prolonged, the spasms are painful and the pain is increased if an attempt is made to overcome it by passive movement.

Laryngospasm is due to a contraction of the laryngeal muscles similar to that of the muscles of the extremities. The respirations are labored and there is prolonged inspiratory stridor. In severe attacks, the child may become unconscious or convulsive seizures may occur. More commonly there are only a few inspiratory "crows" and the child breathes normally until the next spasm develops. Several attacks of laryngospasm may occur daily.

Convulsive seizures are the most common symptoms of active tetany, especially in infants under the age of one year. These seizures are generalized and are accompanied by loss of consciousness. Occasionally the convulsive movements are confined to one side of the body. The seizures may occur with great frequency and in series. A transient hemiplegia may follow repeated unilateral attacks.

Convulsive seizures may occur as the only manifestation of the so-called latent form of tetany. The diagnosis of tetany can be made by the presence of the characteristic Chvostek, Trousseau and Erb signs.

Laboratory Data. In the hypocalcemic forms of tetany, the serum calcium content is less than 8 mg per 100 ml. In hypovitaminosis D and malabsorption syndromes, the serum phosphate content is also decreased, but serum phosphate is increased in hypoparathyroidism and pseudohypoparathyroidism (Table 81). Parathormone is absent in idiopathic hypoparathyroidism but is present in all the other forms. In normal individuals and in patients with idiopathic hypoparathyroidism administration of parathormone is followed by increased urinary excretion of cyclic-AMP. This response is lacking in pseudohypoparathyroidism. In alkalotic tetany, the total calcium and P are normal, but the pH of blood and urine are alkalotic and tetany is present only during periods of high pH.

In all forms of tetany, the peripheral nerves are hyperexcitable as manifest by the reactions to ischemia (Trousseau sign) and percussion (Chvostek sign). The spasms are due to repetitive firing of peripheral nerves, and the iterative discharges tend to occur in groups (doublets, triplets, and multiplets) which occur with increasing frequency until they merge in a spasm of high frequency activity. The EEG is usually diffusely abnormal, with no characteristic pattern.

Diagnosis. Active tetany can be diagnosed without difficulty by the characteristic carpopedal and laryngospasm. In cases where convulsions are the only symptoms, the diagnosis is established by the demonstration of one or more of the clinical signs of tetany and by the low serum calcium.

Laryngeal stridor associated with laryngitis is diagnosed by the presence of cough, hoarse voice, fever and signs of inflammation in the larynx. Parathyroid tetany is distinguished by the late age of incidence and by the elevated phosphorus content of the serum.

Mental deficiency, dementia, psychosis, papilledema, cataracts and ectopic calcification in basal ganglia or subcutaneous tissues may occur in chronic hypocalcemia of any cause. Symptoms of parkin-

Table 81.   Differential Diagnosis of Tetany

	Serum				Urine	
	Ca	P	pH	PTH	Ca	pH
Hypocalcemia						
Hypovitaminosis D	↓	↓	N	↑	↓	—
Resistance to vitamin D	N or ↓	↓	N	↑	↓	—
Malabsorption	↓	↓	N	↑	↓	—
Hypoparathyroidism	↓	↑	N	O	↓	—
Pseudohypoparathyroidism	↓	↑	N	↑		
Alkalosis						
Respiratory	N	N	↑	N	N	↑
Metabolic	N	N	↑	N	N	↑

Symbols: ↓ decreased; ↑ increased.

sonism or chorea may be encountered. Idiopathic hypoparathyroidism is also characterized by ectodermal abnormalities: cutaneous moniliasis, abnormal teeth and fingernails, alopecia, and dry skin. Addison disease and pernicious anemia occur in association with idiopathic hypoparathyroidism.

In addition to the other signs of hypocalcemia, pseudohypoparathyroidism is characterized by short stature, round face, short metacarpal bones (resulting in a characteristic dimple over the head of the affected bone when the fist is clenched). Moniliasis, Addison disease and pernicious anemia do not occur.

Treatment. Acute hypocalcemic tetany is treated by administration of calcium in the form of calcium gluconate given as necessary to control symptoms. Phenobarbital and diphenylhydantoin may also be beneficial. Chronic tetany is treated with at least 2 gm calcium by mouth (15 gm calcium lactate) and vitamin D 50,000 to 100,000 units daily. The amount of vitamin D and calcium may be reduced as the serum content returns to normal. Hyperventilation tetany may be corrected by having the patient rebreathe into a paper bag, with attention to the underlying emotional disorder. Other forms require correction of the underlying pathologic condition.

REFERENCES

Alajouanine, Th., Contanin, F., and Cathala, H. P.: *Le Syndrome Tétaine*, Paris, J.-B.: Baillière et Fils, 1958, 279 pp.
Fishman, R. A.: Neurological Aspects of Magnesium Metabolism, Arch. Neurol., *12*, 562, 1965.
Isgreen, W. P.: Normocalcemic Tetany, Neurology, *26*, 825, 1976.
Robinson, P. K.: The Clinical Effects of Hypocalcemia in the Nervous System, J. Roy. Coll. Phys., *1*, 36, 1966.
Watson, L.: Calcium Metabolism and Neurology, J. Roy. Coll. Phys., *1*, 28, 1966.

COLLAGEN-VASCULAR DISEASES AND SYSTEMIC VASCULITIS

Several different syndromes are commonly linked together because they are characterized by the combination of arthritis, rash and visceral disorders. Since arthritis is common in all of them, and because fibrinoid degeneration of blood vessels is common, they are frequently called "collagen-vascular diseases." However, inflammatory lesions of the blood vessels also characterize syndromes in which the vascular lesions are the dominant pathological change. Periarteritis nodosa was the model vasculitis, but classification of related syndromes depended upon autopsy evaluation of histological changes in the arteries, whether large or small vessels were involved, and which organs were most affected. Similar classifications were applied to clinical diagnosis, but overlap between syndromes and lack of knowledge of

Table 82. Clinical Classification of Vasculitis Syndromes (Christian and Sergent)

Characterized by Necrotizing Vasculitis

Temporal Arteritis	Henoch-Schonlein Purpura
Wegener Granulomatosis	Periarteritis Nodosa
Aortic Arch Arteritis	Cogan Syndrome

Occasionally Complicated by Necrotizing Vasculitis

Rheumatic Diseases: Rheumatoid arthritis; systemic lupus erythematosus; rheumatic fever.

Infections: Hepatitis B; acute respiratory infections; streptococcal infection; post-streptococcal glomerulonephritis; bacterial endocarditis.

Respiratory Diseases: Loeffler syndrome; asthma; serous otitis media.

Hypersensitivity: Serum sickness; drug allergy; amphetamine abuse.

Plasma Cell Dyscrasias: Essential cryoglobulinemia; myeloma; macroglobulinemia.

Others: Dermatomyositis; dermal vasculitis; ulcerative colitis; colon carcinoma.

pathogenesis clouds the area in uncertainty. Some of these diseases seem to be due to the deposition of circulating immune complexes within vessel walls, and some may be due to persistent viral infection. The classification of Christian and Sergent is useful (Table 82), however, and some syndromes have such characteristic clinical and neurologic manifestations that they warrant discussion individually (Table 82A). Clinical disorders of brain, spinal cord, peripheral nerve or muscle are prominent in these diseases.

Periarteritis Nodosa

Periarteritis nodosa is a form of inflammatory arteritis affecting any of the medium-sized and small arteries, characterized by the occurrence of symptoms commonly associated with an acute infection and signs and symptoms of involvement of the thoracic and abdominal viscera, the joints, muscles and the nervous system.

Etiology. The cause of periarteritis nodosa is unknown. The streptococcus, Australia antigen or other virus, or bacterial hyperergy have been suggested as possible causes. The disease is occasionally associated with rheumatic endocarditis, scarlet fever and tonsillitis. The coincidence of the condition with asthma, serum sickness and reactions to drugs speaks strongly for an anaphylactic type of hypersensitivity as the etiological factor. This hypothesis is further supported by the work of Rich, who was able to reproduce the lesions in rabbits by the repeated injection of horse serum. Recent studies suggest that antigen-antibody complexes may be deposited in arterial and arteriolar walls.

Table 82A. Syndromes Associated With Systemic Vasculitis

Syndrome	Systemic Manifestations	Laboratory Abnormalities	Neurological Syndromes
Systemic Vasculitis (Periarteritis Nodosa)	Skin, kidneys, joints, lungs, hypertension; abdominal pain; heart	Serum complement decreased; immune complexes; hepatitis B antigen and antibody; rheumatoid factor	Peripheral neuropathy; mononeuritis multiplex: stroke; polymyositis
Wegener Granulomatosis	Nose, paranasal sinuses, lungs, other viscera	As above; also increased serum IgE	Peripheral or cranial neuropathy; encephalopathy
Churg-Strauss Vasculitis	Lungs, other viscera	As above; also eosinophilia	
Temporal Arteritis (Giant Cell Arteritis)	Fever, malaise, myalgia, weight loss, claudication of chewing	Increased ESR	Visual loss due to lesions of optic nerve or retina; papilledema; stroke rare
Polymyalgia Rheumatica	Fever, malaise; myalgia, weight loss	Increased ESR	None
Cogan Syndrome	Interstitial keratitis, aortic insufficiency; occasionally other viscera	Increased ESR; CSF pleocytosis	Vestibular or auditory loss; peripheral neuropathy; stroke; encephalomyelopathy

Disease	Clinical Features	Laboratory Findings	Neurological Features
Takayasu Syndrome (Aortic Arch Disease; Pulseless Disease)	Cataracts, retinal atrophy; cranial muscular wasting; claudication loss of peripheral pulses; heart.	Increased ESR	Stroke; amaurosis fugax; visual loss
Granulomatous Angiitis of the Brain	None	CSF pleocytosis, increased protein content, normal sugar	Somnolence, confusion; encephalomyelopathy; myeloradiculoneuropathy
Systemic Lupus Erythematosus	Skin, lungs, kidneys, joints, liver, heart, Raynaud, fever	Leukopenia, multiple autoantibodies, increased ESR; evidence of renal or hepatic disease	Organic psychosis; seizures; chorea; myelopathy; peripheral neuropathy; polymyositis; aseptic meningitis
Systemic Sclerosis	Skin, lungs, GI tract, kidneys, heart, joints, Raynaud	None characteristic except disordered mobility of esophagus and bowel	Polymyositis
Rheumatoid Arthritis	Joints; viscera occasionally	Rheumatoid factor	Polymyositis; mononeuritis multiplex, peripheral neuropathy
Dermatomyositis	Skin, by definition; lungs; GI tract, very rare	Inflammatory cells in muscle	Polymyositis
Mixed Connective Tissue Disease (Sclerodermatomyositis?)	Skin lesions of dermatomyositis or scleroderma; joints; Raynaud; lungs; esophagus	Antibody to extractable nuclear ribonucleoprotein	Polymyositis

Pathology. There is a diffuse widespread panarteritis. The adventitia and the vasa vasorum are infiltrated with polymorphonuclear leukocytes, lymphocytes and eosinophiles. There is necrosis of the media and elastic fibers which leads to the formation of multiple small aneurysms. These may become fibrosed, or they may rupture. Proliferation of the intima may lead to thrombosis of the vessels. Repair and fibrosis of the aneurysms and adventitial lesions produce the characteristic nodules which may be felt along the course of the arteries. Although the process is mainly in the arteries, veins may occasionally be affected to a slight degree. Lesions in various organs occur secondary to ischemia or hemorrhage.

Incidence. Periarteritis nodosa is a rare condition. Only a few hundred cases are recorded in the literature, but this does not represent the true incidence of the disease because many isolated cases are unreported. Both sexes are affected. The disease may occur at any age but over 50% of the reported cases were in the third or fourth decades of life.

Signs and Symptoms. The onset may be acute or insidious. Fever, malaise, tachycardia, sweating, fleeting edema, weakness, and pains in the joints, muscles or abdomen are common early symptoms. The blood pressure may be elevated and there may be a moderate or severe anemia with a leukocytosis.

Visceral involvement occurs in practically all cases. Involvement of the kidneys produces a picture similar to that of acute glomerular nephritis. Cutaneous hemorrhages, erythematous eruptions and tender reddened subcutaneous nodules may appear in the skin of the trunk or extremities. Gastrointestinal, hepatic, renal or cardiac symptoms may develop.

Involvement of the nervous system occurs in approximately one half of the cases.

Involvement of the peripheral nerve is most common. This may take the form of mononeuritis multiplex or a diffuse symmetrical polyneuritis. Sympathetic nerves may be affected with changes in the size and shape of the pupils and impairment of their reaction to light. The damage to the nerves is presumably due to ischemia secondary to involvement of the nutrient arteries.

Damage to the arteries in the central nervous system may lead to cerebral thrombosis or to hemorrhage. The large vessels are rarely affected but rupture of the basilar artery has been reported. Symptoms from involvement of the spinal vessels rarely occur.

The most common manifestations of cerebral involvement are headache, convulsions, blurred vision, vertigo, sudden loss of vision in one eye, and confusional states or an organic type of psychosis.

A syndrome characterized by keratitis and deafness in nonsyphilitic individuals was described by Cogan in 1945. The syndrome occurs predominantly in young adults with negative blood and cerebrospinal fluid tests for syphilis and no stigmata of congenital syphilis. The etiology of the syndrome is not known, but a number of cases have been reported in which the syndrome was one of the features of periarteritis nodosa. The symptoms are of sudden onset involving the cornea and both divisions of the eighth nerve. Usually the eye and the eighth nerve are involved simultaneously, but there may be several weeks or months between the onset of symptoms in the eye and the ear. Affection of the eighth nerve is usually signalized by nausea, vomiting, tinnitus and loss of hearing. With progression of the hearing loss to complete deafness, the vestibular symptoms subside.

Laboratory Data. There is a leukocytosis with an inconstant eosinophilia. The serological tests for syphilis may be positive and there may be positive skin and serological tests for trichinosis. The cerebrospinal fluid is normal unless there has been a meningeal hemorrhage.

Diagnosis. The diagnosis of periarteritis nodosa should be considered in all patients with an obscure febrile illness with symptoms of involvement of the nervous system (particularly chronic polyneuritis) and other organs. The diagnosis can often be established by biopsy of sural nerve, muscle, or testicle.

Course and Prognosis. The prognosis is poor. Death usually occurs as result of involvement of kidneys, other abdominal viscera or the heart. Occasionally, lesions in the central nervous system or peripheral nerves may be the cause of death. The duration of life after onset of symptoms varies from a few months to several years. Spontaneous healing of the arteritis may occur and is followed by remission of all symptoms and signs, including those due to involvement of the peripheral nerves.

Treatment. There is no specific therapy. Treatment is chiefly supportive, including blood transfusions and symptomatic therapy for associated conditions. Corticosteroids may be of temporary or permanent benefit in some cases.

REFERENCES

Alarcon-Segovia, D.: The Necrotizing Vasculitides. A New Pathogenetic Classification, Med. Clin. N. A., *61*, 241, 1977.

Bickness, J. M., and Holland, J. V.: Neurologic Manifestations of Cogan Syndrome, Neurology, in press.

Cheson, B. D., Blunming, A. Z., and Alroy, J. A.: Cogan's Syndrome. A Systemic Vasculitis, Am. J. Med., *60*, 549, 1976.

Christian, C. L., and Sergent, J. S.: Vasculitis Syndromes: Clinical and Experimental Models, Am. J. Med., *61*, 511, 1976.

Cogan, D. G.: Syndrome of Nonsyphilitic Interstitial Keratitis and Vestibuloauditory Symptoms, Arch. Ophth., *33*, 144, 1945; *ibid, 42,* 42, 1949.

Ford, R. G., and Siekert, R. G.: Central Nervous System Manifestations of Periarteritis Nodosa, Neurology, 15, 114, 1965.

Lande, A., and Rossi, P.: Total Aortography in Diagnosis of Takayushu's Syndrome, Radiology, 114, 287, 1975.

Lovelace, R. E.: Mononeuritis Multiplex in Polyarteritis Nodosa, Neurology, 14, 434, 1964.

Sairanen, E., and Wasastierna, C.: Periarteritis Nodosa. A 10-year Follow-up Study of 10 Cases, Acta Med. Scand., 191, 501, 1972.

Sergent, J. S., et al.: Vasculitis with Hepatitis B Antigenemia, Medicine, 55, 1, 1975.

Talbott, J. H.: Collagen-Vascular Diseases. New York, Grune & Stratton, 1974.

Temporal Arteritis and Polymyalgia Rheumatica

A special form of periarteritis limited to the temporal artery was described by Horton, Magath and Brown in 1934. Since then, many cases have been recorded. The pathologic condition is similar to that of periarteritis nodosa except that the inflammatory reaction around the vessels is more severe and many multi-nucleated giant cells are found in the media (giant-cell arteritis). It is usually restricted to the temporal arteries, but occasionally other arteries of the head and rarely those elsewhere in the body may be involved. The syndrome occurs in both sexes and is most common in the sixth to eighth decades of life.

The presenting symptoms are headache, centered about the involved temporal artery, together with the general systemic reactions of a low grade infection, i.e., fever, anorexia, weight loss and a leukocytosis in the blood. The erythrocyte sedimentation rate is almost always greater than 50 mm per hour. The affected temporal artery is prominent, nodular, tortuous, tender to pressure, and noncompressible. Blindness occurs in approximately a third of the cases, presumably due to thrombosis of the central artery of the retina. The affected disc may be swollen with retinal hemorrhages, pale and ischemic, or normal. Confusion, hemiplegia or other focal neurological signs may occur when the inflammatory reaction involves the internal carotid artery or its branches. The central nervous system is occasionally affected by giant-cell arteritis without involvement of extracranial arteries.

The course of the disease is self-limited with remission of symptoms after a prolonged course of several months' duration. Partial or complete loss of vision is usually the only residual. Prednisone is apparently of value in shortening the course and preventing blindness in the unaffected eye if started while symptoms are unilateral. Restoration of vision is variable and not clearly benefited by steroid therapy.

Diffuse myalgia may be a prominent symptom in elderly patients with malaise, weight loss, and increased erythrocyte sedimentation rate, a syndrome called "polymyalgia rheumatica." In many of these patients the temporal artery, even when there are no cranial symptoms, may show the same pathological alterations as in temporal arteritis.

These two poorly defined syndromes therefore overlap. (In polymyalgia there is no weakness, the serum enzymes are normal and there are no pathological changes in muscle biopsy or electromyogram; if there were, the syndrome would be indistinguishable from polymyositis.)

REFERENCES

Crompton, M. R.: The Visual Changes in Temporal (Giant-Cell) Arteritis, Brain, *82*, 377, 1959.

Fisher, C. M.: Ocular Palsy in Temporal Arteritis, Minnesota Med., *42*, 1258, 1430, 1617, 1959.

Hamilton, C. R., Jr., Shelley, W. M., and Tumulty, P. A.: Giant Cell Arteritis; Including Temporal Arteritis and Polymyalgia Rheumatica, Medicine, *50*, 1, 1971.

Hollenhorst, R. W., Brown, J. R., Wagener, H. P., and Shick, R. M.: Neurologic Aspects of Temporal Arteritis, Neurology, *10*, 490, 1960.

Horton, B. T., Magath, T. B., and Brown, G. E.: Arteritis of the Temporal Vessels, Arch. Intern. Med., *53*, 400, 1934.

Hunder, G. G., Sheps, S. G., Allen, G. L., and Joyce, J. W.: Daily and Alternate Day Corticosteroid Regimens in Treatment of Giant Cell Arteritis. Comparison in a Prospective Study, Ann. Intern. Med., *82*, 613, 1975.

Itauser, W. A., et al.: Temporal Arteritis in Rochester, Minnesota, 1951–1967, Mayo Clin. Proc., *46*, 597, 1971.

Klein, R. G., Hunder, G. G., Stanson, A. W., and Sheps, S. G.: Large Artery Involvement in Giant Cell (Temporal Arteritis), Ann. Intern. Med., *83*, 806, 1975.

Ostberg, G.: On Arteritis, with Special Reference to Polymyalgia Arterica, Acta Path. Microbiol. Scand. Sect A Suppl. *237*, 1, 1973.

Rewcastle, N. B., and Tom, M. I.: Non-Infectious Granulomatous Angiitis of the Nervous System Associated with Hodgkin's Disease, J. Neurol., Neurosurg., & Psychiat., *25*, 51, 1962.

Wilkinson, I. M. S., and Russell, R. W. R.: Arteritis of the Head and Neck in Giant Cell Arteritis, Arch, Neurol., *27*, 378, 1972.

Granulomatous Giant Cell Arteritis

Various types of granulomatous, giant cell, necrotizing or allergic angiitis have been described in the literature. Various names have been given to the slightly different types of arteritis, including Wegener's granulomatosis, Zeek's necrotizing angiitis and allergic granulomatosis of Strauss, Churg and Zak. Most of the publications have been concerned with the description of the lesions in the upper respiratory tract, the lungs and the kidneys. It is now evident that any of the organ systems may be affected and that symptoms and signs of involvement of the nervous system are not rare. It is postulated that the granulomatous arteritis is allergic in nature and possibly related to bacterial sensitivity, drug or chemical toxicity or autoimmune mechanisms.

The vascular changes may occur at any age, but the vast majority of the patients are between the age of thirty to sixty years. There is a slight predominance of females in the reported cases.

Neurological symptoms may result from involvement of the vessels of the peripheral nerves or central nervous system. Mononeuritis multiplex, polyneuritis, and various focal neurological symptoms and signs may be the result.

In one form of granulomatous angiitis, the clinical manifestations are restricted to the nervous system, primarily the brain, but also the spinal cord in some cases. Several cases have been associated with states of immunological depression, including sarcoidosis or Hodgkin's disease, and a few were associated with herpes zoster infection. Focal cerebral signs may involve the hemispheres, brain stem or cerebellum. Dementia and depressed consciousness are seen in all reported cases. CSF pleocytosis, up to 500 mononuclear cells per high power field, is another consistent abnormality and the CSF protein is increased in almost all cases, exceeding 100 mg/dl in about 75% although the CSF sugar content is normal. Angiography does not show the expected beaded appearance and diagnosis during life would depend upon a cortical biopsy that included meninges. Prednisone therapy has been advocated, but all reported cases have been fatal, half within six weeks and about a third living more than one year.

REFERENCES

Budzilovich, G. W., Feigin, I., and Siegel, H.: Granulomatous Angiitis of the Nervous System, Arch. Path., 76, 250, 1963.
Drachman, D. A.: Neurological Complications of Wegener's Granulomatosis, Arch. Neurol., 8, 145, 1963.
Fauci, A. S., and Wolf, S. M.: Wegener's Granulomatosis; Studies in 18 Patients and Review of Literature. Medicine, 52, 535, 1973.
Harrison, P. R., Jr.: Granulomatous Angiitis of the Central Nervous System, J. Neurol. Sci., 29, 335, 1976.
Nurick, S., Blackwood, W., and Mair, W. G. P.: Giant Cell Granulomatous Angiitis of the Central Nervous System, Brain, 95, 133, 1972.
Russell, R. W. R.: Giant-cell Arteritis: a Review of 35 Cases, Quart. J. Med., 28, 471, 1959.
Stern, G. M., Hoffbrand, A. V., and Urich, H.: The Peripheral Nerves and Skeletal Muscles in Wegener's Granulomatosis, Brain, 88, 151, 1965.
Warrell, D. A., Godfrey, S. and Olsen, E. G. J.: Giant-cell Arteritis with Peripheral Neuropathy, Lancet, 1, 1010, 1968.

Lupus Erythematosus

Lupus erythematosus is a disease complex with widespread inflammatory change in the connective tissue (collagen) of the skin and various organs of the body. The primary damage is to the subendothelial connective tissue of capillaries, small arteries and veins, the endocardium and the synovial and serous membranes.

Etiology and Incidence. The etiology of the disease is not known, but increasing evidence suggests that immune-complexes are deposited within small vessels. The initiating event could be a persistent viral infection, but sometimes serological and clinical manifestations follow administration of drugs, such as procainamide. Although rare, the incidence of the disease may be increasing. Most cases begin between ages twenty and forty, but the disease may be seen in children. Ninety-five per cent of adult patients are women.

Symptoms and Signs. The chief clinical manifestations are: prolonged, irregular fever, with remissions of variable duration (weeks, months or even years); erythematous rash; recurrent attacks with evidence of involvement of synovial and serous membranes (polyarthritis, pleuritis, pericarditis); depression of bone marrow function (leukopenia, hypochromic anemia, moderate thrombopenia); and, in advanced stages, clinical evidence of vascular alterations in the skin, kidneys and other viscera.

Involvement of the nervous system, which is uncommon except in the later stages, may be manifest by convulsions, functional psychosis or organic mental syndrome, cerebral blindness, chorea, cranial nerve palsies, polyneuritis, hemiplegia, transverse myelopathy, or polymyositis (Table 83). These symptoms are attributed to thrombosis of small vessels or multiple petechial hemorrhages.

Laboratory Data. The changes in the blood have been mentioned above. Hematuria, albuminuria and other signs of damage to the kidneys may be present. The serum γ-globulin is often increased and biological false positive serological tests for syphilis may be encountered. Phagocytic polymorphonuclear leukocytes (LE cells), containing masses of chromatin material, which takes a deep purplish color with Wright's or Giemsa's stain, are found in the bone marrow or in the buffy coat of centrifuged heparinized blood of the majority but not all cases. These cells reflect antibody to whole nucleoprotein, one of numerous different antibodies found in the serum of these patients and reacting with autologous tissue constituents. LE cells are present in about 80%

Table 83. Neurological Manifestations in 140 Patients with SLE *

Manifestation	Number of Patients
Psychiatric disorders	24
Organic mental syndrome	22
Seizures	17
Long tract signs	16
Cranial nerve abnormalities	16
Peripheral neuropathy	15
Cerebellar signs	5
Scotomata	4
Papilledema (pseudotumor)	2
Chorea	2
Myelitis	1

* Data from Feinglass, et al. (1976).

of all cases and are considered by some to be pathognomonic of lupus erythematosus, but they may occasionally be found in other diseases. The fluorescent antinuclear-antibody test is present in virtually all cases of SLE, but this greater sensitivity is gained at the expense of specificity since antinuclear antibodies may be encountered in many other diseases. Serum complement may be decreased, especially in patients with renal disease; deposits of globulin and complement may be found in renal biopsies. The cerebrospinal fluid is usually normal, but there may be an increase in the protein content and an abnormal colloidal gold reaction when the peripheral nerves or the central nervous system are involved. For reasons that are not clear, the CSF sugar content may be depressed in patients with myelitis.

Diagnosis. The diagnosis is often extremely difficult. The occurrence of fever, weight loss, arthritis, anemia, leukopenia, pleuritis, cardiac, renal or neurological symptoms in a young woman should lead to a consideration of this diagnosis. The development of an erythematous rash on the bridge of the nose and the malar eminences in a butterfly-like distribution greatly facilitates the diagnosis. The finding of LE cells or antinuclear antibodies in the blood is of value in establishing the diagnosis.

Course and Prognosis. Death usually is the outcome as result of toxemia of the disease, renal failure or intercurrent infection. The course of the disease may be prolonged for many months or years. In some cases there are remissions of months' or years' duration.

Treatment. There is no satisfactory treatment. The administration of corticosteroids may be of value in reducing the severity of the symptoms. Their administration may be followed by a remission of symptoms but more commonly long-term therapy may be needed. The treatment of cerebral manifestations is especially disappointing and has led to the use of large doses which may themselves be deleterious.

REFERENCES

Andrianakos, A. A., Duffy, J., Suzuki, M., and Sharp, J. T.: Transverse Myelopathy in Systemic Lupus Erythematosus, Ann. Intern. Med., *83*, 616, 1973.

Brandt, K. D., Lessell, S., and Cohen, A. S.: Cerebral Disorders of Vision in Systemic Lupus Erythematosus. Ann. Intern. Med., *83*, 163, 1975.

Burton, R. C., McDuffie, F. C. and Mulder, D. W.: Lupus Erythematosus: an Autoimmune Disease of the Nervous System, Res. Publ. Ass. Res. Nerv. Ment. Dis., *49*, 197, 1971.

Canoso, J. J., and Cohen, A. S.: Aseptic Meningitis in Systemic Lupus Erythematosus. Report of 3 Cases, Arth. Rheum., *18*, 369, 1975.

Clark, E. C., and Bailey, A. A.: Neurological and Psychiatric Signs Associated with Systemic Lupus Erythematosus, J.A.M.A., *160*, 455, 1956.

Dubois, E. L.: *Lupus Erythematosus*, New York, Blakiston Division, McGraw-Hill Book Co., 1966.

Estes, D. and Christian, C. L.: The Natural History of Systemic Lupus Erythematosus by Prospective Analysis, Medicine, *50*, 85, 1971.

Feinglass, E. J., et al.: Neuropsychiatric Manifestations of Systemic Lupus Erythematosus; Diagnosis, Clinical Spectrum, and Relations to Other Features of the Disease, Medicine, 55, 323, 1976.

Greenhouse, A. H.: On Chorea, Lupus Erythematosus and Cerebral Arteritis. Arch Intern. Med., 117, 389, 1966.

Johnson, R. T. and Richardson, E. P.: The Neurological Manifestations of Systemic Lupus Erythematosus, Medicine, 47, 337, 1968.

Lewis, D. C.: Systemic Lupus and Polyneuropathy, Arch. Intern. Med., 116, 518, 1965.

Lusins, J. O., and Szilagyi, P. A.: Clinical Features of Chorea Associated with Systemic Lupus Erythematosus, Am. J. Med., 58, 857, 1975.

O'Connor, J. F., and Musher, D. M.: Central Nervous System Involvement in Systemic Lupus Erythematosus, Arch. Neurol., 14, 157, 1966.

Penn, A. S. and Rowan, A. J.: Myelopathy in Systemic Lupus Erythematosus, Arch. Neurol., 18, 337, 1968.

Prockop, L. D.: Myotonia, Procaine Amide and Lupus Like Syndrome, Arch. Neurol., 14, 326, 1966.

Sergent, J. S., et al.: Central Nervous System Disease in Systemic Lupus Erythematosus, Am. J. Med., 58, 644, 1975.

Siekert, R. G., and Clark, E. C.: Neurologic Signs and Symptoms as Early Manifestations of Systemic Lupus Erythematosus, Neurology, 5, 84, 1955.

Dermatomyositis

Dermatomyositis is a disease of unknown etiology characterized by inflammatory changes in the skin, muscles, blood vessels and subcutaneous tissues. There are pain and reddening of the skin, and tenderness, weakness and loss of reflexes in the affected muscles.

Pathology and Pathogenesis. The cause of the changes in the skin and muscles is unknown. Circulating antibodies to muscle have not been found but a similar disorder can be produced in experimental animals immunized with muscle extracts. Sensitized lymphocytes could be responsible for both experimental and human syndromes but this has not been established. Virus-like particles have been seen with the electron microscope but no virus has been isolated. The pathological changes include atrophy and inflammation of the skin, subcutaneous and muscular tissues. There are hyaline and granular degenerative changes in the muscles, with fragmentation of the fibers, proliferation of the sarcolemmal nuclei and fibrous replacement. The walls of blood vessels in the skin, subcutaneous tissue and muscles are thickened and infiltrated with lymphocytes. Inflammatory changes are also present in the interstitial tissues of the muscles and skin.

Incidence. Dermatomyositis is a rare disease. The number of cases reported in the literature, in which both myositis and dermatitis were present, is quite small. The incidence is much greater, however, if the concept of the disease is broadened to include the cases with myositis in the absence of skin manifestations.

The full-blown disease, dermatomyositis, may occur at any age and is about as common in children as it is in young adults. Polymyositis, without the dermatitis, is more common in middle-aged adults. The concidence of myositis or dermatomyositis with cancer has been noted by a number of observers.

Symptoms and Signs. The initial symptoms are usually localized edema and erythema of the skin and weakness of the muscles. Both skin and muscle are usually affected at the same time; the rash may precede weakness by several weeks, but weakness is almost never the first symptom.

The edema and redness may be confined to the skin of the face in a butterfly distribution around the nose and cheeks. Edema and erythema of the eyelids, periungual skin and extensor surfaces of joints are especially characteristic. There are apt to be remissions and exacerbations in the cutaneous changes during the course of the disease. The initial redness of the skin may be replaced by brownish pigmentation. Fibrosis of the subcutaneous tissues and thickening of the skin may produce an appearance indistinguishable from that of scleroderma. Later, calcification may develop in the affected muscles and subcutaneous tissues.

The affected muscles are weak and often tender on pressure. The muscles of the proximal portion of the girdles and the pharyngeal muscles are most commonly affected. There is no clear relationship between the location of the dermatitis and the myositis. The distribution of the muscular weakness is similar to that of progressive muscular dystrophy, but it progresses much more rapidly, and patients may be severely incapacitated within weeks or months. The mass of muscles is normal in the initial stages, but wasting, fibrosis and contractures may develop in the late stages.

Cutaneous sensation is preserved. The tendon reflexes are often reduced or absent in the affected muscles. There are no fibrillations. Other symptoms include an irregular and inconstant fever, tachycardia and hyperhidrosis. Pulmonary fibrosis has been encountered in a few cases and occasionally the heart is involved, but, in general, visceral lesions are lacking.

In about 10% of the cases, the cutaneous manifestations have features of both scleroderma and dermatomyositis, warranting the name "sclerodermatomyositis." In recent years, these cases have been designated as "mixed connective tissue disease," since there is a high incidence of antibody to extractable nuclear antigen. In another unusual syndrome, typical dermatomyositis occurs in children with agammaglobulinemia and echovirus can be isolated from blood or cerebrospinal fluid.

Diagnosis. The diagnosis is made from the appearance of the characteristic symptoms, edema and redness of the skin, tenderness and weakness of the muscles. Diseases, which are to be considered in the differential diagnosis, are lupus erythematosus, periarteritis nodosa, scleroderma, polyneuritis, myasthenia gravis and muscular dystrophy. The differential diagnosis can usually be made from the histological examination of the biopsy of the tissues, but depends primarily on the characteristic clinical disorder of skin and muscle without visceral disease.

Except for signs of inflammation in the biopsy and increased serum activity to CPK or other sarcoplasmic enzymes, there are no characteristic laboratory abnormalities. The EMG usually shows myopathic abnormalities and, in addition, there may be evidence of increased irritability of muscle.

Course. The course of the disease may be progressive but long remissions and complete arrest are not uncommon. In the severe form of the disease, the mortality rate is high and weakness and atrophy may persist as a residual in the recovered cases. Subcutaneous calcinosis may be a serious problem, especially in children who survive childhood dermatomyositis.

Treatment. There is no specific treatment. Analgesics are administered for the pain. Physiotherapy, baking, massage and passive movements are of value. After the acute stage has subsided, manipulation under anesthesia or tenotomies may be necessary to correct deformities produced by contracture of the muscles. Prednisone is effective in the production of remissions in some, but by no means all, of the cases. Immunosuppressive drugs have been tried when steroids fail, but are not always successful either. Diphosphonates may be effective in preventing the extension of calcinosis.

REFERENCES

Banker, B. R., and Victor, M.: Dermatomyositis (Systemic Angiopathy) of Childhood, Medicine, *45*, 261, 1966.

Banker, B. Q.: Dermatomyositis of Childhood. Ultrastructural Alterations of Muscle and Intramuscular Blood Vessels, J. Neuropath. Exp. Neurol., *34*, 46, 1975.

Barnes, B. E. M.: Dermatomyositis and Malignancy. A Review of the Literature, Ann. Intern. Med., *84*, 68, 1976.

Bohan, A., and Peter, J. B.: Polymyositis and Dermatomyositis, N. Engl. J. Med., *292*, 344 and 403, 1975.

Christianson, H. B., Brunsting, L. A., and Perry, H. O.: Dermatomyositis: Unusual Features, Complications, and Treatment, Arch. Dermat., *74*, 581, 1956.

Cram, R. L., et al.: Diphosphonate Treatment of Calcinosis Universalis, N. Engl. J. Med., *285*, 1912, 1971.

Everett, M. A., and Curtis, A. C.: Dermatomyositis: A Review of Nineteen Cases in Adolescents and Children, Arch. Intern. Med., *100*, 70, 1957.

Hashimoto, K., Robinson, L., Velayos, E., and Niizuma, K.: Dermatomyositis. Electron Microscopic, Immunologic and Tissue Culture Studies of Paramyxovirus-like Inclusions, Arch. Derm., *103*, 120, 1971.

Henson, R. A., Russell, D. S., and Wilkinson, M.: Carcinomatous Neuropathy and Myopathy. A Clinical and Pathological Study, Brain, *77*, 82, 1954.

Jerusalem, F., et al.: Morphometric Analysis of Skeletal Muscle Capillary Ultrastructure in Inflammatory Myopathies, J. Neurol. Sci., *23*, 391, 1974.

Metzger, A. L., et al.: Polymyositis and Dermatomyositis: Combined Methotrexate and Corticosteroid Therapy, Ann. Intern. Med., *81*, 182, 1974.

Penn, A. S., Schotland, D. L., and Rowland, L. P.: Immunology of Muscle Disease, Res. Publ. Assoc. Res. Nerv. Ment. Dis., *49*, 215, 1971.

Rowland, L. P., Clark, C., and Olarte, M.: Therapy for Dermatomyositis and Polymyositis. In Griggs, R. C., Moxley, R. T. (Eds.). *Treatment of Neuromuscular Disease.* Adv. Neurol., *17*, 63, 1977.

Schwartz, M. I., et al.: Interstitial Lung Disease in Polymyositis and Dermatomyositis, Medicine, *55*, 89, 1976.

Sharp, G. C., et al.: Mixed Connective Tissue Disease: an Apparently Distinct Rheumatic Disease Syndrome Associated with an Antibody to Extractable Nuclear Antigen, Am. J. Med., *52*, 148, 1972.

Walton, J. N., and Adams, R. D.: *Polymyositis*, Baltimore, Williams & Wilkins, 1958, 280 pp.

Polymyositis

The exact position of polymyositis in the spectrum of muscular disorders is not clear but in view of the nature of the pathological changes in the muscles, it would be reasonable to consider it a variation of dermatomyositis or one of the collagen diseases in which involvement of the skin or other organs is minimal or absent. However, there almost certainly are other etiologies. In some cases a typical syndrome of acute polymyositis is part of systemic infections with influenza or other viruses, toxoplasma, or trichina. Sometimes, polymyositis may follow administration of drugs, such as penicillamine. Chronic hypokalemia of any cause may induce similar changes in muscle. The term polymyositis is often restricted to cases in which such etiology is not recognized, but among the "idiopathic" disorders, the causal factors are also likely to be diverse. In some of the patients the myositis develops in association with carcinoma of lung, breast or other organs of the body. Polymyositis is one of the most common disorders of muscle. It is rated by some as second only to the dystrophies. It may occur at any age, but it is most common in the fourth to seventh decades of life. It is more common in the female than in the male.

Pathology. The pathological changes include focal or diffuse degeneration of muscle fibers, basophilia of some of the fibers and infiltration of the fibers and perivascular spaces with lymphocytes and plasma cells (Fig. 151).

Symptoms and Signs. The symptoms and signs are usually of subacute onset. The girdle muscles are most frequently affected, but the muscles of the distal portion of the extremities may be involved. Dysphagia is a frequent manifestation and slight or moderate weakness of the facial muscles may be present. Muscular pain or tenderness is present in over 50% of the cases. Cutaneous manifestations are present in those patients in whom the myositis is a feature of dermatomyositis or one of the other collagen diseases.

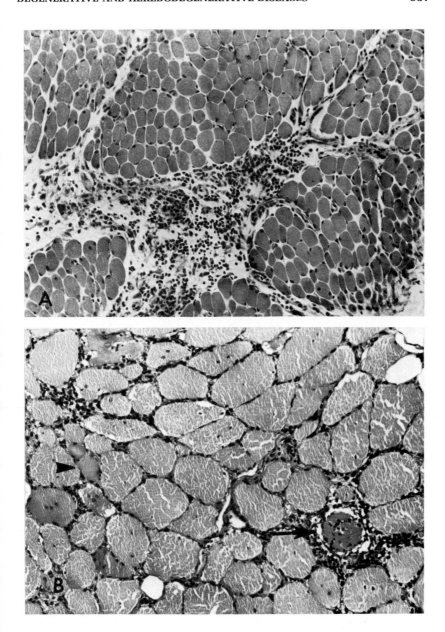

Figure 151. *(A)* Childhood form of dermatomyositis. Mononuclear inflammatory cells are seen chiefly in the perimysium. Atrophic muscle fibers are more frequent at the periphery of fascicles. Magnification, ×150. *(B)* Polymyositis. Mononuclear inflammatory cells are present in the endomysium and surround a single necrotic fiber (arrow) undergoing phagocytosis. Arrow head indicates a basophilic, regenerating fiber. Magnification, ×400.

Laboratory Data. The erythrocyte sedimentation rate is increased in about 40% of the cases, and the gamma globulin content of the serum is increased in 20%. The serum creatine phosphokinase and other enzymes are increased in the majority. The electromyogram shows changes characteristic of myositis in 50% and those of "myopathy" in another 30%. Biopsy of the muscles will show significant changes in most cases.

Differential Diagnosis. Polymyositis must be differentiated from other conditions with muscular weakness. The differential is not difficult when the characteristic clinical history and laboratory findings are present and when the results of muscle biopsy are positive. Many other conditions are associated with myopathy in adults (Table 84).

Course and Treatment. The course of patients with polymyositis is quite variable. The exact mortality rate of untreated cases is not known, but the myopathy is usually less severe than in cases with rash. In some patients the disease runs a slow course with remissions and exacerbations, and in some, spontaneous remissions appear to be permanent. It is more common, however, for the disease, if untreated, to pursue a chronic downhill course with ultimate incapacitation.

The only effective treatment is with the adrenal corticosteroids. The optimum dose is that required to relieve the symptoms and to reduce the serum enzyme levels to normal. The dosage can be gradually reduced after a period of two to three weeks and continued at the level required to relieve the patients of their weakness (usually 7.5 to 15

Table 84.   Differential Diagnosis of The Clinical Syndrome of Polymyositis: Acquired Myopathies

Infections	*Drug-Induced Myopathies*
Trichinosis	Steroids
Toxoplasmosis	Chloroquine
Cysticercosis	Emetine
Viruses (?)	Plasmocid
Collagen Diseases	*Miscellaneous*
Systemic lupus erythematosus	Sarcoidosis
Rheumatoid arthritis	Carcinoma
Progressive systemic sclerosis	Malabsorption syndrome
Giant-cell arteritis	Thymoma
Sjögren's syndrome	Alcoholism
	Amyloidosis
Endocrine Disorders	Senility
Hyperthyroidism	Chronic hypokalemia
Hypothyroidism	
Hyperadrenocorticism	
Hyperparathyroidism	
Osteomalacia	

mg daily). Occasionally the treatment can be temporarily or permanently withdrawn. As in dermatomyositis, immunosuppressive drugs are being tried in cases which do not respond to steroids.

REFERENCES

Chon, S. M., and Gutmann, L.: Picornavirus-like Crystals in Subacute Polymyositis, Neurology, 20, 205, 1970.
Coers, C., Telerman-Toppet, N., and Cremer, M.: Regressive Vacuolar Myopathy in Steatorrhea, Arch. Neurol., 24, 217, 1971.
Devere, R., and Bradley, W. G.: Polymyositis. Its Presentation, Morbidity, and Mortality, Brain, 98, 637, 1975.
Dietzman, D. E., et al.: Acute Myositis Associated with Influenza B Infection, Pediatr., 57, 255, 1976.
Floyd, M., et al.: Myopathy in Chronic Renal Failure, Quart. J. Med., 43, 509, 1974.
Haslock, D. I., Wright, V., and Harriman, D. G. F.: Neuromuscular Disorders in Rheumatoid Arthritis, Quart. J. Med., 39, 335, 1970.
Medsger, T. A., Jr., Robinson, H., and Masi, A. T.: Factors Affecting Survivorship in Polymyositis, Arth., Rheum., 14, 249, 1971.
Perkoff, G. T.: Alcoholic Myopathy, Ann Rev. Med., 22, 125, 1971.
Samuels, B. S., and Rietschel, R. L.: Polymyositis and Toxoplasmosis, J.A.M.A., 235, 60, 1976.
Schott, G. D., and Wills, M. R.: Muscle Weakness in Osteomalacia, Lancet, 1, 626, 1976.
Schraeder, P. L., Peters, H. A., and Dahl, D. S.: Polymyositis and Penicillamine, Arch. Neurol., 27, 456, 1972.
Siegel, R. C.: Scleroderma, Med. Clin. N. A., 61, 283, 1977.
Silverstein, A., and Siltzbach, L. E.: Muscle Involvement in Sarcoidosis, Arch. Nerve, 21, 235, 1969.
Thompson, J. M., et al.: Skeletal Muscle Involvement in Systemic Sclerosis, Ann. Rheum. Dis., 28, 281, 1969.

Myositis Ossificans

The identifying characteristic of this rare disorder is the deposition of true bone in subcutaneous tissue and along fascial planes in muscle. McKusick believes that the primary disorder is in connective tissue and prefers to call the disorder "fibrodysplasia ossificans," rather than its traditional name, which implies a disease of muscle. Nevertheless, in some cases there are myopathic changes in muscle biopsy or electromyogram, and occasionally the serum enzymes are increased.

Symptoms start in the first year or two of life in the majority of cases. Transient and localized swellings of the neck and trunk are the first abnormality. Later, minor bruises are followed by the deposition of solid material beneath the skin and within muscles. Plates and bars of material may be seen and felt in the limbs (Fig. 152), paraspinal tissues, and abdominal wall. These concretions are readily visible on radiographic examination, and when they cross joints, a deforming ankylosis results. The cranial muscles are spared but the remainder of the body may be encased in bone. The extent of disability depends upon

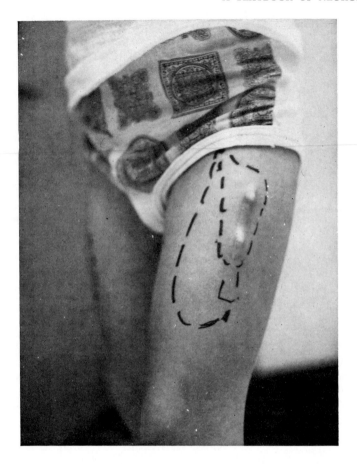

Figure 152. Ossification of muscle biopsy scar in boy with myositis ossificans. The outer border of marks indicates extent of spontaneous ossification.

the extent of ossification, which varies considerably. No abnormality of calcium metabolism has been detected.

Almost all cases are sporadic, but it is suspected that the disease is inherited because minor skeletal abnormalities occur in almost all patients, and these abnormalities seem to be transmitted in the family in an autosomal dominant pattern. The most common deformity is a short great toe (microdactyly) but curved fingers (clinodactyly) and other digital variations are also seen. Restricted ossification at the site of single severe injury may also occur in otherwise normal adults, with no apparent genetic tendency.

In the past, there was no effective treatment, but the recent introduction of diphosphonates has given promise. These compounds seem to prevent the deposition of bone in the pathologic areas without interfering with normal growth. They do not correct established pathologic ossification, however, and the long-range hazards of the drugs are not known.

REFERENCES

Bassett, C. A. L., et al.: Diphosphonates in the Treatment of Myositis Ossificans, Lancet, *2*, 845, 1969.

Frame, B., et al.: Polyostotic Fibrous Dysplasia and Myositis Ossificans Progressiva. A Report of Coexistence, Am. J. Dis. Child., *124*, 120, 1972.

Lutwak, L.: Myositis Ossificans Progressiva, Am. J. Med., *37*, 269, 1964.

Russell, R. G. G., et al.: Treatment of Myositis Ossificans Progressiva with a Diphosphonate, Lancet, *1*, 10, 1972.

Sitzmann, F. C., and Pfaff, U.: Beitrag zum Krankheitsbild der Myositis Ossificans Progressiva, Klin. Padiat., *186*, 384, 1974.

Chapter 7

Metabolic Diseases

HARRY H. WHITE, M.D.

DISEASES DUE TO INBORN METABOLIC DEFECTS

The interest in and study of the inborn errors of metabolism now encompass all disciplines of medical practice. The frequency of these diseases is increasing, mainly due to the interest that has been manifested in them and the availability of biochemical methods for their detection. The majority of these genetically determined diseases become manifest during infancy and childhood and exert a deleterious effect on the growth and development of the nervous system. Mental retardation and seizures are frequent symptoms in many of the multitude of disorders included within the category of inborn errors of metabolism. A detailed biochemical study of these individually rare molecular diseases has taught invaluable lessons concerning normal metabolic events. An understanding of the disturbed metabolism in a particular disease has, in some cases, led to the development of a rational form of therapy for the patient and provided the basis for scientific genetic counseling of the family. It is likely that many of the heredodegenerative diseases of the nervous system will eventually become understandable in terms of their molecular defect and that the rapid advances currently being made in biochemical genetics will soon provide more effective methods of treatment for these patients. Prevention of some genetically-determined diseases has become possible through biochemical studies performed on tissues obtained by amniocentesis, followed by termination of the pregnancy.

No attempt is made to cover the subject comprehensively in this chapter and only the more common entities are discussed.

REFERENCES

Brady, R. O.: Inherited Metabolic Disease of the Nervous System, Science, 193, 733, 1976.
Brady, R. O., Pentcheu, P. G., and Gal, A. E.: Investigations in Enzyme Replacement Therapy in Lipid Storage Diseases, Fed. Proc., 34, 1310, 1975.
Gaull, G. E., et al.: Pathogenesis of Brain Dysfunction in Inborn Errors of Amino Acid Metabolism, in Gaull, G. E. (Ed.): Biology of Brain Dysfunction, Vol. 3, New York, Plenum Press, 1975, p. 47.

Holliday, M. A., et al.: Special Diets for Infants with Inborn Errors of Amino Acid Metabolism, Pediatr., *57*, 783, 1976.

Kolodny, E. H.: Lysosomal Storage Diseases, N. Engl. J. Med., *294*, 1217, 1976.

Menkes, J. H.: Disorders of Amino Acid Metabolism, in Cohen, M. M. (Ed.): *Biochemistry of Neural Disease*, Hagerstown, Harper & Row, 1975, p. 47.

Milunsky, A.: Prenatal Diagnosis of Genetic Disorders, N. Engl. J. Med., *295*, 377, 1976.

Scriver, C. R., and Rosenberg, L. E.: *Aminoacid Metabolism and its Disorders*, Philadelphia, W. B. Saunders Co., 1973, p. 491.

Disorders of Amino Acid Metabolism

Phenylketonuria. "Classical" phenylketonuria is an inborn error in the metabolism of the amino acid, phenylalanine, due to a deficiency of the enzyme phenylalanine hydroxylase in the liver. It is characterized by the development in early infancy of mental retardation, convulsive seizures and other neurological signs. The classical form of the disease must be distinguished from other forms of *hyperphenylalanemia* without *phenylketonuria*. A "mild" variant form with relaxed phenylalanine tolerance and a "transient" form of phenylketonuria are also recognized, indicating the genetic heterogenelity of hyperphenylalanemia.

Pathology and Pathogenesis. Phenylalanine is normally metabolized to tyrosine. When there is a deficiency of phenylalanine hydroxylase, various abnormal metabolites such as phenylpyruvic acid, phenyllactic acid and ortho-hydroxphenylacetic acid are excreted in the urine. There are no constant pathologic findings in the nervous system or other organs although Oteruelo has recently described various inclusions in the oligodendroglial cells thought to be specific for phenylketonuria. Localized or diffuse areas of demyelinization or retarded myelination have been observed in a few cases.

Incidence. The gene involved in the transmission of the disease is a recessive one and the affected individual is homozygous for the gene. The disease is estimated to occur once in every 20,000 births, and approximately one person in every 70 in the United States is a carrier. One per cent of the patients in institutions for the feebleminded are affected. There is no difference in the incidence of the disease in the two sexes. Affected infants are usually normal at birth but develop signs of the disease within the first few weeks of life.

Symptoms and Signs. These include feeblemindedness, usually at the level of idiocy but low normal levels have been reported in a few cases, convulsive seizures, and focal neurological signs such as ataxia, athetoid movements, tremors, and hyperactive reflexes. Convulsive seizures occur in more than one third of the patients. These may be of the grand mal type or there may be minor seizures characterized by brief lapses and quick jerks of the trunk or extremities (infantile spasms). In addition to the neurological findings, there is a tendency for the skin to be light colored and subject to various types of eruption, particularly eczema. The infants are said to have a musty odor. A few cases have been reported in which the mental development is normal and behavior disorders may occur as the only manifestation of the disease.

Laboratory Data. There is an increase in the phenylalanine content of the serum and the presence of phenylketones in the urine. The electroencephalogram is abnormal in the majority of the patients, even in the absence of clinical seizures. The abnormality is frequently of the type described by the term hypsarrhythmia.

Course and Prognosis. Physical development is usually normal but if untreated the mental retardation is permanent. The vast majority of the patients are confined to institutions for the feebleminded. There is a tendency for the convulsive seizures to decrease in frequency with age.

Diagnosis. The diagnosis may be suspected by the demonstration of hyperphenylalaninemia in the newborn period by a number of different biochemical screening methods. A precise diagnosis of classical phenylketonuria, however, depends upon the quantitative determinations of serum phenylalanine and tyrosine and the demonstration of phenylketones (phenylpyruvic acid and ortho-hydroxyphenylacetic acid) in the urine. Sustained serum values greater than 1 mM of phenylalanine while on a normal dietary intake of phenylalanine and normal tyrosine levels after a challenge with phenylalanine are present in the majority of cases. The ferric chloride test on urine has proved to be unreliable because of the occurrence of false negative results. The quantitative tests should be performed in infants when the diagnosis is suspected because early and carefully monitored dietary treatment is essential for the prevention of mental retardation.

Treatment. The only practical method of treatment of phenylketonuria at present is restriction of phenylalanine in the diet. The administration of a diet low in phenylalanine will eliminate the seizures or reduce their frequency with an accompanying improvement in the electroencephalogram. The focal neurological signs tend to disappear and there is an improvement in the mental state. The developing nervous system is particularly vulnerable to the abnormal metabolites, and the end results with regard to mental development are in part related to the age of the infant when treatment is started. It may be possible to discontinue the treatment after the fourth or fifth year of life although adequate studies to make this determination are not available. Improvement in the behavior disorder of retarded phenylketonurics is sometimes possible with prolonged dietary treatment.

Early detection and dietary control of the disease have increased the number of homozygous phenylketonuric women who are of normal intelligence when reaching the childbearing age. The harmful effects of maternal hyperphenylalaninemia in the heterozygous offspring include mental retardation, microcephaly, seizures and congenital heart defects. This damage results from the excessive transport of phenylalanine or other metabolites across the placenta to the developing fetus. A diet low in phenylalanine but sufficient to support a normal pregnancy must be utilized in the pregnant phenylketonuric to prevent this harmful effect.

REFERENCES

Barranger, J. A.: The Implications of Multiple Forms of Phenylalanine Hydroxylase in Phenylketonuria and Related Diseases of Phenylalanine Metabolism, Biochem. Med., 15, 55, 1976.

Blaskovics, M.E., Schaeffler, G. E., and Hack, S.: Phenylalanaemia: Differential Diagnosis, Arch. Dis. Child., 49, 835, 1974.

Brown, E. S., and Waisman, H. A.: Mental Retardation in Four Offspring of a Hyperphenylalaninemic Mother, Pediatr., 48, 401, 1971.

Holtzman, N. A., Welcher, D. W., and Mellits, E. D.: Termination of Restricted Diet in Children with Phenylketonuria: A Randomized Controlled Study, N. Engl. J. Med., 293, 1121, 1975.

Kaufman, S.: The Phenylalanine Hydroxylating System in Phenylketonuria and its Variants, Biochem. Med., 15, 42, 1976.

Kaufman, S., et al.: Phenylketonuria Due to a Deficiency of Dihydropteridine Reductase, N. Engl. J. Med., 293, 785, 1975.

Oteruelo, F. T.: "PKU Bodies": Characteristic Inclusions in the Brain in Phenylketonuria, Acta Neuropath., 36, 295, 1976.

Perry, T. L., et al.: Unrecognized Adult Phenylketonuria, N. Engl. J. Med., 289, 395, 1973.

Scriver, C. R., and Rosenberg, L. E.: Amino Acid Metabolism and its Disorders, Philadelphia, W. B. Saunders Co., 1973, p. 290.

Maple Syrup Urine Disease. Maple syrup urine disease (branched-chain ketoaciduria) is a genetic disorder characterized by anorexia, vomiting, alternating periods of hypertonicity and flaccidity and convulsions appearing during the first week of life. The illness progresses rapidly to decerebrate rigidity and coma, with death occurring during the first month of life. The fundamental defect is an inability to metabolize the keto acids of the branched-chain amino acids leucine, isoleucine and valine. The accumulation of the ketoacids in the urine is responsible for the maple syrup odor. The pathological changes are characterized by a defect in myelin formation with areas of spongy degeneration in the white matter of the cerebral hemispheres. The early institution of a synthetic diet low in the branched-chain amino acids has resulted in a normal growth and development in some cases. Intermittent, intermediate and thiamine-responsive forms of the disease have been reported.

REFERENCES

Crome, L., and Stern, J.: Pathology of Mental Retardation, 2nd. ed., Edinburgh, Churchill Livingstone, 1972, p. 361.

Hambraeus, L., Westphal, O., and Hagberg, B.: Ketotic Hypoglycemia Associated with Transient Branched-Chain Aminoacidemia, Acta Paediat. Scand., 61, 81, 1972.
Kalyanaraman, K., et al.: Maple Syrup Urine Disease (Branched-chain Keto-aciduria) Variant Type Manifesting as Hyperkinetic Behaviour and Mental Retardation, J. Neurol. Sci., 15, 209, 1972.
Scriver, C. R., and Rosenberg, L. E.: Amino Acid Metabolism and its Disorders, Philadelphia, W. B. Saunders Co., 1973, p. 256.
Zee, D. S., Freeman, J. M., and Holtzman, N. A.: Ophthalmoplegia in Maple Syrup Urine Disease, J. Pediatr., 84, 113, 1974.

Hartnup Disease. In 1956 Baron and co-workers described a disease characterized by attacks of cerebellar ataxia, pellagra-like skin rash and psychiatric disturbances in 4 of 8 children in a first-cousin marriage. Over fifty cases have been reported. The basic abnormality is a defect of amino acid transport into the cells of the small intestine and the proximal renal tubules. A renal aminoaciduria of tryptophan, certain neutral amino acids and an excess of urinary indoles are present. Improvement in the dermatitis and neurological signs has usually followed treatment with nicotinamide.

REFERENCES

Baron, D. N., et al.: Hereditary Pellagra-Like Skin Rash with Temporary Cerebellar Ataxia, Constant Renal Amino-Aciduria, and other Bizarre Chemical Features, Lancet, 2, 421, 1956.
Jepson, J. B.: Hartnup Disease, Chapter 61, page 1486, in The Metabolic Basis of Inherited Disease, 3rd ed., J. B. Stanbury, J. B. Wyngaarden, and D. S. Fredrickson (Eds.), New York, The Blakiston Division, McGraw-Hill Book Co., 1972.
Scriver, C. R., and Rosenberg, L. E.: Amino Acid Metabolism and its Disorders, Philadelphia, W. B. Saunders Co., 1973, p. 187.
Tahmousch, A. J., et al.: Hartnup Disease, Arch. Neurol., 33, 797, 1976.
Wilcken, B., Yu, J. S., and Brown, D. A.: Natural History of Hartnup Dsiease, Arch. Dis. Child., 52, 38, 1977.

Homocystinuria (Cystathionine Synthase Deficiency). This inborn error of the metabolism of the sulfur-containing amino acid methionine is characterized by mental retardation and subluxation of the lens. Other features of the disease include: fine hair, malar flush, livedo or cyanosis of the skin, genu valgum, pes cavus and other skeletal changes, systemic (including cerebral) vascular thrombosis and convulsions.

Intimal thickening, necrosis of the media with dilatation and thrombosis are found in the large arteries such as the coronary, renal, subclavian, iliac and carotid. The significant laboratory abnormality is the presence of elevated plasma concentrations of methionine and homocystine and by the excretion of homocystine in the urine.

Both sexes are affected and the mode of inheritance is through an autosomal recessive gene. The symptoms make their appearance in early childhood. The mental retardation is usually of a severe or moderately severe degree but normal mental development has been reported in a number of cases. Some of the reported patients are living at ages of forty-five years or greater, but death during the first or second decade of life is not uncommon. Death usually is due to coronary thrombosis or thrombosis of cerebral arteries or veins. Although the biochemical abnormalities may be reversed by a low-methionine diet or administration of pyridoxine in some cases, the efficacy of these treatments for improvement of the clinical condition is unproven. Other forms of "homocystinuria" due to acquired and inherited blocks of metabolism are discussed by Scriver and Rosenberg.

REFERENCES

Fleisher, L. D., et al.: Homocystinuria: Investigations of Cystathionine Synthase in Cultured Fetal Cells and the Prenatal Determination of Genetic Status, J. Pediatr., 85, 677, 1974.
Freeman, J. M., Finkelstein, J. D., and Mudd, S. H.: Folate-Responsive Homocystinuria and "Schizophrenia," N. Engl. J. Med., 292, 491, 1975.
Gaull, G., Sturman, J. A., and Schaffner, F.: Homocystinuria Due to Cystathionine Synthase Deficiency: Enzymatic and Ultrastructural Studies, J. Pediatr., 84, 381, 1974.
Scriver, C. R., and Rosenberg, L. E.: Amino Acid Metabolism and its Disorders, Philadelphia, W. B. Saunders Co., 1973, p. 207.
Uhlemann, E. R., et al.: Platelet Survival and Morphology in Homocystinuria Due to Cystathionine Synthase Deficiency, N. Engl. J. Med., 295, 1283, 1976.
Uhlendorf, B. W., Conerly, E. B., and Mudd, S. H.: Homocystinuria: Studies in Tissue Culture, Pediat. Res., 7, 645, 1973.

Oculo-Cerebral-Renal Syndrome of Lowe. In 1952, Lowe, Terrey and MacLachlan described a syndrome characterized by involvement of the eye, kidney and the nervous system associated with a generalized aminoaciduria. The amino acid concentration of the serum is normal and it is assumed that the aminoaciduria is due to a renal transport defect. Since the original report more than 50 cases have been reported. The disease occurs in male infants and the inheritance is consistent with a sex-linked recessive pattern. The neurological symptoms in-

Table 85.   Clinical Manifestations of Lowe's Syndrome

(After Chutorian and Rowland, Neurology, 1966)

	Number abnormal/ Number described
Male sex	46/46
Mental deficiency	46/46
Glaucoma or cataract, or both	46/46
Hypotonia (without paresis)	38/38
Areflexia or marked hyporeflexia	29/32
Retarded weight and stature	40/42
Rickets	20/32
Cryptorchidism	16/20

clude mental retardation, convulsions, hypotonia of the muscles and a loss of reflexes. Other symptoms include cataracts, glaucoma, cryptorchidism and evidence of rickets (Table 85). The mental retardation is usually of severe degree and the affected individuals usually die in infancy or early childhood. The nature of the fundamental defect is unknown and no specific treatment is available.

REFERENCES

Abbasi, V., Lowe, C. U., and Calcagno, P. L.: Oculo-Cerebral-Renal Syndrome. A Review, Am. J. Dis. Child., 115, 45, 1968.
Chutorian, A., and Rowland, L. P.: Lowe's Syndrome, Neurology, 16, 115, 1966.
Garzuly, F., et al.: Morbid Changes in Lowe's Oculo-Cerebro-Renal Syndrome, Neuropaediatrie, 4, 304, 1973.
Kornfeld, M., Snyder, R. D., MacGee, J., and Appenzeller, O.: The Oculo-Cerebral-Renal Syndrome of Lowe, Arch. Neurol., 32, 103, 1975.
Lowe, C. U., Terrey, M., and MacLachlan, E. A.: Organic Aciduria, Decreased Renal Ammonia Production, Hydrophthalmos, and Mental Retardation, Am. J. Dis. Child., 83, 164, 1952.
Rosenblatt, D., and Holmes, L. B.: Development of Arthritis in Lowe's Syndrome, J. Pediatr., 84, 924, 1974.

DISORDERS OF PURINE METABOLISM

Hyperuricemia, Mental Retardation and Self-Mutilation Syndrome (Lesch-Nyhan Syndrome). In 1964, Lesch and Nyhan described two brothers with hyperuricemia, mental retardation, choreoathetosis and self-destructive biting of the lips and fingers. Many additional cases have since been described, all in males, and the disease appears to be inherited in an X-linked recessive manner. The basic defect is the absence of an enzyme of purine metabolism, hypoxanthine-guanine phosphoribosyltransferase in all body tissues. As a result of this enzyme deficiency the rate of purine biosynthesis increases and the end product of purine metabolism, uric acid, reaches high levels in blood, urine, and cerebrospinal fluid. Uric acid deposits in the kidneys and joints may result in a progressive nephropathy and gout. The neurological symptoms include severe mental retardation, spasticity, and choreoathetosis developing in the first year of life. The characteristic self-mutilating behavior appears around the second to third year. Death usually results from renal failure but may be delayed until the second or third decade of life. Treatment with allopurinol is beneficial for the renal complications but has no effect on the neurological symptoms. The presence of mild mental retardation or cerebellar ataxia has been associated with a partial deficiency of the enzyme. Hyperuricemia and cerebellar ataxia have also occurred in family members with normal levels of the enzyme.

REFERENCES

deBruyn, C. H. M. M.: Hypoxanthine-guanine Phosphoribosyl Transferase Deficiency, Hum. Genet., 31, 127, 1976.

Emmerson, B. T., and Thompson, L.: The Spectrum of Hypoxanthine-guanine Phosphoribosyltransferase Deficiency, Quart. J. Med., 42, 427, 1973.

Nyhan, W. L.: The Lesch-Nyhan Syndrome, Ann. Rev. Med., 24, 41, 1973.

————: Disorders of Nucleic Acid Metabolism, Chapter 7, in Gaull, G. E. (Ed.), *Biology of Brain Dysfunction*, Vol. 1, New York, Plenum Press, 1973, p. 265.

Rosenberg, A. L., et al.: Hyperuricemia and Neurologic Deficits, N. Engl. J. Med., 282, 992, 1970.

Watts, R. W. E., et al.: Clinical and Biochemical Studies on Treatment of Lesch-Nyhan Syndrome, Arch. Dis. Child., 49, 693, 1974.

DISORDERS OF LIPID METABOLISM

There are a number of diseases in which an inherited disturbance in the lipid metabolism is associated with involvement of the nervous system. In some of these the disorder primarily affects the nervous system and in others the nervous system is only secondarily involved. The latter group includes the various forms of hyperlipoproteinemias. The former group includes disorders in the metabolism of fatty acids (Refsum's disease), cholesterol (cerebrotendinous xanthomatosis), lipoproteins (Bassen-Kornzweig's syndrome and Tangier disease), and the sphingolipids (lipid storage diseases).

REFERENCES

Austin, J.: Metachromatic Leukodystrophy (Sulfatide Lipidosis), Chapter 18 in *Lysosomes and Storage Diseases* edited by H. G. Hers and F. Van Hoof, New York, Academic Press, 1973, p. 411.

Brady, R. O.: Biochemical Genetics in Neurology, Arch. Neurol., 33, 145, 1976.

————: Inherited Metabolic Diseases of the Nervous System, Science, 193, 733, 1976.

Farpour, H., and Mahloudji, M.: Familial Cerebrotendinous Xanthomatosis, Arch. Neurol., 32, 223, 1975.

Fishman, P. H., and Brady, R. O.: Biosynthesis and Function of Gangliosides, Science, 194, 906, 1976.

Grunnett, M. L., and Spilsbury, P. R.: The Central Nervous System in Fabry's Disease. Arch. Neurol., 28, 231, 1973.

Haas, L. F., Austad, W. I., and Bergin, J. D.: Tangier Disease, Brain, 97, 351, 1974.

Harcos, P., Markus, A., Peter, A., and Pucsok, J.: Intermittent Cerebral Symptoms in Type V Hyperlipoproteinemia, Eur. Neurol., 14, 241, 1976.

Hers, H. G., and Van Hoof, F. (Eds.): *Lysosomes and Storage Diseases*, New York, Academic Press, 1973, p. 666.

Kolodny, E. H.: Lysosomal Storage Diseases, N. Engl. J. Med., 294, 1217, 1976.

Lenn, N. J.: Lactosylceramidosis: Light and Electron Microscopic Observations, Neurology, 23, 791, 1973.

Maclaren, N. K., et al.: GM3 Gangliosidosis: A Novel Human Sphingolipodystrophy, Pediatr., 57, 106, 1976.

Mathew, N. T., Davis, D., Meyer, J. S., and Chander, K.: Hyperlipoproteinemia in Occlusive Cerebrovascular Disease, J.A.M.A., 232, 262, 1975.

Salen, G., Meriwether, T. W., and Nicolau, G.: Chenodeoxycholic Acid Inhibits Increased Cholesterol and Cholestanol Synthesis in Patients with Cerebrotendinous Xanthomatosis, Biochem. Med., 14, 57, 1975.

Schreiner, A., Hopen, G., and Skrede, S.: Cerebrotendinous Xanthomatosis (Cholestanolosis), Acta Neurol. Scand., 51, 405, 1975.

Suzuki, Y., and Mizuno, Y.: Juvenile Metachromatic Leukodystrophy: Deficiency of an Arylsulfatase A Component, J. Pediatr., 85, 823, 1974.

Tabira, T., Goto, I., Kuroiwa, Y., and Kikuchi, M.: Neuropatholbgical and Biochemical Studies in Fabry's Disease, Acta Neuropath., 30, 345, 1974.

Sphingolipidoses. Recent and dramatic advancements in the understanding of complex lipid biochemistry have radically altered our approach to the classification of this group of diseases. Previous classifications based upon the age of onset, the presence or absence of specific clinical features and the evolution of the disease have largely been abandoned in favor of one determined by the chemical nature of the stored lipid and delineation of the specific enzyme defect (Table 86). Assays applied to serum, leukocytes or skin biopsies have been developed to confirm the specific enzyme deficiencies and in some cases to detect the heterozygous carrier. A prenatal diagnosis of the ganglioside storage diseases is now possible by enzyme assays performed on amniotic fluid obtained by aminiocentesis. Therapy by replacement of the deficient enzyme in the gangliosidoses is currently under study and encouraging results have been obtained in the case of Fabry's disease and adult Gaucher's disease.

Tay-Sachs Disease. G_{M2}-*Gangliosidosis.* The prototype and most common variety of this group of diseases was first described by Warren Tay in 1881 and Bernard Sachs in 1887 and has been referred to as the infantile form of amaurotic familial idiocy. Tay-Sachs disease (G_{M2}-gangliosidosis, Type 1) is an autosomal recessive disorder characterized by progressive blindness, dementia and paralysis.

Pathology. Although the accumulation of lipid pigment in the liver, spleen and kidney has been reported in a few cases of Tay-Sachs disease, the pathological changes are as a rule limited to the nervous system and retina, affecting in a widespread manner the ganglion cells of the cerebrospinal and autonomic nervous systems. Grossly the brain may be small, but more commonly it is large (megalencephaly), with wide convolutions, and firm in consistency.

The microscopic pathology is primarily present in the ganglion cells. The cell body is distended by stored lipid and its cytoplasm has a reticular network (Fig. 153). The Nissl substance is absent or collected at the periphery in fine granules. The nucleus is displaced and may show varying degrees of disintegration. In the late stages of the disease there is a conspicuous loss of neurons. There is a degeneration of the dendrites and the axons become reduced in number. Demyelination is present in most cases and may become quite extensive. Astrocytes and microglial cells show proliferative changes in the late stages of the disease. With special stains lipid pigment is noted in the swollen ganglion cells, but it does not stain intensely with the usual stains for neutral fat. Electron microscopy reveals the presence of membranous cytoplasmic bodies in the involved neurons, axis cylinders, and dendrites.

Biochemistry. The material which accumulates in brain tissue in Tay-Sachs disease is an acidic glycolipid designated as G_{M2}

Table 86.   Classification of the Sphingolipidoses
(Modified from Brady, Bull. N.Y. Acad. Med., 1971 and O'Brien, N. Engl. J. Med., 1971)

Disease	Lipid Accumulated	Enzyme Defect	Major Clinical Features
G_{M2} gangliosidosis, Type 1 or B variant (Tay-Sachs)	Ganglioside G_{M2}	Hexosaminidase A	Onset 6–9 months age, dementia, blindness, hyperacusis, paralysis, cherry-red spot in macula.
G_{M2} gangliosidosis, Type 2 or O variant (Sandhoff)	Ganglioside G_{M2} plus globoside	Hexosaminidase A & B	Identical to Tay-Sachs, non-Jewish parentage.
G_{M2} gangliosidosis, Type 3 (Juvenile type)	Ganglioside G_{M2}	Partial deficiency of hexosaminidase A	Few cases published, onset 2–6 yrs. age, ataxia, seizures, dementia, pyramidal & extrapyramidal signs, death by 6–15 yrs. age.
G_{M2} gangliosidosis, AB variant	Ganglioside G_{M2}	Hexosaminidase subfraction?	Similar to Tay-Sachs.
G_{M1} gangliosidosis, Type 1 (Generalized gangliosidosis)	Ganglioside G_{M1}	G_{M1} ganglioside galactosyl hydrolase A,B,C (β-galactosidase)	Onset at birth, coarse facies, progressive mental & motor retardation, hepatosplenomegaly, marked skeletal changes, macular red spot, death by 2–3 years of age.
G_{M1} gangliosidosis, Type 2 (Juvenile type)	Ganglioside G_{M1}	G_{M1} ganglioside galactosyl hydrolase B & C (β-galactosidase)	Few cases published, onset 7–14 mos. age, progressive mental and motor deterioration, seizures, normal facies, no visceromegaly, death 3–10 years of age.
G_{M3} gangliosidosis	Ganglioside G_{M3}	G_{M3} n-acetylgalactosaminyl-transferase	Disorder of ganglioside synthesis. Single case reported, onset first days of life, unusual facies, flexor contractures of fingers, hepatosplenomegaly, seizures, hypotonia & reduced spontaneous movements, no skeletal lesions, death at 3½ mos. of age.

Niemann-Pick Disease	Sphingomyelin	Sphingomyelinase	Progressive blindness, mental deterioration, hepatosplenomegaly, macular red spot (some cases) & brownish discoloration of skin.
Gaucher's Disease	Glucocerebroside	Glucosyl ceramide-β-glucosyl hydrolase (β-glucosidase)	Failure of normal mental development, hepatosplenomegaly, motor deterioration, skeletal & hematological abnormalities.
Krabbe's Disease (globoid cell)	Galactocerebroside	Galactosyl ceramide-β-galactosyl hydrolase (β-galactosidase)	Onset first months of life, seizures, blindness, progressive motor deterioration with death 1–2 yrs. age.
Metachromatic Leukodystrophy	Sulfatide	Arylsulfatase A	Mental retardation, peripheral neuropathy, bulbar palsy, pyramidal tract signs.
Lactosyl Ceramidosis (Dawson-Stein)	Lactosyl ceramide	Lactosyl ceramide galactosyl hydrolase (β-galactosidase)	Single case reported, onset 2½ yrs., motor & mental deterioration, hepatosplenomegaly, optic atrophy, death at 50 mos. of age.
Fabry's Disease	Trihexosyl ceramide	Trihexosyl ceramide galactosyl hydrolase	Angiokeratoma of skin, renal failure, cardiac dysfunction, corneal & lenticular opacities, and peripheral neuropathy.
Farber's Disease	Ceramide	Ceramidase	Subcutaneous nodules, progressive arthropathy and psychomotor retardation.

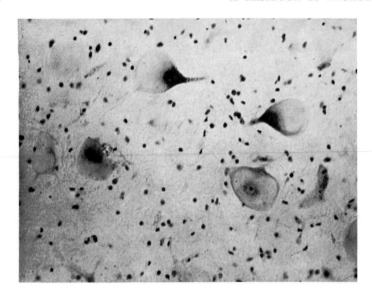

Figure 153.   Tay-Sachs disease. Ballooning of ventral horn cells
in spinal cord. (Courtesy Dr. Abner Wolf.)

ganglioside. It differs from the major monosialoganglioside found in
normal brain in that the terminal molecule of galactose is missing. The
enzyme, hexosaminidase A, is absent in brain, liver, kidney, skin,
serum, leukocytes, and cultured skin fibroblasts. The widespread
absence of this enzyme in the tissues of patients with Tay-Sachs disease
and its partial absence in the heterozygous carriers suggest that it
represents the fundamental defect of the disease.

Incidence. Tay-Sachs disease is rare and occurs predominantly in
infants of Ashkenazic Jewish parentage. The frequency of the disease is
1 in 6,000 to 10,000 births. The age of onset of symptoms in the
majority of cases is in the first six months of life.

Symptoms and Signs. The infant develops normally until the third to
sixth month of life, when weakness of the neck, trunk and extremity
muscles becomes apparent. The child cannot sit up or lift the head from
the bed. There is difficulty in turning over and objects are dropped
from the hands. The weakness increases in severity in the next few
months until there is a generalized paralysis. Coincidental with the
onset of the weakness there is a loss of vision which progresses to
complete amblyopia. The eyes are held wide open and there are roving
or rolling movements of the eyeballs. The pupils are dilated and do not
react to light. There is atrophy of the optic nerve, and an oval or circular
patch of grayish-white atrophy of the macular region of the retina, with

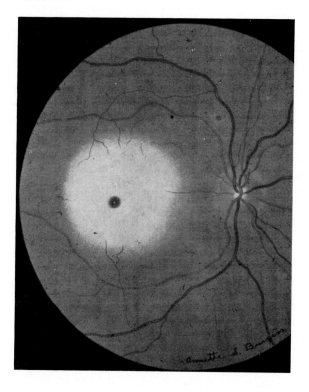

Figure 154. Tay-Sachs disease. Atrophy of macula with
cherry-red spot. (Courtesy Dr. Arnold Gold.)

a cherry-red spot in the center of the atrophic area (Fig. 154). Optic
atrophy may rarely precede the appearance of the cherry-red spot in the
retina.

With the exception of loss of vision the cranial nerves are usually
intact. Deafness may occur but more commonly the hearing is well
preserved and any auditory stimuli provokes a generalized motor
response or startled reaction. Myoclonic jerks and atypical convulsive
seizures are common.

The muscles of the trunk and extremities become progressively
weaker. Varying degrees of flaccidity and spasticity are noted. There is
generalized wasting of the muscles. In the terminal stages of the disease
the child leads a vegetative existence and may require tube feeding.
The tendon reflexes are usually exaggerated and the extensor plantar
responses of infancy persist. The disease is always fatal. Death may
occur within a few months to several years after the onset.

A small number of patients have been studied in whom the clinical
course of the disease has been identical to that of Tay-Sachs disease but

the tissues showed a total deficiency of both components of hexosaminidase, A and B. An additional biochemical feature was the accumulation of globoside in the visceral organs. This entity has been designated as G_{M2}-gangliosidosis, Type 2.

A few cases have been reported in which G_{M2}-ganglioside storage is associated with a *partial* deficiency of hexosaminidase A. The clinical course of the disease (G_{M2}-gangliosidosis, Type 3) in these patients was characterized by the onset of symptoms between two and six years of age, ataxia, seizures, progressive motor impairment, blindness and death by the sixth to fifteenth year of life.

An adult or chronic form of G_{M2}-gangliosidosis has been reported in Jewish siblings who manifested gait disorder, muscle atrophy, spasticity and dystonia. Onset occurred in childhood, running an indolent course into adulthood without producing total disability.

Laboratory Data. There are no significant changes in urine, blood or cerebrospinal fluid by conventional laboratory tests.

Diagnosis. A presumptive diagnosis of Tay-Sachs disease is made without difficulty by the typical clinical course and by examination of the fundi. G_{M2}-gangliosidosis, Type 3 may be suspected by the appearance of ataxia, seizures and dementia commencing between two to six years of age and running a protracted course. A definitive diagnosis of the specific type of G_{M2}-gangliosidoses is established by the demonstration of G_{M2} ganglioside storage in the brain and by the total or partial absence of one or both components of hexosaminidase in the tissues.

Course. The course has been discussed in connection with the various forms of the disease. The disease is fatal in all cases. As a rule the course is less rapid in the juvenile form (Type 3).

Treatment. There is no specific treatment. Reliable enzyme assay methods have been developed which will permit the prenatal diagnosis of Tay-Sachs disease on amniotic fluid and amniotic cells obtained by amniocentesis. Therapeutic abortion may be considered in those cases showing a marked deficiency of hexosaminidase A. Serum assays appear to be equally reliable in detecting the heterozygous carrier so that prevention of the disease by genetic counseling in high-risk matings is now possible.

REFERENCES

deBaecque, C. M., et al.: G_{M2}-gangliosidosis, AB variant, Acta Neuropath., 33, 207, 1975.

Brady, R. O.: The Genetic Management of Complex Lipid Metabolism, Bull. N.Y. Acad. Med., 47, 173, 1971.

Brett, E. M., et al.: Late Onset G_{M2}-Gangliosidosis, Arch. Dis. Child., 48, 775, 1973.

Dreyfus, J-C., Poenaru, L., and Svennerholm, L.: Absence of Hexosaminidase A and B in a Normal Adult, N. Engl. J. Med., 292, 61, 1975.

Fontaine, G., et al.: Gangliosidosis with Total Hexosaminidase Deficiency: Clinical, Biochemical and Ultrastructural Studies and Comparison with Conventional Cases of Tay-Sachs Disease, Acta Neuropath., 23, 118, 1973.

O'Brien, J. S.: Ganglioside-Storage Diseases, N. Engl. J. Med., *284*, 893, 1971.

Okadi, S., McCrea, M., and O'Brien, J. S.: Sandhoff's Disease (GM$_2$ Gangliosidosis Type 2): Clinical, Chemical and Enzyme Studies in Five Patients, Pediat. Res., *6*, 606, 1972.

Rapin, I., Suzuki, K., Suzuki, K., and Valsamis, M. P.: Adult (Chronic) G$_{M2}$ Gangliosidosis, Arch. Neurol., *33*, 120, 1976.

Sachs, B.: On Arrested Cerebral Development, with Special Reference to its Cortical Pathology, J. Nerv. & Ment. Dis., *14*, 541, 1887.

Spence, M. W., et al.: A New Variant of Sandhoff's Disease, Pediat. Res., *8*, 628, 1974.

Suzuki, Y., and Suzuki, K.: Partial Deficiency of Hexosaminidase Component A in Juvenile G$_{M2}$-Gangliosidosis, Neurology, *20*, 848, 1970.

Tay, W.: Symmetrical Changes in the Region of the Yellow Spot in Each Eye of an Infant, Tr. Ophth. Soc. U. Kingdom, 1, 55, 1880–81.

G$_{M1}$-Gangliosidosis. Generalized gangliosidosis (G$_{M1}$-gangliosidosis, type 1) is an inborn error of metabolism resulting in the storage of the G$_{M1}$-ganglioside in brain and the accumulation of ganglioside plus mucopolysaccharides in visceral organs. A deficiency of the enzyme G$_{M1}$ galactoside galactosyl hydrolase (beta galactosidase) A, B and C has been demonstrated in liver, kidney, spleen and brain and is thought to represent the fundamental enzymatic defect in this disease. The clinical characteristics of the disease include a progressive mental and motor deterioration evident shortly after birth, hepatosplenomegaly, peculiar coarse facies, skeletal changes similar to those in Hurler's disease, and death by the second or third year of life. A cherry-red spot in the macula has been present in some cases. MacBrinn and associates believe that the enzyme deficiency results in faulty degradation of both the G$_{M1}$ ganglioside and the mucopolysaccharide which are stored in the tissues.

A small number of cases have been studied in detail in which G$_{M1}$ ganglioside storage was present in the brain but the clinical features of the disease were unlike those in generalized gangliosidosis. The onset of the illness was between seven and fourteen months of life and characterized by a progressive mental and motor deterioration, seizures, and death by three to ten years of age. The facies were normal, no visceromegaly or retinal changes were present and skeletal changes were minor or altogether lacking. O'Brien has referred to this disease as G$_{M1}$-gangliosidosis, Type 2 and has demonstrated the absence of two beta-galactosidase isoenzymes (B and C) with preservation of beta-galactosidase A in liver tissue of an affected patient.

Another variety of G$_{M1}$-gangliosidosis has been reported by Lowden and co-workers. This child developed progressive spasticity and mental deterioration at age five. Two components of β-galactosidase were absent in leukocytes and cultured fibroblasts. The authors propose the designation, G$_{M1}$-gangliosidosis Juvenile O variant for their patient.

REFERENCES

Feldges, A., Müller, H. J., Bühler, E., and Stadler, G.: G$_{M1}$-Gangliosidosis, Helv. Paediat. Acta, 28, 511, 1973.
Fricker, H., et al.: Generalized Gangliosidosis: Acid β-Galactosidase Deficiency with Early Onset, Rapid Mental Deterioration and Minimal Bone Dysplasia, J. Neurol., 213, 273, 1976.
Lowden, J. A., et al.: Juvenile G$_{M1}$-Gangliosidosis, Arch. Neurol., 31, 200, 1974.
MacBrinn, M. C., et al.: Generalized Gangliosidosis: Impaired Cleavage of Galactose from a Mucopolysaccharide and a Glycoprotein, Science, 163, 946, 1969.
O'Brien, J. S.: Ganglioside-Storage Diseases, N. Engl. J. Med., 284, 893, 1971.
O'Brien, J. S., et al.: Spondyloepiphyseal Dysplasia, Corneal Clouding, Normal Intelligence and Acid β-Galactosidase Deficiency, Clin. Genet., 9, 495, 1976.
Patel, V., Goebel, H. H., Watanabe, I., and Zeman, W.: Studies on G$_{M1}$-Gangliosidosis, Type II, Acta Neuropath., 30, 155, 1974.
Percy, A. K., McCormick, U. M., Kabach, M. M., and Herndon, R. M.: Ultrastructure Manifestations of G$_{M1}$ and G$_{M2}$ Gangliosidosis in Fetal Tissues, Arch. Neurol., 28, 417, 1973.

Niemann-Pick Disease. Niemann-Pick disease is a heterogeneous group of clinical disorders in which distinct chemical and enzymatic differences have not been fully elucidated. Crocker has proposed a tentative separation into four groups to which a fifth, or adult form must be added (Table 87). Eighty-five per cent of cases are of the classical infantile type (Type A).

The disease (Type A) has been shown to be associated with the accumulation of sphingomyelin in brain, various visceral organs and reticuloendothelial cells. The enzyme deficiency (sphingomyelinase) reponsible for the lipid storage has been demonstrated in liver, kidney, brain, leukocytes and skin fibroblasts. The gross and microscopic changes in the nervous system are not specific or diagnostic in themselves. Lipid storage is present in the neurons, arachnoidal cells, vascular endothelium, and prominent in microglial cells of the cerebellum. The liver and spleen are enlarged due to the accumulation of lipid-containing "foam cells" which are also present in the bone marrow.

Niemann-Pick disease (Type A) becomes clinically manifest by the development of an enlarged liver and spleen in the first few months of life. Psychomotor retardation soon becomes apparent and is associated with a macular cherry-red spot in one third of cases. Deterioration of general and neurological functions is progressive and death occurs by the second or third year of age.

There is no specific treatment for the disease. The heterozygous carrier can be detected by enzyme assays performed on skin fibroblasts or leukocytes. A prenatal diagnosis can be established using amniotic fluid and fetal cells for enzymatic determinations. Callahan and Khalil have demonstrated the presence of five molecular forms of sphingo-

Table 87. Clinical and Biochemical Types of Niemann-Pick Disease
(Modified from Crocker, J. Neurochem., 1961)

Type	Lipid Accumulation	Enzyme Defect	Major Clinical Features
A (Classical infantile form)	Cerebral & visceral sphingomyelin and cholesterol	Sphingomyelinase virtually absent	Onset first year life, progressive psychomotor retardation; hepatosplenomegaly; macular red spot; death by three years of age.
B (Visceral form)	Visceral storage of sphingomyelin and cholesterol	Sphingomyelinase reduced to 10% normal	Hepatosplenomegaly; no neurological manifestations.
C (Subacute form)	Visceral storage of sphingomyelin and cholesterol	Sphingomyelinase II absent	Onset 2–4 years; hepatosplenomegaly; psychomotor retardation; seizures; macular changes; death between 5–8 years of age.
D (Nova Scotian form)	Visceral storage of lipids cholesterol > sphingomyelin	Sphingomyelinase level reduced or normal	Onset variable (early to middle childhood); hepatosplenomegaly; slowly progressive psychomotor retardation; cerebellar, pyramidal and extrapyramidal signs; death 12–20 years of age.
E (Adult form)	Visceral storage of sphingomyelin & cholesterol	Sphingomyelinase II absent (?)	Few cases reported; asymptomatic? or pulmonary insufficiency

myelinase in liver and brain. Further studies will no doubt clarify the differences seen in the various forms of the disease.

REFERENCES

Anzil, A. P., Blinzinger, K., Mehraein, P., and Dozic, S.: Niemann-Pick Disease Type C: Case Report with Ultrastructural Findings, Neuropädiatrie, 4, 207, 1973.
Brady, R. O., and King, F. M.: Niemann-Pick's Disease, Chapter 19, in H. G. Hers and F. Van Hoff (Eds.), Lysosomes and Storage Diseases, New York, Academic Press, 1973, p. 439.
Callahan, J. W., and Khalil, M.: Sphingomyelinase in Human Tissues: II. Absence of a Specific Enzyme from Liver and Brain of Niemann-Pick's Disease, Type C, Pediat. Res., 9, 908, 1975.
————: Sphingomyelinase in Human Tissues. III. Expression of Niemann-Pick Disease in Cultured Skin Fibroblasts, Pediat. Res., 9, 914, 1975.
————: Sphingomyelinases and the Genetic Defects in Niemann-Pick Disease, in B. W. Volk and L. Schneck (Eds.), Current Trends in Sphingolipidoses and Allied Disorders, New York, Plenum Press, 1976, p. 367.
Crocker, A. C.: The Cerebral Defect in Tay-Sachs Disease and Niemann-Pick Disease, J. Neurochem., 7, 69, 1961.
Fredrickson, D. S., and Sloan, H. R.: Sphingomyelin Lipidosis: Niemann-Pick Disease, Chapter 35, page 783 in The Metabolic Basis of Inherited Disease, 3rd Ed., J. B. Stanbury, J. B. Wyngaarden, and D. S. Fredrickson (Eds.), New York, The Blakiston Division, McGraw-Hill Book Co., 1972.
Gal, A. E., Brady, R. O., Hibbert, S. R., and Pentcheu, P. G.: A Practical Chromogenic Procedure for the Detection of Homozygotes and Heterozygous Carriers of Niemann-Pick Disease, N. Engl. J. Med., 293, 632, 1975.
Niemann, A.: Ein unbekanntes Krankheitsbild, Ann. pediat., 79, 1, 1914.
Pick, L., and Bielschowsky, M.: Ueber lipoidzellige Splenomegalie (Typus Niemann-Pick) und amaurotische Idiotie, Berl. Klin. Wchnschr., 16, 1631, 1927.
Rao, B. G., and Spence, M. W.: Niemann-Pick Disease Type D: Lipid Analyses and Studies on Sphingomyelinases, Ann. Neurol., 1, 385, 1977.

Gaucher's Disease. The eponym Gaucher's disease refers to a group of heterogeneous disorders which have clinical and biochemical features in common (Table 88). With few exceptions the diseases are transmitted by an autosomal recessive gene and characterized by the deposition of glucocerebroside in the reticuloendothelial cells (Gaucher cells) of the spleen, liver, bone marrow and other organs of the body including occasionally the nervous system.

Splenomegaly, anemia, thrombocytopenia, erosion of the cortices of the long bones, pathological fractures and a brownish discoloration of the skin are the common symptoms. Involvement of the nervous system is rare except in the infantile and juvenile forms of the disease. The pathological changes in the nervous system include degeneration of nerve cells, mild distension of ganglion cell cytoplasm with stored cerebroside and neuronophagia. These changes are most pronounced in the nuclei of the basal ganglia and brainstem. In infants the symptoms start in the fourth to fifth month of life with enlargement of the spleen and mental changes. The infant becomes apathetic and

Table 88. Clinical Classification of Gaucher's Disease

Type	Lipid Accumulation	Enzyme Defect	Major Clinical Features
Infantile	Glucocerebroside in liver, spleen, bone marrow and brain	Glucosyl ceramide-β-glucosyl hydrolase (β-glucosidase) 0–9% of normal levels	Onset first 6 mos. life; rapidly progressive neurological deterioration; hepatosplenomegaly; skeletal and hematological changes; death by 2 years age.
Juvenile	Glucocerebroside in viscera and brain	Glucosyl ceramide-β-glucosyl hydrolase (β-glucosidase) 10–17% of normal levels	Onset 6 mos.–1 year of life; hypersplenism followed by slowly progressive neurological deterioration; seizures; death by 8 years of age or older.
Adult	Glucocerebroside in viscera	Glucosyl ceramide-β-glucosyl hydrolase (β-glucosidase) up to 40% of normal levels	Onset late childhood, adolescence, or adulthood; hypersplenism with anemia and thrombocytopenia; skin pigmentation; erosion of long bones; course variable but usually slowly progressive. Neurological symptoms unusual.

listless, the eyes do not fix properly, the head is retracted. The muscles become hypertonic and complete paralysis ensues within a few months. Bulbar symptoms are common with laryngospasm, stridor and difficulty in swallowing. The reflexes are increased.

A deficiency of beta-glucosidase has been found in the spleen of adult cases and in both spleen and brain in the infantile form of the disease. The enzyme defect is also demonstrable in leukocytes and skin fibroblasts. Fetal cells obtained by amniocentesis contain beta-glucosidase so a prenatal diagnosis of the disease is now possible.

The hematological abnormalities frequently respond to splenectomy. Brady and associates have reported encouraging results of treatment by the infusion of highly purified human placental glucocerebrosidase into two patients with Gaucher's disease.

REFERENCES

Brady, R. O., et al.: Replacement Therapy for Inherited Enzyme Deficiency. Case of Purified Glucocerebrosidase in Gaucher's Disease, N. Engl. J. Med., *291*, 989, 1974.
King, J. O.: Progressive Myoclonic Epilepsy Due to Gaucher's Disease in an Adult, J. Neurol. Neurosurg. Psychiat., *38*, 849, 1975.
Melamed, E., Cohen, C., Soffer, D., and Lavy, S.: Central Nervous System Complication in a Patient with Chronic Gaucher's Disease, Eur. Neurol., *13*, 167, 1975.
Petrohelos, M., Tricoulis, D., Kotsiras, I., and Vouzoukos, A.: Ocular Manifestations of Gaucher's Disease, Am. J. Ophth., *80*, 1006, 1975.

Neuronal Ceroid-Lipofuscinosis (Batten's Disease). The specific familial cerebral degeneration associated with macular changes originally described by Batten has been nosologically linked to other forms of "familial amaurotic idiocy," particularly the ganglioside storage diseases. This erroneous association arose because of the presence of storage material in the brain and retina in both the gangliosidoses and neuronal ceroid-lipofuscinosis (NCL). Zeman and his associates have been instrumental in the delineation of NCL as a definite clinical-pathological entity distinct from the disorders of sphingolipid metabolism. Neuronal ceroid-lipofuscinosis is a genetically-determined group of disorders characterized by seizures, visual loss and progressive mental impairment. The majority of cases are inherited by the mutation of an autosomal recessive gene but autosomal dominant inheritance has also been documented.

Pathology. The most characteristic feature of the disease is the widespread deposit of autofluorescent lipopigments in practically all the viscera, being most prominent in the brain. Ceroid and lipofuscin pigments accumulate in the cytoplasm of astrocytes, endothelial cells and neurons of the cerebral cortex, subcortical nuceli, hypothalamus and cerebellum.

Grossly the brain is usually small. The microscopic pathology, in addition to the presence of pleomorphic lipopigment bodies, includes a marked loss of nerve cells and status spongiosus. Many nerve cells show evidence of cell damage and death with only a moderate distention of the cytoplasm by pigment.

Ultrastructural studies have revealed a wide range of variability in the size and internal structure of the lipopigment bodies. Some consist of lamellar aggregates termed curvilinear bodies. Others resemble human finger prints (fingerprint bodies) while some show a nondescript granular matrix surrounded by a limiting membrane. These lipopigment bodies disclose acid phosphatase activity and represent tertiary lysosomes or residual bodies.

The retina shows loss of rod and cone cells, degeneration of the pigment epithelial layer and the presence of lipopigments in various cell types.

Biochemistry. No consistent or significant change is found in the concentration of gangliosides in the brain. Two pigments, designated as ceroid and lipofuscin and having different chemical properties, have been isolated from the brains of affected patients. These pigments are thought to represent cross-linked polymers of the peroxides of polyunsaturated fatty acids. The biochemical abnormality resulting in the excessive accumulation of these lipid peroxides is unknown. No enzyme deficiency has been established as the primary defect responsible for the disease.

Incidence. The precise incidence of the disease is unknown but it has been estimated to occur in 1 per 100,000 population per year. The disease has been described in various racial and ethnic groups. Both sexes are affected equally.

Signs and Symptoms. The onset of the disease may occur at any age from infancy to adulthood. The clinical course is also quite variable but in general those with an early onset of seizures tend to be more rapidly progressive. Convulsions, blindness and dementia are the most prominent clinical signs and are present in almost all cases at some time in the course of the disease, regardless of the age of onset.

Various eponymic designations have traditionally been used which reflect the variable age of onset, the appearance of certain clinical features and the rapidity of the evolution of the disease (Table 89). Their continued use may be helpful in the delineation of the genetic heterogeneity which exists among the various types of NCL. It is probable that different mutant genes account for the various phenotypes.

Motor disorders consisting of spastic weakness (pyramidal tract), rigidity combined with athetosis or dystonia (extrapyramidal dysfunction), and ataxia (cerebellum) invariably appear as the disease pro-

Table 89.   Various Clinical Types of Neuronal Ceroid-Lipofuscinosis
(Modified from Zeman and Siakotos)

	Mode of Inheritance	Age of Onset	Initial Sign	Seizures	Blindness	Dementia	Fundus Changes	Course	Duration	Brain Atrophy
Santavuori or Finnish Type	Auto. Recess.	8 mos.–1½ yrs.	Arrest of mental development, occasionally hypotonia and ataxia.	Myoclonic jerks 4–10 mos. after onset. Generalized convulsions later or absent.	Early amaurosis	Most often is initial symptom	Hypopigmentation of fundus, optic atrophy, brownish discoloration of macula.	Rapidly progressive	3 yrs. to total incapacity	Severe
Jansky-Bielschowsky Type	Auto. Recess.	2–4 yrs., as late as 20 yrs.	Convulsions	Generalized seizures most commonly	Always present	Complete	Optic atrophy; retinitis pigmentosa & macular degeneration later.	Rapidly progressive	Less than 1 to about 6 yrs.	Severe
Spielmeyer-Sjögren Type	Auto. Recess.	1–8 yrs.	Blindness	Appear later in course	Complete	Moderately severe, late onset	Macular degeneration and retinitis pigmentosa	Slowly progressive	Average 11 yrs.	Commensurate with duration of illness
Kufs' Type	Auto. Recess. & Auto. Domin.	After 20 yrs.	Mental changes, occasionally seizures	Myoclonic and generalized seizures	Absent	Often minimal, sometimes complete	Usually none	Slowly progressive	5–35 yrs.	Moderate

gresses. Death usually occurs from the complications of the bedridden vegetative state of the patient in the end-stages of the disease.

Laboratory Data. Conventional laboratory tests have shown no consistent abnormalities. Vacuoles in the lymphocytes and azurophilic hypergranulation of the neutrophils have been observed in the peripheral blood in some patients. These changes are also often found in the parents and siblings of affected individuals. Ultrastructural studies of the lymphocytes and skin show the presence of lipopigment bodies. Autofluorescent material may be present in bone marrow cells. Electron microscopy of urinary sediment has revealed the presence of inclusions similar to those in the brain. Lipopigments may also be demonstrated in peripheral nerve and skeletal muscle. The leukocyte peroxidase deficiency reported by Armstrong has not been substantiated by other investigators.

The electroencephalograms show a wide range of non-specific abnormalities. The electroretinogram is abolished.

Diagnosis. The diagnosis should be considered in patients with progressive intellectual impairment, particularly when accompanied by visual failure due to macular degeneration or retinitis pigmentosa. The diagnosis can be established by the demonstration of stored lipopigments in various tissues including the peripheral lymphocytes, bone marrow, skin, peripheral nerve, skeletal muscle and urinary sediment.

Course. The disease may progress rapidly to death within one year following onset or pursue a more indolent course over ten years.

REFERENCES

Anzil, A. P., Martinius, J., and Blinzinger, K.: Follow-up Study of a Case of Generalized Ceroidlipofuscinosis of Childhood with Special Reference to the Finding of an Abnormal Serum Lecithin Fatty Acid Pattern, Neuropädiatrie, 7, 362, 1976.

Armstrong, D., et al.: Leukocyte Peroxidase Deficiency in a Family with a Dominant Form of Kuf's Disease, Science, 186, 155, 1974.

deBaecque, C.: Diagnosis of Neuronal Ceroid Lipofuscinosis by Electron Microscopy of Urinary Sediment, N. Engl. J. Med., 292, 1408, 1975.

Batten, F. E.: Cerebral Degeneration with Symmetrical Changes in the Macula in Two Members of a Family, Trans. Ophthal. Soc. U.K., 23, 386, 1903.

Boehme, D. H., Cottrell, J. C., Leonberg, S. C., and Zeman, W.: A Dominant Form of Neuronal Ceroid-Lipofuscinosis, Brain, 94, 745, 1971.

Farrell, D. F., and Sumi, M.: Skin Punch Biopsy in the Diagnosis of Juvenile Neuronal Ceroid-Lipofuscinosis, Arch. Neurol., 34, 39, 1977.

Gadoth, N., O'Croinin, P., and Butler, I. J.: Bone Marrow in the Batten-Vogt Syndrome, J. Neurol. Sci., 25, 197, 1975.

Goebel, H. H., Zeman, W., and Damaske, E.: An Ultrastructural Study of the Retina in the Jansky-Bielschowsky Type of Neuronal Ceroid-Lipofuscinosis, Amer. J. Ophth., 83, 70, 1977.

Goebel, H. H., Zeman, W., and Pilz, H.: Significance of Muscle Biopsies in Neuronal Ceroid-Lipofuscinoses, J. Neurol., Neurosurg., Psychiat., 38, 985, 1975.

————.: Ultrastructural Investigations of Peripheral Nerves in Neuronal Ceroid-Lipofuscinoses (NCL), J. Neurol., 213, 295, 1976.

Haltia, M., Rapola, J., Santavuori, P.: Infantile Type of So-Called Neuronal Ceroid-Lipofuscinosis, Acta Neuropath., *26*, 157, 1973.

Haltia, M., Rapola, J., Santavuori, P., and Keranen, A.: Infantile Type of So-Called Neuronal Ceroid-Lipofuscinosis. Morphological and Biochemical Studies, J. Neurol. Sci., *18*, 269, 1973.

Hittner, H. M., and Zeller, R. S.: Ceroid-Lipofuscinosis (Batten Disease), Arch. Ophth., *93*, 178, 1975.

Jakob, H., and Kolkmann, F. W.: Zur Pigment-variante der Adulten Form der Amaurotis-chen Idiotie (KUFS), Acta Neuropath., *26*, 225, 1973.

Lyon, B. B.: Peripheral Nerve Involvement in Batten-Spielmeyer-Vogt's Disease, J. Neurol. Neurosurg. Psychiat., *38*, 1975, 1975.

MacLeod, P. M., and Dolman, C. L.: Neuronal Ceroid-Lipofuscinosis, Arch. Neurol., *34*, 199, 1977.

Pilz, H., Goebel, H. H. and O'Brien, J. S.: Isoelectric Enzyme Patterns of Leukocyte Peroxidase in Normal Controls and Patients with Neuronal Ceroid-Lipofuscinosis, Neuropädiatrie, *7*, 261, 1976.

Santavuori, P., Haltia, M., Rapola, J. and Raitta, C.: Infantile Type of So-Called Neuronal Ceroid-Lipofuscinosis. A Clinical Study of 15 Patients, J. Neurol. Sci., *18*, 257, 1973.

Zeman, W., and Dyken, P.: Neuronal Ceroid-Lipofuscinosis (Batten's Disease): Relation-ship to Amaurotic Family Idiocy? Pediatr., *44*, 570, 1969.

Zeman, W., and Siakotos, A. N.: The Neuronal Ceroid-Lipofuscinoses, Chapter 23 in H.G. Hers and F. Van Hoof (Eds.), *Lysosomes and Storage Diseases*, New York, Academic Press, 1973, p. 519.

Refsum's Disease (Hereditary Ataxic-Polyneuritis). Refsum in 1946 described a syndrome characterized by a diffuse hypertrophic polyneuritis, retinitis pigmentosa, cerebellar ataxia, deafness, electrocardiographic changes, epiphysial dysplasia with skeletal abnormalities, ichthyosis, and an increased protein content in the cerebrospinal fluid. It has been demonstrated that the disease is due to an inborn error of lipid metabolism with storage 3,7,11,15,-tetramethyl hexadeconoic acid (phytanic acid) in the liver, kidney, muscles, neural tissues and other organs of the body. The enzyme deficiency appears to involve the initial step in degradation of phytanic acid: the alpha hydroxylation of phytanic to pristanic acid.

Approximately 50 cases have been reported. The disease is inherited through an autosomal recessive gene. The symptoms, usually those due to the polyneuritis or disease of the retina, commonly make their appearance in the first or second decade of life. The disease is slowly progressive leading to incapacitation, but may be punctuated by incomplete remissions. Periods of clinical deterioration are often associated with intercurrent infection or other stress. Death may occur any time from cardiac or respiratory failure. Some of the reported patients have lived to the age of fifty years. The significant laboratory findings include an increased protein content in the cerebrospinal fluid (values commonly in the range of 100 to 300 mg %), and an increase in the total lipids in the serum due to an excess of phytanic acid.

Restriction from the diet of foods containing phytol and phytanic acid has a beneficial effect on the course of the disease since the stored material appears to have an exogenous origin.

REFERENCES

Blass, J. P., and Steinberg, D.: Disorders of Fatty Acids, Chapter 6 in, G. E. Gaull (Ed.),
Biology of Brain Dysfunction, Vol. 2, New York, Plenum Press, 1973, p. 225.
Fryer, D. G., et al.: Refsum's Disease. A Clinical and Pathological Report, Neurology, 21,
162, 1971.
Refsum, S.: Heredopathia Atactica Polyneuritiformis: Familial Syndrome not Hitherto
Described: Contribution to Clinical Study of Hereditary Disease of Nervous System,
Acta Psychiat. Neurol. Suppl., 38, 303, 1946.
Sahgal, V., and Olsen, W. O.: Heredopathia Atactica Polyneuritiformis (Phytanic Acid
Storage Disease), Arch. Intern. Med., 135, 585, 1975.

DISORDERS OF CARBOHYDRATE METABOLISM

Glycogen Storage Diseases. Abnormal metabolism of glycogen and glucose may occur in a series of genetically determined disorders, each representing a specific enzyme deficiency (Table 90). The signs and symptoms of each disease are largely determined by the site(s) of the deficient enzyme. Those affecting primarily the neuromuscular system are covered in the chapter dealing with muscle diseases.

Severe fasting hypoglycemia may result in periodic episodes of lethargy, coma, convulsions and anoxic brain damage in glucose-6-phosphatase and glycogen synthetase deficiency. Enlargement of the liver is present in both diseases. Clinical manifestations of these diseases tend to become milder in those patients who survive the first few years of life.

Mild to moderate hypoglycemia and hepatomegaly is found in Type III glycogen storage disease. The clinical manifestations are similar to those seen in glucose-6-phosphatase deficiency but tend to be less severe.

REFERENCES

Askansas, V., et al.: Adult-onset Acid Maltase Deficiency, N. Engl. J. Med., 294, 573,
1976.
Dykes, J. R. W., and Spencer-Peet, J.: Hepatic Glycogen Synthetase Deficiency, Arch. Dis.
Child., 47, 558, 1972.
Greene, H. L., Slonim, A. E., O'Neill, J. A., and Burr, I. M.: Continuous Nocturnal
Intragastric Feeding for Management of Type I Glycogen-Storage Disease, N. Engl. J.
Med., 294, 423, 1976.
Hug, G.: Enzyme Therapy and Prenatal Diagnosis in Glycogenosis Type II, Am. J. Dis.
Child., 128, 607, 1974.
Karpati, G., et al.: The Adult Form of Acid Maltase (α-1, 4-Glucosidase) Deficiency, Ann.
Neurol., 1, 276, 1977.
McAdams, A. J., Hug, G., and Bove, K. E.: Glycogen Storage Disease, Types I to X, Human
Path., 5, 463, 1974.
Mehler, M., and DiMauro, S.: Residual Acid Maltase Activity in Late-onset Maltase
Deficiency, Neurology, 27, 178, 1977.
Spencer-Peet, J., et al.: Hepatic Glycogen Storage Disease, Quart. J. Med., 40, 95, 1971.
Takei, Y., and Solitare, G. B.: Infantile Spongy Degeneration of the Central Nervous
System Associated with Glycogen Storage and Markedly Fatty Liver, J. Neurol.
Neurosurg. Psychiat., 35, 11, 1972.

Table 90. Classification of Glycogen Storage Disease

(Modified from Spencer-Peet, et al., Quart. J. Med., 1971 and McAdams, et al., Hum. Path., 1974)

Enzyme Defect	Eponym	Glycogen Accumulation	Major Clinical Features
Glucose-6-phosphatase	Von Gierke Type I	Liver and kidney	Severe hypoglycemia, enlarged liver and kidney, retarded growth
Lysosomal α-1,4 glucosidase (acid maltase)	Pompe Type II	Generalized	Cardiomegaly and neuromuscular symptoms
Lysosomal α-1,4 glucosidase (acid maltase)	Late-onset acid maltase deficiency	Skeletal muscle	Slowly progressive myopathy, onset in childhood or adulthood
Amylo 1,6 glucosidase (debranching enzyme)	Cori; Forbes Type III	Liver, muscle, heart and erythrocytes	Hepatomegaly, mild to moderate hypoglycemia
Amylo-(1,4 → 1,6) transglucosidase (brancher enzyme)	Andersen Type IV	Liver, muscle, heart and erythrocytes	Progressive liver failure
Muscle phosphorylase	McArdle Type V	Skeletal muscle	Muscle cramps after exercise
Hepatic phosphorylase deficiency	Hers Type VI	Liver and leukocytes	Hepatomegaly
Muscle phosphofructokinase	Tarui Type VII	Skeletal muscle	Muscle cramps after exercise
Low hepatic phosphorylase activity	Type VIII	Liver and brain	Progressive central nervous system degeneration, hepatomegaly, death in childhood
Deficient hepatic phosphorylase kinase activity	Type IX	Liver	Hepatomegaly
Deficient activity of cyclic 3'5'-AMP dependent kinase	Type X	Liver, muscle	Hepatomegaly
Glycogen synthetase	—	Liver glycogen reduced	Profound hypoglycemia; hepatomegaly

Galactosemia. Galactosemia is a rare recessively inherited abnormality of galactose metabolism. There is a block in the conversion of galactose to glucose due to inadequate or absent activity of the enzyme, galactose-1-phosphate uridyl transferase from both the liver and red blood cells. Inability to dispose of administered galactose is characteristic of patients and a partial deficiency of the enzyme may be found in the heterozygous carriers.

The clinical picture may appear acutely in the first two weeks of life, with vomiting, diarrhea, jaundice, hepatomegaly, splenomegaly and ascites. Cataracts occur in more than half the cases and may be seen as early as the third week. In less fulminating cases psychomotor development is slow and mental retardation is prominent. Convulsive seizures and evidence of focal brain damage are rarely seen. The mildest cases are manifest only by an aversion to milk and impaired galactose tolerance.

Galactosuria, proteinuria, and aminoaciduria are characteristic of symptomatic cases. Hypoglycemia and laboratory evidence of impaired liver function may be present.

Most of the laboratory abnormalities are reversed if milk, lactose and galactose are rigidly excluded from the diet. Clinical improvement also occurs and normal mental development has been observed in children reared on a strict diet, although once established, mental retardation may be less responsive to therapy. The cataracts have also been noted to disappear on treatment.

Increased blood galactose and galactosuria may be present due to a deficiency of the enzyme galactokinase. Lenticular cataracts but no hepatic or nervous system symptoms result from this defect in metabolism.

REFERENCES

Fensom, A. H., Benson, P. F., and Blunt, S.: Prenatal Diagnosis of Galactosaemia, Br. Med. J., 4, 386, 1974.
Haberland, C., et al.: The Neuropathology of Galactosemia, J. Neuropathol. Exp. Neurol., 30, 431, 1971.
Hammersen, G., Houghton, S., and Levy, H. L.: Rennes-Like Variant of Galactosemia: Clinical and Biochemical Studies, J. Pediatr., 87, 50, 1975.
Kalckar, H. M., Kinoshita, J. H., and Donnell, G. N.: Galactosemia: Biochemistry, Genetics, Pathophysiology, and Developmental Aspects, Chapter 2 in, G. Gaull (Ed.) Biology of Brain Dysfunction, Vol. 1, New York, Plenum Press, 1973, p. 31.
Litman, N., Kanter, A. I., and Finberg, L.: Galactokinase Deficiency Presenting as Pseudotumor Cerebri, J. Pediatr., 86, 410, 1975.
Tedesco, T. A., et al.: The Genetic Defect in Galactosemia, N. Engl. J. Med., 292, 737, 1975.

DISORDERS OF MUCOPOLYSACCHARIDE (GLYCOAMINOGLYCAN) METABOLISM

Mucopolysaccharides. The mucopolysaccharidoses (MPS) represent a group of genetically-determined disorders in which the catabolism of

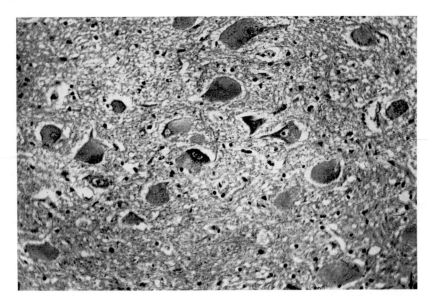

Figure 155. Hurler's disease. Cells of hypoglossal nucleus with abnormal storage
of mucopolysaccharides. (Courtesy Dr. David Cowen.)

certain glycoaminoglycans is defective and results in the storage of
these materials in various tissues of the body and their excretion in
excess amounts in the urine.

Involvement of the skeletal and connective tissue is the most constant feature of the MPS and is responsible for the striking somatic
malformations evident on examination. The cornea, heart, abdominal
viscera and central nervous system are also commonly affected.

The nervous system may be involved by the storage of glycoaminoglycans in neurons of the central nervous system (Fig. 155) or meninges
resulting in mental retardation or hydrocephalus. Other neurological
symptoms such as the carpal tunnel syndrome, deafness and spastic
quadriparesis may result from excess storage of the material in anatomically related connective tissues (carpal tunnel, cervical dura mater) or
bone (vertebral bodies, auditory canal, basilar impression, hypoplasia
of odontoid process with atlanto-axial dislocation).

The enzyme deficiencies responsible for most of the various MPS
phenotypes have now been determined by utilizing cultured fibroblasts
derived from patients in "cross-correction" experiments in vitro.
Neufeld has reviewed these recent and unique biochemical developments. The salient clinical and biochemical features of the MPS are
presented in Table 91.

Mucolipidoses. Spranger and Wiedmann have emphasized the clinical and biochemical features of a group of diseases they designate as mucolipidoses. Patients with these diseases show the dysmorphic skeletal changes seen in the mucopolysaccharidoses, store excessive glycoaminoglycans in the tissues but excrete normal amounts in the urine. In addition to these features, storage of gangliosides, glycolipids or glycoproteins occur in visceral organs and brain. Table 92 enumerates the features of the disorders currently included within this designation.

REFERENCES

Hollister, D. W., Cohen, A. H., Rimoin, D. L., and Silberberg, R.: The Morquio Syndrome (Mucopolysaccharidosis IV): Morphologic and Biochemical Studies, Johns Hopkins Med. J., 137, 176, 1975.
Kelly, T. E.: The Mucopolysaccharidoses and Mucolipidoses, Clin. Orthopaedics Related Res., 114, 116, 1976.
Kousseff, B. G., et al.: Fucosidosis Type 2, Pediatr., 57, 205, 1976.
McKusick, V. A.: Heritable Disorders Of Connective Tissue. 4th ed., St. Louis, C. V. Mosby Co., 1972, p. 521.
Neufeld, E. F.: The Biochemical Basis for Mucopolysaccharidoses and Mucolipidoses, in A. G. Steinberg and A. G. Bearn (Eds.), Progress In Medical Genetics, Vol. X, New York, Grune & Stratton, 1974, p. 81.
Spranger, J. W., and Wiedmann, H. R.: The Genetic Mucolipidoses, Humangenetik, 9, 113, 1970.
Stevenson, R. E., et al.: The Iduronidase-Deficient Mucopolysaccharidoses: Clinical and Roentgenographic Features, Pediatr., 57, 111, 1976.
Tellez-Nagel, I., et al.: Mucolipidosis IV, Arch. Neurol., 33, 828, 1976.
Yunis, J. J., et al.: Clinical Manifestations of Mannosidosis—A Longitudinal Study, Amer. J. Med., 61, 841, 1976.

DISORDERS OF PORPHYRIN METABOLISM

Porphyria. Disturbances of porphyrin metabolism associated with increased excretion of porphyrins in the urine and feces are divided into two groups: acquired and hereditary. In the acquired group the excretion of porphyrin is related to the ingestion of poisons, such as lead, and to certain diseases. Hereditary porphyrias are inborn metabolic defects of heme biosynthesis which may occur in several forms (Table 93). Acute intermittent porphyria (acute hepatic porphyria) is inherited as a Mendelian dominant and is characterized by recurrent gastrointestinal, psychiatric and neurological symptoms and signs occurring singly or in combination. The disease commonly exists in latent or asymptomatic forms.

Pathogenesis. The biochemical abnormality in acute intermittent porphyria consists of an excessive formation and urinary excretion of porphobilinogen and its precursor, delta-aminolevulinic acid. The increased porphyrin precursor excretion results from high levels of the hepatic enzyme, delta-aminolevulinic acid synthetase. The enzyme is

Table 91. The Genetic Mucopolysaccharidoses
(After McKusick, 1972 and Kelly, 1976)

Designation	Clinical Features	Enzyme Defect	Genetics	Mucopoly-sacchariduria	Life Expectancy	Intelligence
MPS I H Hurler syndrome	Early corneal clouding, severe skeletal and cardiac manifestations	α-L-Iduronidase	AR*	DS, HS	6–10 yrs.	MR
MPS I S Scheie syndrome	Stiff joints, cloudy cornea, and aortic regurgitation	α-L-Iduronidase	AR	DS, HS	Normal	Normal
MPS I H/S Hurler-Scheie compound	Phenotype intermediate between Hurler & Scheie	α-L-Iduronidase	AR	DS, HS	20's	Mild MR
MPS II A Hunter syndrome, severe	No corneal clouding, similar to MPS I H but milder course	Sulfo-iduronide sulfatase	X-R**	DS, HS	Teens	MR
MPS II B Hunter syndrome, mild	Mild skeletal manifestations, cardiac symptoms, coarse facies	Sulfo-iduronide sulfatase	X-R	DS, HS	Adulthood	Fair to normal

MPS III A	Sanfilippo syndrome A	Identical phenotype	Sulfo-glucosamine sulfatase	AR	HS	Teens–20's	MR
MPS III B	Sanfilippo syndrome B	Mild somatic, severe central nervous system manifestations	N-Acetyl-β-D-glucosaminidase	AR	HS	Teens–20's	MR
MPS IV	Morquio syndrome (probably more than one allelic form)	Severe bone changes of distinctive type, cloudy cornea, aortic regurgitation	Sulfo-hexosamine sulfatase	AR	KS	20–40	Normal
MPS V	Vacant, formerly the Scheie syndrome						
MPS VI A	Maroteaux-Lamy syndrome, classic form	Severe osseous and corneal changes	Aryl sulfatase B	AR	DS	10–20	Normal
MPS VI B	Maroteaux-Lamy syndrome, mild form	Less severe osseous changes, corneal clouding	Aryl sulfatase B	AR	DS	20–normal	Normal
MPS VII	Sly syndrome (more than one allelic form?)	Hepatosplenomegaly, dysostosis multiplex, white cell inclusions	β-glucuronidase	AR	DS	Restricted (? degree)	MR

*Autosomal recessive   **X-Linked recessive   DH = Dermatan Sulfate   HS = Heparan Sulfate   KS = Keratan Sulfate
MR = Mental Retardation

Table 92. Mucolipidoses

Designation	Clinical Features	Biochemical Features
G G_{M1} gangliosidosis Types 1 and 2	Coarse facies, progressive retardation, macular red spot, marked skeletal changes	Ganglioside storage in brain; keratan sulfate-like material in viscera
Variant or Austin-type of metachromatic leukodystrophy (multiple sulfatase deficiency)	Psychomotor retardation, seizures, deformities of sternum and ribs, occasional hepatosplenomegaly	Sulfatase A, B, C deficiency with increased sulfatides, gangliosides and sulfated glycosaminoglycans in central nervous system. Mucopolysacchariduria
Fucosidosis I. Severe form II. Mild form	Progressive deterioration of central nervous system function, coarse facial features, skeletal changes. Angiokeratoma corporis diffusum in Type II	Absence or deficiency of α-L-fucosidase in liver, brain and other organs. Storage of fucose-glycolipids in the brain and viscera
Mannosidosis	Psychomotor retardation, coarse facial features, mild to moderate skeletal changes	Deficiency of α-D-mannosidase. Excretion of mannose-rich oligosaccharides in urine, storage of mannose-containing glycoprotein
Mucolipidosis I	Mental retardation, Hurler-like appearance, skeletal changes of dysostosis multiplex	Storage of mucopolysaccharides and glycolipids; inclusions in cultured fibroblasts
Mucolipidosis II (I-cell disease)	Hurler-like appearance, more rapid course, striking gingival hyperplasia, mental retardation, hepatosplenomegaly	Dense cytoplasmic inclusions in cultured fibroblasts, defect in lysosomal hydrolase uptake into cells?
Mucolipidosis III (pseudo-Hurler polydystrophy)	Stiffness of joints, coarse facies, short stature, corneal clouding, aortic regurgitation, mild mental retardation and progressive skeletal dysplasia	Similar to Mucolipidosis II
Mucolipidosis IV	Corneal clouding, arrest of mental development, no skeletal abnormalities	Storage of lipid-like and mucopolysaccharide-like material in cornea, brain and lymphocytes

Table 93. Classification of the Porphyrias
(From Meyer, 1976)

Type	Major Clinical Features	Inheritance
Erythropoietic		
Congenital erythropoietic porphyria	Photosensitivity; hemolytic anemia; splenomegaly	Autosomal recessive
Erythropoietic coproporphyria	Mild cutaneous photosensitivity	Unknown
Erythrohepatic		
Protoporphyria	Photosensitivity; hemolytic anemia; liver disease	Autosomal dominant
Hepatic		
Acute intermittent porphyria (Swedish)	Abdominal colic; hypertension; neuropathy; encephalopathy; no photosensitivity	Autosomal dominant
Variegate porphyria (South African)	Cutaneous, abdominal and neurologic symptoms	Autosomal dominant
Hereditary coproporphyria	Similar to variegate porphyria or may be asymptomatic	Autosomal dominant
Porphyria cutanea tarda	Cutaneous and hepatic symptoms	May be genetically-determined
Cutaneous porphyrias	Due to hexachlorobenzene, hepatic tumors or lupus erythematosus	Acquired

induced to high levels because of heme deficiency in the liver secondary to genetic partial deficiency of uroporphyrinogen I synthetase.

Attacks may occur at the time of the menstrual period, during fasting and starvation, with infections, or they may be precipitated by the administration of barbiturates, hormones and related steroids or other drugs.

Pathology. Abnormal findings in the central or peripheral nervous system may be absent in the rapidly fatal cases. In the less acute cases patchy areas of demyelinization, with or without destruction of the axis cylinder, are found in the peripheral nerves and in the central nervous system together with retrograde changes in the motor cells of the spinal cord and brain stem. There may be a mild degree of chronic passive congestion in the viscera and patchy necrosis of the tubules of the kidney.

Incidence. Acute porphyria is probably much more common than one would infer from the relatively small number of cases reported in the literature. Many of the cases with acute abdominal pains and psychotic episodes are not diagnosed. Similarly some of the cases classified as infectious polyneuritis as well as those described by the term recurrent polyneuritis are probably instances of acute porphyria, in which porphyria was absent or overlooked. Although the defect in porphyrin metabolism is present during the entire life of the affected individual, the onset of symptoms is usually in the third to fifth decade. Women are more frequently affected than men.

Symptoms and Signs. The symptoms of acute porphyria are: Pigmentation of the skin, abdominal pains, tachycardia, convulsions, mental symptoms, polyneuritis and the excretion of burgundy-red urine. These may occur singly or in any combination. The abdominal pains, colicky in nature, occur in paroxysms and are often associated with dilatation of the stomach. They may be so severe that laparotomy is performed. Convulsions are rare and usually occur in association with the mental symptoms. The latter may simulate a delirium or any form of psychosis.

The neuritic symptoms may develop alone or follow an attack of abdominal pain or mental symptoms. Paresthesias in the extremities are common at the onset. Weakness of the muscles of the trunk and extremities may rapidly advance to complete paralysis. The weakness is usually greatest in the distal parts of the extremities, but occasionally the proximal muscles may be more severely involved. Any of the cranial nerves may be involved. Dysarthria, dysphagia and facial diplegia are common. Transient amblyopia, which is said to be related to spasm of the retinal vessels, may occur. Cutaneous sensory loss is rare, but there may be a slight hypesthesia in the distal portion of the extremities. The tendon and skin reflexes are diminished or absent.

Laboratory Data. The examination of the blood usually gives normal findings. The cerebrospinal fluid is normal except for a slight or moderate increase in the protein content in a small percentage of cases. The characteristic and diagnostic feature is the urinary excretion of large amounts of porphyrin precursors, porphobilinogen and delta-aminolevulinic acid. The urine may darken on standing due to the formation of various porphyrins or porphobilin.

Porphyrin precursors will usually be found in the urine if several or many examinations are made. Occasionally, however, they may be entirely absent during one of the attacks of abdominal pain or polyneuritis but present in a subsequent attack. Increased delta-aminolevulinic acid synthetase activity may be demonstrated in fresh liver tissue. The primary biochemical defect, a reduced level of uroporphyrinogen I synthetase activity may be demonstrated in liver and erythrocytes.

Course and Prognosis. The neuritic symptoms reach a maximum in most cases within a week of onset of the symptoms. The mortality rate in the reported cases varies between 10 and 50%. It is especially high when the bulbar musculature is involved. In the non-fatal cases, complete recovery is the rule although convalescence may extend over several months. Recurrence of the neuritis is not uncommon.

Diagnosis and Differential Diagnosis. The diagnosis can be made without difficulty when polyneuritis or mental symptoms are preceded by acute abdominal pains and are accompanied by the excretion of burgundy-red urine. The diagnosis may be extremely difficult when porphyria is absent on the initial examination of the urine. Diagnosis in such cases depends on an alertness in considering the diagnosis which should lead to frequent examinations of the urine.

The differential diagnosis between hematoporphyrinuric polyneuritis and infectious polyneuritis can be made only by the demonstration of porphyrin precursors in the urine.

Treatment. There is at present time no treatment that can correct the metabolic disturbance. Asymptomatic and previously undiagnosed cases may be detected by assay of the erythrocytes for the level of uroporphyrinogen I synthase activity. The avoidance of exposure to barbiturates and other drugs known to induce attacks is most important. Treatment of an acute attack is symptomatic. Improved respiratory care of the paralyzed patient has effectively reduced the mortality of the disease. Chlorpromazine can be used for abdominal pain and psychotic manifestations. A high carbohydrate diet has been effective in preventing recurrence in some cases. Watson has reported the disappearance or improvement of nervous system symptons following the intravenous administration of hematin.

REFERENCES

Bloomer, J. R., Bonkowsky, H. L., Ebert, P. S., and Mahoney, M. J.: Inheritance in Protoporphyria, Lancet, 2, 226, 1976.

Elder, G. H., Gray, C. H., and Nicholson, D. C.: The Porphyrias: A Review, J. Clin. Path., 25, 1013, 1972.

Meyer, U. A.: Hepatic Porphyrias: New Findings on the Nature of Metabolic Defects, Chapter 17 in H. Popper and F. Schaffner (Eds.), Progress In Liver Diseases, Vol. 5, New York, Grune & Stratton, 1976, p. 280.

Tschudy, D. P., Valsamis, M., and Magnussen, C. R.: Acute Intermittent Porphyria: Clinical and Selected Research Aspects, Ann. Intern. Med., 83, 851, 1975.

Watson, C. J.: Hematin and Porphyria, N. Engl. J. Med., 293, 605, 1975.

DISORDERS OF METAL METABOLISM

Hepatolenticular Degeneration. Hepatolenticular degeneration (Wilson's disease; pseudosclerosis of Westphal and Strumpell) is a familial disease with signs and symptoms of injury to the basal ganglia accompanied by cirrhosis of the liver. A peculiar rust-colored pigmentation of the cornea near the scleral junction (Kayser-Fleischer ring) is present in the majority of the cases.

In 1912, Wilson described the syndrome of progressive lenticular degeneration in which there was cavitation in the basal ganglia and cirrhosis of the liver. Cases have been reported in which neurological

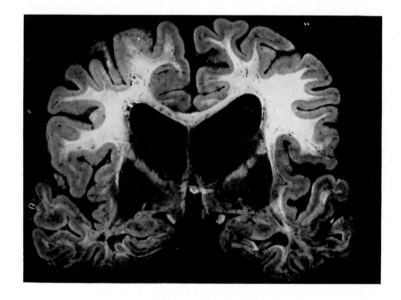

Figure 156.   Wilson's disease. Ventricular dilation, atrophy of caudate nucleus. Cyst in lower half of putamen.

signs were present in combination with cirrhosis of the liver but without gross destruction of the lenticular nucleus. These cases were first described under the terms of pseudosclerosis. Careful examination of this type of case has shown, however, that characteristic histological changes are present in the basal ganglia. At the present time, therefore, the cases without cavitation in the basal ganglia are considered to be examples of hepatolenticular degeneration in which the degenerative changes are less severe and of a slower evolution than in those with cavitation.

Pathology and Pathogenesis. The pathological changes in the nervous system are widespread, involving chiefly the basal ganglia and to a lesser extent the cortex, cerebellum and other parts of the nervous system. The changes in the basal ganglia are of varying degrees of severity. In the rapidly advancing cases there is cavitation in the putamen and the globus pallidus (Fig. 156) and, at times, in the cerebral cortex. In the less rapidly advancing cases the lenticular nucleus is shrunken but there is no cavitation. In the areas of cavitation there is complete loss of neurons, glia and ground substance. In the shrunken areas there is a decrease in the number of neurons and degenerative changes in many of the remaining cells. Characteristic of the disease is a diffuse increase in the glia. Large protoplasmic astrocytes (Alzheimer glia cells) may be found scattered throughout the nervous system. These are more commonly found in the slowly progressing cases but they are present in many of the cases with foci of softening. There may be a diffuse loss of nerve cells in the cortex and other parts of the nervous system and rarely there is a severe degeneration of the white matter of the cerebral cortex.

There is a nodular cirrhosis of the liver. Usually the liver is small and shrunken with nodules of varying size. Ultrastructural studies show specific changes in the mitochondria of the hepatocytes prior to the development of cirrhosis. The spleen is usually enlarged and shows evidence of congestion. In microscopic sections of the cornea there are fine golden yellow granules in Descemet's membrane.

Wilson's disease is due to an inborn defect in the metabolism of copper. Transport and storage of copper is disturbed, resulting in a positive copper balance. There is an increase in the copper content of the tissues, an increased rate of excretion of copper in the urine and a reduction in the copper content in the blood and in the feces. This disturbance in the distribution and excretion of copper is associated with a decrease in the ceruloplasmin content of the serum in most cases. The pathogenesis of the disease is unknown although all available evidence indicates that the copper overload bears a direct relationship to the production of the signs and symptoms. The decreased biliary excretion of copper is thought to be due to a defect in hepatic lysosomes. Accumulation of copper in the kidneys results in characteristic renal lesions with aminoaciduria, phosphaturia and uricosuria. The lesions in the brain, cornea and in the liver are also presumably due to the accumulation of copper in these organs.

Incidence. Hepatolenticular degeneration is a rare disease but is more frequent than commonly considered. Many cases have been recorded in the literature since Wilson's report in 1912. The disease was considered by Wilson to be familial because of its frequent occurrence in two or more members of one family, and it is now known that the disease is inherited through an autosomal recessive gene.

In the vast majority of patients the symptoms have their onset between the ages of eleven and twenty-five years. Onset at the age of four and as late as the fifth decade have been recorded. In the reported cases, there is a slight preponderance of the male sex over the female.

Symptoms and Signs. The signs and symptoms of hepatolenticular degeneration are those of damage to the liver and to the nervous system.

Although it was formerly thought that the cirrhosis of the liver was always asymptomatic, it is now known that signs of liver damage. ascites or jaundice may occur at any stage of the disease. They have been observed in a small percentage of the cases several or many years before the onset of neurological symptoms.

The neurological manifestations are so varied that it is impossible to describe a clinical picture which is characteristic. Symptoms of basal ganglia damage usually predominate, but occasionally cerebellar symptoms may be in the foreground. Tremors and rigidity are the most common early signs. The tremor may be of the intention type, or the alternating tremor of Parkinson's syndrome. More commonly, however, it is a bizarre tremor, localized to the upper extremities, which is best described by the term "wing-beating" (Fig. 157). This tremor is usually absent when the arms are at rest and develops after a short latent period when the arms are held extended. The beating movements may be confined to the muscles of the wrist but more commonly the arm is thrown up and down in a wide arc. The movements increase in severity and may become so violent that the patient is thrown off balance. Changing the posture of the outstretched arms may alter the severity of the tremor. The tremor may affect both upper extremities but is usually more severe in one. Occasionally the tremor may be present even when the extremity is at rest. A fixed, open-mouthed smile is present in many patients.

Rigidity and spasms of the muscles are often present in varying degrees. In some cases a typical parkinsonian rigidity may involve all of the muscles. Torticollis, tortipelvis and other dystonic movements are not uncommon. Spasticity of the laryngeal and pharnygeal muscles

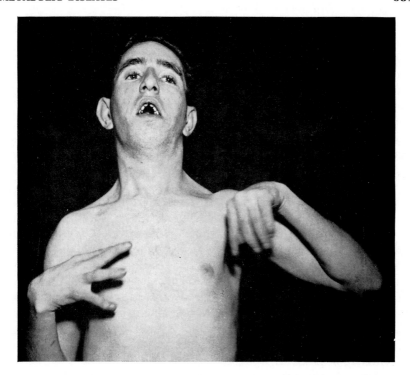

Figure 157.   Wilson's disease. Open mouth, athetoid posture of arms
and wing-beating movements of the left hand.

may lead to dysarthria and dysphagia. Drooping of the lower jaw and
excess salivation are common. Other symptoms include convulsions,
transient periods of coma and mental changes. Mental symptoms may
dominate the clinical course for varying periods of time and simulate
an affective disorder or functional psychosis.

The sensory examination is usually normal. The tendon reflexes are
increased and an extensor plantar response is present in a small
percentage of the cases.

A rust-colored ring of pigment is present in the cornea at the junction
with the sclera in over 50% of the cases. The incidence of this finding
would probably be greater if the eyes of all cases were examined with
the slit lamp.

Laboratory Data. The examination of the blood and spinal fluid is
usually normal. Tests of liver function are apt to be negative unless
they are performed coincidental with an episode of increased activity
in the liver pathology. Evidence of impaired liver function can be
found in the majority of the cases if the tests are repeated at frequent

intervals during the course of the disease. There is an abnormality in the pattern of the amino acid excretion and an increase in copper excretion in the urine. The ceruloplasmin content of the serum is reduced in almost all of the cases. The uric acid content of the serum is decreased. The frequency of this finding in Wilson's disease makes the determination of the uric acid content of the serum a valuable aid in the screening of patients.

Diagnosis. The diagnosis of hepatolenticular degeneration can be made without difficulty in the well-advanced case when there is a combination of familial incidence, signs of basal ganglia disease (parkinsonism, dystonia or wing-beating tremor) and pigmentation of the scleral margin of the cornea. The diagnosis can be confirmed by the finding of a low ceruloplasmin content in the serum (<20 mg per 100 ml) and an elevated concentration of hepatic copper (>250μg per gm dry liver). The differentiation between dystonia musculorum deformans or juvenile paralysis agitans cannot be made in the absence of a history of family incidence, corneal pigmentation or signs of cirrhosis of the liver.

The diagnosis can be made before the onset of clinical symptoms in siblings of affected cases by the findings of a decreased serum ceruloplasmin, an increased urinary copper excretion, and the finding of copper storage in biopsy specimens of the liver. These findings are of importance because early treatment may prevent damage to the liver and brain and the later development of the clinical syndrome.

Course and Prognosis. The onset of the disease is usually insidious and the progress slow. Partial remissions and acute exacerbations are not uncommon. The untreated disease is almost always fatal. The duration of life from onset of symptoms varies from a few weeks to many years (forty-three years in 1 reported case). Survival for more than ten years is uncommon in untreated cases and the average duration of the disease is four to six years. Febrile episodes may occur in the course of the disease possibly due to acute exacerbations of the cirrhotic process in the liver and to acute cerebral damage. Death may occur from intercurrent infections or as direct result of the disease.

Treatment. The treatment recommended by Scheinberg is based on the hypothesis that the degenerative changes are the result of the deposition of copper in the tissues. A copper-poor diet and potassium sulfide, 20 mg with each meal, are recommended to minimize copper absorption. Penicillamine, 1 to 4 gm daily in divided doses, on an empty stomach, is given to promote urinary excretion of copper. Improvement of neurological symptoms and signs and fading of the Kayser-Fleischer rings result from this form of therapy and there may be improvement in the hepatic disturbance. Survival for many years with complete or almost complete remission of symptoms has been reported.

REFERENCES

Grand, R. J., and Vawter, G. F.: Juvenile Wilson Disease: Histologic and Functional Studies During Penicillamine Therapy, J. Pediatr., 87, 1161, 1975.

Levi, A. J., et al.: Presymptomatic Wilson's Disease, Lancet, 2, 575, 1967.

Scheinberg, I. H.: The Effects of Heredity and Environment on Copper Metabolism, Med. Clin. North Am., 60, 705, 1976.

————, and Sternlieb, I.: Wilson's Disease, Chapter 5 in G. E. Gaull (Ed.), Biology of Brain Dysfunction, Vol. 3, New York, Plenum Press, 1975, p. 247.

————, and ————.: Pregnancy in Penicillamine-treated Patients with Wilson's Disease, N. Engl. J. Med., 293, 1300, 1975.

Schulman, S., and Barbeau, A.: Wilson's Disease: A Case with Almost Total Loss of Cerebral White Matter, J. Neuropathol. Exp. Neurol., 22, 105, 1963.

Slovis, T. L., et al.: The Varied Manifestations of Wilson's Disease, J. Pediatr., 78, 578, 1971.

Sternlieb, I., Bennett, B., and Scheinberg, I. H.: D-Penicillamine Induced Goodpasture's Syndrome in Wilson's Disease, Ann. Intern. Med., 82, 673, 1975.

Sternlieb, I., and Scheinberg, I. H.: Prevention of Wilson's Disease in Asymptomatic Patients, N. Engl. J. Med., 278, 352, 1968.

Strickland, G. T., and Leu, M-L.: Wilson's Disease, Medicine, 54, 113, 1975.

Walshe, J. M.: The Biochemistry of Copper in Man and Its Role in the Pathogenesis of Wilson's Disease (Hepatolenticular Degeneration), Chapter 4 in, J. N. Cumings (Ed.), Biochemical Aspects of Nervous Diseases, New York, Plenum Press, 1972, p. 111.

Wilson, S. A. K.: Progressive Lenticular Degeneration: Familial Nervous Disease Associated with Cirrhosis of the Liver, Brain, 34, 295, 1912.

DISORDERS OF THE ENDOCRINE GLANDS

H. Houston Merritt, M.D.

The secretions of the endocrine glands have a profound influence on the metabolism of the nervous system. Disturbances of consciousness and mental activity as well as various neurological symptoms may occur with dysfunction of the glands. It is the purpose of this chapter to consider the clinical manifestations which occur with hyper- and hypofunction of these glands.

Pituitary

Hypopituitarism

Hypofunction of the pituitary may occur as the result of undersecretion of unknown cause or damage to the gland by tumors, inflammatory processes, vascular lesions or trauma.

The syndromes produced by hypofunction of the pituitary include Simmonds' disease, pituitary dwarfism and diabetes insipidus. Adiposogenital dystrophy (Fröhlich's syndrome) is also attributed to a deficiency of pituitary function, but it doubtful whether this syndrome has any relationship to pituitary dysfunction.

Simmonds' Disease. Simmonds' disease or pituitary cachexia is the result of total destruction of the anterior lobe. Destruction of the gland may result from infarction, hemorrhage, trauma, tuberculosis and other infections. Rarely it may be due to damage to functional portions of the gland by pituitary adenomas or other tumors in the region of the sella turcica.

Pituitary cachexia occurs most commonly in middle life and in women of childbearing age, especially after parturition. The syndrome has a pluriglandular nature, probably due to hypofunction of the thyroid, adrenal and gonads, as a consequence of loss of the trophic hormones of the pituitary.

Symptoms include severe asthenia and progressive wasting of fat and subcutaneous tissue. The skin becomes thin, dry and wrinkled, the nails brittle, the hair is shed and the teeth fall out. Body temperature is sub-normal, the blood pressure may be low, the basal metabolic rate reduced and the blood sugar content decreased. Psychotic symptoms may develop.

The syndrome of pituitary cachexia is closely imitated by that of anorexia nervosa. The latter condition occurs in young females who abstain from eating.

The course of patients with Simmonds' disease is subject to some variation. Death may result when the failure of function of the anterior pituitary is of severe degree. The treatment of pituitary cachexia consists of a high protein, high salt diet and replacement therapy with prednisolone, thyroid and testosterone.

Pituitary Dwarfism. Retardation of growth may occur as a result of a reduction in the secretion of the growth hormone. The degree of retardation of growth varies from frank dwarfing to a slightly less than normal degree of development. Stunting of development may occur in children in whom the gland is injured by tumors in the suprasellar region.

So-called pituitary dwarfs may be normal in size at birth or they may be abnormally small when born. They are usually the children of normal-sized parents and their mental development is normal. In infancy and childhood, except for the smallness, the body configuration is normal. With increasing age they develop the wizened appearance of a dwarfish old man (progeria). The genitals are underdeveloped and there is a lack of development of the secondary sexual characteristics. Occasionally, however, sexual development is normal and the dwarf is able to produce offspring, for example, Barnum's famous dwarf, Tom Thumb.

Other forms of dwarfism not related to hypofunction of the pituitary gland include achondroplasia, and those associated with Pott's disease and nutritional disorders of infancy (pancreatic insufficiency or celiac disease). The dwarfing of cretinism is attributed to primary hypofunction of the thyroid, but it is likely that associated pituitary dysfunction is partly responsible for the underdevelopment in these cases.

Adiposogenital Dystrophy. Adiposogenital dystrophy (Fröhlich's syndrome) may occur in patients with tumors in the suprasellar region, but more commonly the term Fröhlich's syndrome is used to describe a child, usually a boy, who is obese and in whom development of the secondary sex characteristics is retarded. There is no evidence that pituitary dysfunction is present in such patients and with progress of time, sexual development will be normal and frequently the patients will cease to be fat after puberty.

Diabetes Insipidus. Diabetes insipidus is a clinical syndrome characterized by the excessive excretion of urine and an abnormally large fluid intake.

Etiology. Diabetes insipidus is caused by a deficiency in the production of the antidiuretic hormone (arginine vasopressin) of the posterior lobe of the pituitary. There are two general groups of cases: The so-called primary type in which there is no known lesion in the pituitary or hypothalamus; and the secondary type, which is associated with lesions in the hypothalamus, either in the supraoptic nucleus or in the tract from this nucleus to the pituitary. Among the conditions which may cause lesions in this region are tumors (pituitary adenomas, craniopharyngiomas, meningiomas and aneurysms), xanthomatosis (Schüller-Christian disease), sarcoidosis, trauma, infections and vascular lesions.

Incidence. Primary diabetes insipidus is a rare condition. It affects chiefly young people and is seen in males more frequently than in females. Heredity is a factor in some of the cases. Secondary or symptomatic diabetes insipidus is also rare. It is present in a large percentage of patients with xanthomatosis and in a small percentage of those with tumors or other lesions in the hypothalamic region.

Symptoms and Signs. Unless complicated by symptoms associated with the lesion which is also the cause of the diabetes insipidus, the symptoms are limited to polyuria and polydipsia. Eight to 20 liters or even more of urine are passed in twenty-four hours and there is a comparable high level of water intake. The necessity of frequent voiding and the excessive water intake may interfere with normal activities and disturb sleep. Usually, however, the general health is maintained. The symptoms and signs in patients with tumors or other lesions in the hypothalamic region are those usually associated with these conditions and are considered elsewhere.

Laboratory Data. The laboratory findings are normal with the exception of the low specific gravity of the urine (1.001 to 1.005) and an increase in the osmolality of the serum in many of the cases.

Diagnosis. The diagnosis of diabetes insipidus is made on basis of the excretion of the large amount of urine and the insatiable thirst. It is distinguished from the polyuria of diabetes mellitus by the glucosuria and high specific gravity of the urine in the latter disease. A large amount of urine may be passed by patients with chronic nephritis, but the presence of albumin and casts in the urine as well as the other associated findings in this condition should prevent any confusion in the diagnosis. Hysterical polydipsia may simulate diabetes insipidus, and must be differentiated by tests described below and by a psychological study of the patient.

There is no significant change in the specific gravity of the urine of patients with diabetes insipidus when fluids are withheld for twelve hours, whereas the urine of patients with hysterical polydipsia will become concentrated.

The functional integrity of the supraoptico-hypophyseal system can be tested by the response to the injection of saline. Sodium chloride in 2.5% solution is injected in dose of 0.25 ml per kg of body weight per minute for forty-five minutes. In diabetes insipidus, the polyuria is increased by the procedure; in hysterical polydipsia, the pituitrin released from the normal pituitary causes a sharp decrease in the urinary output.

A rare cause of diabetes insipidus is the failure of the kidney to respond to pitressin. This has been reported as a hereditary defect in male infants and is diagnosed by the injection of 0.1 unit of pitressin. It has been suggested that the defect in some of the familial cases of diabetes insipidus may be in the osmoreceptor mechanism.

The diagnosis of diabetes insipidus carries with it the necessity of determining, if possible, the cause. This means a thorough examination of the nervous system with particular attention to the visual acuity and the fields of vision. Roentgenograms of the skull and a CAT brain scan should be a routine part of the examination.

Cause. Diabetes insipidus of the primary type may persist for years. Diabetes insipidus secondary to known lesions in the hypothalamus may also be permanent but remissions with complete cessation of symptoms are not infrequent.

Treatment. The treatment of patients with diabetes insipidus associated with tumors or other remediable lesions in the hypothalamus is that appropriate to the lesion, *i.e.,* surgical removal or radiation therapy. Symptomatic therapy of the diabetes insipidus if it persists in these cases and in the patients with diabetes insipidus of unknown cause is directed toward suppression of the diuresis. No efforts should be made to limit the fluid intake. Dietary restrictions are not necessary with the exception of limitation of salt intake to the minimum requirement. Aqueous pitressin can be administered hypodermically in doses of 1 ml, 1 to 3 times daily; it may be sprayed intranasally or placed high in the nasopharynx on cotton pledgets. Pitressin tannate in oil injected intramuscularly is slowly absorbed and may be effective for several days. Dried posterior pituitary extract may be inhaled as a snuff.

REFERENCES

Atkins, L.: Progeria. Report of a Case With Post-Mortem Findings, N. Engl. J. Med., *250*, 1065, 1954.
Coggins, C. H., and Leaf, A.: Diabetes Insipidus, Am. J. Med., *42*, 807, 1967.
Dingman, J. F., Benirschke, K., and Thorn, G. W.: Studies of Neurohypophyseal Function in Man. Diabetes and Psychogenic Polydipsia, Am. J. Med., *23*, 226, 1957.
Farquharson, R. F.: *Simmonds' Disease; Extreme Insufficiency of the Adenohypophysis*, Springfield, Charles C Thomas, 1950, 93 pp.
Hickey, R. C., and Hare, K.: The Renal Excretion of Chloride and Water in Diabetes Insipidus, J. Clin. Invest., *23*, 768, 1944.
Kunstadter, R. H., and Tanman, F.: Diabetes Insipidus, Pediatrics, *28*, 679, 1961.
Locke, S., and Tyler, H. R.: Pituitary Apoplexy, Am. J. Med., *30*, 643, 1961.
Martin, F. I. R.: Familial Diabetes Insipidus, Quart. J. Med., *28*, 573, 1959.
Stevko, R. M., Balsley, M., and Segar, W. F.: Primary Polydipsia-Compulsive Water Drinking, J. Pediatr. *73*, 845, 1968.
Todd, J.: Simmonds' Disease with Mental Symptoms, Br. M. J., *2*, 569, 1951.
Warkany, J., and Mitchell, A. G.: Diabetes Insipidus in Children, Am. J. Dis. Child., *57*, 603, 1939.

Excessive Secretion of Antidiuretic Hormone. Inappropriate secretion of the antidiuretic hormone (cerebral salt wasting) may occur with injury to the hypothalamohypophyseal system, by head injury, infections, tumors and other causes. It has been reported in association with carcinomas of the lung which elaborate vasopressin.

The salient features of the syndrome are: hyponatremia and hypotonicity of the body fluids; urinary excretion of significant quantities of sodium despite hyponatremia; normal renal and adrenal function; absence of edema, hypotension, azotemia or dehydration; and improvement of the electrolyte disturbance and clinical symptoms on restriction of fluids.

Evidence of cerebral dysfunction related to the electrolyte disturbance may occur. Headache, confusion, somnolence, coma, convulsive seizures, weakness or transient focal neurological signs and an abnormal electroencephalogram have been reported in a few of the cases. The symptoms clear with fluid restriction.

REFERENCES

Forest, J. N., et al.: Superiority of Demeclocycline over Lithium in the Treatment of Chronic Syndrome of Inappropriate Secretion of Antidiuretic Hormone, N. Engl. J. Med., *298*, 174, 1977.
Lockwood, A. H.: Shy-Drager Syndrome with Abnormal Respirations and Antidiuretic Hormone Release, Arch. Neurol., *33*, 292, 1976.
Matuk, F.: Syndrome of Inappropriate Secretion of Antidiuretic Hormone in Patients Treated with Psychotherapeutic Drugs, Arch. Neurol., *34*, 374, 1977.

Hyperpituitarism

The symptoms of hyperfunction of the pituitary gland may be divided into two classes, according to whether there is overfunction of the acidophilic or basophilic cells. Hyperfunction of the acidophilic cells is usually due to a tumor and results in the syndromes of acromegaly or gigantism. Overactivity of the basophilic cells produces the syndrome described by Cushing. These are described in Chapter 3.

Cerebral Gigantism in Childhood (Sotas Syndrome)

Sotas and his associates in 1964 described five children with a syndrome characterized by gigantism which had its onset *in utero* or in the first few years of life and was thought to be of cerebral origin. Other features of the syndrome in addition to high stature include macrocrania, hypertelorism, dolichocephaly, high arched palate, macroglossia, large hands and feet, and syndactyly of toes and scoliosis.

The neurological abnormalities which are nonprogressive include clumsiness, convulsive seizures and mental retardation. The ventricles are enlarged without evidence of cortical atrophy.

The overgrowth is presumably due to abnormal secretion of the growth hormone, but the values are usually normal at the time the patients are presented for study.

REFERENCES

Abraham, J. M., and Snodgrass, G. J. A. I.: Sotas Syndrome of Cerebral Gigantism, Arch. Dis. Child., *44*, 203, 1969.
Hook, F. B., and Reynolds, J. W.: Cerebral Gigantism. Endocrinological and Clinical Observations of Six Patients, J. Pediatr., *70*, 900, 1967.
Milansky, A., et al.: Cerebral Gigantism in Childhood, Pediatr., *40*, 395, 1967.
Ott, J. E., and Robinson, A.: Cerebral Gigantism, Am. J. Dis. Child., *177*, 357, 1969.
Sotas, J. F., et al.: Cerebral Gigantism, N. Engl. J. Med., *271*, 108, 1964.

Thyroid

Hypothyroidism. Hypothyroidism is the functional state which results from a deficiency or complete lack of the thyroid hormone. It may develop before birth, in infancy, childhood or adult life. The thyroid hormone is important in early growth and development and the syndromes which occur as a result of deficiency depend upon the age of the patient at the time of the onset of the deficiency. These can be divided into three categories: cretinism, juvenile myxedema and adult myxedema.

When severe thyroid deficiency develops *in utero* or in early life, there is retardation of physical and mental development. Soon after birth there is thickening of the subcutaneous tissue, hoarseness of the cry, enlargement of the tongue, widely spaced eyes, pot-belly and an umbilical hernia. If treatment is not given promptly, dwarfism and a severe degree of mental deficiency results.

The clinical picture in juvenile myxedema is similar to that of cretinism with variations depending upon the age of onset of the thyroid deficiency. The degree of physical and mental retardation is usually less severe than in infantile myxedema. Enlargement of the sella turcica has been reported in juvenile myxedema.

Adult myxedema is characterized by lethargy, weakness, slowness of speech, non-pitting edema of the subcutaneous tissues, coarse, pale skin, dry brittle hair, thick lips, enlargement of the tongue, decreased sweating and excessive sensitivity to cold.

The neurological complications of myxedema include: headache, cranial nerve palsies, peripheral neuritis, myopathy, reflex changes, psychotic episodes, and coma with convulsions.

The incidence of cranial nerve palsies is relatively low. Diminution of auditory acuity is estimated to occur in about 15% of the patients. Vertigo and tinnitus may also be present. Unilateral or bilateral facial palsy is recorded in a higher percentage of patients than would be expected by the coincidence of the two conditions. Dysarthria or hoarseness of the voice commonly occurs, but this is probably related to myxedematous infiltration of the tongue and palate and not to involvement of the twelfth or tenth cranial nerves.

A mild polyneuritis has been reported in a few patients. This is characterized mainly by paresthesia in the extremities. Paresthesias accompanied by thenar atrophy are usually due to involvement of the median nerve in the carpal tunnel. A mild generalized myotonia or slow relaxation of muscles and myoedema (mounding phenomenon) on percussion of the muscles is not infrequent. A striking degree of generalized enlargement or "hypertrophy" of the muscles most marked in the extremities and the girdle accompanied by weakness has been reported in a few children and an occasional adult (Kocher-Débre-Sémélaigne syndrome). The enlarged muscles give the affected individual an athletic appearance (infant Hercules, Fig. 158). The muscular weakness improves and the size of the muscles decreases with replacement therapy.

Characteristic of the hypothyroid state is the slow relaxation of the tendons, particularly the Achilles, on testing the reflexes.

Episodes of delirium, uncontrolled excitability, depression, and other psychotic states are infrequent complications. Coma of sudden or rapid onset is a rare complication. If untreated, this complication has a high mortality rate. Cerebellar ataxia and choreoathetosis have been reported in a few cases.

The coincidence of myxedema and myasthenia gravis has been noted in a few patients.

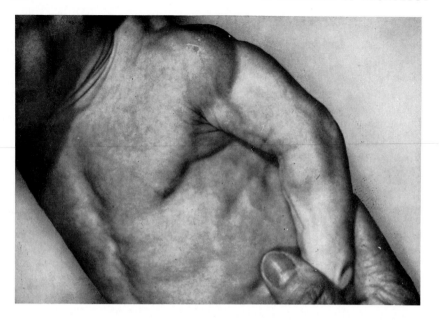

Figure 158.   Enlargement of muscles in myxedema, Kocher-Débre-Sémélaigne
syndrome. (Courtesy Dr. Arnold Gold.)

The characteristic laboratory findings in myxedema are elevated serum cholesterol (300 to 700 gm), low serum protein-bound iodine (less than 3 μgm), a low radioiodine uptake and an increased protein content in the spinal fluid. An absence of alpha waves and a decrease in the amplitude of the waves in the electroencephalogram have been reported. The protein content of the cerebrospinal fluid is increased. Values in excess of 100 mg per cmm are not uncommon. All of the laboratory findings revert to normal after adequate therapy.

The diagnosis of myxedema can usually be made from the characteristic appearance of the patient and the results of laboratory tests. Any physical or mental retardation in infants should lead to a consideration of hypothyroidism. Since basal metabolic rates cannot be reliably determined in infants and young children, the level of the cholesterol in the serum is of great diagnostic value. The diagnosis of myxedema in adults should not be made on the basis of a low basal metabolic rate alone. The level of the serum cholesterol, serum protein-bound iodine and the uptake of radioiodine should be measured to establish or exclude this diagnosis before treatment is instituted.

The treatment of myxedema is thyroid extract (U.S.P.) in dosages varying from 6 mg daily in infants under two months to 180 mg in adults. The initial dose should be small and increased after a period of one to two weeks if there are no toxic symptoms and the desired effects are not obtained with the previous dose. Prophylactic treatment of cretinism is important in goiter districts, where iodine should be given to all pregnant women.

Hyperthyroidism (Graves' Disease). Hyperthyroidism is the condition which results from an excessive secretion of the thyroid gland. Clinically it is associated with an increased metabolic rate, disturbances in the vegetative nervous system, tremors, exophthalmos, other ocular abnormalities and a disturbance in creatine metabolism.

The neurological symptoms are usually limited to tremors of the hands, exophthalmos, lid lag, infrequency of winking, weakness of convergence and a mild or moderately severe weakness of the muscles of the trunk and extremities. Mental disturbances may occur ranging from mild emotional instability to a variety of psychotic syndromes.

In addition to the common signs of Graves' disease, various neurological syndromes may occur in association with thyrotoxicosis, namely, myasthenia gravis, chronic thyrotoxic myopathy, familial periodic paralysis and exophthalmic ophthalmoplegia.

It is clear that there is no etiological relationship between hyperthyroidism and myasthenia gravis, but the coincidence of the two diseases is relatively frequent (5% in the series of Millikan and Haines). In some patients, the two diseases may occur simultaneously, in others myasthenia gravis may precede or follow the thyrotoxicosis by months or years. The differential diagnosis between the muscular weakness of hyperthyroidism and myasthenia gravis is made on the basis of responses to neostigmine and curare. The muscular weakness of hyperthyroidism is not alleviated by neostigmine, whereas a significant degree of improvement results in practically all cases of myasthenia gravis. Conversely, the weakness in patients with myasthenia is greatly increased by small doses of curare, whereas patients with hyperthyroidism do not have an increased sensitivity to this toxin. Treatment of patients with hyperthyroidism and myasthenia gravis consists of a combination of the modern therapies for each of the two diseases. Neostigmine is preferred for the treatment of the myasthenia gravis. Thyroidectomy is hazardous in the presence of difficulty in swallowing, coughing or breathing and the administration of ^{131}I is the preferred form of therapy for the hyperthyroidism.

The term *thyrotoxic myopathy* appeared in the medical literature about forty years ago. The subject has been confused by the fact that adequate studies were not performed in a number of the reported cases. Millikan and Haines reported 9 cases and state that the condition is more frequent than is commonly supposed. The myopathy occurs most commonly in males at the time there are other signs of thyrotoxicosis.

The weakness and wasting are greatest in the muscles of the pelvic girdle, particularly the iliopsoas, and to a lesser extent in the muscles of the shoulder girdle. The distal muscles of the extremities are usually spared or only slightly affected. The reflexes are normal or hyperactive and the sensory examination is normal. Gross muscular twitchings may be seen, but fibrillation potentials are not seen in the electromyogram. The diagnosis is made from the characteristic distribution of the muscular weakness and wasting in a patient with thyrotoxicosis. Myasthenia gravis is excluded by the neostigmine and curare tests, and myositis by histological examination of a specimen of the muscle. Improvement in the strength and nutrition of the affected muscles follows effective treatment of the hyperthyroidism.

The occurrence of *hyperthyroidism and periodic paralysis* in the same patient is rare but is much more frequent than would be anticipated on chance occurrence. Millikan and Haines state that more than 400 cases of familial periodic paralysis are reported in the literature and that less than 30 of them had concurrent hyperthyroidism. The attacks of weakness in the cases with hyperthyroidism are similar to those in the usual cases. Millikan and Haines conclude that clinical and laboratory evidence indicates that periodic paralysis and hyperthyroidism are separate diseases but that the former may exist in a latent form and become manifest with the development of thyrotoxicosis. In such cases the treatment is control of the hyperthyroidism.

Exophthalmic ophthalmoplegia is a rare syndrome in which there is a combination of exophthalmos and paralysis of the extraocular muscles. In addition, there may be chemosis of the lids, edema of the conjunctiva and choking of the optic disks.

The relationship of exophthalmic ophthalmoplegia to diseases of the thyroid is not clear. The condition may develop in patients with hyperthyroidism, in patients who have had a thyroidectomy but who are euthyroid, and in euthyroid patients with no previous history of hyperthyroidism. Brain contends that exophthalmic ophthalmoplegia is a syndrome distinct from exophthalmic goiter. He states that it differs from the latter in age incidence and greater frequency in the male sex.

The pathological changes are confined to the orbit. There is an increase in the orbital contents with edema, hypertrophy, infiltration and fibrosis of the extraocular muscles.

The onset of symptoms is gradual, with exophthalmos accompanied by diplopia due to paresis of one or more ocular muscles. Both eyes may be involved at the same time or the exophthalmos in one eye may precede that in the other by several months. With advance of exophthalmos, paresis of the extrinsic muscles of the eye increases until finally the eyeball is almost totally fixed. Occasionally the optic disk may be choked, and ulcerations of the cornea may develop due to failure of the lid to protect the eye. The paralysis may involve all of the eye muscles or those muscles concerned with the movement of the eyes in a particular plane, particularly upward and outward. The symptoms progress rapidly for a few months and only rarely do they arrest before the development of complete ophthalmoplegia. Occasionally there is spontaneous improvement, but as a rule the symptoms persist unchanged throughout the life of the patient unless they are relieved by surgical therapy.

Radiation therapy of the pituitary or thyroid has no effect on the syndrome, nor does the surgical removal of the thyroid produce any amelioration. The roof of the orbit and canal of the optic nerve can be removed from above, through an anterior craniotomy. The exophthalmos may be relieved by this operation but if the condition has been of extended duration, little improvement in the ophthalmoplegia will result since irreversible changes have already developed in the extraocular muscles. Some authors state that the operation is rarely needed, because the exophthalmos usually does not progress to a serious degree before it comes to a spontaneous arrest. Partial suturing of the lids is recommended in order to protect the eyeball.

Brown and his associates report improvement of chemosis and injection in all of 101 patients treated with prednisone. Improvement in ocular mobility and decrease of proptosis occurred in only a small percentage of patients. Improvement in vision was obtained in all of the patients with severe degree of visual loss.

REFERENCES

Barnard, R. D., Campbell, M. J. and McDonald, M. I.: Pathological Findings in a Case of Hypothyroidism with Ataxia, J. Neurol. Neurosurg. Psychiat., 34, 755, 1971.

Brain, W. R.: Exophthalmic Ophthalmoplegia, Quart. J. Med., 7, 293, 1938.

Brody, I. E., and Dudley, A. W., Jr.: Thyrotoxic Hypokalemic Periodic Paralysis, Arch. Neurol., 21, 1, 1969.

Brown, J., et al.: Adrenal Steroid Therapy of Severe Infiltrative Ophthalmopathy of Graves' Disease, Am. J. Med., 34, 786, 1963.

Burstein, B.: Psychoses Associated with Thyrotoxicosis, Arch. Gen. Psych., 4, 267, 1961.

Catz, B., and Russell, S.: Myxedema, Shock and Coma, Arch. Intern. Med., 108, 407, 1961.

Condon, J. V., Becka, D. R., and Gibbs, F. A.: Electroencephalographic Abnormalities in Hyperthyroidism, J. Clin. Endocrin, 14, 1511, 1954.

Cronstedt, J., Carling, L., and Ostbert, H.: Hypothyroidism with Subacute Pseudomyotonia. An Early Form of Hoffman's Syndrome? Acta Med. Scand., 198, 137, 1975.

Day, R. M., and Carroll, F. G.: Corticosteroids in Treatment of Optic Nerve Involvement Associated with Thyroid Dysfunction, Tr. Am. Ophth. Soc., 65, 40, 1967.

Dyck, P. J., and Lambert, E. H.: Polyneuropathy Associated with Hypothyroidism, J. Neuropathol. Exp. Neurol., 29, 631, 1970.

Fidler, S. M., O'Rourke, R. A., and Buchsbaum, A. W.: Choreoathetosis as a Manifestation of Thyrotoxicosis, Neurology, 21, 55, 1971.

Fincham, R. W. and Cape, C. A.: Neuropathy in Myxedema, Arch. Neurol., 19, 464, 1968.

Forester, C. F.: Coma in Myxedema. Report of Case and Review of World Literature, Arch. Intern. Med., *111*, 734, 1963.

Gorman, C. M., DeSanto, L. W., et al.: Optic Neuropathy of Grave's Disease, N. Engl. J. Med., *290*, 70, 1974.

Hagberg, B., and Westphal, O.: Ataxic Syndrome in Congenital Hypothyroidism, Acta paediat. Scand., *59*, 323, 1970.

Havard, C. W. H., Campbell, E. D. R., Ross, H. B., and Spence, A. W.: Electromyographic and Histological Findings in the Muscles of Patients with thyrotoxicosis, Quart. J. Med., *32*, 145, 1963.

Lindberger, K.: Myxoedema Coma, Acta Med. Scand., *198*, 87, 1975.

McFarland, K. F., and Schumacher, O. P.: Enlargement of the Sella Turcica Secondary to Juvenile Myxedema, Cleveland Clin. Quart., *38*, 195, 1971.

Millikan, C. H., and Haines, S. F.: Thyroid Gland in Relation to Neuromuscular Diseases, Arch. Intern. Med., *92*, 5, 1953.

————: Thyroid Gland in Relation to Metabolic Disorders of the Nervous System, Assoc. Res. Nerv. & Ment. Dis., Proc., *32*, 61, 1953.

Nordgren, L. and von Scheele, C.: Myxedematous Madness without Myxedema, Acta Med. Scand., *199*, 233, 1976.

Norris, F. H., Jr., and Panner, B. J.: Hypothyroid Myopathy. Clinical, Electromyographic and Ultrastructural Observations, Arch. Neurol., *14*, 574, 1966.

Rosman, N. D.: Neurological and Muscular Aspects of Thyroid Dysfunction in Childhood, Pediat. Clin. North Am., *23*, 575, 1976.

Sanders, V.: Neurologic Manifestations of Myxedema, N. Engl. J. Med., *266*, 547 and 599, 1962.

Satoyoshi, E., et al.: Periodic Paralysis in Hyperthyroidism, Neurology, *13*, 746, 1963.

Solomon, D. H., Chopra, I. J., et al.: Identification of Subgroups of Euthyroid Graves's Ophthalmopathy, N. Engl. J. Med., *296*, 181, 1977.

Spiro, A. J., et al.: Cretinism with Muscular Hypertrophy (Kocher-Débre-Sémélaigne), Arch. Neurol., *23*, 340, 1970.

Taher, Y., et al.: Electro-Encephalographic Changes in Cretinism, Clin. Electroenceph., *1*, 6, 1970.

Teng, C. S. and Yeo, P. P. B.: Ophthalmic Graves's Disease: Natural History and Detailed Thyroid Function Studies, Br. Med. J., *1*, 273, 1977.

Werner, S. C.: Prednisone in Emergency Treatment of Malignant Exophthalmos, Lancet, *1*, 1004, 1966.

Parathyroid

Hypoparathyroidism. The disturbance in the calcium and phosphorus metabolism which results from a deficiency in the activity of the parathyroid gland produces a train of neurological symptoms described by the term parathyroid tetany.

Incidence. Hypoparathyroidism may be due to the removal of the glands in the course of a thyroid operation. Rarely, hypoparathyroidism may occur without any obvious cause or it may be associated with either Addison's disease or moniliasis. Idiopathic hypoparathyroidism may develop at any age, but is uncommon in children. A form of hypoparathyroidism (pseudohypoparathyroidism), described in 1942 by Albright and his associates, is characterized by hyperphosphatemia and hypocalcemia, similar to that of true hypoparathyroidism, but the parathyroids are histologically normal or hyperplastic, and the administration of parathyroid hormone does not cause significant phosphaturia or an increase in the serum calcium content. In addition to the usual signs of hypocalcemia there is a characteristic habitus in these patients. There is shortening of the stature, the body build is stocky, the face is round and there is shortening of the metacarpal and metatarsal bones. Occasionally subcutaneous ossification also occurs. Convulsive seizures occur in over two-thirds of these cases. A form of pseudohypoparathyroidism has been described in which the serum calcium and phosphorus are normal and tetany is absent. This has been described by the unwieldy term pseudopseudohypoparathyroidism and probably represents a forme fruste of pseudohypoparathyroidism.

Symptoms. The symptoms of hypoparathyroidism include numbness and cramps in the extremities, carpopedal spasm, laryngeal stridor and convulsive seizures. All of the above symptoms may be present or any one or two of them alone. The convulsive seizures of hypoparathyroidism are usually of the grand mal type. Sometimes, however, they are quite bizarre and are apt to be called hysterical attacks. They tend to occur frequently and their frequency is not influenced by the administration of anticonvulsive drugs. Although hypoparathyroidism is a rare cause of seizures, this diagnosis should be considered in patients with frequent or bizarre seizures that do not respond to anticonvulsive medication, even though no signs of tetany can be elicited. Psychotic manifestations may occur in connection with or independent of the convulsive seizures.

Signs. Tetany is present in practically all of the patients. It may be manifested by carpopedal spasm or it may be present only in latent form. Latent tetany can be demonstrated by: Contraction of the facial muscles on tapping the facial nerve in front of the ear (Chvostek's sign); the production of carpal spasm by reducing the circulation in the arm by means of a blood pressure cuff (Trousseau's sign); and lowered threshold of electrical excitability of the nerve (Erb's sign).

Other findings in patients with hypoparathyroidism include cataracts, symmetrical bilateral punctate calcifications in the basal ganglia, multiple ectodermal lesions (dry scaly skin, alopecia, and atrophic changes in the nails) and aplasia or hypoplasia of the teeth. Choked discs and increased intracranial pressure have been reported in a few cases, but the mechanism is unexplained. Chorea, torticollis, athetosis, dystonia, paralysis agitans, oculogyric crises and other basal ganglia symptoms have been reported in isolated cases. These symptoms do not appear to have any relationship to the presence or absence of calcifications in the basal ganglia.

Laboratory Data. The level of the blood calcium depends upon the degree of hypofunction of the glands. It will fall as low as 4.5 mg per 100 ml with complete absence of activity of the parathyroids, but values in the range of 6 to 8 mg are most commonly encountered. These figures are below the threshold for calcium excretion and there will be an absence of calcium in the urine. The serum phosphorus is elevated. Values in adults are considerably lower than those in children, in whom the serum phosphorus content may be as high as 12 mg per 100 ml. The serum phosphatase is usually low. The cerebrospinal fluid findings are normal except in rare cases with choked disc, where the pressure may be moderately increased. The electroencephalogram shows various abnormalities, particularly 2 to 5 per second waves occurring in short bursts. Minute symmetrical areas of calcification in the cerebral substance may be seen in the roentgenograms of the skull.

Diagnosis. The diagnosis of hypoparathyroidism is made on basis of the clinical symptoms, the hypocalcemia and the absence of calcium in the urine by the Sulkowitch test.

Hypoparathyroidism must be differentiated from other causes of tetany and hypocalcemia. In patients with convulsive seizures or choked discs, the differential must include other causes of these signs. The relationship of these signs to the hypocalcemia is determined by the effects of therapy with dihydrotachysterol.

Tetany may occur in association with alkalosis resulting from excessive loss of gastric content or the ingestion of large amounts of alkali. The tetany of these conditions is distinguished from that of hypoparathyroidism by the presence of calcium in the urine, the normal serum calcium content and changes in the carbon dioxide content of the blood or the carbon dioxide-combining power of the serum.

Other causes of hypocalcemia are rickets, osteomalacia and renal insufficiency with urea and phosphate retention. In rickets and osteomalacia the decrease in the serum calcium is not accompanied by an increase in the phosphorus content. Rickets can also be diagnosed by the characteristic findings of this condition. The hypocalcemia of renal insufficiency is of a lesser degree in comparison to the level of serum phosphorus than that of hypoparthyroidism.

Course and Prognosis. The hypoparathyroidism which follows damage to the gland by thyroidectomy is frequently transient, the symptoms disappearing with regeneration of the damaged glands. The symptoms and signs of idiopathic hypoparathyroidism may be mild and occur only in connection with active exercise, gastrointestinal disturbances or acute infections. In other cases, the symptoms are constant. Fatalities are rare but mental deterioration may occur, particularly in patients with convulsive seizures.

Treatment. Parathormone is effective in relieving the symptoms and in restoring the serum levels of calcium and phosphorus to normal, but its effect diminishes with prolonged administration. In addition, it is entirely ineffective in the rare form of hypoparathyroidism labeled by Albright as pseudohypoparathyroidism.

Dihydrotachysterol (A.T. 10), a substance closely related to vitamin D, aids in the absorption of calcium from the intestines and increases the excretion of phosphorus. It is effective in relieving the symptoms of tetany and restoring the serum calcium and phosphorus level to normal. The dose should be regulated according to the needs of the patient. Overdosage will result in abnormally high levels of calcium in the serum. Dihydrotachysterol is administered by mouth in dosage of 1.25 mg 3 times daily until the blood calcium is normal. The drug is then administered in a suitable dosage to maintain the serum calcium at a normal level as determined by direct estimation of the serum content or the excretion of calcium in the urine.

Hyperparathyroidism (Osteitis Fibrosa Cystica). An excess of the parathyroid hormone causes thinning of the bones, muscular weakness and the formation of renal stones.

Etiology. It was not until 1925 that the role of the parathyroid as the cause of the bone disease in von Recklinghausen's osteitis fibrosa cystica was known. It soon became obvious that all of the symptoms were related to the presence of a tumor or hyperplasia of the gland. Albright postulated that hyperplasia or adenoma formation may be the result of some situation tending to lower the serum calcium levels with stimulation of germinal centers which lose their property of being controlled by normal stimuli. Adenomas or hyperplasia of the gland have been reported in association with eosinophilic or basophilic adenomas of the pituitary, adenomas of the islets of Langerhans, pancreatitis and gastric ulcers.

Pathology. Overactivity of the parathyroids is due to the presence of an adenoma or to a diffuse enlargement of the glands. The tumors are usually simple adenomas but carcinomatous involvement of the gland has been reported. The adenomas usually occur singly, but two or more tumors were found in 6% of the 89 cases collected by Albright. In simple hyperplasia, all of the parathyroids are enlarged as the result of proliferation of the "Wasserhelle" cells.

The changes in the bones are described by the term osteitis fibrosa cystica. The bones are decalcified and there is a great increase in the number of osteoclasts. As a result, there may be bone tumors (osteoclastomas) or multiple cysts with fibrous walls. Nephrolithiasis is present in over three fourths of the cases and nephrocalcinosis in a much smaller percentage.

Incidence. The disease was formerly considered to be quite rare, but Cope and his associates have collected 343 cases at the Massachusetts

General Hospital. The condition may occur at any age, but it is rare before the age of twenty. Females are affected approximately twice as frequently as males.

Symptoms. The initial symptoms (Table 94) may be pains in the back and extremities and hypotonic weakness of the skeletal muscles. Loss of appetite, nausea or constipation may occur as result of hypotonia of the smooth muscles of the intestines. Spontaneous fractures and shortening of stature may occur as result of changes in the bones. Renal stones are common and symptoms of chronic nephritis develop when calcium is deposited in the renal tubules. Polyuria and polydipsia are common.

Signs. The muscles of the trunk and extremities are weak and hypotonic. Sometimes this is so severe that the diagnosis of myasthenia gravis or Addison's disease may be suggested. The muscles may show a mild or moderate degree of atrophy. The electrical excitability of the muscles is diminished and the tendon reflexes are decreased or absent. Psychotic episodes or periods of coma may occur.

All kinds of bone deformities may occur. The long bones may be bent, the pelvis deformed, or various deformities of the vertebral column may develop. In advanced cases, the stature is shortened, the neck disappears into the thorax and the chest takes on a pigeon-breast appearance. Cyst formation in the vertebrae is a rare cause of spinal cord or root compression.

Laboratory Data. The blood calcium content is high, usually over 12 mg per 100 ml, the phosphorus content is low or normal except when the renal function is impaired. A determination of the renal tubular reabsorption of phosphate may be of additional value in borderline cases. The serum phosphatase is elevated. Anemia and leukopenia may

Table 94.   Clues to the Diagnosis of Hyperparathyroidism in the First 343 Cases at the Massachusetts General Hospital

(After Cope, N. Engl. J. Med., 1966)

Clue	No. of Cases
Bone disease	80
Renal stones	195
Peptic ulcer	27
Pancreatitis	9
Fatigue	10
Hypertension	6
Mental disturbance	3
Central nervous system signs	7
Multiple endocrine abnormalities	3
Lumps in neck	1
No symptoms	2

occur when there is extensive fibrosis in the bone marrow. The volume of the urine is increased. Albumin and casts may be present.

The changes in the bones in the roentgenograms are characteristic. There is a general decalcification except for the teeth. The thickness of the skull is not affected but the calvarium has an even ground glass appearance in the roentgenograms. Tumor and cysts of the bone may be seen in roentgenograms of the bones.

Diagnosis. Hyperparathyroidism may manifest itself by the combination of bone and kidney disease or by either one of these alone. The development of typical skeletal deformities or recurrent attacks of nephrolithiasis should lead to the consideration of hyperparathyroidism. The diagnosis is confirmed by the findings of a high calcium and low phosphorus content in the serum.

The differential diagnosis includes diseases of the bone with changes which may be mistaken for those for hyperparathyroidism and other causes of hypercalcemia. These can usually be distinguished without difficulty from the clinical picture, the character and distribution of the roentgenographic changes and the blood chemistry.

Course. When the disease is discovered early and treated, there is a prompt improvement of symptoms. The giant cell tumors disappear and the bone cysts fill in slowly.

If untreated, the disease progresses slowly. The bones become thin, there are spontaneous fractures and collapse of the vertebrae. The patients become bedridden and die of renal failure.

Treatment. The treatment is surgical removal of the adenomas. All of the glands should be visualized on the possibility that more than one adenoma is present or that the condition is due to hyperplasia of the glands. In the latter case subtotal resection should be performed. Postoperative tetany may develop in patients with severe bone decalcification. This complication is treated by a high-calcium, low-phosphorus regimen.

REFERENCES

Albright, F., and Reifenstein, E. C., Jr.: *The Parathyroid Gland and Metabolic Bone Disease,* Baltimore, Williams & Wilkins, 1948. 406 pp.

Beal, M. G., et al.: Vitamin D: Discovery of its Metabolites and Their Therapeutic Applications, Pediatr., *57,* 729, 1976.

Cullen, D. R., and Pearce, J. M. S.: Spinal Cord Compression in Pseudohypoparathyroidism, J. Neurol., Neurosurg., and Psychiat, *27,* 459, 1964.

Cope, O.: the Story of Hyperparathyroidism at the Massachusetts General Hospital, N. Engl. J. Med., *274,* 1174, 1966.

Dudley, A. W., and Hawkins, H.: Mineralization of the Central Nervous System in Pseudopseudohypoparathyroidism, J. Neurol., Neurosurg., and Psychiat., *33,* 147, 1970.

Editorial: Anticonvulsant Osteomalacia, Br. Med. J., *2,* 1340, 1976.

Frame, B., et al.: Myopathy in Primary Hyperparathyroidism, Ann. Intern. Med., *68,* 1022, 1968.

Hossain, M.: Neurological and Psychiatric Manifestations in Idiopathic Hypopara-
    thyroidism: Response to Treatment, J. Neurol., Neurosurg., and Psychiat., *33*, 153,
    1970.
Mautalen, C. A., Dymling, J. F., and Horwith, M.: Pseudohypoparathyroidism 1942-1966,
    Am. J. Med., *42*, 977, 1967.
McKinney, A. S.: Idiopathic Hypoparathyroidism Presenting as Chorea, Neurology, *12*,
    485, 1962.
Mallette, L. E., et al.: Primary Hyperparathyroidism. Clinical and Biochemical Features,
    Medicine, *53*, 127, 1974.
Mallette, L. F., Patten, R. M. and Engel, W. K.: Neuromuscular Disease in Secondary
    Hyperparathyroidism, Ann. Intern. Med., *82*, 474, 1975.
Nusynowitz, M. L., Frame, B., and Kolb, P. O.: The Spectrum of Hypoparathyroid States,
    Medicine, *53*, 127, 1974.
Patten, B. M., et al.: Neuromuscular Disease in Primary Hyperparathyroidism, Ann.
    Intern. Med., *80*, 182, 1974.
Roberts, P. D.: Familial Calcification of the Cerebral Basal Ganglia and Its Relation to
    Hypoparathyroidism, Brain, *82*, 599, 1959.
Schott, G. D. and Wills, M. R.: Muscle Weakness in Osteomalacia, Lancet, *1*, 626. 1976.
Smith, R., and Stern, G.: Muscular Weakness in Osteomalacia and Hyperparathyroidism,
    J. Neurol. Sci., *8*, 511, 1969.

Pancreas

Hyperinsulinism. The nervous system depends entirely on glucose
for its metabolism, and dysfunction develops rapidly whenever the
amount of glucose in the blood falls below critical levels. Low blood
sugar levels may be associated with overdosage of insulin in the
treatment of diabetes mellitus. Spontaneous hypoglycemia is usually
the result of an excessive secretion of insulin by the pancreas (hyperinsulinism).

Etiology. According to Conn, approximately 80 to 90% of all cases of
spontaneous hypoglycemia are due to one of three causes: functional
hypoglycemia, hyperinsulinism with demonstrable pancreatic lesion,
or organic disease of the liver. Hypoglycemia may occur with tumors of
the islet cells, or it may be associated with functional overactivity of the
cells. In the 27 cases reported by Hoefer, Guttman and Sands, an
adenoma was present in 21, carcinoma in 4 and hyperplasia in 2. Islet
cell tumors occur most frequently in the body or tail of the pancreas.
Multiple tumors which are present in over 10% of the cases are in rare
instances associated with adenomas of the parathyroid. The tumors are
usually small, 1 to 2 cm in diameter, but occasionally they are much
larger.

Hypoglycemia may occur when the function of the liver is severely
impaired or when the pituitary or adrenal is seriously damaged. Little
is known in regard to the etiology of the functional hypoglycemia
which occurs in patients with no demonstrable lesion of the pancreas,
liver or other endocrine glands.

Spontaneous hypoglycemia occasionally occurs in infants. The cause is as yet unknown. In approximately half of the cases the fall in the blood glucose level can be related to the administration of case in hydrolysate or L-leucine ("leucine sensitive hypoglycemia"). It is probable that the appearance of spontaneous hypoglycemia in some of these infants may be an early manifestation of an inherited metabolic abnormality associated with diabetes mellitus. The symptoms associated with the hypoglycemia include muscular twitchings, myoclonic jerks and convulsive seizures. Failure of mental development results if the condition is not recognized and adequately treated at the onset.

Pathology. The pathological changes associated with hypoglycemia include those related to the underlying cause and include: Tumors of the pancreas; tumors and atrophy of the pituitary; cirrhosis and other diseases of the liver; and atrophy of the adrenals. In addition, there may be degenerative changes in the brain of patients who have been subject to one or more severe and prolonged attacks of hypoglycemia. In such cases there is a loss of neurons of the third and fourth layers of the cortex of the cerebral hemispheres. There is glial proliferation in the affected areas.

Incidence. Hyperinsulinism is rare. Whipple collected 32 cases at the Presbyterian Hospital in New York. Islet cell tumors were present in 27 of the 32 cases. The age at time of operation in Whipple's patients varied between twenty and sixty-five years. The duration of symptoms before operation varied from a few months to twenty years. Females were affected twice as frequently as males.

The symptoms in infantile hypoglycemia usually have their onset in the first six to twelve months of life. There is a tendency for the condition to have a familial occurrence.

Symptoms and Signs. The symptoms of hyperinsulinism are paroxysmal in nature, tending to occur at periods when the blood sugar could be expected to be low, that is, in the morning before breakfast, after a fast of several or many hours and after heavy exercise. Occasionally, however, the symptoms may occur only a few hours after an apparently adequate meal. The duration of symptoms is subject to great variation. They may last only a few minutes or they may be prolonged for hours. Their severity is also quite variable. There may be only nervousness, anxiety or tremulousness, readily relieved by the ingestion of food. Severe attacks last for several hours during which the patient may perform automatic activity with complete amnesia for the entire period, or there may be convulsive seizures, followed by a prolonged coma. The latter, in rare instances, may be entirely unresponsive to therapy. The frequency of attacks varies from several a day to one in several or many months.

The symptoms manifested by the patients during the period of hypoglycemia may be divided into two groups: (1) disturbances of the activity of the sympathetic nervous system; (2) symptoms of dysfunction of the central nervous system.

Sympathetic disturbances are present in most of the patients at the onset of the hypoglycemia and usually precede the development of the more serious symptoms of central nervous system dysfunction. They include lightheadedness, sweating, nausea, vomiting, pallor, palpitation, precordial oppression, headache, abdominal pain and ravenous hunger.

Symptoms of dysfunction of the central nervous system usually occur in association with the sympathetic phenomena, but in a few cases they may be the only manifestations of the hypoglycemia. The most common symptoms are paresthesias in the extremities or face and diplopia or blurred vision. These may be followed by generalized weakness, tremors, transient hemiplegia, aphasia, periods of abnormal behavior, mental confusion, incoherence, irritability, minor or major convulsive seizures, or periods of coma without a preceding convulsive seizure. The periods of confusion and abnormal behavior may simulate the attacks of so-called psychomotor epilepsy. Convulsive seizures, when they occur, may be of the jacksonian or grand mal type. Although convulsions are a common manifestation of severe hypoglycemia, hyperinsulinism is a rare cause of recurrent convulsive seizures (epilepsy), probably representing less than 0.1% of the cases.

Signs. The neurological examination is usually normal except during the attacks of hypoglycemia when there may be oculomotor weakness, nystagmus, hemiparesis or hemianesthesia. The reflexes may be hyperactive or depressed. The plantar responses are extensor in type, whenever convulsive seizures or coma occur. Amyotrophy as result of damage to ventral horn cells has been reported. Retardation of mental development is common in untreated cases of infantile hypoglycemia.

Laboratory Data. The fasting blood sugar is usually low, but it may be normal and remain normal for many days or months in the patients with infrequent attacks. In the 27 cases with proven lesions of the pancreas reported by Hoefer, Guttman and Sands, the fasting blood sugar level varied between 30 and 71 mg per 100 ml. It was below 40 mg in 28% and below 50 mg in 68%. The blood sugar is always low at the onset of an attack. It may have returned to normal if the specimen is not withdrawn until after a convulsive seizure or the patient has been in coma for several hours. The level at which symptoms appear varies; some patients do not develop any symptoms until the level is below 40 mg and others present classical symptoms with blood levels between 50 and 60 mg. The glucose tolerance test gives variable results. It may be flat or of the diabetic type, but more commonly low values will be found especially if specimens are taken five to eight hours after the stimulating dose of glucose. The electroencephalogram shows focal or widespread dysrhythmia during an attack of hypoglycemia and in some cases even in the interval between attacks.

Diagnosis. The diagnosis of hyperinsulinism is made by the paroxysmal appearance of signs of dysfunction of the sympathetic and central nervous system in association with a low blood sugar. The paroxysms usually appear at a time when the blood sugar could be expected to be low and practically all of the patients know that their symptoms can be relieved by eating.

If it is not possible to obtain a specimen of blood during an attack, the blood should be tested after a fast of twenty-four hours. As noted, the glucose tolerance, unless prolonged for five to eight hours, is not of much value in the diagnosis.

The differential diagnosis includes other causes of symptoms of sympathetic overactivity and convulsive seizures. These are usually excluded by the lack of relationship of the attacks to fasting and by the normal blood sugar.

Hypoglycemia associated with diseases of the liver, pituitary or adrenal can usually be distinguished by the other signs and symptoms of disease in these organs.

The differential between tumors of the islet cells and functional hyperinsulinism cannot be made except by surgical exploration. A negative exploration does not absolutely exclude the presence of a tumor because small adenomas can be present in the depth of the gland and not be palpated by the surgeon.

Course. Mild attacks of spontaneous hypoglycemia may occur at infrequent intervals for many years, but as a rule they tend to become more frequent and severe with the passage of years. There may occasionally be remission of the attacks for months or years. Death may occur in one of the attacks of coma. Rarely, the patient may remain in coma for many days or weeks although the blood sugar returns to normal. This coma is due to severe irreversible damage to the cerebral cortex. This sequence of events is also a rare occurrence in psychotic patients treated with large doses of insulin.

Treatment. The treatment of spontaneous hypoglycemia is separated into the treatment of the acute attack and the treatment of the underlying cause.

Early and intensive treatment of an acute attack is important in order to prevent anoxic damage to the brain. If the patient is conscious, sugar can be administered by mouth in the form of candy, orange juice or milk. Comatose patients should be given 0.5 to 1.0 mg of epinephrine subcutaneously and 10 to 20 gm of glucose intravenously. Glucose should be given by hypodermoclysis and by stomach tube when the coma is prolonged.

When the episodes of hypoglycemia cannot be explained on any other basis, the presumptive diagnosis is adenoma of the islets of Langerhans and exploratory operation is indicated. This should not be delayed because the frequent feedings which are needed to ward off the attacks often lead to obesity. The attacks of hypoglycemia usually disappear after operative removal of the tumor. A second operation may be necessary if two or more tumors are present and are not all removed at the first operation.

Functional hyperinsulinism is treated by a diet high in proteins and low in carbohydrates in order to avoid the stimulatory effect of the latter on the pancreas.

Corticosteroids and extra carbohydrates in the diet are recommended for the treatment of infantile hypoglycemia. A low-leucine diet should be given to the infants who are found to be sensitive to leucine. Partial pancreatectomy has been suggested for patients who do not respond to conservative therapy.

Hypoinsulinism. Hypoinsulinism, or diabetes mellitus, may be accompanied by a variety of lesions in the nervous system. These are mainly in the form of a mono- or polyneuritis. Other neurological complications include diabetic coma associated with an extreme degree of hyperglycemia and acidosis. Vascular lesions may occur in the brain as result of the vascular disease associated with diabetes mellitus.

REFERENCES

Anderson, J. M., Milner, R. D. G., and Strich, S. J.: Effects of Neonatal Hypoglycemia on the Nervous System: A Pathological Study, J. Neurol., Neurosurg. and Psychiat., 30, 295, 1967.
Bell, W. E., Samaan, W. A., and Longnecker, D. S.: Hypoglycemia Due to Organic Hyperinsulinism in Infant, Arch. Neurol., 23, 330, 1971.
Conn, J. W., and Pek, S.: Current Concepts of Spontaneous Hypoglycemia. Kalamazoo, Upjohn Co., 1970.
Courville, C. B.: Late Cerebral Changes Incident to Severe Hypoglycemia (Insulin Shock): Their Relation to Cerebral Anoxia, Arch. Psychiat., 78, 1, 1957.
Harrison, M. J. G.: Muscle Wasting after Prolonged Hypoglycemic Coma: Case Report with Electrophysiological Data, J. Neurol. Neurosurg., Psychiat., 30, 465. 1976.
Hoefer, P. F. A., Guttman, S. A., and Sands, I. J.: Convulsive States and Coma in Cases of Islet Cell Adenoma of the Pancreas, Am. J. Psychiat., 102, 486, 1946.
Mabry, C. C., DiGeorge, A. M., and Auerbach, V. H.: Leucine-Induced Hypoglycemia, J. Ped., 57, 526, 1960.
Merimee, T. J.: Spontaneous Hypoglycemia in Man, Arch. Intern. Med., 22, 301, 1977.
Mulder, D. W., Bastron, J. A., and Lambert, E. H.: Hyperinsulin Neuronopathy, Neurology, 6, 627, 1956.
Pagliara, A. S., et al.: Hypoglycemia in Childhood, Pediatrics, 82, 365, and 82, 558, 1973.
Richardson, J. C., Chambers, R. A., and Heywood, P. M.: Encephalopathies of Anoxia and Hypoglycemia, Arch. Neurol., 1, 178, 1959.
Turkington, R. W.: Encephalopathy Induced by Oral Hypoglycemic Drugs, Arch. Intern. Med., 136, 136, 137:1082, 1977.
Whipple, A. O.: Hyperinsulinism in Relation to Pancreatic Tumors, Surgery, 16, 289, 1944.

Adrenal

The adrenal is composed of two portions, the cortex and the medulla. The cortex elaborates approximately 26 steroids which are concerned with: the regulation, distribution and excretion of sodium, potassium and chloride; regulation of water balance by opposing the action of the posterior pituitary antidiuretic hormone; regulation of carbohydrate utilization; regulation of the number of circulating eosinophils, lymphoid tissue and thymus by promoting their lysis; stimulation of certain androgenic functions such as axillary hair growth in women and nitrogen retention in both sexes; and the prevention of excessive melanin deposits in the pigment layers of the skin.

The hormone elaborated by the adrenal medulla is composed of two fractions, epinephrine and norepinephrine. Epinephrine has a stimulatory effect on the central nervous system and acts as a vasodilator of peripheral blood vessels. Norepinephrine constricts peripheral blood vessels and elevates the systemic blood pressure.

Adrenal Hypofunction: Addison's Disease. There is no known disease which results from hypofunction of the adrenal medulla. Adrenal cortical hypofunction may develop acutely in the presence of severe overwhelming infections, particularly meningococcemia or staphylococcemia. Acute or chronic adrenal cortical insufficiency may also be a feature of hypofunction of the pituitary.

Hypofunction of the adrenal cortex is usually due to an atrophy of the gland of unknown cause. The gland may be destroyed by tuberculosis, neoplasms, amyloidosis, hemachromatosis and fungal infections. Chronic insufficiency of the adrenal cortex, Addison's disease, is characterized by weakness, easy fatigability, weight loss, increased pigmentation of the skin, hypotension, anorexia, nausea, vomiting, diarrhea, irritability, anxiety, and episodes of hypoglycemia. Psychotic symptoms develop in a few of the cases. The syndrome of pseudotumor cerebri has been reported as a complication of Addison's disease. Addison's disease is quite rare and the symptoms usually have their onset in middle or late life. The diagnosis is suggested by the appearance of the characteristic symptoms. It can be confirmed by the failure of an injection of corticotropin to produce a reduction in the number of circulating eosinophils, and by a decrease in the twenty-four hour urinary output of 17-ketosteroids.

The prognosis of Addison's disease without substitution therapy is poor. The average life expectancy is one to two years. The course is punctuated by a series of crises, which may be precipitated by overexertion, acute infections, surgical procedures or administration of laxatives. Death is often due to severe hypoglycemia. With adequate hormone therapy, the symptoms can be relieved and the life expectancy greatly increased.

The treatment of Addison's disease consists of regulation of sodium metabolism by the administration of deoxycorticosterone, fludrohydrocortisone, or high-salt diet. Hydrocortisone is also given to maintain strength and create a sense of well-being.

REFERENCES

Abbas, D. H., Schlagenhauff, R. E., and Strong, H. H.: Polyradiculoneuropathy in Addison's Disease: Case Report and Review of the Literature, Neurology, 27, 494, 1977.
Addison, T.: On the Constitutional and Local Effects of Diseases of the Suprarenal Capsules, London, D. Highley, 1855.
Christy, N. P.: The Human Adrenal Cortex, New York, Harper & Row, 1971.
Drake, F. R.: Neuropsychiatric-Like Symptomatology of Addison's Disease: A Review of the Literature, Am. J. Med. Sci., 234, 106, 1957.
Van Dellen, R. G., and Purnell, D. C.: Hyperkalemic Paralysis in Addison's Disease, Mayo Clin. Proc., 44, 904, 1969.

Adrenal Hyperfunction

Adrenal Virilism and Adrenogenital Syndrome. Hyperfunction of the adrenal cortex produces the syndrome described by Cushing and attributed by him to the presence of a basophilic adenoma of the pituitary.

The clinical symptoms of Cushing's disease can be reproduced by the administration of the corticosteroids. In addition myopathy or increased intracranial pressure may result. The syndrome of pseudotumor with headache, nausea, vomiting and choked disc tends to occur on withdrawal of therapy, particularly in children who were given steroid therapy for asthma, eczema, arthritis and nephrosis. Treatment is reinstated with later gradual withdrawal of the steroid therapy.

Overproduction of the steroid hormones with androgenic activity by hyperplasia or tumors of the adrenal cortex may produce the syndrome of masculinization in women. Its biological counterpart, a tumor with excessive production of estrogenic substances causing feminization in men, has been recognized but is extremely rare. Adrenal virilism is relatively rare but may occur at any time from the prenatal period to old age. The syndromes which develop depend upon the sex of the patient and the age at the time of onset.

Androgenic hyperplasia of the adrenal cortex before birth results in pseudohermaphroditism in the female and pubertas praecox with macrogenitosomia in the male. Precocious puberty may result from injury to the hypothalamus by hamartomas or other tumors in that region. Tumor or hyperplasia of the gland before the age of puberty causes macrogenitosomia in the male and virilization in the female. Virilization in young females is characterized by enlargement of the clitoris, hirsutism, retarded breast development, rapid growth, amenorrhea and an increase in the excretion of the 17-ketosteroids. Virilism after the age of puberty is not uncommon. Symptoms may vary widely, from that of the classical adrenogenital syndrome to a moderate degree of hirsutism.

Adrenal virilism is usually suspected from the history and physical examination. There is invariably an increased excretion of urinary 17-ketosteroids. In tumors associated with feminization, there is an increase in the excretion of estrogenic substances in the urine. In some cases a tumor in the adrenal region can be palpated. Changes in the pyelogram are often of value in establishing the diagnosis. Arrhenoblastoma of the ovary, tumors of the testes, pineal tumors and Cushing's syndrome are to be considered in the differential diagnosis.

Treatment is surgical removal of the tumor. Corticotropin should be given preoperatively and cortisone in dose of 50 to 200 mg daily for the first few days following the operation.

REFERENCES

Askari, A., Vignos, P. J., Jr., and Moskowitz, R. W.: Steroid Myopathy in Connective Tissue Disease, Am. J. Med., 61, 485, 1976.
Azarnoff, D. L. (Ed.): Steroid Therapy. Philadelphia, W. B. Saunders Co., 1975.
Cohn, G. A.: Pseudotumor Cerebri in Children Secondary to Administration of Adrenal Steroids, J. Neurosurg., 20, 784, 1963.
Gabrilove, J. L., et al.: Feminizing Adrenocortical Tumors in the Male. A Review of 52 Cases Including a Case Report, Medicine, 44, 37, 1965.
Krieger, D. T.: The Central Nervous System and Cushing's Syndrome, Mt. Sinai J. Med., N.Y., 39, 416, 1972.
List, C. F., et al.: Posterior Hypothalamic Hamartomas and Gangliogliomas Causing Precocious Puberty, Neurology, 8, 164, 1958.
Orth, D. N., and Liddle, G. W.: Results of Treatment in 108 Patients with Cushing's Syndrome, N. Engl. J. Med., 285, 243, 1971.
Walker, A. E., and Adamkiewicz, J. J.: Pseudotumor Cerebri Associated with Prolonged Corticosteroid Therapy, J.A.M.A., 188, 779, 1964.

Primary Aldosteronism. In 1955, Conn reported a new syndrome due to production of aldosterone by a tumor of the adrenal cortex. Since the original report a small number of cases have been recorded in the literature. The clinical syndrome is characterized by recurrent attacks of severe muscular weakness simulating familial periodic paralysis, tetany, polyuria, hypertension, inability of the kidneys to concentrate urine, and a striking imbalance of serum electrolytes with hypokalemia, hypernatremia and alkalosis. Changes consistent with those of hypokalemia are found in the electrocardiogram. An excessive amount of aldosterone is excreted in the urine.

The treatment is removal of the adrenal tumor or subtotal adrenalectomy in the cases where the hyperaldosteronism is due to functional overactivity of the gland. Conn has reported that essential hypertension can result from adrenocortical tumors which produce hyperaldosteronism without a concomitant hypokalemia.

REFERENCES

Conn, J. W.: Presidential Address: II Primary Aldosteronism, New Clinical Syndrome, J. Lab. & Clin. Med., 45, 6, 1955.
Conn, J. W., Rovner, D. R., Cohen, E. L., and Nesbit, R. M.: Normokalemic Primary Aldosteronism. Its Masquerade as "Essential" Hypertension, J.A.M.A., 195, 21, 1966.
Hewlett, J. S., et al.: Aldosterone-Producing Tumor of the Adrenal Gland; Report of Three Cases, J.A.M.A., 164, 179, 1957.

Pheochromocytoma. Hyperfunction of the adrenal medulla as result of tumor of the chromaffin cells is characterized by an increased secretion of epinephrine and norepinephrine with signs and symptoms of hyperadrenalism. Tumors of the chromaffin cells of the adrenal medulla are rare, but they are important because they are one cause of hypertension that can be cured. They may occur in association with von Recklinghausen's disease, tuberous sclerosis and tumors of other endocrine glands.

Hypertension of a moderate or severe degree is the characteristic feature. This may be sustained or intercurrent in nature. The persistent hypertension is indistinguishable on routine examinations from other types of benign or malignant hypertension. The intercurrent type is characterized by paroxysmal attacks of palpitation, precordial pain, severe headache, dizziness, sweating, weakness, anxiety, nausea, vomiting, diarrhea, dilated pupils, paresthesias, rapid pulse, and a rise in blood pressure which may attain levels between 200 and 300 mm Hg. Death may result from cerebral hemorrhage, pulmonary edema or cardiac failure in one of the acute attacks or as a result of one of these complications in the sustained type.

The diagnosis of the intercurrent type is suggested by the paroxysmal occurrence of the symptoms of hyperadrenalism. Differentiation from acute anxiety attacks can be made when an attack can be precipitated by massaging the abdomen in the region of the adrenals or by the histamine test of Roth and Kvale. In this test a severe rise in blood pressure occurs following the intravenous injection of 0.025 to 0.050 mg of histamine base. The persistent type of hypertension associated with a pheochromocytoma can be diagnosed by the benzodioxan or Regitine test. Determination of the catecholamines, norepinephrine or epinephrine (or both) in urine or blood is invaluable in the establishment of the diagnosis. The catecholamines are increased in the urine and blood of the cases with sustained hypertension. They are increased in the blood during spontaneous or induced attacks of paroxysmal hypertension associated with a pheochromocytoma.

The treatment is surgical removal of the tumor.

REFERENCES

Anderson, W. H., Rolufs, L. S., and Doerner, A. A.: Use of Pharmacological Tests in Diagnosis of Pheochromocytoma, Am. Heart J., 43, 252, 1952.
Axelrod, J., and Weinshilbroom, R.: Physiology in Medicine: Catecholamines, N. Engl. J. Med., 287, 237, 1972.
Cahill, G. F.: Pheochromocytomas, J.A.M.A., 138, 180, 1948.
Goldenberg, M., et al.: The Hemodynamic Response of Man to Norepinephrine and Epinephrine and Its Relation to the Problem of Hypertension, Am. J. Med., 5, 792, 1948.
Howard, J. E., and Barker, W. H.: Paroxysmal Hypertension and Other Clinical Manifestations Associated with Benign Chromaffin Cell Tumors, Bull. Johns Hopkins Hosp., 61, 371, 1937.
Iance, J. W. and Hinterberger, H.: Symptoms of Pheochromocytoma with Particular Reference to Headache, Correlated with Catecholamine Production, Arch. Neurol., 3, 4, 1976.
Iseri, L. T., Henderson, H. W., and Derr, J. W.: Use of Adrenolytic Drug, Regitine, in Pheochromocytoma, Am. Heart J., 42, 129, 1951.
Masson, G. M., Corcoran, A. C., and Humphrey, D. C.: Diagnostic Procedures for Pheochromocytoma. Technique of Assay of Urine in Rat and Demonstration of Piperoxan Hydrochloride-Antidiuresis During Normotensive Phase, J.A.M.A., 165, 1555, 1957.
Moorehead, E. L., et al.: The Diagnosis of Pheochromocytoma, J.A.M.A., 196, 1107, 1966.
Paloyan, E., et al.: Familial Pheochromocytoma, Medullary Thyroid Carcinoma and Parathyroid Adenomas, J.A.M.A., 214, 1443, 1970.
Reutter, F. W., Zileli, M. S., Hamlin, J. T., Thorn, G. W., and Friend, Dale, G.: Importance of Detecting Rapid Changes in Blood Catecholamine Levels in the Diagnosis of Pheochromocytoma, N. Engl. J. Med., 257, 323, 1957.
Sjoerdsam, A., et al.: Pheochromocytoma: Current Concepts of Diagnosis and Treatment, Ann. Intern. Med., 65, 1302, 1966.
Smithwick, R. H., Greer, W. E. R., Robertson, C. W., and Wilkins, R. W.: Pheochromocytoma, N. Engl. J. Med., 242, 252, 1950.
Thomas, J. E., Rooke, E. D., and Kuale, W. F.: The Neurologist's Experience with Pheochromocytoma: A Review of 100 Cases, J.A.M.A., 197, 754, 1966.
Thorn, G. W., Hindle, J. A., and Sandmeyer, J. A.: Pheochromocytoma of the Adrenal Associated with Persistent Hypertension, Ann. Intern. Med., 21, 122, 1944.

Ovary: Complications of Administration of Contraceptive Hormones

Estrogen-containing compounds have been widely used as contraceptives for more than ten years and there are many reports in the literature on the untoward side effects. These include hypertension, migraine, cerebral vascular lesions, optic neuritis and choked discs with increased intracranial pressure (pseudotumor cerebri).

In view of the large number of patients taking these hormones and the occasional occurrence of all of these conditions in women of the age groups concerned, it is difficult to assess the role of the hormone in the development of the morbid condition under consideration.

There is no doubt, however, that the taking of estrogenic hormones for contraceptive purpose is accompanied by the risk of certain complications. This risk must be measured against the importance of prevention of pregnancy.

REFERENCES

Collaborative Group for the Study of Stroke in Young Women: Oral Contraception and Increased Risk of Cerebral Ischemia or Thrombosis, N. Engl. J. Med., 288, 871, 1973.
Collaborative Group for the Study of Stroke in Young Women: Oral Contraceptive and Stroke in Young Women: Associated Risk Factors, J.A.M.A., 231, 718, 1975.
Heyman, A., Hurtig, H.: Clinical Complications of Oral Contraceptives, Disease-A-Month, August, 1975.
Masi, A. T., and Dugdale, M.: Cerebrovascular Diseases Associated with the Use of Oral Contraceptives, Ann. Intern. Med., 72, 111, 1970.
Shoenberg, B. S., et al.: Strokes in Women of Childbearing Age. A Population Study, Neurology, 20, 181, 1970.

DISEASES OF THE BLOOD

Primary Anemia

Subacute Combined Degeneration of the Spinal Cord. The neurological manifestations of primary (pernicious) anemia are the result of degenerative changes in the peripheral nerves and central nervous system. They have been described under the terms subacute combined degeneration of the cord, combined system disease and funicular myelitis. The characteristic early clinical symptoms are paresthesias in the distal parts of the extremities and a spastic, ataxic weakness of the legs.

Neurological symptoms, similar to those which are present in the patient with pernicious anemia, have been reported with other types of anemia or nutritional deficiency. The symptoms in these latter conditions are usually related to changes in the peripheral nerves and not to degeneration of the spinal cord.

Etiology. The anemia and the changes in the nervous system are the result of a deficiency of vitamin B_{12}, a cobalt-containing vitamin which is present in many foods of animal origin. Patients with pernicious anemia have a defect of the gastric secretion which deprives them of an enzyme (so-called intrinsic factor) specifically required for the absorption of vitamin B_{12} (extrinsic factor) which is present in low concentration in most foods. The disease is usually related to an inborn defect in the secretion of intrinsic factor by the parietal cells of the stomach. It may occur when there is malabsorption of vitamin B_{12} from other causes or after total gastrectomy.

Pathology. The pathological changes in the nervous system are essentially degenerative in nature and involve the white matter to a much greater extent than the gray. Peripheral nerves, tracts in the

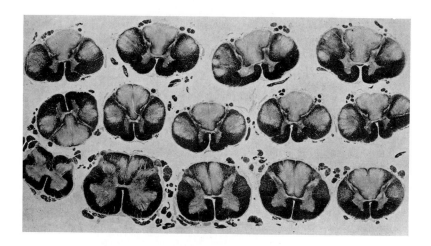

Figure 159. Combined system disease. Sections of spinal cord at various levels showing diffuse degeneration, but most intense in dorsal and lateral funiculi. (Myelin sheath stain.)

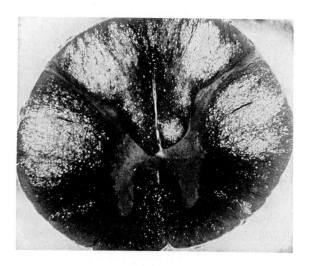

Figure 160. Combined system disease. Destruction of myelin and ground substance (status spongiosus.)

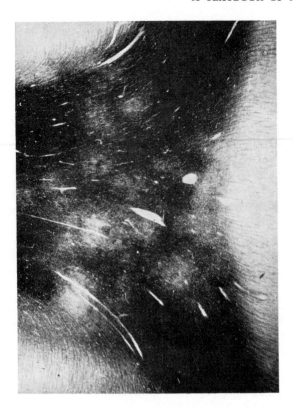

Figure 161. Combined system disease. Partial loss of myelin in punctate areas
in white matter of frontal lobe. (Myelin sheath stain.) (Courtesy Dr. L. Roizin.)

spinal cord and the white matter of the brain all show varying degrees
of degeneration (Figs. 159, 160, and 161). Changes in the nerve cells are
inconstant and of a minor nature. The anterior horn cells may show the
changes characteristic of the axonal reaction when there is a moderate
or severe degree of peripheral nerve degeneration. Similar changes may
be found in cortical neurons and demyelinating lesions may be present
in the cerebral white matter (Fig. 161).

Incidence. The incidence of subacute combined system disease
parallels that of pernicious anemia. The figures in the old literature
indicated that the spinal cord was involved in a high percentage of the
cases with primary anemia. Neurological symptoms usually developed
shortly after the onset of the anemia, but occasionally their onset
preceded the anemia. At the present time subacute combined system
disease due to deficiency of vitamin B_{12} is a clinical rarity. This is due
to the fact that vitamin B_{12} is now present in the diet of most people.

Symptoms and Signs. Sensory and motor symptoms are present in varying proportion depending upon the degree of damage to the individual tracts in the spinal cord. When there is extensive damage to the posterior funiculi, there is an ataxic weakness, severe loss of vibratory and position sense and loss of the tendon reflexes in the legs, with only an extensor plantar response as evidence of lateral tract degeneration. In the cases with preponderance of lesions in the lateral tracts, there is spastic weakness and hyperactivity of the reflexes and impairment of vibratory sense.

Other Neurological Symptoms. Cranial nerve palsies are rare. Visual symptoms may occur as result of changes in the retina secondary to the anemia and optic atrophy occurs as a rare manifestation of the degenerative process in the nerves.

Mental Symptoms. Mental symptoms are present in a large percentage of cases and are considered by some authors as characteristic of the disease. Irritability, refusal to cooperate in treatment, paranoid trends, nocturnal confusion and some impairment of memory are common. Frank psychotic episodes are infrequent. There is considerable disagreement as to the relationship of the mental symptoms to the pathological process. In view of the frequency of their occurrence and the presence of degenerative changes in the cerebral cortex, it is most probable that the mental symptoms are an integral part of the disease.

Laboratory Data. The laboratory findings are those of primary anemia and need not be discussed in detail here.

Diagnosis. The diagnosis of subacute combined degeneration of the cord is made without difficulty by the appearance of the characteristic neurological signs in a patient with achylia gastrica and the findings of pernicious anemia in the blood and bone marrow. Difficulties in diagnosis occur when the onset of the neurological manifestations precedes the blood changes or when the blood picture has been obscured by inadequate therapy with folic acid or vitamin B_{12}. The responses of the neurological symptoms to adequate therapy should establish the diagnosis. The diagnosis can be established by the failure of absorption of orally administered radioactive vitamin B_{12} (Schilling test). More recently attempts have been made to substantiate the diagnosis by determining the presence of antibodies to gastric parietal cells in the serum.

Peripheral neuritis associated with nutritional deficiency or liver disease may cause some difficulty in differential diagnosis, particularly if anemia and achylia gastrica are also present. The absence of evidence of involvement of the lateral tracts in the cord and the response of the symptoms to dietary therapy, without the administration of vitamin B_{12}, should serve to establish the diagnosis.

Course. Although spontaneous remissions of the anemia are not infrequent, it is uncommon for any spontaneous improvement to occur in the neurological signs once they are fully developed. Without treatment these are usually steadily progressive and lead inevitably to death. With adequate therapy there is a prompt remission of the gastrointestinal symptoms and of the anemia within the course of a few weeks. Improvement in the neurological symptoms is slower but should occur within two months of the start of treatment.

Treatment. The treatment is that for pernicious anemia. Vitamin B_{12} should be given intramuscularly daily or every other day for ten days, and once or twice weekly for the next two months. The subsequent schedule of therapy should be adjusted so that the red blood count is maintained at a level of over 5,000,000 per cu mm. This may require the intramuscular injection of 30 μg of vitamin B_{12} at intervals varying from one to several weeks. Treatment should be continued for the duration of the life of the individual. Increase in the frequency of the dosage is indicated if there is a fall in the red blood count or if neurological symptoms recur. Lapse from treatment will invariably result in a recurrence of the symptoms after a period of several to many months. The administration of iron is of value when there is evidence of iron deficiency. Physiotherapy, massage, passive movement, muscle training and re-education are necessary for the maximum recovery.

Treatment with pteroylglutamic acid (folic acid) is contraindicated because the neurological symptoms may progress or develop de novo in patients treated with this compound alone, even when there is improvement in the anemia.

REFERENCES

Baldwin, J. W., and Dalessio, D. J.: Folic Acid Therapy and Cord Degeneration in Pernicious Anemia, N. Engl. J. Med., 264, 1339, 1961.
DeBoer, W. G. R. M., Nairn, R. C., and Maxwell, A.: Pernicious Anemia Autoantibody to Gastric Parietal Cells, J. Clin. Path., 18, 456, 1965.
Ferraro, A., Arieti, S., and English, W. H.: Cerebral Changes in the Course of Pernicious Anemia and Their Relationship to Psychic Symptoms, J. Neuropathol. Exp. Neurol., 4, 217, 1945.
Freeman, A. G., and Heaton, J. M.: The Aetiology of Retrobulbar Neuritis in Addisonian Pernicious Anaemia, Lancet, 1, 908, 1961.
Leiken, S. L.: Pernicious Anemia in Childhood, Pediatrics, 25, 91, 1960.
Minot, G. R., and Murphy, W. P.: Treatment of Pernicious Anemia by a Special Diet, J.A.M.A., 87, 470, 1926.
Robertson, D. M., Dinsdale, H. B., and Campbell, R. J.: Subacute Combined Degeneration of the Spinal Cord, Arch. Neurol., 24, 203, 1971.
Schilling, R. F.: Vitamin B_{12} Absorption, Am. J. Clin. Nutrition, 6, 322, 1958.
Spurling, C. L., Sacks, M. S., and Jiji, R. M.: Juvenile Pernicious Anemia, N. Engl. J. Med., 271, 995, 1964.
Strachan, R. W., and Henderson, J. G.: Psychiatric Syndromes Due to Avitaminosis B_{12} with Normal Blood and Marrow, Quart. J. Med. n.s. 34, 303, 1965.
Weir, D. G., and Gatenby, P. B. B.: Subacute Combined Degeneration of the Cord after Partial Gastrectomy, Br. Med. J., 2, 1175, 1963.

West, R., and Reisner, E. H., Jr.: Treatment of Pernicious Anemia with Crystalline Vitamin B_{12}, Am. J. Med., 6, 643, 1949.
Williams, J. A., et al.: Neurological Disease after Partial Gastrectomy, Br. Med. J., 3, 210, 1969.

Polycythemia Vera

(Erythremia, Osler-Vaquez Disease)

Polycythemia vera is a chronic progressive disease of unknown origin characterized by excessive activity of the bone marrow with a persistent elevation of the number of red blood cells in the circulation and splenomegaly.

Etiology. The nature of the stimulus which causes an increased rate of formation of red cells is unknown. Tenable theories regard the disease either as a neoplastic condition of the erythropoietic tissues analogous to leukemia or as a response to diffuse stagnant anoxia of the bone marrow. There is insufficient evidence to prove either of these theories.

Incidence. Polycythemia vera is a rare disease. It occurs in all races. The onset of symptoms is usually in the fifth to sixth decades of life. Rarely young adults or children are affected. Men are affected more frequently than women.

Symptoms and Signs. In addition to the plethoric facies, and reddish or purple color of the mucous membranes and skin of the neck and extremities, there is a varied and diffuse symptomatology: Lassitude, increased sweating, loss of weight, headache, vertigo, tinnitus, visual disturbances, paresthesias in the extremities, dyspnea, various gastrointestinal symptoms, enlargement of the spleen and an increased metabolic rate.

Hemiplegia, aphasia or other focal neurological signs may occur when there is thrombosis or rupture of intracranial vessels. Papilledema may occur as result of changes in the circulation of the retina or as result of increased intracranial pressure possibly due to thrombosis of one of the dural sinuses. Symptoms commonly attributed to insufficiency of the cerebral circulation are not uncommon in patients with polycythemia.

Laboratory Data. The total volume of the blood is increased. The red cell mass per kg of body weight is constantly high in contrast to symptomatic polycythemia in which it is normal. The blood is abnormally dark and thick with delay in the clotting time. The red count is usually in the range of 7 to 11 million per cu mm. The hemoglobin content is proportionately increased but occasionally it is less markedly elevated than the red count as result of an achromia of the red cells. The white cell count is commonly in the neighborhood of 15,000 per cu mm and the number of platelets is increased. Immature red cells and leukocytes may be present in the blood.

The cerebrospinal fluid is normal unless there has been an intracranial hemorrhage. The fluid may then be bloody. The pressure is increased when there is papilledema associated with venous sinus thrombosis.

Diagnosis. The diagnosis of polycythemia vera as the cause of neurological symptoms can usually be made without difficulty on the basis of the plethoric appearance of the patient, the splenomegaly and the examination of the blood. Occasionally tumors of the brain, particularly cerebellar hemangioblastomas, may be accompanied by a high red cell count in the blood. Distinction between these and cases of polycythemia vera with choked discs may be difficult. CAT brain scan may be necessary to establish the diagnosis if there is no enlargement of the spleen.

Course. Polycythemia vera is a slowly progressive disease which usually leads to death in five to twenty years. There may be spontaneous remissions. Death may occur as result of the vascular complications in the nervous system or in other organs of the body.

Treatment. Venisection, phenylhydrazine hydrochloride, "spray x-ray therapy" and radioactive phosphorus have all been used in the therapy. Adequate treatment by one or more of these various types of treatment results in alleviation of symptoms and a prolongation of the life span. Anti-coagulant therapy is indicated when the red count is high and there are signs or symptoms suggesting insufficiency of the circulation of one or more of the cerebral vessels.

REFERENCES

Christian, H. A.: The Nervous Symptoms of Polycythemia Vera, Am. J. Med. Sci., 154, 547, 1917.
D'Agostino, A. N., Pease, G. L., and Kernohan, J. W.: Cerebral Demyelination Associated with Polycythemia Vera, J. Neuropathol. Exp. Neurol., 22, 138, 1963.
Lawrence, J. H., Berlin, N. I., and Huff, R. L.: The Nature and Treatment of Polycythemia, Medicine, 32, 323, 1953.
Loman, J., and Dameshek, W.: Plethora of Intracranial Venous Circulation in Case of Polycythemia, N. Engl. J. Med., 232, 394, 1945.
Millikan, C. H., Siekert, R. G., and Whisnant, J. P.: Intermittent Carotid and Vertebral-Basilar Insufficiency Associated with Polycythemia, Neurology, 10, 188, 1960.
Pike, G. M.: Polycythemia Vera, N. Engl. J. Med., 258, 1250 and 1297, 1958.
Silverstein, A., Gilbert, H., and Wasserman, L. R.: Neurologic Complications of Polycythemia, Ann. Intern. Med., 57, 909, 1962.
Winkelman, N. W., and Burns, M. A.: Polycythemia Vera and Its Neuropsychiatric Features, J. Nerv. & Ment. Dis., 78, 597, 1933.

Sickle Cell Anemia

Sickle cell anemia is an inherited disease of the blood related to the presence of abnormal hemoglobin patterns in which the red cells assume a "sickle" or oat-shaped form. It occurs predominantly in the colored race. Symptoms develop in only a small proportion of the individuals whose blood exhibits the characteristic anomaly. Affected subjects are frequently of asthenic habitus and are prone to develop chronic ulcers on the legs. The clinical course is punctuated by so-called "crises" characterized by fever and pains in abdomen or extremities. Multiple thromboses and infarct formation in the bones and viscera may give rise to a variety of clinical manifestations.

Symptoms of the disease may occur in childhood or may be delayed to late adult life. Involvement of the nervous system may be manifested by thrombosis of the dural sinuses, subdural or subarachnoid hemorrhage and hemorrhage from or thromboses of the large vessels in the cranium or the smaller vessels in the substance of the brain. According to Wertham, Mitchell and Angrist the essential features of the cerebral lesions include: Small areas of necrosis on a vascular basis, diffusely distributed, with predilection for the border between the cortex and subcortical white matter; large vascular lesions (softening, thromboses, etc.); and small hemorrhages and extravasations.

The neurological manifestations, which are usually those of an acute cerebral vascular lesion, may develop coincidental with or independent of the crises. Psychotic manifestations and convulsion may occur.

The diagnosis of sickle cell anemia should be suspected when signs and symptoms of an acute cerebral vascular accident occur in a young colored person. The usual stained blood smear may not reveal the typical anomaly of the red cells. This will be evident if a drop of blood is mixed with a drop of 2% solution of sodium metabisulfate on a glass slide under a cover slip and allowed to stand for ten to fifteen minutes. The diagnosis should be suspected when there are roentgenographic findings of infarcts in the bones, particularly in the skull where the extension of the marrow through the outer table of the skull gives the characteristic hair-on-end appearance.

REFERENCES

Bridges, W. H.: Cerebral Vascular Disease Accompanying Sickle Cell Anemia, Am. J. Path., 15, 353, 1939.

Greer, M., and Schotland, D.: Abnormal Hemoglobin as a Cause of Neurologic Disease, Neurology, 12, 114, 1962.

Hughes, J. G., Diggs, L. W., and Gillespie, C. E.: Involvement of the Nervous System in Sickle Cell Anemia, J. Pediatr., 17, 166, 1940.

Rowland, L. P.: Neurological Manifestations in Sickle Cell Disease, J. Nerv. & Ment. Dis., 115, 456, 1952.

Stockman, J. A., et al.: Occlusion of Large Intracerebral Vessels in Sickle-Cell Anemia, N.
Engl. J. Med., *287*, 846, 1972.
Wertham, F., Mitchell, N., and Angrist, A.: The Brain in Sickle Cell Anemia, Arch.
Neurol. & Psychiat., *47*, 752, 1942.

Macroglobulinemia

Waldenström, in 1944, described a disease of unknown etiology
characterized by the presence in the serum of globulins of enormous
molecular size. Since the original report, several hundred cases have
been reported, usually in middle-aged adults. The disease is usually
fatal within two to ten years. In addition to the large globulins there are
relative lymphocytosis, thrombopenia, splenomegaly, and lymphoid
hyperplasia. The symptoms include weakness, weight loss, and those
associated with hemorrhage. The neurological complications include
hemorrhagic and ischemic lesions and collections of reticulum cells in
the central nervous system, and polyneuritis. Improvement of
symptoms and decrease in the abnormal globulins have been reported
with the administration of chlorambucil or cyclophosphamide.

REFERENCES

Bouroncle, B. A., Datta, P., and Frajola, W. J.: Waldenström's Macroglobulinemia. Report
of Three Patients Treated with Cyclophosphamide, J.A.M.A., *189*, 729, 1964.
Edgar, R., and Dutcher, T. F.: Histopathology of the Bing-Neel Syndrome, Neurology, *11*,
239, 1961.
Waldenström, J.: Incipient Myelomatosis or "Essential" Hyperglobulinemia with Fibro-
genopenia: A New Syndrome? Acta Med. Scand., *117*, 216, 1944.

Hodgkin's Disease

Involvement of the nervous system in Hodgkin's disease usually
takes the form of invasion of the meninges by granulomatous masses
which compress the spinal cord or occlude its blood supply. Invasion
of the parenchyma of the brain or spinal cord is rare.

Pathology. Cerebral involvement in Hodgkin's disease is so rare that
for many years its existence was doubted. Isolated cases with convulsions or other cerebral symptoms have been recorded in the literature,
but in most of these the symptoms were due to the presence of nodules
in the dura. A few cases with lesion within the brain have been
reported. In the three cases reported by Jackson and Parker, the lesions
were in the cerebellum, with invasion of the brainstem.

The spinal cord may be damaged by the lesions of Hodgkin's disease
by direct compression of its substance, by compression of its vascular
supply or by collapse of affected vertebrae.

Involvement of the peripheral nerves is due to compression by tumor masses. Cranial nerve paralysis and cerebral symptoms are usually related to growth of the tumor through the foramen magnum, over, around and under the dura. The coincidence of herpes zoster and Hodgkin's disease is high. The occurrence of the herpes zoster is explained by some as due to mechanical compression of the dorsal root ganglia by the granulomatous masses, but it is more likely that the tumor serves in some way to activate a latent virus.

Areas of demyelination in the brain and spinal cord have been reported in a number of cases. These lesions are quite similar to those of multiple sclerosis or Schilder's disease and vary in size from small microscopic lesions to areas of demyelination involving a major portion of one lobe of the hemisphere or a cross section of the spinal cord. The term progressive multifocal leukoencephalopathy has been used to describe the lesions. The pathogenesis is unknown. It was thought that they may be related to previous radiation therapy but it is most likely that they are due to infection by a virus of the papova group.

Incidence. Spinal cord involvement occurred in 9 and brain involvement in 3 of the 174 cases reported by Jackson and Parker. Diamond found neurological complications in 205 of 1,593 cases, divided as follows: Herpes zoster 52; spinal cord compression 50; cranial nerve paralyses in 20; peripheral nerve paralyses in 48; and cerebral involvement in 25. In the 403 cases reported by Thies and his associates, the nervous system was involved in 12%.

Signs and Symptoms. In the majority of the cases, the involvement of the spinal cord is due to compression of its vascular supply by the granulomatous masses. The dorsal region of the cord is most frequently the site of these lesions with resulting flaccid paraplegia, complete sensory loss and paralysis of the sphincters. Spastic paraplegia with an incomplete sensory loss below the level of the lesion is the rule when the injury to the cord is due to compression by the granulomatous masses in the subdural or epidural spaces.

Rarely, there may be a diffuse involvement of the meninges by Hodgkin's disease with signs or symptoms of a subacute meningitis and a lymphocytic pleocytosis in the cerebrospinal fluid.

The symptoms in the patients with diffuse encephalopathy are similar to those which occur in multifocal leukoencephalopathy of other causes. The lesions are apt to be widely disseminated with resultant evidences of involvement of the cerebral hemispheres, brainstem, cerebellum or spinal cord. Parenchymatous cerebellar degeneration may occur in association with Hodgkin's disease.

The cerebrospinal fluid dynamics are normal and the fluid shows no significant abnormalities when the damage to the cord is the result of vascular occlusion. Dynamic block and increased protein content in the fluid are the characteristic findings when the symptoms are due to compression of the cord.

Diagnosis. The diagnosis of Hodgkin's disease as the cause of the neurological symptoms is usually made without difficulty in the majority of cases on the basis of the other characteristic features of the disease. In doubtful cases, the diagnosis can be established by the microscopic examination of involved lymph nodes.

Prognosis. The prognosis is poor in all cases of Hodgkin's disease with involvement of the nervous system. Death from sepsis or urinary complication is the rule when flaccid paraplegia develops. Patients with Hodgkin's disease are particularly susceptible to infection with cryptococci and other fungal infections.

Treatment. The treatment of Hodgkin's disease is radiation therapy to the affected areas. Improvement in the symptoms of spinal cord damage can be expected except when the damage is due to occlusion of the spinal vessels. Laminectomy with removal of the granulomatous masses is indicated only when there is a spastic paraplegia and evidence of spinal subarachnoid block at lumbar puncture.

REFERENCES

Diamond, H. D.: Hodgkin's Disease: Neurologic Sequelae, Missouri Med., 54, 945, 1957.
Dolman, C. L., and Cairns, A. R. M.: Leukoencephalopathy Associated with Hodgkin's Disease, Neurology, 11, 349, 1961.
Horwich, L., Buxton, P. H., and Ryan, G. M. S.: Cerebellar Degeneration with Hodgkin's Disease, J. Neurol., Neurosurg. & Psychiat., 29, 45, 1966.
Jackson, H., Jr., and Parker, F., Jr.: Hodgkin's Disease; Involvement of Certain Other Organs, N. Engl. J. Med., 233, 369, 1945.
Sohn, D., Valensi, Q., and Miller, S. P.: Neurological Manifestations of Hodgkin's Disease. Intracerebral Hodgkin's Granuloma, Arch. Neurol., 17, 429, 1967.
Thies, H., Kiefer, H., and Noetzel, H.: The Neurological Complications of Hodgkin's Disease, German Medical Monthly, 6, 356, 1961.
Williams, H. M., et al.: *Neurological Complications of Lymphomas and Leukemias*, Springfield, Charles C Thomas, 1959.

Leukemia

Symptoms of injury to the nervous system develop when the meninges or parenchyma is the site of leukemic infiltrations.

Pathology. Foci of infiltration may be found in the peripheral or cranial nerves, epidural space, meninges or the parenchyma of the central nervous system. The lesions in the parenchyma are usually microscopic in size and only rarely are they large enough to produce focal neurological signs. They may be associated with large or petechial hemorrhages. Leukemic infiltrations of the meninges may obstruct the outflow of cerebrospinal fluid from the basal cisterns.

Small or large hemorrhages may be found in the brain as result of the bleeding tendency associated with the reduced platelet content of the blood. Symptoms of a progressive multifocal encephalopathy, similar to that described for Hodgkin's disease, occur in a small percentage of the cases of both acute and chronic leukemia. Patients with leukemia are particularly susceptible to infections with cryptococci and other fungi.

Incidence. Pathological reports indicate that the meninges or parenchyma of the nervous system are invaded by leukemia infiltrations in over two-thirds of the cases. The incidence does not seem to be related to the cell type or to the acuteness or chronicity of the disease. Although there are no clinical signs of nervous system disease in many of these cases, there is some evidence to indicate that symptomatic involvement of the nervous system has increased in recent years. It is thought that this may be due to the fact that lesions in the nervous system are more resistant to therapy than those in other parts of the body.

Symptoms and Signs. Cranial nerve paralysis, particularly the seventh nerve, is probably the most common symptom of focal damage to the nervous system. Hemiplegia, aphasia or other signs of focal cerebral damage are infrequent. Increased intracranial pressure, with papilledema and separation of sutures, is not an uncommon sign with diffuse infiltration of the meninges in infants or young children. Paraplegia may occur with leukemic infiltration of the spinal epidural space.

Laboratory Signs. The findings in the blood are those associated with leukemia. With infiltration of the meninges the cerebrospinal fluid pressure is increased. The protein content of the fluid is increased and there is a pleocytosis in the fluid. The cells are usually normal lymphocytes or polymorphonuclear leukocytes. Only rarely are leukemia cells present in the fluid. The sugar content of the fluid may be moderately or greatly reduced.

Course and Prognosis. The prognosis is poor when there is clinical evidence of involvement of the meninges or the central nervous system. Although remission in symptoms may occur spontaneously or as result of treatment, death usually occurs within a year. Meningeal or intracerebral hemorrhages may be the immediate cause of death.

Treatment. Radiation therapy to the entire skull and spine and therapy with adrenal steroid hormones are of value in relieving the symptoms and prolonging the course of the disease. Beneficial results have been reported as result of administration of 6-mercaptopurine or amethopterin. Improvement of the neurological symptoms has been reported as the result of the removal of spinal fluid by lumbar puncture or the intrathecal injection of methotrexate or aminopterin.

REFERENCES

Annotation: Encephalitis and Encephalopathy in Childhood Leukemia, Develop. Med. Child. Neurol., *18*, 90, 1976.
Baker, R. D.: Leukopenia and Therapy in Leukemia as Factors Predisposing to Fatal Mycoses, Am. J. Clin. Path., *37*, 358, 1962.
Bergevin, P. R.: Central Nervous System Leukemia, N.Y. State J. Med., *75*, 367, 1975.
Dritschilo, A., Cassady, S. R., Camitta, B., Jaffe, N., Paed, D., Furman, L., Traggis, D.: The Role of Irradiation in Central Nervous System Treatment and Prophylaxis for Acute Lymphoblastic Leukemia, Cancer, *37*, 2729, 1976.
Fritz, R. D., et al.: The Association of Intracranial Hemorrhage and "Blastic Crisis" in Patients with Acute Leukemia, N. Engl. J. Med., *261*, 59, 1959.
Geiser, C. F., Bishop, Y., Jaffe, N., Furman, L., Traggis, D., Frei, E.: Adverse Effects of Intrathecal Methotrexate in Children with Acute Leukemia in Remission, Blood, *45*, 189, 1975.
Haghbin, M., and Zeulzer, W. W.: A Long-Term Study of Cerebrospinal Leukemia, J. Pediatr., *67*, 23, 1965.
Hyman, C. B., et al.: Central Nervous System Involvement by Leukemia in Children, I. Relationship to Systemic Leukemia and Description of Clinical and Laboratory Manifestations, Blood, *25*, 1, 1965.
Moore, E. W., Thomas, L. B., Shaw, R. K., and Freireich, E. J.: The Central Nervous System in Acute Leukemia, Arch. Intern. Med., *105*, 451, 1960.
Nies, B. A., Thomas, L. B., and Freireich, E. J.: Meningeal Leukemia. A Follow-up Study, Cancer, *18*, 546, 1965.
Phair, J. P., Anderson, R. E., and Namiki, H.: The Central Nervous System in Leukemia, Ann. Intern. Med., *67*, 863, 1964.
Pochedly, C.: Neurologic Manifestations in Acute Leukemia, N.Y. State J. Med., *75*, 575, 715, 878, 1975.
Price, R. A., Johnson, W. W.: The Central Nervous System in Childhood Leukemia, I. The Arachnoid, Cancer, *31*,520, 533, 1973; II. Subacute Leukoencephalopathy, Cancer, *35*, 306, 1975.
Richardson, E. P.: Progressive Multifocal Leukoencephalopathy. N. Engl. J. Med., *265*, 815, 1961.
Rubinstein, L. J., Herman, M. M., Long, T. F., Wilbur, J. R.: Disseminated Necrotizing Leukoencephalopathy: a Complication of Treated Central Nervous System Leukemia and Lymphoma, Cancer, *35*, 291, 1975.
Shanbrom, E., Miller, S., and Fairbanks, V. F.: Intrathecal Administration of Amethopterin in Leukemic Encephalopathy of Young Adults, N. Engl. J. Med., *265*, 169, 1961.
Shapiro, W. R., Young, D. F., Mehta, B. M.: Methotrexate: Distribution in Cerebrospinal Fluid after Intravenous, Ventricular and Lumbar Injections, New Engl. J. Med., *293*, 161, 1975.
Sibley, W. A., and Weisberger, A. S.: Demyelinating Disease of the Brain in Chronic Lymphatic Leukemia, Arch. Neurol., *5*, 300, 1961.
Sullivan, M. P.: Leukemic Infiltration of Meninges and Spinal Nerve Roots, Pediatr., *32*, 63, 1963.
Wilhyde, D. E., Jane, J. A., and Mullan, S.: Spinal Epidural Leukemia, Am. J. Med., *34*, 281, 1963.
Williams, H. M., et al.: *Neurological Complications of Lymphomas and Leukemias*, Springfield, Charles C Thomas, 1959.

Thrombotic Thrombocytopenic Purpura

Thrombotic thrombocytopenic purpura is a rare disorder of unknown etiology in which three pathogenetic mechanisms have been identified: (1) Occlusion of arteries, arterioles and capillaries by amorphous hyaline material (Fig. 162) of uncertain nature, especially in heart,

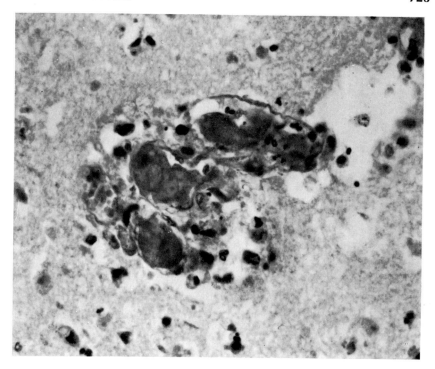

Figure 162. Thrombotic thrombocytopenic purpura. Occlusion of small cerebral vessels by amorphous hyaline material. (Courtesy Dr. Abner Wolf.)

kidney and brain; (2) hemolytic anemia, probably due to an extracorpuscular mechanism although also associated with increased mechanical and osmotic fragility of the red blood cells; and (3) thrombocytopenia. In a few cases pathological features have suggested a relationship to lupus erythematosus or periarteritis nodosa.

The disease is usually acute, lasting from a few days to several months. The hematological abnormalities give rise to pallor, hematuria, purpura and jaundice. Vascular thrombi cause cerebral symptoms in nearly all cases, as well as fever, abdominal pain, nausea, vomiting and arthralgia.

The cerebral symptoms in order of frequency are: mental confusion progressing to coma; seizures usually generalized but occasionally focal; aphasia; hemiplegia; and papilledema. The focal neurological signs are apt to be transient lasting for only a few days. Within a few days or weeks similar or other symptoms may occur.

Diagnosis is based upon the triad of hemolytic anemia, thrombocytopenia and cerebral symptoms and signs. The platelets are almost always decreased, but the platelet count may be normal in the interval between attacks. This disorder must be differentiated from the symptomatic hemolytic anemias of malignancy, leukemia, Hodgkin's disease, bacteremia and lupus erythematosus. Clinical features and appropriate laboratory studies usually identify these conditions. Bacteremia is excluded by negative results of culture of the blood.

Treatment is unsatisfactory although the use of cortisone and its derivatives is still being evaluated. Transfusions of blood and platelets are of some supportive value, but benefit is only transient. The value of anticoagulant drugs directed against the thrombi is limited because of the hazard of bleeding in the presence of thrombocytopenia. Almost all of the reported cases have run a brief course terminating in death.

REFERENCES

Amorosi, E. L., and Ultmann, J. E.: Thrombotic Thrombocytopenic Purpura: Report of 16 Cases and Review of the Literature, Medicine, 45, 139, 1966.
Antes, E. H.: Thrombotic Thrombocytopenic Purpura, Ann. Intern. Med., 48, 512, 1958.
Bornstein, B., Boss, J. H., Casper, J., and Behor, M.: Thrombotic Thrombocytopenic Purpura, J. Clin. Path., 13, 124, 1960.
Cahalane, S. F., and Horn, R. C.: Thrombotic Thrombocytopenic Purpura of Long Duration, Am. J. Med., 27, 333, 1959.
McKay, D. G.: Disseminated Intravascular Coagulation, New York, Hoeber Medical Division of Harper & Row, 1965.
Moschowitz, E.: An Acute Febrile Pleiochromic Anemia with Hyaline Thrombosis of the Terminal Arterioles and Capillaries, Arch. Intern. Med., 36, 89, 1925.
O'Brien, J. L., and Sibley, W. A.: Neurologic Manifestations of Thrombotic Thrombocytopenic Purpura, Neurology, 8, 55, 1958.

Chediak-Higashi Disease

Chediak-Higashi disease is a rare inherited metabolic disorder with onset in early childhood. Giant peroxidase-positive cytoplasmic granules occur in leukocytes. Disseminated focal infiltrations by lymphocytes and large mononuclears with similar inclusions may be present in many organs. Cytoplasmic inclusions probably of a complex glyco-lipoprotein have recently been described in neurons of the central and peripheral nervous systems. Symptoms include albinism, photophobia, generalized lymphadenopathy and hepatosplenomegaly. Cranial and peripheral polyneuropathy may develop. Anemia, leukopenia and thrombocytopenia are frequently noted. The administration of prednisone and vincristine has been reported to be of value in the acute phases. Death usually occurs in childhood as a result of recurrent pyogenic infections or the development of malignant lymphomas.

REFERENCES

Blume, R. S., and Wolff, S. M.: The Chediak-Higashi Syndrome: Studies in Four Patients and a Review of the Literature, Medicine, 51, 247, 1972.

Donohue, W. L., and Bain, H. W.: Chediak-Higashi Syndrome: A Lethal Familial Disease with Anomalous Inclusions in the Leukocytes and Constitutional Stigmata: Report of a Case with Necropsy, Pediatr., 20, 416, 1957.

Higashi, O.: Congenital Gigantism of Peroxidase Granules: First Case Ever Reported of Qualitative Abnormality of Peroxidase, Tohoku J. Exp. Med., 59, 315, 1954.

Lockman, L. A., Kennedy, W. R., and White, J. G.: The Chediak-Higashi Syndrome Electrophysiological and Electron Microscopic Observation on the Peripheral Neuropathy, J. Pediat., 70, 942, 1967.

Myers, J. P., Sung, J. M., Cowen, D., and Wolf, A.: Pathological Findings in the Central and Peripheral Nervous Systems in Chediak-Higashi's Disease: The Finding of Cytoplasmic Neuronal Inclusions, J. Neuropathol. Exp. Neurol., 22, 357, 1963.

Histiocytosis (Xanthomatosis or Histiocytosis X). Histiocytosis X is the term proposed by Lichtenstein to include eosinophilic granuloma of bone, Hand-Schüller-Christian disease and Letterer-Siwe disease. The unified concept that these diseases represent only varied clinical manifestations of a single nosologic entity has received widespread although not universal acceptance.

Pathology and Pathogenesis. The cause of the disease is unknown. An infectious agent has been suggested as the most likely etiology. The essential feature of the pathological changes is the presence of focal or widespread chronic inflammatory granuloma in the involved organs. The microscopic pathology consists of proliferation of the histiocytic cells with an associated proliferation of fibroblasts and an infiltration of lymphocytes, eosinophilic leukocytes and mature plasma cells. In the chronic stages of the disease large collections of foamy macrophages containing cholesterol are conspicuous within the granulation tissue.

Table 95.   The Frequency of Clinical Manifestations in 180 Cases of
Schüller-Christian Disease
(Modified from Avioli, Lasersohn, and Lopresti, Medicine, 1963)

	No. of Cases	%
Skeletal lesions	147	81
Diabetes insipidus	102	56
Exophthalmos	89	49
Growth retardation	54	30
Skin	45	25
Gingivitis	42	23
Adenopathy	32	18
Otitis media	28	15
Splenomegaly	27	15
Pulmonary infiltration	26	15
Hepatomegaly	26	15
Anemia	22	12

These lipid-laden macrophages represent a secondary effect of the destructive process and not a primary storage of lipid.

Incidence. The disease is relatively rare. There is no evidence that it is inherited but familial occurrence has been reported. The onset of symptoms in the Letterer-Siwe form is usually in infancy. The majority of cases with the Hand-Schüller-Christian variant begin in childhood or adolescence while eosinophilic granuloma of bone usually becomes symptomatic in young adult life.

Symptoms and Signs. The signs and symptoms of the disease are dependent upon the location of the granulomas (Table 95). A solitary focus in one of the long bones produces a painful bony swelling (eosinophilic granuloma of bone). Widespread, destructive granulomas of the spleen, liver, bone marrow, lymph nodes and skin produce hepatosplenomegaly, a hemorrhagic diathesis, lymphadenopathy, anemia, sepsis and chronic ulcerations of the skin (Letterer-Siwe disease). When the histiocytic lesions are localized in the membranous bones, defects in the skull (Fig. 163), exophthalmos and diabetes insipidus are the principal features of the disease (Hand-Schüller-

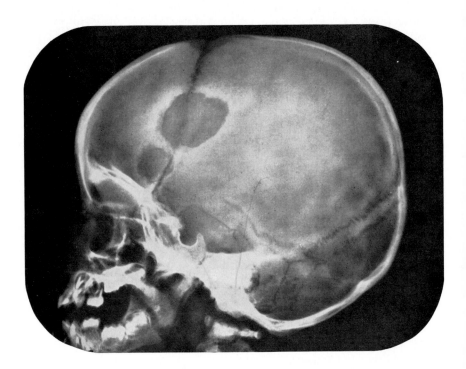

Figure 163.   Histiocytosis. Defects in skull associated with lesions in the bone.
(Courtesy Dr. Juan Taveras.)

Christian disease). Involvement of the alveolar process may result in loss of the teeth and spontaneous pneumothorax has been reported with the development of granulomas in the lungs.

Neurological signs may be produced by nodular infiltration of the dura with extension to the underlying brain or by the development of histiocytic granulomas within the substance of the nervous system. Granulomas within the hypothalamus and third ventricle may result in retardation of growth, diabetes insipidus and an organic mental syndrome. Pyramidal tract signs, cranial nerve palsies and cerebellar ataxia may be present and related to corresponding lesions in the base of the skull, cerebellum and brainstem. Increased intracranial pressure and hydrocephalus may result from granulomas and chronic inflammatory changes in the dural sinuses, ventricular cavities and subarachnoid cisterns. Kepes and Kepes have emphasized cases showing only involvement of the nervous system with no evidence of visceral or skeletal lesions.

Laboratory Data. A mild or moderate degree of anemia may occur. The cerebrospinal fluid may be normal or show an elevated protein content and increased cells, usually lymphocytes.

Diagnosis. Little difficulty is encountered when visceral and skeletal lesions are present. Roentgenograms of the skull and other bones and biopsy of the liver, spleen or lymph nodes are usually sufficient to establish the diagnosis. Surgical biopsy may be necessary in those cases showing only involvement of the nervous system. Histiocytosis must be differentiated from the malignant diseases of the reticuloendothelial system.

Course. The course of the disease, when untreated, is variable but progressive. Remissions may occur.

Treatment. Lesions of the bone respond to radiation therapy or surgical curettage. Corticosteroid therapy is advised for the systemic manifestations of the disease. Nitrogen mustard, methotrexate and the Vinca alkaloids should be used with caution in the treatment of the nonmalignant reticuloendothelioses (histiocytosis). Diabetes insipidus and septicemia are treated by standard techniques.

REFERENCES

Avioli, L. V., Lasersohn, J. T., and Lopresti, J. M.: Histiocytosis X (Schüller-Christian Disease): Clinico-Pathological Survey, Review of Ten Patients and the Results of Prednisone Therapy, Medicine, 42, 119, 1963.

Beard, W., et al.: Xanthomatosis of the Central Nervous System. Clinical and Pathological Observations of a Case with a Posterior Fossa Syndrome, Neurology, 20, 305, 1970.

Braustein, G. D., and Kohler, P. O.: Deficient Growth Hormone Release in Hand-Schüller-Christian Disease, N. Engl. J. Med., 286, 1225, 1972.

Christian, H. A.: *Defects in Membranous Bones, Exophthalmos and Diabetes Insipidus, Contributions to Medical and Biological Research,* Vol. 1, New York, Paul B. Hoeber, 1919, 390 pp.

Elian, M., et al.: Neurological Manifestations of General Xanthomatosis, Arch. Neurol., 21, 115, 1969.

Feinberg, S. B., and Langer, L. O.: Roentgen Findings of Increased Intracranial Pressure and Communicating Hydrocephalus as Insidious Manifestations of Chronic Histiocytosis-X, Am. J. Roentgen., 95, 41, 1965.

Hand, A., Jr.: Polyuria and Tuberculosis, Arch. Pediatr., 10, 673, 1893.

Kepes, J. H., and Kepes, M.: Predominantly Cerebral Forms of Histiocytosis-X, Acta Neuropath., 14, 77, 1969.

Lahey, M. E.: Prognosis in Reticuloendotheliosis in Children, J. Pediatr., 60, 664, 1962.

Lichtenstein, L.: Histiocytosis X (Eosinophilic Granuloma of Bone, Letterer-Siwe Disease and Schüller-Christian Disease), J. Bone Jt. Surg., 46–A, 76, 1964.

Lieberman, P. H., et al.: A Reappraisal of Eosinophilic Granuloma of Bone, Hand-Schüller-Christian Syndrome and Letterer-Siwe Syndrome, Medicine, 48, 375, 1969.

Oberman, H. A.: Idiopathic Histiocytosis. A Clinicopathologic Study of 40 Cases and Review of the Literature on Eosinophilic Granuloma of Bone, Hand-Schüller-Christian Disease and Letterer-Siwe Disease, Pediatrics, 28, 307, 1961.

Price, D. L., et al.: Familial Lymphohistiocytosis of the Nervous System, Arch. Neurol., 24, 270, 1971.

Schüller, A.: Ueber eigenartige Schädeldefekte im Jugendalter, Fortschr. a. d. Geb. d. Röntgenstrahlen, 23, 12, 1916.

DISEASES OF THE LIVER

Myelopathy and encephalopathy may occur in association with inherited or acquired liver disease or after portal-systemic shunts. Clinical symptoms are accompanied by an increased ammonia content of the serum and are apt to follow attacks of hepatic coma. The clinical syndromes which develop consist of dementia of varying degrees of severity, dysarthria, ataxia of gait, intention tremor, choreoathetosis, spastic paraplegia or other evidence of damage to the spinal cord.

The pathological changes in the nervous system include necrosis of the neurons in the cerebral cortex, basal ganglia and cerebellum, increase in the size and number of the protoplasmic astrocytes and degeneration of the white matter of the brain and spinal cord. There are diffuse changes in the electroencephalogram. The blood ammonia level is increased and serum ceruloplasmin is normal and there is no disturbance of copper metabolism.

The development of neurological complications in patients with liver disease is usually followed by a fatal outcome, but amelioration or disappearance of the symptoms has been reported following ileosigmoidostomy with exclusion of the rest of the colon.

REFERENCES

Gardner, D. L., Macpherson, A. I. S., Maloney, A. F. J., and Richmond, J.: Leucoencephalopathy after Portacaval Anastomosis in a Patient with Hepatic Cirrhosis, J. Neurol., Neurosurg., & Psychiat., 27, 530, 1964.

Gardner, W. A., Jr., and Konigsmark, B. W.: Familial Nonhemolytic Jaundice: Bilirubinosis and Encephalopathy, Pediatr., 43, 365, 1969.

Jellinger, K., Minauf, M., and Weissenbacher, G.: Hirnveränderungen bei kongenitelem nichthämolytischen Ikterus (Crigler-Najjar-Syndrom), Acta Neuropath., 16, 141, 1970.
Liversedge, L. A., and Rawson, M. D.: Myelopathy in Hepatic Disease and Portosystemic Venous Anastomosis, Lancet, 1, 277, 1966.
McDermott, W. V., Jr., Victor, M., and Point, W. W.: Exclusion of the Colon in the Treatment of Hepatic Encephalopathy, N. Engl. J. Med., 267, 850, 1962.
McDonald, R., and de la Harpe, P. L.: Hepatic Coma in Childhood, J. Pediatr., 63, 916, 1963.
Raskin, N. H., Price, J. B., and Fishman, R. A.: Portal-Systemic Encephalopathy Due to Congenital Intrahepatic Shunts, N. Engl. J. Med., 270, 225, 1964.
Read, A. E., et al.: The Neuropsychiatric Syndrome Associated with Chronic Liver Disease and an Extensive Portal-Systemic Collateral Circulation, Quart. J. Med., 141, 135, 1967.
Scobie, B. A., and Summerskill, W. H. J.: Permanent Paraplegia with Cirrhosis, Arch. Intern. Med., 113, 805, 1964.

DISEASES OF BONE

Osteitis Deformans (Paget's Disease)

Osteitis deformans is a chronic disease of the adult skeleton characterized by bowing and irregular flattening of the bones. Any or all of the bones of the skeleton may be affected, but the tibia, skull and pelvic bones are the most frequent site of the changes. Except for the production of skeletal deformities and pain, the disease produces disability only when there is involvement of the skull or spine.

Pathology. In the affected bones there is imbalance between the process of bone formation and bone resorption. In most cases there is a mixture of excessive bone formation and bone destruction. The areas of bone destruction are filled with hyperplastic vascular connective tissue. New bone formation may take place in the destroyed areas in an irregular disorganized manner. The metabolic disturbance, which is the cause of the abnormality in the bones, is unknown.

Incidence. Osteitis deformans is a common affection of bones in adult life. A postmortem incidence of 3% in patients over forty years of age was reported by Schmorl. Males and females are equally affected. The common age of onset is in the fourth to sixth decades and it is extremely rare before the age of thirty years.

Symptoms and Signs. The neurological symptoms which appear in patients with Paget's disease are of two types: (1) those due to the abnormalities in the bone, and (2) those which are the result of arteriosclerosis which is a common accompaniment. The cerebral signs and symptoms which occur with the latter are no different from those which occur in patients with arteriosclerosis in the absence of Paget's disease.

The neurological defects which are the result of the bony disease are usually related to pressure on the central nervous system or the nerve roots by the overgrowth of bone. Convulsive seizures, pains in the head, generalized or neuralgic in type, cranial nerve palsies and paraplegia occur in a small percentage of the cases. Deafness as result of pressure on the auditory nerves is the most common symptom. Unilateral facial palsy is the next most common symptom. Loss of vision in one eye, visual field defects or exophthalmos may occur when the sphenoid bone is affected. Compression of the cerebral substance by the bony overgrowth is extremely rare except when there is sarcomatous degeneration of the lesions. Compression of the spinal cord is more common. Platybasia may occur in advanced cases.

Laboratory Data. The serum calcium content is normal and the serum phosphorus is normal or only slightly increased. The serum phosphatase is increased, the level varying with the extent and activity of the process. It may be only slightly elevated when the disease is localized to one or two bones.

Diagnosis. The diagnosis of Paget's disease is made from the appearance of the patient and the characteristic changes in the roentgenograms. Involvement of the skull in the advanced cases is manifested by a generalized enlargement of the calvarium, anteroflexion of the head and depression of the chin on the chest. When the spine is involved, the stature is shortened, the spine is flexed forward and its mobility greatly reduced.

The roentgenographic features (Fig. 164) of osteitis deformans in the skull are areas of increased density of the bone with loss of normal architecture, mingled with areas in which the density of the bone is decreased. The margins of the bones are fuzzy and indistinct. The general appearance is that of an enormous skull with a "cotton wool" appearance of the bones of the vault. In advanced cases there may be a flattening of the base of the skull on the cervical vertebrae (platybasia) with signs of damage to the lower cranial nerves, medulla or cerebellum.

Difficulties in diagnosis are encountered in the cases where the clinical symptoms are mainly of a neurological nature. In these instances, roentgenograms of the pelvis, the lower extremities or a general survey of the entire skeleton may serve to establish the diagnosis. Rarely, it may be impossible to distinguish monophasic Paget's disease of the skull from osteoblastic metastases. A careful search for a primary neoplasm, particularly in the prostate, or biopsy of one of the lesions in the skull may be necessary in these cases.

Course. The course of Paget's disease is quite variable, but usually extends over several decades. The neurological lesions seldom lead to any serious degree of disability except that which is due to deafness, convulsive seizures or compression of the spinal cord.

Treatment. There is no specific therapy. Radiation therapy for the

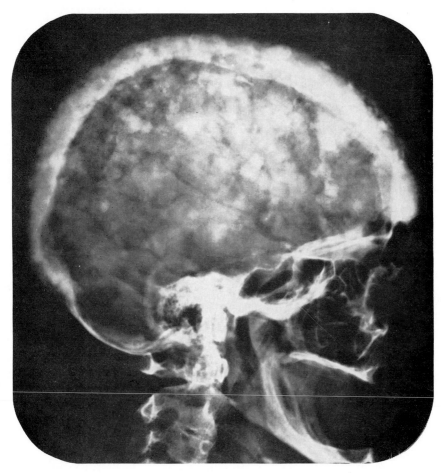

Figure 164.   Paget's disease of the skull. (Courtesy Dr. Juan Taveras.)

affected bones may temporarily relieve the pains. Bauer recommended the administration of a high-calcium, high-vitamin diet with the addition of large doses of vitamin D and cevitamic acid to aid in the formation of new bone. The latter is especially important when there is involvement of the weight-bearing bones. Thyrocalcitonin is now being given to inhibit the osteolytic process. Decompression of the cord may be necessary when it is compressed by involved vertebrae. Decompression of the posterior fossa gives temporary relief of symptoms in cases with platybasia associated with Paget's disease of the skull.

REFERENCES

Allison, F. G., and Penner, D. W.: Paget's Disease of the Skull with Basilar Invagination (Platybasia) and Internal Hydrocephalus, Canad. M. A. J., 65, 476, 1951.

Feldman, F., and Seaman, W. B.: The Neurologic Complications of Paget's Disease in the Cervical Spine, Am. J. Roentg. Rad. Therapy and Nucl. Med., 105, 375, 1969.

Finney, H. L., and Roberts, J. S.: Fibrous Dysplasia of the Skull with Progressive Cranial Nerve Involvement, Surg. Neurol., 6, 341, 1976.

Grunthal, E.: The Brain in Paget's Disease of the Skull, Ztschr. f. d. ges. Neurol. u. Psychiat., 136, 656, 1931. Abstracted in Arch. Neurol. & Psychiat., 28, 1425, 1932.

Gurdjian, E. S., Webster, J. E., and Latimer, F. R.: Paget's Disease of the Spine with Compression of the Spinal Cord, Tr. Am. Neurol. A., 77, 243, 1952.

Haddad, J. G., Jr., et al.: Effects of Prolonged Thyrocalcitonin Administration on Paget's Disease of Bone, N. Engl. J. Med., 283, 549, 1970.

Knaggs, R. L.: The Inflammatory and Toxic Diseases of Bone, New York, William Wood, 1926.

Paget, J., Fricker, G., and ver Brugghen, A.: Osteitis Fibrosa Cystica Localisata of the Skull, J. Neurosurg., 7, 447, 1950.

Palmer, H. D., Harrow, R., and Schwartz, L. A.: Osteitis Fibrosa Cystica of the Skull Associated with Hemianopia and Psychotic Symptoms, Arch. Neurol. & Psychiat., 27, 45, 1932.

Pyke, R., Cope, J. R., and Dosh, R.: Fibrous Dysplasia Mimicking Intracranial Tumor, J. Laryngol. Otol., 87, 1233, 1973.

Wyllie, W. G.: The Occurrence in Osteitis Deformans of Lesions of the Central Nervous System, Brain, 46, 336, 1923.

Fibrous Dysplasia

The skull and the bones in other parts of the body are occasionally involved in a process characterized by small areas of bone destruction or massive sclerotic overgrowth.

The clinical picture is related to the site and extent of the bony overgrowth. Sassin and Rosenberg reported on the incidence of involvement of the various bones of the skull in 50 cases: frontal 28, sphenoid 24, frontal and sphenoid in 18, temporal 8, facial 15, parietal 6 and occipital 8. Diffuse involvement of the entire skull produces a condition described as leontiasis ossea. In this condition there is exophthalmos, optic atrophy and other cranial nerve palsies.

In addition to the disfiguration of the appearance of the skull in the polyostotic form, symptoms of the monostotic form of the disease include headache, convulsions, exophthalmos, optic atrophy and deafness. The onset of symptoms may be at any age, but is usually in early adult life. The family history is negative and there is no racial or sexual predominance.

A polyostotic form of the disease characterized by café-au-lait spots, endocrine dysfunction with precocious puberty in girls, and involvement of the femur (shepherd's crook deformity) was described by Albright and his associates.

REFERENCES

Albright, F.: Polyostotic Fibrous Dysplasia: A Defence of the Entity, J. Clin. Endocr., 7, 307, 1947.
Harris, W. H., Dudley, H. R., and Barry, R. J.: The Natural History of Fibrous Dysplasia, J. Bone Joint Surg., 44–A, 207, 1962.
Leeds, N., and Seaman, W. B.: Fibrous Dysplasia of the Skull and Its Differential Diagnosis, Radiol., 78, 570, 1962.
Sassin, J. F., and Rosenberg, R. N.: Neurologic Complications of Fibrous Dysplasia of the Skull, Arch. Neurol., 18, 363, 1968.

Achondroplasia

Achondroplasia (chondrodystrophy) is a form of dwarfism characterized by short arms and legs, lumbar lordosis and enlargement of the head due to an inherited defect in the ossification of cartilage.

The disease is quite rare and is estimated to occur in 15 of 1,000,000 births in the United States. It is usually inherited as an autosomal dominant trait.

Symptoms of involvement of the nervous system develop in a few patients as result of hydrocephalus, compression of the medulla and cervical cord at the level of the foramen magnum and compression of the spinal cord by ruptured intervertebral disc or bony compression of the lower thoracic or lumbar cord. Convulsive seizures, ataxia and paraplegia are the most common symptoms. Mental development is usually normal.

The diagnosis is made from the characteristic body configuration of short arms and legs, normal sized trunk, enlargement of the head and the changes in the roentgenograms of the skeleton.

Many of the affected individuals die in utero in the last month of pregnancy or shortly after birth. A normal life span is possible in patients with a less severe degree of involvement of the bones.

Shunting procedures may be necessary in patients with hydrocephalus as result of involvement of the bones at the base of the skull. Laminectomy is indicated when signs of cord compression appear.

REFERENCES

Cohen, M. E., Rosenthal, A. D., and Matson, D. D.: Neurologic Abnormalities in Achondroplastic Children, J. Pediatr., 71, 367, 1967.
Dandy, W. F.: Hydrocephalus in Chondrodystrophy, Bull. Johns Hopkins Hosp., 32, 5, 1921.
Denis, J. P., Rosenberg, H. S., and Ellsworth, C. A., Jr.: Megalocephaly, Hydrocephalus and other Neurological Aspects of Achondroplasia, Brain, 84, 427, 1961.
Duvosin, R. C., and Yahr, M. D.: Compressive Spinal Cord and Root Symptoms in Achondroplastic Dwarfs, Neurology, 12, 202, 1962.
Langer, L. O., Jr., Bauman, P. A., and Gorlin, R. J.: Achondroplasia, Am. J. Roentgen. Rad. Ther. and Nuc. Med., 100, 12, 1967.

Cervical Spondylosis

In recent years attention has been called to the effect of degenerative and arthritic changes in the cervical spine on nerve roots and the spinal cord. The term cervical spondylosis has been used to describe a combination of pathological changes including: (1) narrowing of the intervertebral disc spaces by herniation of the nucleus pulposus or by desiccation and degeneration consequent upon age: (2) osteophyte and spur formation on the vertebrae; and (3) partial subluxation of one or more cervical vertebrae.

Pathogenesis of Symptoms. The symptoms and signs which result are due to injury to the nerves by narrowing of the foramina, and damage to the cord by compression and possibly by other factors. It has been postulated that damage to the cord may be due, in part at least, to interference with its circulation.

Incidence. Degenerative changes in the cervical spine are common in middle and late life, but in the majority of the cases they are productive of few or no symptoms. The age at onset in the patients who develop symptoms varies from thirty to seventy years with an average of fifty years. Men are more frequently affected than women.

Symptoms and Signs. Pains in the neck, shoulders and arms and stiffness of the neck are common presenting symptoms. These are due to pressure on the nerve roots. There may be weakness of one or both legs, which gradually increases and extends to involve the arms. Sensory symptoms in the form of paresthesias and dysesthesias are common in the arms and in the lower extremities. Cutaneous sensory loss in one or more dermatomes in one or both upper extremities may occur. A slight degree of impairment of cutaneous sensation below the second to fifth thoracic level occurs in a few cases. Loss or impairment of the vibratory sense in the lower extremities is present in about one half of the cases.

The reflexes in the lower extremities are increased, with unilateral or bilateral extensor plantar responses. The arm reflexes may be increased, decreased or absent, depending on the level of the cord lesion and the presence or absence of root lesions.

Urinary urgency, hesitancy and incontinence are present in a small percentage of the cases as a relatively late symptom. Osteophytes on the cervical vertebrae may compress the vertebral artery and produce symptoms of vertebral or basilar insufficiency.

Laboratory Data. The significant findings in the laboratory examinations are those obtained by lumbar puncture and by roentgenograms of the spine. Complete subarachnoid block is rarely present but incomplete block is found in about 15%. The spinal fluid content is normal in about two thirds of the cases. A moderate increase is present in the remainder with values over 100 ml in only a small percentage. Abnormal findings in roentgenograms of the cervical spine (Figs. 165 and 166) include narrowing of the disc spaces, slight degrees of vertebral subluxation, loss of cervical lordosis, and anterior and posterior osteophytes on the vertebral rims. There is no distinct clinical correlation between the severity of the bony changes and the clinical signs. On myelography, there are indentations adjacent to one or more disc spaces, filling defects opposite the body of a vertebra, narrowing of the cervical canal, and interruption of the flow of the dye.

Diagnosis and Differential Diagnosis. The diagnosis of cervical spondylosis should be entertained when symptoms and signs of nerve

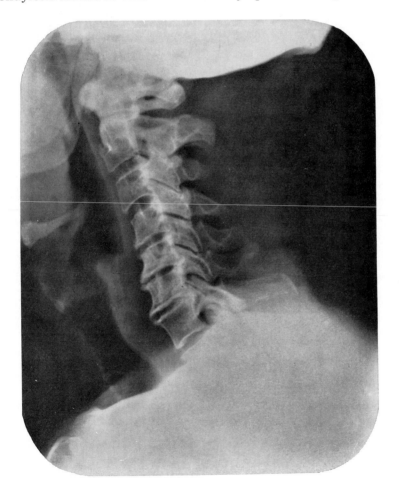

Figure 165. Cervical osteoarthritis. Narrowing of intervertebral spaces, spur formation on the vertebral bodies, and reversal of normal curve. (Courtesy Dr. Juan Taveras.)

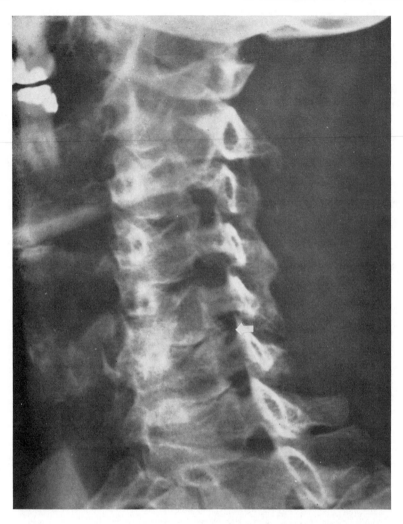

Figure 166. Cervical osteoarthritis. In oblique view the left C 5–6 intervertebral foramen is reduced to less than half normal size by spur formation (arrow). (Courtesy Dr. Ernest Wood.)

root injury and cord compression develop in a middle-aged patient with roentgenographic evidences of severe disease of the cervical spine. The presence of arthritic and degenerative changes in the cervical spine cannot be accepted as meaning that the symptoms and signs are due to these changes and the diagnosis must be confirmed by myelography.

The differential diagnosis includes multiple sclerosis, spinal cord tumor, syringomyelia, amyotrophic lateral sclerosis and the spinal cord degeneration of pernicious anemia. Cervical spondylosis may be a complicating factor in any of these diseases, but the differential diagnosis should not be difficult if the clinical features of the various diseases are considered and interpreted in connection with the findings at myelography if the latter is considered necessary.

Course. The course of the condition is subject to considerable variation. Long periods of non-progressive disability are the rule and a progressively deteriorating course is exceptional. Symptoms of damage to the spinal cord are not apt to develop if they are not present in the early stage of the disease.

Treatment. Medical treatment includes bed rest, immobilization of the neck by a collar, neck traction, and diathermy, ultrasound, or radiation therapy to the cervical spine. There are no clear-cut indications for surgical therapy or for the extent of the operative procedures. In general, operation is indicated when: (1) differential diagnosis between cervical spondylosis and spinal cord tumor cannot be made on the clinical data; (2) when there is complete spinal block on myelography; and (3) when medical therapy has failed to arrest the progress of the paraplegia or to relieve severe pains in arms and neck.

The operation should be limited to a laminectomy, with sectioning of the dentate ligaments and unroofing of appropriate foramina. No attempt should be made to remove centrally placed osteophytic bars. Soft midline protrusions or dorsolateral protrusions which stretch nerve roots can be removed or pared away.

REFERENCES

Bradshaw, P.: Some Aspects of Cervical Spondylosis, Quart. J. Med., 25, 177, 1957.

Braham, J., and Herzberger, E. E.: Cervical Spondylosis and Compression of the Spinal Cord, J.A.M.A., 161, 1560, 1956.

Brain, W. R.: Some Unsolved Problems of Cervical Spondylosis, Br. Med. J., 1, 771, 1963.

Brain, W. R., Northfield, D., and Wilkinson, M.: The Neurological Manifestations of Cervical Spondylosis, Brain, 75, 187, 1952.

Brooker, A. E. W., and Barter, R. W.: Cervical Spondylosis—A Clinical Study with Comparative Radiology, Brain, 88, 925, 1965.

Clarke, E., and Robinson, P. K.: Cervical Myelopathy: A Complication of Cervical Spondylosis, Brain, 79, 483, 1956.

Lees, F., and Turner, J. W. A.: Natural History and Prognosis of Cervical Spondylosis, Br. Med. J., 2, 1607, 1963.

Nugent, G. R.: Clinicopathologic Correlations in Cervical Spondylosis, Neurology, 9, 273, 1959.

Sheehan, S., Bauer, R. B., and Meyer, J. S.: Vertebral Artery Compression in Cervical Spondylosis, Neurology, 10, 968, 1960.

Teng, P.: Spondylosis of the Cervical Spine with Compression of the Spinal Cord and Nerve Roots, J. Bone Joint Surg., 42A, 392, 1960

Teng, P., and Papatheodorou, C.: Lumbar Spondylosis with Compression of Cauda Equina, Arch. Neurol., 8, 221, 1963.

POLYNEURITIS

General Considerations

Polyneuritis (multiple peripheral neuritis) is the term used to describe the clinical syndrome produced by widespread involvement of the peripheral nerves, with resultant weakness, sensory loss and impairment of reflexes.

Etiology. For practical purposes the conditions with which a polyneuritis is related can be divided into two groups: toxic and metabolic. In the majority of the cases the exact cause of the degenerative changes in the peripheral nerves is unknown. It is probable that impairment of the vascular supply of the nerves is responsible for the degeneration in periarteritis nodosa, lupus erythematosus and in the mononeuritides of diabetes mellitus. The vascular factor is not of significance, however, in the polyneuritides associated with toxic or metabolic disturbances. It is possible that the damage to the nerves in these conditions is due to a disturbance in the system of enzymes concerned with the nutrition of the nerves. For example, the polyneuritis which accompanies the administration of isoniazid and hydralazine is presumed to be due to an interference with the metabolism of pyridoxine.

Any listing of the toxic substances which have been reported to damage the peripheral nerves would be inadequate since additions are being made constantly. This list would include: Many of the heavy metals; chemical compounds used in industry and in medical therapy; bacterial toxins; and other substances.

The metabolic disturbances which may be accompanied by a polyneuritis are also quite diverse and include: General dietary deficiency; lack of specific nutritional factors or vitamins; cachexia of wasting diseases such as tuberculosis or cancer (particularly carcinoma of the lung); infectious diseases; uremia; endocrine disturbances; amyloidosis; and diseases of unknown etiology such as sarcoidosis.

The polyneuritis associated with many of these conditions has been considered in previous chapters. The discussion in this section will be confined to the forms of polyneuritis which are most commonly encountered in general practice.

Pathology. In the majority of the forms of polyneuritis, the pathology is mainly a non-inflammatory degeneration (Fig. 167) of the peripheral nerves. In the initial stages there are swelling and fragmentation of the myelin. With progress of the destructive process the axis cylinders are also injured. Retrograde changes may be found in the cells of the ventral horns (axonal reaction) and in chronic cases, there is a degeneration of the fibers of the posterior funiculi.

Occasionally, there is no obvious damage to the myelin sheath or axis

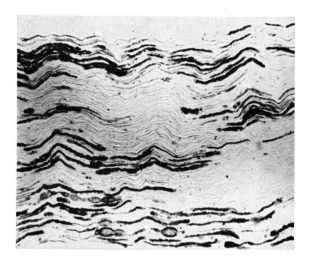

Figure 167. Multiple peripheral neuritis. Degeneration of myelin sheath. (Myelin sheath stain.)

cylinder. Conduction through the axis cylinder is apparently interrupted by swelling of either the axis cylinder or the myelin sheath. As would be expected, rapid recovery is possible in such cases. Whenever there has been actual destruction of myelin sheaths and axis cylinders, recovery will be slow. The rate of recovery is dependent on the extent of damage to the axon. The process of regeneration of the nerves in multiple peripheral neuritis is similar to that following injury to individual nerves by trauma.

Symptoms and Signs. The clinical picture of polyneuritis is similar regardless of the cause, but there may be variations in the distribution of paralysis and in the degree of sensory loss, which are related in some way to the underlying cause. Cases of polyneuritis may be divided into three groups according to the severity of the damage to the nerve: (1) Mild, with subjective pains and paresthesias, but with little or no weakness, sensory loss or reflex disturbances; (2) moderate, with subjective pain and paresthesias, slight weakness of the lower or upper extremities, diminution of vibratory sense and hypesthesia in the distal portion of the extremities, and decrease or loss of the tendon reflexes; and (3) severe, with complete paralysis of the muscles of the extremities, weakness of the muscles of the trunk and occasionally of the facial, palatal and pharyngeal muscles, loss of sensation in the distal portions of the extremities and absence of all tendon and skin reflexes.

Polyneuritis may occur at any age but it is most common in young or middle-aged adults. Men are much more frequently affected than women. The symptoms develop slowly over a period of several weeks in the majority of cases, although the onset is apparently sudden in a few cases of alcohol-vitamin deficiency polyneuritis, and rapid evolution of symptoms, i.e., within twenty-four to seventy-two hours, is the rule in "infectious or allergic" polyneuritis.

The symptoms of polyneuritis are pains, paresthesias, weakness and sensory loss. Pains are usually mild in character, but occasionally they may be sharp and burning. The paresthesias are usually a sensation of numbness or tingling. The paresthetic areas are sometimes exquisitely sensitive to touch or pressure.

Muscular weakness is greatest in the distal part of the extremities in the majority of the cases. Rarely, the proximal muscles of the extremities may be more severely affected than the distal muscles. In the moderately severe cases, there is paralysis of the digits and weakness of the movements at the ankle and wrist joint with wrist and foot drop. In the severe cases, the patient is completely bedridden with paralysis of all four extremities and weakness of the trunk muscles. Involvement of the cranial nerves is rare but paralysis of the facial, pharyngeal and other cranial muscles is not uncommon in diphtheritic or in so-called "infectious" polyneuritis. Weakness of the muscles of accommodation occurs frequently and is characteristic of the diphtheritic form. Sphincter disturbances may be present in the severe cases.

A mild sensory deficit, especially for vibration, is common in all forms of polyneuritis but an extensive loss of cutaneous sensation is most frequent in arsenical or the alcohol-vitamin deficiency types of polyneuritis. The cutaneous sensory loss, when present, consists of a hypesthesia or anesthesia to all forms of sensation in an irregular glove or stocking-like fashion. Frequently, there is a diminution of the threshold to painful stimuli but a delayed and greater than normal reaction to such stimuli. Pressure along the course of the nerve produces pain and the muscles are tender to pressure.

The reflexes are absent with a polyneuritis of moderate or severe degree. The plantar response is absent when the toes are paralyzed and the abdominal skin reflexes are diminished or absent when there is weakness of the abdominal muscles. Vasomotor and trophic disturbances may also be present. The skin may be smooth and shiny and the secretion of sweat may be disturbed.

Confusion, disorientation, amnesia and confabulation (Korsakoff's psychosis) are occasionally seen in any form of polyneuritis, but are most common in the alcohol-vitamin deficiency form and that which occurs with pregnancy.

The clinical features characteristic of special forms of polyneuritis are discussed in detail below.

Laboratory Data. The cerebrospinal fluid may be altered in any form of polyneuritis. The most common abnormalities are a slight increase in pressure when there is weakness of the muscles of respiration and an increase in the protein content. Rarely there is a slight pleocytosis. The increase in protein, when present, is usually only of a slight degree (45 to 75 mg per 100 ml), but occasionally the protein values may be over 100 mg and values greater than 1000 mg per 100 ml may occur. High values are most common in the diabetic, diphtheritic and so-called infectious type, but they may occur in any form of polyneuritis.

Other than the changes in the cerebrospinal fluid noted above there are no clinical pathological abnormalities in the majority of the cases of polyneuritis. Specific changes in the blood or urine are present in certain forms, for example, the excretion of porphyrins in the neuritis of acute porphyria, an elevated blood sugar in the diabetic polyneuritis or an excessive amount of lead or arsenic in the blood and urine of patients with polyneuritis associated with poisoning by these metals. These changes are considered in connection with the discussion of these entities.

Course. Complete or incomplete recovery is the rule in most cases of polyneuritis. The mortality rate is high in the "infectious" or acute porphyric forms, but death is infrequent in the other types unless complicated by bronchopneumonia, severe vitamin deficiency, or cerebral changes. i.e., Korsakoff's psychosis or polioencephalitis hemorrhagica superior. The course of patients with polyneuritis depends upon the extent to which the destruction of the nerves has progressed before treatment is instituted. With removal of the toxic agent or correction of the metabolic defects which are responsible for the neuritis, recovery may be fairly rapid if the continuity of the nerves has not been interrupted. On the other hand, the signs and symptoms may continue to progress for some days or weeks and recovery will be delayed for many months when the myelin sheaths and axis cylinders have been destroyed. In the latter case muscular wasting is severe and recovery is incomplete; there may be a residual weakness, muscular wasting and diminution of reflexes.

Treatment. The treatment of patients with polyneuritis can be divided into two phases: (1) Removal or treatment of the condition which is responsible for the development of the neuritis; and (2) symptomatic therapy.

The former will be considered with the discussion of the individual forms of polyneuritis. The administration of corticosteroids is recommended by some authors for all forms of polyneuritis. There is no evidence, however, that they are of any value except in the patients with polyneuritis associated with collagen diseases. The symptomatic treatment of the patient with polyneuritis consists of general supportive measures and physiotherapy. The patient should be kept in bed with the extremities protected from the bed clothes by means of a cradle. The diet should be nutritious and palatable. Tube feeding may occasionally be necessary. It is customary to supplement the diet with vitamins. This is essential when the neuritis is associated with dietary and vitamin deficiency but there is no evidence to indicate that vitamins in excess of that contained in a well-balanced diet has any appreciable effect on the clinical course of other forms of polyneuritis. Artificial respiration may be needed in patients with paralysis of the diaphragm and intercostal muscles. The bed should be kept clean and the sheets smooth to prevent injury to the anesthetic skin, although pressure sores rarely develop. The paralyzed extremities should be splinted to prevent stretching of paralyzed muscles. Physiotherapy should include daily or twice-daily massage of all the weak muscles and passive movements of all joints to their fullest extent. When voluntary movements begin to return, muscle training exercises should be given daily. Care should be taken not to overstrain weak muscles. It is, therefore, unwise to allow the patient to get out of bed or attempt to walk before the results of muscle testing indicate that he is prepared for these exertions.

REFERENCES

Cobb, S., and Coggeshall, H. C.: Neuritis, J.A.M.A., 103, 1608, 1934.
Gamstorp, I.: Polyneuropathy in Childhood, Acta Paediat., 57, 230, 1968.
Miller, H.: Polyneuritis, Br. Med. J., 2, 1219, 1966.
Simpson, J. A.: Biology and Disease of the Peripheral Nerves, Br. Med. J., 2, 709, 1964.
Tasker, W., and Chutorian, A. M.: Chronic Polyneuritis of Childhood, J. Pediatr., 74, 669, 1969.
Watters, G. V., and Barlow, C. F.: Acute and Subacute Neuropathies, Pediatr. Clin. North Am., 14, 997, 1967.

Alcohol-Vitamin Deficiency Polyneuritis

Etiology. The cause of this type of polyneuritis is disputed. It occurs in patients who have been addicted to the use of large amounts of alcoholic beverages for many years. The dietary intake of these patients is also apt to be inadequate. Since it is not clear whether the damage to the nerves is due to the toxic action of the ingested alcohol or whether it is due to the associated nutritional deficiency, it is customary to speak of the disease as alcohol-vitamin deficiency polyneuritis.

Incidence. Alcohol-vitamin deficiency polyneuritis is the most common form of polyneuritis. The figures for large municipal hospitals indicate that it is more frequent than all other forms combined. It is most common in the fourth to seventh decades of life, but it is occasionally seen in the third or eighth decades. It occurs about five or six times as frequently in the male as in the female.

Symptoms and Signs. The development of symptoms is usually slow, extending over a period of several weeks or months. Occasionally, however, the symptoms appear to develop rapidly, *i.e.,* within the course of a few days. The first symptoms are pain in the legs and paresthesia in the hands and feet. These symptoms are soon followed by weakness of the legs, foot drop and ataxia in walking. Unless the process is arrested by treatment, the legs gradually become paralyzed and the weakness spreads to involve the muscles of the upper extremities and the trunk. In extreme cases there may be optic neuritis, paresis of the ocular, facial, palatal and pharyngeal muscles and paralysis of the urinary and rectal sphincters. Dryness, scaling and pigmentation of the skin on the back of the wrists and hands, similar to that seen in patients with pellagra and vitamin A deficiency, are often present. The muscular weakness is greatest in the distal part of the extremities and extensors are more severely affected than the flexors. There is anesthesia or hypesthesia in the distal parts of the extremities, merging gradually with normal sensibility in the middle or proximal portion of the limbs. Vibratory and kinesthetic sensibilities are impaired. The nerves are sensitive to pressure and the muscles are painful when squeezed. In some patients, stroking the soles of the feet produces exquisitely painful paresthesias. The reflexes are absent in the legs and they may also be lost in the arms when the disease is unusually severe. The plantar responses are absent and the abdominal skin reflexes are decreased or absent.

The vital signs are normal except that the pulse rate may be increased.

Laboratory Data. A secondary type of anemia and a moderate leukocytosis are present in a large number of the cases. Alcohol may be found in the blood and cerebrospinal fluid if these are examined at the time of the patient's admission to the hospital. There is a decrease or absence of hydrochloric acid in the gastric juice in approximately one third of the cases. In an analysis of the cerebrospinal fluid from 56 cases, we found that the pressure was increased in 20% and there was a slight pleocytosis in the fluid in 8%. The protein content was increased in 20%, but it was not greater than 100 mg per 100 ml in any fluid.

Course. The course of alcoholic polyneuritis is prolonged, particularly if paralysis is present before treatment is instituted. Not infrequently there will be an increase in the severity of the signs and symptoms after treatment is begun. The mortality rate is low in uncomplicated cases, but is increased greatly when there are associated mental symptoms, or signs of involvement of the hypothalamus and midbrain (hemorrhagic polioencephalitis) are present. In the severe cases which recover, it is usually several months before the patient is able to get out of bed and six months to two years before the patient has recovered sufficiently to return to work.

Complications—Korsakoff's Syndrome. The combination of polyneuritis with a mental state characterized by confusion, disorientation, loss of memory and tendency to confabulate was described by Korsakoff in 1887. The syndrome is most frequently found in connection with the alcoholic form of polyneuritis but it may occur with the polyneuritis of pregnancy as well as with other forms. The mental symptoms characteristic of Korsakoff's syndrome can occur also in alcoholics in the absence of polyneuritis, and they may be present in non-alcoholic patients with brain tumors, meningitis or who have suffered a severe head injury or a spontaneous subarachnoid hemorrhage. The syndrome is fairly common in connection with alcoholic polyneuritis. The age incidence is similar to that for alcoholic polyneuritis in general. The male is affected approximately twice as often as the female. The relatively high incidence of the syndrome in women is well recognized and is much greater than the ratio of female to male admissions for chronic alcoholism. The duration of the symptoms before admission to the hospital varies between less than one week to more than six months. The vast majority of the patients have been addicted to the use of strong alcoholic beverages for many years and the dietary intake is usually grossly inadequate. Although Korsakoff's syndrome may develop in patients with only minor evidences of damage to the peripheral nerves, it most frequently is associated with a severe or moderately severe polyneuritis. Signs and symptoms of liver damage are present in about one fifth of the cases and convulsive seizures are not uncommon.

A moderate anemia is present in one half and a severe anemia is seen in about 10% of the cases. A leukocytosis greater than 11,000 is present in 30%. The cerebrospinal fluid findings are similar to those described for alcoholic polyneuritis except that increase in the protein content is more common and values higher than 100 mg are not rare.

The mortality rate in untreated cases is approximately 50% and does not appear to be related to the severity of the polyneuritis. Death usually occurs within the first few weeks after the symptoms become severe enough to require hospitalization. Recovery is slow and often incomplete in the patients who survive. Residual mental defects may be incapacitating enough to necessitate confinement in a mental institution.

The treatment is the same as that of alcoholic polyneuritis. Thiamine and vitamin B complex should be given intravenously in large doses. The mortality rate is low in patients who receive this form of treatment.

Polioencephalitis Superior of Wernicke. In 1881, Wernicke described an illness characterized by the sudden onset of paralysis of eye movements, ataxic gait and disturbances in the state of consciousness. Two of Wernicke's patients were chronic alcoholics and the third was a young woman with persistent vomiting associated with the ingestion of sulfuric acid.

In the vast majority of cases recorded in the literature since Wernicke's original report, the syndrome has been associated with chronic alcoholism, but isolated cases have been reported in association with pernicious vomiting of pregnancy and with various states of undernutrition or avitaminosis. It is now generally considered that the lesions in Wernicke's syndrome are not the result of injury to the nervous system by alcohol but to the associated nutritional deficiency.

At necropsy the lesions are concentrated in the hypothalamus, in the neighborhood of the third ventricle and in the peri-aqueductal gray (Fig. 168). The small vessels are hyperplastic and tortuous, with numerous petechial hemorrhages, and there is necrosis of nerve cells.

Although Wernicke's syndrome was considered at one time to be relatively rare and highly fatal, the concept has been broadened and it is now known that many cases with a mild or moderate degree of damage may recover.

The clinical syndrome includes various types of oculomotor palsies, nystagmus, ataxia, tremor, and alterations in the state of consciousness, varying from coma to a mild confusion. Symptoms and signs of

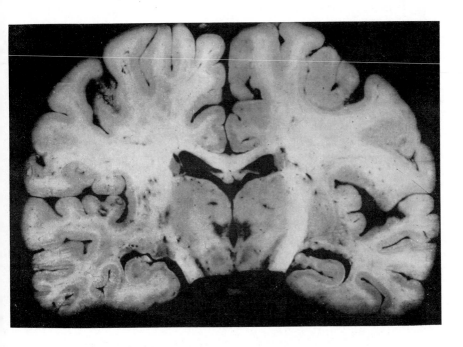

Figure 168.   Wernicke's syndrome. Petechial hemorrhages in the hypothalamus near the third ventricle.

polyneuritis and the Korsakoff's type of psychosis are present in over one half of the cases. Other complications of alcoholism or nutritional deficiency are present in a small percentage of the cases. These include convulsive seizures, optic neuritis, anemia and liver disease.

The ocular symptoms and the ataxia usually clear within a few days or a few weeks with adequate therapy but the mental symptoms and the polyneuritis persist for several or many months.

Therapy includes bed rest, withdrawal of alcohol, high-calorie, high-vitamin diet with addition of thiamine parenterally in large dosages.

Diagnosis and Differential Diagnosis. The diagnosis of alcoholic polyneuritis can usually be made without difficulty when the typical symptoms develop in an individual who is addicted to the use of alcoholic beverages in large amounts. Difficulty is encountered only when some other form of polyneuritis develops in a patient who also takes alcohol in moderate amounts.

Treatment. The treatment of alcoholic polyneuritis is the same as that for other forms of polyneuritis. Since signs of vitamin deficiency are present in a high percentage of the cases, the patient should be given a high-calorie diet supplemented by concentrated vitamins parenterally and by mouth.

REFERENCES

Bailey, F. W.: Histopathology of Polioencephalitis Hemorrhagica Superior, Arch. Neurol. & Psychiat., 56, 609, 1946.
Campbell, A. C. P., and Biggart, J. H.: Wernicke's Encephalopathy (Polioencephalitis Hemorrhagica Superior); Its Alcoholic and Non-alcoholic Incidence, J. Path. & Bact., 48, 245, 1939.
Cravioto, H., Korein, J., and Silberman, J.: Wernicke's Encephalopathy, Arch. Neurol., 4, 510, 1961.
Kahn, E. A., and Crosby, E. G.: Korsakoff's Syndrome Associated with Surgical Lesion Involving the Mammillary Bodies, Neurology, 22, 117, 1972.
Korsakoff, S.: Razstoistro psichich, dejatel. pri alkohol. paraliche. (Psychical derangement active in alcoholic paralysis), Vestnik klin; sudebnoi psichiat. i nevropatol., St. Petersb., 4, pt. 2, 1887.
Malamud, N. and Skillicorn, S. A.: Relationship Between the Wernicke and the Korsakoff Syndrome, Arch. Neurol. & Psychiat., 76, 585, 1956.
Minot, G. R., Strauss, M. B., and Cobb, S.: "Alcoholic" Polyneuritis; Dietary Deficiency as a Factor in Its Production, N. Engl. J. Med., 208, 1244, 1933.
Phillips, G. B., Victor, M., Adams, R. D., and Davidson, C. S.: A Study of the Nutritional Defect in Wernicke's Syndrome; the Effect of a Purified Diet, Thiamine, and Other Vitamins on the Clinical Manifestations, J. Clin. Invest., 31, 859, 1952.
Rosenbaum, M., and Merritt, H. H.: Korsakoff's Syndrome, Arch. Neurol. & Psychiat., 41, 978, 1939.
Strauss, M. B.: Etiology of "Alcoholic" Polyneuritis, Am. J. Med. Sci., 189, 378, 1935.
Victor, M., and Adams, R. D.: The Effect of Alcohol on the Nervous System, A. Res. Nev. & Ment. Dis., Proc., 32, 526, 1953.
Victor, M., Adams, R. D., and Collins, G. H.: *The Wernicke-Korsakoff Syndrome*, Philadelphia, F. A. Davis Co., 1971.

Arsenical Polyneuritis

Damage to the peripheral nerves may develop following chronic exposure to small amounts of arsenic or after the ingestion or parenteral administration of a large amount of the metal.

Etiology. Arsenical polyneuritis, which was formerly quite common as the result of ingestion of small amounts of inorganic arsenic in foods or beverages, is now relatively rare.

Arsenical poisoning occasionally occurs following the accidental ingestion of rat poison or excessive exposure to arsenate sprays or dust. The peripheral neuropathy is thought to be due to an interference with the pyruvate oxidase system by the arsenic.

Gastrointestinal symptoms, vomiting and diarrhea, occur when a toxic amount of arsenic is ingested. These symptoms may be entirely absent if the arsenic is given parenterally or if taken in small amounts over long periods of time. In acute poisoning the onset of the neuritis is delayed for four to eight weeks, but once the symptoms develop they reach their maximum intensity within a few days. The evolution of the neuritic symptoms is much slower in patients with chronic arsenical poisoning.

Symptoms and Signs. The symptomatology of arsenical polyneuritis is so similar to that of alcoholic polyneuritis that many attempts have been made to explain the neuritis which occurs in chronic alcoholics on basis of chronic arsenical poisoning. Sensory symptoms are prominent in the early stages. Pains and paresthesias in the lower extremities may be present for several days or weeks before the onset of motor weakness. The weakness progresses slowly to a complete flaccid paralysis of the lower extremities with extension to the upper extremities in the severe cases. Cutaneous sensation is impaired or lost in a stocking or glove distribution. The tendon reflexes and the plantar reflexes are lost. Pigmentation and hyperkeratosis of the skin and changes in the nails are frequently present.

Laboratory Data. Arsenic is present in the urine in the acute stage of the poisoning and it may be found in the hair or nails in the late stages. It must be remembered, however, that a trace of arsenic is not an uncommon finding in the urine of healthy individuals.

Prognosis. Complete or almost complete recovery is the rule if the source of poisoning is removed. The duration of convalescence depends upon the degree of damage to the nerves. Acute hemorrhagic encephalitis, a rare complication of arsphenamine therapy, is discussed elsewhere.

Treatment. British anti-lewisite should be administered in doses of 3 mg per kg of body weight every four to six hours for two to three days and then twice daily for ten days. Arsenical polyneuritis can also be treated with penicillamine in dose of 250 mg four times a day. It is not known whether BAL or penicillamine has any significant effect on the course of neuritis.

REFERENCES

Chuttani, P. N., et al.: Arsenical Neuropathy, Neurology, *17*, 269, 1967.
Hassin, G. B.: Symptomatology of Arsenical Polyneuritis, J. Nerv. & Ment. Dis., *72*, 628, 1930.
Heyman, A., Pfeiffer, J. B., Jr., Willett, R. W. and Taylor, H. M.: Peripheral Neuropathy Caused by Arsenical Intoxication, N. Engl. J. Med., *254*, 401, 1956.
Longcope, W. T., and Luetscher, J. A.: The Use of BAL (British Anti-Lewisite) in the Treatment of the Injurious Effects of Arsenic, Mercury and Other Metallic Poisons, Ann. Intern. Med., *31*, 545, 1949.

Lead Polyneuritis

The polyneuritis associated with lead poisoning is essentially a motor neuritis with a predilection for the extensor muscles of the fingers and wrist. It occurs almost exclusively in adults. Lead poisoning in infants usually causes an encephalopathy rather than a neuritis. When neuritis does occur in infants, it is more apt to be generalized rather than the "radial nerve type" of adults.

Etiology. Lead may enter the body through the skin, lungs and alimentary tract, and cases of poisoning can be divided into two groups: occupational and accidental. In the former, lead is absorbed mainly through the lungs and skin in such occupations as lead-workers, painters, pottery glaziers and the like. Accidental poisoning follows the ingestion of lead in food or beverages which have been in contact with lead. In infants poisoning may result from the ingestion of lead paint on toys or cribs. Precautionary measures in industry and the elimination of lead from the paint on furniture have greatly reduced the incidence of lead poisoning.

Pathology. The pathology of lead polyneuritis is similar to that of other forms of polyneuritis. There are no adequate pathological studies of the cases with muscular wasting and lateral tract signs which have been reported as following lead poisoning.

Symptoms and Signs. The polyneuritis of lead poisoning commonly begins as a weakness of extensors of the fingers and wrist. The weakness is usually bilateral, but one arm may be affected before the other. The weakness may extend to other muscles of the upper extremity and, rarely, to those of the lower extremity. Sensory symptoms and signs are usually absent. The initial weakness in lead polyneuritis is quite similar to that of radial nerve palsy with the exception that the brachioradialis muscle is spared.

Other signs and symptoms of lead poisoning are common in children but are less conspicuous in adults. Lead colic, anemia with basophilic stippling of the red cells, lead line in the bones and the deposition of lead pigment at the gingival margins are frequent concomitant findings.

Laboratory Data. Lead can be found in the urine, feces and cerebrospinal fluid. In addition the protein content of the cerebrospinal fluid may be increased with values sometimes greater than 100 mg per 100 ml.

Course and Prognosis. The polyneuritic symptoms usually reach their maximum intensity within the course of several days or weeks. With the removal of the exposure to lead and institution of proper treatment, complete or nearly complete recovery takes place in the course of several to many months. Fatalities are rare except in infants with coincidental encephalopathy. A few cases are reported in which the polyneuritis is followed by muscular wasting, fibrillation and lateral tract signs, similar to amyotrophic lateral sclerosis.

Treatment. In general, the treatment of lead polyneuritis is similar to that of other forms of polyneuritis. Specifically, however, one of the primary aims is to precipitate the lead which is present in the blood stream into the bones; this can be done by the administration of milk, calcium salts, basic disodium phosphate and viosterol. The question of the advisability of removing the lead from the body after the patient has recovered is still under debate. The lead can be removed by the administration of iodides, acid salts and citrates or the parenteral injection of parathormone. The danger of recurrence of symptoms with this treatment has led some authors to advise that no attempts be made to de-lead the patient, but rather allow it to be slowly excreted over the course of years. British anti-lewisite is of doubtful value in the treatment of lead poisoning. Experience with the use of chelating agents such as versene is too limited to evaluate their effectiveness.

REFERENCES

Aring, C. D., and Trufant, S. A.: Effects of Heavy Metals on the Central Nervous System, A. Res. Nerv. & Ment. Dis., Proc., *32*, 463, 1953.
Aub, J. C.: Biochemical Behavior of Lead in the Body, J.A.M.A., *104*, 87, 1935.
Chisolm, J. J., Jr.: Treatment of Acute Lead Intoxication; Choice Chelating Agents and Supportive Therapeutic Measures, Clin. Toxicol., *3*, 527, 1970.
Haley, T. J.: Saturnism, Pediatric and Adult Lead Poisoning, Clin. Toxicol., *4*, 11, 1971.
Seto, D. S. Y., and Freeman, J. M.: Lead Neuropathy in Childhood, Am. J. Dis. Child., *107*, 337, 1964.

Polyneuritis Associated with Deficiency States

The spinal or cranial nerves may be damaged in patients who have had an inadequate food intake, particularly if the diet has been low in the essential vitamins. Attempts have been made to explain the neuritis on basis of a deficiency of single factors. These have not been entirely successful for various reasons. First, experimental deficiencies in animals have not always given clear-cut results; second, deficient diets in humans are usually lacking in multiple factors; and third, the failure of symptoms to improve with the administration of a specific vitamin cannot be taken as evidence that this substance is not the chief etiologic factor. This is particularly true when the neuritis is of moderate or severe degree and there has been actual degeneration of myelin or axons.

Dietary deficiency is generally considered to be the cause of the polyneuritis associated with beriberi, pellagra, chronic malnutrition, chronic gastrointestinal diseases such as sprue, chronic colitis, chronic bacillary dysentery and pernicious vomiting, and with cachectic states of cancer, tuberculosis and senility. It is believed by some that the polyneuritis associated with cancer is due to the action of some toxin which interferes with the metabolism of nerves. There is evidence to indicate that infiltration of the nerves by the neoplasm is the cause of the polyneuritis in at least some of the cases.

Beriberi. Beriberi is endemic in hot climates, but it is occasionally seen in the temperate zones. The cases with beriberi are commonly divided into the wet and dry forms, dependent upon the presence or absence of edema and serous effusion. It is now agreed that the edema and serous effusions are due to cardiac failure and that these symptoms respond to treatment with vitamin B_1. The evidence in regard to the role of deficiency of vitamin B_1 in the production of the neuritic symptoms is less clear.

The symptoms and signs of beriberi polyneuritis are similar to those previously described for alcoholic polyneuritis. Pains and paresthesias are present for several days or weeks before the onset of motor weakness. The latter is quite severe, with paralysis of the muscles of the distal part of the lower extremities and, in advanced stages, also those of the upper extremities. There is cutaneous sensory loss below the wrists and knees and absence of the tendon reflexes.

Fatalities, not uncommon in the tropical form of beriberi, are rare in the sporadic cases which occur in temperate climates. Recovery is slow and there may be residual muscular weakness and atrophy.

The treatment is the same as that of other forms of polyneuritis with the addition of the vitamin B complex parenterally. The intravenous administration of vitamin B_1 or co-carboxylase will often result in a dramatic relief of the pains and some improvement in the weakness, but there is little change in the signs which are due to peripheral nerve damage. Relief of pain, according to Aring and Spies, is due to a humoral action of vitamin B_1 which cannot be expected to affect parenchymatous changes in the nerves.

Pellagra. Pellagra is a deficiency disease characterized by the occurrence of gastrointestinal symptoms, symmetrical skin eruptions, and symptoms due to injury to the central and peripheral nervous system.

Etiology. The evidence at the present time indicates that the signs and symptoms of pellagra can be explained on basis of a dietary deficiency which involves mainly the vitamin B complex. The gastrointestinal, mental and cutaneous symptoms are due to a deficiency of nicotinic acid, while the neuritic symptoms are more closely related to a deficiency of thiamine.

Pathology. The pathological changes in the nervous system in pellagra include degenerative changes in the peripheral nerves, in the white matter of the dorsal and to a lesser extent in the lateral funiculi of the spinal cord. Retrograde degenerative changes are seen in the nerve cells of the spinal cord and brain.

Incidence. Pellagra is a widespread disease, occurring in most parts of the world. In the United States, the form which was formerly common in the southern states is almost purely a deficiency state, whereas that which is found in the northern and eastern sections is usually associated with chronic alcoholism. Although pellagra may occur at any age, it is most common in the third and fourth decades of life. The incidence in the two sexes is approximately equal, except in the alcoholic form where males predominate.

Symptoms and Signs. The gastrointestinal symptoms are usually first to appear. These include anorexia, vomiting and diarrhea. The latter is often the most prominent and earliest symptom. In addition there may be fissuring of the skin around the corners of the mouth, glossitis and stomatitis.

The extent of the skin eruption is variable. In mild cases, it may be limited to the skin on the wrist and dorsum of the hands, appearing after exposure to the sun, and often attributed to sunburn. In severe cases, the dermatitis may also involve the skin of the neck (Casal's collar), face, dorsum of the feet and areas which are not commonly exposed to the sun.

Any part of the neuraxis may be damaged. Involvement of the cerebrum is manifested by the development of mental symptoms, which include acute confusional states, mania, melancholia, dementia and neurasthenic-like states. Peripheral neuritis is the most common neurological sign, but there may be evidence of involvement of the spinal cord, brainstem, cerebellum or basal ganglia.

Laboratory Data. A mild or moderate degree of anemia and achlorhydria are present in approximately 50% of the cases. The cerebrospinal fluid is normal except for a slight increase in the protein content in a small percentage of the cases.

Course. The course of pellagra depends upon the degree to which the disease has progressed before treatment is instituted. The cutaneous and gastrointestinal symptoms respond readily to treatment. Minor mental or neurological symptoms can often be relieved by treatment, but permanent mental loss is to be expected in cases of long standing dementia and improvement will be slow when the neuritic symptoms are severe.

Treatment. The treatment is essentially directed toward correction of the dietary deficiency. It should include a balanced diet together with large doses of nicotinic acid and thiamine parenterally or by mouth.

Chronic Malnutrition. Malnutrition in prisoners of war and in concentration camps in Japan and the Far East resulted in the development of various symptoms, such as spastic paraplegia, nerve deafness, amblyopia and "burning feet." These symptoms developed in various combinations and in some instances were associated with other well-known syndromes, such as beriberi, pellagra or Wernicke's encephalopathy. Smith studied the incidence of these complications in a large concentration camp in China. The frequency of symptoms was related to the level of vitamin B intake. Treatment was effective in relieving the symptoms in the early stages, but recovery was slow or there were permanent residuals in patients whose symptoms were of long duration before adequate treatment could be instituted.

REFERENCES

Crawford, J. N., and Reid, J. A. C.: Nutritional Disease Affecting Canadian Troops Held Prisoners of War by the Japanese, Can. J. Res. Sect. E. 25, 53, 1947.

Lewy, F. H., Spies, T. D., and Aring, C. D.: Incidence of Neuropathy in Pellagra; the Effect of Cocarboxylase upon Its Neurologic Signs, Am. J. Med. Sci., 199, 840, 1940.

Montgomery, R. D., Cruickshank, E. K., Robertson, W. B., and McMenemey, W. H.: Clinical and Pathological Observations on Jamaican Neuropathy—A Report of 206 Cases, Brain, 87, 425, 1964.

Olivarius, B. def.: Neurological Sequelae of Partial Gastrectomy, Acta Neurol. Scand., Suppl. 43, 204, 1970.

Ridley, H.: Ocular Manifestations of Malnutrition in Released Prisoners of War from Thailand, Brit. J. Ophth., 29, 613, 1945.

Rowland, L. P., and Schneck, S. A.: Neuromuscular Disorders Associated with Malignant Neoplastic Disease, J. Chron. Dis., 16, 777, 1963.

Smith, D. A.: Nutritional Neuropathies in the Civilian Internment Camp, Hong Kong, January, 1942-August, 1945, Brain, 69, 209, 1946.

Spies, T. D., Aring, C. D., Gelperin, J., and Bean, W. B.: The Mental Symptoms of Pellagra; Their Relief with Nicotinic Acid, Am. J. Med. Sci., 196, 461, 1938.

Spillane, J. D.: *Nutritional Disorders of the Nervous System*, Baltimore, Williams & Wilkins, 1947, 280 pp.

Victor, M., and Dreyfus, P. M.: Nutritional Diseases of the Nervous System, World Neurology, 2, 862, 1961.

Williams, A. D., and Osuntokun, B. O.: Peripheral Neuropathy in Tropical Nutritional Ataxia in Nigeria, Arch. Neurol., 21, 475, 1969.
Zimmerman, H. M.: Neuropathies Due to Vitamin Deficiency, J. Neuropathol. Exp. Neurol., 51, 335, 1956.

Diphtheritic Polyneuritis

Diphtheritic polyneuritis, formerly a common complication of infection with Corynebacterium diphtheriae, is now relatively rare in the United States. This is due to the widespread passive immunization of the population and the early use of serum when infection occurs.

Etiology and Pathology. Involvement of the nerves in diphtheria is presumably due to the action of the diphtheritic toxin on peripheral nerves and nerve roots. It may follow diphtheritic infections in any part of the body. The pathology is the same as that of other forms of polyneuritis, *i.e.,* degenerative changes in the myelin sheaths and axons of peripheral nerves and retrograde changes in the motor cells in the spinal cord and brainstem.

Incidence. Neuritis following faucial diphtheria occurs predominantly in childhood, but is rare before the age of one year. The two sexes are about equally affected. Neuritis following cutaneous diphtheria, which is frequent in the tropics, is most common in adult males.

The neuritis may follow an infection of the throat which is so slight that it has been overlooked. As a rule, however, the frequency of the incidence of nerve involvement is proportional to the severity of the infection, and to the delay in the administration of antitoxin for the original infection.

Symptoms and Signs. The symptoms of the neuritis rarely appear before the third week after the onset of infection but evidence of involvement of the palatal muscles may occur in the first or second week. It is commonly thought that this is due to local injury to the nerves. Against this hypothesis, however, is the fact that palatal weakness may be the initial symptom of the neuritis following cutaneous diphtheria.

In the vast majority of cases palatal weakness and blurring of vision due to paralysis of accommodation are the first symptoms. The voice has a nasal quality and the patient is unable to read unless the book is held at some distance from the eyes. These symptoms are followed in the course of the next few days or weeks by evidence of involvement of other cranial and peripheral nerves with paralysis of pharyngeal, facial, external ocular muscles and the muscles of the extremities. Occasionally, the peripheral nerves may be initially involved with paresthesias in the extremities as the first symptom.

Progress of the symptoms is slow and variable. In some instances, the paralysis may be confined to the cranial nerves and in others to the muscles of the extremities. Occasionally, the signs and symptoms of involvement of the extremities will appear coincidental with improvement in the weakness of the palatal and ciliary muscles. Rarely, the disease may assume an ataxic form with paresthesias, loss of proprioceptive sensations and absence of reflexes.

The clinical signs of diphtheritic polyneuritis are similar to those of other forms of polyneuritis except for the high incidence of paralysis of muscles supplied by the cranial nerves. The usual clinical syndrome is closely simulated by that of so-called infectious polyneuritis, with the exception that palatal and ciliary muscle weakness is rarely, if ever, the initial symptom in the latter form of polyneuritis.

Laboratory Data. Corynebacterium diphtheriae can be isolated from the nasopharynx or from the cutaneous sores in a small percentage of the cases as long as several weeks or months after the infection. The protein content of the cerebrospinal fluid is practically always increased. Values between 100 and 400 mg per 100 ml are not uncommon. This increase in protein may persist for many months and is considered by some authors as an indication of persistence of the active process.

Course. The mortality rate is high (approximately 30%) in the neuritis following faucial diphtheria. This is probably due to the high incidence of cardiac involvement in such cases.

The paralysis usually reaches its maximum within several weeks after the onset of the first symptoms of involvement of the nervous system. After this time there is gradual improvement, but it may be many months before recovery is complete. Permanent residuals are uncommon, but there may be some weakness or atrophy of the affected muscles.

Diagnosis and Differential Diagnosis. The diagnosis of diphtheritic polyneuritis is not difficult when the symptoms follow directly upon a proven diphtheritic infection. The diagnosis may be difficult when the initial diphtheritic infection was slight or not detected. The occurrence of paralysis of accommodation or palatal weakness as the initial symptom of a slowly progressing polyneuritis should lead to the consideration of diphtheria as the cause of the symptoms.

Diphtheritic polyneuritis must be distinguished from other forms of polyneuritis, particularly the so-called infectious form. Involvement of the cranial nerves and an increased protein content in the cerebrospinal fluid are common to both of these forms of polyneuritis. In addition, a minor upper respiratory infection often precedes the onset of symptoms in the latter form. Absolute differential diagnosis between the two may not be possible in some cases. Examination of the bacterial flora of the pharynx may be of value. In addition, the symptoms in "infectious" polyneuritis usually develop within five to twelve days after the upper respiratory infection, while those of diphtheritic polyneuritis most commonly occur after an interval of two to four weeks.

Treatment. There is no specific treatment once the neuritis has developed. Early treatment of the diphtheritic infection is of great importance in preventing the development of nerve damage. The administration of vitamins has no effect on the course of the neuritis. Physiotherapy and muscle training are important in obtaining maximum return of function of weakened muscles.

REFERENCES

DiFiore, J. A.: Polyneuritis following Cutaneous Diphtheria, J. Nerv. & Ment. Dis., 114, 333, 1951.

Fisher, C. M., and Adams, R. D.: Diphtheritic Polyneuritis—A Pathological Study, J. Neuropathol. Exp. Neurol., 15, 243, 1956.

Gaskill, H. S., and Korb, M.: Occurrence of Multiple Neuritis in Cases of Cutaneous Diphtheria, Arch. Neurol. & Psychiat., 55, 559, 1946.

Hertz, M., and Thygesen, P.: Postdiphtheric Nervous Complications, and a Comparison between Polyradiculitis of Diphtheric Origin and That Due to Other Causes, Acta Psychiat. et Neurol., Suppl., 44, 1947.

———: Nervous Complications in Diphtheria, Acta. Med. Scand., Suppl., 206, 541, 1948.

Perkins, R. F., and Laufer, M. W.: Clinical Study of Postidiphtheritic Polyneuritis, J. Nerv. & Ment. Dis., 104, 59, 1946.

Ronaldson, G. W. and Kelleher, W. H.: Palatal Paralysis in Extrafaucial Diphtheria, Br. Med. J., 1, 1019, 1935.

Infectious Polyneuritis

(Infectious Neuronitis; Polyneuritis with Facial Diplegia; Landry-Guillain-Barré Syndrome)

Infectious polyneuritis is a clinical syndrome of unknown etiology characterized by the acute onset of symptoms of involvement of the peripheral and cranial nerves. A history of a preceding infection of the upper respiratory or gastrointestinal tract is obtained from about two thirds of the patients.

Isolated cases were reported in the literature before attention was directed to this syndrome by the studies of Guillain, Barré, and Strohl and others in the second and third decades of this century. Since that time there have been many articles reporting the clinical and pathological findings in a large number of cases. There is no convincing evidence, however, that these cases constitute a new syndrome or that they differ significantly from those reported by Landry in 1859.

Etiology. The cause of this type of polyneuritis is unknown. Indeed, there is some doubt whether the reported cases constitute a clinical entity since a similar syndrome may be present in polyneuritis of diverse causes. The clinical picture in typical cases is sufficiently characteristic to justify the conviction that there may be some common etiological factor, although all attempts to isolate this factor have been unsuccessful. Alcohol, the common metallic poisons and dietary deficiency have been excluded as causative factors. Since the onset of the neuritic symptoms in many of the cases follows an upper respiratory infection, it was natural to assume that a filtrable virus might be the causative agent. In fact, Bradford, Bashford and Wilson in 1919 claimed to have isolated such a virus. This finding has never been confirmed and all of the attempts of modern workers to isolate a virus from the blood, cerebrospinal fluid, brain or spinal cord of these patients have yielded negative results. In addition, the pathological changes are unlike those of any known viral disease of the nervous system. At the present time, we can only state that infectious polyneuritis is in all probability not due to an infection of the nervous system by any known bacterium or virus. The most plausible hypothesis is that the neuritis is of allergic origin. This hypothesis is supported by the fact that polyneuritis can be produced in animals by the injection of extracts of peripheral nerves.

Pathology. The pathological changes are confined to degenerative changes in the spinal and cranial nerves with retrograde changes in the motor cells of the spinal cord and medulla. In the patients who die within a few days of the onset of the neuritis, the pathological findings may be quite meager, with only a questionable edema of the nerves or roots. There is no inflammatory reaction in the central or peripheral nervous system. Reports of secondary degeneration of the ascending tracts in the spinal cord are rare, mainly because death, in the fatal cases, occurs before these changes can develop.

Incidence. Although few cases were reported before 1916, infectious polyneuritis is now second only to alcoholic polyneuritis in frequency. In fact, it is now the most frequent form of polyneuritis that is seen in general hospitals which do not admit chronic alcoholics.

The disease may occur at any age. It is slightly more common in the third and fourth decades, but may be seen as early as the second year of life and as late as the ninth decade. The sexes are equally affected.

Symptoms and Signs. A mild upper respiratory infection, or less commonly a gastroenteritis, precedes the onset of the neuritis in approximately two thirds of the cases. No diagnostic studies have been made to determine the exact nature of these infections. The symptoms of the infection usually last only a few days and subside before the onset of the neuritic symptoms, which usually develop after an interval of five to twelve days.

Table 96. Involvement of the Cranial Nerves in 26 Cases of Infectious Polyneuritis

Nerves Involved	No. of Cases
Seventh alone	6
Seventh with tenth	5
Seventh with ninth and tenth	2
Seventh with fifth, ninth and tenth	2
Seventh with fifth, ninth, tenth, eleventh and twelfth	2
Seventh with ninth, tenth and eleventh	2
Seventh with third, fifth, ninth and tenth	1
Seventh with fifth, eleventh and twelfth	1
Seventh with sixth, ninth, tenth, eleventh and twelfth	1
None	4

The initial neurological symptom is usually weakness of the lower extremities which extends within twenty-four to seventy-two hours to the upper extremities and the facial muscles. Occasionally, paresthesias in the extremities may precede the weakness. The paralysis usually reaches its maximum within a few days of the onset, but occasionally there may be an increase in the weakness for two to three weeks. Paralysis of the cranial nerves is frequent (Table 96). Facial diplegia is present in 85%, dysphagia or dysarthria in 50%, and paralysis or weakness of the muscles supplied by the eleventh cranial nerve in 20%. Involvement of the extraocular or jaw muscles occurs infrequently. Choked discs, due to increased intracranial pressure resulting from respiratory embarrassment or interference with the absorptive mechanism of the cerebrospinal fluid by the high protein content of the fluid, are occasionally seen. Motor weakness in the muscles of the trunk and extremities is usually quite severe. Occasionally, it is greater in the proximal part of the limb than in the distal muscles. A flaccid quadriplegia is not uncommon and weakness of the muscles of respiration requiring the use of a respirator develops in about one fourth of the cases. The interim between the onset of symptoms and the development of respiratory failure ranges between two and twenty-one days, with an average of twelve days.

Sensory changes are usually not a prominent part of the clinical picture. Cutaneous hypesthesia in the distal parts of the extremities is present in about a third of the cases and a slight or moderate diminution of vibratory sense occurs in a similar percentage. Occasionally, the degree of impairment of cutaneous sensibility may be quite severe. In a few cases the loss of position and vibratory senses in the extremities is out of proportion to the cutaneous sensory loss or the muscular weakness (ataxic form). Muscle tenderness or sensitivity of the nerves to pressure of a slight or moderate degree is present in the majority of cases.

The tendon reflexes are diminished or absent. The plantar and abdominal skin reflexes are usually absent. Rapid pulse, low grade fever and a moderate degree of hypertension are common findings in the severe cases.

An unusual type of polyneuritis, which is considered by some to be an atypical form of post-infectious polyneuritis, was reported by Fisher in 1956. The clinical symptoms and signs are restricted to ataxia of gait, absence of tendon reflexes and partial ophthalmoplegia. The course is benign with complete recovery within one to three months. The cerebrospinal fluid is normal except for a slight or moderate increase in the cerebrospinal protein in about 50% of the cases.

Laboratory Data. Routine examination of the blood and urine usually gives normal results. A slight anemia, probably not related to the neuritis, is present in a small percentage of the cases. A leukocytosis together with elevation of the body temperature may occur in association with complicating infections. The changes in the blood characteristic of infectious mononucleosis are found in the cases in which the neuritis is associated with this disease. The cerebrospinal fluid pressure is elevated in the severe cases. A slight pleocytosis (10 to 100 cells per cu mm) is present in approximately 20%. The most common finding, however, is an increase in the protein content, with values as high as 1000 mg per 1000 ml in some cases. The protein content is not always increased however, and values below 75 mg are present at the onset in 39% (Table 97).

This protein increase, when present, is usually found in the early stages but occasionally the protein content of the fluid may be normal in the early stages and increased in the later stages.

Course and Prognosis. The symptoms usually reach their maximum extent within a week of the onset, but rarely there may be progression of the disease for three weeks or more. Although infectious polyneuritis

Table 97.   The Protein Content of the Cerebrospinal Fluid Removed at First Puncture in 26 Cases of Infectious Polyneuritis

Protein Content (mg/100 ml)	No. of Cases	%
Less than 45	7	27
45–75	3	12
75–200	12	46
200 or above	4*	15
	26	100

*354, 363, 399 and 750 mg

was formerly considered a benign syndrome, the mortality rate in the series reported in recent years has varied between 15 and 60%. The prognosis does not appear to be related to the presence or absence of an infection prior to the onset of the neuritis nor to the level of the protein content in the cerebrospinal fluid. Although fatalities have been reported in children, the mortality rate is higher in adults. Death is usually due to respiratory failure or to intercurrent infection and commonly occurs within three weeks of the onset.

The rate of recovery in patients who survive is variable. In some it is quite rapid with complete restoration to normal within a few days or weeks. In the majority, however, recovery is slow and is not complete for many months. Residuals are infrequent, but a slight weakness of the facial muscles or weakness and atrophy of the muscles of the extremities may persist.

Diagnosis and Differential Diagnosis. Since there is no specific diagnostic test the diagnosis rests entirely upon the presence of the typical clinical picture and the exclusion of other diseases characterized by a widespread paralysis of acute onset. The difficulties in the delineation of the syndrome have been increased by the fact that many of the reports in the literature include in this category all diseases of the nervous system with two common features, i.e., widespread paralysis and an increased protein content in the cerebrospinal fluid. Many of these cases, labeled as the Guillain-Barré syndrome, could more properly be classified as cases of acute myelitis, encephalomyelitis, or polyneuritis due to other causes. Great stress has been laid on the increased protein content in the cerebrospinal fluid in the absence of a pleocytosis. This so-called albuminocytological dissociation is not of value in the differential diagnosis because it is common in the diphtheritic and diabetic form of polyneuritis and is occasionally present in any form of polyneuritis, in acute encephalomyelitis and in a high percentage of the cases of acute anterior poliomyelitis after the second week of the infection.

Diphtheritic polyneuritis can usually be distinguished by the long latent period between the upper respiratory infection and the onset of neuritis, the frequency of paralysis of accommodation and by the relatively slow evolution of the neuritic symptoms. The neuritis of acute porphyria can be differentiated by the prodromal abdominal pains, the frequency of mental symptoms or convulsions and the presence of porphyria. Acute anterior poliomyelitis can usually be distinguished by the asymmetry of the paralysis, and by the presence of a pleocytosis in the cerebrospinal fluid if the puncture is performed within the first week of the infection. Acute involvement of the peripheral nerves following vaccination is diagnosed from the history. Asbury and his colleagues described in 1969 a form of polyneuritis characterized pathologically by an acute or subacute inflammatory reaction in the nerve roots and peripheral nerves. They considered these changes to be related to those of acute allergic neuritis produced in animals. A distinction on a clinical basis between these cases and the usual case classified under the term Guillain-Barré syndrome does not seem possible at the present time.

Treatment. There is no specific therapy. The treatment for the muscular weakness is the same as that for other forms of polyneuritis. The use of the artificial respirator is necessary in the cases with paralysis of the respiratory muscles. Good results have been reported with the administration of corticosteroids. The duration of the paralysis in untreated cases is so variable that it is impossible to determine whether this form of therapy is of any value.

REFERENCES

Asbury, A. K., Arnason, B. G., and Adams, R. D.: The Inflammatory Lesions in Idiopathic Polyneuritis, Medicine, 48, 173, 1969.

Bradford, J. R., Bashford, E. F., and Wilson, J. A.: Acute Infective Polyneuritis, Quart. J. Med., 12, 88, 1918.

Dowling, P. C., Menonna, J. P., Cook, S. D.: Guillain-Barré Syndrome in Greater New York-New Jersey, JAMA, 238, 317, 1977.

Drew, A. L., and Magee, K. R.: Papilledema in the Guillain-Barré Syndrome, Arch. Neurol. & Psychiat., 66, 744, 1951.

Fisher, M.: An Unusual Variant of Acute Idiopathic Polyneuritis (Syndrome of Ophthalmoplegia, Ataxia and Areflexia), N. Engl. J. Med., 255, 57, 1956.

Forster, F. M., Brown, M., and Merritt, H. H.: Polyneuritis with Facial Diplegia, N. Engl. J. Med., 225, 51, 1941.

Gibberd, F. B.: Ophthalmoplegia in Acute Polyneuritis, Arch. Neurol., 23, 161, 1970.

Goodall, J. A. D., Kosmidis, J. C., Geddes, A. M.: Effect of Corticosteroids on Course of Guillain-Barré Syndrome, Lancet, 1, 524, 1974.

Guillain, G., Barré, J. A., and Strohl, A.: Sur un syndrome de radiculonévrite avec hyperalbuminose due liquide céphalo-rachidien sans reaction cellulaire. Remarques sur les caractères cliniques et graphiques des réflexes tendineux, Bull. et mém. Soc. méd. d. hôp. de Paris, 40, 1462, 1916.

Haymaker, W., and Kernohan, J. W.: The Landry-Guillain-Barré Syndrome, Medicine, 28, 59, 1949.

Hewer, L., et al.: Acute Polyneuritis Requiring Artificial Respiration, Quart. J. Med., 33, 479, 1968.

Leneman, F.: The Guillain-Barré Syndrome. Definition, Etiology and Review of 1,100 Cases, Arch. Intern. Med., 118, 139, 1966.

Lisak, R. P., et al.: Guillain-Barré Syndrome and Hodgkin's Disease: Three Cases with Immunological Studies, Arch. Neurol., 1, 72, 1977.

Marshall, J.: The Landry-Guillain-Barré Syndrome, Brain, 80, 55, 1963.

Munsat, T. L., and Barnes, J. E.: Relation of Multiple Cranial Nerve Dysfunction to the Guillain-Barré Syndrome, J. Neurol. Neurosurg. & Psychiat., 28, 115, 1965.

Primeas, J. W., and McLeod, J. G.: Chronic Relapsing Polyneuritis, J. Neurol. Sci., 27, 427, 1976.

Richter, R. B.: The Ataxic Form of Polyradiculoneuritis (Landry-Guillain-Barré Syndrome), J. Neuropathol. Exp. Neurol., 21, 171, 1962.

Schmitz, H., and Enders, G.: Cytomegalovirus as a Frequent Cause of Guillain-Barré Syndrome, J. Med. Virol., 1, 21, 1977.

Sullivan, R. L., Jr., and Reeves, A. G.: Normal Cerebrospinal Fluid Protein, Increased Intracranial Pressure, and the Guillain-Barré Syndrome, Ann. Neurol., 1, 108, 1977.

Wahren, B., and Link, H.: Antibodies to Epstein-Barr Virus and Cytomegalovirus in Guillain-Barré Syndrome, J. Neurol. Sci., 28, 129, 1976.
Wiederholt, W. C., and Mulder, D. W.: Cerebrospinal Fluid Findings in the Landry-Guillain-Barré-Strohl Syndrome, Neurology, 15, 184, 1965.

Polyneuritis of Pregnancy
(Gestational Polyneuritis)

Etiology and Incidence. Polyneuritis is a rare complication of pregnancy. Berkowitz and Lufkin collected a total of 52 cases from the literature up to 1932. The neuritic symptoms develop slowly during the middle or later months of pregnancy or they may not appear until after delivery. They are usually preceded by signs and symptoms of toxemia of pregnancy, particularly pernicious vomiting. For this reason, Strauss and McDonald considered the neuritis as due to a dietary deficiency. A few cases have been reported, however, in the absence of signs or symptoms of toxemia. The neuritis occurs more commonly in the first or second pregnancy.

Symptoms and Signs. The symptomatology and clinical course (including the frequent occurrence of mental symptoms and Korsakoff's syndrome) of polyneuritis of pregnancy are similar to those of the alcoholic form of polyneuritis. Tachycardia and a hypochromic or macrocytic anemia are frequently present.

Course and Prognosis. The severity of the polyneuritis, the frequency of signs of toxemia of pregnancy and the high incidence of mental symptoms all contribute to the high mortality rate of this form of polyneuritis (68% in the cases collected by Plass and Mengert). In patients who survive, recovery from the polyneuritis is slow and residual defects are not uncommon.

Treatment. The treatment is the same as that of other forms of polyneuritis. A high-calorie, high-vitamin diet, supplemented with vitamins parenterally, should be given in the hope of lowering the high mortality rate. There is no evidence to indicate that termination of pregnancy is of any value.

REFERENCES

Berkowitz, N. J., and Lufkin, N. H.: Toxic Neuronitis of Pregnancy, Surg., Gynec. & Obst., 54, 743, 1932.
Maisel, J. J., and Woltman, H. W.: Neuronitis of Pregnancy without Vomiting, J.A.M.A., 103, 1930, 1934.
Plass, E. D., and Mengert, W. F.: Gestational Polyneuritis, J.A.M.A., 101, 2020, 1933.
Strauss, M. B., and McDonald, W. J.: Polyneuritis of Pregnancy; a Dietary Deficiency Disorder, J.A.M.A., 100, 1320, 1933.

Diabetic Polyneuritis

Signs and symptoms of involvement of the peripheral nerves in the form of pains, paresthesias, motor weakness and reflex loss, develop in a fairly large percentage of the patients with diabetes mellitus. A severe degree of polyneuritis is uncommon.

Etiology. The cause of the neuritis in patients with diabetes is unknown. Attempts have been made to explain the symptoms on basis of arteriosclerotic changes in the nerve, vitamin deficiency or an interference with carbohydrate metabolism. None of these theories has received general acceptance as applicable to all cases. Mononeuritis or mononeuritis multiplex is generally considered to be due to occlusion of the nutrient vessels to the nerves. The neuritis develops most commonly in patients in whom the diabetes is inadequately controlled.

Pathology. The pathology in the nervous system consists of degenerative changes in the peripheral nerves, nerve roots and posterior columns of the spinal cord. Retrograde or degenerative changes may be found in the ventral horn cells.

Incidence. The frequency of polyneuritis in diabetes mellitus is variously estimated from 0.5 to over 50%, depending upon the criteria for diagnosis. The figure given by Rundles (125 cases of polyneuritis in 3,000 diabetics or 4%) is probably representative. Males and females are approximately equally affected. The neuritis may develop at any age but is most common in the fifth to seventh decades (Table 98). It is not rare in children.

Symptoms and Signs. In the majority of cases, sensory symptoms predominate. Paresthesias or severe pains in the lower extremities are the initial symptoms. A mild or moderate weakness of the legs soon develops and rarely this may progress to a complete paralysis. The

Table 98.   Age Incidence of Diabetic Polyneuritis and Duration of
Preceding Diabetes Mellitus
(Modified from Rundles, Medicine, 1945)

Age	No. of Cases	%	Average Duration of Diabetes
17 to 20	8	6	2.9
21 to 30	11	9	4.5
31 to 40	14	11	5.0
41 to 50	26	21	6.5
51 to 60	44	35	6.0
61 to 70	19	15	2.7
Over 70	3	3	15.0
Total	125	100	

Achilles reflex is absent in the majority of the cases and patellar reflexes in approximately 50%. Cutaneous sensation may be impaired in the distal part of the legs. The muscles and nerves are tender to pressure. Vibratory and position sense is frequently impaired. The loss of proprioceptive sensation together with the absent reflexes produces a clinical picture superficially similar to that of tabes dorsalis, which has been described as diabetic pseudotabes. Sphincter disturbances and changes in the size, shape and reaction of the pupils are not infrequent. Rarely, there may be oculomotor palsies or facial diplegia. Paralysis of either the third, fourth or sixth cranial nerves on one or both sides may occur in patients with diabetes in the absence of other signs of polyneuritis. The paralysis in these cases is presumed to be due to a small vascular lesion (hemorrhage) in the brainstem. Isolated mononeuritic paralysis of the obturator, femoral, sciatic, median, ulnar or other nerves is occasionally seen.

Attempts have been made to delineate a spinal cord syndrome associated with diabetes. The symptom complex in the patients considered to have spinal cord involvement consists of proximal weakness of the legs, various changes in the tendon reflexes in the legs, minimal cutaneous sensory loss in the legs and abnormal plantar responses. These cases have been labeled with such terms as diabetic myelopathy, diabetic amyotrophy and diabetic pseudotabes. There is insufficient pathological evidence to implicate the spinal cord in this condition and it is more probable that the symptoms are due to degenerative changes in the nerves and muscles.

The complications of diabetic polyneuritis include orthostatic hypotension and tachycardia and those commonly associated with diabetes, *i.e.*, retinitis and peripheral vascular disease. Arthropathies (Charcot joint) similar to those of tabes dorsalis may occur.

Course. Symptoms may continue to advance for a short while after the diabetes is controlled. As a rule, however, there is gradual improvement of the neuritis when the diabetes is adequately treated. The paralysis in the mononeuritic form may, however, be permanent.

Laboratory Data. The findings in the blood and urine are those usually associated with diabetes mellitus. The cerebrospinal fluid is normal except for an increase in the glucose and protein content. The protein content is increased in approximately two thirds of the cases and values between 100 and 500 mg per 100 ml are found in more than 15%.

Diagnosis. The diagnosis of diabetic polyneuritis can be made without difficulty when the typical symptoms, paresthesia, pain, mild weakness and reflex loss, occur in patients with diabetes mellitus. Confusion with tabetic neurosyphilis can be avoided by examination of the cerebrospinal fluid.

Treatment. The treatment of diabetic polyneuritis is that of the underlying diabetes mellitus, together with physiotherapy. Analgesics should be given to control the pains.

REFERENCES

Colby, A. O.: Neurologic Disorders of Diabetes Mellitus, Diabetes, *14*, 424 and 516, 1965.
Eeg-Olofsson, O., and Petersén, I.: Childhood Diabetic Neuropathy, Acta Paed. Scand., *55*, 163, 1966.
Ewing, D. J., Campbell, I. W. and Clark, B. F.: Mortality in Diabetic Autonomic Neuropathy. Lancet, *1*, 601, 1976.
Greenbaum, D.: Observations on the Homogeneous Nature and Pathogenesis of Diabetic Neuropathy, Brain, *87*, 215, 1964.
Lippmann, H. I., Perotto, A., and Farrar, R.: The Neuropathic Foot of the Diabetic, Bull. New York Acad. Med., *52*, 1159, 1976.
Locke, S., Lawrence, D. G., and Legg, M. A.: Diabetic Amyotrophy, Am. J. Med., *34*, 775, 1963.
Raff, M. C., and Asbury, A. K.: Ischemic Mononeuropathy and Mononeuropathy Multiplex in Diabetes Mellitus, N. Engl. J. Med., *279*, 17, 1968.
Ross, A. T.: Recurrent Cranial Nerve Palsies in Diabetes Mellitus, Neurology, *12*, 180, 1962.
Rundles, R. W.: Diabetic Neuropathy, Medicine, *24*, 111, 1945.
Winegrad, A. I., and Greene, D. A.: Diabetic Polyneuropathy. The Importance of Insulin Deficiency, Hyperglycemia and Alterations in Myoinositol Metabolism in its Pathogenesis, N. Engl. J. Med., *295*, 1416, 1976.

Polyneuritis Associated with Carcinoma and Other Malignant Neoplasms

The occurrence of polyneuritis in the terminal stages of cancer has been recognized for many years. Recently attention has been directed to the fact that the symptoms of neuritis may appear before there is any clinical evidence of the primary tumor. This is most common with carcinoma of the lung but may occur with carcinoma of any organ of the body or with other malignant processes, such as multiple myeloma, lymphoma, Hodgkin's disease and leukemia.

The mechanism of the damage to the peripheral nerves is not clear. In some of the patients the nerves or nerve roots are infiltrated with neoplastic cells. In others there is no evidence of damage to the nerves by the neoplasm. In these cases, dietary deficiency, chronic malnutrition, and metabolic or toxic factors are considered to be of etiological significance.

The clinical picture is similar to that of other forms of polyneuritis. Occasionally, sensory defects will predominate, but more commonly there is a mixture of motor weakness, sensory loss and absence of reflexes in the extremities. Occasionally, the protein content of the fluid may be moderately increased (100 to 200 mg per 100 ml). Mental symptoms—confusion and memory loss and dementia—may also occur related to the presence of multifocal leukoencephalopathy or so-called central neuronitis. Remission of symptoms may occur, but more commonly the course is progressive until death ensues as result of the primary malignancy or the neuritis.

A syndrome of motor neuron disease similar to that of amyotrophic lateral sclerosis with muscle wasting and fibrillation and extensor plantar responses has been described in patients with carcinoma in various organs. The syndrome differs from that of amyotrophic lateral sclerosis in the benign course if the tumor is recognized and removed.

The diagnosis of malignancy should be suspected in a middle-aged or elderly patient with a polyneuritis of obscure causes. Occasionally the diagnosis can be confirmed by the findings of metastatic infiltrations in nerves removed at biopsy.

REFERENCES

Barron, K. D., Rowland, L. P., and Zimmerman, H.: Neuropathy with Malignant Tumor Metastases, J. Nerv. & Ment. Dis., 131, 10, 1960.
Brain, Lord, Croft, P. B., and Wilkinson, M.: Motor Neurone Disease as a Manifestation of Neoplasm (With a Note on the Course of Classical Motor Neurone Disease), Brain, 88, 479, 1965.
Croft, P. B., Henson, R. A., Urich, H., and Wilkinson, P. C.: Sensory Neuropathy with Bronchial Carcinoma: A Study of Four Cases Showing Serological Abnormalities, Brain, 88, 501, 1965.
Fisher, C. M., Williams, H. W., and Wing, E. S., Jr.: Combined Encephalopathy and Neuropathy with Carcinoma, J. Neuropathol. Exp. Neurol., 20 535, 1961.
Holt, G. W.: Idiopathic Neuropathy in Cancer. A First Sign in Multiple System Syndromes Associated with Malignancy, Am. J. Med. Sci., 242, 93, 1961.
Klingon, G. H.: The Guillain-Barré Syndrome Associated with Cancer, Cancer, 18, 157, 1965.
Moore, R. Y., and Oda, Y.: Malignant Lymphoma with Diffuse Involvement of the Peripheral Nervous System, Neurology, 12, 186, 1962.
Victor, M., Banker, B. Q., and Adams, R. D.: The Neuropathy of Multiple Myeloma, J. Neurol., Neurosurg. & Psychiat., 21, 73, 1958.

Amyloid Polyneuritis

Primary amyloidosis, a disease of unknown etiology, is characterized by deposition of amorphous hyaline-like material around blood vessels and extending through connective tissue. The heart, tongue, gastrointestinal tract, skeletal muscle and kidneys are most commonly affected. Peripheral nerve involvement may occur, but brain and spinal cord are usually spared. Various familial forms of polyneuritis related to amyloidosis have been reported in Portugal, Japan, Sweden, and in various parts of the United States. The carpal tunnel syndrome is a prominent feature of many cases.

Peripheral neuropathy may result from direct infiltration in amyloidosis complicating multiple myeloma. Neurological symptoms are rare in secondary amyloidosis associated with chronic suppurative or inflammatory processes.

REFERENCES

Andersson, R.: Hereditary Amyloidosis with Polyneuropathy, Acta Med. Scand., *88*, 85, 1970.
Andrade, A., et al.: Hereditary Amyloidosis, Arth. Rheum., *13*, 902, 1970.
French, J. M., Hall, G., Parish, D. J., and Smith, W. T.: Peripheral and Autonomic Nerve Involvement in Primary Amyloidosis Associated with Uncontrollable Diarrhea and Steatorrhea, Am. J. Med., *39*, 277, 1965.
Haberland, C.: Primary Systemic Amyloidosis. Cerebral Involvement and Senile Plaque Formation, J. Neuropathol. Exp. Neurol., *23*, 135, 1964.
Mahloudji, M., et al.: The Genetic Amyloidoses, Medicine, *48*, 1, 1969.
Munsat, T. L., and Poussaint, A. F.: Clinical Manifestations and Diagnosis of Amyloid Polyneuropathy, Neurology, *12*, 413, 1962.
Osserman, E. F.: Plasma-cell Myeloma, N. Engl. J. Med., *261*, 1006, 1959.
Rukavina, J. G., et al.: Primary Systemic Amyloidosis: A Review and an Experimental Genetic and Clinical Study of 29 Cases with Particular Emphasis on the Familial Form, Medicine, *35*, 239, 1956.
Van Allen, M. W., et al.: Inherited Predisposition to Generalized Amyloidosis, Neurology, *19*, 10, 1969.

Chapter 8

Diseases of the Myelin Sheath

Charles M. Poser, M. D.

INTRODUCTION

Demyelination is a characteristic response of the white matter to pathologic stimuli not severe enough to cause full necrosis of nervous tissue. Almost any traumatic, infectious or toxic disorder can, under appropriate circumstances, result in destruction of myelin.

One way to define the diseases of the myelin sheath described in this chapter is to say that they are diseases in which there is widespread failure of the myelin sheath to stain by the usually accepted methods and in which no known or suspected etiologic agent such as trauma, infection, neoplasia or metabolic disturbances can be discovered.

In most conditions affecting the nervous system demyelination is usually only one feature of the pathologic process and is accompanied by destructive changes in other elements of the nervous system. The group of diseases of the nervous system which are considered in the first part of this chapter represent those for which no definitive etiologic basis has yet been established and, for lack of a better term, have been called primary diseases of the myelin sheath.

It is important to remember that myelin is a complex protein-lipid carbohydrate structure, which forms part of the cell membrane of the oligodendroglia (or of the Schwann cell in the peripheral nervous system). The formation, and the maintenance of its structure are dependent not only on the oligodendroglia, but also on the axon around which it is wrapped. Destruction of the axon inevitably results in demyelination, the so-called Wallerian degeneration. Oligodendroglia or Schwann cells cannot form myelin in tissue culture in the absence of an axon. The formation and the maintenance of myelin are also dependent upon the integrity of its vascular supply. It might therefore be better to speak of a *myelin system* which includes the myelin sheath itself, the oligodendroglial cell of which it is a part, the axon without which it cannot exist and the blood vessels. In diseases of the myelin sheath it is known in only very few circumstances which part of this myelin system is the primary target of the injurious agent.

Diseases of the myelin system can be divided into two large groups: First the myelinoclastic (or demyelinizing) conditions. In these it is assumed that myelin was normally formed and is subsequently injured or destroyed by either endogenous or exogenous agents, or a combination of both. Secondly, the dysmyelinating diseases in which some enzymatic disturbance interferes either with formation of myelin or with its maintenance.

The prototype for the first group is multiple sclerosis with such variants as transitional sclerosis, myelinoclastic diffuse sclerosis (Schilder 1912 type), neuromyelitis optica (Devic's disease), and concentric sclerosis (Balo's disease). While dysmyelination is a common feature of a large number of inborn errors of metabolism, a special, rather heterogeneous group in which the myelin sheath appears to be most severely involved has been called the leukodystrophies.

In general, the differentiation between the myelinoclastic and the dysmyelinating diseases is made on basis of histopathologic changes. The pathologic characteristics of myelinoclasia are essentially the same regardless of etiologic factors. An important characteristic of "primary" myelinoclastic diseases is the dissociation between the degree of destruction of the myelin sheath and that of the axon, leading to what has been called periaxial demyelination, or relative sparing of the axon. The dysmyelinating diseases can be differentiated from myelinoclastic conditions by a number of specific histopathologic features as well as by the fact that in many instances there is strong evidence for genetic determination and a frequently positive family history.

This chapter will describe both the myelinoclastic and the dysmyelinating conditions which will be examined separately.

THE MYELINOCLASTIC DISEASES

Multiple Sclerosis

Multiple sclerosis (disseminated sclerosis, insular sclerosis [sclérose en plaques]) is a chronic disease characterized pathologically by the presence of numerous areas of demyelination in the central nervous system (the peripheral nervous system is never involved), and clinically by a variety of neurological symptoms and signs, which have a tendency toward remission and exacerbation. There is a variation in the number and character of symptoms and signs from time to time, and at any one time there is usually evidence of multiple lesions. The term multiple sclerosis gives no inkling that the myelin sheath bears the brunt of the disease. The term was coined by neuropathologists who, with limited methods of study, could only describe the end stage of the

lesions which are indeed characterized by scarring or sclerosis resulting from glial overgrowth in the areas that had been involved.

   Pathogenesis. The cause of multiple sclerosis is unknown. Attempts
have been made to explain the lesions on the basis of a wide variety of
causes ranging from infections, nutritional deficiencies, overindulgence in animal fats, endogenous or exogenous poisons, vascular
disturbances, and allergic reactions.

   Multiple sclerosis is a disease which affects only man since, as far as
is known, it has never been found to occur spontaneously in animals
nor has it ever been produced experimentally in laboratory animals in
the form known in man. It may well be, therefore, that man is indeed
the only experimental animal in which the disease can be produced.

   While pathologic lesions identical to those seen in multiple sclerosis
have been demonstrated in patients dying of complications of measles,
German measles and varicella, as well as the result of vaccination
against rabies, the classical, intermittent clinical course has never been
seen.

   At the present time, two major theories which are not necessarily
mutually exclusive are being pursued. The first one rests upon the
concept of an infection (presumably by a viral agent) with a long
incubation period. The development of the clinical manifestations of
the disease would be influenced by environmental factors. Support for
this theory is derived from the fact that antibodies to measles (but also
to other viral agents such as rubella) have been found to be elevated
much more frequently in patients with multiple sclerosis than in
controls. On the other hand, these antibodies are also found to be
significantly elevated in the siblings of patients with multiple sclerosis.
While several investigators have reported the presence of viral-like
particles in M.S. brains, similar particles have not only been found in
other diseases of the nervous system, but it has also been suggested that
these presumed viral particles represent nothing more than degenerated nuclear proteins. In spite of long and numerous attempts a virus
(parainfluenza I) has been isolated from only a single M.S. brain;
immunologic studies, however, have failed to substantiate the possible
etiologic significance of this organism. Other investigators have reported finding what has been called a multiple sclerosis associated
agent from a variety of biological fluids and tissues from patients with
multiple sclerosis, but these findings have not yet been confirmed. On
the basis of the available data, while the possibility of a slow viral
infection has not been effectively ruled out, the possibility of a single,
specific etiologic agent such as a slow virus appears extremely unlikely.

   The other major theory proposes that multiple sclerosis results from
alterations in the individual's immune system. Initial support for this

theory has been derived from the superficial similarity between the lesions of multiple sclerosis and those seen as a result of experimental allergic encephalomyelitis in animals. Such a model, however, when closely scrutinized, differs in many important respects from multiple sclerosis. The ultrastructure of the lesions is totally different; the immunologic parameters are not applicable to multiple sclerosis and the classical remittent clinical course of multiple sclerosis does not occur as a result of experimental allergic encephalomyelitis.

Immunologic studies have given contradictory results. Some would point to the existence of a hyperergic state such as the elevated antibody titers to a number of common viruses, the elevation of immunoglobulin G in the cerebrospinal fluid of many M.S. patients, the alteration of lymphocyte responses to a number of viral antigens, etc. On the other hand, studies reporting relative decrease and ineffi-cacy of T-lymphocytes would suggest a cellular immunodeficiency. In fact, these data are reconcilable if one considers that the humoral immune response may represent an ineffectual attempt by the body to compensate for a cellular immunodeficiency.

Of major importance has been the demonstration that the serologi-cally determined histocompatibility antigens HLA-A3 and HLA-B7 are found with significantly higher frequency in multiple sclerosis patients in northern Europe and North America. Even more important is the association between multiple sclerosis and the HLA-DW2 (LD-7a) antigen, a cellular immunity marker also found to be significantly more common in similar populations. Finally, a B-lymphocyte alloantigen (group 4 or BT 101) has also been reported to have a high frequency among such patients. The association between HLA antigens and multiple sclerosis may be a secondary effect due to linkage disequilibrium—the tendency of certain alleles of linked but different genetic loci to occur in association. Thus, another gene or genes may well exist within the HLA region of the sixth chromosome which should consistently show a very high degree of association with multiple sclerosis. While the significance of these findings remains unclear, they suggest that immunogenetic determinants may identify groups of individuals who, when exposed to the appropriate environ-mental factors, are more prone to develop multiple sclerosis. Further-more, it now has been demonstrated that the striking elevation of antibody titers to measles and other viruses which has been found in such large numbers of patients with multiple sclerosis and their siblings, appears to be better related to the histocompatibility antigens than to the presence of the disease. This would mean that not only is a constitutional factor important in determining susceptibility to multi-ple sclerosis, but this same factor may determine the level of antiviral antibodies in the multiple sclerosis patient.

The epidemiologic data which strongly support the existence of environmental factors accord rather well with the immunogenetic information available. In brief, a viral infection, be it measles or another common virus, would initiate, in an individual with the appropriate immunogenetic factors, an alteration of the immune system, be it humoral hyperimmunity or cellular immunodeficiency or a combination of both; at a later date, exposure to similar viral antigens or closely related ones, would precipitate a recall phenomenon manifested by a clinical exacerbation.

While the pathogenesis of the initial swelling and eventual destruction of the myelin sheath remains unexplained, a better understanding exists regarding the possible mechanism for the very transient symptoms so characteristic of this disease: demyelination in the fiber tract, e.g., the optic nerve, reduces what has been called the margin of safety or its functional reserve, for the transmission of nerve impulses. Thus physiologic alterations of conduction capability by raising body temperature or increasing calcium ion concentration, may result in the appearance of symptoms from a fiber tract in which a plaque had reduced the physiologic reserve but not the minimum number of fibers necessary for normal function. The physiologic alterations in a system devoid of its normal margin of safety, would then cause a significant reduction in function and the appearance of clinical symptoms. The demonstration of an unidentified substance in the serum of multiple sclerosis patients which interfere with synaptic transmission in tissue culture has been suggested as an alternative explanation, but the extremely short duration of some symptoms, lasting no longer than a few minutes, would be difficult to explain on that basis.

The initial attack of multiple sclerosis, or relapses in the course of the disease, may follow an acute infection of any type, trauma, unusual fatigue, vaccination, the injection of serum, severe emotional upsets or may occur during the course of a pregnancy. It is difficult to evaluate the role of these and other factors which have been presumed to affect the course of the disease.

Numerous cases have been cited to support the claim that trauma to the head or distant parts of the body precipitated or aggravated the disease. The pathologic findings, the epidemiologic and immunologic data as well as numerous clinical studies all militate strongly against trauma to the head or body as having any etiologic significance whatsoever in the causation of multiple sclerosis. It must be kept in mind that patients with an incipient nervous disorder may be especially likely to suffer trauma; and that all of us are prone to attribute disease to injury, or to date the onset of a symptom to a well-remembered, concrete event such as an accident, an injury or an unexpected, unpleasant emotional upset!

It is difficult to evaluate the effect of pregnancy on the disease. It is true that the first symptoms may develop or that a relapse may occur during pregnancy. The age period at which the symptoms of multiple sclerosis are apt to develop roughly parallels the childbearing period, but there is no evidence to indicate that the first attack occurs more frequently in pregnant women than in other women of similar age. Pregnancy does not always exert a deleterious effect on the course of the disease. It has been our policy to consider the general condition of the patient, the clinical course of the disease, the ability of the patient or family to care for the child after delivery, and the desires of the patient and her husband for a child before deciding whether pregnancy is contraindicated or whether it should be terminated in any given case.

Pathology. The gross appearance of the external surface of the brain is usually normal. Occasionally there is atrophy of the cerebral convolutions with enlargement of the lateral and third ventricles. On sectioning the brain there are numerous small irregular grayish areas in the cerebral hemispheres, particularly in the white matter and in the periventricular regions (Fig. 169). The white matter forming the

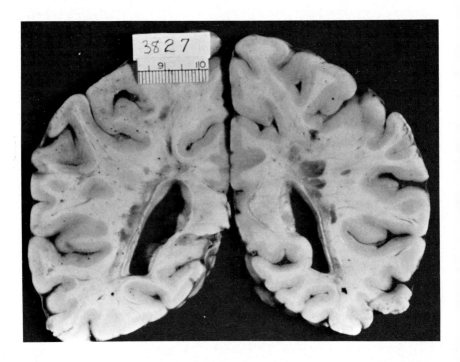

Figure 169. Gross appearance, coronal section, occipital lobe. Note extensive periventricular lesions. Several small lesions are scattered elsewhere in the white matter. (Courtesy Dr. Daniel Perl.)

superior lateral angle of the body of the lateral ventricles is frequently and characteristically affected. Similar areas of discoloration are also found in the brainstem and cerebellum. These are the plaques of multiple sclerosis.

The external appearance of the spinal cord is usually normal. In a small percentage of cases the cord may be slightly shrunken and the pia arachnoid thickened. Rarely, the cord may be swollen over several segments if death follows soon after the onset of an acute transverse lesion of the cord. Plaques similar to those in the cerebellum can occasionally be seen on the external surface of the cord but they are most easily recognized on cross sections. The optic nerves may be shrunken but the external appearance of the other cranial nerves and the peripheral nerves is usually normal. In rare instances, necrotic areas may be present.

Myelin sheath stains of sections of the nervous system show areas of demyelination in the regions which were visibly discolored in the unstained specimen. In addition, many more plaques are apparent. These plaques are sharply circumscribed and are diffusely scattered throughout all parts of the brain and spinal cord. They are most numerous in the white matter of the cerebrum (Fig. 170), brainstem, cerebellum and spinal cord. The lesions in the brain tend to be grouped

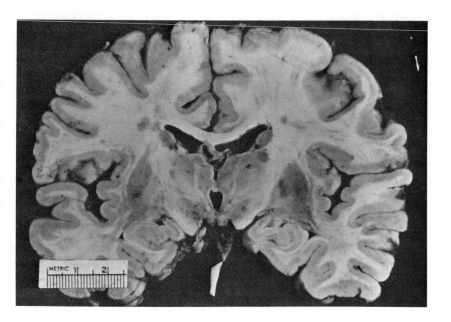

Figure 170. Gross appearance, coronal section; scattered plaques in the subcortical white matter and in several areas of the basal ganglia and thalamus.

around the lateral and third ventricles. The lesions in the cerebral hemisphere vary in size from that of a pinhead to huge areas encompassing the major portion of one lobe of the hemisphere. Small lesions may be found in the gray matter and in the zone between the gray and white matter. Lesions in the corpus callosum are not uncommon (Fig. 171). Plaques of varying sizes may be found in the optic nerves, chiasm, or tracts (Fig. 172). The lesions in the brainstem are usually quite numerous and sections from this area when stained by Weigert's method have a characteristic "Holstein cow" appearance (Fig. 173).

In sections of the spinal cord the areas of demyelination vary in size from small lesions involving a portion of the posterior or lateral funiculi to an almost complete loss of myelin in an entire cross section of the cord (Figs. 174, 176).

Each individual lesion is characterized by its sharp delimitation from the surrounding normal tissue (Figs. 173, 175). Within the lesion there is a complete or incomplete destruction of the myelin, a characteristically lesser degree of damage to the axis cylinders or neurons, proliferation of the glial cells, changes in the blood vessels, and relatively good preservation of the ground structure. Only rarely is the damage severe enough to affect the latter and produce a cyst (Fig. 174).

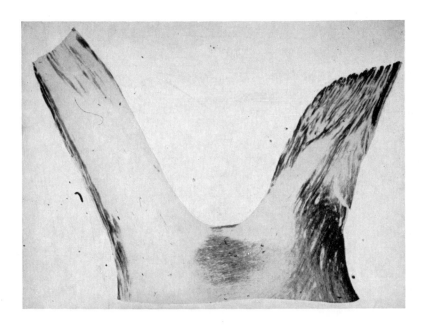

Figure 171.   Multiple sclerosis. Demyelinization of optic nerves and chiasm.
(Courtesy Dr. Abner Wolf.)

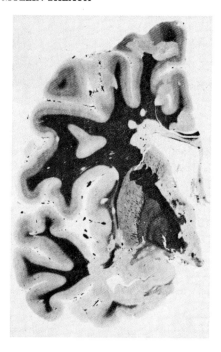

Figure 172. Myelin sheath stain in multiple sclerosis. Note lesions in corpus callosum, periventricular areas, white matter of the hemisphere and in the gray matter of superior frontal and temporal gyri.

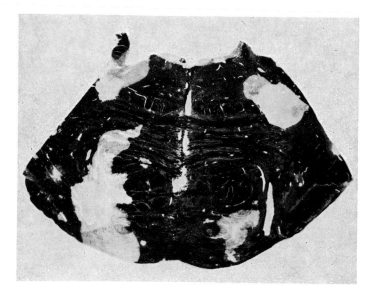

Figure 173.   Myelin sheath stain of brainstem in multiple sclerosis. Note sharp demarcation of lesions.

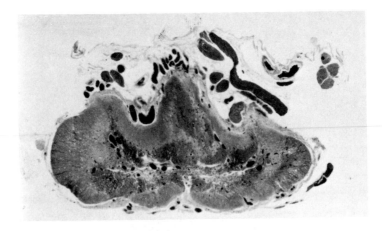

Figure 174. Myelin sheath stain: 10th thoracic segment of spinal cord. Almost complete demyelination of the entire section. The gray matter is severely involved and there is cystic degeneration, causing obliteration of normal architecture.

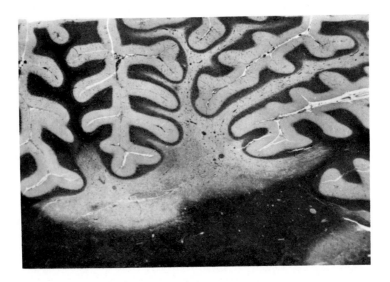

Figure 175. Myelin sheath stain: sharply demarcated lesion in the cerebellar white matter.

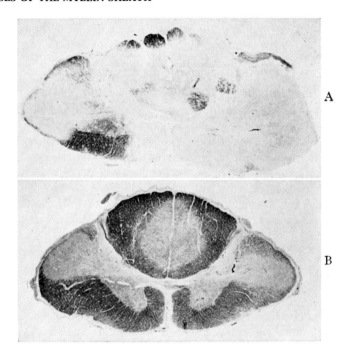

Figure 176. Multiple sclerosis. A, Almost complete loss of myelin in transverse section of cord. B, Symmetrical lesions in the posterior and lateral funiculi simulating distribution of lesions in combined system disease. (Merritt, H. H., Mettler, F. A., Putnam, T. J.: Fundamentals of Clinical Neurology, courtesy The Blakiston Co.)

The majority of myelin sheaths within a lesion are destroyed and there is swelling and fragmentation of many of those that remain. The degree of damage to the axis cylinders is variable. In the more severe lesions these may be entirely destroyed, but more commonly only a few are severely injured and the remainder are normal or show only minor changes. Secondary degeneration of long tracts occurs when the axis cylinders have been destroyed.

When the lesion involves the gray matter, the nerve cells are affected to a lesser degree than the myelin, but some of the cells may be completely destroyed and others show various degenerative changes.

The microglial cells proliferate and migrate into the lesion to phagocytize the debris. Compound granular cells laden with cholesterol esters (which have traditionally, although erroneously, been referred to as neutral fat) are present in great numbers in fresh lesions, in the perivascular spaces of the vessels and in the tissue adjacent to them. In older lesions these cells are found chiefly in the perivascular spaces in and around the lesion. In ordinary cell stains (hematoxylin-eosin or Nissl's) this perivascular accumulation of cells gives the appearance of a mild inflammatory reaction. The macroglia proliferate and produce fibrils which give the older lesions their characteristic sclerotic appearance and make them visible to the naked eye. Occasionally the extent of the gliosis exceeds the area of myelin loss.

Electronmicroscopic examination of brain tissue obtained by cerebral biopsy in patients with multiple sclerosis reveals the following findings: there is evidence of both primary and segmental demyelination with short internodes, and wide nodes of Ranvier; the myelin sheaths appear to be thin in relation to the axon diameter; there is evidence of remyelination including unusual node of Ranvier configurations. The oligodendroglia reveal accumulation of dense bodies and myelin figures as well as vacuolization of cyto-membrane systems. The astrocytes also show accumulation of dense bodies and myelin figures, increased numbers of glial filaments and scattered cytoplasmic vacuoles. The endothelium of blood vessels contains dense bodies and "lipid" droplets. The same dense bodies are also seen in pericytes and, rarely, in the perivascular inflammatory cells as well as in the axons. There is a general increase in the extracellular spaces. There is no evidence of platelet or other thrombi in blood vessels nor are there any structural abnormalities of capillary or basement membrane. There is no evidence of "peeling" away of myelin lamellae by phagocytic cells and no unequivocal virus particles are seen. There are no myelin sheaths of the peripheral type.

Neurochemistry. The changes that are most consistently found in the biochemical analysis of demyelinated areas of the brain are identical with those found in secondary demyelination and in experimental Wallerian degeneration. There is a general decrease of all the characteristic myelin lipids, *i.e.*, cerebrosides, sphingomyelin and cholesterol. In addition, there is a change in cholesterol from the free form, which is the only one normally found in white matter, to esterified cholesterol. This change is actually the earliest and most characteristic biochemical feature of myelinoclasia. Some authors have also stressed the reduction of plasmalogens, out of proportion to the loss of other phospholipids.

A high concentration of immunoglobulin G has been demonstrated in plaque tissue as opposed to noninvolved cerebral white matter. It has also been clearly demonstrated that lymphocytes within the central nervous system, including those found in and around M.S. plaques, are capable of synthesizing immunoglobulin G. Nevertheless, the role of immunoglobulin G remains unclear because it contains neither antimyelin nor antiviral antibodies, and it can easily be washed away from brain tissue. Thus it is possible that it represents a by-product of tissue destruction.

Incidence and Epidemiology. The correct incidence or prevalence of multiple sclerosis is somewhat difficult to estimate. In the absence of a completely reliable, definitive, laboratory test for this disease, as well as the relative paucity of autopsy material, these estimates must be based upon clinical considerations. Nevertheless, while absolute incidence or prevalence may be difficult to obtain, comparative figures appear to be reliable.

With some remarkable exceptions, the disease is more common in the higher latitudes than in those countries closer to the equator but no definite relationship has been established with the climatic characteristics of latitude. This is true for the United States, Europe, Australia and New Zealand from where accurate data have been accumulated. Kurland estimates that the prevalence rate in the United States varies from 6 to 14 per 100,000 in the southern states to about 40 to 60 per 100,000 in the northern states and that at any time there are about 75,000 to 100,000 persons with clinically identifiable multiple sclerosis in the United States. These rates are similar for Canada, Great Britain, the Scandinavian countries, France, Belgium, Germany, Switzerland and Austria while the southern and central European countries have lower rates. Practically no reliable data are available for such large land masses as most of Latin America, the Soviet Union, continental Asia and practically all of Africa with the notable exception of the white population of South Africa.

No reliably documented instance of multiple sclerosis has ever been found in the native-born African. The disease is quite rare (and somewhat different clinically) in Japan, Taiwan, India and Colombia.

In the United States the incidence rate is equal in the white and nonwhite races in any given region with the exception of Hawaii where it is significantly lower among the Hawaiian-born orientals. Recent studies suggest that occupation and social status may play a role in the incidence of this disease. Reports from England point out that there were significantly more members of the professional and managerial classes than expected from general population percentages. It would appear that the disease is somewhat more common in urban than rural areas and there are indications that the level of development of sanitary facilities may parallel the incidence and prevalence of multiple sclerosis.

Detailed epidemiologic studies have revealed some rather unusual "pockets" of the disease which have cast some doubts about the relationship between latitude (which *per se* may be meaningless but may signify a number of environmental factors) and the incidence and prevalence of multiple sclerosis. For example, in the Orkney-Shetland Islands the prevalence of multiple sclerosis is 153 per 100,000 while in the Faroe Islands situated at almost the same latitude, the prevalence is only 48 per 100,000. The most immediately conspicuous difference between the populations of these climatically similar but geologically different islands are the predominantly Celtic and Scandinavian origins of their respective inhabitants and a higher content in the Faroe diet of fish and its products, a possible relationship already noted by Norwegian neurologists in connection with an apparently higher prevalence in inland as compared to seaboard Norway.

It has also been pointed out that there are differences in the nature of the disease relating to locality: acute syndromes of massive monophasic demyelination are uncommon in temperate countries but not uncommon in tropical east Asia. Chronic, remittent multiple sclerosis is common in England but most series of acute and hyperacute cases have been reported from central Europe.

Exhaustive studies of immigrants to Israel on the one hand, and to South Africa on the other, have provided interesting results which may be of possible etiologic significance. In both countries it was found that the rate of incidence of the disease among various immigrant groups reflected that of the area of origin of the immigrant: thus, while the disease is rare among the native Israeli and among immigrants from other Near East countries and north Africa, it was considerably higher among immigrants from central Europe, and even higher among those from northern Europe. More recent studies have shown that the children of these immigrants now have essentially the same prevalence of multiple sclerosis, regardless of the country of origin of their parents, a situation which gives added significance to environmental factors. Similar differences were noted among the native-born South African whites with a relatively low incidence, as opposed to the high incidence of immigrants from Great Britain. Refinement of these studies then revealed that age at immigration appeared to play an important role in that an immigrant leaving his country of origin roughly before the age of fifteen would have the risk of acquiring multiple sclerosis similar to that of the native born Israeli or South African; an individual immigrating after that age would "carry" with him the risk factor of his country of origin. These findings have been confirmed by studies among various ethnic groups in Hawaii. These now well-established data relating to the critical importance of the period at, or immediately after, puberty have been variously interpreted in terms of the acquisition at a critical period of an infectious agent with long latency, or, conversely, the acquisition prior to that critical period of some temporarily effective protective, possibly immune mechanism. A remarkably close correlation, with some exceptions, has been found between the geographic distribution of multiple sclerosis and that of certain histocompatibility antigens (HLA-A3, B7): in fact, Japanese multiple sclerosis patients do not have a higher incidence of these antigens. In a study in Philadelphia, HLA-A3, B7 and DW2 were found to be elevated in both Caucasian and black M.S. patients while in Israel there was no difference in these antigens between the high M.S. immigrant group from northern Europe and the low M.S. immigrant group from Afro-Asian countries.

While the basic facts regarding the remarkable direct correlation between latitude and M.S. prevalence, and the interesting studies of immigrants to Israel and South Africa are incontrovertible, their significance remains unclear except to reinforce the idea that multiple sclerosis results from the interplay between genetic and environmental factors, the importance of each being variable in different groups.

Recently, an attempt has been made to correlate the epidemiologic-geographic data with the ingestion of dairy products and fats. The major stumbling block in this regard is the fact that the native born Afrikaner who has a high consumption of these products also has a relatively low incidence of multiple sclerosis.

The disease shows a somewhat higher prevalence in women (Table 98) although the data vary in this respect from country to country. Conjugal incidence is extremely rare and is of no statistical significance. On the other hand, several studies would seem to indicate that the incidence among siblings is much higher than can be expected by chance alone: among siblings of patients, the frequency of the disease ranged from 19 to 42 times that of the general population and among parents from 12- to 32-fold. Even distant relatives seem to be more

Table 98. Age and Sex Distribution of Autopsy-Proved Multiple Sclerosis

| | Country of Origin | | | |
	England	Norway	U.S.	Total
Number of Patients	55	31	71	157
Sex: Male (%)	33	61	60	47
Female (%)	67	39	40	53
Age of Onset: Range (Years)	14–64	17–49	18–57	14–64
Mean (Years)	34	31	28	32
Males	37	32	28	33
Females	33	29	27	31
Age Groups:				
Under 20 (%)	15	13	14	14
21–30 (%)	22	42	51	35
31–40 (%)	38	26	25	29
41–50 (%)	18	19	10	14
51–60 (%)	5	0	3	4
61–70 (%)	2	0	0	1
Duration of Disease				
Mean (Years)	12	17	14	14
Range	2 mo. to 36 yrs.	3 mo. to 37 yrs.	2 mo. to 32 yrs.	2 mo. to 37 yrs.

prone, the prevalence among cousins being from 5 to 12 times that in the general population. Studies with twins have essentially ruled out simple genetic determination. Some evidence has been adduced to suggest the operation of a common environmental factor. On the other hand, it is also entirely possible that genetic factors are involved in the etiology of multiple sclerosis but that these must be subjected to exogenous, environmental agents without whose operation the phenotype could not be produced.

Multiple sclerosis is predominantly a disease of young adults. The age incidence in 157 autopsy-proved cases is given in Table 98. While cases have been reported with the onset of symptoms before the age of ten and after the age of sixty, these are extremely rare and in the vast majority the initial symptoms occur in the period between twenty and forty years of age. Although some series have reported as many as 3% of patients having the onset of their symptoms before the age of ten, pathologic verification has been obtained in only a few instances. The onset of symptoms in middle life is not rare. In one series, the onset of symptoms occurred after the age of forty in 13% of 310 clinically studied cases and in 21% of 42 cases proved by necropsy. The oldest age at onset of symptoms in that series was sixty-three years. In a series of 111 autopsy-proved cases, the oldest age of onset was sixty-four years.

Symptoms and Signs. The disease has been characterized by many authors as having dissemination of lesions in both time and space. The former relates to the fact that exacerbations and remissions occur

Table 99.   Frequency of Various Symptoms in 157 Autopsy-Proved Cases of Multiple Sclerosis

	Country of Origin			
	England	Norway	U.S.	Total
Number of Patients	55	31	71	157
	Percentage of Occurrence			
Muscle Weakness	95	100	96	96
Ocular Disturbance	84	81	92	85
Urinary Disturbance	93	87	70	82
Gait Ataxia	45	68	60	60
Paresthesiae	69	55	52	60
Dysarthria or Scanning Speech	53	61	52	54
Mental Disturbance	42	52	50	47
Pain	13	19	32	19
Vertigo	7	26	20	17
Dysphagia	14	13	9	12
Convulsions	5	6	7	6
Decreased Hearing	3	6	10	6
Tinnitus	—	3	7	5

frequently while the inability to explain the patient's signs and symptoms on the basis of a single lesion refers to the latter portion of the statement. Another characteristic of the disease is that symptoms and signs may be very transient and some of its manifestations extremely bizarre. The patient may experience unusual subjective sensations which are both difficult to describe and impossible to verify objectively by even the most experienced and conscientious examiner.

The symptoms and signs of multiple sclerosis are (Tables 99 and 100) so diverse that their enumeration would include all of the symptoms which can result from injury to any part of the neuraxis from the spinal roots to the cerebral cortex. The chief characteristics of the symptoms of multiple sclerosis are their multiplicity, and tendency to vary in nature and severity with the passage of time. Complete remission of the initial symptoms occurs frequently but with subsequent attacks, remissions do not occur or are incomplete. The clinical course extends over a period of one or many decades in the majority of cases, but in a few the disease may terminate in death within a few months of the onset.

There is no classical form of multiple sclerosis and the clinical manifestations naturally depend upon the particular areas of the nervous system which are involved. For reasons which remain unknown, the disease frequently involves certain areas and systems in preference to others so that manifestations of lesions in the optic chiasm and nerves, brainstem and cerebellum and the spinal cord, in particular the corticospinal tracts and the posterior columns are most frequent.

Table 100. Frequency of Signs in 157 Autopsy-Proved Cases of Multiple Sclerosis

	Country of Origin			
	England	Norway	U.S.	Total
Number of Patients	55	31	71	157
	Percentage of Occurrence			
Spasticity or Hyperreflexia, or both	96	100	99	98
Babinski's Sign	95	100	86	92
Absent Abdominal Reflexes	73	94	84	82
Dysmetria or Intention Tremor	80	81	76	79
Nystagmus	73	68	73	71
Impairment of Vibratory Sensation	65	55	60	61
Impairment of Position Sensation	62	49	48	52
Impairment of Pain Sensation	51	39	43	44
Facial Weakness	27	52	46	42
Impairment of Touch Sensation	22	29	36	29
Impairment of Temperature Sensation	16	19	20	17
Changes in State of Consciousness	—	3	6	5

Since multiple sclerosis is primarily a disease of white matter, although the lesions may spill over into gray matter, signs and symptoms of nuclear involvement are relatively uncommon and signs and symptoms of basal ganglia involvement are quite rare. While many clinicians like to classify multiple sclerosis into spinal, brainstem and cerebellar and cerebral forms, there are so many cases in which these forms are combined as to make that classification of little clinical value. Is is the combination of anatomically unrelated signs and symptoms which most commonly forms the basis for the clinical diagnosis of multiple sclerosis.

Visual disturbances may include diplopia, blurring of vision, diminution or loss of visual acuity either unilaterally or bilaterally, visual field defects which may range from a unilateral central scotoma or field contraction (Fig. 177) to a homonymous hemianopsia. In early or very mild optic or retrobulbar neuritis, color vision may be decreased to some degree while black and white vision may remain normal. Examination of the visual fields with a red or green test object may reveal a relative central scotoma or field contraction which will not be apparent with the usual white test object. Optic neuritis must be differentiated from papilledema since both may look similar, on funduscopic examination, but the former is characterized by a more severe impairment of

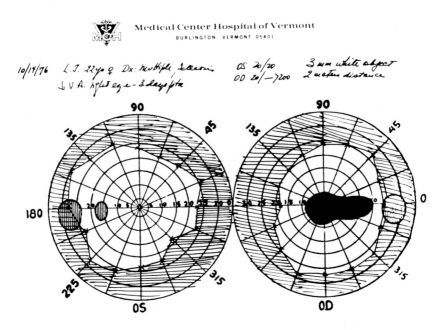

Figure 177.   Cecocentral scotoma in patient with acute right optic neuropathy; multiple sclerosis of 3 years' duration.

visual acuity. A central or cecocentral scotoma is most characteristic. Retrobulbar neuritis, a very common manifestation of multiple sclerosis, may not be associated with any funduscopic abnormalities but is always manifested by loss or diminution of visual acuity.

Diplopia in multiple sclerosis may be caused by involvement of the medial longitudinal fasciculus resulting in internuclear ophthalmoplegia. Although internuclear ophthalmoplegia is present in only a small percentage of the cases of multiple sclerosis, it is uncommon in any other condition and therefore constitutes a very important sign in the diagnosis of this disease. It is a disturbance of the lateral movements of the eyes which is characterized by an apparent paralysis of the internal rectus on one side and weakness of the external rectus on the other side, together with nystagmoid jerks of the outwardly deviating eye (monocular nystagmus). This impairment of gaze may be present on attempt to deviate the eyes to one or both sides. In uncomplicated lesions of the medial longitudinal fasciculus, the intactness of the internal rectus muscle can be demonstrated by the preservation of its action in convergence.

The sudden onset of optic or retrobulbar neuritis, without any other associated sign or symptom of central nervous system involvement, is often interpreted as being the first symptom of multiple sclerosis. It should be remembered, however, that such a condition may also result from a postinfectious or postvaccinal reaction and other conditions. It is often impossible, on the basis of history and physical examination, to differentiate between these various conditions except in the relatively rare cases of intoxication causing optic neuritis. It may thus be either the first attack of multiple sclerosis, or the only one. Several long-term followup studies indicate that approximately 20% of patients with optic or retrobulbar neuritis will ultimately develop other signs and symptoms indicative of multiple sclerosis.

The most common pupillary abnormalities are irregularity in the outline of the pupil, partial constriction and partial loss of the light reflex.

Involvement of the descending root of the fith cranial nerve occurs in a very small percentage of the cases. In these cases there may be an impairment of the pain sensation in the face, diminution or loss of the corneal reflex and, rarely, pains in the face which are indistinguishable from those of trigeminal neuralgia.

Weakness of the facial muscles of the lower half of one side of the face is a common finding, but a complete peripheral facial palsy is rare. The dysarthria, and, rarely the dysphagia, seen in advanced cases of multiple sclerosis are most commonly due to the associated cerebellar involvement, or to lesions in the corticobulbar tracts in the nature of pseudobulbar palsy. In those instances, emotional incontinence, forced laughing or crying without the accompanying emotional affect may also be present.

Weakness of the extremities is the most common sign of the disease and may be manifested as a monoplegia, hemiplegia or quadriplegia (or pareses). Asthenia which is out of proportion to the demonstrable muscular weakness is a common complaint.

In some patients, in particular those with a relatively late onset, the disease may appear under the guise of a slowly progressive spastic paraplegia. These patients have a slowly progressive spastic weakness involving the lower extremities and may show no neurologic signs except evidence of pyramidal tract signs (spasticity, hyperreflexia and bilateral Babinski signs) and a slight impairment of proprioceptive sensation.

The cerebellum or its connections with the brainstem are involved in the majority of the cases, with speech disturbance, ataxia of gait, tremors and incoordination of the muscles of the trunk and extremities. The characteristic scanning speech of multiple sclerosis is a result of cerebellar incoordination of the palatal and labial muscles combined with dysarthria of corticobulbar origin.

Urinary disturbances are also extremely common, including incontinence, frequency or urgency of urination which must be differentiated from those disturbances resulting from urinary tract infections or local conditions. Loss of libido and impotence are frequently found in male patients.

Paresthesiae include spontaneous feelings of numbness and tingling in the extremities, trunk or face. Lhermitte's sign, while frequently considered to be pathognomonic of multiple sclerosis, describes the sensation of "electricity" felt by the patient on passive or active flexion of the neck. It simply indicates that a lesion of the posterior columns is present in the cervical portion of the spinal cord and may be seen in other diseases. In rare instances, Lhermitte's sign can be elicited by flexion of the trunk. Sharp shooting pains in the legs or in the abdomen, identical to those seen in tabes dorsalis may also be encountered.

Mental symptoms occur much more frequently than suspected. Depression may occur as frequently if not more so than the euphoria which is said to be characteristic of the disease. Disturbances of memory, subtle aphasic manifestations of various types as well as fairly widespread cognitive defect may be elicited. Most important is the fact that hysterical symptoms may be found in addition to those unquestionably due to anatomic lesions or physiologic alterations. A purely psychiatric presentation may occur; dementia due to multiple sclerosis may be more common than suspected.

The psychologic manifestations of multiple sclerosis assume a particular importance in the genesis of the exacerbations: whenever a previously experienced symptom recurs, serious consideration must be given to the possibility that this may represent the result of a physiologic alteration secondary to heat or some kind of systemic or metabolic dysfunction or, alternately, that it may represent what can be called a psychologically induced recall phenomenon. It is probable that the former may well explain some of the recurrences of symptoms associated with systemic illness while the latter may follow emotional upsets and tension, or physical trauma. The very nature of multiple sclerosis, affecting relatively young individuals, very often at the threshold of life-determining decisions, or at the peak of professional productivity, faced with the possibility of serious disability, increases the likelihood of psychologic alterations. The lack of specific treatment, the uncertainty about long term prognosis, as well as the difficulty, in many instances, of establishing a definitive diagnosis early in the course of the disease, all complicate this serious problem.

As the disease progresses, either with remissions and exacerbations, or with a steadily progressive course, the vast majority of patients with multiple sclerosis will eventually exhibit signs or symptoms which will point to the involvement of many different systems and areas within the neuraxis.

In terms of frequency of signs and symptoms combinations, the following are found to occur in more than three-fourths of the patients at some time during the course of the illness (Tables 99 and 100): ocular disturbances, muscle weakness, spasticity and hyperreflexia, Babinski sign, absent abdominal reflexes, dysmetria or intention tremor and urinary disturbances. Other combinations which occur in approximately one-half to three-fourths of the patients include nystagmus, gait ataxia, dysarthria or scanning speech, paresthesiae, objective alterations of vibratory and position senses. Mental disturbances of some kind, including both euphoria and depression, are seen in almost half the patients (Table 101).

Table 101. Frequency of Mental Disturbances in Multiple Sclerosis in 46 Autopsy-Controlled Cases

(After Carter, Sciarra and Merritt, A. Res. Nerv. & Ment. Dis., Proc., 1950)

Symptom		% of Cases
Disturbances of affect		54
Euphoria	31%	
Depression	7%	
Lability of mood	16%	
Psychotic episodes		4
Mental deterioration		26

One of the characteristics of symptoms of multiple sclerosis is the fact that they may be extremely transient. Diplopia may last for a matter of minutes, paresthesiae may last for anywhere from seconds to hours, and diminution of visual acuity may be equally short-lived. An interesting symptom is that of transient loss of color vision which may presage the development of optic or retrobulbar neuritis. Because of the transient and bizarre nature of some of these complaints, they are not infrequently called hysterical.

While remissions are a characteristic feature of the disease, it is somewhat difficult for clinicians to agree on the nature or duration of these remissions. If one includes only the complete, or almost complete, disappearance of a major symptom such as loss of vision, marked weakness of an extremity, diplopia and the like, significant clinical remissions occur in approximately 70% of the patients with multiple sclerosis.

Mode of Onset. The onset of multiple sclerosis is usually acute or subacute. While there is no characteristic mode of onset, there are several symptoms and signs which frequently occur at the onset. Various combinations of these are often helpful in establishing the presumptive diagnosis. Not infrequently, however, a thorough review of the past history reveals the existence, either remote or recent, of other manifestations of the disease hitherto ignored or not considered significant by patient or physician. This is particularly true of transient paresthesiae, mild urinary disturbances (which are often and erroneously diagnosed and treated as painless urinary tract infections) and mild ocular manifestations such as blurring of vision or transient diminutions of monocular visual acuity. Muscle weakness, paresthesiae, ocular and cerebellar disturbances constitute the most commonly observed symptoms of the onset bout of multiple sclerosis.

Laboratory Data. The only significant, reasonably consistent abnormalities in the laboratory examination are in the cerebrospinal fluid.

The protein content of the fluid is slightly increased in 40% of the cases and the white cell count is slightly increased in 30%. A mild pleocytosis is often interpreted as signifying "activity" of the demyelinizing process.

The most significant finding is an increase in the globulin fractions of the spinal fluid protein. The colloidal gold curve is found to be abnormal in approximately half the cases.

In most routine clinical laboratories the determination of CSF immunoglobulin G by either electroimmunodiffusion or radioimmunodiffusion will show elevation of this fraction (above 13 to 15% of the total protein) in 40 to 60% of cases of multiple sclerosis. In some research laboratories, this percentage rises to 75 to 85%. The presence of oligoclonal bands of IgG in several laboratories is said to occur in as high as 98% of patients with multiple sclerosis.

The elevation of CSF IgG is not pathognomonic: other conditions such as syphilis and other infections, postinfectious or postvaccinal myelinopathies, collagenopathies, certain dysproteinemias, subacute sclerosing panencephalitis, etc. may also show a similar elevation (Table 101A). As a general rule, the elevation of the CSF IgG is significant only if the CSF sample is blood free and the serum IgG is within normal limits. The CSF IgG becomes more reliable as a diagnostic test when the disease has been present for at least one year; unfortunately, it gives no indications regarding the state of activity of the disease, since no significant variations have been found in its level during exacerbations or remissions.

A number of other diagnostic tests for multiple sclerosis have been proposed, but have not yet gained clinical acceptance: the formation of lymphocyte rosettes from M.S. serum around measles infected cells; the decreased serum/CSF protein serine ratio; a relative decrease in the number of CSF T-lymphocytes, etc.

In regard to the laboratory determination of activity of the disease process, the measurement by radioimmunoassay of myelin basic protein in CSF and the alterations of the serum/CSF protein serine ratio are the only tests that appear to be promising.

At this time, however, no single, absolutely reliable or completely pathognomonic laboratory examination exists for this disease. The determination of cerebrospinal fluid IgG when coupled with the history and the clinical examination, appears to be the most valuable diagnostic aid.

With the possible exception of pleocytosis in the spinal fluid (which is lymphocytic in nature and rarely exceeds 40 cells per cu mm), there are no laboratory findings indicative of progress of the disease. Elevation of the IgG cannot be considered as an indication of activity of the disease process.

Table 101A.   CSF Immunoglobulins in Multiple Sclerosis
(Schneck & Claman, 1969)
Electroimmunodiffusion

Elevated IgG (> 14% TP)

Multiple Sclerosis (54 pts.)	55.6%*
(Normal CSF protein 71.4%)	
(Elevated CSF protein [> 50 mg%] 26.3%)	
Other "demyelinating" diseases	12.5%
Optic & retrobular neuritis	20.0%
Guillain-Barré syndrome	50.0%
Neurosyphilis	60.0%
Miscellaneous	12.7%

*IgG absolute value elevated in 74.1%

Electroencephalographic abnormalities are found in about one-third of the cases in the acute state of the disease while slight changes may also be present in other stages. The abnormalities are chiefly in the form of slow waves and are considered to be a nonspecific reaction of the brain to an acute local pathological process.

The recording of cortical evoked responses from visual, auditory and somatosensory stimulation has proved to be of great value in demonstrating the existence of clinically unsuspected lesions. Visual evoked responses to both flash and pattern reversal stimuli have demonstrated abnormalities in relatively large numbers of multiple sclerosis patients without history or signs of visual impairment. Similarly, auditory evoked responses have demonstrated such unsuspected lesions in brainstem structures, while somatosensory evoked responses have suggested the presence of lesions in the spinal cord. Measurement of the delay of the blink reflex following electrical stimulation of the supraorbital nerve indicates the presence of a pontine lesion. The main advantage of these procedures is that they are simple, noninvasive, harmless and relatively inexpensive with a remarkably high yield.

Radioactive isotope brain scanning is found to be positive in rare cases and only when the lesion measures at least 1½ to 2 cm in diameter. This is more likely, of course, to occur in patients with diffuse or transitional sclerosis.

Computer assisted tomography (CT brain scanning) has already been shown to be of some value in demonstrating the presence of cerebral involvement by multiple sclerosis. Rather nonspecific ventricular enlargement and/or cortical atrophy has been demonstrated in as many as 44% of patients. More important is the fact that the classical periventricular plaques can be found in a relatively large number of patients (36% in one series). Isolated subcortical plaques are found with extreme rarity.

Psychologic testing, in particular in patients without clinical symptoms of mental or intellectual involvement, has revealed significant impairment of cognitive functions in a surprisingly large number of patients (47% in one series). These tests can, therefore, also be used in appropriate situations to demonstrate the existence of clinically unsuspected multiple lesions.

Diagnosis. Since there is no specific test for multiple sclerosis, the diagnosis rests on the appearance of multiple signs and symptoms of central nervous system involvement and the occurrence of the characteristic remissions and exacerbations. The diagnosis can rarely be made with any degree of assurance at the time of the first attack. In day to day clinical practice, the diagnosis of multiple sclerosis is based upon the ability to demonstrate, on the basis of the history and the neurologic examination, the existence of lesions involving different parts of the nervous system. Thus, eliciting from the patient a history of relatively mild, transient, and often overlooked or forgotten symptoms, such as transient diplopia or diminution of visual acuity, urinary urgency, weakness or numbness of a limb lasting for a day or two, may provide such evidence. The old aphorism that multiple sclerosis is a disease characterized by dissemination in time and space remains very much the keystone of clinical diagnosis.

Examination for monocular (and thus asymptomatic) disturbances of color vision with isochromatic Ishihara or AO color plates may demonstrate evidence of unsuspected subclinical optic neuropathy. The hot bath test, carried out by immersing the patient in water at 104° F may bring out otherwise undetectable neurologic signs such as nystagmus, weakness and sensory changes, decreased visual acuity and specific color blindness, dysconjugate gaze, abnormal reflexes and cerebellar incoordination. This is an extremely valuable and totally harmless diagnostic technique which should be used routinely in order to either confirm undocumented symptoms or demonstrate hitherto unsuspected neurologic signs. The recording of visual, auditory or somatosensory evoked responses (Fig. 178) will also add to the diagnostic capability by demonstrating the existence of poorly documented or unsuspected lesions of the visual system, brain stem and spinal cord. Careful and expert psychologic evaluations may also reveal evidence of cerebral dysfunction not apparent on clinical neurologic examination and thus provide evidence of the existence of multiple lesions. Similarly, CT brain scanning, although rarely necessary, may provide such data. The presence of an elevated CSF immunoglobulin-G and especially oligoclonal bands, other conditions producing these laboratory changes having been excluded, can be interpreted as strong supportive evidence for the diagnosis.

While a suspicion of multiple sclerosis, or a presumptive diagnosis of the disease can be made reasonably early in the course of the disease, a more definitive diagnosis must often depend upon continued observation and numerous re-examinations over a period of months or years.

Differential Diagnosis. Since multiple sclerosis is almost exclusively a disease of the white matter of the central nervous system, signs and symptoms indicating involvement of the basal ganglia, the cranial nerve nuclei, the anterior horn cells or of the roots and peripheral nerves militate strongly against the diagnosis.

It is extremely difficult, if not impossible, to clearly differentiate between the first attack of multiple sclerosis and a postinfectious or postimmunization myelinoclastic encephalomyelopathy. What has often been referred to as acute disseminated encephalomyelitis, most commonly considered to be postinfectious or postimmunization in nature, turns out to be the first episode of multiple sclerosis in about 1

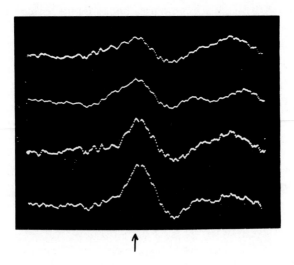

Left eye- Lower field

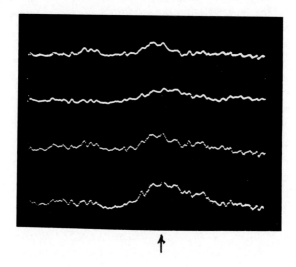

Right eye- Lower field

Figure 178. Visual evoked responses elicited by checkerboard pattern reversal. Right optic neuropathy. There is a 20-msec delay (arrows) in the first major peak, as well as a marked decrease in the amplitude of that peak, (Courtesy Dr. Joseph McSherry.)

out of 4 patients. A familial incidence, being quite unusual, also should be considered as evidence against the diagnosis as should age of onset beyond the sixth decade.

Other conditions which may closely resemble the intermittent course of multiple sclerosis along with the dissemination of lesions include: collagen diseases such as disseminated lupus erythematosus or polyarteritis nodosa; vascular malformation or hemangiomas involving the brainstem and spinal cord; gliomas of the brainstem; cervical cord neoplasms; syringomyelia; cervical discs and spondylosis; and some of the diseases in the lymphoma group.

Progressive multifocal leukoencephalopathy, which is usually associated with a leukemia or a lymphoma, may mimic an acute attack of multiple sclerosis.

Other conditions which need occasionally be ruled out include neurosyphilis, the spinocerebellar ataxias, malformations of the cervical spine, the base of the skull and the cerebellum, tumors in the region of the foramen magnum, cerebellopontine angle tumors, tumors of the cerebral hemispheres, and combined system disease secondary to vitamin B_{12} deficiency.

One of the most difficult differential diagnoses is that of conversion reaction. Because of the fleeting nature of symptoms, the absence or paucity of neurologic signs, in particular at the onset of the disease, the not uncommon emotional disturbance and the fact that the disease may become manifested following physical or emotional trauma, this differential may tax the ingenuity of even the most astute physician. On the other hand, psychologic symptoms may mask the underlying disease for a long time and delay the establishment of the correct diagnosis.

Course and Prognosis. Multiple sclerosis is so often inevitably progressive, despite its remissions, that both the public and the medical profession have come to consider it uniformly hopeless. In fact, if a neurologic disease seems at length to be nonprogressive, the diagnosis of multiple sclerosis is more than likely to be discarded. Yet, a wide clinical experience with this exceedingly pleomorphic disease strongly suggests that it may on occasion be a mild disorder indeed— mild in its onset, in its pattern of evolution, or in its ultimate results. It may even remain "clinically silent" for years—or rarely forever. There are indeed instances of multiple sclerosis that have been discovered as an incidental finding at autopsy. Some individuals have symptoms so mild and so transient that they have not sought medical advice or the disease may be unrecognized because it has not caused any significant degree of disability.

The course of the disease is extremely variable, ranging from a matter of days or weeks between onset and death to as long as forty or more years. One well-documented case had a "remission" lasting sixty-four years!

The average duration of the disease in autopsy-proven cases is about fourteen years, but this represents a highly selected group of cases which includes many cases with extremely short courses.

In a study of 476 cases of "definite" multiple sclerosis in men given this diagnosis in Army hospitals during World War II, calculation by life table methods revealed that survival is 76% twenty years after onset and 69% twenty-five years after onset. The indication is that half of 527 patients (the definite group plus the probables) whose average age at onset was twenty-five will live some thirty-five years following onset. These findings reveal a much more optimistic outlook than has generally been given for multiple sclerosis.

Keeping in mind the concept of benign and subclinical multiple sclerosis, in general, the prognosis is not as frightening as it is usually considered to be. Equally as important in regard to prognosis as survival, is the degree of disability, or better put, of interference with normal activities. The estimates for "incapacitation" range from one-fourth to one-half the patients after the first few years of the disease. As a rough rule of thumb it can be stated that approximately one-third of the patients with evidence of disseminated lesions will continue to be able to carry out their usual way of life without significant disability; that an additional one-third will eventually become somewhat disabled and will have to alter their way of life to some degree while the remaining one-third will become so severely disabled as to become unable to carry out these activities in any way.

The direct cause of death in multiple sclerosis is usually intercurrent disease. Death from the disease itself is extremely rare and is usually seen in those patients with acute and severe involvement of the lower brainstem and medulla. Infection of the urinary tract, respiratory infections and septicemia secondary to decubiti are the most common causes of death. As patients get into the older age groups, they may succumb to any of the common death-causing illnesses such as heart failure, coronary occlusions, neoplastic disease and cerebrovascular accidents.

Multiple Sclerosis in Children. By all accounts disseminated sclerosis is extremely rare in childhood. Exactly how rare is somewhat difficult to determine, in particular in the absence of an adequate number of postmortem studies. Onset before the age of five has never been proved; it is exceedingly rare under the age of ten but onset between fifteen and twenty accounts for 7 to 8% in large series.

Treatment. The list of therapeutic regimens that have been tried is long, and the results of their use extremely disappointing. There is as yet no fully accepted treatment of multiple sclerosis. It is unrealistic to expect that any therapeutic agent or regimen will result in a reversal of well-established neurologic signs and symptoms due to irreparable damage to the nervous system. It is, of course, impossible to say at any one time in the course of the disease if the neurologic deficit or complaint represents swelling of the myelin sheath, its destruction or the presence of a scar. It is thus also equally unrealistic to think in terms of a cure for the lesions of multiple sclerosis once they have become established.

Since the etiology and the pathogenesis remain unknown, preventive measures—the only really effective method of treatment for a disease resulting in destruction of nervous tissue—cannot yet be considered. Therapeutic measures, perforce based on improved hypotheses, can be applied only after the disease has become manifest and should be aimed at shortening bouts, or interrupting the progress of the disease for as long as possible, ideally permanently.

Another aspect of therapy must be symptomatic: alleviating distressing or disabling neurologic deficits, and returning patients to normal life styles and occupations.

While practically all of the various therapeutic agents which have been tried have been discarded, ACTH and the adrenal corticosteroids remain in use, albeit with considerable controversy. The rationale for their use is poorly established but is essentially based upon the belief that a hyperimmune component exists in the disease, that there is a well-demonstrated inflammatory component in many instances, and that edema of the myelin sheath appears to be an early pathologic finding. These agents have been successfully used to combat all three of these components in other conditions. Large numbers of neurologists have reported beneficial effects in inducing remissions in patients with multiple sclerosis using ACTH or a number of the corticosteroids, primarily prednisone and dexamethasone.

A cooperative study in the evaluation of the use of ACTH versus placebo on the course of patients in acute exacerbations of the disease was carried out jointly by a number of American investigators and involved a total of 197 patients of which 103 were treated with ACTH and 94 with placebo. The conclusion of the study was that the value of this treatment was very questionable in view of the fact that a significant number of patients also improved while on placebo therapy. The value of hospitalization per se must not be underestimated: with our better understanding of the physiologic and psychologic induction of symptoms, removing M.S. patients from the stresses and strains of daily living may in fact have a beneficial effect.

While anecdotal results are often denigrated, in the absence of any definitive therapy, and in the presence of a potentially disabling disease, the use of ACTH or steroids may be justified, particularly in the acute cases. The major criticism of the use of these agents is that in fact they do not prevent exacerbations of the disease.

The use of intrathecal corticosteroids is contraindicated because of the danger of adhesive arachnoiditis. Immunosuppressant agents such as methotrexate, 6-mercaptopurine, cytosine-arabinoside and massive X-irradiation have also been tried but have proved to be most disappointing.

These treatments have been based upon the concept of multiple sclerosis as a hyperimmune disease. Conversely, the use of transfer factor, based upon the concept of immunodeficiency in this illness, has only recently been tried. Because the goal of such treatment is prevention of exacerbations, only a long term follow-up study can give indications regarding its efficacy. This information is not yet available from the small group of patients receiving such treatment.

There has recently been a renewed interest in the dietary treatment based upon the controversial discovery of reduced serum linoleate concentration in M.S. patients. Supplementation with sunflower seed oil emulsion has been tried, again with less than impressive results. From all that is known of multiple sclerosis, it would appear rather unlikely that any form of dietary therapy would have any more than possibly psychologic beneficial effects.

In general, the treatment at present must remain symptomatic. Diplopia can be relieved by as simple a measure as prescribing an eye patch. Urinary frequency and urgency often respond to judiciously timed dose of methantheline or propantheline bromide (Banthine or Pro-Banthine). The severe cerebellar tremor has been abolished in some patients by cryothalamotomy.

A number of agents have been employed with some success for the relief of spasticity. Diazepam (Valium) has been of some value, but may have a significant sedative effect. Dantrolene (Dantrium) may be of value; however, too much of this drug will so reduce muscle tone as to make the patient unable to lock hips and knees in order to stand. Another such agent, now available in the United States is baclofen (Lioresal) which is similar to dantrolene in its action, but is said to be better tolerated by most patients. Intrathecal selective phenol injections, particularly useful for the relief of severe tonic spasms, can be considered as well as obturator nerve crush or section for severe adductor spasm of the lower extremities. The rarer but disabling spasms of trigeminal neuralgia which occasionally are seen in multiple sclerosis respond dramatically to the administration of carbamazepine (Tegretol). Dorsal column stimulation, again for the relief of spasticity and, according to some clinicians, for improvement of bladder dysfunction, has proved to be of only transient benefit in a small number of patients.

Physical therapy is advisable for the rehabilitation of patients in whom there is long remission or in whom the course appears to be static. Prevention or control of urinary bladder infection is of the most utmost importance: in patients with chronic bladder disturbance, cystometrography should be carried out in order to determine if the bladder is atonic or hypertonic. The use of tidal drainage, while no longer popular, should, however, be considered in order to attempt to establish automaticity of micturition. When dribbling or frank incontinence cannot be controlled and in particular if it is complicated by chronic bladder infection, suprapubic cystostomy or ileal conduit should be considered. The patient who is bedridden or chair-ridden because of paraplegia requires special consideration including care of the skin to prevent the development of decubitus ulcers, monitoring of calcium metabolism to prevent renal and bladder calculi and bony demineralization, protein nutrition, prevention of contractures, regulation of bowel function and prevention of impactions.

Whenever possible, the patient should continue to carry out his usual activities and occupation. The so-called mood elevating drugs such as amitriptyline (Elavil), perphenazine (Trilafon) and imipramine (Tofranil) have been of value in the treatment of the depression which occurs as frequently as the euphoria. Good nutrition as well as prevention, and prompt treatment, of intercurrent infections of all types are important. The question of bedrest during the acute exacerbation of the disease has never been adequately settled, although in the balance it would seem to be indicated but the development of chronic invalidism should be discouraged. The recommendation that patients with multiple sclerosis move to a warm, dry climate has little basis in fact but extreme heat or cold should be avoided. Psychologic support, in particular from the physician, plays an important role in management; involvement of the patient's family in the management program is imperative. In those individuals with physical disability, simple and inexpensive modifications and alterations of the home may prove to be extremely important. In general, there are few diseases in which sympathy and compassion on the part of the physician play a more important role than medicinal therapy.

REFERENCES

Alter, M.: Is Multiple Sclerosis an Age-Dependent Host Response to Measles, Lancet, 1, 456, 1976.
Brody, J., et al.: Virus Antibody Titers in Multiple Sclerosis Patients, Siblings and Controls, J.A.M.A., 216, 1441, 1971.
Cohen, S., et al.: Radioimmunoassay of Myelin Basic Protein in Spinal Fluid, N. Engl. J. Med., 295, 1455, 1976.
Compston, D., et al.: B-lymphocyte Alloantigens Associated with Multiple Sclerosis, Lancet, 2, 1261, 1976.
Dean, G. and Kurtzke, J.: On the Risk of Multiple Sclerosis According to Immigration to South Africa, Br. Med. J., 3, 725, 1971.

Feinsod, M., and Hoyt, W.: Subclinical Optic Neuropathy in Multiple Sclerosis, J. Neurol. Neurosurg. Psychiat., *38*, 1109, 1975.

Field, E.: Multiple Sclerosis: Relationship to Scrapie and Slow Infection: Ageing and Measles, Acta Neurol. Scand., *51*, 285, 1975.

Gyldensted, C.: Computer Tomography of the Cerebrum in Multiple Sclerosis, J. Neuroradiol., *12*, 33, 1976.

Kempe, C., et al.: Elevated CSF Vaccinia Antibodies in Multiple Sclerosis, Arch. Neurol., *28*, 278, 1973.

Kimura, J.: Electrically Elicited Blink Reflex in Diagnosis of Multiple Sclerosis, Brain, *98*, 413, 1975.

Kurtzke, J.: A Reassessment of the Distribution of Multiple Sclerosis, Acta Neurol. Scand., *51*, 137, 1975.

Lampert, F., and Lampert, P.: Multiple Sclerosis: Morphologic Evidence of Intranuclear Paramyxovirus or Altered Chromatin Fibers? Arch. Neurol., *32*, 425, 1975.

Leibowitz, V.: Multiple Sclerosis: Progress in Epidemiology and Experimental Research, J. Neurol. Sci., *12*, 307, 1971.

Mackay, R., and Hirano, A.: Forms of Benign Multiple Sclerosis, Arch. Neurol., *17*, 588, 1967.

McFarlin, D., and McFarland, H.: Histocompatibility Studies and Multiple Sclerosis, Arch. Neurol., *33*, 395, 1976.

Olsson, J., et al.: Immunoglobulin Abnormalities in Multiple Sclerosis, J. Neurol. Sci., *27*, 233, 1976.

Opelz, G., et al.: The Association of HLA Antigens A3, B7 and DW2 with 330 Multiple Sclerosis Patients in the United States, Tissue Antigens, *9*, 54, 1977.

Paty, D., et al.: Measles Antibodies as Related to HLA Types and Multiple Sclerosis, Neurology, *26*, 651, 1976.

Périer, O., and Grégoire, A.: Electronmicroscopic Features of Multiple Sclerosis Brains, Brain, *88*, 937, 1965.

Porterfield, J. (ed.): Multiple Sclerosis, Br. Med. Bull., *33*, 1, 1977.

Poser, C., et al.: Clinical Characteristics of Autopsy-proved Multiple Sclerosis, Neurology, *16*, 791, 1966.

Poser, C.: Recent Advances in Multiple Sclerosis, Med. Clin. N. A., *56*, 1343, 1972.

Poser, C.: Multiple Sclerosis. In Tower, D. (ed.): *The Nervous System*, New York, Raven Press, 1975, Vol. 2, p. 337.

Reddy, M., and Goh, K.: B and T Lymphocytes in Man, Neurology, *26*, 997, 1976.

Robinson, K., and Rudge, P.: Auditory Evoked Responses in Multiple Sclerosis, Lancet, *1*, 1164, 1975.

Schumacher, G.: Critique of Experimental Trials of Therapy in Multiple Sclerosis, Neurology, *24*, 1010, 1974.

NEUROMYELITIS OPTICA
(Devic's disease)

Neuromyelitis optica is a clinical syndrome characterized by the acute occurrence of optic neuritis and transverse myelitis. In the past many authors have considered it to be a separate clinical and pathologic entity but all evidence points to it being nothing more than a variant of multiple sclerosis. The combination of optic neuritis and transverse myelitis may occur as the initial bout of multiple sclerosis or may develop at any time in the course of this disease. There is little justification for continuing to consider it as a separate entity.

For some unknown reason, the combination of acute involvement of the optic system and the spinal cord is more common in Japan, Taiwan,

India and Colombia than the disseminated forms of the disease seen in the United States and western Europe.

Clinically it is extremely difficult if not impossible to differentiate this condition from a postinfectious or postimmunization myelinopathy.

Because of the fact that the disease usually assumes an acute form, necrosis of the spinal cord is not uncommon. This may be associated with swelling of the spinal cord leading to spinal subarachnoid block. When the visual symptoms are absent, an exploratory laminectomy may be justified although the beneficial effects of this procedure claimed by some have been quite doubtful.

The prognosis for recovery from the transverse myelitis is usually quite poor while on the other hand recurrences after partial recovery are quite rare.

REFERENCE

Cloys, D. E., and Netsky, M. G.: Neuromyelitis Optica. In *Handbook of Clinical Neurology*, ed. by Vinken, P. J. and Bruyn, G. W. Amsterdam, North Holland Publishing Company, Vol. 9, pp. 426–436, 1970.

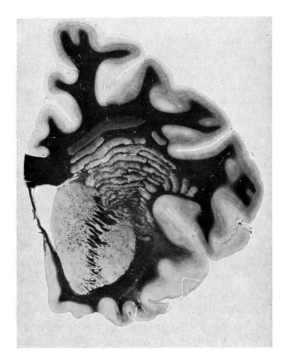

Figure 179. Concentric areas of demyelination in centrum ovale. Myelin sheath stain of Balo's disease. (Courtesy of Dr. H. Shiraki, Tokyo.)

CONCENTRIC SCLEROSIS
(Balo's disease)

Concentric sclerosis is considered to be a variant of multiple (or by some, of diffuse) sclerosis. It cannot be differentiated clinically from either multiple or diffuse sclerosis and the characteristic histologic picture of concentric areas of myelinoclasia may represent a peculiar local tissue reaction. Only a few cases have been reported in which a single, extensive area of demyelination exists with the characteristic concentric areas of alternating normal and demyelinized tissue (Fig. 179). Areas with such concentric appearance have been found in more classical cases of diffuse or disseminated sclerosis. In essence, it is strictly a histologic diagnosis without recognizable clinical concomitant.

REFERENCE

Courville, C. B.: Concentric Sclerosis. In *Handbook of Clinical Neurology*, ed. by Vinken, P. J. and Bruyn, G. W. Amsterdam, North Holland Publishing Company, Vol. 9, pp. 437–451, 1970.

Diffuse and Transitional Sclerosis

Loose and indiscriminate use of the term diffuse sclerosis has led to a great deal of confusion in the nomenclature and terminology of this complex and heterogeneous group of diseases. Since many authors have used the term diffuse sclerosis as being equivalent with Schilder's disease, the latter eponymic designation deserves some clarification.

In 1912, Schilder described the brain of a girl in which large areas of the white matter of the cerebral hemispheres had been affected by a condition which appeared to primarily involve the myelin sheath while relatively sparing the axons. He named this condition *encephalitis periaxialis diffusa* or diffuse sclerosis. The following year, in 1913, he published the results of a thorough study of another brain which he also included in his newly established category of *encephalitis periaxialis diffusa*, not stressing the fact that a sibling of the patient had died of a similar disease at an earlier date and that some of the staining characteristics of the brain were somewhat unusual. This second case has now been recognized as being an example of a leukodystrophy, *i.e.* a dysmyelinating condition rather than a myelinoclastic one. Finally, in 1924 Schilder published the last of his three *princeps* cases. In this instance, the pathologic examination revealed extensive areas of diffuse demyelination without sharply demarcated borders but with extensive glial proliferation, with an enormous accumulation of phagocytes and many giant astrocytes as well as intensive perivascular lymphocytic infiltration and capillary proliferation. It was later pointed out by Lumsden that this third case almost certainly belonged to the group of the subacute sclerosing leukoencephalitides.

Following Schilder's example, many authors used the term diffuse sclerosis to describe a host of unrelated disease entities. The problem of classification and of differentiation has been further complicated by the fact that it is extremely difficult in many instances to differentiate on pathologic grounds, as well as on clinical grounds, between diffuse demyelination and sclerosis resulting from so-called primary demyelination on the one hand, and the result of vascular and toxic conditions on the other. Two examples of this are the *maladie de Schilder-Foix* which is clearly an instance of bilateral involvement of the posterior cerebral arteries and Binswanger's disease which is now well accepted as being a manifestation of arteriosclerosis mainly affecting the small vessels serving the gray-white matter junction.

The myelinoclastic type of diffuse sclerosis is exemplified by Schilder's 1912 case. For historical reasons and to continue to give Schilder due credit, the eponymic designation *Schilder's disease* should be reserved for the myelinoclastic diffuse sclerosis. The term Schilder's cerebral sclerosis has been proposed as a substitute.

The matter of classification of Schilder's disease has been further complicated by the recognition that the combination of extensive dysmyelinating or myelinoclastic involvement of the brain associated with adrenal insufficency, what is now called adrenoleukodystrophy, is a distinct entity which has now been well shown to belong to the group of leukodystrophies or dysmyelinating diseases. It is quite likely that many, but probably not all the cases of Schilder's myelinoclastic diffuse sclerosis occurring in boys are in fact instances of adrenoleukodystrophy.

Pathogenesis and Pathology. The pathogenesis is considered to be identical with that of multiple sclerosis. Myelinoclastic diffuse sclerosis is a variant form of multiple sclerosis, the difference resulting, perhaps, from a difference in the terrain, *i.e.*, the cerebral tissue in which the disease process occurs. It has been suggested that the large areas of demyelination might be due to the fact that the child's nervous system, being still immature, is more susceptible to the injurious agent. The etiology, as in multiple sclerosis, remains unknown.

The close relationship to multiple sclerosis is further illustrated by the existence of another condition which has been given the name of transitional sclerosis or diffuse-disseminated sclerosis. In this condition, the areas of myelinoclasia vary in size from the very large ones characteristic of diffuse sclerosis to small, scattered ones seen in multiple sclerosis. The close relationship between these two conditions was illustrated by the fact that in a survey of 105 reported cases of Schilder's myelinoclastic diffuse sclerosis, only 33 were found in which the only lesions present were bilateral, symmetrical areas of demyelination involving a large area of the centrum ovale while in the other 72 there were several, or many, small isolated plaques as seen in classical multiple sclerosis in addition to the large bilateral lesions.

There are large sharply demarcated areas of demyelination in the centrum ovale of the cerebral hemispheres (Fig. 180). The axons are usually affected but to a lesser degree than the myelin. The subcortical U fibers are usually spared. The glial reaction is similar to that of any cerebral inflammatory condition with formation of giant multinucleated or swollen astrocytes. In the acute stages there is severe perivascular cuffing with lymphocytes and phagocytes. Areas of frank tissue necrosis may occur in the severe lesions indicating that the process may go beyond simple myelinoclasia.

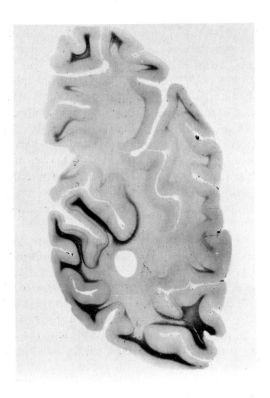

Figure 180.   Diffuse myelinoclastic sclerosis. Myelin sheath stain: almost complete loss of myelin in occipital white matter. U-fibers are irregularly involved. (Courtesy Dr. H. Shiraki, Tokyo.)

Table 102. Diseases of the Myelin Sheath
Histopathologic Characteristics

	Myelinoclasia	Dysmyelination
Symmetry	Rare	Frequent
Edge of lesion	Sharply demarcated	Diffuse (to U fibers)
U fibers	Often involved	Usually spared
Gliosis	Anisomorphic	Isomorphic
Axons	Usually spared	Involved early
Inflammatory reaction	Mild to moderate	Usually absent
Myelinogenesis	Normal	Abnormal
Myelin breakdown	Classical Wallerian degeneration to cholesterol esters	

Electronmicroscopic observations of myelinoclastic diffuse sclerosis have shown that the pattern of demyelination appears to be primary and similar to that in multiple sclerosis. Evidence of Wallerian degeneration is common, and there are features suggesting abortive remyelination. There are many naked axons and axons partially covered with thin layers of myelin (segmental demyelination).

Because the differentiation between the myelinoclastic diffuse scleroses and the dysmyelinating diseases is based to a great extent on histopathologic characteristics, these differences have been summarized in Table 102.

Essentially, it is assumed that in the myelinoclastic diffuse scleroses myelin had originally been normally constituted and is then secondarily destroyed as the result of either endogenous or exogenous factors. The disease process produces a periaxial demyelination, relatively sparing the axons. The gliosis is a true reactive or inflammatory response and the myelin breakdown proceeds in the usual fashion, similar to that seen in the classical Wallerian degeneration, ending in cholesterol esters which are phagocytized. In summary, the lesions have the same pathologic characteristics of those seen in multiple sclerosis.

Incidence. Myelinoclastic diffuse sclerosis is clearly a disease of children: on the basis of 33 autopsy-proven cases of the classical form of the disease, almost half started before the age of ten. The disease may rarely be seen in adulthood. The age incidence of transitional sclerosis on the other hand follows a distribution curve which closely resembles that for autopsy-proven multiple sclerosis; most cases of myelinoclastic diffuse sclerosis seen in the adult probably belong to the transitional sclerosis group.

The number of definitively diagnosed cases is too small to establish any racial, ethnic or geographic predilection, but it is probably similar to that of multiple sclerosis. The incidence between the sexes would appear to be roughly the same.

Familial Incidence. Many cases of familial Schilder's disease have been reported in the literature. In most instances, close examination of the original reports indicates that the authors were describing instances of leukodystrophy. In others, the diagnosis was made purely on clinical grounds and thus it was impossible to tell from the published reports if they were dealing with a myelinoclastic or a dysmyelinating condition. With our current knowledge, it is probable that some of these cases represent instances of adrenoleukodystrophy. There is only one well-documented instance of the familial incidence of myelinoclastic diffuse sclerosis involving a woman with transitional sclerosis and her daughter with diffuse sclerosis. These extraordinarily rare instances might best be explained on the basis of coincidence.

Signs and Symptoms. It is difficult to delineate a typical clinical picture for myelinoclastic diffuse sclerosis primarily because in two-thirds of the cases, one may well be dealing with transitional sclerosis rather than true diffuse sclerosis, and the additional, scattered small lesions would modify the clinical signs and symptoms.

Basically, the clinical course is that of subacute or chronic mental and neurologic deterioration after a period of normal development. As a general rule, the disease progresses slowly and relentlessly and is manifested by intellectual deterioration, increasing spasticity with signs of pyramidal tract involvement, blindness and deafness. In the rare adult cases, the clinical presentation may be purely psychiatric. A list of all the signs and symptoms that might be observed during the clinical course of this disease would include the following: headache, vertigo, convulsive seizures, optic neuritis and atrophy, true papilledema, hemianopsia, cortical blindness, extraocular muscle paralysis, internuclear ophthalmoplegia, nystagmus, facial palsy, deafness, hemiparesis, cortical sensory deficits, cerebellar and rarely extrapyramidal signs and symptoms, dysarthria, dysphagia, aphasic disturbances, memory impairment, dullness, irritability, change in personality, confusion, disorientation, dementia, generalized spasticity, bladder and bowel incontinence, fever of unknown origin, general malnutrition and cachexia. Death is usually due to intercurrent pulmonary, skin, or urinary tract infection.

Increased intracranial pressure suggesting a mass lesion is not uncommon and is due to the fact that the large subcortical areas of myelinoclasia are usually associated with a considerable degree of cerebral edema.

Laboratory Data. As in multiple sclerosis, the only reasonably reliable, although clearly not definitive laboratory test, is the elevation of the spinal fluid gamma globulin or IgG fractions.

Because of the size of the lesions, radioisotope and CT brain scan may be positive. This may turn out to be an exceedingly valuable diagnostic index in view of the rarity of lateralized, supratentorial cerebral neoplasms in the usual age group for this disease.

The electroencephalogram may be quite helpful in showing a large slow wave focus corresponding to the clinical localization of the myelinoclastic lesion.

Diagnosis and Differential Diagnosis. The early clinical symptomatology is so nonspecific that it is difficult to differentiate from other degenerative diseases of childhood. It is almost impossible to pose this diagnosis with any degree of reliability beyond the childhood years. The absence of positive family history; the relatively early appearance of the combination of optic atrophy, pyramidal tract signs and, in particular, deafness; the nonspecific but often large, focal electroencephalographic abnormalities and the relatively infrequent occurrence of convulsive seizures are most helpful.

The single most important condition to be differentiated is adrenoleukodystrophy: this can be done on the basis of adrenal function studies.

The differential diagnosis includes subacute sclerosing panencephalitis which can be identified by means of high or rising measles antibody titers in the serum and spinal fluid, unusually high level of spinal fluid IgG and the characteristic electroencephalographic changes, when present. Progressive multifocal leukoencephalopathy is practically always associated with the presence of chronic leukemia or lymphoma.

Of the dysmyelinating diseases, metachromatic leukodystrophy (sulfatide lipidosis) frequently has a history of familial incidence, and specific diagnostic signs such as consistently elevated spinal fluid protein with normal gamma globulin and IgG fractions, the significantly decreased peripheral nerve conduction time and nonfilling gallbladder in addition to some specific biochemical tests (see below) can establish that diagnosis. The gangliosidoses of the late infantile and juvenile types can now be identified by biochemical procedures.

There have been isolated reports of myelinoclastic diffuse sclerosis following lead encephalopathy, ergotamine intoxication as well as a number of cases of carbon monoxide intoxication.

In the adult, the major problem in differential diagnosis is cerebral neoplasm. In the absence of elevation of spinal fluid gamma globulin or IgG, it may be impossible to differentiate between these conditions except by CT scanning, angiography or cerebral biopsy.

Course and Prognosis. In the 29 cases of Schilder's myelinoclastic diffuse sclerosis collected from the medical literature, the mean duration of the disease was 3.2 years with extremes ranging from fifteen days to twenty-five years. In 62% of the cases, the disease lasted one year or less. As far as is known, the disease is invariably fatal.

Of the 72 cases of transitional sclerosis, the duration of the disease was known in 70. The mean duration was 6.2 years with extremes ranging from three days to forty-five years. It lasted ten years in 23% of the cases. In general, transitional sclerosis leads to death much more quickly than multiple sclerosis but not as fast as in diffuse sclerosis.

Treatment. ACTH and corticosteroids have been used for the treatment of this disease but here again the number of cases available for review is too small to permit any conclusions as to the effectiveness of the treatment. Nevertheless, it appears that these agents are probably of little value.

REFERENCES

Nelson, E., et al.: Electronmicroscopic and Histochemical Studies in Diffuse Sclerosis, Neurology, *12*, 896, 1962.
Poser, C. M.: Myelinoclastic Diffuse and Transitional Sclerosis. In *Handbook of Clinical Neurology*, ed. by Vinken, P. J. and Bruyn, G. W., Amsterdam, North Holland Publishing Company, Vol. 9, pp. 469–484, 1970.
Poser, C. M., and van Bogaert, L.: Natural History and Evolution of the Concept of Schilder's Diffuse Sclerosis, Acta Psychiat. Neurol. Scand., *31*, 285, 1956.
Schilder, P.: Zur Kenntnis der sogenannten diffusen Sklerose (Ueber Encephalitis periaxialis diffusa), Ztschr. f. d. ges Neurol. u. Psychiat., *10*, 1, 1912.

THE DYSMYELINATING DISEASES

The Leukodystrophies

Introduction. Definition. The term dysmyelination is used to signify the existence of an enzymatic disturbance in the mechanisms of both myelinogenesis and myelin maintenance. Therefore, it includes conditions in which there is absence, or delay of myelin formation; formation of biochemically or physically abnormal myelin; as well as conditions in which there exists what one might call a true abiotrophy of the myelin system resulting in eventual destruction of either normally or abnormally formed myelin. Thus, while an alteration of myelinogenetic mechanisms exists in most of the dysmyelinating diseases, in others a metabolic defect may persist once myelinogenesis has been completed and the myelin itself may be more susceptible to catabolic processes, both normal and abnormal. It should therefore not be surprising that in some of the dysmyelinating diseases, one may encounter features of both dysmyelination and myelinoclasia. Adrenoleukodystrophy is a good example of this particular situation.

Pathogenesis. Dysmyelination is a condition which is found in a large and disparate number of conditions: thus, in addition to what have been termed the leukodystrophies to be discussed here, it characterizes a number of lipid storage diseases such as Tay-Sachs disease and hematosidosis; Niemann-Pick's disease; a large number of aminoacidopathies such as phenylketonuria, maple syrup urine disease and oasthouse disease; but also a condition due to copper deficiency, Menkes' kinky-hair disease. Obviously, there must be a number of different pathogenetic mechanisms, and therefore enzymatic disturbances, which can result in dysmyelination. As a matter of fact, it is important to note that even in those dysmyelinating conditions in which a specific enzyme deficiency has been documented, the latter fails to provide a complete explanation for the observed pathologic and neurochemical alterations. It is impossible at this time to pinpoint the site of impairment of enzymatic mechanisms responsible for the disturbance of myelinogenesis which leads to dysmyelination. Until the role of the axon is understood, it may be somewhat naïve to point to the oligodendroglia as the only culprit. One of the histologic characteristics of dysmyelinating conditions is the invariable involvement of axons; electronmicroscopic examination has also revealed axonal changes which are strongly suggestive of a disturbance in axonal transport mechanisms. While neurochemical studies have emphasized abnormalities in glycosphingolipid (cerebroside and sulfatide) metabolism, one of the classic examples of dysmyelination is found in Tay-Sachs disease, a disturbance of ganglioside GM2 catabolism, characterized by neuronal storage of this material as well as a striking absence of myelin in the central nervous system. Klenk pointed out many years ago that the close structural similarity between gangliosides, cerebrosides and sphingomyelin suggested that an abnormality of ganglioside metabolism might lead to alterations in cerebroside and sphingomyelin synthesis; a precursor-product relationship might exist between gangliosides and these important constituents of myelin. While the important role of the oligodendroglia in myelination and myelin maintenance cannot be ignored, a similar role for the neuron and the axon has received little attention. In a number of the dysmyelinating diseases, the neurochemical data point to this role consisting of an as yet unexplained utilization of axonal gangliosides or of their degradative products in the formation of cerebrosides and sphingomyelin. Even a more direct role in myelinogenesis may be postulated on the basis of the fact that GM1 ganglioside is now known to be a normal constituent of myelin.

In addition to a disturbance in myelination, there is a characteristic concurrent overgrowth of astrocytes. It should be clearly understood that the gliosis, which is an obligatory finding in the leukodystrophies is not a reactive phenomenon, i.e. there is no causal relationship between dysmyelination and gliosis in contrast to what happens in the myelinoclastic diseases where there is indeed a simply reactive gliosis. The gliosis of the dysmyelinating diseaes is a parallel phenomenon.

Classification. The leukodystrophies constitute a group of diseases with a basic pathogenesis and pathology as well as many clinical similarities. There are in addition, some pathognomonic histologic features which are superimposed upon the general picture of dysmyelination. A number of the leukodystrophies are characterized by their age at onset. Since they are all presumably genetically determined diseases, the incidence of positive familial history is quite high.

In general, these are extremely rare diseases. They are true degenerative conditions since they manifest themselves as a true decline of nervous function in a previously normal infant or child.

The leukodystrophies constitute a heterogeneous group linked together only by the fundamental pathologic feature of dysmyelination of the central, and often peripheral, nervous system. On the other hand, this same feature is characteristic of many other conditions such as some of the gangliosidoses and aminoacidopathies. It thus seems clear that to continue to maintain the leukodystrophies as a separate group is no longer justified: at least two of them, metachromatic and globoid cell leukodystrophy are clearly lipidoses; spongy sclerosis is seen in a large number of aminoacidopathies, while adrenoleukodystrophy has now been shown to result from a direct or indirect disturbance of fatty acid metabolism. One logical classificatory scheme could be based upon what appears to be the predominant metabolic abnormality: metachromatic leukodystrophy is a sulfatide storage disease; globoid cell leukodystrophy is characterized by a relative accumulation of galactocerebrosides; spongy sclerosis may result from a disturbance of phenylalanine, methionine or GM3 ganglioside (hematoside) metabolism. Unfortunately, the metabolic defect remains unknown in a number of cases. Another possible scheme would be to classify dysmyelinating diseases on the basis of neuropathologic features such as the associated neuronal storage, (e.g., Tay-Sachs disease, Niemann-Pick's disease, sulfatidosis, etc.); extraneuronal storage (globoid cell leukodystrophy, metachromatic leukodystrophy); absence of stored material (phenylketonuria, adrenoleukodystrophy, etc.); presence of status spongiosus; etc. This classification is of limited value since a number of entities would have to be represented in more than one subgroup. For historical reasons, and for lack of a satisfactory classification, the traditional grouping of the leukodystrophies will be continued for purposes of this discussion.

The classification in Table 103 includes a number of the eponymic designations which have appeared in the literature in order to clarify what is an extremely confusing nomenclature.

Pathology. The histopathologic appearance in general is rather uniform. The main features have been summarized in Table 102. The

Table 103. The Leukodystrophies

I. METACHROMATIC TYPE
   Glial insufficiency type of Bielschowsky and Henneberg
   Prelipoid type of Scholz
   Metachromatic type of Einarson and Neel, and Greenfield
   Metachromatic type of von Hirsch and Peiffer
   Late adult metachromatic type of van Bogaert and Nyssen
   Sulfatide lipidosis of Jatzkewitz, Austin and Jervis
   Simple storage type (Poser)
II. GLOBOID CELL TYPE (COLLIER AND GREENFIELD)
   Krabbe's disease
III. SPONGY SCLEROSIS (WOLMAN)
   Familial idiocy with spongy degeneration of the neuraxis of
      van Bogaert and Bertrand
   Canavan's disease
IV. SUDANOPHILIC TYPE (NORMAN)
   A. Adrenoleukodystrophy
   B. Pelizaeus-Merzbacher's disease
      Classical type
      Seitelberger type
      Lowenberg-Hill type
   C. Neutral fat leukodystrophy (Hallervorden)
      Orthochromatic leukodystrophy (Peiffer)
V. FIBRINOID TYPE (PEIFFER)
   Alexander's disease
   Leukodystrophy with hyaline bodies
   Leukodystrophy with Rosenthal fibers
   Dysmyelinogenic leukodystrophy of Wohlwill, Bernstein, and Yakovlev

failure of the myelin sheath to stain is diffuse, quite symmetrical and habitually involves both the cerebral and cerebellar hemisphere white matter. In some of the leukodystrophies the myelin sheath of the peripheral nerves is also involved. The edges of the lesion in the white matter are poorly demarcated except when it reaches the subcortical U-fibers which are either preferentially spared (Fig. 181), or, in one particular type—spongy sclerosis—appear to be preferentially involved. The cortex is seldom affected. The myelin-axonal dissociation is lacking, the axons being almost always involved to the same degree as the myelin sheath, thus leading to early tract degeneration. Perivascular inflammatory reaction is minimal or completely absent. There is extensive, isomorphic gliosis without intensification around blood vessels. A characteristic feature of the leukodystrophies is the fact that extensive gliosis may be found in areas of the white matter where the myelin sheath appears to be normal by the usual staining techniques (Fig. 182).

The leukodystrophies are grouped on the basis of additional, rather special histopathologic features which will be discussed below.

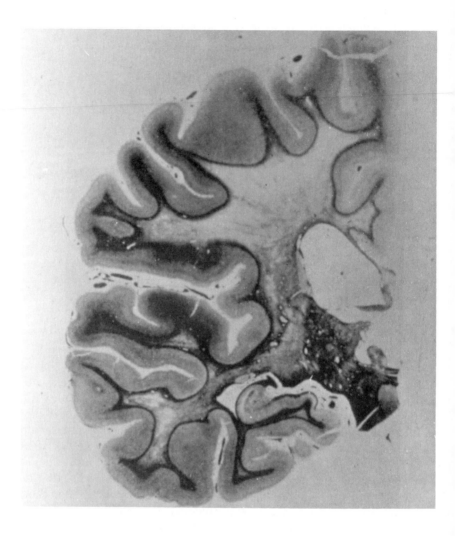

Figure 181. Myelin sheath stain: metachromatic leukodystrophy. Almost complete absence of myelin in subcortical white matter. U-fibers are spared. The edge of the lesion is poorly demarcated. This is the typical appearance of dysmyelination of the brain.

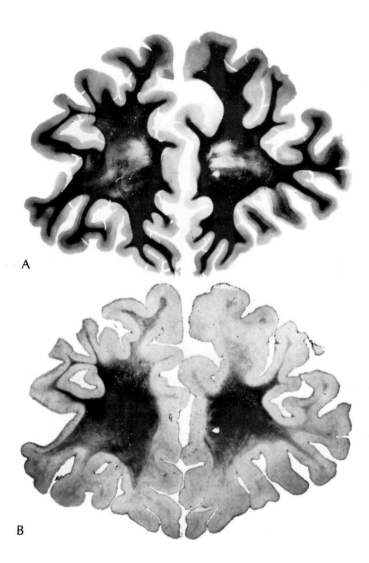

Figure 182. Leukodystrophy: (A) Myelin sheath stain: symmetrical dysmyelinating lesion in deep frontal white matter; the edges of the lesion are diffuse. (B) Holzer stain of same section: note that the gliosis extends to the entire white matter of the frontal lobe, beyond the area of dysmyelination.

REFERENCES

Einarson, L., and Neel, A. V.: Contribution to the Study of Diffuse Brain Sclerosis with a
    Comprehensive Review of the Problem in General, Acta Jutland., 14, 1, 1942.
Norman, R. M.: Lipid Diseases of the Brain. In Modern Trends in Neurology, ed. by
    Williams, D. Washington, Butterworths, Vol. 3, pp. 173–199, 1962.
Poser, C. M.: The Differential Diagnosis of Diffuse Sclerosis in Children, Am. J. Dis.
    Child., 100, 380, 1960.
————: Leukodystrophy and the Concept of Dysmyelination, Arch. Neurol., 4, 323, 1961.
————: Diseases of the Myelin Sheath. In Pathology of the Nervous System, ed. by
    Minckler, J. New York, McGraw-Hill Book Co., Vol. 1, pp. 767–821, 1968.
Poser, C. M., and van Bogaert, L.: Neuropathologic Observations in Phenylketonuria,
    Brain, 82, 1, 1959.

Metachromatic Leukodystrophy
(Sulfatide lipidosis)

Pathogenesis and Pathology. Myelin has been found to be abnormally constituted because of the presence of unusually short chain fatty
acids in the sphingolipid constituents. The specific enzymatic defect
which has been identified in this condition consists of the absence or
severe deficiency of aryl sulfatase-A. This enzyme is necessary for the
normal breakdown of sulfatide (cerebroside sulfuric acid ester) into
cerebroside. This enzyme defect does not, however, account for the
demonstrated failure of chain elongation of myelin fatty acids. Sulfatide is a constituent of normal myelin but since there appears to be an
overabundance of this material, it accumulates and is found deposited
in the white matter parenchyma, in glial cells and phagocytes as well as
in neurons. The material is also found in peripheral nerves and even in
the neural fibers in muscle as well as in the myenteric plexus of the
intestine. In addition, and indicating that this is a general, systemic
disturbance, the material can also be found in the interstitial cells of the
testis, the wall of the gallbladder, the retinal ganglion cells, the capsule
of the pituitary gland, and, clinically most important, in the renal
tubules.

While credit should be given to Greenfield for the first pathologic
description of this disease, the term metachromatic leukoencephalopathy was first introduced by Einarson and Neel in 1942. The
term metachromatic refers to the fact that sulfatide has the peculiar
property of changing the color of certain tissue stains: toluidine blue or
thionine will produce a color other than blue, usually reddish-purple
(although green and orange have also been reported) and an acetic
acid-crystal violet mixture will give a brown stain instead of the usual
purple one. It is this last named reaction which is now commonly used
for demonstrating metachromasia.

Incidence. No racial, ethnic or geographic predilection for this
disease has been noted. More than 200 cases of metachromatic

leukodystrophy have been published but it is likely that the number of known cases is much larger because of the many cases diagnosed by biopsy and biochemical techniques. The total number of cases is estimated to be over 350.

Four different forms of the disease based upon the age of onset have been recognized: the congenital, late infantile, juvenile and adult forms. The late infantile form is by far the most common, age of onset being usually between one and four years. Sex incidence is approximately equal. Genetic transmission is most commonly as autosomal recessive, although other possibilities must be considered in individual families.

A rare variant of this disease, mucosulfatidosis, characterized by a disturbance of ganglioside, mucopolysaccharide and sulfatide metabolism has also been described. It forms an interesting link with both the gangliosidoses and the mucopolysaccharidoses.

Signs and Symptoms. The disease is characterized by severe mental regression and loss of neurologic function, hypertonia, flaccid paraplegia associated with signs of pyramidal tract involvement, peripheral neuropathy and optic atrophy. A macular cherry red spot has been reported in a few cases. The clinical picture depends considerably upon the age of onset. In the infantile cases there is normal development until the first and second year of life. Early symptoms include progressive loss of the ability to walk, a tendency to fall, and weakness of the muscles of the legs. Early signs include nystagmus, then ptosis or strabismus and then inability to walk or stand. Dysarthria, loss of bladder control, muscle hypotonia and severe ataxia occur subsequently. In the early stages in most patients the tendon reflexes are absent. Later pyramidal signs usually appear and spasticity or rigidity is noted terminally.

Laboratory Data. The cerebrospinal fluid findings are quite characteristic in that the protein is always significantly elevated and is frequently above 100 mg %. Electrophoretic or electroimmunodiffusion examinations of the protein have shown no consistent abnormalities. Because of the presence of peripheral nerve involvement, nerve conduction studies often reveal slow values which may be extremely helpful. The wall of the gallbladder may contain an excess of sulfatide, and cholecystography will often reveal a nonfilling gallbladder, a sign which is practically pathognomonic for this disease in this age group.

The nitrocatechol sulfate test can be considered as completely reliable and definitive for metachromatic leukodystrophy. It can be performed not only on urine, but also with serum, and with fibroblasts and leukocytes grown in tissue culture. The test is based upon the fact that in an alkaline medium, and in the presence of aryl sulfatase-A, nitrocatechol sulfate will split and the nitrocatechol will produce a reddish color. In the absence of the enzyme, no color will develop. Biopsies of intestinal mucosa (either rectal or appendix), of kidney, of peripheral nerve (e.g. the sural), and of brain have all been used to confirm the diagnosis but are rarely necessary to establish the diagnosis.

Diagnosis and Differential Diagnosis. The diagnosis has been rendered quite easy by the fact that a number of laboratory procedures give quite characteristic results. The combination of a slowly progressive neurologic disease in a child with a positive family history, coupled with an elevation of the spinal fluid protein, a nonfilling gallbladder and a decreased nerve conduction time is tantamount to making the diagnosis of metachromatic leukodystrophy. Absolute confirmation of the diagnosis must depend upon the nitrocatechol sulfate test, which is unfortunately rather complex and difficult to carry out, or biopsy with appropriate histochemical study of either rectal mucosa, appendix or sural nerve.

The differential diagnosis depends essentially upon the age of onset. In the infant, it includes other leukodystrophies, the amaurotic idiocies which can now be rather easily diagnosed, Niemann-Pick's disease, Gaucher's disease, poliodystrophy, and a variety of other degenerative conditions including a number of aminoacidopathies. The last named can usually be identified by means of chromatographic analysis of blood or urine. In the childhood age group, myelinoclastic diffuse sclerosis, subacute sclerosing panencephalitis, sudanophilic leukodystrophy and Pelizaeus-Merzbacher disease should be considered. In the extremely rare cases of this disease in the adult, only the most unusual index of suspicion can lead to the appropriate laboratory investigations and the correct diagnosis.

Course and Prognosis. The disease is relentlessly progressive inevitably leading to death. It rarely lasts for more than three or five years from date of onset although longer courses have been described.

Treatment. No treatment is available.

Since it is possible to detect heterozygotes by means of determinations of the aryl sulfatase activity in cultured skin fibroblasts, genetic counseling can be recommended. It is also possible to make a prenatal diagnosis by means of a similar examination of cells obtained by amniocentesis. Therapeutic abortion might thus be recommended on that basis.

REFERENCES

Austin, J., et al.: Metachromatic Form of Diffuse Sclerosis. VI. A Rapid Test for the Sulfatase A Deficiency in Metachromatic Leukodystrophy Urine, Arch. Neurol., *14,* 259, 1966.
Austin, J., et al.: Metachromatic Form of Diffuse Cerebral Sclerosis. The Nature and Significance of Low Sulfatase Activity, Arch. Neurol., *15,* 13, 1966.

Bass, N., et al.: A Pedigree Study of Metachromatic Leukodystrophy, Neurology, 20, 52, 1970.

Beratis, N., et al.: Metachromatic Leukodystrophy: Detection in Serum, J. Pediatr., 83, 824, 1973.

Dubois, G., et al.: Absence of ASA Activity in a Healthy Father of a Patient with Metachromatic Leukodystrophy, N. Engl. J. Med., 293, 302, 1975.

Fullerton, P.: Peripheral Nerve Conduction in Metachromatic Leukodystrophy, J. Neurol. Neurosurg. Psychiat., 27, 100, 1964.

Hagberg, B., et al.: Sulfatide Lipidosis in Childhood, Am. J. Dis. Child., 104, 644, 1962.

Hirose, G., and Bass, N. : Adult and Late Infantile Metachromatic Leukodystrophy, Neurology, 21, 443, 1971.

O'Brien, J., and Sampson, E.: Myelin Membrane: A Molecular Abnormality, Science, 150, 1613, 1965.

Percy, A., and Kaback, M.: Infantile and Adult Onset Metachromatic Leukodystrophy: Biochemical Comparison and Predictive Diagnosis, N. Engl. J. Med., 285, 785, 1971.

Pilz, H.: Late Adult Metachromatic Leukodystrophy, Arch. Neurol., 27, 87, 1972.

Rampini, S., et al.: Mukosulfatidose, Helv. Paediat. Acta, 25, 436, 1970.

Globoid Cell Leukodystrophy
(Krabbe's disease)

This extremely rare condition is characterized by loss of neurologic function and progressive spasticity and blindness starting in late infancy. It was first described by Krabbe in 1916 but the presence of the characteristic globoid cells was not emphasized until 1923 by Collier and Greenfield.

Pathologically, in addition to widespread dysmyelination, there is a characteristic accumulation in the white matter of large multinucleated, multilobulated giant cells (Fig. 183). These may be scattered throughout the parenchyma as well as accumulate around blood vessels. They have been demonstrated to be derived from mesodermal phagocytes. Peripheral neuropathy also occurs.

Electronmicroscopic studies of the globoid cells in the parenchyma appear essentially identical to those in the periventricular space. They contain pleomorphic laminated crystals and spicules, some of which represent cerebrosides, others which are more characteristic of lactosylceramide.

Two possible enzymatic disturbances have been identified: First, a deficiency of beta galactosidase. This enzyme is necessary for the catabolic breakdown of cerebrosides and splits galactoside into galactose and ceramide. Second, another enzyme, sulfotransferase, which conjugates cerebroside and phosphoadenosine to form sulfatide, has also been implicated in that it has been found to be significantly low in this disease.

On the basis of the deficiency of beta galactosidase, an enzymatic disturbance which is absolutely pathognomonic for this disease, it has been postulated that the accumulation of cerebrosides in globoid cells

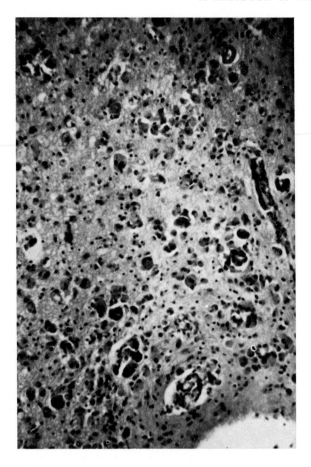

Figure 183. Globoid cell leukodystrophy; H&E stain. Globoid cells in white matter.

establishes a metabolic basis for this disease. The situation, however, is considerably more complex: it has been shown that many other sphingolipids and related substances are found in increased concentrations in this condition, including glucocerebrosides, lactosylceramide, as well as a number of gangliosides. The presence of lactosylceramide, a degradative product of ganglioside metabolism within globoid cells, raises the important question regarding the role of ganglioside mechanism in this condition. While the lack of beta galactosidase constitutes an exceedingly important and diagnostically useful indicator, it cannot possibly be regarded as the only, or even a significant, explanation for the pathologic and biochemical findings. Of great theoretical and practical interest is the fact that a case has now been diagnosed on the basis of the enzyme deficiency, but without the presence of the heretofore characteristic globoid cells.

This particular type of leukodystrophy is an example of a disease in which a specific enzyme disturbance has been identified, has proved to be extremely useful in characterization, but contributes little to our understanding of the biochemical pathogenesis. It is more than likely that additional enzyme deficiencies including almost certainly one or more necessary for ganglioside metabolism will be discovered in this disease. Equally important, it emphasizes the fact that specific neurochemical investigation of still unclassifiable dysmyelinating diseases, e.g., sudanophilic leukodystrophy and idiopathic spongy sclerosis, may lead to a more definitive classification.

Incidence. This is a rare disease with less than 100 pathologically verified cases. The overwhelming majority have been of the infantile type with a few occurring in late childhood and early adolescence.

There does not seem to be a preference for either sex, for any ethnic-racial group or for any geographic distribution. The disease is presumed to be transmitted as an autosomal recessive.

Signs and Symptoms. Hagberg *et al.* have provided an excellent review of the clinical course of this disease based upon a study of 32 confirmed instances. They have divided the disease into three stages. The first one is characterized by hyperirritability and/or arrest of previously normal psychomotor development. The infants seem to be extremely sensitive to light and noise which brings them into violent tonic spasms. They also have periods of unexplained fever. Muscular tone increases but, coincidentally because of peripheral neuropathy, deep tendon reflexes become difficult to elicit and then disappear. The second stage is characterized by constant opisthotonos with generalized neurologic deterioration. Myoclonic jerks of arms and legs as well as other atypical seizures are common. Optic atrophy and blindness usually start at this stage. The third and final stage is characterized by mental and neurologic decerebration, hypotonicity, blindness and cachexia.

Irritability, mental regression, hypertonicity, unexplained fever, and decerebration are found in all cases followed by hypotonicity and areflexia. Blindness is also present in all cases.

Laboratory Data. There is elevation of the spinal fluid protein, almost always above 100 mg %, occasionally as high as 500 mg %.

The CT scan may reveal the extensive cerebral dysmyelination. The EEG is usually normal at the onset but then becomes abnormal in a nonspecific way. Conduction velocities of peripheral nerves have been recorded in a number of cases and regularly found to be markedly reduced.

Determination of deficiency of beta galactosidase activity, using the natural substrate galactocerebroside, in serum or leukocytes, is pathognomonic.

Diagnosis and Differential Diagnosis. Arrest and regression of normal psychomotor development in mid-infancy should immediately bring the diagnosis to mind. The combination of opisthotonos, hypo- or areflexia and markedly elevated spinal fluid protein strongly suggests the diagnosis. Reduced nerve conduction velocities help confirm the suspicion which can be established definitively on the basis of cerebral biopsy alone.

The major disease to be considered in the differential diagnosis is spongy sclerosis (see below). In that disease, however, the children usually have a large head and the cerebrospinal protein is within normal limits. It is nearly impossible to differentiate globoid cell leukodystrophy from the rare form of infantile metachromatic leukodystrophy.

Course and Prognosis. Age of onset ranges between one and one-half months and one year, the mean age of onset in one series being four months. In Hagberg's series, death occurred at ages varying between five and one-half months and two years nine months, the mean age at death being 1.2 years, the longest duration being about two and one-half years. The disease is invariably fatal.

Treatment. There is no known treatment for this disease. Genetic counseling should be seriously considered once the diagnosis has been established in a child. Determination of beta galactosidase activity of serum, leukocytes and fibroblasts can be used for the identification of heterozygotes as well as for prenatal diagnosis using cells obtained by amniocentesis.

REFERENCES

Austin, J., et al.: Studies in Globoid (Krabbe) Leukodystrophy: V. Controlled Enzymic Studies in Ten Human Cases, Arch. Neurol., 23, 502, 1970.
Dunn, H., et al.: The Neuropathy of Krabbe's Infantile Cerebral Sclerosis, Brain, 92, 329, 1969.
Dunn, H., et al.: Krabbe's Leukodystrophy without Globoid Cells, Neurology, 26, 1035, 1976.
Hagberg, B., et al.: Infantile Globoid Cell Leukodystrophy, Neuropaediat., 1, 74, 1969.
Malone, M., et al.: Globoid Leukodystrophy, Arch. Neurol., 32, 606, 613. 1975.
Schochet, S., et al.: Krabbe's Disease: a Light and Electronmicroscopic Study, Acta Neuropathol., 36. 153, 1976.
Suzuki, Y. and Suzuki, K.: Krabbe's Globoid Cell Leukodystrophy; Deficiency of Galactocerebrosidase in Serum, Leukocytes and Fibroblasts, Science, 171, 73, 1971.
Vanier, M., and Svennerholm, L.: Chemical Pathology of Krabbe's Disease, Acta Paediat. Scand., 64, 641, 1975.
Wenger, D., et al.: Globoid Cell Leukodystrophy: Deficiency of Lactosylceramide Beta Galactosidase, Proc. Nat. Acad. Sci., 71, 854, 1974.

Spongy Sclerosis

This condition was described as a clinical and pathologic entity by van Bogaert and Bertrand in 1959 under the name familial idiocy with spongy degeneration of the neuraxis. The disease is often referred to as Canavan's disease in the Anglo-Saxon literature.

A great deal of controversy exists regarding the exact classification of this very rare condition. Because the brain shows all the histopathologic characteristics of a dysmyelinating disease, it is retained in the group of leukodystrophies by most authors.

Pathology and Pathogenesis. The brain shows an almost total lack of stainable myelin involving the entire nervous system (Fig. 184). In addition, there is a spongy state characterized by multiple vacuoles

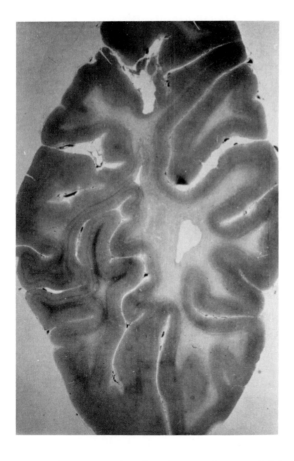

Figure 184. Spongy sclerosis. Myelin sheath stain of occipital lobe with almost complete absence of stainable myelin. (Courtesy Dr. D. S. Buchanan, Washington, DC.)

which appear to preferentially involve the deep layers of the cortex and the subcortical U-fibers. This spongy degeneration is also seen in the cerebellum. Another characteristic is the presence in the white matter of large numbers of Alzheimer type II astrocytes, a particular cell type which has long been associated with metabolic disturbances. The brain is usually somewhat larger and heavier than expected for age.

Electronmicroscopic studies have demonstrated abnormal organelles in the astrocytic cytoplasm and processes. The mitochondria were frequently enormously elongated and showed distension and distortion of the cristae and striation of the matrix.

The exact pathogenetic mechanism remains unknown. It must be emphasized that the extensive dysmyelination is always present and is probably pathogenetically unrelated to the characteristic spongy state. The combination of dysmyelination and status spongiosus has been described in a variety of conditions including phenylketonuria, maple syrup urine disease, homocystinuria, oasthouse disease, hyperprolinemia; a newly described disturbance of ganglioside synthesis, GM3 gangliosidosis or hematosidosis; a peculiar glycogen disease; carbamyl phosphate synthetase deficiency, and in a number of cases of idiopathic infantile spasms with hypsarrhythmia. Spongy degeneration with dysmyelination probably represents a generalized, nonspecific manifestation of a number of diverse metabolic disturbances. A number of investigators have demonstrated that the abnormal astrocytic mitochondria have decreased or absent histochemical reactions to ATPase. No abnormality, however, has been proposed to explain the dysmyelination which extends far beyond the subcortical areas of spongy degeneration.

Incidence. Approximately 90 cases of this rare disease have been published. There is no definite sex predominance. Consanguinity of the parents is not unusual. There is a striking predilection for Jewish children of eastern European origin. The disease is transmitted as an autosomal recessive.

Signs and Symptoms. The disease is characterized by progressive enlargement of the head with apathy, generalized flaccidity and inability to control the head, followed by blindness and decorticate rigidity, cachexia and death. Convulsions are frequent, spasticity often follows the initial hypotonia.

Laboratory Data. No characteristic laboratory findings, in particular the cerebrospinal fluid is completely normal. The CT brain scan has been positive in one case. Nerve conduction may be decreased in some instances.

Diagnosis and Differential Diagnosis. The megalocephaly is quite characteristic for this disease as is the high incidence in Jewish children. No specific laboratory tests exist and the definitive diagnosis requires a cerebral biopsy.

Differential diagnosis includes globoid cell leukodystrophy, infantile amaurotic familial idiocy (Tay-Sachs) disease, which can easily be ruled out by the absence of the pathognomonic cherry red spot, and other infantile lipidoses such as Niemann-Pick and Gaucher's disease. More difficult is the differentiation from fibrinoid leukodystrophy (Alexander's disease) which is also characterized by an enlarging head.

An important differential diagnostic problem is that of necrotizing encephalomyelopathy (Leigh's disease) which is usually sporadic but may be familial.

Course and Prognosis. The disease starts before the sixth month of life and may be present at birth. While in most instances the patient usually dies within the first three years of life, one patient survived to the age of eleven years two months. The disease is invariably fatal.

Treatment. There is no known treatment.

REFERENCES

Adachi, M., et al.: Spongy Degeneration of the Central Nervous System, Hum. Pathol., 4, 331, 1973.
Adornato, B., et al.: Cerebral Spongy Degeneration of Infancy, Neurology, 22, 202, 1972.
Martin, J. and Schlote, W.: Central Nervous System Lesions in Disorders of Amino Acid Metabolism, J. Neurol. Sci., 15, 49, 1972.
Mirimanoff, P.: La Dystrophie Spongieuse Héréditaire des Enfants, J. Neurol. Sci., 28, 159, 1976.
Tanaka, J., et al.: Cerebral Sponginess and GM3 Gangliosidosis, J. Neuropath. Exp. Neurol., 34, 249, 1975.

Sudanophilic Leukodystrophy

In the traditional classifications, this group has included a number of exceedingly rare conditions which are characterized by widespread dysmyelination (Fig. 184), but lack other characteristic histopathologic findings. In a few instances, a small amount of sudanophilic cholesterol esters may be found in periadventitial phagocytes.

Three subtypes have been proposed, although the validity of this subclassification is doubtful. It is quite likely that neurochemical and enzymatic studies will enable relocation of these cases in other groups.

Adrenoleukodystrophy
(Melanodermic leukodystrophy, Addison-Schilder's disease)

The association of diffuse cerebral sclerosis with skin pigmentation and, in some cases, evidence of adrenal insufficiency has been reported in approximately 60 cases. This condition has been found to occur only in boys and suggests a sex-linked recessive hereditary transmission.

From a review of the published cases, it is clear that *both* myelino-clastic as well as dysmyelinating diffuse scleroses have been found in

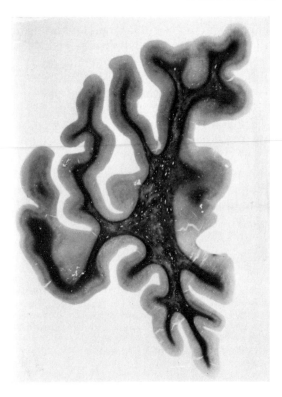

Figure 185. Sudanophilic leukodystrophy, type undetermined. Frontal pole; myelin sheath stain. Note mottled aspect of dysmyelination in the entire subcortical white matter, poorly demarcated edges, sparing of U-fibers; severe cerebral atrophy.

association with adrenal insufficiency. The signs and symptoms of adrenal insufficiency tend to precede the neurological disturbance. Correction of the Addisonian state does not alter the inevitable progression of the diffuse sclerosis.

It must be noted that neither clinical nor laboratory evidence of adrenocortical insufficiency may be present, the diagnosis being based upon the existence of a positive family history of male blood relatives with clinical manifestations of idiopathic Addison's disease.

The pathologic examination of the brain reveals the findings of either myelinoclastic diffuse sclerosis or of extensive dysmyelination. In addition, however, there are distinctive cytoplasmic inclusions in the macrophages: these curvilinear bodies consist of paired electrondense leaflets. In some of the cases, demyelination of peripheral nerves was seen, a finding which emphasizes the fact that this is a dysmyelinating rather than a myelinoclastic disease. Distinctive and pathognomonic changes are also found in the adrenal cortex, consisting of nests of large, often ballooned, cortical cells with eosinophilic cytoplasm and eccentric hypochromatic nuclei. Ultrastructurally, the characteristic striations within these abnormal cortical cells are similar to those found in the brain.

The disease has also been characterized biochemically: cholesterol esters of both brain and adrenal contain substantially higher proportions of fatty acids longer than C22; gangliosides from cerebral white matter also showed increased proportions of long chain fatty acids, as well as an abnormal increase of GD2 and GD3 gangliosides.

The CSF protein is elevated in the majority of the cases. Interestingly enough, the CSF IgG has been found to be elevated in a few cases, suggesting that this finding may represent myelin destruction.

Age of onset (for neurologic symptoms) ranged from five to fourteen and one-half years, the duration of disease ranging from six months to four years.

While in the majority of instances, the combination of diffuse sclerosis and adrenal insufficiency has been found in the same individual, there are at least two families known in which well-documented Addison's disease was found in some children who had no suggestion whatsoever of neurologic involvement, while another sibling had the combination of Addison's disease and signs and symptoms suggestive of diffuse sclerosis. This would strongly suggest that rather than a direct causal relationship existing between the two conditions, they might simply represent two phenotypic expressions of a single, complex genotype.

REFERENCES

Domagk, J., et al.: Adrenoleukodystrophy, Neuropaediat., 6, 41, 1975.
Igarashi, M., et al.: Fatty Acid Abnormality in Adrenoleukodystrophy, J. Neurochem., 26, 851, 1976.
Powell, H., et al.: Adrenoleukodystrophy, Arch. Neurol., 32, 250, 1975.
Schaumburg, H., et al.: Adrenoleukodystrophy, Arch. Neurol., 33, 577, 1975.

Pelizaeus-Merzbacher's Disease

Pelizaeus-Merzbacher's disease was originally characterized as a genetically determined, familial disease with extensive involvement of myelin, probably resulting from an aplasia of the myelin sheath, but having a very prolonged course. The disease started in infancy but went on for as long as thirty years. A number of subtypes have been proposed on the basis of the genetic transmission pattern ranging from possible dominant transmission through sex-linked recessive, to autosomal recessive. The close relationship of this disease, if indeed it exists as an entity, to Cockayne's syndrome should be noted.

The disease is eventually fatal.

Seitelberger, F.: Pelizaeus-Merzbacher Disease. In *Handbook of Clinical Neurology*, ed. by Vinken, P. J. and Bruyn, G. W. Amsterdam, North Holland Publishing Company, Vol. 10, pp. 150–202, 1970.
Watanabe, I., et al.: Early Lesions of Pelizaeus-Merzbacher's Disease, J. Neuropath. Exp. Neurol., *32*, 313, 1973.
Zeman, W., et al.: Pelizaeus-Merzbacher's Disease, J. Neuropath. Exp. Neurol., *23*, 334, 1964.

Fibrinoid Leukodystrophy
(Alexander's disease)

This is the rarest of all leukodystrophies, only 11 cases having been reported.

The brain shows the usual characteristics of dysmyelination with almost complete, symmetrical absence of stainable myelin but with a very striking feature consisting of deposits of eosinophilic hyaline bodies which are most numerous beneath the pia and around blood vessels. These bodies have been identified as being similar to Rosenthal fibers. Confusion regarding the classification of this disease has arisen from the fact that some authors have used the term Alexander's disease to describe a number of other conditions, including multiple sclerosis, simply because of the presence of Rosenthal fibers. It is more than likely that in fibrinoid leukodystrophy, the dysmyelination and the accumulation of Rosenthal fibers may be parallel expressions of the underlying pathogenetic mechanism.

Clinically, the disease is characterized by mental and neurologic deterioration occurring early in infancy and associated with a rapidly enlarging head. Muscle weakness, pyramidal signs and convulsions are characteristic. Ridigity and opisthotonos may occur terminally.

Nothing is known regarding the pathogenesis of this condition. It is believed to be genetically determined. The age of onset ranges from zero to twenty-four months with a mean of six months. No treatment is known.

REFERENCES

Herndon, R., et al.: Light and Electronmicroscopic Observations on Rosenthal Fibers in Alexander's Disease and in Multiple Sclerosis, J. Neuropath. Exp. Neurol., *29*, 524, 1970.
Russo, L. et al.: Alexander's Disease: a Report and Reappraisal, Neurology, *26*, 607, 1976.

Chapter 9

Paroxysmal Disorders

MIGRAINE AND OTHER TYPES OF HEADACHE

Arnold P. Friedman

It has been estimated that headache is a complaint in more than half of the patients who seek medical advice or attention from a physician. Headache is a symptom which may indicate an intracranial or systemic disease, a personality or situational problem, or a combination of these factors. Chronic recurring headaches are usually vascular headaches of the migraine or muscle-contraction (tension) type, or a combination of these two types. If clinical data are clear and fit into a specific entity, the diagnosis of headache can be a simple one. Otherwise, it can be difficult to appreciate variations in the principal symptoms of the attacks because the story may be obscure or in part misleading. Headache always demands careful differential study; it may signal the presence of an underlying disease process that deserves treatment or even constitutes a threat to life, or it may represent the disruptive effects of a psychological disorder.

The clinical approach must take into account the whole patient, not only medically and psychologically, but also his family, occupational, and social problems. To make a correct diagnosis and to treat effectively a patient with headache, the physician must understand the basic physiology and mechanisms of headache as well as the clinical aspects of the problem.

Pathophysiology. Headache may have its origin in stimulation of extracranial or intracranial structures. The extracranial pain-sensitive structures of the head include the scalp, extracranial arteries, mucous membranes of the nasal and paranasal spaces, external and middle ear, teeth, and muscles of the scalp, face, and neck. Pain due to disease of these structures is usually well localized, but it can spread to include a relatively wide area of the head.

Intracranial pain-sensitive structures in the head include the intracranial venous sinuses and their tributaries; parts of the dura at the base of the skull; dural arteries (anterior and middle meningeal); large arteries at the base of the brain (proximal 20%) leading to and coming

825

from the circle of Willis; upper cervical nerves; and fifth, ninth, and tenth cranial nerves. The brain parenchyma, much of the dura, arachnoid, and pia mater, the ependyma of the ventricles, the choroid plexus, and the cranium are insensitive to pain. The periosteum is locally sensitive to stretch.

Basic Mechanisms. The basic mechanisms in intracranial disease are traction due to direct or indirect displacement of pain-sensitive structures, distention and dilatation of intracranial arteries, inflammation in or about the pain-sensitive structures of the head, distortion of pain-sensitive areas due to increased intraventricular pressure caused by lesions that obstruct cerebrospinal fluid flow, or direct pressure by an intracranial mass on certain cranial and cervical nerves. One or more of the mechanisms may be operating in any given patient with headaches.

Raised intracranial pressure in itself does not cause headache. Headache cannot be provoked by raising the pressure in the cerebrospinal system, by injecting saline solution, or by breathing carbon dioxide.

The basic extracranial headache mechanisms are distention of scalp arteries, sustained muscle contraction, and inflammation in and about these structures.

Pain Pathways. If the pain is supratentorial in origin, it is felt anteriorly in the distribution of the fifth cranial nerve in front of a line drawn vertically from the ears across the top of the head. Pain arising from structures below the tentorium cerebelli and the posterior fossa is felt posteriorly to this line and is conveyed by the glossopharyngeal and vagus nerves and by the upper cervical spinal roots. Pain arising from the posterior half of the sagittal sinus or the upper surface of the transverse sinus is transmitted over a branch of the first division (Arnold's nerve) of the trigeminal nerve and is referred to the frontal area; it is commonly retro-orbital. Gardner et al. and White and Sweet have suggested that an accessory pathway for pain from the supratentorial structures referred to the ear or to frontotemporal areas may lie in the nervus intermedius of the facial nerve.

Although early reports indicated that dural stimulation elicits strictly unilateral referral of head pain, further investigations have indicated that head pain of dural origin has limited clinical significance because of a lack of consistent specificity in its referral pattern.

Pain fibers carried in the intraspinal portion of the descending trigeminal tract and nucleus descend into the upper two segments of the cervical cord where they are joined by similar fibers from the facial seventh, ninth, and tenth cranial nerves. Sensory fibers from the first three cervical dorsal roots ramify throughout this center and connect with trigeminal neurons in the nucleus of the spinal tract. After synapsing, the second order of neurons cross the midline and terminate in the opposite dorsal horn. This mechanism explains referral of pain from the upper neck to the head and vice versa.

There is some evidence that pain fibers descend with the periarterial nerve plexuses in the neck to reach the lower cervical and upper thoracic spinal cord but the role of these fibers in headache is uncertain.

Clinical Approach. The history is all important in treating the patient whose sole complaint is headache, especially since physical signs are rarely seen in such a patient. Correct evaluation of a complete history will establish the diagnosis in most types of chronic, recurring headache, particularly in different types of migraine and tension headache.

Different possibilities are raised by the patient who presents himself with an acute onset of headache for the first time in his life. A severe headache of sudden onset, particularly if it is followed by impairment of consciousness or focal neurological signs, suggests a serious condition, such as hemorrhage, or an illness, such as meningitis. Headache appearing for the first time in the aged is probably not migraine or tension, nor does it usually reflect a primary psychiatric disorder. The headache here, if it recurs or is continuous, suggests cranial arteritis, glaucoma, carotid artery or vascular insufficiency disease, or hypertension.

Relationship of the onset of headache with time of day may indicate the underlying cause of the headache. For example, a headache resulting entirely from hypertension (210 mm Hg systolic over 100 mm Hg diastolic) is usually present on wakening. Space-occupying lesions and migraine may cause headache early in the morning, while cluster headaches are frequently nocturnal, wakening the patient after only a few hours of sleep. Headaches associated with frontal sinusitis may commence early in the morning; those due to maxillary sinusitis usually commence in the afternoon. Chronic sinusitis does not cause persistent headache. Onset of tension headache is generally not related to time of day; the patient may go to bed with the headache and wake up with it, or it may occur upon wakening or later in the day.

Location of the headache may be significant. Migraine tends to vary from side to side with different attacks and is commonly anterior. It is unilateral in two thirds of the patients and bilateral in the other third. The possibility of an intracranial mass must be considered if a recurring headache is always localized to the same side. The site of pain is usually not a reliable means of localizing cerebral tumors and can be misleading. As a broad generalization, intracranial lesions in the posterior fossa initially produce pain in the occipital nuchal region, whereas supratentorial lesions produce pain in the frontal, temporal and parietal region. In the absence of papilledema, if the headache is one sided, the side of the headaches is the site of the lesion. The headaches of space-occupying lesions become bilateral if cerebrospinal fluid pressure increases, but they may be unilateral earlier in their course. Disease of the paranasal sinuses, teeth, eyes, or upper cervical vertebrae induces pain that is referred in a regional but not sharply localized distribution that is fairly constant.

The quality of the pain should be carefully studied. A pulsatile, throbbing headache is of vascular origin whether due to vasodilatation of migraine or to hypertension or fever. The pain of neuralgia occurs as transient, shock-like stabs of intense pain. Headaches associated with brain tumors are usually of a steady aching quality and tend to be intermittent early in the course of the disease. The patient with tension (muscle-contraction) headache usually complains of a constant, tight, pressing or band-like ache; throbbing is conspicuously absent.

Intensity of the headache is not a reliable indication of the seriousness of the underlying cause; pain may be moderate with an intracranial lesion and severe in a chronic anxiety state. An extremely severe headache of sudden onset must always give rise to the suspicion of a subarachnoid hemorrhage.

The symptoms accompanying the headache may be an important guide to the underlying cause or type of headache.

Neurological deficits usually accompany a headache due to intracranial lesions. An infiltrating glioma, however, may extend throughout the hemisphere without causing headache because the larger blood vessels remain undisturbed until the late stage of this disease process, whereas compression of the brain from a meningioma is more likely to cause seizures, focal cerebral symptoms, or progressive impairment of intellectual function before headache appears. Patients with subdural hematomas almost invariably present with headache, because the increase in the size of the hemorrhage displaces the brain downward stimulating pain-sensitive structures.

Headache associated with tumors metastatic to the brain can be deceptive; while it is one of the most common associated manifestations, it is not necessarily constant or severe. Headache is a common symptom with carcinomatosis of the meninges and may be the presenting symptom for several months before mental and other symptoms develop.

Chronic meningitides, such as fungal, parasitic, or tuberculous, commonly have headache as an early complaint. Signs of meningeal involvement will point toward the need for further study, including examination of spinal fluid.

Vasculitis due to collagen tissue disorders may present with headaches and bizarre and varied focal or generalized neurological signs.

The patient should be carefully questioned about the relationship of his headache to his daily pattern of living or to recent experiences. An intracranial vascular disturbance and accompanying headache, whether caused by "hangover", fever, or intracranial tumor, will be aggravated by jarring, sudden movements of the head, coughing, sneezing, or straining at stool. Sexual intercourse may bring on a combined muscle-contraction and vascular headache and has occasionally been known to precipitate a subarachnoid hemorrhage.

Many headaches are precipitated by psychological or environmental or situational stress factors. But before the clinician places his patient in this diagnostic category, it should be clear from the symptoms and motivations that psychological factors are present. The exclusion of physical symptoms or signs and atypical features of the headache are not in themselves diagnostic of a headache of this type. A direct relationship between the headache and emotional conflict or situational difficulties should be determined.

Examination of the head and neck, including inspection, palpation, percussion, and auscultation, must be performed on all headache patients. The neurological examination must be complete. The cervical spine should be tested for tenderness and mobility. Examination of the skull for local infections, hardened or tender arteries, bony swelling, and sensitive areas should be part of the routine examination. Palpation and auscultation of the major cranial arteries should be done. There is some question about the diagnostic value of bruits, which are normally heard in children and sometimes heard in adults with no symptoms of cerebrovascular disease. Nevertheless, they may indicate cerebral atherosclerosis or cerebral angiomatous malformation.

As part of the initial examination, a number of ancillary studies are advisable for all headache patients. Initially noninvasive tests may be chosen; these may include simple radiographic examination of the skull and cervical spine, computerized axial tomographic (CAT) examination of the head, echoencephalography, and thermography. At times radionuclide imaging is included in the atraumatic group of studies.

Principal Varieties of Headache. There are several ways of classifying headache. The most useful classification is the one based as far as possible on the mechanism of the pain. The pathophysiology of certain specific categories of headaches and their clinical examples based on general mechanism will be briefly considered.

Headaches from intracranial sources are most often produced by traction, displacement of intracranial arteries, or inflammation in or about pain-sensitive intracranial structures, chiefly the large arteries, veins, venous sinuses, and certain cranial nerves. This form of headache is evoked by an intracranial mass (tumor, abscess, aneurysm), nonspecific brain edema, meningitis, and other infections.

Headache may result from distention and dilatation of intracranial arteries associated with a number of systemic conditions, including fever, infection, hypoxia, nitrite and foreign protein administration, hypertension, electrolyte imbalance, and metabolic disorders.

Disease of the extracranial structures of the head that may give rise to headache and head pain include glaucoma, errors of refraction, inflammatory processes in the eyes, nose and ears, and cranial and neck structures that include involvement of the ligaments, muscles, and cervical nerve roots.

One of the most common causes of headaches is contraction of the cervical muscles as a manifestation of emotional stress. This type of headache is called tension, muscular contraction or psychogenic. The headache results from long-sustained contraction of the skeletal muscles of scalp, face, neck, and shoulders. Concurrent vascular and local chemical changes within the skeletal muscles are factors in producing the pain.

Headaches may occur with no demonstrable evidence of any physiological disturbance as a manifestation of conversion mechanisms, hypochondriacal reactions, and delusional states.

A common sequela of minor or severe head injuries is headache. It may present intermittently for months or even years after a head trauma; however, it usually tends to disappear with the passage of time. A headache localized to the site of the skull or scalp injury may be due to stimulation of traumatized nerve endings in the contused scalp. A variety of extracranial and intracranial mechanisms may be responsible, including sustained contraction of the muscles of the neck and scalp, vasodilatation, scar formation in the scalp or cranium, injury to structures of the neck, tissue distortion, contusion or bleeding in the meninges, and subdural hematoma. Psychological mechanisms, including anxiety, fear, worry over loss of income or permanent disability, and compensation neurosis, may play an important part.

Migraine

The most extensively studied common headache syndrome is vascular headache of the migraine type. Migraine, often familial, is characterized by recurrent attacks of headache variable in intensity, frequency, and duration. Attacks are commonly unilateral and are usually associated with anorexia, nausea, and vomiting. They may be preceded by or associated with neurological and mood disturbances. All these characteristics are not necessarily present in each attack or in every patient.

Etiology of Migraine. The primary cause of migraine still eludes us; but there can be no doubt that the attack itself is associated with changes in the intracranial and extracranial arteries. The evidence for this, though largely indirect, is nevertheless overwhelming. Direct measurements of cerebral blood flow, though relatively sparse, point to a phase of cortical vasoconstriction during the aura followed by a phase of vasodilatation affecting both cortical and extracranial vessels. Reduction of cortical perfusion rates is shown by use of xenon-133 inhalation and intracarotid flow measurements, and angiograms taken during the aura reveal constriction of the cerebral arteries. The two phases are not sharply separated; some corfical areas show vasodilatation at a stage when vessels in other areas are still constricted. This would account for those cases of migraine in which the usual temporal profile of an aura followed by a headache is disturbed. The symptoms of the aura may continue into the headache phase, or the headache may precede the aura.

It has been demonstrated that cervical sympathectomy does not provide any lasting benefit in migraine. At present there is no convincing evidence that the neural control of blood vessels is impaired in migraine or that migraine is caused by abnormal neural discharge. Operations on every relevant nerve pathway have not interrupted the course of the migraine attack.

An adequate theory of the pathogenesis of migraine must take in account biochemical changes associated with the syndrome, particularly the role of the endogenous or exogenous vasomotor agents that influence the tone of vascular smooth muscle and alter the caliber of its vessels. Among the substances that could be involved are the amines (serotonin), catecholamines (epinephrine or norepinephine), histamine, and tyramine; heparin, the polypeptides (bradykinin, angiotensin), the free fatty acids (prostaglandins), and prolactin; gamma aminobutyric acid (GABA—inhibitory transmitter). The exact role of the platelets in migraine and the significance of platelet aggregation are unknown.

An important factor in the production of pain vessels appears to be the accumulation around the dilated arteries of various substances that are capable of sensitizing them to pain. During a headache the temporal artery on the painful side shows a greater catechol uptake capacity than the same artery on the pain-free side. It has been suggested by Harold Wolff and his co-workers that a sterile, local, inflammatory reaction occurs. In this view, this combination of vasodilatation and sterile inflammation is needed if the clinical syndrome of migraine is to become manifest.

At the onset of a migraine attack serotonin levels of the plasma fall, but an increase in the major metabolite of serotonin, 5-hydroxyindole acetic acid (5-HIAA), has been inconsistently demonstrated during a migraine attack. Serotonin will constrict scalp arteries in man, and its fall may play a part in the extracranial vasodilation character of migraine.

Prostaglandin EI will trigger migraine in subjects who have never previously experienced migrainous headache, and reserpine will precipitate an attack in patients who have migraine headaches. Hovrobin has presented laboratory evidence that suggests the biochemical changes and clinical observations associated with migraine can be explained by the concept that a prostaglandin-like material is the final common cause of all types of migraine.

Tyramine, a pressor amine found in certain foods (red wines, cheese), can evoke migraine in susceptible subjects. It is postulated that in dietary (tyramine) migraine the patient lacks the enzyme responsible for sulfate conjugation and that we may be dealing with an inborn error of metabolism.

It is of interest that a number of the vasoactive substances are associated with inflammation and have a wide range of pharmacologic activity at low concentrations. However, their physiologic roles cannot be stated with assurance except for a few. They are known to be important in the function of the body, and their discovery has provided new possibilities for therapeutic intervention in migraine by the use of drugs that antagonize either their direction action or their metabolism.

We must be cautious about interpreting changes in amines and other humoral agents found in venous blood as being primary factors in the initiation of an attack of migraine. Many of the humoral changes may result from dilatation of the vessels. The mechanism underlying all trigger factors appears to be some sudden rate of change in the external or internal milieu.

During the last decade these and other biochemical approaches to migraine have been vigorously investigated. It is fair to conclude that no clear picture has been evoked particularly as regards events in how the human organism responds biochemically to the stress that precedes and possibly provokes migraine.

Incidence. The incidence of migraine in the general population is difficult to evaluate, because perhaps half the migraine sufferers do not consult a physician. Estimates for the general population run from 5 to 10%.

Certain general characteristics may be shared by all types of vascular headaches of the migraine type, especially classic and common migraine. Women are more frequently affected by migraine than are men, but the ratio varies considerably in published reports. In early childhood, motion sickness and cyclic vomiting may be present without the headache. The period in a life-span when migraine first appears is extremely variable. The attack may start in infancy and continue until the later years of life (eighth decade), may begin in puberty and terminate at menopause, or may occasionally start in the forties and terminate in the sixties. In most patients, the headaches start in the second or third decade. At the time of menopause, the attacks may have an exacerbation after many years of remission or may begin at this time. Migraine may start at certain peak points, either psychologic or physiologic, in the patient's life, and long periods of unpredictable remissions may occur. In some women the attacks may occur only during or immediately preceding menstruation. As a rule, migraine sufferers lose their headache during pregnancy, especially after the first trimester, although occasionally the severity of the headache may increase with pregnancy. There are reports that migraine attacks may follow minor or severe head injuries, but in my experience these patients had migraine prior to trauma.

Many patients with migraine also have muscle-contraction (tension) headache, which may occur at various periods between their migraine attacks. Attacks of migraine may be precipitated or their frequency increased by the administration of oral contraceptives.

Diagnosis. Migraine attacks, which can occur in many complex patterns and setting, can be classified into the following types.

Classic Migraine. The headache of classic migraine is recurrent and periodic. Familial and personality factors are of great importance in its pathogenesis. As a rule, the prodromes are sharply defined. Contralateral neurologic manifestations, usually visual but occasionally motor or sensory, are common. The visual symptoms include scotomata, fortification spectra, field defects, and transient amblyopia. The pre-headache symptoms of classic migraine may appear transiently, inconstantly, or regularly, developing over ten to twenty minutes. Visual prodromes may be accompanied by electroencephalographic changes consisting of a slowing of rhythm in the affected occipital lobe.

There is a high incidence of ophthalmic migraine in individuals over fifty years of age, and unless the physician is acquainted with this partial syndrome and pursues the patient's description of the visual phenomena, he will be likely to make the wrong diagnosis, usually that of transient ischemic attacks. The usual ischemic attacks of transitory blindness (amaurosis fugax) are shorter in duration (seconds to three to five minutes), usually monocular, rarely hemianopic, and are not accompanied by a hemianopic fortification spectrum. The monocular visual loss may be total or partial, and occasionally photopsias consisting of showers of stationary flecks of light that disappear quickly may occur, as well as other types of scotomata. On the other hand, the older patient with migraine may have internal carotid artery disease with severe stenosis, and early recognition of the cause of these visual phenomena is of importance before a catastrophe occurs. Intraoptic disorders (visual phenomena of retinal disorders) and episodic blindness of giant-cell arteritis are other considerations in differential diagnosis. In some patients sensory disturbances may develop simultaneously in the fingers and tongue. In about 20% of adult patients, the headache may occur on the same side as the visual or sensory deficit or be bilateral. The quality of the pain is throbbing and unilateral, in the later stages often spreading to other parts of the head. Anorexia, nausea, and vomiting are concomitant features. Classic migraine occurs in about 10% of patients with migraine.

Common Migraine. This is the most frequent type of migraine, occurring in over 80% of migraine sufferers. The prodromes of common migraine are not sharply defined, and they may precede the attack by several hours or days. These vary widely from patient to patient and include psychic disturbances, fatigue, gastrointestinal manifestations (nausea, vomiting), and changes in fluid balance. The actual headache episode is frequently longer than in the classic type; it may last from many hours to several days. The pain is steady, unilateral or bilateral, and aching or throbbing in quality. Symptoms common to both types include irritability, chills, pallor, localized or general edema, sweating, and diuresis. The occurrence of nasal signs and symptoms may lead the physician to ascribe the headache to involvement of nasal structures. Sensitivity to light and noise are prominent features. This type of migraine commonly occurs on weekends and holidays.

Cluster Headache. Cluster headache (ciliary or migrainous neuralgia, histamine cephalalgia, petrosal neuralgia) occurs in a series of closely spaced attacks occurring several or many times daily for a number of days or weeks. These clusters may be followed by remissions of months or even years. Prodromes are uncommon. The pain may occur suddenly and wake the patient after an hour or two of sleep. Congestion of the conjunctivae, lacrimation, occasionally ptosis of the eyelids and sweating are associated manifestations. After twenty to ninety minutes the pain stops as suddenly as it began. Cluster migraine is more common in men but may occur in women. Not all agree that this type of headache should be classified under migraine.

In a few patients attacks of paroxysmal and neuralgic pain occur, mainly in the distribution of the first division of the fifth cranial nerve with Horner's syndrome (paratrigeminal syndrome), that resemble cluster migraine. The exact mechanism is unknown, but it may be due to inflammation in the region of the eye, nose, and internal carotid artery or edema in and about the walls of the internal carotid artery.

A unique spotted pattern of hypothermia has been found by thermography in two thirds of patients with cluster headache. The pattern appears to be the result of a fixed vascular state since it does not change even over a period of years. The findings are not altered by the presence or absence of headache, nor by the administration of vasoconstricting or vasodilating drugs. This thermographic picture is not found in other types of vascular headache.

Hemiplegic and Ophthalmoplegic Migraine. This rare type of migraine may occur in the young adult. In ophthalmoplegic migraine the pain is severe, on the same side as the ophthalmoplegia, and is accompanied by extraocular muscle palsies involving the third cranial nerve (internal as well as external ophthalmoplegia) and other oculomotor nerves. Often the paralysis occurs as the headache subsides—three to five days after the onset of a persisting headache. Recurrent attacks over years or months may occur. Repeated ophthalmoplegic attacks may cause permanent injury to the third cranial nerve. One should be alert for the presence of a sphenoidal mucocele or an intracranial aneurysm on the main trunk of the internal carotid or at its junction with the posterior communicating artery. The hemiplegic migraine complex is characterized by neurologic deficits, hemiparesis, or even hemiplegia. The neurologic phenomena of both hemiplegic and ophthalmoplegic migraine may persist for some time after the headache has subsided.

Basilar Artery Migraine. Bickerstaff introduced the term "basilar artery migraine," which is a fairly well-recognized clinical entity but can be a difficult diagnostic problem. This type of migraine occurs in young women and girls, often in relation to their menstrual periods. The first prodromal symptoms are usually visual and include visual loss and scintillations throughout both halves of the visual fields. This is quickly followed by vertigo, ataxia, dysarthria, and, occasionally, tinnitus and tingling and numbness in the toes and fingers, not necessarily all or in this order. Disturbances of consciousness may occur in some patients. The symptoms last from several minutes to forty-five minutes and are followed by a severe, throbbing occipital headache with vomiting. Sometimes the symptom pattern is similar to that of classic or common migraine.

Migraine Equivalents. Some patients who have had migraine attacks may have these replaced by the periodic occurrence of other bodily disturbances which have been called migraine equivalents. These may consist of abdominal pain associated with nausea, vomiting, and diarrhea (abdominal migraine); pain localized in the thorax, pelvis, or extremities; bouts of fever; attacks of tachycardia; benign paroxysmal vertigo; and cyclic edema. Impairment of consciousness, altered mental states, confusion, lethargy, and disorders of mood, sleep, and behavior have been reported as psychic equivalents of migraine.

Complications. In some patients, permanent sequelae may occur after severe attacks of migraine. Occasionally an attack precipitates major or minor cerebrovascular accidents. These include infarction or thrombosis of cerebral or retinal vessels as a sequela of the vasoconstrictor phase and hemorrhage resulting from rupture or diapedesis of the intracranial or extracranial vessels during the vasodilatation phase.

Many years ago, Charcot observed that the transient neurologic disturbances of migraine could become permanent. Recent arteriographic studies, which have excluded the presence of malformations, also indicated that permanent damage of neurologic structures may be associated with migraine. Lesions of the retina, cerebral hemispheres, and brain stem have been found in patients with migraine. The ages of these patients were below the usual age of onset of cerebrovascular disease. As a rule, the area most frequently affected is the occipital cortex, and a permanent hemianopsia may occur. Recent reports of studies with CAT scanning have indicated that local changes, including edema and infarction of the cerebral hemisphere, may be observed during severe migraine attacks.

Differential Diagnosis. Migraine must be differentiated from other conditions that may produce chronic recurring headache. A headache that continues for weeks or months suggests that it is caused by underlying anxiety and depression.

Migraine appears to be independent of the presence or absence of aneurysm or angioma in which the recurrent headaches are always on the same side of the head and focal neurologic signs as well as bleeding may be present. Typical periodic headache that occurs for years is never caused by saccular aneurysm; that is, an aneurysm de novo will not cause or predispose to migraine headache and is coincidental when the two are associated. The occurrence of migraine in patients with unruptured angioma is not frequent. It is possible that migraine with or without aura exists with angioma but is not related to this condition.

Except for brain tumors in the occipital lobe, expanding lesions in the cranium, neoplasms, abscesses, and hematomas are rarely accompanied by a headache that simulates migraine. The finding of choked disks, focal neurological signs, and abnormalities by the ancillary studies will serve to direct attention to the possibility of an expanding lesion and the need for further study.

Headache associated with temporal arteritis, carotid and basilar insufficiency, hypertension, and glaucoma must be considered in the differential diagnosis of migraine in older patients.

The existence of a relationship between migraine and epilepsy is still controversial. Reports in the literature indicate that there is a higher incidence of epilepsy in unselected migraine sufferers than in the population as a whole. Headache is common after a convulsion in epilepsy. Migraine differs from epilepsy in the timing of the attack; the onset of a migraine attack is rarely accompanied by loss of consciousness, although it may be followed by drowsiness or sleep. In epilepsy, the electroencephalogram frequently reveals specific abnormalities, whereas in migraine it is usually normal or shows nonspecific irregularities. Ergot preparations, which are specific in the treatment of acute migraine headache, are of no help in epilepsy. Viewing the problem from a broad perspective, there are some people with convulsive disorders who may have in their family history either epilepsy or migraine, and there are some similarities in these attacks but in only a small number of patients.

Although allergy is common in migraine patients, it is also common in the general population. There is no good evidence that inhaled or ingested allergens play any but an occasional role in producing a migraine attack.

Treatment and Management of Headache. In the treatment and management of a patient with headache we are concerned with a broad spectrum of medical, surgical, and psychological problems or combinations of these factors. As common to all problems of treatment, diagnosis is the first step in the management of headache. Treatment of headache as a symptom in the course of an already recognized disease is directed toward the fundamental pathophysiology. The choice of therapy and its degree of intensity will depend upon the specific problem presented and may entail operative therapy for remediable lesions, chemotherapy for infectious processes, treatment of metabolic disturbances, or removal of an allergic factor. Once the underlying cause has been determined and treatment started, the headache itself usually requires the appropriate analgesic.

The nonaddictive analgesics are effective for head pain of low intensity. For attacks of severe, persistent muscle-contraction headache the use of a non-narcotic analgesic sedative and tranquilizer combination is more effective. In combination, these drugs raise the pain threshold and reduce the anxiety and reaction to pain. Codeine sulfate (0.03 gm) may be used alone or in combination with acetylsalicylic acid (0.3 to 0.6 gm) if the pains are severe. Tranquilizers and sedatives in small doses are effective in treating the associated anxiety and tension. Antidepressants are most helpful in anxious and depressed patients. Physical dependence on these agents may develop, and it is therefore necessary that these patients be followed closely. The lack of sufficient data, including control studies, makes it wise to withhold judgment as to the degree of temporary or permanent success of acupuncture with headache patients.

Surgical procedures for relief of chronic recurring headache are usually not helpful or recommended; these include dorsal column stimulators, sensory rhizotomy, and the like.

A variety of autoregulatory techniques have been recently introduced for treatment of chronic recurring headache, particularly migraine and muscle-contraction (tension) headache. One of the major ones is biofeedback. There are a variety of other relaxation techniques from which some individuals secure temporary relief from their tension states. However, in all these techniques the underlying factors that produce the tensions are not usually understood by the patient, so that rather than getting at the cause of tension, a reconditioning or, in some instances, covering technique is used rather than insight into and working through of the patient's problem. The long-term results of these approaches to headaches need further evaluation.

Treatment of Migraine. The array of therapeutic approaches proposed for migraine is more remarkable for diversity than for therapeutic results. The management of the patient with migraine can, for practical purposes, be divided into three parts: general principles, symptomatic treatment of the acute attack, and prophylactic treatment.

General principles include elimination of the factors of importance in precipitating or provoking an attack and general mental and physical hygiene. The elimination of the factors of importance in precipitating migraine requires treatment of all underlying physiological or structural abnormalities that have been discovered in the examination of the patient. Treatment includes correction of medical disorders, such as anemia, metabolic disorders, or intercurrent infection, refractive errors, and dental problems, and removal or reduction of provoking factors. Examples of the latter are overload in environmental stress at home, at work, or in social situations; ingestion of foods containing tyramine (cheese or wine) or monosodium glutamate (i.e., "Chinese restaurant syndrome"), nitrites, particularly in hot dogs; phenylethyl amine (chocolate); offending allergens; missing of meals; exposure to glare or flickering lights; and certain drugs, such as oral contraceptives. It should be understood that the elimination of these provoking factors will not result in a complete disappearance of attacks in most patients.

Physical activity of the patient should be regulated so as to provide daily routine exercise, wholesome well-balanced meals, and general avoidance of food or beverages that may trigger migraine attacks. The patient should have a set time for retiring and arising and should not stay in bed later on weekends than during the week. Adequate social activities and periods of relaxation should be encouraged.

Symptomatic Therapy for an Acute Attack. Symptomatic therapy for migraine includes analgesics, sedatives, and antianxiety agents. Of all the agents used and studied, ergotamine tartrate is the most effective in the treatment of an acute attack. Analgesics combined with sedatives or tranquilizers may be helpful in the late stages of an attack of migraine or in mild attacks. If the pain is a mild, dull, aching headache, it may respond to acetylsalicylic acid in doses of 0.3 to 0.6 gm or to various combinations of this agent with 0.3 to 0.6 gm of phenacetin or acetaminophen and 50 mg of caffeine. A moderately severe headache may be relieved by 60 mg of codeine phosphate when ergotamine is contraindicated due to nausea and vomiting. For patients who cannot take ergotamine or for whom the drug is not effective, meperidine hydrochloride (Demerol) may be necessary, especially in severe attacks in which the headache has been present for hours. The danger of addiction in the migraine patient who uses this agent must always be considered.

It is important that medication be administered early in the course of an attack and that the dosage be adjusted to each patient. However, caution should be used in giving ergotamine to patients who have experienced prolonged specific neurologic phenomena (visual, sensory, motor). Patients vary greatly in their response to ergotamine, as they do to other drugs. Even in one individual, different physiologic states can cause different responses to the agent at various times. The improper use of this drug has caused many failures in therapy.

Caffeine acts synergistically with the ergot alkaloids by potentiating the vasoconstrictor effect of the ergot, as well as by producing faster and more complete intestinal absorption. This reduces the total dosage of ergotamine necessary to control an attack of migraine. Sedatives and antiemetics may be used to help control the nausea and vomiting that occur during the migraine attack or are induced by the ergotamine itself. Sedatives plus salicylates are of special value in treatment of a migraine attack in children.

Ergotamine tartrate can be given orally, sublingually, parenterally, or rectally. The recommended oral or rectal dose is 1 to 2 mg at the onset of headache, followed by 2 mg within the hour, but not more than 6 mg for any single attack. The intramuscular dosage is 0.25 mg to 0.5 mg at onset. Rectal suppositories have a higher degree of efficacy than oral preparations.

It is important to titrate the drug for each patient to find the appropriate dose for subsequent attacks. Most patients tolerate ergotamine tartrate well, but side effects may occur; these include aching muscles, paresthesiae, nausea, vomiting, and occasionally ischemia of the extremities, angina pectoris, and thrombophlebitis.

The problem of drug dependence in migraine patients must be considered in the management of this disorder. This is particularly noticeable in patients who take ergotamine or narcotics daily for many years. Manifestations of withdrawal are a possible complication in patients who use the drug daily and use it with increasing dosage for long periods of time. For most of these patients, gradual withdrawal of the drug and management of the underlying depression form the basis of proper treatment.

Dihydroergotamine, an ergot derivative, moderately constricts the extracranial arteries; its side effects (nausea and vomiting) are less severe than those of ergotamine tartrate, but its results are less predictable. It is administered only parenterally.

Occasionally, an acute attack is relieved by the inhalation of 100%

oxygen. The basis of this relief may be the reduction of the cerebral blood flow after inhalation of the oxygen.

Prophylactic or Interim Treatment of Migraine. There is no wholly effective treatment for prevention of migraine. The response to various treatments is highly individual and for each patient the treatment must be tailored to his needs. In prophylaxis or interval treatment, pharmacotherapy and psychotherapy are fundamental to success. Pharmacologic treatment is essentially the same for all types of migraine, including cluster headache.

The effect of drugs is difficult to assess; in some studies a placebo has reduced the frequency of migraine in over 40% of patients. Methysergide maleate (Sansert) has proved to be an effective prophylactic agent in migraine. Methysergide is chemically related to methylergonovine and is a potent antagonist of 5-hydroxytryptamine (serotonin). It may act by maintaining tonic vasoconstriction of scalp arteries if the plasma serotonin level drops during a migraine attack.

Daily administration of 2 to 6 mg of methysergide will suppress migraine completely or partially in approximately 60% of migrainous patients. However, from 20 to 40% of these patients experience such adverse side effects as abdominal discomfort, muscle cramps, and, in some, edema, numbness, tingling of extremities, or depression. Of this group, about 10% are unable to tolerate methysergide because of symptoms of peripheral vasoconstriction, intermittent claudication or rarely, angina pectoris. These last symptoms disappear when medication is discontinued. The medication should be discontinued after two months of use and then after a month off resumed in the same sequence.

In addition to the above early side effects, a syndrome resembling retroperitoneal fibrosis and pleuropulmonary and cardiac fibrosis occasionally develops during long-term therapy with methysergide.

Cyproheptadine hydrochloride (Periactin), which is antagonistic to both serotonin and histamine, has reduced the frequency and severity of headache in some patients. The side effects include drowsiness, the most common, with stimulation of appetite and weight gain as secondary effects.

Propranolol hydrochloride (Inderal), a beta-adrenergic blocker, has been used in the prophylaxis of migraine with limited success. The dilatation of peripheral arteries in response to adrenalin is thought to be due to the uptake of adrenalin by beta receptors in the vessel wall. Beta blockade could therefore prevent dilatation in response to any humoral agent employing these receptors.

Pizotifen is a benzocycloheptathioprene derivative which is structurally closely related to cyproheptadine. Initial pharmacologic reports suggest that it has marked antiserotonin and antihistaminic effects. In clinical trials the drugs appear to be safe and effective in the prevention of migraine.

Amitriptyline has been reported by Couch et al. as effective in the prophylactic treatment of intractable migraine. Beneficial results do not appear to have any relationship to the presence of symptoms of depression.

Barbiturates and minor tranquilizers may be beneficial in reducing anxiety, and they may temporarily improve the patient's ability to handle stress. These chemical agents should be used only on an intermittent basis. The benzodiazepines (Librium, Valium) appear to have a more specific action against anxiety and are preferable to the barbiturates or to meprobamate.

For migrainous patients who are also subject to depression, antidepressants, such as imipramine hydrochloride (Tofranil) and amitryptyline hydrochloride (Elavil), are more effective than the anxiety-reducing drugs.

Diuretics have not proved useful in the treatment of migraine, although the patient with edema (especially before menses) feels more comfortable following fluid loss. There is no evidence that retention of water is related to the migraine attack.

Daily use of ergotamine for migraine prophylaxis is not advisable. However, for patients suffering from nocturnal attacks of cluster headache, an oral dose of 1 to 2 mg before retiring, taken for a period of ten to 14 days, may help terminate the series of headaches.

Psychotherapy. The personality structure of the migraine patient, which needs careful evaluation, has been described as compulsive, with outstanding performance because of the emphasis on perfection, overconscientiousness, and ambition. No doubt some migraine patients have anxiety, neurotic depressive reactions, conversion, and dissociative and phobic reactions. No one personality type describes all migraine patients.

It is not surprising that if the situations in which some headaches occur and recur are analyzed in relation to their psychological, social, and emotional significance to the patient, the occurrence of headache may be related to a psychological or emotional stress. For these patients, the supportive doctor-patient relationship during the initial phase of therapy is a key step in treatment. The physician should limit himself to supportive therapy, guidance, counseling, and situational insight. Interpretive insight, uncovering transference, and long-term intensive therapy should be done only by the psychiatrist. Some physicians can receive useful advice from a psychiatrist in difficult management problems.

REFERENCES

Adams, C. W. M., Orton, C. C., and Zilkha, K. J.: Arterial Catecholamine and Enzyme Histochemistry in Migraine, J. Neurol. Neurosurg. & Psychiat., *31*, 50, 1968.

Albadran, R. H., Weir, R. J., and McGuinness, J. B.: Hypertension and Headache, Scot. Med. J., *15*, 481, 1970.

Bickerstaff, E. R.: Basilar Artery Migraine, Lancet, *1*, 15, 1961.

Bille, B.: Migraine in School Children, Acta Paidiatrica, *51*, 31, 1962.

Bradshaw, P., and Parsons, M.: Hemiplegic Migraine, A Clinical Study, Quart. J. Med., *34*, 65, 1965.

Chapman, L. F., et al.: A Humoral Agent Implicated in Vascular Headache of the Migraine Type, Arch. Neurol., *3*, 223, 1960.

Charcot, J. M.: Sur un Case de Migraine, Ophtalmoplegique (Paralysie Oculomotrice Periodique), Progr. Med. (Paris) 2nd Series, Vol. XII, *83*, 99, 1890.

Couch, J. R. et al.: Amitriptyline in the Prophylaxis of Migraine, Neurolgy, *26*, 121, 1976.

Fields, W., and Sahs, A. L.: *Intracranial Aneurysms and Subarachnoid Hemorrhage.* Springfield, Charles C Thomas, 1965, pp. 6–7.

Frazier, S. H.: Headache. In Friedman, A. P., ed.: *Research and Clinical Studies in Headache:* An International Review, Vol. II, Basle, Karger, 1969, pp. 195–215.

Friedman, A. P.: Part I, Migraine Headaches, J.A.M.A., *222*, 1399, 1972.

Friedman, A. P. et al.: Classification of Headache. J.A.M.A., *179*, 717, 1962.

Friedman, A. P., Harter, D., and Merritt, H. H.: Ophthalmoplegic Migraine, Arch. Neurol., *7*, 320, 1962.

Friedman, A. P., and Merritt, H. H.: *Headache; Diagnosis and Treatment.* Philadelphia, F. A. Davis Co., 1959, pp. 401.

Graham, J. R.: Methysergide for Prevention of Headache. Experiences in Five Hundred Patients over Three Years, N. Engl. J. Med., *270*, 67, 1964.

Graham, J. R., Suby, H. I., LeCompte, P. R., and Sadowsky, N. L.: Fibrotic Disorders Associated with Methysergide Therapy for Headache, N. Engl. J. Med., *274*, 359, 1966.

Haas, D. C., and Sovner, R. D.: Migraine Attacks Triggered by Mild Head Trauma, and Their Relationship to Certain Post-traumatic Disorders of Childhood, J. Neurol., Neurosurg. & Psychiat., *32*, 548, 1969.

Hanington, E., and Harper, A. M.: The Role of Tyramine in the Etiology of Migraine and Related Studies on the Cerebral and Extracerebral Circulation, Headache, *3*, 67, 1963.

Hovrobin, D. F.: The Role of Prostaglandins in Migraine. American Association for the Study of Headache, 19th Annual Meeting. June, 1977. Personal Communications (In Press).

Lance, J. W., Anthony, M., and Hinterberger, H.: The Possible Relationship of Serotonin to the Migraine Syndrome. In: *Research and Clinical Studies in Headache,* Basle, Karger, Vol. II, 1969, pp. 29–59.

Marshall, John: Cerebral Blood Flow in Migraine. Proceedings of the First International Migraine Symposium, London, September 17, 1976. (In Press).

O'Brien, M. D.: Cerebral Cortex Perfusion Rates in Migraine, Lancet, *1*, 1036, 1967.

Ostfield, A. M., Goodell, H., and Wolff, H. G.: Studies in Headache Mechanisms, Arch. Intern. Med., *101*, 755, 1958.

Pearce, J.: The Ophthalmologic Complications of Migraine, J. Neurol. Sci., *6*, 73, 1968.

Sicuteri, F.: Prophylactic and Therapeutic Properties of 1-methyl Lysergic Acid Butanolamide in Migraine, Int. Arch. Allergy, *15*, 300, 1959.

Sicuteri, F.: Headache Biochemistry and Pharmacology, Archivos De NeuroBiologia, *37*, 26–27, 1974.

Skinhj, E., and Paulson, O. B.: Regional Blood Flow in Internal Carotid Distribution during Migraine Attack, Br. Med. J., *2*, 569, 1969.

Tourtellotte, W., et al.: *Post-Lumbar Puncture Headaches.* Springfield, Charles C Thomas 1964, p. 69.

VanPelt, W. and Andermann, F.: On the Early Onset of Ophthalmoplegic Migraine, Am. J. Dis. Child., *107*, 628, 1964.

Wainscott, Gillian: Prolactin Levels During a Migraine Attack. Proceedings of the First International Migraine Symposium, London, September 17, 1976. (In Press).

Whitty, C. W. M.: Migraine Without Headache, Lancet, 2, 283, 1967.
Whitty, C. W. M., Hockaday, J. M., and Whitty, M. M.: The Effects of Oral Contraceptives on Migraine, Lancet, 1, 856, 1966.
Wolff, H. G.: Personality Features and Reactions of Subjects with Migraine, Arch. Neurol. & Psychiat., 37, 895, 1937.
Wolff, H. G.: Headache and Other Head Pain, 3rd Ed., New York, Oxford University Press, 1972, p. 57.

CONVULSIVE DISORDERS
(Epilepsy)

GILBERT H. GLASER, M.D.

Definition. Although epilepsy has been known since antiquity, it is difficult to define the disorder in terms which will cover its manifold features. Epilepsy has been defined as a paroxysmal disorder of the nervous system characterized by recurrent attacks usually with alteration of consciousness, with or without convulsive movement. This definition is inadequate because it does not cover the variety of manifestations which may occur in patients with recurrent seizures, in the category of the convulsive disorders or the "epilepsies."

Classification. In general, there are two ways of classifying patients with convulsive seizures; neither of these is entirely satisfactory but both have some merit. The first method classifies patients into two groups, symptomatic and idiopathic, according to the presence or absence of known organic factors which may be of importance in the occurrence of the attacks. This method of division is of value in calling attention to the necessity of a thorough study of each patient before initiating treatment. It is a fallacious method of division because it presumes that seizures in the patient with symptomatic epilepsy are due solely to the organic lesion. Conversely, it assumes that there is no lesion in the patients with so-called idiopathic epilepsy. This latter assumption is not justified. All that we can say is that we cannot demonstrate any pathology in these cases by the methods which are available at the present time.

The second method of dividing patients with seizures is that of separating them into several groups according to the manifestations which occur during the attack. This method of classifying the patients is of value because it calls attention to the areas or regions of the brain which are involved in the seizure and serves as a guide in the direction of the therapy.

Incidence. There are no totally accurate figures on the number of individuals who suffer with recurrent convulsive seizures. Estimates based on various epidemiologic studies indicate that approximately one half to 1% of the population or about one million people in the

United States are affected. Kurland estimates that the annual incidence rate in the United States is 48 per 100,000 population. The incidence rate is highest in the age group under five years (152 per 100,000) and drops to a lower level (40 per 100,000) between the ages of twenty and seventy years. In old age the rate rises to 74 per 100,000 population for ages eighty and over. The prevalence rate is about 650 per 100,000. There is little difference in the prevalence rate for age groups between ten and sixty years.

Seizures of unknown cause or those which accompany organic disease of the brain occur in all races and climates. The incidence of seizures is relatively greater in the male than in the female. In the 1500 noninstitutional cases studied by Lennox, the ratio of males to females was 100 to 77. This ratio varied quite significantly according to the age of the onset of seizures (Table 104). Late onset of seizures in the male sex is possibly related to the frequency of minor or severe head injuries in this sex.

As a rule, convulsive seizures have their onset early in life but they may start at any age. In the vast majority, seizures start before the age of twenty-five, but from this age to senility there is a small but fairly constant percentage for each decade in which seizures of unknown origin occur for the first time. Contrary to the general opinion no gross lesion can be demonstrated by clinical examination in many of the patients who develop seizures after the age of twenty years. As a rule, however, the later the onset of seizures the greater the probability that they are associated with some gross organic lesions of the brain. There are two peaks in the curve for the onset of seizures. The first peak is in the first two years of life and the second is at the age of puberty. The first peak is highest in the patients in institutions for epileptics and the second peak is highest in the noninstitutionalized cases.

Convulsive seizures associated with organic lesions of the brain may have their onset at any age of life. The distribution of the curve of the

Table 104.   The Frequency of Convulsive Seizures in the Two Sexes According to the Age of Onset in 1500 Noninstitutional Cases
(After Lennox)

Age at Onset of Seizures	No. of Females per 100 Males
Before 5 years	106
5 to 9 years	100
10 to 19 years	77
Over 20 years	59
Total	77

age of incidence is more even in these cases than in the cases of unknown cause, but like the latter, there are two peaks. The first is in the early years of life and the second after the third decade of life. The first peak is related to the fact that the developing brain of the infant or young child is much more apt to react with convulsive seizures when it is injured by trauma, by infections of the nervous system or by simple febrile illnesses. The second peak is related to severe head injuries and the neurological diseases of adult life (brain tumors, cerebral trauma and the like).

Inheritance. There remains considerable dispute as to the actual role of inheritance in the occurrence of convulsive seizure. Statistics which offer definitive information in regard to the role of inherited factors in the causation of epilepsy are relatively meager. Lennox found a high degree of concordance of epilepsy in similar twins. He also found that a history of recurrent seizures was present in 2.7% of the 12,119 near relatives (parents, siblings and children) of 2,130 epileptic patients. This incidence of 2.7% in near relatives is approximately five times as great as the incidence of the disease in the general population. According to Lennox, these figures would indicate that any given child of the average epileptic has about 39 chances out of 40 of being normal.

Various conditions may modify the weight of heredity. The incidence of a family history of epilepsy is lower (1.4%) in patients whose seizures developed following an injury than in those without a history of brain injury (3.0%). Familial incidence of epilepsy is greater in patients whose seizures started early in life and in female patients (Table 105).

Lennox considered the electroencephalogram to be of value in determining the "predisposition" to epilepsy. He found "some degree" of abnormality in the electroencephalogram in 50% of near relatives in contrast to the finding of such abnormalities in 16% of the adult normal population. However, the incidence of actual epileptiform abnormality is much lower. Yet, the Metrakoses have found a higher occurrence of

Table 105. The Incidence of Seizures in Blood Relatives of Patients with Epilepsy

(After Lennox, Am. J. Psychiat., 1946–47)

Age of Patient at First Seizure	Male Patients		Female Patients	
	No. of Relatives	% Epileptic	No. of Relatives	% Epileptic
0–4 years	1440	3.4	1307	5.8
5–19 years	2796	2.2	2374	2.9
20 years or over	2864	1.2	1633	1.2

epileptiform discharges in the EEG's of relatives of patients with epilepsy and spike-wave discharges, and others are finding similar "genetic" backgrounds in family members of patients with focal epilepsy.

On the other hand Lilienfeld and Pasamanick found significantly more abnormalities during the mother's pregnancy and delivery and in the neonatal period, in the records of 564 epileptic children than in a similar number of matched controls. They state that these findings raise doubts as to the significance of the genetic basis of convulsive disorders. They postulate a continuum of reproductive casualty composed of a lethal component, consisting of abortions, stillbirths and neonatal deaths, and a sublethal component consisting of cerebral palsy, epilepsy and mental deficiency.

Etiology of Convulsions. A great number of biochemical and physiological studies have been made on patients with convulsive seizures but the pathophysiology of convulsive seizures is still unknown.

Convulsions may result from an acute cerebral anoxemia of whatever cause, disturbances of calcium-phosphorus metabolism, hypoglycemia, excessive hydration and other metabolic disturbances, but it has not been shown that any of these disturbances is present in any significant number of patients with epilepsy.

The high incidence of seizures in patients with organic lesions in the brain makes it seem probable that the presence of damage to cerebral tissue is of great importance in the occurrence of seizures. Evidence of gross damage to the brain is lacking, however, in the majority of patients with seizures. It, therefore, must be concluded that other factors are responsible for the development of the abnormal discharge which precipitates the seizure. It is, of course, obvious that a cerebral abnormality, when present, cannot be the sole cause of the seizure. This abnormality is constant, but the seizures occur only at irregular intervals. Similarly, it cannot be presumed that inert tissues are the focus of an abnormal discharge, and it is more likely that the normal or nearly normal tissue adjacent to the injury is the site of origin of the epileptic discharges, *i.e.* the aggregate of abnormally excitable neurons, according to Jackson. An undue susceptibility, of the normal or relatively normal tissue in the neighborhood of destroyed or damaged nervous tissue, to various stimuli or metabolic disturbances would explain the high incidence of seizures in patients with organic lesions in the nervous system. The spread of seizure is through normal tissue.

It has been demonstrated that the application of acetylcholine to the cerebral cortex is followed by the development of abnormal cortical discharges, and that convulsive seizures can be produced by the injection of acetylcholine intravenously or intracisternally. Abnormal discharges which spread to adjacent and remote portions of the cerebral hemispheres are more easily produced by the application of acetylcholine when the underlying cortex has been partially isolated by severing a portion of its connections. Since acetylcholine is a normal constituent of nervous tissue and is important in the transmission of the nerve impulse, it is suggested that various endogenous and exogenous stimuli may release acetylcholine and thus excite a seizure discharge in an irritable focus. This also may be related to a shift in cationic balance in the neuronal environment. Reduction in inhibitory transmitter, gamma-amino butyric acid (GABA), also may be a factor.

Convulsive seizures may be produced in normal individuals by the injection of camphor, Metrazol, strychnine and by electrical stimulation. It could be said that a seizure is the normal mode of expression of the nervous system to overwhelming stimuli. In addition it has been shown that the electrical activity of the cortex may be influenced by afferent stimuli such as light and sound. In fact, in susceptible individuals, seizures may be rarely precipitated by these stimuli. Thus it may be postulated that the cerebral cortex, particularly any partially damaged or sensitive area, can be activated to produce a violent discharge sufficient to cause a seizure, by various internal or external stimuli without any inherent metabolic defect being present.

Conditions Accompanied by Seizures. From the foregoing it is clear that seizures are much more apt to occur in patients with organic lesions in the brain than in patients with a normal central nervous system. There are, however, certain diseases and injuries to the brain which have a relatively high incidence of seizures and others in which the incidence is only slightly greater than that of the general population.

The list of diseases and conditions which are frequently accompanied by seizures is extensive and includes developmental and congenital defects, cerebral aplasias, birth injuries, acute infectious diseases of childhood, meningitis, encephalitis, cerebral trauma, tumors, abscesses, granulomas, parasitic cysts, degenerative diseases of the nervous system, metabolic disturbances or intoxications such as uremia, water, and alcoholic intoxication, cerebral edema, cerebral vascular lesions, polycythemia, asphyxia, carbon monoxide poisoning, protein shock, anaphylaxis, Raynaud's disease, Stokes-Adam's syndrome, carotid sinus sensitivity, tetany, insulin shock, hyperventilation and the ingestion of convulsant drugs. The seizures associated with alcoholic intoxication usually appear within forty-eight hours after cessation of drinking, *i.e.* withdrawal seizures. The frequency of the association of various organic diseases with convulsive seizures is given in Table 106 for children and in Table 107 for all ages. It is noteworthy that the occurrence of convulsions is relatively rare (28%)

Table 106.   The Frequency of the Various Causes of Convulsion at Different Ages of Childhood

	Number of Cases at Age of					
Presumed Cause of Seizures	Less than 6 Months	6 to 36 Months	3 to 10 Years	10 to 16 Years	Total	%
Acute infections	67	201	62	0	330	34
Idiopathic epilepsy	8	66	110	37	221	23
Birth injury	79	49	22	3	153	16
Spasmophilia or tetany	22	57	0	0	79	8
Cerebral malformations	13	10	3	2	28	3
Meningitis or encephalitis	2	33	19	9	63	6
Post-natal trauma	1	4	11	0	16	2
Miscellaneous	3	5	17	5	30	3
Unknown	22	17	7	0	46	5
Total	217	442	251	56	966	100

Table 107.   The Frequency of the Various Causes of Recurrent Convulsive Seizures in 2,000 Noninstitutional Cases of Epilepsy at all Ages
(After Lennox)

Presumed Cause of Seizures	% of Cases
None demonstrated	77.6
Cerebral trauma	5.7
Birth injury or congenital defect	5.6
Brain infection	4.2
Brain tumor	2.6
Cerebral circulatory defect	1.9
Extracerebral causes	0.9

in infants and children in the absence of acute infections or clinical evidence of organic injury to the brain.

It should be noted that an isolated seizure, i.e. such as occurring after drug withdrawal or other accidental cause, does not mean a diagnosis of epilepsy. Such a diagnosis requires the recurrence of spontaneous seizures.

It is likely that the figure of 77.6% given in Table 107 for no demonstrable lesion is excessively high. Falconer and his associates, for example, found obvious organic lesions (mesial temporal sclerosis, small tumors, scars or infarcts) in 78 of 100 patients subjected to operation for temporal lobe epilepsy (see Table 113, page 879).

It is of interest to note at this point that the frequency of convulsive seizures in organic diseases of the central nervous system is not directly related to the severity or degree of cerebral damage. The incidence of convulsive seizures, although significantly greater than in the general population, is relatively low in certain diseases of the nervous system in which there is extensive cortical or subcortical damage. Examples of such conditions are uncomplicated cases of cerebral arteriosclerosis, with or without areas of encephalomalacia, and multiple sclerosis.

The incidence of seizures is particularly high when damage to the cerebral cortex is followed by the formation of a scar which is composed of fibroblasts and glia (penetrating wounds), and in abscesses and slowly growing tumors of the brain.

Pathology. There is no specific pathology of epilepsy. Seizures are common in patients with various organic lesions of the nervous system. The incidence of cerebral lesions or abnormalities in the nervous system is relatively high in patients who die in epileptic colonies. There is, however, a large number of patients who have suffered with seizures for many years in whose brains no gross abnormalities can be demonstrated. Lesions such as sclerosis of the Ammon's horn or minute areas of cortical cellular loss are considered by some to be the result of rather than the cause of seizures, but this remains the subject of continued research.

Symptoms. The clinical manifestations of seizures are so varied that an entirely satisfactory classification is difficult. The division which is used in this chapter is one that has been found to be useful in the clinical management of the patients with seizures.

Patients with seizures may be divided into four groups according to the manifestations which occur during the attacks: (1) Grand mal or generalized seizures. (2) Focal or partal seizures—jacksonian and generalized seizures with a focal onset. (3) Petit mal or minor attacks. (4) Psychomotor-temporal lobe attacks.

Grand mal is the most frequent type of seizure if numbers of affected patients are considered (Tables 108–110). Petit mal seizures are the next most frequent and psychomotor-temporal lobe attacks are the least common though they are being found more frequently. It is not unusual for a patient to have two or even all three types of attacks.

In a study of 586 patients (Table 110) treated in out-patient clinics, 434 were subject to only one type of seizure and the remaining 152 patients were subject to two or more types of attacks. Grand mal attacks occurred as the only type of seizure in 372 or 61%, and alone or in combination with other types of seizures in 524 or 89%; petit mal occurred as the only type of seizure in about 4% and alone or in combination with other types in 21%; psychomotor attacks were the

Table 108.   The Frequency of the Various Types of Convulsive
Seizures in 966 Patients of Various Ages with
Only One Type of Seizure
(After Gibbs, Gibbs and Lennox, Arch. Neurol. & Psychiat., 1943)

Ages	Grand Mal	Petit Mal	Psycho-motor	Focal	Total
0–9	77	36	7	14	134
10–19	184	42	25	18	269
20–29	172	10	30	9	221
30–39	128	4	18	7	157
40–49	76	1	10	12	99
50 and over	74	0	5	7	86
Total	711	93	95	67	966

Table 109.   The Incidence of the Combination of Grand Mal and
Other Types of Seizure at Various Ages in 294 Patients
(After Gibbs, Gibbs and Lennox, Arch. Neurol. & Psychiat., 1943)

Ages	Grand Mal and			Total
	Petit Mal	Psychomotor	Petit Mal and Psychomotor	
0–9	15	3	1	19
10–19	81	21	6	108
20–29	57	24	9	90
30–39	17	29	2	48
40–49	7	11	1	19
50 and over	4	6	0	10
Total	181	94	19	294

Table 110.   The Frequency of Various Types of Seizures
in 586 Patients

Type of Seizure	Alone	Associated with Other Types	Total	% of 586 Cases
Grand mal	372	152	524	89
Petit mal	25	100	125	21
Psychomotor	37	33	70	12

sole type of seizure in 6% and occurred alone or in combination with other types in 12%.

If the number of attacks is considered, petit mal is the most common seizure because it is not unusual for many attacks to occur daily in patients who are subject to this form.

Grand Mal Seizures. Approximately 90% of patients with convulsions suffer with seizures of the grand mal type. In the classical form the grand mal attack consists of an aura which is followed by a shrill cry, loss of consciousness and generalized tonic and clonic movements. During the convulsive phase of the attack there may be tongue-biting, urinary or fecal incontinence and, rarely, ejaculation. During the tonic phase of the attack the respirations may be suspended and the face becomes cyanotic. With the onset of the clonic phase respirations are jerky and stertorous. Saliva, mixed with blood if the tongue or inside of the cheek has been bitten, is blown from the mouth. After cessation of the convulsive movements, the patient relaxes. Consciousness may return within a few minutes or the patient may lapse into a heavy sleep to awaken several hours later. On awakening the patient may complain of headache, nausea, stiffness of the muscles and general fatigue. A period of mental confusion and behavioral automatism of several hours' or days' duration may follow a severe attack. Patients usually know that they have had an attack, except when they are nocturnal. In the latter case, the occurrence of an attack may be unknown to the patient unless he awakens on the floor with bruises on his body, has bitten his tongue or voided in bed.

At times, residual neurologic symptoms such as hemiparesis, monoparesis, sensory disturbances or dysphasia may exist after the seizure *i.e.* post-ictally. Such post-ictal paralysis has been called Todd's paralysis; it ordinarily lasts several minutes to hours, and may be a relevant clue to the focal origin of a generalized seizure.

There are many variations in the severity and duration of the attacks. The aura may be entirely absent and either the tonic or clonic phase may be so brief as to pass unnoticed. There may be no muscular contraction, the attack simulating simple syncope.

The duration of an individual attack varies from less than a minute to thirty minutes or more. The frequency varies from many in one day to one in several years. It is uncommon for more than one or two attacks to occur in twenty-four hours, but in some patients with infrequent attacks, one attack may be followed within a few hours by a second one. The occurrence of a series of attacks at intervals so short that consciousness from the first attack is not regained before the next attack supervenes is known as status epilepticus. This is unusual except in institutional cases, but many non-institutional cases have one or more episodes of status during the course of their disease, usually precipitated by a lapse in medication.

Grand mal seizures may occur at any time of day or night and there is no evidence of seasonal incidence. In some patients, there is an apparent periodicity to the attacks, particularly in women in whom they may be associated with the menstrual periods. In a small percentage, the attacks occur only at night or while the patient is sleeping, but in most patients the attacks are evenly distributed during the twenty-four hours. Spontaneous variations in the frequency of attacks are not uncommon. In some patients whose attacks occur at regular intervals, they may disappear entirely for several or many years. In others, there may be transient periods when the attacks are much more frequent than usual.

Aura. The aura is not something apart from the seizure, but is an integral part of the attack. Approximately 50% of the patients experience some sort of aura. Sometimes the aura is not followed by the full-blown attack. The duration of the aura may be long enough to allow the patient to lie down, but more commonly it is only a few seconds before other manifestations of a seizure develop. The aura is usually an ill-defined sensation described as a feeling of "weakness," "dizziness," "fear," "numbness," a "peculiar sensation" or rarely pain in the abdomen. Patients with focal lesions in the cortex are apt to have an aura which can be related to the damaged area. Occasionally, attacks may be preceded by a prodromal period of several hours' or even days' duration, during which the patient does not feel well or is mentally confused.

Jacksonian and Focal (Partial) Seizures. Jacksonian and focal seizures occur almost exclusively in patients with an organic lesion in the cortex. This lesion may be of macroscopic or microscopic size. It is commonly thought that the occurrence of jacksonian or focal convulsive seizures is pathognomonic of tumors of the brain, but in most of the cases these attacks are associated with lesions due to other causes (birth injury, trauma, infections and vascular lesions).

The focal seizures described by Jackson are associated with lesions in the motor cortex. The seizure starts with convulsive twitchings of one portion of the body, usually the distal part of one extremity. If the seizure starts in the fingers, the spread is to the wrist, the forearm, arm, the face and then to the homolateral leg. If the movements spread to the opposite half of the body, consciousness is lost and the further manifestations are similar to those of a grand mal seizure. The power of speech may be impaired or lost when the focal discharge arises in the dominant temporal or frontal lobe.

Lesions in other portions of the cerebral cortex may be accompanied by focal seizures (Table 111), but with the exception of the focal

Table 111.   Epileptic Seizures—Clinical and Anatomical Classification

(After Penfield and Erickson, *Epilepsy and Cerebral Localization,* Charles C Thomas, 1941)

Clinical Type	Localization
Somatic Motor	
1. General Seizure (Grand Mal)	Complete Motor
2. Jacksonian Seizure (Local Motor)	Pre-Rolandic Gyrus
3. Masticatory Seizure	Lower Rolandic
4. Simple Adversive Seizure	Frontal
5. Tonic Postural Seizure	Brain Stem
Somatic Sensory (Auras)	
6. Somatosensory Seizure	Post-Rolandic Gyrus
7. Visual Seizure	Occipital
8. Auditory Seizure	Temporal
9. Vertiginous Seizure	Temporal
10. Olfactory Seizure	Infra-temporal
Visceral	
11. Autonomic Seizure	Diencephalic
Psychical	
12. Dreamy State Seizure	Temporal
13. Petit Mal	
14. Automatism (Ictal and Post-ictal)	
15. Psychotic States (Secondary)	

sensory seizures which are characterized by a sensation of numbness or tingling in one extremity or one half of the body, they do not have the specific localizing value of a jacksonian seizure. They do, however, localize the lesion to one hemisphere and sometimes to a restricted portion of the hemisphere.

Psychomotor Seizures. A special type of focal or partial seizure is the psychomotor or temporal lobe (limbic) seizure. The temporal lobe and its deeper nuclear masses, the amygdala and hippocampus and their associated limbic structures, are vulnerable to many pathologic processes and a relatively high proportion of seizure states probably originates in these areas. Such seizures may well appear in at least 25% of all patients in childhood and over 50% in adult life, along with the coexistence of other seizures such as grand mal. In over 60% of such cases, a structural lesion is present in this anatomical system, either clearly diagnosable or confirmed from a history of trauma or encephalitis. Some patients with psychomotor seizures have been found with diffuse cerebral disease or focal lesions in other than temporal lobe structures (such as orbitofrontal) but even in these there is evidence that the clinical manifestations are due to propagation of epileptic discharges through temporal-limbic regions. In a number of cases a significant history of status epilepticus in infancy has been reported (Ounsted, et al.), indicating the importance of control of this condition as promptly as possible.

The most simple, but relatively rare type of focal temporal lobe seizure, due to a lesion involving the dominant lobe, is manifest by a paroxysmal dysphasic speech disturbance, either an inability to form speech components or a blocking of the ideation necessary to produce speech. Psychomotor-temporal lobe-limbic seizures usually are characterized by an aura of anxiety and visceral symptoms, especially a peculiar epigastric sensation welling up into the throat; this is followed by an alteration in consciousness but not a loss and is associated with many varied complex feeling and thinking states and automatic somatic and autonomic motor behavior. These phenomena are associated with at least a partial amnesia, particularly for the automatism. During the seizure itself, there first may be an arrest or suspension of activity followed by simple movements such as chewing, swallowing, sucking, lip smacking, and aimless motions of the arms and legs. These are followed by repetitive, usually stereotyped, automatisms of varying complexity which involve partially purposeful or inappropriate, often bizarre behavior associated in interplay with the environment and occasionally determined by psychological factors. The occurrence of unpleasant olfactory hallucinations associated with lesions of the mesial portions of the temporal lobe, the uncus, was called "uncinate" seizure by Jackson, who also described the "dreamy and confused" state of the patient during the seizure and occasionally post-ictally. Many varieties of such seizure patterns are encountered. In the young patients there is emphasis on visceral manifestations with expressions of hunger, nausea, vomiting, and abdominal pain. Destructive, aggressive behavior may occur, but usually is not goal directed. Affective disturbances, particularly expressions of fear, anger and depression, may be present. Occasionally, prolonged fugue-like states with running or wandering about may last many minutes. During some psychomotor seizures patients experience hallucinations, both visual and auditory, as well as interpretive illusions involving their own bodies or the immediate environment. These symptoms frequently are associated with ideational blocking and forced thinking, as well as peculiar feelings of déjà vu and déjà pensé.

The electroencephalographic concomitants (Fig. 186) of psychomotor-temporal lobe seizures are characterized by discharges of spikes, complexes, sharp and slow waves localized from the involved temporal lobe in at least 75% of instances, and often enhanced by sleep. Frequently, however, the abnormalities are bitemporal or more generalized and asynchronous representing transmission and diffusion of the paroxysmal discharges. This is particularly so in the electroencephalograms of children with this type of epilepsy.

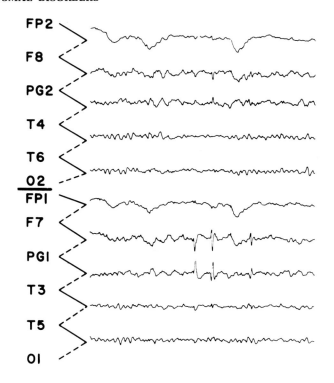

Figure 186. Temporal lobe seizures. A spike focus in the left anterior medial-temporal area is highly localized to a nasopharyngeal electrode (PGl) which is common to channels 7 and 8. (Courtesy Dr. Eli S. Goldensohn.)

Petit Mal Seizures. Petit mal seizures are a manifestation of epilepsy in childhood and rarely, if ever, have their onset after the age of twenty. They are also characteristic of so-called idiopathic epilepsy. They may occur in patients with birth injuries or developmental defects or may develop following acute febrile illnesses in childhood, but they are most commonly seen in children with no gross lesion in the nervous system and practically never appear for the first time in adult patients with cerebral tumors, abscesses or following cerebral trauma. It is thought by some that the focus of the abnormal discharge which precipitates a petit mal is subcortical.

According to Lennox, the syndrome of petit mal epilepsy consists of a triad of symptoms, myoclonic jerks, akinetic seizures and the typical petit mal attacks—transient absences or loss of contact with the environment. These three symptoms were classified together by Lennox on account of similarity of the electroencephalographic changes and also because they may be refractory to the drugs which are effective in the control of grand mal seizures.

Myoclonus consists of sudden involuntary contraction of the muscles of the trunk or extremities. The movements produced by these contractions may be slight or they may be so violent as to cause the patient to drop or throw an object held in the hands or they may upset equilibrium if the muscles of the trunk or lower extremities are affected. Myoclonic jerks (Fig. 187) may occur in patients with petit mal seizures, but they are equally as frequent in patients whose seizures are of the grand mal type. In some patients, myoclonic jerks may occur at irregular intervals for several hours or days, increasing in frequency and severity until a grand mal seizure occurs. Myoclonus is also a symptom of an organic disease of the cerebellum, brainstem and cerebral cortex known as myoclonus epilepsy.

Akinetic seizures are characterized by sudden loss of tone in all of the muscles of the body of such severity that the patients falls to the

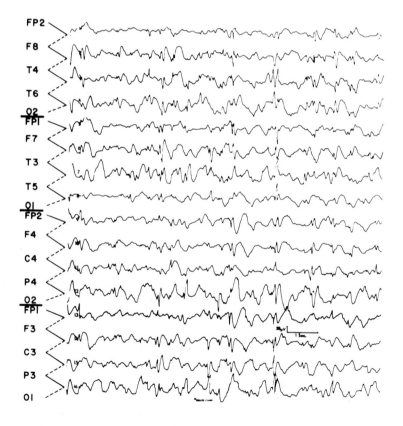

Figure 187. Myoclonic seizures in a patient with progressive degenerative disease. Bursts of multiple spikes shown are sometimes associated with observable myoclonic jerks. (Courtesy Dr. Eli S. Goldensohn.)

ground. The fall is sometimes so violent that the patient may seriously injure himself. It is difficult to determine whether there is loss of consciousness at the onset of the akinetic seizures. If there is any loss of consciousness, it is extremely brief, because the patients immediately arise from the fall and most of them claim that there was no lapse in consciousness. Akinetic seizures may occur in patients who have typical petit mal attacks, but they also occur in patients whose clinical seizures are of the grand mal type.

Petit mal attacks are characterized by a brief loss of consciousness with little or no tonic or clonic movement. In some patients, the attack may last for only a second or two and consist of a fixation of the gaze and blankness of expression which is unnoticed except by the most careful observer. In others, the attacks are of longer duration, lasting from fifteen to ninety seconds. In these attacks, the patient is out of contact with the environment and there may be a few clonic jerks of the arms or of the eye muscles. It is rare for the patient to fall in even the most severe attacks. There may be a drooping of the head, the patient may stagger a few steps or there may be a loss of control of the urinary sphincter. At the termination of the attack, the patient is immediately alert and continues previous activities. This immediate alertness makes it difficult to determine whether the patient actually suffered any loss of consciousness. The length of the lapse can be determined by talking to the patient during the attack and asking him to repeat what was said. If a nonsensical list of names of animals, followed by a few letters of the alphabet is recited to the patient during the attack, it can be shown that there has been a loss of consciousness and a rough estimation of its duration can be determined. The length of the loss of consciousness can be monitored by taking numerous serial pictures of the patient's face and the electroencephalogram.

Unlike grand mal seizures, petit mal attacks may occur with great frequency in the afflicted subjects. In some patients there may be only a few attacks daily but in others there may be as many as 20 or 30 in the course of a single hour. As a rule, they are most frequent in the first few hours after arising, or when the patient is sitting quietly while eating or reading. They are relatively infrequent during active exercise or attention. Spontaneous variations in the frequency of attacks are not uncommon. In some patients they may be infrequent or entirely disappear for several to many months. Cases of so-called petit mal status have been reported. In these unusual cases there is a prolonged alteration in the state of consciousness lasting for several or many hours. During this period the patient appears confused, forgetful and is incoherent. Associated with this state, there is a more or less constant spike and slow wave abnormality in the electroencephalogram.

Petit mal epilepsy is a disease of childhood. In the majority of cases the onset of seizures is in the first decade, but in some it may be delayed to the time of puberty. Some patients may continue to have petit mal attacks in adult life, but it is not uncommon for the seizures to become less frequent as the child grows older and in many cases they disappear before the age of twenty. Grand mal or psychomotor seizures may develop at any time in patients who had only petit mal seizures at the onset, and may persist in adult life in the patient who ceases to have petit mal attacks.

The occurrence of frequent petit mal seizures in childhood with cessation in adult life has been described as a separate syndrome known as pyknolepsy. There is no justification for this classification, since these patients do not differ from the usual case of petit mal. There are no criteria which are of value in separating the patients who will cease to have their seizures from those who will develop grand mal or psychomotor attacks.

Atypical Seizures. Prolonged periods of mental cloudiness or automatic behavior with complete amnesia for the entire period are also described under the term of psychic equivalent attacks. These seizures, or rather periods of abnormal behavior, are poorly understood. They are extremely rare but are of considerable medico-legal importance since patients may commit some misdemeanor or serious crime while they are in such attacks. Their behavior usually is not goal-directed, however.

Pain in the abdomen may occur as an aura in patients with seizures, and it is claimed by some authors that paroxysmal attacks of abdominal pain may be the only manifestation of the convulsive seizures. These cases have been described as a clinical entity under the term of abdominal epilepsy. The evidence in support of the claim that the abdominal pain is an epileptic manifestation consists of the finding of an abnormal electroencephalogram at the time of the occurrence of the pain, the favorable results of treatment with anticonvulsant drugs or the development of recurrent convulsive seizures in later years.

In some patients there are brief periods in which the patient experiences minor motor movements and partially loses contact with the environment. This type of attack is apt to occur in patients with grand mal seizures, who are receiving anticonvulsant therapy. These so-called minor or fragmentary seizures are probably manifestations of a disturbance in the cerebral cortex which remains localized and does not spread to other portions of the cortex.

A syndrome known as infantile spasms is characterized by the occurrence of lightning-fast akinetic and myoclonic seizures, associated with moderate to severe mental retardation. The electroencephalographic findings are quite characteristic and are described by the term hypsarhythmia. There are high sharp irregularly occurring

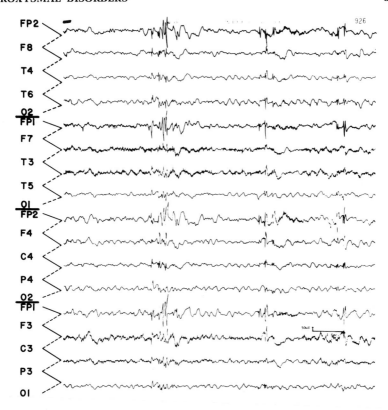

Figure 188. Tonic spasms of infancy. High voltage rhythmic and arrhythmic slow waves in the delta range and spikes and irregular spike and wave discharges in generalized and random distribution appear in all areas. This constellation of abnormalities is referred to as hypsarrhythmia. (Calibration: 50 μV and 1 second.) (Courtesy Dr. Eli S. Goldensohn.)

spikes in all leads, interspersed with many high voltage slow waves (Fig. 188). This syndrome has been found in association with phenylketonuria or hypoglycemia and with developmental defects or organic diseases of the nervous system in infants. Nonspecific degenerative changes in the gray and white matter of the cerebral cortex have been found in autopsied cases. Corticotropin and adrenal steroids are of value in the control of the spasms but do not seem to have any effect on the mental defect.

Laughter, as one of the manifestations of an attack, has been reported in patients with psychomotor seizures (gelastic epilepsy).

Precipitating Factors. In the majority of patients, the attacks occur without any obvious precipitating factor. In isolated cases, however, the attacks may be always related to some specific stimulus and in many others, an occasional attack can be attributed to some precipitating factor. This is not surprising when it is remembered that abnormalities in the activity of the cerebral cortex of epileptics can be activated by a wide variety of stimuli, including drugs, sleep, sound, light, and the like. The term "reflex" epilepsy may be applied to some of these cases.

The electroencephalographic abnormalities and the characteristic clinical attacks can be regularly precipitated by hyperventilation in patients who are subject to petit mal attacks. Grand mal or focal seizures can be produced by the administration of sub-convulsive doses of the convulsant drugs and grand mal seizures can be precipitated by excessive hydration by the drinking of water and the prevention of diuresis by the injection of pitressin. Rarely, seizures of akinetic or grand mal type may be precipitated by a sudden loud noise. A few cases have been reported in which the seizures occur only when the patient is listening to music (musicogenic epilepsy). Although these cases are extremely rare, a number of well-authenticated cases have been recorded and most workers in the field of epilepsy have seen one or more cases. In another form seizures are precipitated by light—usually of a flickering nature. Experimentally petit mal and occasionally grand mal seizures can be precipitated by stroboscopic light. Grand mal seizures may be produced by viewing television in susceptible patients, particularly if the set is defective and there is flickering of the intensity of the light or rapid horizontal or vertical shifting of the picture (television epilepsy).

Localized convulsive movements and loss of consciousness sometimes occur in amputees when a sensitive point on the stump is stimulated (stump epilepsy). Forster and Penfield reported the case of a young girl with a small tumor in the parietal cortex in whom localized abnormal cortical activity in the electroencephalogram and focal seizures could be precipitated by tapping the shoulder on the side opposite to that of the cerebral tumor. Fainting attacks or convulsions may follow a prolonged bout of coughing (laryngeal epilepsy). The physiological mechanism of these attacks has not been clearly elucidated. Occasionally grand mal seizures may be precipitated by prolonged reading (reading epilepsy). Seizures may occur in infants as a result of apnea in crying.

The role of emotional stimuli in the precipitation of seizures is often unclear. There is no doubt that in patients with many seizures an occasional attack may follow immediately upon some acute emotional experience. The coincidence of attacks with acute emotional stimuli is not sufficiently frequent, however, to make the latter a significant factor in the course of the disease in other patients.

In some patients, seizures occur only during sleep at night or when they take a nap in the daytime. It is known that sleep produces changes in the electroencephalogram and in these individuals, the changes must be of a sufficient degree of severity to precipitate an attack. The mechanism of this is not understood.

Signs. There are no physical findings that are diagnostic of epilepsy. Scars on the tongue or lips may result from lacerations which occur during attacks. Subconjunctival and subcutaneous hemorrhages in the face and neck may occur as result of vascular congestion during a seizure, especially in men who wear tight collars. Fractures of the skull or other bones may result from falls against hard objects and compression fractures of the spine are not an infrequent complication of the violent muscular movements.

Abnormal neurological findings may be present in the patients in whom the convulsive seizures accompany organic lesions or disease of the nervous system. These abnormal findings are characteristic of the underlying pathologic condition and are exactly the same as those which occur in patients having similar lesions without convulsive seizures. Abnormal neurological findings may be found in patients with so-called idiopathic epilepsy: (1) during an attack, (2) as a result of injuries sustained during seizures, and (3) as the result of untoward side action of anticonvulsant medicines. Extensor plantar responses and loss of pupillary reflexes are the most common abnormal findings during a seizure. Cerebral contusion, cerebral laceration, cranial nerve damage and subdural hematoma are some of the complications which occur as the result of falls during seizures. The neurological symptoms and signs which result from drug therapy are discussed later.

There is considerable controversy regarding the subject of mental deterioration in patients with convulsive seizures. The impression is widespread that mental deterioration is inevitable. This impression arose because the majority of statistics on this subject were compiled from institutional cases. The findings of the studies on institutional cases, which constitute only a small portion of the patients with epilepsy, are not applicable to non-institutionalized cases. In the study of over 2,000 patients who were seen in clinics or in private practice, Lennox found that 67% were mentally normal, 23% slightly deteriorated and only 10% definitely deteriorated. Mental deterioration was more common in patients whose seizures were associated with organic lesions of the brain. Mental deterioration was most frequently seen in patients in whom damage to the brain occurred in the first year of life and it was also more common in patients with injury to the nervous system in adult life than in the group of patients with no known lesion in the brain, although seizures in the latter group were more frequent and had occurred for many more years.

The mental level of the patients in the group without organic lesions in the brain was related to the mental level in the first years of life, the frequency and type of seizures and the duration of the period during which the patient had been subject to attacks. Seventy-five per cent of the patients who were mentally normal in infancy were normal at the time of examination. Mental deterioration, when present, was commonly associated with the occurrence of frequent seizures over a period of many years. Psychomotor seizures, grand mal and petit mal attacks appeared to be harmful in regard to the development of mental impairment in the order named. The role of status epilepticus in infancy is significant.

Keith and his co-workers found a greater incidence of mental retardation in 296 children with epilepsy than in the control group. The percentage of retardation was not related to seizure type, but was much greater in the group in which the convulsive disorder was associated with an organic lesion in the nervous system.

There is a great deal of discussion regarding the existence of a personality type which is characteristic of patients with epilepsy. It is claimed by some that the epileptic patient is egocentric, pedantic and emotionally impoverished. It is quite true that some patients with seizures show these personality traits and others show various personality features which are considered to be deviations from the normal. It has not been shown, however, that such personality traits are due to the seizures. They may be related to the underlying cerebral pathologic lesions, when such exists, and they are due in part to the difficulties which these patients encounter in their progress through life. Abnormal personality traits are uncommon in patients whose seizures are controlled by treatment and who are able to engage in the usual activities of life.

Mental disturbances and psychotic episodes in the interseizure period are not uncommon in the course of epilepsy, particularly in patients whose seizures are not controlled by treatment. These psychotic episodes are, in general, of three types: Transient episodes of uncontrolled behavior; psychotic episodes of several days' or weeks' duration, characterized by confusion, delusions and mental clouding; and a prolonged or permanent psychosis, similar in character to that of schizophrenia.

When mental symptoms occur as a paroxysmal outburst of brief duration, they are considered by some to be an atypical seizure in the nature of a psychic equivalent. Psychotic episodes which are prolonged for several days or weeks may follow immediately upon a seizure or a series of seizures or their onset may have no relation to an attack. The cause of these psychotic episodes is not known. They may be in some way related to a disturbance in cerebral activity associated with the disease or secondary to the administration of anticonvulsants. In the majority of cases, these episodes disappear spontaneously regardless of whether the type of anticonvulsant medicine is changed. It is not known whether prolonged states of psychotic behavior in a patient with seizures are related to the epileptic process or whether there may be a coincidence of epilepsy and schizophrenia in the same individual. There is evidence that these states are more frequent in patients with psychomotor-temporal lobe epilepsy.

Laboratory Data. With the exception of the electroencephalogram, laboratory findings are within normal limits in the majority of the patients with seizures of unknown cause. When the seizures are associated with some metabolic disturbance such as hyperinsulinism or hypoparathyroidism, there will be a low sugar or calcium content in the blood. When seizures are associated with brain tumor, brain abscess or other organic diseases of the nervous system, the laboratory findings will be those which are characteristic of the underlying disease process.

Although the cerebrospinal fluid is normal in the majority of patients with seizures of unknown cause, slight deviations from the normal are present in a small percentage of the cases. A brief discussion of these abnormalities is advisable because of the importance that is placed upon the examination of the cerebrospinal fluid in the determination of the cause of seizures in any given patient. In a series of over 800 cases, the only abnormalities were slight pleocytosis (4 to 10 cells per cu mm) in 4%, an increased protein content in 10% (see Table 112) and a pressure between 200 and 330 mm of water in 9%. The increased pressure in the majority of these cases could be related to failure of the patient to relax during the measurement of the pressure. If care is taken to secure complete relaxation, the pressure should be normal. The slight pleocytosis and increased protein content which are found in a small percentage of cases are probably related to the presence of small areas of cerebral contusion and laceration which resulted from falls in recent seizures. This can be proven by repeating the examination

Table 112.   The Protein Content of the Cerebrospinal Fluid in 793 Patients with Convulsive Seizures of Unknown Cause

Protein Content (mg per 100 ml)	No. of Patients	%
7 to 45	710	90
45 to 85	80	10
85 to 100	2	0
100 to 200	1	0

several weeks later. The cerebrospinal fluid should then be normal unless additional seizures with falls have occurred in the interval.

Electroencephalograms. The electroencephalogram is of value in establishing the diagnosis of epilepsy and is an aid in determining the type of seizure. The factors which influence the frequency of abnormalities in the electroencephalographic tracings of patients with seizures are discussed later. It must be remembered that a normal electroencephalogram does not exclude the diagnosis of epilepsy, nor does the finding of minor abnormalities confirm the diagnosis. Nonspecific abnormalities similar to those found in seizure-free intervals in a large percentage of the epileptics are found in 10 to 15% of the population

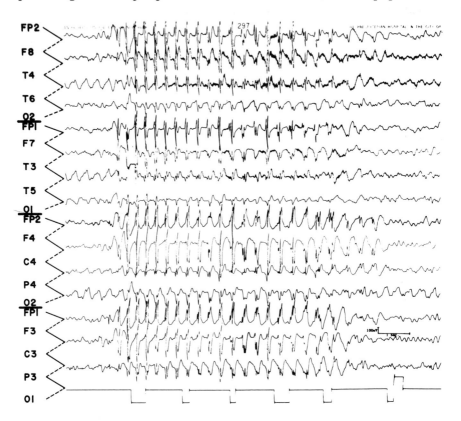

Figure 189. Absence with 3 per second spike and wave complexes (petit mal). Three per second spike and wave discharges in generalized distribution begin and end abruptly. The patient involuntarily stopped hyperventilating at the beginning of the discharge and resumed hyperventilation when it was over. In the lowest line, auditory stimuli are signalled by a downward deflection of the pen. When the patient recognizes the stimulus she presses a button which deflects the pen upward. During the attack the patient is unable to signal recognition of the sound stimuli until the 3/sec spike and wave discharge has subsided. (Courtesy Dr. Eli S. Goldensohn.)

who have never been subject to seizures. The occurrence of abnormalities of a specific type, known as seizure discharges and which are described below, are distinctly rare except in patients who are subject to seizures.

In their earlier studies, the Gibbses and Lennox found that electroencephalographic records taken during a clinical seizure showed abnormalities which were characteristic for each of three clinical types of seizures and that short bursts of abnormal activity were not infrequently found in the tracings which were taken in the interval between attacks.

The petit mal seizure (Fig. 189) is characterized by the bilaterally synchronous occurrence in all leads of high voltage rounded waves occurring at the rate of 3 per second, usually with a spike superimposed on each wave. Short bursts of this type of abnormality are common in all patients with petit mal epilepsy in the interval between attacks, and when it persists for more than a few seconds there is a depression of consciousness, as manifested by a delayed or lack of response to visual or auditory stimuli.

Characteristic of psychomotor epilepsy is the occurrence of spike discharges from the temporal lobe, particularly during sleep. These discharges may be bilateral, especially in children.

Grand mal seizures (Fig. 190) are characterized by the rapid or

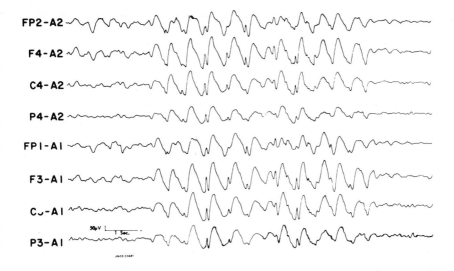

Figure 190. Generalized major and atonic seizures with mental retardation. Slow spike and wave discharges at 2 cycles per second are superimposed on a poorly organized background. This is typical of the clinical condition sometimes referred to as the Lennox-Gastaut syndrome.

sudden development of high-voltage spikes occurring at the rate of 20 to 30 per second. During the clonic phase of the seizure the voltage increases but the frequency decreases. Immediately following the seizure the tracing is almost flat with little or no evidence of cortical activity. Short bursts of abnormal activity characteristic of grand mal attacks are found only rarely in the seizure-free intervals in patients who are subject to grand mal attacks.

In addition to short bursts of abnormal activity of the types described above, the electroencephalogram of patients with epilepsy may show other abnormalities in the interval between seizures. Variation in the frequency or voltage may be found. While such abnormalities are not specific for epilepsy, their occurrence is an indication of an instability of cortical activity and are, therefore, of some diagnostic value.

During a seizure the abnormalities in the electroencephalogram may involve all portions of the cortex. In the interval between seizures focal abnormalities are present in a high percentage of the patients with a focal lesion in the cortex and are of value in establishing the diagnosis of cortical injury resulting from trauma, infections, tumors, or vascular accidents. Focal abnormalities in the temporal lobes are relatively common in the records of patients with seizures of the psychomotor type if the records are taken during sleep or after sleep deprivation. It is not known whether focal abnormalities, when present, are always indicative of a focal lesion or whether they may be due to an excessive irritability of apparently normal cortex. In addition, the presence of a focus in one region of the cortex does not necessarily indicate that this area of the cortex is the site of the original discharge. In some cases the electroencephalographic abnormality is a reflection of activity in some adjacent or remote or subcortical focus.

Abnormalities are found in the electroencephalographic tracings in practically all patients with seizures if the record is taken during an attack. The reports in regard to the incidence of abnormalities in the tracings which are taken in the interval between attacks vary from a low of 50% to a high of over 85%. These variations are due to a number of factors including the type and frequency of seizures to which the patient is subject, the duration of the tracing and the physiological state of the patients.

Abnormal tracings can be obtained in almost all children who are subject to frequent attacks of the petit mal type if the record extends over several hours or if the patient breathes deeply and rapidly for two to three minutes. On the other hand, normal records may be obtained in as high as 50% of adult patients with infrequent grand mal or psychomotor seizures when a single short record is taken while the patient is awake. The Gibbses have reported that the incidence of "seizure discharges" of a focal or generalized nature increased from

36% when the record was taken while the patients were awake to 82% when the patient fell into a natural sleep. A similar increase in the frequency of abnormalities in the electroencephalographic tracings can be obtained if sleep is induced by hypnotic drugs. An increase in the frequency of certain abnormalities in the electroencephalogram can also be produced by photic simulation (Fig. 191). This so-called activation of the electroencephalogram has been used as an aid in the diagnosis, but its chief value is in the activation of a focalized abnormality in patients with organic lesions in the brain, which could serve as a guide to the neurosurgeon in operative treatment.

Diagnosis. The diagnosis of convulsive seizures can be made without difficulty if the patient is observed during an attack, or if an adequate description of the attack can be given by a reliable witness. More difficult, however, is the determination of whether there is some

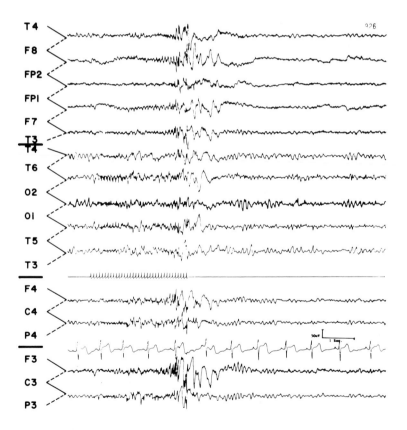

Figure 191. Photic sensitive epilepsy. Stimuli at 10 flashes per second (line 11) precipitate generalized multiple spikes followed by spike and wave discharges which outlast the photic stimulation. (Courtesy Dr. Eli S. Goldensohn.)

abnormality which may be playing a role in the occurrence of the seizures. For this reason, every patient with seizures should be subjected to a thorough study including a complete history, general physical and neurological examination, roentgenograms of the skull, determination of the glucose, non-protein nitrogen, and calcium content of the blood, electroencephalogram, examination of the cerebrospinal fluid and radioisotope brain scanning. Other diagnostic tests of value are echoencephalography, pneumoencephalography and cerebral angiography, and especially the new computerized axial tomography (CAT brain scan) of the brain.

The history and the results of the preliminary examinations will determine whether pneumoencephalography or cerebral angiography is indicated. If the attacks are of a focal nature or if focal neurological abnormalities are found which cannot be adequately explained, one or both of these may be indicated. However, the use of the CAT scan is reducing markedly any need for pneumoencephalography and angiography.

Differential Diagnosis. The differential diagnosis in patients with seizures is mainly concerned with the question as to whether there is a focal lesion in the brain or a metabolic defect which is amenable to treatment. Brain tumor, brain abscess, vascular malformations, adenomas of the pancreas, hypoparathyroidism are among the conditions which it is important to exclude. These can be diagnosed from the results of routine and special examinations previously discussed.

Convulsive seizures must be distinguished from hysterical attacks. This differential is not difficult if the patient is observed during an attack. The manifestations of convulsive seizures are extremely varied and the absence of tongue biting, incontinence or other isolated features of a seizure cannot be taken as an indication that the attack is of hysterical nature. In addition, the bizarre behavior and automatic activity of patients in psychomotor-temporal lobe attacks may appear to the inexperienced observer to be the simulation of an attack. There are no absolute criteria for the differentiation of an hysterical attack from an epileptic seizure. Perhaps the best guide is the state of consciousness of the patient. If the patient can be aroused from a "major" seizure by a noxious stimulus or if the events which transpired during the attack can be recalled fully, it is unlikely that a real seizure has occurred. Hysterical attacks usually occur in the presence of an audience and are frequently precipitated by emotional situations and are not followed by headache, muscle soreness or mental cloudiness. It must be remembered, however, that emotional stimuli may act as a precipitating factor of convulsive seizures. The electroencephalogram may be of value, but the final diagnosis is usually dependent on a thorough psychological study of the patient or the effect of anticonvulsant therapy on the seizures. Finally, it should be noted that major hysterical seizures are uncommon at the present time.

Clinical Course. Once the pattern of epileptic seizures has been established for a number of years, the chances of complete remission are poor. It is true that remissions for several or many years do occur spontaneously in a small percentage of cases and therapeutically induced remissions can be obtained in a much larger percentage. We cannot speak, however, of a clinical cure since seizures may return after an interval of ten to twenty years in patients with spontaneous remissions, and recurrence of seizures in therapeutically induced remissions of three to five years' duration is not unusual if treatment is withdrawn.

According to Lennox, spontaneous remissions of one to five years' duration occur in 23% and remissions greater than five years occur in 6% of the patients. Probably the percentage of remissions is higher than these statistics indicate. In taking the history of patients with seizures, it is not infrequently found that a relative had seizures for a number of years but they stopped after a certain age.

There are certain features which offer a more favorable prognosis in regard to remission of seizures. The probability of a spontaneous or therapeutically induced remission is good if there have been only a few seizures, if the seizures have their onset after childhood, if there is no gross brain injury, and the electroencephalogram becomes and remains normal.

It has been generally assumed that the prognosis with regard to relief of seizures is poor in patients with post-traumatic epilepsy. It is our experience that these patients respond as readily to anticonvulsive therapy as those with no known organic lesion. Walker reports that more than one-third of a group of 246 cases with post-traumatic epilepsy were free of seizures five to ten years after injury. Less than half of these patients were receiving anticonvulsant therapy.

The relationship of febrile convulsions in infants and young children to the development of epilepsy merits special discussion. According to Lennox-Buchthal seizures occur in approximately 5% of all children under the age of five. In approximately one half of these patients the seizures are related to some febrile illness. Severe, prolonged seizures in infants can produce serious damage to the brain which may result in retardation of mental development. It is generally agreed that the occurrence of seizures in young children with febrile illnesses does not necessarily presage the later development of epilepsy but the likelihood of this eventuality is great if the seizures recur with every febrile illness, if there are multiple seizures, or if there are paroxysmal abnormalities in the electroencephalogram in the seizure-free interval. The probability of the ultimate development of epilepsy is, of course, great when the seizures are "explained" on the basis of teething, dietary indiscretions or other such nonspecific factors. According to Millichap the height of the body temperature is an important factor in the occurrence of seizures. Such febrile seizures may be the precursors of mesial temporal sclerosis and psychomotor-temporal lobe epilepsy (Lennox-Buchthal, Falconer, et al.). The prevention of recurrent febrile seizures is, therefore, an important consideration.

Although longevity is compatible with the diagnosis of epilepsy, the mortality rate is higher than that of the general population. With modern methods of treatment this mortality rate is rapidly decreasing. The principal causes of death in patients with epilepsy are similar to those of the general population and include heart disease, pneumonia, tuberculosis and cerebral vascular lesions. In addition death may occur as a direct or indirect result of the seizures. Exhaustion in status epilepticus, suffocation in single seizures and fatal injuries in falls are several of the more common causes of death of patients with epilepsy.

Treatment. The treatment of patients with convulsive seizures can be divided into four parts: (1) Elimination of the factors of importance in the causation or precipitation of attacks; (2) general mental and physical hygiene; (3) medical therapy directed toward elevations of the convulsive threshold and thus the prevention of attacks; and (4) surgical therapy in carefully selected patients with focal epilepsy.

1. *The elimination of the factors of importance in the causation of seizures* requires treatment of all underlying physiological or structural abnormalities which have been discovered in the examination of the patient. This includes surgical removal of operable tumors of the brain, evacuation of brain abscess, treatment of infections or endocrine abnormalities such as hypoparathyroidism or hyperinsulinism, and the correction of any physical defects. The question of the advisability of removing scar tissue resulting from traumatic or vascular injuries to the brain will be discussed more fully later.

2. *Mental and Physical Hygiene.* It is only rarely that the elimination of causative factors indicated above will result in the disappearance of attacks; in the vast majority of patients, control of the attacks requires, in addition, regulation of physical and mental hygiene and the administration of anticonvulsive drugs. The period of treatment in the majority of patients is measured in terms of years or in a lifetime. Patients must be encouraged to use all of their resources to overcome their feelings of inferiority and self-consciousness resulting from the attacks. Adults should be assisted in obtaining productive work which will occupy their time and give them remuneration. Children should be kept in school unless the frequency of attacks unduly disturbs the routine of the classroom, or unless mental deficiency requires special facilities. A long-continued schedule of psychotherapy is of value in

some patients in aiding them to adjust to their difficulties, and may have in some instances a significant effect on the frequency of the attacks. Education of other members of the family in regard to their attitude toward the patient's illness is of great importance. Excessive attention and over-solicitousness should be avoided and the family should not be allowed to make a chronic invalid of the patient.

Physical activity of the patient should be regulated so that there is a set time for eating and sleeping and regular exercises every day. These exercises should be of a moderate nature and the patient should not participate in competitive sports to the point of exhaustion. Meals should be wholesome and of a simple nature with the proper amount of carbohydrates and proteins and an abundance of fresh fruits and vegetables. Alcoholic beverages are to be avoided. Bowels can be regulated by training and, if necessary, by the judicious use of mild laxatives. The patient should have a set time for retiring and arising and should not be allowed to stay in bed after the other members of the household have arisen. Special activities, such as parties, dancing, moving pictures, and so on, should be encouraged. Swimming, horseback riding and otherwise dangerous sports can be permitted when there are proper safeguards. The risk involved in these activities is justified in most instances in order to prevent the development of chronic invalidism. Activities which endanger the lives of others, such as driving of automobiles, should be under appropriate regulation when seizures are not controlled. Commitment of the patient to an institution is not desirable unless mental deterioration or unduly violent or frequent attacks not controllable by treatment make it necessary. On the other hand, definitely deteriorated, destructive or psychotic patients should not be kept at home and allowed to disturb seriously the lives of other members of the family.

3. *Medical Therapy.* The efforts directed toward the social and mental hygiene of the patient are of great importance, but the success of such measures depends to a large extent upon the ability of the physician to prevent the occurrence of seizures. There are effective measures at hand for the prevention of seizures and they should be given an adequate, thorough trial in each individual patient. The most effective method for the control of seizures is the use of the anticonvulsive drugs; namely, phenobarbital, mephobarbital (Mebaral), phenytoin or diphenylhydantoin sodium (Dilantin, Epamin, Epanutin), mephenytoin (Mesantoin), primidone (Mysoline), carbamazepine (Tegretol), trimethadione (Tridione), paramethadione (Paradione), ethosuximide (Zarontin), phensuximide (Milontin), methsuximide (Celontin), dextroamphetamine (Dexedrine), acetazolamide (Diamox), and bromides.

The ketogenic diet, which was formerly used extensively in the treatment of petit mal seizures in children, has fallen into disuse because of the difficulties inherent in its use and because medical therapy is effective in a high percentage of the patients with this type of attack. It is still of value, however, in selected cases.

The decision regarding which drugs should be used in a given case depends mainly on the nature of the attacks. It is important to remember that, if satisfactory results are not obtained with one of these drugs, others should be tried. In some patients, a combination of two or more drugs will yield much better results than the use of one alone. A sudden change in the type of therapy may be accompanied by an increase in the frequency of attacks or the precipitation of status epilepticus. For this reason the old drug should be continued for several days while the full dosage of the new drug is gradually established.

Indications for the Use of Specific Drugs. Phenobarbital or phenytoin (diphenylhydantoin) sodium are the drugs of choice in the treatment of patients with grand mal seizures because of their high therapeutic index. If satisfactory results are not obtained, primidone (Mysoline) can be utilized. Mephenytoin (Mesantoin) should be reserved only for the most resistant cases because of its high incidence of toxic reactions. A combination of phenytoin with phenobarbital or primidone is often more effective than any one of these drugs when used alone. When used in combination, a full therapeutic dose of each drug must be used. Primidone is oxidized *in vivo* to phenobarbital in significant quantities; therefore, primidone and phenobarbital should not be used in combination.

In patients with psychomotor-temporal lobe or psychic equivalent seizures, phenytoin sodium and primidone or carbamazepine are the drugs of choice. For petit mal seizures, ethosuximide (Zarontin) is the drug of choice, followed by trimethadione (Tridione), paramethadione (Paradione) and phensuximide (Milontin). If patients are subject to petit mal seizures and grand mal or psychomotor attacks, one of the "anti petit mal" drugs should be given in combination with phenytoin sodium, phenobarbital or primidone. Acetazolamide (Diamox) is often an effective adjunctive medication for these types of seizures, but may have to be administered intermittently because of the development of tolerance.

Serum anticonvulsant drug levels now can be determined and utilized in adjusting the proper dose of medication for each patient. These measurements also allow the physician to verify that the medications are being taken or whether there may be a problem in absorption, metabolism or excretion. Previously, the dose of medication was adjusted on the basis of therapeutic effect or toxicity. These criteria still are appropriate, but in a significant number of cases tolerance to clinical manifestations of toxic drug concentrations may exist, for example, making clinical assessment alone not an efficient indicator of drug concentrations capable of exerting untoward reactions in nervous system, bone marrow, liver, etc. These reactions now can be avoided by monitoring the serum concentration of each drug at appropriate intervals. A range of therapeutic serum concentrations now has been established for most of the major anticonvulsants (i.e., phenytoin, phenobarbital, primidone, ethosuximide) (see below). To a certain extent these concentrations are those at which minimal toxicity exists rather than maximal therapeutic benefit, and there is relatively wide variation among patients. Dosages should used in a thoughtful manner in each case, rather than as absolute guidelines. For example, a patient with completely controlled seizures and a low serum concentration of the anticonvulsant used should not have the dosage raised merely to achieve a "therapeutic level." Some patients may exhibit toxic reactions at relatively low serum concentrations of a drug.

Dosages to Be Used—Phenobarbital. For the average adult the initial dose of phenobarbital should be 0.1 gm daily. This can be given at bed time. After a trial period of several weeks or as long as is necessary to determine whether this dose is effective, further increases can be made in the dosage until the patient is taking as much as 0.3 gm per day. If this amount of the drug is not sufficient to control the seizures, it is probable that a further increase will not be of value. In children, the dose of phenobarbital should be in proportion to weight, but it has been found that children are able to tolerate and require almost as large a dose as adults. It is, therefore, advisable to give children, over six or seven years of age, the minimum dose of 0.1 gm per day. However, some children become hyperkinetic when taking phenobarbital, even at low dosage, necessitating discontinuation of the drug, and substitution of non-barbiturate medication.

In infants and young children, phenobarbital has been found the most effective drug to prevent recurrent febrile seizures. The useful therapeutic range in the serum is from 15 to 25 μg/ml, with increasing central nervous system depression occurring with higher serum concentration. Doses above 50 μg/ml are definitely toxic, although some patients on chronic dosage tolerate this manifesting but a slowness of thought processes. Drowsiness is common at the start of the treatment but this disappears with continued use of the medicine in the majority of patients, and it is only occasionally necessary to discontinue this treatment because of its persistence.

Phenytoin sodium (5,5-Diphenyl Glycolyl Urea, diphenylhydantoin, Dilantin Sodium, Epanutin, Epamin). This drug is particularly valuable in the treatment of psychomotor and grand mal attacks. It has the advantage over phenobarbital and the bromides in that it has little or no hypnotic activity. Regulation of the dosage is more difficult, however, and minor toxic symptoms are frequent. The toxic symptoms are usually not serious and it is almost impossible for a patient to take a fatal dose of the medicine.

The principle of administration of phenytoin sodium is similar to that of phenobarbital, that is, the establishment and maintenance of a reservoir of the drug sufficient to control the seizures. In the average adult, the initial dose should be 0.1 gm, three times daily. If any seizures occur after two weeks of this dosage, it should be increased to 0.4 gm daily. Further increases in the dosage should be by increments of 0.1 gm until the maximum dose of 0.6 gm daily is reached. In the majority of adults, 0.4 gm is the optimum dose. In children over twelve or fourteen years, the average dose is 0.3 to 0.4 gm and in younger children 0.2 to 0.3 gm. The medicine can be given in divided doses spread out through the day or twice daily. The drug may cause gastric upsets; this can be prevented by giving it along with meals or with some food. The effective therapeutic range of serum concentration is from 10 to 25 mg/ml with increasing incidence of toxicity as the concentration exceeds 25 mg/ml. At 45 to 50 mg/ml almost everyone will have toxic symptoms. After oral administration of the drug, effective levels usually are not reached until after thirty-six to forty-eight hours.

The toxic symptoms of phenytoin sodium are different from those of phenobarbital in that nervousness or sleeplessness rather than drowsiness is more commonly an early symptom. Other toxic symptoms are gastric distress, nausea and vomiting, unsteadiness of gait, hypertrophy of the gums, dermatitis, hyperchromic anemia, adenopathy, and occasionally encephalopathic symptoms.

The minor toxic symptoms are frequently transient and may disappear with continuation of the therapy or when the dosage is temporarily reduced. Nystagmus and ataxia can be produced in practically all patients if the dosage is raised sufficiently high. A few adults will tolerate as much as 0.6 to 0.8 gm, but toxic symptoms usually develop when the dose is increased beyond 0.5 gm. The appearance of these symptoms calls for a temporary or permanent reduction of the dosage. If the reduced dose is not effective in controlling the seizures and attempts to increase the dose again result in the appearance of toxic symptoms, a combination of phenytoin sodium and phenobarbital or primidone should be tried, or one of the other hydantoins, such as mephenytoin, should be substituted.

Gastric discomfort, nausea and vomiting may be controlled by the administration of the drug alone with a little bicarbonate of soda or at meal time. Dermatitis occurs within two weeks of institution of therapy in approximately 5 to 10% of the patients and is usually of a scarlatiniform or morbilliform nature and may be accompanied by fever. The rash usually disappears within a few days after withdrawal of the drug. Recurrence of the rash when treatment is reinstituted or the development of an exfoliative dermatitis precludes further use of the medicine.

One of the troublesome toxic symptoms of the drugs is hypertrophy of the gums. This is most common in children and varies from a slight swelling of the gums to a marked hyperplasia with almost a total covering of the teeth. The hyperplastic tissue is usually quite firm without any tendency to bleeding and is not related to any disturbance in the absorption or utilization of vitamin C. This swelling of the gums can be retarded by daily massage of the gums. Excessive growth of the gum tissue can be excised by electric cautery.

The development of encephalopathic symptoms in patients under therapy with phenytoin sodium is unusual. These may be manifested by increase in seizures, a confusional state or delirium and slowing of the electroencephalogram. Reduction in dosage ordinarily relieves the symptoms. Actual psychotic states are rare and preclude the continual use of the drug.

Primidone (5-Phenyl-5-ethyl-hexohydropyrimidine-4, 6-dione) (Mysoline). This compound is of value in the control of grand mal and psychomotor seizures when given alone or in combination with phenytoin sodium. The average dose for adults is 0.75 to 1.5 gm daily. The dosage for children varies from 0.125 to 0.75 gm daily. Because of the relatively high incidence of early side effects and toxicity it is recommended that the initial dosage be low; *i.e.* in an adult, 125 mg twice daily with gradual increments to therapeutic effect.

Primidone is actually a desoxybarbiturate, and significant amounts of phenobarbital are derived from it metabolically. However, the overall anticonvulsant effects are different from and may be more than those of phenobarbital, since primidone often is effective in cases not responding to phenobarbital alone. Some of this additional effect may be due to the derived metabolite phenylethylmalonamide (PEMA). The range of effective blood levels are 5 to 15 μg/ml for primidone, and for PEMA, 5 to 15 μg/ml. Toxic reactions to primidone include nausea, vomiting, dizziness, somnolence, headache and minor psychic disturbances. These disappear with withdrawal of the drug or proper regulation of dosage.

Carbamazepine (5-carbamyl-dibenz (b, f)-azepine), (Tegretol). Originally used in the treatment of trigeminal and glossopharyngeal neuralgia, carbamazepine is regarded now as often effective in the control of complex partial seizures of the temporal-lobe-psychomotor type. As with other similar medications, combination with phenytoin may be more useful than either drug alone. The dosage of carbamazepine should begin with 100 μg (one-half tablet) and be increased gradually to 200 mg 3 times daily, as an average. Peak plasma level per dose is reached within 2.5 hours and the therapeutic range is regarded to be 2 to 4 μg/ml, but there is much individual variation. The toxic range is 8.5 to 10 μg/ml and manifestations include dizziness, unsteadiness, drowsiness, diplopia, nausea, rashes, and rarely renal dysfunction. Leukopenia and aplastic anemia occurred and periodic blood counts are recommended. The drug should not be administered to patients sensitive to tricyclic substances or taking monoamine oxidase inhibitors.

Trimethadione (Tridione) (3,5,5-Trimethyloxazolidine-2,4-dione). The use of this drug is accompanied by a cessation or reduction in frequency of petit mal attacks in more than 50% of the cases. In a few patients, the cessation of attacks is accompanied by a decrease in the abnormalities in the electroencephalogram. If this occurs, it may be possible to discontinue the use of the drug without recurrence of the petit mal seizures. The drug is of no value in the control of grand mal or psychomotor seizures. If patients are subject to one of the latter types of seizures, as well as petit mal, phenytoin sodium or phenobarbital should be given along with trimethadione.

The dosage of trimethadione for the treatment of petit mal varies from 0.3 to 3.0 gm daily, starting with 0.3 gm and gradually increasing the dose until the seizures are controlled or toxic symptoms appear. Among the toxic symptoms are skin rashes, which require a cessation of the treatment, and visual symptoms—an unusual sensitivity to light or hemerolapia. This latter symptom is apt to develop in adolescent or adult patients and is uncommon in young children. The "photophobia" is not accompanied by any change in visual acuity and disappears when the medicine is discontinued.

Several cases of fatal aplastic anemia and several cases of nephrosis following the administration of trimethadione for periods of several months have been reported. An unusual myasthenic syndrome also has occurred. Prolonged use of the drug may also be accompanied by a decrease in the percentage of polymorphonuclear leukocytes in the blood without an absolute decrease in the total number of leukocytes. Although it is not known whether the observation of precautions will make it possible to prevent serious or fatal changes in the blood, it is recommended that routine blood counts be made monthly in patients using trimethadione. Owing to its potential dangers, the use of trimethadione should be restricted to those cases with frequent petit mal attacks and the drug should be discontinued if any toxic symptoms develop. Paramethadione (Paradione) may be substituted for trimethadione, but the toxic effects of the two drugs are almost identical.

Mephenytoin (Mesantoin). Various derivatives of the hydantoins have anticonvulsive properties. In some patients, some of these hydantoin derivatives may be more effective in controlling grand mal or psychomotor seizures than either phenobarbital or phenytoin sodium. Work on the majority of these drugs is still in the experimental stage with the exception of mephenytoin, 3-methyl,5-phenyl,5-ethyl hydantoin, which has been given an extensive clinical trial. The average dose for children is 0.4 gm daily, and for adults is 0.6 gm. The maximum daily dose is 1.0 gm. The drug can be used in combination with phenytoin sodium. The most common symptoms of overdose are drowsiness and ataxia. Toxic rash may also develop. Fatal agranulocytosis or pancytopenia has been recorded in a number of cases treated with mephenytoin. Complete blood counts should be made at monthly intervals in patients receiving mephenytoin. The severe toxicity of this drug usually limits its usefulness.

Mephobarbital (Mebaral) (3 Methyl, 5 phenyl ethyl barbital). Various barbiturates have anticonvulsant activity, but only phenobarbital and mephobarbital are used to any extent. Mephobarbital is equally as effective as phenobarbital in the control of seizures; it is actually totally transformed into phenobarbital by liver metabolism. We have not seen any appreciable difference in the action of the two compounds and prefer phenobarbital on account of its lower cost. The dosage of mephobarbital for adults is 0.2 to 0.6 gm daily, and 0.1 to 0.4 gm for children.

Phensuximide (Milontin) (N-Methyl-a-phenylsuccinimide). This drug has been reported to be effective in the control of petit mal seizures in some patients who are not benefitted by trimethadione. The daily dosage varies from 0.75 to 3.0 gm, the average for adults being about 2.4 gm. Toxic side effects in the nature of nausea, dizziness, drowsiness, hematuria, vomiting and dream-like states are seen in about 20% of the patients receiving this drug. These symptoms clear when the drug is discontinued or the dosage sufficiently reduced. Ethosuximide (Zarontin) has almost entirely replaced phensuximide in the treatment of petit mal seizures.

Ethosuximide (Zarontin). This is the drug of choice in the treatment of petit mal seizures. The therapeutic effects are equal to those obtained with trimethadione, and the side effects are less serious. The drug is marketed in the form of gelatin capsules (250 mg) or as a liquid (50 mg per ml). The dose in young children is 250 mg 2 or 3 times daily. In older children the drug can be given in dose of 250 mg 4 times a day. Larger doses may occasionally be necessary. The reported side effects include abdominal discomfort, headache, drowsiness, mental changes and dermatitis. Most of these side effects will disappear as the medication is continued or on reduction of the dosage. The drug should be withdrawn if rash occurs.

Amphetamine Sulfate (Benzedrine). Amphetamine sulfate or other sympathomimetic compounds are useful as an adjuvant in the treatment of patients with convulsive seizures. They have no apparent direct anticonvulsant action, but they are useful in combatting the lethargy produced by phenobarbital or primidone. Their stimulative effect may be of value in reducing the frequency of petit mal attacks in children. The dose of amphetamine varies from 5 to 20 mg daily according to the needs of the patient. The toxic side effects of these compounds are anorexia, insomnia, and overstimulation.

Bromides. Bromides, which were formerly the main therapeutic agent in epilepsy, have been replaced almost entirely by phenobarbital and the hydantoins. They are, however, occasionally effective when other forms of therapy fail. Although any of the salts may be used, the drug is most commonly given as the sodium or potassium salt, in tablets or aqueous solution. The average dose for an adult is 1 gm three times daily with proportionate doses to children according to size. In the absence of toxic symptoms this dose can be increased to a maximum of 2 gm three times daily. The chloride intake must be kept at an adequate level to prevent undue replacement of chloride ion in the body fluid by the bromide. Facilities for the determination of the bromide content of the serum should be available. The effective level may be as low as 100 mg/100 ml in some patients, whereas 300 mg/100 ml may not be effective in others. Toxic symptoms usually develop with a concentration of 150 mg or greater. The chief objections to the use of bromides lie in the frequency of the development of skin rash, toxic psychosis and their reputed tendency to product mental dullness.

Combination of Phenytoin Sodium with Phenobarbital or Primidone. Since phenytoin sodium has little sedative effect, it is particularly adapted to use in combination with phenobarbital or primidone. Various combinations can be used when one drug is not effective in controlling seizures or when the effective dose of phenytoin sodium alone produces toxic symptoms. The doses of the combination must be worked out according to the tolerance of each patient. Three to five doses a day of a combination of 0.1 gm phenytoin sodium with either 0.03 gm of phenobarbital, or 0.25 gm primidone, are usually required in the more resistant cases.

Other Forms of Therapy—Ketogenic Diet. It has been shown that a shift in the acid-base balance of the body fluid to the acid side tends to prevent seizures. This can be accomplished by the ingestion of acid or acid-forming salts but the use of such substances for long periods is not desirable. A satisfactory acidosis can be produced by a diet which contains an excess of fats over carbohydrates. Good results in the control of seizures by this diet have been reported by numerous observers. As stated before, however, patients who respond to this form of therapy usually respond to phenobarbital, ethosuximide or phenytoin sodium therapy, and since the administration of these drugs is a simpler procedure than the establishment of ketosis, the ketogenic diet is reserved for those patients who are refractory to medical drug therapy.

Surgical Treatment. Whenever convulsive seizures are associated with a surgically removable lesion of the brain, such as tumor or abscess, removal of the lesion is indicated. Relief of convulsive seizures will result in only about 50% of cases of meningioma of the brain and in a much smaller percentage of cases of glioma or abscess of the brain. In such cases, further treatment with drugs is necessary.

In addition to the removal of the expanding lesions, favorable results have been obtained by the removal of cortical scars secondary to cerebral trauma, vascular lesions and birth injuries. The rationale of this mode of therapy is that such scars, or the brain adjacent to the scar, act as a trigger mechanism for the production of seizures. This form of treatment should be limited to the group of patients with focal attacks who do not respond to medical therapy. In addition, the excision of such lesions should be performed only by neurosurgeons who have facilities for adequate localization of the abnormal focus in the cortex which is acting as the trigger mechanism for the seizures. This focus may not be in the actual scar but in apparently normal brain tissue several centimeters removed from the scar. Medical treatment must also be used in these patients after operation.

The anterior portion of the temporal lobe has been removed in patients with temporal lobe epilepsy. Decrease in the frequency of the seizures and improvement in the psychiatric disturbance have been reported in over 50% of the operated patients. The percentage of the patients showing improvement is related to the presence of structural lesions in the excised cortical tissue (Table 113).

Table 113.   The Relationship of Pathological Findings to Clinical Results of Temporal Lobectomy in the Treatment of Temporal Lobe Seizures

(After Falconer and Serafetinides, J. Neurol., Neurosurg. & Psychiat., 1963)

	Free or Almost Free of Seizures	Worthwhile Improvement	Not Improved	Totals
Mesial temporal lobe sclerosis	28	15	4	47
Small focal tumors or angiomas	14[1]	8[3]	2	24[1,3]
Miscellaneous lesions (scars, infarcts, etc.)	7[2]	3	3	13[2]
Equivocal changes	8	6	8	22
Totals	53	30	17	100

[1] Includes 1 patient with mesial temporal lobe sclerosis.
[2] Includes 3 patients who also had mesial temporal lobe sclerosis.
[3] Includes 2 patients who also had mesial temporal lobe sclerosis.

Hemispherectomy has been performed for the relief of intractable seizures in children with hemiplegia as result of birth injury or developmental defect. Good results have been obtained with regard to relief of seizures, without any increase in the neurological deficit.

Operations other than on the central nervous system are not advisable unless indicated for reasons apart from the occurrence of convulsive seizures. Removal of the cervical sympathetics or portions of the large intestine, operation on the sinuses, and the like have no effect on the ultimate course of the seizures. Removal of tumors of the pancreas is, of course, necessary when attacks are definitely proved to be related to hyperinsulinism. Denervation of the carotid sinus may be of benefit in patients with carotid sinus syncope.

Status Epilepticus. Patients who are subject to seizures may have attacks so frequently that they do not recover from the coma produced by one attack before the next attack supervenes. The patient remains in coma for twelve to twenty-four hours, during which time there may be many convulsive seizures. The attacks may cease spontaneously and the patient recover consciousness after a period of twenty-four to forty-eight hours, or death may occur as the result of the repeated attacks. The likelihood of the latter eventuality is so great that vigorous therapeutic methods aimed at terminating the seizures are justified. Good results can sometimes be obtained by anesthetizing the patient with one of the volatile anesthetics, such as chloroform or ether. Termination of the seizure is more certain with the injection of sodium phenobarbital, phenytoin or paraldehyde intravenously and there is less risk of pulmonary complications. It is important that a large dose be given at the first injection because best results are obtained when the full amount is given in one rather than in divided doses. For status epilepticus in adults, 0.4 to 0.8 gm of sodium phenobarbital dissolved in distilled water, 0.3 to 0.4 gm phenytoin or 3 to 6 ml of paraldehyde (diluted in saline) should be injected intravenously. The dosage for children is 0.2 to 0.4 gm of sodium phenobarbital or 2 to 4 ml of paraldehyde according to the size of the child. Diazepam (Valium) has been recommended as the drug of choice, 2.5 to 10 mg given intravenously. It often is effective, but repeated dosages may have to be administered, occasionally limiting its usefulness. Also, if effects of excessive muscle metabolism and apnea, as occur in the severe generalized seizures of status epilepticus, are reduced or eliminated by assisted respiration and administration of oxygen, severe cerebral hypoxia does not occur. Actually, under these conditions cerebral blood flow increases to meet cerebral oxygen demands during seizures.

Results of Treatment. Grand mal seizures with or without focal onset are more amenable to therapy than petit mal or psychomotor attacks. Our experience, relying chiefly on phenytoin sodium, phenobarbital and Zarontin has been as follows: grand mal seizures can be controlled in 50% of the cases, and the seizures greatly reduced in frequency in another 35%; petit mal seizures are controlled in 60% and 33% are greatly improved; 28% of the patients with psychomotor seizures are controlled and another 50% are greatly improved. The use of primidone and carbamazepine is enhancing the latter results.

Complete withdrawal of medication, after two or more years' freedom from attacks while on medication, is possible in only a small percentage of cases. The seizures tend to recur in at least two-thirds of the patients, even after slow withdrawal of medication and despite normality of the electroencephalogram.

REFERENCES

Brazier, M. A. B. (Ed).: Epilepsy. Its Phenomena in Man. New York, Academic Press, 1973, pp. 391.
Caveness, W. F.: Onset and Cessation of Fits Following Craniocerebral Trauma, J. Neurosurg., 20, 570, 1963.
Charlton M. H., and Hoefer, P. F. A.: Television and Epilepsy, Arch. Neurol., 11, 239, 1964.
Critchley, M., Cobb, W., and Sears, T. A.: On Reading Epilepsy, Epilepsia, 1, 403, 1960.
Currier, R. D., Kooi, K. A., and Saidman, L. J.: Prognosis of "Pure" Petit Mal, Neurology, 13, 959, 1963.
Daly, D. D. and Mulder, D. W.: Gelastic Epilepsy, Neurology, 7, 189, 1957.
Daube, J. R.: Sensory Precipitated Seizures. A Review, J. Nerv. & Ment. Dis., 141, 524, 1966.
Echlin, F. A.: Supersensitivity of Chronically Isolated Cerebral Cortex as a Mechanism in Focal Epilepsy, Electroenceph. & Clin. Neurophysiol., 11, 697, 1959.
Falconer, M. A., and Serafetinides, E. A.: A Follow-up of Surgery in Temporal Lobe Epilepsy, J. Neurol., Neurosurg., & Psychiat., 26, 154, 1963.
Falconer, M. and, Taylor, D. C.: Surgical Treatment of Drug-resistant Temporal Lobe Epilepsy due to Mesial Temporal Sclerosis: Etiology and Significance, Arch. Neurol., 18, 353, 1968.
Gastaut, H.: Clinical and Electroencephalographic Classification of Epileptic Seizures, Epilepsia, 11, 102, 1970.
Gastaut, H., and Tassinari, C. A.: Triggering Mechanisms in Epilepsy: The Electroclinical Point of View, Epilepsia, 7, 85, 1966.
Gibbs, E. L., and Gibbs, F. A.: Diagnostic and Localizing Value of Electroencephalographic Studies in Sleep, A. Res. Nerv. & Ment. Dis. Proc., 26, 366, 1947.
Gibbs, F. A., Gibbs, E. L., and Lennox, W. G.: Electroencephalographic Classification of Epileptic Patients and Control Subjects, Arch. Neurol. & Psychiat., 50, 111, 1943.
Gibbs, F. A., and Gibbs, E. L.: Atlas of Electroencephalography, Vol. II, Epilepsy, 2nd Ed., Reading, Mass., Addison-Wesley Publishing Co., 1952, pp. 426.
Glaser, G. H.: Limbic Epilepsy in Childhood, J. Nerv. Ment. Dis., 144 391, 1967.
Goldensohn, E. A. and Gold, A. P.: Prolonged Behavioral Disturbances as Ictal Phenomena, Neurology, 10, 1, 1960.
Hauser, H. A. and, Kurland, T. T.: The Epidemiology of Epilepsy in Rochester, Minnesota, 1935 Through 1967, Epilepsia, 16, 1, 1975.
Hoefer, P. F. A., Schlesinger, E. G., and Pennes, H. H.: Seizures in Patients With Brain Tumors, A. Res. Nerv. & Ment. Dis. Proc., 26, 50, 1947.
Holowach, J., Thurston, D. L., and O'Leary, J. L.: Prognosis in Childhood Epilepsy, N. Engl. J. Med., 286, 169, 1972.
Jasper, H. H., Ward, A. A., and Pope, A. (Editors): Basic Mechanisms of the Epilepsies. Boston, Little, Brown & Co., 1969, 835 pp.

Jeavons, P. M. and Harding, G. F. A.: *Photosensitive Epilepsy.* London, William Heinemann Medical Books, Ltd., 1975, 121 pp.

Jeavons, P. M., Harper, J. R., and Bower, B. D.: Long-Term Prognosis in Infantile Spasms: A Follow-up Report on 112 Cases, Develop. Med. Child Neurol., *12*, 413, 1970.

Joynt, R. J., Green, D., and Green, R.: Musicogenic Epilepsy, J.A.M.A., *179*, 501, 1962.

Keith, H. M., Ewert, J. C., Green, M. W., and Gage, R. P.: Mental Status of Children With Convulsive Disorders, Neurology, *5*, 419, 1955.

Kutt, H. and McDowell, F.: Management of Epilepsy With Diphenylhydantoin Sodium, J.A.M.A., *203*, 969, 1968.

Lacy, J. R. and Penry, J. K.: *Infantile Spasms.* New York, Raven Press, 1976. 169 pp.

Lennox-Buchthal, M. A.: *Febrile Convulsions.* A Reappraisal. Amsterdam, Elsevier Publ. Co., 1973. 138 pp. (Also, Suppl. Na32. Electroenceph. Clin. Neurophysiol.)

Lennox, W. G.: Brain Injury, Drugs, and Environment as Causes of Mental Decay in Epilepsy, Am. J. Psychiat., *99*, 174, 1942.

————: The Petit Mal Epilepsies: Their Treatment With Tridione, J.A.M.A., *129*, 1069, 1945.

————: The Genetics of Epilepsy, Am. J. Psychiat., *103*, 457, 1947.

————: Heredity of Epilepsy as Told by Relatives and Twins, J.A.M.A., *146*, 529, 1951.

————: Phenomena and Correlates of the Psychomotor Triad, Neurology, *1*, 357, 1951.

Lennox, W. G. and Lennox, M. A.: *Epilepsy and Related Disorders.* Boston, Little, Brown & Co., 1960, 2 Vols., 1100 pp.

Lennox, W. G. and Merritt, H. H.: The Cerebrospinal Fluid in "Essential" Epilepsy, J. Neurol. & Psychopath., *17*, 97, 1936.

Lilienfeld, A. M. and Pasamanick, B.: Association of Maternal and Fetal Factors With the Development of Epilepsy. 1. Abnormalities in the Prenatal and Paranatal Periods, J.A.M.A., *155*, 719, 1954.

Livingston, S.: Etiologic Factors in Adult Convulsions. An Analysis of 698 Patients Whose Attacks Began After Twenty Years of Age, N. Engl. J. Med., *254*, 1211, 1956.

Margerison, J. H. and Corsellis, J. A.: Epilepsy and the Temporal Lobes. A Clinical, Electroencephalographic and Neuropathological Study of the Brain in Epilepsy, With Particular Reference to the Temporal Lobes, Brain, *89*, 499, 1966.

Merritt, H. H. and Putnam, T. J.: Sodium Diphenyl Hydantoinate in the Treatment of Convulsive Disorders, J.A.M.A., *111*, 1068, 1938.

Metrakos, J. D. and Metrakos, K.: Genetic Studies in Clinical Epilepsy. In: Jasper, H. H., Ward, A. D. and Pope, A. Op. Cit. 1969. pp 700–708.

Millichap, J. G.: *Febrile Convulsions.* New York, The Macmillan Co., 1968.

Ounsted, C., Lindsay, J., and Norman, R.: *Biological Factors in Temporal Lobe Epilepsy.* London, William Heinemann Medical Books Ltd., 1966, 135 pp.

Penfield, W. and Erickson, T. C.: *Epilepsy and Cerebral Localization.* Springfield, Charles C Thomas, 1941, 623 pp.

Penfield, W. and Jasper, H. H.: *Epilepsy and the Functional Anatomy of the Human Brain.* Boston, Little, Brown & Co., 1953, 912 pp.

Penry, J. K. and Daly, D. D. (Eds): *Complex Partial Seizures and Their Treatment.* Advances in Neurology. Volume II. Raven Press, New York, 1975.

Poser, C. M. and Low, N. L.: Autopsy Findings in Three Cases of Hypsarhythmia (Infantile Spasms With Mental Retardation), Acta Paediat., *49*, 695, 1960.

Posner, J. B., Plum, F., and Van Poznak, A.: Cerebral Metabolism During Electrically Induced Seizures in Man, Arch. Neurol., *20*, 388, 1969.

Prensky, A. L., Raff, M. C., Moore, M. J., and Schwab, R.: Intravenous Diazepam in the Treatment of Prolonged Seizure Activity, N. Engl. J. Med., *276*, 779, 1967.

Putnam, T. J. and Merritt, H. H.: Dullness as an Epileptic Equivalent, Arch. Neurol. & Psychiat., *45*, 797, 1941.

Ransohoff, J. and Carter, S.: Hemispherectomy in the Treatment of Convulsive Seizures Associated With Infantile Hemiplegia, A. Res. Nerv. & Ment. Dis. Proc., *34*, 176, 1956.

Reynolds, E. H.: Mental Effects of Anticonvulsant Drugs and Folate Metabolism, Brain, *91*, 197, 1968.

Rodin, E. A.: *The Prognosis of Patients With Epilepsy.* Springfield, Charles C Thomas, 1968, 455 pp.

Rook, A. F.: Coughing and Unconsciousness: The "So-Called" Laryngeal Epilepsy, Brain, 69, 138, 1946.

Stevens, H.: Reading Epilepsy, N. Engl. J. Med., 257, 165, 1957.

Walker, A. E.: Prognosis in Post-Traumatic Epilepsy: A Ten-Year Follow-up of Craniocerebral Injuries of World War II, J.A.M.A., 164, 1636, 1957.

Walker, A. E.: Post-Traumatic Epilepsy. Springfield, Charles C Thomas, 1949, 86 pp.

Weber, R.: Musikogene Epilepsie, Nervenarzt, 27, 337, 1956.

White, H. H.: Cerebral Hemispherectomy in the Treatment of Infantile Hemiplegia, Confinia Neurologica, 21, 1, 1960.

White, P. T., Bailey, A. A., and Bickford, R. G.: Epileptic Disorders in the Aged, Neurology, 3, 674, 1953.

Williams, D.: The Thalamus and Epilepsy, Brain, 88, 539, 1965.

Woodbury, D. M., Penry, J. K., and Schmidt, R. P.: Antiepileptic Drugs. New York, Raven Press, 1972, 520 pp.

Yahr, M. D. and Merritt, H. H.: Current Status of the Drug Therapy of Epileptic Seizures, J.A.M.A., 161, 333, 1956.

Yahr, M. D., Sciarra, D., Carter, S. and Merritt, H. H.: Evaluation of Standard Anticonvulsant Therapy in 319 Patients, J.A.M.A., 150, 663, 1952.

Syncope

H. Houston Merritt

Definition. Syncope (fainting) is defined as a transient loss of consciousness due to cerebral ischemia. Syncope usually occurs when the patient is standing. It is uncommon when the patient is seated and practically never occurs in the recumbent position.

Prodromal symptoms are present in almost all of the cases. Weakness, sweating, dizziness, light-headedness and epigastric discomfort are common. Less frequently there may be vertigo, blurred vision, paresthesias in extremities, headache or pallor. The duration of the premonitory symptoms varies from a few seconds to a minute or two.

During the period of unconsciousness the pulse is feeble, the pupils dilated and the skin is cold, pale or ashen in color, and covered with perspiration. Clonic movements of the extremities and incontinence may rarely occur especially after twenty–twenty-five seconds. The duration of the state varies from a few seconds to a minute or two. The patient is usually mentally clear immediately on recovering consciousness but may feel weak. Unconsciousness of more than two or three minutes or mental confusion on recovery of consciousness should lead to the consideration of some cause for the severity of the disturbance other than simple syncope.

Causes. The causes of syncope are numerous, but they can be divided into five large groups: cardiac, vasopressor, orthostatic hypotension, cough syncope, and carotid sinus syncope. In the vast majority of the cases the fainting is due to a sudden decrease in the circulation to the brain.

The various causes of syncope as determined by Wayne in 510 patients are listed in Table 114, Epilepsy, cerebral vascular disease,

Table 114.   Causes of Syncope in 510 Patients
(After Wayne, Am. J. Med., 1961)

Cause of Fainting	No. of Patients	%
Vasovagal	298	58
Orthostatic hypotension	28	5.5
Epilepsy	26	5
Cerebral vascular disease	24	5
Unknown etiology	23	4.5
Post-micturition	17	3
Adams-Stokes syndrome	17	3
Hyperventilation	15	3
Hypersensitive carotid sinus	15	3
Tussive	13	2.5
Aortic stenosis	9	2
Paroxysmal tachycardia	8	1.5
Angina pectoris	4	1
Hysteria	4	1
Myocardial infarction	3	0.5
Pulmonary hypertension	2	0.5
Migraine	2	0.5
Hypertensive encephalopathy	2	0.5
Total	510	100

hysteria, migraine and hypertensive encephalopathy, included in this table, could well be omitted because the loss of consciousness in these patients is due to factors other than a general diminution of cerebral circulation.

Vasovagal Syncope. The most common cause of fainting is vasovagal syncope which is the result of a sudden loss of resistance in the peripheral circulation. Vasovagal syncope is common in normal healthy individuals of all ages and it may occur in association with anxiety tension states, gastrointestinal disturbances and the like. The episode of fainting is usually precipitated by some stress-producing emotional or environmental factor. Fear, apprehension, fatigue, lack of sleep, mild trauma, hot or close room, instrumentation, sight of blood and sight of others fainting are a few of the precipitating factors.

Orthostatic Hypotension. The next most common cause of fainting is orthostatic hypotension. A mild degree of hypotension on assuming the erect posture is not uncommon in normal individuals. In some patients the cardiovascular reflexes are impaired and the fall in blood pressure is excessive and results in cerebral ischemia.

Orthostatic hypotension has been reported without any accompanying disease, but it is most often associated with organic disease of the central or peripheral nervous system (Table 115) and diabetes mellitus. It is possible that involvement of the autonomic fibers in the peripheral nerves may be responsible for the hypotension in the patients with diabetes mellitus.

Table 115. Diseases of the Nervous System Associated with
Orthostatic Hypotension

Sympathectomy	Parkinsonism
Polyneuritis	Idiopathic, Shy-Drager Syndrome
	Parkinson's Disease
Tabes Dorsalis	Other Cerebral or Spinal Cord Disease
Syringomyelia	Diabetes Mellitus (Neuritis)

Orthostatic hypotension may occur following the administration of drugs, such as the tranquilizers, antidepressants, antihypertensives, and levodopa.

Micturition syncope is probably due to a combination of orthostatic hypotension and the reflex action of a distended bladder. The fainting which occurs with coughing or laughing has never been adequately explained, but it is thought by some to be due to fall in blood pressure secondary to pooling of the blood in the splanchnic bed. Others state that it is due to interference with the cerebral circulation as a result of the increase in intracranial pressure secondary to the enormous increase in intrathoracic pressure.

The so-called idiopathic form of orthostatic hypotension is accompanied by signs and symptoms of disease of the central nervous system including dysarthria, monotonous speech, diplegia, pupillary irregularities, vertigo, rigidity, tremor, cerebellar ataxia and incontinence. Various changes in the nervous system have been described. Degenerative changes in the autonomic ganglia with inclusion bodies in the cells, loss of neurons in the intermediolateral columns and degenerative changes in the neurons of the cortex, basal ganglia have been reported on examination of the nervous system.

Cardiac Syncope. Syncope is not uncommon when there is a sudden decrease in the circulation secondary to cardiac disturbances such as Stokes-Adams syndrome, paroxysmal tachycardia, auricular fibrillation or aortic stenosis.

Carotid Sinus Syndrome. Pressure on the carotid sinus will produce a reflex slowing of the heart and a slight fall in blood pressure in normal subjects. If the sinus is especially sensitive, syncope may result from asystole or a great decrease in the blood pressure. Weiss and Baker in their thorough study of the carotid sinus postulated that syncope could occur from pressure on an irritable carotid sinus without any significant change in heart rate or fall in blood pressure (cerebral type of carotid sinus reflex). They thought that localized changes in the cerebral circulation were responsible for the syncope in these cases. There is considerable doubt that syncope which occurs in these so-called cerebral cases is related to stimulation of the sinus. It is now known that pressure on or massage of one carotid artery can produce syncope if the other carotid artery is occluded or partially stenosed. It is also possible that posturing the head in performing the test may occlude one of the vertebral arteries at atlantoaxial junction.

Treatment. When syncope is associated with organic disease, the underlying disease should be treated. Patients with vasovagal syncope should lie down or sit down with the head bent forward at the immediate onset of symptoms. Patients with orthostatic hypotension should be cautioned with regard to arising suddenly from the recumbent position. They should be instructed to exercise the extremities before sitting on the edge of the bed and exercise them further in this position. In the severe cases the legs should be bandaged and an abdominal support should be worn. Ephedrine, in dose of 25 mg 3 times daily, is often of value in preventing the syncopal attacks. If this is not effective, fludrocortisone acetate can be tried, starting with 0.1 mg daily and gradually increasing over a period of three to four weeks until orthostatic hypotension does not occur. Occasionally daily dose of 1 mg or greater may be required. Close observation is necessary for the development of edema, severe hypertension in the supine position or exacerbation of existing diabetes mellitus.

Syncope with the carotid sinus syndrome is treated by atropine in doses of 0.3 mg or amphetamine sulfate in doses of 5 to 10 mg, once to three times daily. If medical therapy is not effective, denervation of the sensitive carotid sinus is indicated.

REFERENCES

Bickelmann, A. G., Lippschutz, E. J., and Brunjes, C. F.: Hemodynamics of Idiopathic Orthostatic Hypotension, Am. J. Med., *30*, 26, 1961.
Engel, G. L. *Fainting.* 2nd Ed., Springfield, Charles C Thomas, 1962. pp. 196.
Gurdjian, E. S., Webster, J. E., Hardy, W. G., and Lindner, D. W.: Nonexistence of the So-Called Cerebral Form of Carotid Sinus Syncope, Neurology, *8*, 818, 1958.
Hutchinson, E. G., and Stock, J. P. P.: The Carotid-Sinus Syndrome, Lancet, *2*, 445, 1960.
Jonas, S., Klein, I., and Dimant, J. D.: Importance of Holter Monitoring in Patients with Periodic Cerebral Symptoms, Ann. Neurol., *1*, 470, 1977.
Roesman, U., van den Noort, S., and McFarland, D. E.: Idiopathic Orthostatic Hypotension, Arch. Neurol., *24*, 503, 1971.
Thomas, J. E., and Schirger, A.: Idiopathic Orthostatic Hypotension. Study of Its Natural History in 57 Neurologically Affected Patients, Arch. Neurol., *22*, 289, 1970.
Toole, J. F., and Weeks, S. D.: Stimulation of Carotid Sinus in Man. I. The Cerebral Response. II. Significance of Head Positioning, Am. J. Med., *27*, 952, 1959.
Vanderhaeghen, J. J., Perier, O., and Sternan, J. E.: Pathological Findings in Orthostatic Hypotension, Arch. Neurol., *22*, 207, 1970.
Wayne, H. H.: Syncope. Physiological Considerations and an Analysis of the Clinical Characteristics in 510 Patients, Am. J. Med., *30*, 418, 1961.
Weiss, S., and Baker, J.: The Carotid Sinus Reflex in Health and Disease, Medicine, *12*, 297, 1933.

MÉNIÈRE'S SYNDROME

H. Houston Merritt

Ménière's syndrome or paroxysmal labyrinthine vertigo is a symptom complex characterized by recurrent attacks of severe vertigo accompanied by tinnitus and loss of hearing. The attacks of vertigo are the cardinal feature of the syndrome. Tinnitus and loss of hearing are often present in the interval between the attacks and may be increased in severity during the paroxysms. The symptom complex was first described by Prosper Ménière in 1861 and since that date thousands of cases have been reported.

Pathogenesis and Pathology. The pathogenesis of the syndrome is unknown. It may follow infections of the middle ear, or trauma to the head, but in the majority of the cases it develops without any antecedent injury to the ear or the nervous system. Attempts have been made to explain the attacks on basis of an acute hydrops of the labyrinth, vasoconstriction, allergy and anomalies of the internal auditory artery, but the arguments which are used to support any of these various hypotheses are not convincing.

The pathology of Ménière's syndrome is unknown. Necropsy observations are rare and the findings scant. Hallpike and his co-workers found a gross distention of the endolymphatic system together with degenerative changes in the sensory element in 3 cases. Dandy reported a few cases in which a loop of the internal auditory artery either elevated or indented the auditory nerve but sections of the nerve which have been removed at operation have not shown any significant abnormalities.

Incidence. Ménière's syndrome is common as attested by the fact that large numbers of cases are used by various authors as basis for their claims regarding the efficacy of varied forms of surgical and medical therapy. The syndrome is primarily a disease of middle life. The symptoms develop during the fifth or sixth decades in approximately two thirds of the patients, and occur only rarely before the third or after the seventh decade. Males are affected approximately two to three times as frequently as females.

Symptoms. The vertigo of Ménière's syndrome is intermittent. Its onset is sudden and occasionally of such a violent nature as to throw the patient to the ground. Loss of consciousness of a few seconds' duration occurs in a small percentage of the cases. Whirling or spinning of objects in the environment is described by the majority of the patients, but occasionally they complain of only a severe sensation of giddiness. Accompanying the vertigo, there may be nausea and vomiting and profuse perspiration. The duration of the symptoms of an attack, although fairly constant for each individual, varies widely in different patients. In some, they last for only a few minutes but in others, they may be prolonged for several hours. The attacks are irregular in their occurrence. In some patients, they may occur once or several times a day for several weeks with a free interval of weeks or months. In less severe cases, the attacks may occur only two or three times a year. Tinnitus and hearing loss are present in practically all cases during the acute attacks of vertigo and they persist in the interval between attacks in the majority of cases. The occurrence of the characteristic attacks of vertigo without tinnitus or hearing loss has been described by some authors as pseudo-Ménière's syndrome. Hearing loss, when present, is progressive and is more severe or confined to one ear in approximately two thirds of the cases. Headaches are common following the attack and rarely there may be diplopia or paresthesias in the extremities.

Signs. With the exception of the signs of involvement of the eighth nerve, the findings on general physical and neurological examinations are within normal limits in the interval between attacks. Nystagmus may be present during the attacks of vertigo. The impairment of hearing, which is bilateral in approximately one third of the cases, varies in severity. It is of the nerve type in 75%, conduction type in 10% and of the mixed type in 15%. Caloric or Bárány tests of the labyrinthine functions give normal results in approximately one half of the cases. In the remaining one half the tests may show a hypo- or hyperactive labyrinth with a complete absence of response in about 5%.

Laboratory Data. The results of the routine examinations of the blood, urine and cerebrospinal fluid are normal. Complete studies of the acid-base constituents of the blood have not shown any consistent deviation from normal during the attacks or in the interval between the attacks.

Course and Prognosis. Ménière's syndrome is a chronic disease with recurrence of symptoms over a period of many years. Temporary or complete remission of the attacks of vertigo occurs not infrequently, either spontaneously or after various forms of treatment, but the hearing loss and tinnitus are usually permanent. Progression of hearing loss may be slow and may be arrested before there is complete deafness in the affected ear. Complete loss of hearing is sometimes followed by a cessation of the attacks of vertigo.

Diagnosis. The diagnosis of Ménière's syndrome can be made without difficulty in most cases on basis of the characteristic history of acute transient attacks of vertigo, associated with tinnitus and impairment of hearing in the absence of evidence of involvement of any part of the nervous system other than the eighth nerve.

Differential Diagnosis. Ménière's syndrome must be differentiated from other diseases with similar symptomatology. The vertigo of acute labyrinthitis is more prolonged and is not usually recurrent. Tumors of the posterior fossa, especially neuromas of the acoustic nerve, may have tinnitus, hearing loss and vertigo as a part of their symptomatology. In these cases, the vertigo rarely occurs in explosive attacks but is present constantly to a more or less severe degree. In addition, other cranial nerve palsies, signs of involvement of the brainstem and increased intracranial pressure are usually present. Considerable difficulty is often experienced in differentiating between the dizziness which may accompany attacks of anxiety neurosis and the vertigo of Ménière's syndrome. The diagnosis is further complicated by the fact that the emotional reaction of patients subject to acute attacks of vertigo is such that they are apt to be classed as neurotics. When hearing loss and tinnitus are present, the diagnosis of Ménière's syndrome should be made.

Treatment. Since there is no satisfactory pathological physiology of the attacks in Ménière's syndrome, there is no specific medical treatment. Attempts have been made to relieve the acute attacks of vertigo by destruction of the labyrinth, section of the vestibular branch of the auditory nerve or by various forms of medical therapy. Destruction of the labyrinth or surgical section of the nerve results in a cessation of the attacks of vertigo in a high percentage of the cases, and good results are obtained with the various forms of medical therapy in about two thirds of the cases. The fairly uniform percentage of remissions which are reported with radically different forms of medical treatment suggests that some other factor, such as spontaneous variation in the frequency of the attacks, is playing a contributing role in the results obtained.

Medical Treatment. The various forms of medical treatment which have been recommended include restriction of fluid and sodium intake, administration of potassium salts, ammonium chloride, and diuretics. These often are not effective, however.

Reduction in the frequency and severity of attacks may follow the prophylactic administration of one of the antihistamines, dimenhydrinate (Dramamine) in dose of 50 mg 2 or 3 times daily. Other similar useful drugs are cyclizine (Marezine) and meclizine (Antivert, Bonamine).

Surgical Treatment. Various procedures are used to destroy the labyrinth or the vestibular ganglion. In addition, the vestibular branch or the entire acoustic nerve on the affected side can be sectioned in the posterior cranial fossa. When the tinnitus and hearing loss are bilateral, the operation should be performed on the side with the greatest degree of hearing loss. Occasionally it may be necessary to section the vestibular branch of the acoustic nerve on both sides. The disturbance of equilibrium, which follows this operation, is temporary.

Operative treatment is effective in preventing attacks of vertigo in a large percentage, but not all, of the patients. Tinnitus is apt to persist but may be decreased in intensity. Complete section of the nerve is preferred to section of the vestibular portion by some neurosurgeons because the results are better in regard to the relief both from attacks of vertigo and from tinnitus. Total section of the nerve results in a complete loss of hearing in the homolateral ear, but this is apt to occur spontaneously or after partial section of the nerve. Operative treatment is indicated in all patients with Ménière's disease in whom severe attacks of vertigo are not prevented by medical therapy.

REFERENCES

Dandy, W. E.: Treatment of Ménière's Disease by Section of Only the Vestibular Portion of the Acoustic Nerve, Bull. Johns Hopkins Hosp., 53, 52, 1933.
Drachman, D. A.: An Approach to the Dizzy Patient, Neurology, 22, 323, 1972.
Fürstenberg, A. C., Lashment, F. H., and Lathrop, F.: Ménière's Symptom Complex, Ann. Otol., Rhin. & Laryng., 43, 1035, 1934.
Green, R. E., and Douglass, C. C.: Intracranial Division of Eighth Nerve for Ménière's Disease. Follow-up Study of Patients Operated on by Dr. Walter E. Dandy, Ann. Otol., Rhin. & Laryng., 60, 610, 1951.
Ménière, P.: Sur une forme particulière de surdité de surdité grave dépendant d'une lésion de l'oreille interne, Gaz. med. de Paris, 16, 29, 1861.

NARCOLEPSY

H. Houston Merritt

Narcolepsy is a clinical syndrome of unknown etiology characterized by recurrent attacks of an uncontrollable desire to sleep, sudden transient loss of tone in the muscles of the extremities or trunk (cataplexy), pathological weakness of the muscles during emotional reactions, such as laughing (lachschlag) or crying, attacks of inability to move developing in the transition between sleep and arousal (sleep paralysis), and vivid visual or auditory sensations at the onset of sleep (hypnogogic hallucinations).

The first description of the syndrome is credited to Westphal (1877), although Bright reported in 1836 a case with the characteristic features of the disease which he attributed to disease of the arteries of the brain. The name narcolepsy was applied to the syndrome by Gelineau in 1880.

Etiology. In the majority of the cases the symptoms start without antecedent injury to the nervous system. In a few cases the onset of symptoms has followed acute epidemic encephalitis, trauma to the head, or acute infections such as pneumonia or scarlet fever. Psychological disturbances are reported to play a role in the onset of the symptoms in some cases.

It has been postulated that narcolepsy may be related to a disturbance in the reticular activating system. Some authors divide the cases into idiopathic and secondary types depending upon the relationship of the symptoms to some organic disease and use the term narcolepsies to describe the entire group. This division serves no useful purpose and there should be no confusion in nomenclature if the term narcolepsy is used to describe the cases with the characteristic short periods of forced but apparently normal sleep with or without catalepsy, sleep paralysis, or the other associated symptoms. Prolonged drowsiness or somnolence associated with such conditions as tumor of the brain, uremia, cerebral trauma or psychoses should be excluded.

Pathology. There is no known clinical or anatomical pathologic condition to explain the symptoms of narcolepsy.

Incidence. Narcolepsy was a rare condition and only a few cases were reported before 1920. Since that date the frequency of the disease has been increasing, as attested by the reports from the group of Dement at Stanford and those at the Mayo Clinic (Yoss and Daly). The age at onset of symptoms is usually in the second to the fourth decade of life, but it may be in the first or after the fifth decade. The ratio of men to women is about 3:2. There is a strong tendency for the familial occurrence of the disease and it is postulated that its transmission is by a single dominant gene with relatively slight penetrance.

Symptoms–Sleep Attacks. The attacks of sleep vary in frequency from one to many times daily and their duration from a few minutes to several hours. The sleep differs from that of so-called normal sleep only in its occurrence at inappropriate times. The desire to sleep can be resisted by great effort but in most cases it is only temporarily postponed. The attacks of sleep frequently occur under circumstances conducive to normal sleep, such as after a heavy meal or while the patient is sitting in a relaxed position. On the other hand, sleep may overtake the patient while pursuing such hazardous occupations as driving an auto or on sentry duty on the battlefield. When the desire for sleep overtakes the patient, he usually seeks a bed or chair, but in some cases the patient may be walking on the streets and awake to find that he walked several blocks while asleep. Similarly one patient would fall asleep while driving an automobile and find herself some miles away when she awoke. This is a rare occurrence, however, since most narcoleptics who fall asleep while driving an automobile wake up after running into another car or off the road.

When the patient awakes from one of his attacks of sleep, or is aroused by external stimuli, which need not be violent, he feels refreshed, but may fall into sleep again within a short while. It is not uncommon for patients to have 6 to 20 naps during the course of the day in addition to a full night's sleep. The nocturnal sleep of the patient is usually of normal duration but in many cases may be interrupted by disturbing dreams. The diurnal attacks of sleep are also occasionally accompanied by similar dreams.

Transient Attacks of Weakness and Loss of Muscular Tone. Weakness or loss of tone of muscle sudden or rapid onset occurs in over 50% of the patients. Commonly the weakness involves the leg muscles causing the patient to fall to the ground, so-called cataplectic attacks. In addition to the cataplectic attacks, the patients may have transient paralysis of an extremity or the head may slump on the chest as result of weakness of the neck muscles. Occasionally the weakness of the muscles may be accompanied by twitchings.

The precipitating causes of the attacks of muscular weakness and atonia are usually some emotional stimuli, such as mirth, anger, fear, surprise, joy or amusement. A mild degree of muscular weakness under such emotional stimuli is a common phenomenon in the normal individual but its severity is not such as to cause him to fall helplessly to the ground as is common in patients with narcolepsy when they laugh (lachschlag). An element of surprise in the emotional situation is important in precipitating the muscular weakness.

Sleep Paralysis. Paralysis of the extremities concomitant with falling to sleep or on awakening occurs in about one third of the patients. Loss of speech and the ability to open the eyes may also occur. These are of brief duration, lasting only a few seconds. They can be terminated by touching an object in proximity, being touched by someone or by "jerking the eyes."

Hypnogogic Hallucinations. Hallucinations in association with falling to sleep occur in about one third of the patients. At times it is difficult for patients to distinguish these sensations from vivid dreams. At times they occur in association with sleep paralysis.

Signs. The general physical and neurological examinations are usually within normal limits except for a moderate or severe degree of obesity in about a third of the cases. Not infrequently, in such cases, a gain in weight coincides with or immediately precedes the onset of the narcoleptic symptoms.

Laboratory Data. The findings in the urine, blood and cerebrospinal fluid are within normal limits. The electroencephalogram is usually normal if taken when the patient is awake. Dynes and Finley found normal records in 17 of 22 patients when they were awake. During one of the attacks of narcoleptic sleep, the brain potentials became modified in the manner that is commonly seen in normal physiological sleep. In 5 patients they obtained abnormal records while the patients were awake. There was no constant or specific alteration in the character of brain potentials in these 5 cases. According to Dement and his associates the sleep episodes are characterized by the immediate onset of full-blown "rapid eye movement" sleep in a high percentage of the patients in whom narcolepsy is associated with catalepsy.

Prognosis. Narcolepsy is a chronic syndrome. Too few cases have been followed for a long enough period to know the ultimate outcome, but in the majority of the cases the symptoms persist throughout the life of the individual unless relieved by treatment.

Diagnosis. The diagnosis of narcolepsy is made from the history. The combination of irresistible attacks of sleep with transient episodes of muscular weakness and atonia is so characteristic that, when present together, they are sufficient to make the diagnosis. The diagnosis is less secure when only the sleep attacks are present, and should be made with caution in such cases.

Differential Diagnosis. Some of the symptoms of narcolepsy are present in other diseases of the nervous system. The excessive somnolence or stupor which may be seen in patients with tumors of the brain, uremia, cerebral arteriosclerotic states or in psychotic patients can be readily differentiated from the sleep of narcolepsy by the prolonged nature of the somnolence or stupor and the associated physical and laboratory findings. The weakness of the muscles has a superficial resemblance to that of familial periodic paralysis, but the long duration of the paralysis and the disturbance of potassium metabolism in the latter should prevent any confusion in the diagnosis.

Muscular twitchings and cataplectic attacks may occur in patients with epilepsy. Clouding of consciousness and electroencephalographic abnormalities during the attacks serve to establish the diagnosis of epilepsy. It must be remembered, however, that the combination of narcolepsy and epilepsy in the same patient may rarely occur.

Treatment. The treatment of narcolepsy is an empirical one directed toward the prevention of the attacks of somnolence. Janota in 1931 and Doyle and Daniels in the same year reported that ephedrine prevented these attacks. Prinzmetal and Bloomberg in 1935 demonstrated that amphetamine sulfate was more effective than ephedrine. In recent years, Dexedrine (dextroamphetamine) or other sympathomimetic drugs have replaced amphetamine sulfate in the treatment of narcolepsy. Yoss and Daly recommend methylphenidate (Ritalin hydrochloride) in dose of 40 to 60 mg as a substitute for Dexedrine. The somnolence can be relieved in practically all cases, but the cataplexy and the attacks of generalized muscular weakness which accompany laughing or crying are not improved in all of the cases in which these symptoms are present. Recently, Shapiro has found that clomipramine in doses of 25 to 75 mg per day will relieve attacks of cataplexy, sleep paralysis and hypnogogic hallucinations.

REFERENCES

Bright, R.: Cases Illustrative of the Effects Produced when the Arteries of the Brain Are Diseased, Guy's Hosp. Rep., *1*, 9, 1836.

Dement, W., Rechtschaffen, A., and Gulevich, G.: The Nature of Narcoleptic Sleep Attack, Neurology, *16*, 18, 1966.

Dynes, J. B., and Finley, K. H.: The Electroencephalograph as an Aid in the Study of Narcolepsy, Arch. Neurol. & Psychiat., *46*, 598, 1941.

Ganado, W.: The Narcolepsy Syndrome, Neurology, *8*, 487, 1958.

Guilleminault, C. and Dement, W.: Pathologies of Excessive Sleep. In: *Advances in Sleep Research*, Vol. 1. (Weitzman, E. Ed). New York, Spectrum Publications, 1974. Chapter 8: pp. 345–390.

Janota, O.: Symptomatische Behandlung der pathologischen Schlafsucht, besonders der Narkolepsie, Medizinische Klinik., *27*, 278, 1931.

Kamman, G. R.: Narcolepsy following Epidemic Encephalitis, J.A.M.A., *93*, 29, 1929.

Krabbe, E., and Magnussen, G.: On Narcolepsy: Familial Narcolepsy, Acta Psychiat. et Neurol., *17*, 149, 1942.

Levin, M.: Narcolepsy (Gelineau's Syndrome) and Other Varieties of Morbid Somnolence, Arch. Neurol. and Psychiat., *22*, 1172, 1929.

Prinzmetal, M., and Bloomberg, W.: The Use of Benzedrine for the Treatment of Narcolepsy, J.A.M.A., *105*, 2051, 1935.

Shapiro, W. R.: Treatment of Cataplexy with Clomipramine. Arch. Neurol. *35*, 653, 1975.

Sours, J. A.: Narcolepsy and Other Disturbances in the Sleep-Waking Rhythm: A Study of 115 Cases with Review of the Literature, J. Nerv. & Ment. Dis., *137*, 525, 1963.

Yoss, R. E., and Daly, D. D.: Narcolepsy in Children, Pediatrics, *5*, 1025, 1960.

SYNDROME OF HYPERSOMNIA AND BULIMIA

(Kleine-Levin Syndrome)

H. Houston Merritt

A syndrome characterized by the episodic occurrence of excessive hunger (bulimia) and sleep was described by Kleine in 1925 and further elucidated by Levin in 1936. Less than 50 cases have been described since these original reports. In a review, Gallinek stresses the fact that psychic phenomena are an integral part of the syndrome. The symptoms usually develop in young males. There are periodic attacks of somnolence, in which the patient may sleep for several days or weeks, awakening only for short intervals during which he eats ravenously and in excessive amounts and takes care of the urinary and bowel functions. When awake the sensorium may be clouded, and on recovery there is partial or total amnesia for certain periods of the attacks. Symptoms of a minor or moderately severe depression may follow the attacks. An intense craving for sweet foods has been reported.

There is no known pathology and routine laboratory investigations are negative. Attempts have been made to relate the syndrome to migraine because of the occurrence of severe headache preceding the attack in several of the cases. Critchley has stated that the syndrome has four hallmarks: Occurrence preponderantly if not exclusively in the male; onset in adolescence; spontaneous eventual disappearance of the syndrome; and the possibility that the megaphagia is in the nature of a compulsive eating rather than bulimia. A few cases have been reported in females. Gallinek has treated 2 patients with amphetamine sulfate and states that there was a reduction in the frequency and severity of the attacks. He suggests that the syndrome may be related to narcolepsy.

REFERENCES

Critchley, M.: Periodic Hypersomnia and Megaphagia in Adolescent Males, Brain, 85, 627, 1962.
Gallinek, A.: The Syndrome of Episodes of Hypersomnia, Bulimia and Abnormal Mental States, J.A.M.A., 154, 1081, 1954.
————: The Kleine-Levin Syndrome, Dis. of Nerv. Syst., 28, 1, 1967.
Garland, H., Sumner, D., and Fourman, P.: The Kleine-Levin Syndrome. Some Further Observations, Neurology, 15, 1161, 1965.
Gilbert, G. J.: Periodic Hypersomnia and Bulimia. The Kleine-Levin Syndrome, Neurology, 14, 844, 1964.
Kleine, W.: Periodische Schlafsucht, Monatschr. f. Psychiat. u. Neurol., 57, 285, 1925.
Levin, M.: Periodic Somnolence and Morbid Hunger: A New Syndrome, Brain, 59, 494, 1936.

Chapter 10

Diseases Due to Toxins

H. Houston Merritt

BACTERIAL TOXINS

The toxins elaborated by several of the pathogenic bacteria have a special predilection for the nervous system. The exotoxin of the diphtheria bacillus affects chiefly the peripheral nerves; tetanus the activity of the neurons in the central nervous system; and botulism presumably interferes with conduction at the myoneural junction.

Diphtheria

The mode of action of the exotoxin of Corynbacterium diphtheriae on the peripheral nerves is unknown. It has been suggested that the toxin interferes with the synthesis of cytochrome B or related enzymes, but direct proof for this is lacking. The toxin spreads from the site of infection into the blood and cerebrospinal fluid. It has a predilection for the sensory and motor nerves of the limbs and to a lesser extent the ciliary muscle or nerve. The frequency of palatal and pharyngo-laryngo-esophageal involvement is possibly a result in part of local action of toxin since the incidence of involvement of these structures is less in cutaneous diphtheria than in faucial diphtheria. The resistance of other cranial nerves and the brain is unexplained since they are all susceptible to an adequate dose.

The symptomatology and the course of patients with diphtheritic neuritis are considered on page 753.

Tetanus

Tetanus (lock jaw) is an infectious disease in which there is localized or generalized spasm of muscle due to the toxin produced by the causative organism, Clostridium tetani.

Etiology. Clostridium tetani is present in the excreta of humans and most animals and is present in dirt and putrefying liquids. It is especially prevalent in fertilized or contaminated soil. The organisms usually gain entrance to the human body through puncture wounds, compound fractures, or wounds from blank cartridges and fireworks. Infection has been reported from contamination of operative wounds, burns, parenteral injections (particularly in heroin addicts) and through the umbilicus of the newborn. The mere deposition of spores of the organism is not sufficient for infection. Necrotic tissue and an associated pyogenic infection are necessary for growth of the organism and production of the toxin.

The symptoms are due to a toxin elaborated by the organism. The toxin has a local effect at the site of inoculation and travels through the blood and the perineural connective tissue. When the spread is through the nerves, the symptoms are those of localized tetanus. The toxin acts on the muscles or motor nerve endings as well as on the spinal cord and brainstem.

Pathology. There are no pathological changes in the central or peripheral nervous system.

Incidence. The disease is found in all portions of the world. In the United States, it is most commonly due to puncture wounds of the extremities by nails or splinters contaminated by human or animal excreta or by wounds inflicted by cap-pistols and fireworks. The incidence of infection in soldiers by wounds received in combat was high until the introduction of active immunization of all recruits and passive immunization of all wounded soldiers. In the United States, the infection is most common in narcotic addicts. This is possibly related to the fact that the narcotic is "cut" by admixing with quinine which favors the growth of the organisms at the site of the injection.

Symptoms. The incubation period is usually between five and ten days. Occasionally, it may be as short as three days or as long as three weeks. As a rule, the severity of the disease is greater when the incubation period is short.

The symptoms may be localized or generalized. In the localized form, the muscular spasms and contractions are confined to the injured extremity. This form is relatively rare and is most commonly seen in patients who have been partially protected by prophylactic doses of antitetanic serum. When the portal of entrance is in the head (face, ear, tonsils, etc.), the symptoms may be localized to that region (cephalic tetanus). Trismus, facial paralysis and ophthalmoplegia are characteristic of this rare form of tetanus.

In the generalized form, the presenting symptom is usually stiffness of the jaw (trismus). This is followed by stiffness of the neck, irritability and restlessness. As the disease progresses, stiffness of the muscles becomes generalized. Rigidity of the back muscles may become so extreme that the patient assumes the position of opisthotonos. Rigidity of the facial muscles gives a characteristic facial expression, the so-called risus sardonicus. Added to the stiffness of the muscles are paroxysmal tonic spasms or generalized convulsions. These may occur spontaneously or be precipitated by an external stimulus. Dysphagia may develop from spasm of the pharyngeal muscles and cyanosis and asphyxia from spasm of the glottis or respiratory muscles. Consciousness is preserved except during convulsions. The pulse and respiratory rates are elevated. The temperature may be normal, but more commonly it is elevated to 101° to 103° F.

Laboratory Data. There are no specific changes in blood, urine or cerebrospinal fluid.

Diagnosis. The diagnosis of tetanus is made on the appearance of the characteristic signs of the disease, trismus, risus sardonicus, tonic spasms and generalized convulsions, in a patient who has received a wound of the skin and deeper tissues. The symptoms of strychnine poisoning differ from those of tetanus in that the muscles are relaxed between spasms and the jaw muscles are rarely involved.

Course and Prognosis. The outlook is grave in all cases of tetanus. The mortality rate is over 50%. Prognosis is best when the incubation period is long or when generalized convulsive seizures are either absent or do not develop until several days after the onset. The mortality rate is reduced by the prompt administration of serum. In fatal cases, death usually occurs in three to ten days. Death is most commonly due to paralysis of respiration. In the patients who recover there is a gradual reduction in the frequency of seizures and in the severity of muscular contractions.

Treatment. The patient should be hospitalized in a special care unit. The wound should be surgically cleaned. Antiserum does not neutralize toxins that have been fixed in the nervous system but it is administered on the chance that it will neutralize toxin which has not yet entered the nervous system. It is customary to administer antiserum as soon as diagnosis is made. Human tetanus immune globulin (TIG) is given intravenously in dose of 3,000 to 6,000 units. Penicillin G is the most effective antibiotic for inhibiting the growth of the organisms, and should be given intramuscularly. Tracheostomy should be performed to assure adequate ventilation. Sedatives, muscular relaxants and anticonvulsants should be given to combat the muscular spasms and convulsions. Paraldehyde, diphenylhydantoin and curare should be given in sufficient dosage to prevent muscular spasms and convulsions. Fluid and electrolyte balance should be maintained by indwelling gastric tube if necessary.

Pascale and his associates report that hyperbaric oxygenation is effective in the treatment of tetanus and obviates the necessity for tetanus antitoxin or tracheotomy.

In prophylactic treatment, tetanus toxoid or 1500 units of antitetanic serum should be injected intramuscularly to all patients with perforating or contaminated wounds. Children, farmers and all military personnel should be actively immunized by the injection of toxoid.

Botulism

Botulism, a type of poisoning due to the ingestion of food contaminated with the toxin of Clostridium botulinum, is characterized by weakness of the striated and smooth muscles.

Etiology and Pathology. Six immunologic types of Clostridium botulinum have been identified. Botulism in man usually results from ingestion of toxin produced by types A, B, and E. Types A and B botulism follow the eating of inadequately processed vegetables or meat. Type E is associated with fish and marine mammal products.

The toxin is thermolabile and is easily destroyed by heat. Poisoning occurs when the preserved food is served uncooked and the rancid taste obscured by acid dressings. The disease is a clinical rarity in the United States.

There are no significant pathological changes in the nervous system and it is probable that the toxin interferes with the action of acetylcholine at the myoneural junction.

Symptoms and Signs. The symptoms of poisoning by the toxin appear twelve to forty-eight hours after the ingestion of contaminated food and may or may not be preceded by nausea, vomiting, or diarrhea. The initial symptom is usually difficulty in convergence of the eyes. This is soon followed by ptosis and paralysis of the extraocular muscles. The pupils are dilated and may not react to light. The ocular symptoms are followed by weakness of the jaw muscles, difficulty in swallowing, and dysarthria. The weakness spreads to involve muscles of the trunk and extremities. The smooth muscle of the intestines and bladder is occasionally affected, with resulting constipation and retention of urine. The mental faculties are usually preserved but convulsions and coma may develop terminally. The results of the examination of the blood and cerebrospinal fluid are normal. In the severe cases the presenting symptoms may be those of cardiac and respiratory failure.

Diagnosis. The diagnosis is not difficult when several members of one household are affected or if samples of the contaminated food can be obtained for testing. Bulbar palsy in acute anterior poliomyelitis can be excluded by the normal cerebrospinal fluid.

Course. The course depends upon the amount of toxin ingested. The symptoms are mild and there is complete recovery if only a small amount is taken. When large amounts are ingested, death usually occurs within four to eight days from circulatory failure, respiratory paralysis or the development of pulmonary complications.

Treatment. Botulism can be prevented by taking proper precautions in the preparation of canned foods and discarding (without sampling) any canned food with a rancid odor in which gas has formed. The toxin is destroyed by cooking.

Patients who have been poisoned by the ingestion of contaminated food should be given botulinum antitoxin in dosage of 20,000 to 40,000 units 2 to 3 times daily. The antitoxin commercially available in this country is bivalent (type A and B). Attempts should be made to obtain type E or a trivalent antitoxin if fish is suspected as the source of the toxin. The stomach should be washed and the gastrointestinal tract cleansed as thoroughly as possibly by enemas and saline purges. The patient should be given artificial respiration if there is any embarrassment of respiration. Feedings should be given through a nasal tube. Although the symptoms of botulism are similar to those of myasthenia gravis, neostigmine is of no value in the treatment of botulism. Some beneficial results have been reported with the use of guanidine hydrochloride.

REFERENCES

Abel, J. J., Hampil, B., and Jonas, A. F., Jr.: Researches on Tetanus; Further Experiments to Prove that Tetanus Toxin is Not Carried in the Peripheral Nerves to Central Nervous System, Bull. Johns Hopkins Hosp., 56, 317, 1935.
Brown, H.: Tetanus, J.A.M.A., 204, 614, 1968.
Cherington, M., and Ryan, D. W.: Botulism, N. Engl. J. Med., 278, 931, 1969.
Cole, L.: Treatment of Tetanus, Lancet, 1, 1017, 1969.
Illis, L. S.: Neurological and Electroencephalographic Sequelae of Tetanus, Lancet, 1, 826, 1971.
Koenig, M. G., et al.: Type B Botulism in Man, Am. J. Med., 42, 208, 1967.
Koenig, M. G., Spickard, A., Cardella, M. A., and Rogers, D. E.: Clinical and Laboratory Observations on Type E Botulism in Man, Medicine, 43, 517, 1964.
La Force, F. M., Young, L. S., and Bennett, J. V.: Tetanus in the United States (1965–1966). Epidemiologic and Clinical Features, N. Engl. J. Med., 280, 569, 1969.
Pascale, L. R., Wallyn, R. J., Goldfein, S., and Gumbiner, S. H.: Treatment of Tetanus by Hyperbaric Oxygenation, J.A.M.A., 189, 408, 1964.
Ryan, D. W., and Cherington, M.: Human Type A Botulism, J.A.M.A., 261, 513, 1971.
Sanchez-Longo, L. P., and Schlezinger, N. S.: Cephalic Tetanus, Neurology, 5, 381, 1955.

METALLIC POISONS

Arsenic

Poisoning may result from the accidental ingestion of arsenical compounds commonly used as insecticides, rat poisoning or weed killers, or the medical administration of Fowler's solution or organic arsenical compounds.

The symptoms of arsenical poisoning are related chiefly to the gastrointestinal tract and the nervous system. Involvement of the nervous system is most commonly in the form of a polyneuritis, but an acute hemorrhagic encephalopathy may follow the intravenous injection of organic arsenical compounds. Optic neuritis is not uncommon with the administration of the pentavalent arsenical compounds tryparsamide, stovarsol and acetarsone. The pathological changes, clinical symptoms and therapy of the neurological complications have been previously considered as noted above.

The accidental or intentional ingestion of large doses of arsenic by mouth causes acute gastrointestinal irritation with vomiting and diarrhea. Convulsive seizures and death may result if the dose is sufficiently large. Polyneuritis may develop after an interval of several weeks in the patients who recover.

The treatment of acute poisoning includes gastric lavage, the feeding of milk and eggs by mouth, supportive therapy and the administration of 2,3-dimercaptopropanol (BAL) in dose of 3 mg per kg of body weight every four hours for the first two days, four injections on the third day and twice daily injections for ten days or until complete recovery.

REFERENCES

Alpers, B.: So-called "Brain Purpura" or "Hemorrhagic Encephalitis," Arch. Neurol. & Psychiat., 20, 497, 1928.
Globus, J. H., and Ginsburg, S. W.: Pericapillary Encephalorrhagia Due to Arsphenamine; So-called Arsphenamine Encephalitis, Arch. Neurol. & Psychiat., 30, 1226, 1933.
Longcope, W. T., and Luetscher, J. A., Jr.: The Use of BAL (British Anti-lewisite) in the Treatment of the Injurious Effects of Arsenic, Mercury and Other Metallic Poisons, Ann. Intern. Med., 31, 545, 1949.
Randall, R. V., and Seeler, A. O.: BAL, N. Engl. J. Med., 239, 1004 and 1040, 1948.

Bismuth

Bismuth is a relatively non-toxic, heavy metal, which was formerly used extensively in the treatment of syphilis and for the relief of the diarrhea of gastrointestinal diseases. Complications of bismuth therapy include stomatitis, pigmentation of the buccal mucous membrane and a dark line on the gum similar to that of lead poisoning. The sciatic nerve may be accidentally injured with the injection of bismuth preparations into the buttocks. Herpes zoster and polyneuritis have been reported as complications of bismuth therapy, but there is no evidence to indicate that the occurrence of these complications is anything more than coincidental.

REFERENCE

Becker, S. W.: Herpes Zoster and Polyneuritis following Administration of Bismuth, Am. J. Syph., 16, 313, 1932.

Lead

Lead poisoning may result from industrial or occupational exposure, accidental ingestion of lead compounds or lead-containing paint, or the administration of lead compounds in medical therapy. Lead may be absorbed from the skin, inhaled through the lungs and ingested into the gastrointestinal tract.

Acute lead poisoning may result from the sudden absorption of large amounts of the metal. With acute poisoning there may be vomiting, abdominal pain, diarrhea or constipation, headaches, weakness, prostration and an acute anemia.

Chronic lead poisoning affects almost all of the organs of the body. Stomatitis, lead line in the gums, gastrointestinal symptoms, constipation and cramps (lead colic), changes in the bones and a chronic anemia are the more common manifestations of lead poisoning. Involvement of the nervous system by lead takes the form of a chronic polyneuritis or an acute encephalopathy.

Lead Encephalopathy. Lead encephalopathy occurs almost exclusively in children or infants and is most frequently due to the ingestion of lead from nipple shields and the gnawing of the lead paint on cribs, toys, and walls. It has become less common since the use of lead paint has been discontinued in the painting of household furniture but the danger of poisoning is still present in tenement houses where lead-containing paint has been covered by one or more coats of supposedly lead-free paint.

Pathology. Lead encephalopathy is characterized by an intense cerebral edema and damage to the capillaries. The convolutions of the cerebral cortex are flattened, the parenchyma is permeated with a serous exudate, causing the tissue to be distended and spongy. The capillaries may be necrotic. Degenerative changes are found in the nerve cells and myelin sheaths, and there is proliferation of the glial cells. The ventricles are usually small, apparently compressed by the cerebral edema.

Symptoms and Signs. The onset of cerebral symptoms is usually abrupt and may be coincidental with the onset of acidosis. Convulsive seizures of a generalized or focal nature are common. Paralysis may follow the seizures. Any type of neurological sign may develop, including cerebellar ataxia, hemiplegia or decerebrate rigidity. Lethargy, coma and delirium are not uncommon. The optic discs may be choked or there may be an optic atrophy. Cranial nerve palsies are uncommon, but facial or oculomotor paralysis may develop. The sutures of the skull are separated and the fontanelles, if still open, are full and bulging. Polyneuritis may accompany the encephalopathy in older children but in infants there is usually no evidence of neuritis. The temperature is usually normal, but hyperpyrexia may occur in association with convulsions or in the terminal stages of the disease.

Laboratory Data. The urine contains albumin and in many cases glucose and coproporphyrin are also present. The cerebrospinal fluid pressure is greatly increased. The protein content of the fluid is increased and there is an inconstant pleocytosis. The cell count may be normal but more commonly is in the range of 20 to 40 per cu mm. Cell counts of several hundred may occur. There is a hypochromic anemia with basophilic stippling of the red blood cells. The epiphyseal ends of the bones show a dense line by roentgenography. Lead can be found in the urine and demonstrated in the blood by the spectroscope. Roentgenogram of the abdomen may show lead in the intestines when the poisoning is the result of ingestion of the metal.

Diagnosis. The diagnosis of lead encephalopathy in infants is made from the history of ingestion of lead paint or other exposure to lead, the anemia, the characteristic changes in the roentgen-ray films of the long bones, and the presence of lead in the blood and urine. Brain tumor, subdural hematoma, tetany and other causes of convulsions and paralyses should be considered in differential diagnosis.

Treatment and Prognosis. The treatment of choice at the present time is the administration of a short course of 2,3,dimercapto-1-propanol (BAL) and edathamil calcium disodium (Ca EDTA) followed by the long-term administration of oral D-penicillamine for one to six months. Supportive therapy before the administration of chelating therapy includes restriction of fluid intake for two to three days and the infusion of 10% dextrose or mannitol in order to initiate the flow of urine which has been interfered with by the inappropriate secretion of antidiuretic hormone. Paraldehyde is given to control the convulsive seizures in the initial stages. The use of phenobarbital and diphenylhydantoin is reserved for the long-term control of seizure. Body temperature is reduced to normal by the use of oxygen tents and cooling blankets. The use of steroids for control of cerebral edema and reduction of intracranial pressure is recommended by some.

With this mode of therapy the mortality rate has been greatly reduced from a level of over 50% to zero in the series of 24 cases treated by Chisolm with some reduction in the late incidence of convulsions and the severity of the retardation of mental development in the children who recover.

The long-term control of lead poisoning includes measures by health departments to insure early case finding, the removal of lead-containing paint from the homes, and the educational measures to eliminate pica.

REFERENCES

American Academy of Pediatrics Subcommittee on Accidental Poisoning: Prevention, Diagnosis and Treatment of Lead Poisoning in Childhood, Pediatr., 44, 291, 1969.
Aub, J. C., et al.: Lead Poisoning, Medicine, 4, 1, 1925.
Byers, R. K.: Lead Poisoning, Review of the Literature and Report of 45 Cases, Pediatr., 23, 585, 1959.
Byers, R. K., and Lord, E. E.: Late Effects of Lead Poisoning on Mental Development, Am. J. Dis. Child., 66, 471, 1943.
Chisolm, J. J., Jr.: The Use of Chelating Agents in the Treatment of Acute and Chronic Lead Intoxication in Childhood, J. Pediatr., 73, 1, 1968.
——: Lead Poisoning, Scientific American, 224, 15, 1971.
Chisolm, J. J., Jr., and Kaplan, E.: Lead Poisoning in Childhood—Comprehensive Management and Prevention, J. Pediatr., 73, 942, 1968.
Klein, M., et al.: Earthenware Containers as a Source of Fatal Lead Poisoning, N. Engl. J. Med., 283, 669, 1970.
Kopits, L., Byers, R. K., and Schwachman, H.: Lead in Hair of Children with Chronic Lead Poisoning, N. Engl. J. Med., 276, 949, 1967.
Smith, H. S., King, L. R., and Margolin, E. G.: Treatment of Lead Encephalopathy, Am. J. Dis. Child., 109, 322, 1965.
Weissberg, J. B., Lipschultz, F., and Oski, F. A.: Delta Aminolevulinic Acid Dehydralase Activity in Circulatory Blood Cells in Lead Poisoning. A Sensitive Laboratory Test for the Detection of Childhood Lead Poisoning, N. Engl. J. Med., 284, 565, 1971.
White, H. H., and Fowler, F. D.: Chronic Lead Encephalopathy, a Diagnostic Consideration in Mental Retardation, Pediatr., 25, 369, 1960.

Manganese

Manganese usually gains entrance into the body through the lungs. The dust is coughed up, swallowed and eventually absorbed through the gastrointestinal tract.

The pathological changes of chronic manganese poisoning in man include cirrhosis of the liver and degenerative changes in the neurons of the cerebral cortex and basal ganglia. Similar changes in the brains of animals poisoned by manganese were reported by Mella.

There is no clear-cut neurological syndrome associated with exposure to manganese in man. The parkinsonian syndrome, which is reported to result from chronic poisoning with manganese, is indistinguishable from that which develops of unknown cause or follows other types of injury to the basal ganglia. The occurrence of these symptoms in a middle-aged or elderly male who is exposed to manganese raises a difficult medicolegal problem. The course, prognosis and treatment are those of parkinsonism due to other causes.

REFERENCES

Abd El Naby, S., and Hassanein, M.: Neuropsychiatric Manifestations of Chronic Manganese Poisoning, J. Neurol., Neurosurg., & Psychiat., 28, 282, 1965.
Canavan, M. M., Cobb, S., and Drinker, C. K.: Chronic Manganese Poisoning, Arch. Neurol. & Psychiat., 32, 501, 1934.

Edsall, D. L., Wilbur, F. P., and Drinker, C. K.: Chronic Manganese Poisoning, J. Indust. Hyg., 1, 183, 1919.
Rosenstock, H. A., Simons, D. G., and Meyer, J. S.: Chronic Manganism. Neurologic and Laboratory Studies During Treatment with Levodopa, J.A.M.A., 217, 1354, 1971.
Szobor, A.: Contribution à la Question du Manganisme, Psychiat. et Neurol., 133, 221, 1957.

Mercury

There is usually no evidence of direct injury to the nervous system in acute poisoning with metallic mercury. The brunt of the damage is sustained by the kidneys resulting in uremia with delirium, coma and convulsions. If the patient recovers, there is no evidence of damage to the nervous system.

Chronic metallic mercury poisoning may result from exposure in industry and the administration of mercurial drugs. Chronic mercurial poisoning except in the milder forms is quite rare. In the milder form of intoxication, the symptoms are confined to the gastrointestinal tract with gingivitis, stomatitis, excessive salivation, anorexia, abdominal pains, constipation, and diarrhea. Neurological complications are rare and usually take the form of irregular tremor of the muscles of the face and extremities. The tremors may increase in intensity with voluntary movements and they sometimes assume the character of choreiform movements. Various personality changes are reported as characteristic of chronic mercurial poisoning; shyness, lack of self-confidence, irritability, apathy and mental deterioration. Pathological studies have shown various degrees of degeneration in the nerve cells of the cortex and basal ganglia. The occurrence of muscular atrophy, fibrillations and signs of involvement of the pyramidal tract, as result of chronic ingestion of mercury, has been reported by Kantarjian.

In recent years there have been a number of small endemics of poisoning with alkyl mercury compounds, particularly with methyl mercury. These have occurred as the result of ingestion of shellfish or free-swimming fish which have been contaminated by methyl mercury discharged into the waters as industrial waste. The first endemic occurred in Minamata Bay, Japan in 1953. The symptoms, described by the term Minamata disease, have also developed as the result of eating animals (hogs) fed with seed grain that had been treated with a methyl mercury fungicide or by eating the poisoned grain. The fetus may absorb through the placenta sufficient amounts of the toxin to produce severe symptoms.

Fears have been expressed that the eating of certain foodstuffs particularly tuna or swordfish, which have a high methyl mercury content, may also produce symptoms. This is rare because it is unlikely that sufficient amounts will be ingested daily over a long enough period of time to raise the blood content of mercury to toxic levels.

Symptoms, which may develop several weeks or months after the ingestion of methyl mercury compounds, include paresthesias of the mouth, tongue and extremities, visual loss (constriction of visual fields, blindness), hearing loss, weakness, inability to concentrate, dysarthria, tremors and cerebellar incoordination. When large amounts have been ingested, there may be a generalized spastic weakness followed by coma and death.

Mercury is found in blood and hair and is present in large amounts in the brain, kidney and liver of the fatal cases. There are diffuse, sometimes severe, changes in the electroencephalogram.

In the fatal cases there are severe degenerative changes in the cerebellum and the cerebral cortex, particularly in the calcarine, pre- and post-central areas.

Acute mercurial poisoning is treated by stomach lavage and the administration of BAL as given for arsenic poisoning. No treatment is needed for chronic metallic mercury poisoning. Improvement of symptoms will follow withdrawal from exposure. There is no specific treatment for organic mercury poisoning. The fatality rate is high in the patients who are severely poisoned and residuals are common in those who recover.

REFERENCES

Eyl, T. B.: Organic-Mercury Food Poisoning, N. Engl. J. Med., 284, 706, 1971.
Hay, W. J., Rickards, A. G., McMenemey, W. H., and Cumings, J. N.: Organic Mercurial Encephalopathy, J. Neurol. Neurosurg. & Psychiat., 26, 199, 1963.
Kantarjian, A. D.: A Syndrome Clinically Resembling Amyotrophic Lateral Sclerosis Following Chronic Mercurialism, Neurology, 11, 639, 1961.
Kurland, L. T., Faro, S. N., and Siedler, H.: Minamata Disease, World Neurology, 1, 370, 1960.
Likosky, W. H., Hinman, A. R., and Barthol, W. F.: Organic Mercury Poisoning in New Mexico, Neurology, 20, 401, 1970.
Pierce, P. E., et al.: Alkyl Mercury Poisoning in Humans. Report of an Outbreak, J.A.M.A., 220, 1439, 1972.
Snyder, R. D.: Congenital Mercury Poisoning, N. Engl. J. Med., 284, 1014, 1971.

Thallium

Thallium poisoning in many cases may result from the accidental ingestion of the metal in rat poisons or the use of salves in the treatment of ringworm or depilatory creams containing thallium acetate.

The accidental ingestion of large amounts of the metal in rat poisons usually causes death. Gastrointestinal symptoms, epigastric pain, colic, nausea, vomiting and diarrhea develop within twenty-four hours. The gastrointestinal symptoms are followed within two to five days by numbness and weakness of the extremities, delirium, convulsions, cranial nerve palsies and blindness. The hair falls out, ecchymoses appear in the skin and bleeding may develop from the skin. The urine contains albumin and casts. Death usually ensues within a few days.

In the chronic form of intoxication where only small amounts of the poisons are absorbed from the skin, the most common symptoms are alopecia and optic neuritis or a generalized polyneuritis. Blurring or dimness of vision develops after several weeks or months of use of the drug. There is a loss of central vision with some constriction of the peripheral fields. The optic discs, which are normal in appearance at the onset, later undergo atrophy.

A generalized polyneuritis may develop coincidental with the optic neuritis or either the optic neuritis or the generalized polyneuritis may occur independently. Paresthesias in the extremities, motor weakness, loss of reflexes with little or no impairment of the cutaneous sensibility are characteristic of involvement of the peripheral nerves by thallium.

The prognosis is poor and death usually occurs in acute poisoning when large amounts of the toxin are ingested. In the chronic form of poisoning the prognosis for life is good. The polyneuritis is usually only of a mild or moderate degree and complete recovery is the rule. There may be improvement in vision in the patients with optic neuritis, but there is always some reduction in visual acuity. The treatment includes discontinuing the use of all salves and creams which contain thallium and the administration of British anti-lewisite.

REFERENCES

Bank, W, J., et al.: Thallium Poisoning, Arch. Neurol., 26, 456, 1972.
Chamberlain, P. H., Stavinoha, W. B., Davis, H., Kniker, W. T., and Panos, T. C.: Thallium Poisoning, Pediatr., 22, 1170, 1958.
Gleich, M.: Thallium Acetate Poisoning in the Treatment of Ring Worm of the Scalp, J.A.M.A., 97, 851, 1931.
Mahoney, W.: Retrobulbar Neuritis Due to Thallium Poisoning from Depilatory Cream, J.A.M.A., 98, 618, 1932.
Passarge, C., and Wieck, H. H.: Thallium Polyneuritis, Fortschr. der Neurologie-Psychiatrie, 33, 477, 1965.
Rambar. A. C.: Acute Thallium Poisoning, J.A.M.A., 98, 1372, 1932.
Smith, D. H., and Doherty, R. A.: Thallitoxicosis: Report of Three Cases in Massachusetts, Pediatr., 34, 480, 1964.
Stein, M. D., and Perlstein, M. A.: Thallium Poisoning, Am. J. Dis. Child., 98, 80, 1959.
Stine, G. H.: Optic Neuritis and Optic Atrophy Due to Thallium Poisoning following Prolonged Use of Koremlu Cream, Am. J. Ophth., 15, 949, 1932.

ORGANIC COMPOUNDS

Ethyl Alcohol

Ethyl alcohol is a depressant of the central nervous system. The apparent stimulating effect is probably related to suppression of inhibitions.

Table 116.   An Analysis of 266 Consecutive Patients Admitted with Obvious Alcoholic Complications to the Boston City Hospital over a 60-day Period

(After Victor and Adams, A. Res. Nerv & Ment. Dis. Proc., 1953)

	Number	%
Acute inebriation	56	21.0
Intoxication (14)		
Stupor or coma (27)		
Combative (15)		
Acute alcoholic tremulousness	92	34.6
Tremor and transitory hallucinations	30	11.3
Acute auditory hallucinosis	6	2.3
Typical delirium tremens	14	5.3
Atypical delirious-hallucinatory states	11	4.1
Nutritional diseases (Wernicke's—Korsakoff's neuropathy)	8	3.0
Other	49	18.4
Total	266*	100

*Convulsive seizures occurred in 12% of the cases:

The effects of a single large dose is an acute intoxication. This usually occurs when the level of alcohol in the blood reaches 150 mg%. Coma develops with levels above 250 mg and a fatal outcome is common when the level is greater than 400 to 500 mg%.

The complications of chronic intoxication with alcohol (Table 116) include delirium tremens, acute auditory hallucinosis, alcoholic convulsive seizures, peripheral neuritis, Korsakoff's psychosis, Wernicke's polioencephalitis, parenchymatous cerebellar degeneration and mental deterioration.

According to Victor and Adams the majority of the symptoms which result from overindulgence in alcohol, usually develop twenty-four to ninety-six hours after cessation of drinking. There is as yet no satisfactory explanation of the mode of action of alcohol on the central nervous system and the peripheral nerve. There is no doubt that alcohol has a toxic, anesthetic action on nerve cells and that long-continued use of the drug can produce permanent damage to nervous tissues. The role of nutritional deficiency and vitamin deprivation in the polyneuritis and other complications of chronic alcoholism is not clear.

REFERENCES

Victor, M., and Adams, R. D.: The Effect of Alcohol on the Nervous System, A Res Nerv. & Ment. Dis. Proc., 32, 526, 1953.
Victor, M., Adams, R. D., and Collins, G. H.: The Wernicke-Korsakoff Syndrome, Philadelphia, F. A. Davis Co., 1971.

Methyl Alcohol

Methyl alcohol poisoning may occur from ingestion or from exposure in industry. It is used as a solvent in industry and formerly as an adulterant in ethyl alcohol. Toxic effects are due to the oxidation of the methyl alcohol to formaldehyde and formic acid. The toxic dose of methyl alcohol may be as little as 10 ml. The lethal dose is usually in range of 100 to 250 ml. Methyl alcohol produces a depression of the central nervous system, cerebral edema and acidosis. It has a specific toxic effect on the optic nerve and the respiratory centers.

The symptoms of poisoning, which usually develop within a few hours of ingestion, are drunkenness, drowsiness, headache, blurring of vision, nausea, vomiting, abdominal pain, dyspnea and cyanosis. Delirium and coma may ensue if a large amount has been ingested. Blindness is the most common symptom to persist after recovery from the acute intoxication. The occurrence of visual loss is probably related in part to individual idiosyncrasy to the drug, because it does not occur in all cases of intoxication.

When large amounts of the poison are ingested, death usually occurs within one to three days. Recovery has occurred after a coma of three or four days. Visual loss is the only neurological sequel in patients who recover from acute poisoning. The visual acuity is greatly reduced. There is a central scotoma with constriction of the peripheral fields. The pupils may be large and react poorly to light. The optic disc may be congested or normal in appearance. There is usually complete or nearly complete restoration of vision in the course of a few months.

The diagnosis of methyl alcohol poisoning in a patient admitted to the hospital in coma is difficult unless there is a history of ingestion of the poison or its odor can be detected on the breath. The diagnosis is not difficult in the patients with visual loss following acute intoxication.

Treatment includes gastric lavage, high saline enema, and intravenous administration of 15 gm of sodium bicarbonate or sodium lactate in 1000 ml of 5% glucose in saline solution. This should be repeated if necessary. Pain and restlessness can be combatted by the use of opiates or scopolamine. Oxygen or oxygen-carbon dioxide mixtures should be given if respirations are depressed. Caffeine and sodium benzoate, amphetamine or coramine may also be of benefit.

REFERENCES

Bennett, I. L., Jr., et al.: Acute Methyl Alcohol Poisoning: A Review Based on Experience in an Outbreak of 323 Cases, Medicine, 32, 431, 1953.
Harrop, G.A., Jr., and Benedict, E. M.: Acute Methyl Alcohol Poisoning Associated with Acidosis, J.A.M.A., 74, 25, 1920.

Barbiturates

Many derivatives of barbituric acid are used in medical therapy as sedatives, hypnotics and in the treatment of convulsive disorders. The ready availability of these compounds has led to their uncontrolled use with the creation of a form of addiction. In addition, the ingestion of barbiturates is perhaps the most common method of attempting suicide.

Long continued use of the barbiturates often leads to a partial tolerance to their sedative and hypnotic effects, and if the administration is controlled, it is frequently possible for patients with convulsive seizures to take as much as 0.3 to 0.4 gm of phenobarbital daily without manifesting any untoward side effects. Dosages of phenobarbital or other barbiturates in excess of this amount or even with lesser dosages in susceptible individuals are usually accompanied by lethargy or drowsiness, headache, thickness of speech, ataxia of the gait, slowness of mental process, nystagmus and psychotic states. These symptoms usually disappear within forty-eight to seventy-two hours after withdrawal of the drug, but convulsive seizures may occur as a withdrawal symptom, regardless of whether the patient has been subject to convulsive seizures or not. For this reason, the process of withdrawal should be slow, reducing the dosage by 0.1 to 0.2 gm every twenty-four to forty-eight hours. Psychotic states have occasionally been reported in patients addicted to the use of the barbiturates.

Acute poisoning with the barbiturates is usually due to accidental or suicidal overdosage. The lethal dose is quite variable. Death has occurred in patients who have ingested less than 2 gm and others have survived after dosages as high as 20 gm. Acute poisoning with large doses is characterized by deep coma, slowness of the respirations, cyanosis, slow weak pulse, subnormal temperatures, loss of the tendon reflexes, loss of the corneal and pupillary reflexes and extensor plantar responses. Recovery has been reported in patients with an isoelectric encephalogram lasting more than twenty-four hours. Death may ensue as result of respiratory failure or the development of pulmonary complications. In the patients who recover, there are usually no residuals even when the coma has persisted for five to seven days.

The treatment of the patient in the acute stage is mainly supportive. The immediate danger is respiratory and circulatory failure. The airway must be kept clear by suction and tracheotomy, if necessary. Oxygen is administered by nasal catheter. The patient should be placed in a respirator if there is cyanosis or the respirations are slow and labored. Intravenous infusion should be started immediately. Plasma expanders and vasopressor drugs can be added to keep the systolic blood pressure at level of 90 to 100 mm Hg.

Pictrotoxin, strychnine and other analeptic drugs, as well as electrical stimulation and the so-called barbiturate antagonist, Megimide, have been recommended. There is no evidence that their administration has any effect on the ultimate outcome.

Hemodialysis by the artificial kidney, if available, is of value in reducing the length of the coma in severe cases.

REFERENCES

Curran, F. J.: The Symptoms and Treatment of Barbiturate Intoxication and Psychoses, Am. J. Psychiat., 95, 73, 1938.
———: Current Views on Neuropsychiatric Effects of Barbiturates and Bromides, J. Nerv. & Ment. Dis., 100, 142, 1944.
Ferguson, M. J., and Grace, W. J.: The Conservative Management of Barbiturate Intoxication: Experience with 95 Unconscious Patients, Ann. Intern. Med., 54, 726, 1961.
Plum, F.: Recovery from Barbiturate Overdose Coma with a Prolonged Isoelectric Electroencephalogram, Neurology, 18, 456, 1968.
Plum, F., and Swanson, A. G.: Barbiturate Poisoning Treated by Physiological Methods, With Observations on Effect of Beta, Beta-methylglutarimide and Electrical Stimulation, J.A.M.A., 163, 827, 1957.
Tatum, A. L.: The Present Status of the Barbiturate Problem, Physiol. Rev., 19, 472, 1939.
Wikler, A.: Neurophysiological Aspects of Opiate and Barbiturate Abstinence Syndromes, A. Res. Nerv. & Ment. Dis., Proc., 32, 269, 1953.

Belladonna

Toxic symptoms may develop from the ingestion of excessive doses of any of the belladonna alkaloids including atropine, hyoscine, hyoscyamus and stramonium. Toxic symptoms occasionally develop from the administration of therapeutic dosages of these alkaloids to susceptible or elderly individuals.

Dryness of the mouth, dilatation of the pupils and difficulty in convergence of the eyes are the usual accompaniments of use of the belladonna drugs in small or moderate dosages. With larger dosages or in susceptible individuals there may be restlessness, mental confusion, hallucinations, delusions and acute psychotic states. The symptoms usually disappear within twenty-four to forty-eight hours after withdrawal and fatalities are rare even after the ingestion of large dosages. Long continued use of belladonna drugs or belladonna-like compounds (Artane, Cogentin, etc.) may be accompanied by acute psychosis with visual hallucinations which may persist for weeks or months after the use of these drugs is discontinued.

Bromides

Bromides, formerly used extensively in the treatment of epilepsy and as a mild hypnotic or sedative, frequently produce toxic manifestations. An acneiform skin rash develops in almost all of the patients receiving this drug. Headache, somnolence, lassitude, ataxia, urinary incontinence and confusional psychotic states develop in a high percentage of the patients who use bromides in large amounts over an extended period of time. These symptoms may develop when the level of bromides in the serum is as low as 125 to 150 mg per 100 ml, but occasionally they may be absent in patients with more than 300 gm per 100 ml in the blood. Psychoses associated with bromide intoxication accounted for approximately 4% of the admissions to psychopathic hospitals fifty years ago. They are relatively uncommon at the present time.

The diagnosis of psychosis due to bromide intoxication is made from the history of the ingestion of the drug, the acneiform skin rash and the presence of bromides in the serum in concentrations greater than 150 mg per 100 ml.

The treatment of bromide intoxication is immediate withdrawal of the drug and the administration of sodium chloride in dose of 10 gm daily along with the forcing of fluids.

The prognosis, of bromide intoxication is good, but psychotic symptoms which necessitate hospitalization may persist for several weeks. Psychotherapy is essential in the care of patients with personality disturbances which were the underlying factors in the habituation to bromides.

REFERENCES

Claiborne, T. S.: Bromide Intoxication, N. Engl. J. Med., 212, 1214, 1935.
Levin, M.: Bromide Psychoses, Ann. Intern. Med., 7, 709, 1933.
Sensenbach, W.: Bromide Intoxication, J.A.M.A., 125, 769, 1944.
Wagner, C. P., and Bunbury, D. E.: Incidence of Bromide Intoxication among Psychotic Patients, J.A.M.A., 95, 1725, 1930.

Hydantoins

The hydantoins most commonly used in the therapy of patients with convulsive seizures are the diphenyl and the phenyl ethyl methyl derivatives. An allergic rash with fever and eosinophilia in the blood occurs in approximately 5% of the patients who receive either of these two compounds. The phenyl ethyl methyl derivative (Mesantoin) has a mild hypnotic action and pancytopenia has developed in a few patients. The toxic effect of Mesantoin on the bone marrow is not related to the dosage and may be irreversible and there is no method of detecting with certainty which individual patient will suffer this serious untoward complication. It is recommended that blood counts be made at periodic intervals in patients receiving Mesantoin, but there is insufficient evidence to indicate that damage to the bone marrow can be detected from the examination of the peripheral blood before it is irreversible.

The diphenyl derivatives of hydantoin (Dilantin, Phenytoin, Epanutin, Epamin) have little or no sedative action and it is almost impossible to take a fatal dose. Minor toxic side effects of the administration of Dilantin include, (1) ataxia and nystagmus, which develop in practically all patients taking more than 0.6 gm daily, and with a lower dose in the patients who are sensitive to the drug; (2) gingival hyperplasia develops in practically all children taking the drug. It is usually of a mild degree and only rarely is it severe enough to require excision of the excess tissue; (3) a mild degree of hirsutism particularly in young females; and (4) psychotic states have developed in epileptic patients under therapy with diphenyl hydantoin. The exact causal relationship of the drug to the psychotic manifestation is not clear, since similar symptoms may occasionally appear in epileptics who are receiving other forms of therapy or no therapy at all. Rare complications of the long-term administration of the drug include: hyperchromic anemia as result of inhibition of folic acid metabolism; lymphadenopathy, clinically similar to malignant lymphoma; mild polyneuritis; and depression of the protein-bound iodine content in the serum without any other clinical or laboratory evidence of hypothyroidism. Acute cerebellar ataxia with permanent signs and symptoms of cerebellar degeneration has been reported as the result of the administration of larger dosages.

In spite of the variety of side effects of the administration of Dilantin, there have been few serious complications and almost no mortality. The majority of the toxic symptoms will disappear within a few days after discontinuing the drug.

The phenyl ethyl derivative of hydantoin (Nirvanol), which was formerly used in the therapy of Sydenham's chorea, was accompanied by an allergic skin rash with fever, leukocytosis and eosinophilia in the blood in over half of the cases.

REFERENCES

Abbott, J. A., and Schwab, R. S.: Medical Progress: Serious Side Effects of Newer Antiepileptic Drugs, N. Engl. J. Med., 242, 943, 1950.
De Jong, R. N.: Neurologic Complications of Drugs with Primary Action on Nervous System, N.Y. State J. Med., 70, 1857, 1970.
Durskin, M. S., Wallen, M. H. and Bonagura, L.: Anticonvulsant-Associated Megaloblastic Anemia: Response to 25 Microgm. of Folic Acid Administered by Mouth Daily, N. Engl. J. Med., 267, 483, 1962.
Flexner, J. M., and Hartmann, R. C.: Megaloblastic Anemia Associated with Anticonvulsant Drugs, Am. J. Med., 28. 386, 1960.
Merritt, H. H., and Putnam, T. J.: Sodium Diphenyl Hydantoinate in Treatment of Convulsive Seizures, Arch. Neurol. & Psychiat., 42, 1053, 1939.

Recant, L., and Hartroft, W. S.: Lymphoma or Drug Reaction Occurring During Hydantoin Therapy for Epilepsy, Am. J. Med., 32, 286, 1962.
Sparberg, T.: Diagnostically Confusing Complications of Diphenylhydantoin Therapy, Ann. Intern. Med., 59, 914, 1963.
Tenckhoff, H., et al.: Acute Diphenyl Hydantoin Intoxication, Am. J. Dis. Child., 116, 422, 1968.

Penicillin

It has been known for some years that convulsive seizures could occur following the intraventricular, intrathecal, or cortical application of penicillin. Recently attention has been called to the fact that myoclonic jerks, convulsive seizures and death may occur in patients treated with penicillin intravenously. This is especially apt to occur when massive dosages are given for the treatment of resistant infection and in patients with uremia or with cardiopulmonary bypass in open heart surgery.

REFERENCES

Bloomer, H. A., Barton, L. J., and Maddock, R. K., Jr.: Penicillin-Induced Encephalopathy in Uremic Patients, J.A.M.A., 200, 131, 1967.
Cohill, D, F., et al.: Central Nervous System Toxicity Secondary to Massive Doses of Penicillin 'G' in the Treatment of Overwhelming Infections, Am. J. Med. Sci., 254, 692, 1967.
Seamans, K. B., et al.: Penicillin Induced Seizures During Cardiopulmonary Bypass, N. Engl. J. Med., 278, 861, 1968.
Smith, H., et al.: Neurotoxicity and "Massive" Intravenous Therapy with Penicillin, Arch. Intern. Med., 120, 47, 1967.

Phenothiazines

The phenothiazines and other tranquilizers are used extensively in the treatment of schizophrenia and other psychoses, psychoneurosis, and in the treatment of vertigo, nausea and vomiting. Untoward effects include: (1) parkinsonism-like syndrome which is produced in the majority of the patients who are given large doses of the drugs. This side effect is not serious becaue it will disappear when the drug is withdrawn; (2) less frequent but more troublesome are the dystonic or choreic movements which appear in a small percentage of the cases. The movements are apt to involve the mouth, tongue or shoulder girdle. They usually disappear when the drug is withdrawn but in a few cases the symptoms have persisted; (3) acute hypotensive episodes which may simulate coronary thrombosis, and (4) convulsive seizures. The seizures may be due to direct action of the drugs or they may occur as a withdrawal symptom. Tardive dyskinesia (orobuccal dyskinesia) may develop in elderly patients after long continued use of the tranquilizers. This is apt to be persistent and does not respond to any form of therapy.

REFERENCES

Dabbous, I. A., and Bergman, A. B.: Neurological Damage Associated with Phenothiazine, Am. J. Dis. Child., *111*, 291, 1966.
Grünthal, E., und Walther-Büel, H.: Ueber Schädigung der Oliva inferior durch Chlor-perphenazin (Trilafon), Psychiatria et Neurologia, *140*, 249, 1960.
Jus, A., et al.: Epidemiology of Tardive Dyskinesias, Part I, Dis. Neuro. Sys., *37*, 310, 1976, Part 2, *37*, 257, 1976.
Kazamatsuri, H., Chien, C. P. and Cole, J. O.: Therapeutic Approach to Tardive Dyskinesias, A Review of the Literature, Arch. Gen. Psychiat., *37*, 44. 1972.
Schmidt, W. R., and Jarcho, L. W.: Persistent Dyskinesias Following Phenothiazine Therapy, Arch. Neurol., *14*, 369, 1966.

Carbon Monoxide

Carbon monoxide poisoning usually results from the accidental or intentional inhalation of illuminating gases, the exhaust of automobiles or fumes from the defective burning of coal in home furnaces or stoves. Minor degrees of intoxication produce headache, drowsinese, fatigue and mental confusion. Severe degrees of intoxication result in coma and death. Recovery from a severe degree of intoxication may be accompanied by various signs of cerebral damage or the later development of parkinsonism.

Pathology. The combination of carbon monoxide with hemoglobin forms carboxyhemoglobin, a relatively stable compound, which interferes with the ability of the blood to absorb oxygen. The pathological changes in the nervous system in the cases that die within a few hours include edema and congestion and multiple minute perivascular hemorrhages. In the fatal cases which survive for several days, there are ischemic changes in the neurons and small or large areas of softening in the cerebral cortex and in the basal ganglia. The changes in the nervous system are secondary to anoxemia.

Symptoms and Signs. The majority of the patients with coma due to acute carbon monoxide poisoning either die or recover without residual. In a small percentage of the cases, various neurological defects are present when the patient recovers consciousness. After recovery from the coma, which may persist for several days, the patient is confused. When the mental faculties are regained, there may be amnesia for the period immediately prior to loss of consciousness. Occasionally hemiplegia, aphasia, apraxia, cortical blindness or athetoid and choreiform movements may be present as a result of damage to the brain. These symptoms gradually improve in the course of the next few days or weeks. Occasionally the typical signs of parkinsonism may develop in the ensuing months or years. Multiple neuritis has also been reported as a sequel to carbon monoxide poisoning.

Diagnosis. The diagnosis is made from the history of exposure to the gas, the cherry red color of the skin, and the demonstration of carboxyhemoglobin in the blood by the spectroscope.

Prognosis. The prognosis depends upon the severity of the poisoning. Complete recovery is the rule when there was no or only a short period of coma. Death usually occurs when the coma is prolonged beyond forty-eight to seventy-two hours. Recovery of consciousness in these cases is usually accompanied by mental confusion, loss of memory and focal signs of damage to the brain. These focal symptoms tend to improve or completely disappear but parkinsonism may develop later.

Treatment. The treatment is supportive together with transfusions of whole blood.

REFERENCES

Ferraro, A., and Morrison, L. R.: Illuminating Gas as Poisoning; an Experimental Study of Lesions of the Nervous System in Acute and Chronic Stages, Psychiatric Quart., *2*, 506, 1928.

Gilbert, G. J., and Glaser, G. H.: Neurologic Manifestations of Chronic Carbon Monoxide Poisoning, N. Engl. J. Med., *261*, 1217, 1959.

Grinker, R. R.: Parkinsonism following Carbon Monoxide Poisoning, J. Nerv. & Ment. Dis., *64*, 18, 1926.

Hiller, F.: Uber die krankhaften Veränderungen im Zentralnervensystem nach Kohlenoxydvergiftung, Ztschr. f. d. ges. Neurol., u. Psychiat., *93*, 594, 1924.

Shillito, F. H., Drinker, C. K., and Shaughnessy, T. J.: The Provlem of Nervous and Mental Sequelae in Carbon Monoxide Poisoning, J.A.M.A., *106*, 669. 1936.

Schwenderg, T. H.: Leukoencephalopathy Following Carbon Monoxide Asphyxia, J. Neuropathol. Exp. Med., *18*, 597, 1959.

Strecker, E. A., Taft, A. E., and Willey, G. F.: Mental Sequelae of Carbon Monoxide Poisoning, Arch. Neurol. & Psychiat., *17*, 552, 1927.

Wilson, G., and Winkleman, N. W.: Multiple Neuritis following Carbon Monoxide Poisoning, J.A.M.A., *82*, 1407, 1924.

TICK PARALYSIS

Tick paralysis is a reversible disorder of the central nervous system of man or animal which is due to a toxin injected by a tick while living on the host.

Pathogenesis. The paralysis is due to a toxin which is injected by gravid female ticks. The toxin has its action primarily on neuromuscular conduction without producing any morphological changes. It is apparently excreted or destroyed rapidly because the symptoms clear shortly after the tick or ticks are removed. The wood tick, *Dermacentor andersoni,* and the dog tick, *Dermacentor variabilis,* have been responsible for the reported cases in the United States and Canada. The tick must feed for five to seven days before symptoms develop.

Incidence. Tick paralysis is relatively rare. It has been reported from Australia, South Africa, Crete, Yugoslavia, United States and Canada. Domestic animals or man may be affected. Children, usually girls, seem most susceptible. The tick is usually attached to the scalp and hidden by the hair, but it may be attached to any part of the body.

Symptoms and Signs. Irritability or diarrhea occasionally precedes the onset of paralysis by twenty-four hours but the cardinal symptom is motor weakness. This appears as an ataxia or weakness of the legs with a staggering gait. If the tick is not removed, the weakness advances within twenty-four to forty-eight hours to a flaccid paralysis of the extremities, trunk and the muscles innervated by the bulbar nuclei. Sensory changes are usually absent but there may be paresthesias and hyperesthesia in the extremities. The deep tendon reflexes, the abdominal skin reflex and the plantar responses are absent. Nystagmus, strabismus and convulsive seizures have been reported in infants. There is no fever unless a secondary infection is present.

Laboratory Data. The leukocyte count in the blood is normal and there are no changes in the cerebrospinal fluid.

Diagnosis. The diagnosis should be considered when an acute flaccid paralysis develops in an individual who lives in a tick-infested area and has recently been exposed to them. The diagnosis is confirmed by the finding of the tick and the disappearance of symptoms when it is removed.

Acute anterior poliomyelitis is excluded by the absence of fever or stiffness of the neck and the normal cerebrospinal fluid findings. Polyneuritis of the so-called infectious type (Guillain-Barré syndrome) may offer considerable difficulty in diagnosis. Sensory loss or an increased protein content in the cerebrospinal fluid are findings which favor the diagnosis of polyneuritis.

Course and Prognosis. If the diagnosis is made before signs of bulbar involvement develop, the prognosis is good. Removal of the tick is followed by rapid improvement with complete recovery within a few days. If the tick is not removed, death may result from respiratory paralysis.

Treatment. Treatment is the removal of the ticks. A careful search of all parts of the body, particularly the scalp, should be made, in order to be certain that all ticks are found. It may be necessary to excise retained mouth parts. Respiratory paralysis requires the use of the artificial respirator and tracheotomy.

REFERENCES

Cherington, M., and Snyder, R. D.: Tick Paralysis. Neurophysiological Studies, N. Engl. J. Med., *278*, 95, 1968.
Henderson, F. W.: Tick Paralysis, J.A.M.A., *175*, 615, 1961.

Lagos, J. C., and Thies, R. E.: Tick Paralysis without Muscle Weakness, Arch. Neurol., *21*, 471, 1969.
Schmitt, N., Bowmer, E. J., and Gregson, J. D.: Tick Paralysis in British Columbia, Can. Med. J., *100*, 417, 1969.
Stanbury, J. B., and Huyck, J. H.: Tick Paralysis, Medicine, *24*, 219, 1945.

Index

Page numbers in *italics* refer to illustrations; numbers followed by t refer to tables.

921